Nutrition and Nutritional Therapy in Nursing

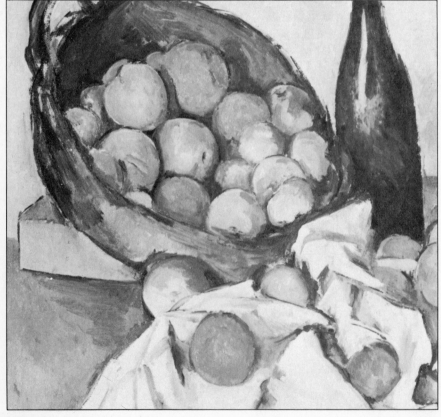

Paul Cézanne *The Basket of Apples*

With contributions by:

Mary C. Dowe, R.N., Ed.D.
Associate Professor
School of Nursing
University of North Carolina
Chapel Hill, North Carolina

Laurel Mellin, M.A., R.D.
Assistant Clinical Professor
  of Pediatrics
Nutritionist, Division of
  Adolescent Medicine
School of Medicine
University of California
San Francisco, California

Rachel E. Spector, R.N., Ph.D.
Associate Professor
School of Nursing
Boston College
Chestnut Hill, Massachusetts

Nutrition and Nutritional Therapy in Nursing

Clara Mixon Lewis, R.D., M.S.
Associate Professor
School of Nursing
University of North Carolina
Chapel Hill, North Carolina

APPLETON-CENTURY-CROFTS/Norwalk, Connecticut

0-8385-7076-3

86 87 88 89 90 / 10 9 8 7 6 5 4 3 2 1

Prentice-Hall of Australia, Pty. Ltd., Sydney
Prentice-Hall Canada, Inc.
Prentice-Hall Hispanoamericana, S.A., Mexico
Prentice-Hall of India Private Limited, New Delhi
Prentice-Hall International (UK) Limited, London
Prentice-Hall of Japan, Inc., Tokyo
Prentice-Hall of Southeast Asia (Pte.) Ltd., Singapore
Whitehall Books Ltd., Wellington, New Zealand
Editora Prentice-Hall do Brasil Ltda., Rio de Janeiro

Library of Congress Cataloging-in-Publication Data

Lewis, Clara M., 1932–
  Nutrition and nutritional therapy in nursing.

  Includes bibliographies and index.
  1. Diet therapy. 2. Nutrition. 3. Nursing.
I. Title. [DNLM: 1. Diet Therapy—nurses'
instruction. 2. Nutrition—nurses' instruction.
WB 400 L673n]
RM215.L48 1985   615.8′54   85–18670
ISBN 0-8385-7076-3

Design: Jean M. Sabato-Morley

PRINTED IN THE UNITED STATES OF AMERICA

To my family,
my husband, Walter
our children, Roger and Glenn
for their long-enduring patience, encouragement, and help
which contributed greatly toward making
this project a reality.

Contents

Preface

This book is designed to serve as a basic nutrition textbook for nursing students and was planned to meet the following objectives: (1) provide a comprehensive but concise background in normal and therapeutic nutrition to serve as a basis for decision making in assisting clients to maintain or achieve optimal nutritional status; (2) provide a framework for integrating nutritional care into the total nursing care process; and (3) identify the role of nutrition in the etiology, treatment, and prevention of health problems. Although this text was written specifically for nursing students, the content should also be of interest to students and practitioners in other health disciplines who share the responsibility for nutritional care and counseling of individuals and families.

The text is organized into four parts. In Part I, which deals primarily with the food nutrients and their utilization, there is a discussion of the current nutritional environment in the United States and of current dietary guidelines. Reference is made throughout this section to situations that nurses are likely to encounter in their clinical practice. Part II addresses nutritional care as an integral part of the nursing process. Emphasis is given to nutritional assessment and nursing diagnosis and an example of a nursing care plan is included. Nutrition education is also a part of this section. Part III focuses on nutrition during the life cycle and describes the physiologic and psycho-socio-cultural aspects of the growth stages and health problems common to each stage, each with its related nutritional aspects. Cultural influences on food habits and alternative dietary practices are included in this part. The final part of the book contains a discussion of the various health problems in which nutrition has a role in etiology, prevention, and management. The first chapter of Part IV provides content related to the effects of hospitalization on nutritional status, methods of nutritional support for hospitalized clients, and diet–drug interactions.

The topical organization is designed to progress from lesser to greater complexity. Moreover, the content from Parts I and

II is applicable to all of the clinical situations presented in Parts III and IV.

Each chapter includes behaviorally stated objectives, review questions and activities (including case studies for some of the chapters), references, and bibliography. Many terms are defined within the text; some terms are highlighted with bold face type, and these highlighted terms are defined in a glossary at the end of the book. A variety of summary tables and illustrative materials is included throughout the book, and a listing of foods allowed and not allowed is provided for therapeutic diets. Extensive reference materials, such as food composition tables, are included in the appendices.

The topical coverage is broad, yet concise. A concerted effort was made to keep content from other science-related areas such as anatomy and physiology to a minimum in order to avoid repetition for students, and at the same time to emphasize nutrition-related content and aspects of its clinical application. Emphasis is given to the assessment and intervention phases of the nursing process in providing nutritional care in relevant sections of the book. Controversial issues are presented as such.

The level of sophistication and writing style assume a science background such as that common to nursing education. Lack of a background in areas such as biology or chemistry will not be a major handicap in following most of the facts and principles discussed in Parts I, II, and III. However, a science background would definitely be a benefit in following the content of Part IV.

Acknowledgments

The author wishes to express her sincere appreciation to the following people for their generous help during the preparation of this book:

Margaret M. Ball, University of Colorado at Denver, for reviewing the manuscript and assisting me to shape it into the final product.

Mary C. Dowe, University of North Carolina at Chapel Hill, for contributing her extensive expertise in nursing education as a co-author for Chapter 11, "The Nutritional Care Process in the Nursing Process."

Rachel E. Spector, Boston College, for providing valuable contributions toward Chapters 19 and 20, "Cultural Influences on Dietary Practices" and "Alternative Dietary Practices."

Laurel Mellin, University of California at San Francisco, also for providing valuable contributions to Chapter 19, "Cultural Influences on Dietary Practices."

The editorial staff of Appleton-Century-Crofts, particularly Marion Kalstein-Welch, Donna Frassetto, and Terry Sternberg, for providing the expertise, encouragement, and patience needed to convert the manuscript into a book.

Joyce Senter, Chapel Hill, North Carolina, for making the tireless and relentless effort needed to type the manuscript.

Elizabeth Tornquist, University of North Carolina at Chapel Hill, for editing the initial manuscript and providing invaluable encouragement throughout.

The library staff at the Health Sciences Library, University of North Carolina at Chapel Hill, for assisting with reference material in a kind and willing manner.

The various investigators, authors, and publishers, for granting permission to quote from their research and work.

My students, for stimulating and enriching my life.

PART I
Foundations of Nutrition

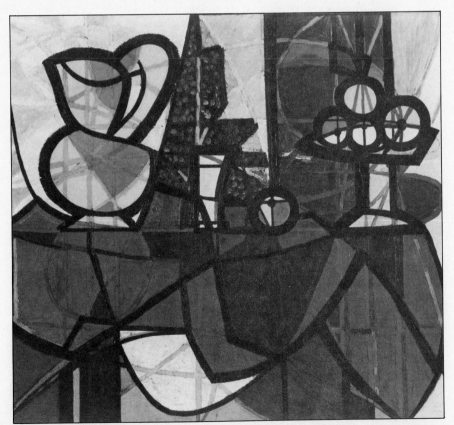

Pablo Picasso *Pitcher and Bowl of Fruit*

CHAPTER 1

Introduction

Objectives

After completion of this chapter, the student will be able to:

1. Assess changes that have occurred in dietary consumption patterns of Americans as they possibly relate to current patterns of disease.

2. Compare and contrast the findings of the major nutritional status surveys that have been conducted in recent years and differentiate between the *types* of information provided by these surveys and food consumption surveys.

3. Distinguish among the roles of each health team member in providing nutritional care.

Why is the study of nutrition important? What does it mean to you as an individual and as a nurse?

When we speak of nutrition, we immediately think of food since food is the source of nutrients. How do you feel about food? What associations does food have for you? What are some of your favorite foods? Why do you like them? What foods do you not like? Why? Feelings, beliefs, and behaviors regarding food and eating are very individualized, personal experiences. Food and eating have much more significance than merely being the means to obtain the nutrients necessary to live.

Food can be used to express feelings: it can make us feel secure, loved, and cared for. It can also be used to express displeasure: foods can remind us of pleasant experiences or unpleasant ones. Food is used as a means of sharing happy occasions with others and as a source of comfort when we are sad or upset. Meals are also social occasions—a time when we interact with family members or friends.

The act of eating can be very pleasurable, as when foods that we especially like are properly prepared and attractively served, or it can be unpleasant if the food is improperly or unattractively prepared or if we do not like the particular food served. Since eating involves all the senses, the number of

ways in which it can be perceived as pleasant or unpleasant are many. Some foods may please all our senses whereas others may not; for example, we may feel that a certain dish looks unappetizing but tastes very good, or vice versa.

Since our bodies must receive nourishment to live, food and eating are essential to life itself. However, nutrition is much more than just "staying alive"; it has numerous influences on our daily lives. For example, proper nutrition is necessary to keep our bodies healthy, to promote growth and development, to facilitate wound healing, to prevent illness, and to aid in the treatment of diseases. Also important is the fact that nutrition affects us mentally and emotionally—proper nutrition helps us feel alert, energetic, and more capable of handling life's situations, whereas improper nutrition can make us feel tired, run down, irritable, depressed, and unable to handle the activities of everyday life. In addition to these general considerations, there are many specific disorders that result from underconsumption or overconsumption of particular nutrients. The effects of improper nutrition can be long-lasting.

Thus, nutrition is very important to you as an individual and as a provider of health care. It is important to you as an individual to help you fulfill your own optimum developmental potential physically, mentally, and emotionally. It is also important to you as a provider of health care because it affects your clients' current health status, their potential for optimum health, and their ability to cope with disease. Nutrition must be considered in assessing, planning, implementing, and evaluating all aspects of health care.

In order to effectively provide nutritional care, it is necessary to have an understanding of the overall nutritional situation in America today. Thus, this chapter presents an overview of the changes in food patterns in America during this century, the nutritional status of Americans, current nutritional concerns, barriers to optimum nutrition, the role of health care providers, and perspectives for improving health care.

ASSESSMENT

Changes in Food Consumption Patterns

Since the beginning of the century, many changes have occurred in the food consumption patterns of Americans. While the quantity of protein consumed has remained relatively constant, carbohydrate consumption has declined by approximately 10 percent and fat consumption has increased by approximately 10 percent. During this period, the total energy level has fluctuated. However, it is slightly higher in 1980 than it was in the early 1900s.[1]

Changes have also occurred in specific types of foods chosen from all three of these nutrient classes. While total carbohydrate consumption has declined, the percentage of total kilocalories (kcal) provided by sugar has increased, and consumption of foods containing starch and fiber has declined. There has been a notable decline in the consumption of grain products and potatoes. The decline in grain consumption, along with the refinement of cereal and flour, has reduced fiber intake from these sources (Fig. 1–1).

As total fat consumption has increased, there has been a shift in the types of fat consumed. While the proportion of saturated fat has declined slightly, the consumption of unsaturated fat has increased in association with the greater use of salad and cooking oils.

Consistent with the pattern of affluent societies in the Western world, the consumption of animal sources of protein has increased, and consumption of plant sources has declined. Beef consumption has increased markedly, and there has been some increase in the use of poultry.

The nutritional quality of the food supply has also undergone changes. Many fabricated foods are available. Some supply primarily kilocalories, whereas others (such as meat analogs) are manufac-

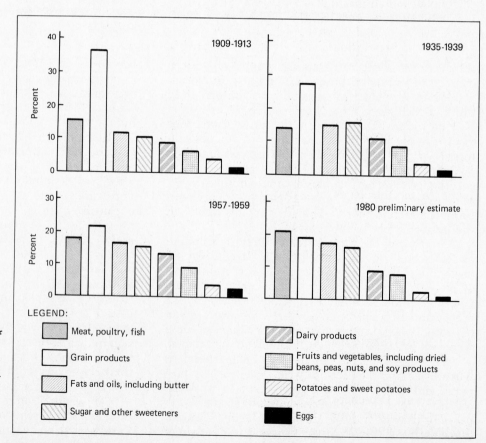

Figure 1–1
Contribution of various food groups to per capita supply of food energy (calories).
(*Source: Committee on Diet, Nutrition and Cancer: Diet, Nutrition and Cancer. Washington, DC, National Academy Press, 1982, p A-3, reproduced with permission.*)

tured to contain the same nutrients as the foods they are designed to replace. At present, however, vitamin and mineral content may differ from the meats they simulate.

A number of chronic diseases are associated with the overconsumption of certain types of foods. Six of the ten leading causes of death in the United States—heart disease, cancer, cerebrovascular disease, diabetes, arteriosclerosis, and cirrhosis of the liver—have been connected with the diet pattern.[2] These disorders have been related to the overconsumption of fat, sugar, salt, and alcohol. Further, it has been estimated that about 20 percent of all adults in the United States are overweight to a degree that may interfere with optimal health and longevity.[3] In particular, obesity is a risk factor for such diseases as cancer, heart diseases, hypertension, and arthritis. There are also relationships between diets low in fiber and heart disease and certain gastrointestinal disorders, such as cancer of the colon and diverticular disease.[4] Sugar is implicated in tooth decay, which may be the most widespread disease related to nutrition.

Along with the overconsumption of some foods, current dietary trends may be leading to malnutrition through undernourishment. Sugar and fat from shortenings and oils (which together account for approximately one third of total energy consumption) contribute little toward meeting essential nutrient needs, and the remaining diet must be carefully selected to assure nutrient adequacy. Thus, persons consuming a high fat/high sugar diet may be meeting their energy needs but may be seriously malnourished in regard to necessary nutrients.

Other factors influencing food consumption patterns include changes in lifestyles and food-processing procedures. As more and more women are employed outside the home, prepackaged or convenience foods are used more frequently. Many products that used to be made at home are now available in convenience form, such as canned or frozen. The proliferation of fast food establishments makes it very tempting to use them for an increasing number of meals rather than preparing meals at home. While fast foods can be incorporated into a balanced diet, many consumers regard taste, price, and convenience as more important than nutritional quality. Activities outside the home may also make demands on people's time, and meals may be skipped or a quick snack substituted for a meal. Excessively sweet or salty snack foods with very little nutritional value are increasingly available and are often eaten in place of more nutritional foods.

Nutritional Status Surveys and Surveys of Food Consumption

In recent years, four national surveys of nutritional status have been conducted: The Ten-State Nutrition Survey, Preschool Nutrition Survey, and National Health and Nutrition Examination Surveys (NHANES I and NHANES II). These surveys provided information about the nutritional status of three different segments of the population. The Ten-State Survey focused on low-income groups of all ages in 10 designated states, the Preschool Survey on children ages 1 through 6 from all socioeconomic and ethnic groups in the population, and NHANES I and NHANES II on all age, ethnic, and socioeconomic groups in the general population. Each survey provided medical, biochemical, and dietary data from which an evaluation of nutritional status was made. A brief description and the most important findings are summarized below.

Ten-State Nutrition Survey (1968–1970). The Ten-State Nutrition Survey was originally envisioned as a national survey. However, time and money constraints limited its implementation to 10 states—Washington, California, Texas, Louisiana, South Carolina, Kentucky, West Virginia, Michigan, Massachusetts, and New York (with separate data gathered for New York City)—distributed throughout the nation to reflect the various ethnic and social groups in the population.

The large proportion of families living at or below the poverty level selected for study was considered to be a representative sample of the low-income families. However, some middle- and upper-income families who resided in districts having a low average income were also included in the study. Because these two groups were not considered representative of the overall middle- and high-income population, the study sample was not representative of the entire population within a county or state. The largest percentage of the sample was white; the next largest black, and the smallest percentage Spanish-American. The latter group included both Puerto Ricans (predominantly in New York City) and Mexican-Americans (in Texas and California).

States were designated as low-income-ratio states or high-income-ratio states based on the numbers of families living below and above the poverty level. Half the states fell into each category and were evaluated separately to allow for comparisons reflecting the effects of regional and economic factors.

An evaluation of the findings of the dietary data is shown in Table 1–1. The results of the survey indicated that a significant proportion of the population surveyed was malnourished or was at high risk of developing nutritional problems. The malnutrition varied in severity and in regard to specific nutrients in different segments of the population. While income tended to be a major determinant of nutritional status, other factors, such as social, cultural, and geographic differences, also appeared to affect the nutritional status of a population group. The highest prevalence of unsatisfactory nutritional status was observed in children and adolescents, ages 10 through 16 years, and problems were greater in male than in female adolescents. Undernutrition was also significant in persons over age 60 and was

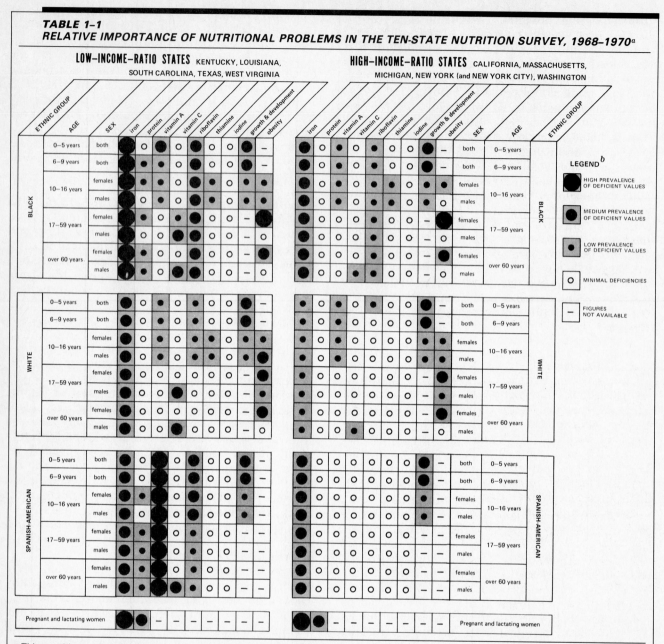

TABLE 1-1
RELATIVE IMPORTANCE OF NUTRITIONAL PROBLEMS IN THE TEN-STATE NUTRITION SURVEY, 1968–1970[a]

a This graphic presentation summarizes the relative importance of those nutritional problems identified by the Ten-State Nutrition Survey. The presentation involves some judgments and generalizations that cannot reflect all the finer differences among various subgroups of the population.
b The symbols represent relative degrees of importance as public health problems.
(*Source: U.S. Department of Health, Education, and Welfare; Health Services and Mental Health Administration; Centers for Disease Control, Atlanta, Ga.*)

not restricted to the very poor or to any single ethnic group.

Among specific findings were these:

Problems Related to Kilocalorie Intake. Significant numbers of people had kilocalorie intake below the standard for age, size, and weight, indicating an inadequate quantity of food intake. In this regard, there was considerable evidence of retarded growth in children 0 through 9 years of age in both sexes

and in all states and ethnic groups. The overall nutritional deficiencies identified can be related basically to consumption of inadequate amounts of nutritious food. In spite of observed kilocalorie deficits, obesity was an important nutritional problem, especially in women of all ethnic groups. Black women showed the highest prevalence of obesity, exceeding 50 percent in the 45- to 55-year-old age group. White women demonstrated the next highest prevalence of obesity, with more than 40 percent of them obese in the 45- to 55-year-old group.[5]

Anemia. A high prevalence of low hemoglobin and hematocrit values was noted in all age and ethnic groups. The black population in both categories of states had the poorest hemoglobin status, whereas the best hemoglobin status was observed in the white population. For all ethnic groups, hemoglobin status was less satisfactory in the low-income-ratio states than in the high-income-ratio states. Although hemoglobin status tended to improve with an increase in income level, hemoglobin status did not appear to be solely income dependent. In many instances, males had a higher percentage of deficient or low hemoglobin values than had females of the same age and ethnic group. This finding was not consistent with general clinical experience indicating that women are at greater risk than men with regard to iron nutriture. Although these data appear to indicate that iron deficiency indicated by a lowered hemoglobin level is a significant problem, questions have been raised about the standards used in the survey, and the problem needs further investigation.[6]

Dental Problems. Poor dental health associated with a low level of dental care was encountered in many segments of the population surveyed, indicating that a major health problem in regard to the delivery of dental care exists. Data on decayed, missing, and filled teeth indicated that Spanish-Americans in the low-income-ratio states appeared to have the lowest level of dental care, although a large percentage of all children showed evidence of receiving little or no dental care. In adults, periodontal disease was the major dental problem seen, and periodontal disease and poor oral hygiene appeared to have some relationship to income status. The amount of carbohydrate from desserts and foods high in sugar was calculated and compared with the caries experience of adolescents. It was found that between-meal snacks of high carbohydrate foods, such as candy, soft drinks, and pastries, were associated with the development of dental caries. Little relationship was seen between selected biochemical parameters (such as serum levels of selected nutrients) and dental disease.[7]

Specific Nutrients. Most groups had a sufficient intake of protein, but there was some suggestive evidence of marginal protein nutriture in a relatively large proportion of pregnant and lactating women. These women demonstrated low serum albumin levels. Spanish-Americans (primarily Mexican-Americans in Texas) exhibited evidence of inadequate vitamin A intake. Vitamin C deficiency was not a major problem among any groups studied, although the prevalence of poor vitamin C status increased with age. Among the B-complex vitamins, riboflavin status was poor among blacks and young people of all ages. There was no evidence that iodine deficiency was a problem in any group studied.

Preschool Nutrition Survey (1968–1970). The findings of this survey were not dissimilar to those of the Ten-State Survey, that is, the highest prevalence of nutritional problems was among the population sample (in this case, preschool children) of lower socioeconomic status. Evidence of nutritional risk in these children—lower dietary intakes, lower biochemical indices, and smaller physical size for age in comparison with the other subjects—was associated with consumption of an insufficient quantity of food. Although more than half of the children in the survey consumed an inadequate amount of iron, the level of protein intake did not pose a nutritional problem. However, approximately one third of children in the lowest socioeconomic group consumed diets containing inadequate kilocalories.

National Health and Nutrition Examination Surveys (NHANES I and NHANES II). Since 1956, information about the health status of the population has been provided through the Health Examination Survey conducted by the National Center for Health Statistics. In 1971, this survey was expanded to include a system for measuring nutritional status and monitoring changes in this status over time and was renamed the National Health and Nutrition Examination Survey (NHANES). NHANES I, conducted from 1971 to 1974, was the first of its kind to collect measures of nutritional status for a scientifically designed sample representative of the civilian, noninstitutionalized population ages 1 to 74 years. The population was classified racially as "white," "Negro," or "other." Findings, though not as dramatic as the Ten-State Survey, point to the same areas of nutritional concern.[8]

A substantial proportion of individuals had low kilocalorie intakes, with the lowest intakes observed in blacks in lower-income groups. Children in the income groups above the poverty level were taller and heavier, and whereas no significant differences were noted in height and weight between white and black groups, black youths exhibited a relatively greater leanness than whites. Again, adult obesity was prevalent, especially in women, and particularly in black women.

As in the Ten-State Survey, iron deficiency was found to be prevalent. While more common in children ages 1 through 5, the deficiency was observed in all age and income groups. With a few exceptions, there was a fairly low prevalence of other observable clinical signs that placed individuals at high or moderate risk for specific nutrient deficiency or imbalances. Notable exceptions were for vitamins (A, some of the B-complex, C, and D), some of the minerals (iodine—in contrast to the Ten-State Survey—and calcium–phosphorus), and protein.

Older people showed a generally higher prevalence of more of the clinical signs possibly indicative of nutrient deficiency than did the young. When compared with persons above the poverty level over the different age groups, persons with incomes below the poverty level had a generally higher prevalence of clinical signs possibly indicating deficiencies of vitamins A and C and calcium–phosphorus imbalance. Blacks, regardless of age and income level, showed a generally higher prevalence rate than whites for clinical signs indicating possible deficiencies of vitamins A, C, and D, thiamin, calcium–phosphorus, and iodine. Males had generally higher prevalence rates than did females for clinical signs indicating possible deficiencies of protein, vitamin C, and vitamin D, whereas females had higher rates than males for signs suggesting deficiencies of vitamin A, niacin, and iodine, and calcium–phosphorus imbalance.[9]

Findings from NHANES II, conducted in 1976–1980 on individuals ages 6 months to 74 years are becoming available.[10] Analysis and synthesis of these survey results will allow for assessment of changes in nutritional status since NHANES I. Other findings from the Survey will be published periodically. Early release of selected findings are reported in *Advance Data from Vital and Health Statistics of the National Center for Health Statistics.* Detailed reports follow in the *Vital and Health Statistics, Series II,* and can be obtained from these sources.

Household Food Consumption Surveys

The U.S. Department of Agriculture surveys food consumption of a representative sample of U.S. households at periodic intervals and uses the survey results to evaluate the nutritive quality of diets consumed. Findings from the lastest survey conducted in 1977–1978 indicate that of the nutrients studied, calcium, iron, magnesium, and vitamin B_6 were most often consumed in inadequate amounts (Table 1–2). Substantial numbers of individuals also consumed inadequate vitamin A and vitamin C.

Unlike the nutritional status surveys, which provide information on all aspects of nutritional status, food consumption surveys provide information only about what foods are consumed by the public.

CURRENT NUTRITIONAL CONCERNS

Nutritional issues that are currently of national concern include the short-term and long-term effects of malnutrition, the need for techniques of improving nutritional status through long-term (education) and short-term (food enrichment) approaches, the safety of the current food supply, the need for improvement in the system of providing assistance to low-income groups, and the need to expand research efforts in all of the above areas.

Each of these concerns relates to the nutritional status of individuals and groups, or that condition of the body resulting from the intake and use of the essential food nutrients. Observe for overt effects of nutritional deficiency, such as a deficiency of protein, vitamins, or minerals, and, equally important,

TABLE 1–2
PERCENTAGE DISTRIBUTION OF 37,785 INDIVIDUALS WITH NUTRIENT INTAKES AT SPECIFIED LEVELS OF 1980 RDAs

Nutrient	% of Individuals Receiving		
	100% and over of RDA	70–99% of RDA	Less than 70% of RDA
Energy	24	44	32
Protein	88	9	3
Calcium	32	26	42
Iron	43	25	32
Magnesium	25	36	39
Phosphorus	73	19	8
Vitamin A value	50	19	31
Thiamine	55	28	17
Riboflavin	66	22	12
Preformed niacin[a]	67	24	9
Vitamin B_6	20	29	51
Vitamin B_{12}	66	19	15
Vitamin C	59	15	26

[a] Based on RDA values as milligrams of preformed niacin
(*Source: USDA: Food and nutrient intakes of individuals in 1 day in the United States, Spring, 1977. Nationwide Food Consumption Survey, 1977–1978. Preliminary Report No. 2, USDA, Consumer Nutrition Center, Hyattsville, Md, 1980.*)

observe for the more subtle and long-term effects of diet, for example, in its relationship to the degenerative diseases, infant mortality, adaptive behavior of schoolchildren, and work capacity of adults.

Malnutrition can be defined at several levels. ▶ **Primary malnutrition** occurs when an individual receives a deficit or excess of kilocalories or essential nutrients for a period of time sufficient to compromise health. Malnutrition may also exist in individuals who experience periods of prolonged hunger, even though nutritional deficiency may not be manifest. Finally, malnutrition may exist in those who are unable to acquire those foods that are common to their society or culture.

INTERVENTION

Optimum Nutritional Care

The following barriers to sound nutritional care have been listed by the American Dietetic Association.[11]

1. There is little or no public recognition of the role of nutrition education in health promotion, the need for ongoing support of nutrition research, and the necessity for nutritional care.
2. Funding for nutritional services is inadequate. Except during hospitalization for crisis care, nutrition services tend to be less accessible to the working poor and to middle-

income persons than to the affluent (who can afford the service for a fee) and the indigent (who are eligible for a variety of public health programs). Mechanisms for providing nutrition services to ambulatory clients are very limited.

3. Acceleration is needed in the expansion of the role of the dietitian as a primary caretaker and physician extender in providing nutritional care on a continuing basis in primary care settings. Organizational structures in which dietitians can work in teams with other health professionals are lacking or deficient.

4. Basic and continuing education in nutrition is not provided in the curricula for many health professionals, such as physicians, dentists, and others.

5. Routine screening efforts often omit indices of nutritional status (such as history of dietary intake and physical and biochemical assessment data). Even when these are available, they are often not used to initiate needed referrals.

6. Health insurance plans seldom include dietary counseling as a reimbursable service.

Because of the importance of nutrition in the promotion of growth, health maintenance, and treatment and rehabilitation following illness, a comprehensive health care delivery system should include an identifiable nutrition component.

Providers of Nutritional Care

In providing nutritional care, apply the science and art of human nutrition in assisting individuals, families, and groups to obtain and select food for nourishing their bodies in health and disease throughout the life cycle. Give emphasis to emotional as well as physical needs in providing this care. In providing nutritional care, first, assess nutritional needs, second, develop and implement a nutritional care plan, and, finally, evaluate and report the results. Provide dietary counseling on an individualized basis as needed to assist people to adjust their daily food consumption to their health needs. One individual may need assistance in selecting proper foods from the supermarket, another with food preparation techniques when facilities are meager or a physical handicap is present, another with techniques for feeding a handicapped child, and so forth.

▶ Given the multidisciplinary nature of the science of nutrition and the multiple causes of many health problems, use the **interdisciplinary team approach** to nutritional care that combines the expertise of a variety of disciplines to provide the most comprehensive approach to improving the health of individuals and groups through nutritional improvement. Members of the health team who assume a primary role in nutritional care are the physician, dietitian or nutritionist, and nurse. Supportive roles

are played by other team members, such as the physical therapist, occupational therapist, and social worker.

The physician prescribes diets and may assume other aspects of nutritional care, such as diet counseling. More frequently, however, the physician refers the client to the appropriate team member for counseling. Dietitian–nutritionists and nurses provide valuable input concerning the nutritional status of the patient in assisting the physician to prescribe a diet tailored to specific nutritional needs.

The dietitian or nutritionist is the one team member whose primary role is providing nutritional care. Providing nutritional care is only one component of the services provided by other members. The responsibility for the quality of nutritional care provided by any health care team ultimately rests with the physician and dietitian–nutritionist.

Nurses assume a variety of roles relative to nutritional care—they provide input into the development of a realistic nutritional care plan, assist the client to accept and understand it, assist the client to maintain an adequate nutritional intake, and assist in educating the client in principles of nutrition related to the specific diet.

The social worker may become involved with the socioeconomic and psychologic aspects of nutrition care. Supportive services provided by the physical therapist and occupational therapist include the introduction of exercises that strengthen muscles and counteract some of the negative nutritional effects of immobilization, and the provision of self-help devices for feeding and aids for food preparation for the physically handicapped.

Other team members who extend or supplement nutritional health care services are health educators and nutrition aides. Some health care facilities also maintain a patient education center that provides teaching aids and resource materials on diet as related to specific health problems. Health planners assist with the delivery of all health care services by identifying needs and resources and by structuring the environment for health care delivery.

To cope with the problem of malnutrition among hospitalized patients, some hospitals have assembled a specialized team—the nutritional support team. This team usually includes a physician, nurse, dietitian–nutritionist, pharmacist, and a clinical coordinator. However, in larger hospitals a team with larger numbers, types, and time commitments of personnel may be desirable. The functions of this team are to monitor the nutritional status of hospitalized patients, to initiate and supervise appropriate nutritional support measures, and to provide a multidisciplinary approach to nutritional problems that arise in the hospital.

Current Perspectives for Improving Health Care

According to some authorities, further expansion of the nation's current health system is likely to produce only marginal improvements in overall health status. The greatest benefits are likely to accrue from techniques designed for the prevention and early detection of disease.[12] There is much research to indicate that the incidence of cardiovascular disease, some types of cancer, and some other chronic diseases may be significantly reduced through preventive care. In the etiology of most of the major chronic illnesses that plague modern society, there are both behavioral and environmental components. For example, educational level, housing pattern, employment opportunities, access to health services, nutritional status, and other factors influence disease patterns. Many current health problems are associated with the lifestyle of affluence—sedentary living; overconsumption of food, alcohol, cigarettes; and so on. Because of this multifaceted etiology, a multifaceted approach that requires modifications of both personal health habits and the environment for prevention should be applied.

To look at health in this manner may require a new orientation for health professionals. Additionally, the involvement of nonhealth professionals, such as those in law, urban planning, environmental technology, and management, will be increasingly required. For example, highway accidents are not prevented by increasing the number of trauma centers or helicopters available for emergency transport of the injured, but accidents and the risk of injury may be reduced by such measures as surveillance of alcohol consumption, improved passenger restraints, and lower speed limits.

Some diseases may be avoided through primary prevention—improvement of personal health habits or modifications in the environment—and the progression of a disease may be limited by secondary prevention—early detection and subsequent treatment. Stimulate personal responsibility and motivation in the improvement of personal health habits to increase the potential for success in any primary prevention program. While this tactic is applicable to the entire population, apply it particularly to target groups including young children and those adults who have been identified as being at high risk for the development of certain diseases. Introduce preventive measures in such areas as nutrition as early in life as practicable to assure maximum effectiveness in the establishment of behavior patterns that are likely to carry over into adult life. At the same time, adapt suggested changes to various ethnic, sociocultural, and age categories. To achieve this end, work toward improvement in the current system for providing health education, including nutrition education, for both children and adults.

Use outreach efforts as necessary to identify individuals at high risk of developing a particular health problem. Once they are identified, assist them to reduce the risk factors by providing access to an appropriate control program whether it be for nu-

trition, smoking, alcohol abuse, or hypertension. Again, control programs designed for the prevention of health problems require expansion if these preventive techniques are to be effective.

While personal health preventive techniques can be applied on an individual basis, many of the environmental components of primary prevention require cooperative action. For example, malaria has been controlled in the United States primarily as a result of clearing the swamps and wetlands that were in close proximity to populous areas, and goiter has largely been controlled by the addition of iodine to salt. Many of the current concerns related to health, such as the quality and safety of the food supply, the air we breathe, and the water we drink, are in varying degrees subject to group decision via the legislative process. In order to express opinions in any of these areas, become active in the political decision-making process.

Early detection of disease through selective screening followed by early treatment is the focus of secondary prevention. This differs from risk factor detection in that nurses look for the earliest possible evidence of diseases rather than identifying a probability of developing an illness (risk). When nurses assist with periodic health examinations, hypertension screening clinics, and screening tests for cancer of the breast and cervix, they are practicing secondary prevention.

ROLE OF NUTRITIONAL CARE

Nutritional care is an essential component of both the prevention and treatment of disease. Although nutrition as a single therapeutic modality can serve a curative function as in treatment of deficiency diseases, its greatest usefulness is in combination with other modalities in the prevention and treatment of health problems. Preventive nutrition means nutritional balance—on the one hand, assurance of an adequate supply of nutrients to maintain normal metabolic processes at all stages of development and, on the other hand, avoidance of nutrient excesses that can lead to pathologic changes.

Dietary modifications are an essential component of the treatment of a number of disease states, such as hypertension, cardiac disease, renal disease, and diabetes. Further, concern about the poor nutritional status of hospitalized patients gives a new emphasis to the importance of nutrition as supportive therapy for clients who cannot ingest or use an adequate amount of food because of illness.

REVIEW QUESTIONS AND ACTIVITIES

1. Compare the current pattern of consumption of total energy, carbohydrate, protein, and fat with the consumption pattern of each of these during the early 1900s.

2. Describe the association between current dietary consumption patterns and occurrences of certain chronic diseases.
3. Describe the major findings from the three major nutritional status surveys and the one major food consumption survey that have been conducted in recent years.
4. Identify the roles of each of the following health team members in providing nutritional care: physician, dietitian–nutritionist, nurse, social worker, physical therapist, and occupational therapist.

REFERENCES

1. Welsh SO, Marston R: Review of trends in food use in the United States, 1909–1980. J Am Diet Assoc 81:120, 1982.
2. Select Committee on Nutrition and Human Needs: Dietary Goals for the United States. Washington, DC, U.S. Government Printing Office, Feb 1977, pp 9–14.
3. Ibid, p 9.
4. Trowell H: Definition of dietary fiber and hypothesis that it is a protective factor in certain diseases. Am J Clin Nutr 29:417, 1976.
5. DHEW: Ten-State Nutrition Survey, 1968–1970, III. Clinical, Anthropometric, Dental. Publication No. (HSM) 72–8131, Atlanta, p III-15.
6. Ibid, IV. Biochemical. Publication No. (HSM) 72–8132, pp IV-7–8.
7. Ibid, III. Clinical, Anthropometric, Dental. Publication No. (HSM) 72–8131, pp III-87–93.
8. DHEW: Preliminary Findings of the First Health and Nutrition Examination Survey, United States, 1971–1972. Dietary Intake and Biochemical Findings. Publication No. (HRA) 74–1219–1. Anthropometric and Clinical Findings. Publication No. (HRA) 75–1229. Rockville, Md, 1975.
9. Ibid, Anthropometric and Clinical Findings, pp 27–28.
10. USDHHS, National Center for Health Statistics: Hematological and Nutritional Biochemistry Reference Data for Persons 6 Months–74 Years of Age: United States, 1976–80. DHHS Publication No. (PHS) 83–1682, Hyattsville, Md, 1982; Dietary Intake Source Data: United States 1976–80. DHHS Publication No. (PHS) 83–1681, Hyattsville, Md, 1983.
11. The dietitian in primary health care. J Am Diet Assoc 70:589, 1977.
12. U.S. Public Health Services: The Forward Plan for Health 1978–82. Washington, DC, U.S. Government Printing Office, 1976, p 69.

BIBLIOGRAPHY

American Dietetic Association: Costs and Benefits of Nutritional Care, Phase I. Chicago, American Dietetic Association, 1979.

Connor WE: Too little or too much: The case for preventive nutrition. Am J Clin Nutr 32:1975, 1979.

Harper AE: Healthy people: Critique of the nutrition segments of the Surgeon General's Report on Health Promotion and Disease Prevention. Am J Clin Nutr 33:1703, 1980.

McGinnis JM: Prevention—Today's dietary challenges. J Am Diet Assoc 77:129, 1980.

Shannon BM, Parks SC: Fast foods: A perspective on their nutritional impact. J Am Diet Assoc 76:242, 1980.

Windham CT, Wyse BW, Hansen RG, Hurst RL: Nutrient density of diets in the USDA Nationwide Food Consumption Survey, 1977–1978: I. Impact of socioeconomic status on dietary density. J Am Diet Assoc 82:28, 1983.

Windham CT, Wyse BW, Hansen RG, Hurst RL: Nutrient density of diets in the USDA Nationwide Food Consumption Survey, 1977–1978: II. Adequacy of nutrient density consumption practices. J Am Diet Assoc 82:34, 1983.

USDA: Food Consumption: Households in the United States, Spring, 1977, Nationwide Food Consumption Survey 1977–78. Report No. H-1. Washington, DC, U.S. Government Printing Office, 1982.

USDHEW: The Surgeon General's Report on Health Promotion and Disease Prevention. Publication No. 79–55071. Washington, DC, U.S. Government Printing Office, 1979.

CHAPTER 2

Dietary Guidelines

Objectives

After completion of this chapter, the student will be able to:

1. Differentiate between the Recommended Dietary Allowances, the Basic Four Food Groups, and the six Food Exchange Lists.

2. Distinguish among three uses of the Recommended Dietary Allowances.

3. Assess the nutritional adequacy of a day's meals for an adult female client.

4. Plan a menu for one day for an adult that meets the Basic Four recommendations (including amounts of foods) and adjust the menu to include only low-cost foods.

5. Develop a teaching plan for a client on the topic of low-cost meal planning and adjust the plan so that it is appropriate for a client with limited time, limited food preparation facilities, and limited skills in storing and preparing foods.

6. Compare and contrast the dietary guidelines offered by the Senate Select Committee on Nutrition and Human Needs, the USDA–USDHEW, and the Food and Nutrition Board.

To assist families and individuals of all ages to meet nutritional needs, nurses must be familiar with what these needs are and must be able to translate nutrient needs into specific foods that will supply these nutrients.[1] Tools currently available to assist in this task include the Recommended Dietary Allowances (RDA), the Basic Four Food Groups, food composition tables, and the six Food Exchange Lists.

ASSESSMENT TOOLS

Recommended Dietary Allowances

Meals and snacks planned for an individual or family should provide adequate amounts of approxi-

mately 50 nutrients that are known to be essential for humans. Of these 50 nutrients, sufficient knowledge is presently available to make specific recommendations for amounts needed for only 17 of these nutrients.[2] The RDAs are compiled by the Food and Nutrition Board of the National Academy of Sciences–National Research Council.[3] The RDAs are widely recognized as the authoritative standard of dietary adequacy in the United States and are generally revised every 5 years to incorporate new research findings. Specific recommendations are made for the following:[2]

1. Kilocalories
2. Protein
3. Fat-soluble vitamins
   a. Vitamin A
   b. Vitamin D
   c. Vitamin E

Content in this chapter has been adapted from Lewis CM: Basic and Family Nutrition, A Self-Instructional Approach, ed 2. Philadelphia, FA Davis, 1984.

4. Water-soluble vitamins
   a. Vitamin C (ascorbic acid)
   b. Vitamin B complex
      (1) Folacin (folic acid)
      (2) Niacin
      (3) Riboflavin
      (4) Thiamine
      (5) B$_6$ (pyridoxine)
      (6) B$_{12}$
5. Minerals
   a. Calcium
   b. Phosphorus
   c. Iodine
   d. Iron
   e. Magnesium
   f. Zinc

Recommended amounts of kilocalories and nutrients are given for individuals of a specified weight and height in 15 sex–age categories (17 in the case of kilocalories) and for pregnant and lactating women. Table 2–1 provides recommendations for kilocalories, and nutrient recommendations are found in Table 2–2.

The RDAs for nutrients specify the level of intake of essential nutrients considered to be adequate to meet the known nutritional needs of practically all healthy persons who live in the United States under the usual environmental stresses. They reflect the best available estimate of the amount of essential nutrients that should be consumed by each person in a healthy population in order to be reasonably assured that the physiologic needs of all persons in the population will be met. In determining the RDAs, actual nutritional requirements and individual variations in these requirements are considered. Except for kilocalories, the amount recommended for each nutrient is intended to provide a margin above actual physiologic requirements to cover variations among individuals in the general population. Although the nutrient needs for most individuals are overstated, there is no practical way of predicting whose requirements are below, equal to, or above the RDA. The recommendations for kilocalories represent the average needs of people in each category.

The RDAs are expressed in terms of the amount of nutrients that should be consumed daily. Therefore, consider the nutrient losses that occur in food processing, storage, and preparation when evaluating the nutritional content of a diet using data ac-

TABLE 2–1
MEAN HEIGHTS AND WEIGHTS AND RECOMMENDED ENERGY INTAKE[a]

	Age (years)	Weight (kg)	Weight (lb)	Height (cm)	Height (in)	Energy Needs (with range) (kcal)	Energy Needs (with range) (MJ)
Infants	0.0–0.5	6	13	60	24	kg × 115 (95–145)	kg × 0.48
	0.5–1.0	9	20	71	28	kg × 105 (80–135)	kg × 0.44
Children	1–3	13	29	90	35	1300 (900–1800)	5.5
	4–6	20	44	112	44	1700 (1300–2300)	7.1
	7–10	28	62	132	52	2400 (1650–3300)	10.1
Males	11–14	45	99	157	62	2700 (2000–3700)	11.3
	15–18	66	145	176	69	2800 (2100–3900)	11.8
	19–22	70	154	177	70	2900 (2500–3300)	12.2
	23–50	70	154	178	70	2700 (2300–3100)	11.3
	51–75	70	154	178	70	2400 (2000–2800)	10.1
	76 +	70	154	178	70	2050 (1650–2450)	8.6
Females	11–14	46	101	157	62	2200 (1500–3000)	9.2
	15–18	55	120	163	64	2100 (1200–3000)	8.8
	19–22	55	120	163	64	2100 (1700–2500)	8.8
	23–50	55	120	163	64	2000 (1600–2400)	8.4
	51–75	55	120	163	64	1800 (1400–2200)	7.6
	76 +	55	120	163	64	1600 (1200–2000)	6.7
Pregnancy						+300	
Lactation						+500	

[a] The data in this table have been assembled from the observed median heights and weights of children, together with desirable weights for adults for the mean heights of men (70 in) and women (64 in) between the ages of 18 and 34 years as surveyed in the U.S. population (HEW/NCHS data).

The energy allowances for the young adults are for men and women doing light work. The allowances for the two older age groups represent mean energy needs over these age spans, allowing for a 2% decrease in basal (resting) metabolic rate per decade and a reduction in activity of 200 kcal/day for men and women between 51 and 75 years, 500 kcal for men over 75 years, and 400 kcal for women over 75. The customary range of daily energy output is shown for adults in parentheses and is based on a variation in energy needs of ± 400 kcal at any one age, emphasizing the wide range of energy intakes appropriate for any group of people.

Energy allowances for children through age 18 are based on median energy intakes of children these ages followed in longitudinal growth studies. The values in parentheses are 10th and 90th percentiles of energy intake, to indicate the range of energy consumption among children of these ages.

(*Source: National Research Council: Recommended Dietary Allowances, ed 9. Washington, DC, National Academy Press, 1980.*)

TABLE 2–2
RECOMMENDED DAILY DIETARY ALLOWANCES[a]

Age (years)	Weight (kg)	Weight (lb)	Height (cm)	Height (in)	Protein (g)	Vitamin A (μg RE)[b]	Vitamin D (μg)[c]	Vitamin E (mg α-TE)[d]	Vitamin C (mg)	Thiamine (mg)	Riboflavin (mg)	Niacin (mg NE)[e]	Vitamin B6 (mg)	Folacin (μg)[f]	Vitamin B12 (μg)	Calcium (mg)	Phosphorus (mg)	Magnesium (mg)	Iron (mg)	Zinc (mg)	Iodine (μg)
Infants																					
0.0–0.5	6	13	60	24	kg × 2.2	420	10	3	35	0.3	0.4	6	0.3	30	0.5[g]	360	240	50	10	3	40
0.5–1.0	9	20	71	28	kg × 2.0	400	10	4	35	0.5	0.6	8	0.6	45	1.5	540	360	70	15	5	50
Children																					
1–3	13	29	90	35	23	400	10	5	45	0.7	0.8	9	0.9	100	2.0	800	800	150	15	10	70
4–6	20	44	112	44	30	500	10	6	45	0.9	1.0	11	1.3	200	2.5	800	800	200	10	10	90
7–10	28	62	132	52	34	700	10	7	45	1.2	1.4	16	1.6	300	3.0	800	800	250	10	10	120
Males																					
11–14	45	99	157	62	45	1000	10	8	50	1.4	1.6	18	1.8	400	3.0	1200	1200	350	18	15	150
15–18	66	145	176	69	56	1000	10	10	60	1.4	1.7	18	2.0	400	3.0	1200	1200	400	18	15	150
19–22	70	154	177	70	56	1000	7.5	10	60	1.5	1.7	19	2.2	400	3.0	800	800	350	10	15	150
23–50	70	154	178	70	56	1000	5	10	60	1.4	1.6	18	2.2	400	3.0	800	800	350	10	15	150
51+	70	154	178	70	56	1000	5	10	60	1.2	1.4	16	2.2	400	3.0	800	800	350	10	15	150
Females																					
11–14	46	101	157	62	46	800	10	8	50	1.1	1.3	15	1.8	400	3.0	1200	1200	300	18	15	150
15–18	55	120	163	64	46	800	10	8	60	1.1	1.3	14	2.0	400	3.0	1200	1200	300	18	15	150
19–22	55	120	163	64	44	800	7.5	8	60	1.1	1.3	14	2.0	400	3.0	800	800	300	18	15	150
23–50	55	120	163	64	44	800	5	8	60	1.0	1.2	13	2.0	400	3.0	800	800	300	18	15	150
51+	55	120	163	64	44	800	5	8	60	1.0	1.2	13	2.0	400	3.0	800	800	300	10	15	150
Pregnant					+30	+200	+5	+2	+20	+0.4	+0.3	+2	+0.6	+400	+1.0	+400	+400	+150	h	+5	+25
Lactating					+20	+400	+5	+3	+40	+0.5	+0.5	+5	+0.5	+100	+1.0	+400	+400	+150	h	+10	+50

[a] The allowances are intended to provide for individual variations among most normal persons as they live in the United States under environmental stresses. Diets should be based on a variety of common foods in order to provide other nutrients for which human requirements have been less well defined. See preceding table for weights and heights by year of age and for suggested average energy intake.

[b] Retinol equivalents. 1 retinol equivalent = 1 μg retinol or 6 μg β carotene.

[c] As cholecalciferol. 10 μg cholecalciferol = 400 IU of vitamin D.

[d] α-tocopherol equivalents. 1 mg d-α tocopherol = 1α-TE.

[e] 1 NE (niacin equivalent) is equal to 1 mg of niacin or 60 mg of dietary tryptophan.

[f] The folacin allowances refer to dietary sources as determined by Lactobacillus casei assay after treatment with enzymes (conjugases) to make polyglutamyl forms of the vitamin available to the test organism.

[g] The recommended dietary allowance for vitamin B12 in infants is based on average concentration of the vitamin in human milk. The allowances after weaning are based on energy intake (as recommended by the American Academy of Pediatrics) and consideration of other factors, such as intestinal absorption.

[h] The increased requirement during pregnancy cannot be met by the iron content of habitual American diets nor by the existing iron stores of many women; therefore the use of 30–60 mg of supplemental iron is recommended. Iron needs during lactation are not substantially different from those of nonpregnant women, but continued supplementation of the mother for 2–3 months after parturition is advisable in order to replenish stores depleted by pregnancy.

(Source: National Research Council: Recommended Dietary Allowances, ed 9. Washington, DC, National Academy Press, 1980.)

Data in Tables 2–2 and 2–3 are based on the 1980 Recommended Dietary Allowances, the most recent at the time of publication. New data will be available in early 1986. If you desire updates of these tables, please contact the publisher.

TABLE 2–3
ESTIMATED SAFE AND ADEQUATE DAILY DIETARY INTAKES OF ADDITIONAL SELECTED VITAMINS AND MINERALS[a]

		Vitamins			Trace Elements[b]					
	Age (years)	Vitamin K (µg)	Biotin (µg)	Pantothenic Acid (mg)	Copper (mg)	Manganese (mg)	Fluoride (mg)	Chromium (mg)	Selenium (mg)	Molybdenum (mg)
Infants	0–0.5	12	35	2	0.5–0.7	0.5–0.7	0.1–0.5	0.01–0.04	0.01–0.04	0.03–0.06
	0.5–1	10–20	50	3	0.7–1.0	0.7–1.0	0.2–1.0	0.02–0.06	0.02–0.06	0.04–0.08
Children	1–3	15–30	65	3	1.0–1.5	1.0–1.5	0.5–1.5	0.02–0.08	0.02–0.08	0.05–0.1
and	4–6	20–40	85	3–4	1.5–2.0	1.5–2.0	1.0–2.5	0.03–0.12	0.03–0.12	0.06–0.15
Adolescents	7–10	30–60	120	4–5	2.0–2.5	2.0–3.0	1.5–2.5	0.05–0.2	0.05–0.2	0.1–0.3
	11+	50–100	100–200	4–7	2.0–3.0	2.5–5.0	1.5–2.5	0.05–0.2	0.05–0.2	0.15–0.5
Adults		70–140	100–200	4–7	2.0–3.0	2.5–5.0	1.5–4.0	0.05–0.2	0.05–0.2	0.15–0.5

[a] Because there is less information on which to base allowances, these figures are not given in the main table of the RDA and are provided here in the form of ranges of recommended intakes.
[b] Since the toxic levels for many trace elements may be only several times the usual intakes, the upper levels for the trace elements given in this table should not be habitually exceeded.
(*Source: National Research Council: Recommended Dietary Allowances, ed 9. Washington, DC, National Academy Press, 1980.*)

quired from tables of food composition (see Appendix 1). Assess nutritional requirements on an individual basis for persons with disease conditions, those subjected to prolonged stress, or those taking certain medications, since these situations alter nutritional requirements.

The 1980 revision of the RDA also provides provisional allowances for additional selected vitamins (vitamin K, biotin, and pantothenic acid) and minerals (copper, manganese, fluoride, chromium, selenium, molybdenum, sodium, potassium, and chloride). Ranges of safe and adequate intakes of these nutrients are given for three age categories: infants, children and adolescents, and adults (Table 2–3). At present, knowledge of human requirements for these nutrients is not sufficiently refined to state a recommended intake. These provisional allowances are intended to serve as guidelines to the public and food manufacturers to ensure a supply of the nutrients sufficient to prevent a marginal deficiency and, at the same time, provide safety from chronic toxicity.

To assure an adequate intake of other nutrients that are essential but not listed in the RDA, a varied diet should be consumed. Since foods provide nutrients only if eaten, be sensitive to the social and psychologic significance of food by assisting clients to meet the RDA with foods that are both acceptable and palatable. Some individuals believe that ingesting excessive amounts of some nutrients (such as vitamins A, C, and E) provides additional health benefits. However, advise clients that excessive doses of a number of nutrients are known to exert a chemical action in the body that is totally unrelated to nutritional (metabolic) function. In some cases, this chemical action is toxic to the body. Except in certain pathologic conditions that may require large doses of some nutrients, use the RDA (and the ranges given for the provisional allowances) as a standard in the event that nutrient supplementation is necessary.

The RDA is sometimes used by nurses and dietitian–nutritionists to assess the nutritional adequacy of diets of individuals. A modification of the RDA, the U.S. RDA, is also used as a standard for providing nutritional information on food labels, and the RDA is being investigated for use as a standard for expressing nutrient density, i.e., the relationship of the nutrient content of a food to its energy content.

U.S. RDA and Nutritional Labeling

Nutritional labeling, which is regulated by the Food and Drug Administration, provides information about the content of energy and selected nutrients on packaged food labels. The information provided must be based on laboratory analysis of the product, not calculated from food composition tables. The practice is *mandatory* for two classes of foods shipped in interstate commerce: (1) those for which a claim about nutritional properties is made on the label or in advertising, e.g., "low in kilocalories," "high in vitamin C," (2) those that are fortified or enriched by the addition of nutrients, such as enriched bread or fortified milk. For other foods, nutritional labeling is *voluntary*. However, some foods, such as those prepared for institutional food service, are exempt.

The standard used for nutritional labeling is the U.S. RDA derived from the RDA. Like the RDA, the U.S. RDA provides a considerable margin of safety above actual requirements, and, therefore, the allowances are overstated for many people. There are four distinct sets of U.S. RDAs to correspond to the various age–sex characteristics of the population: infants (0 to 12 months), children under 4 years, children above 4 years and adults, and pregnant and lactating women. To assure an allowance high enough to cover the needs of practically everyone in these categories, the figure selected for each nutrient (except calcium and phosphorus) is the highest RDA figure value for each age–sex category.

Electrolytes		
Sodium (mg)	Potassium (mg)	Chloride (mg)
115–350	350–925	275–700
250–750	425–1275	400–1200
325–975	550–1650	500–1500
450–1350	775–2325	700–2100
600–1800	1000–3000	925–2775
900–2700	1525–4575	1400–4200
110–3300	1875–5625	1700–5100

```
               NUTRITION INFORMATION
                    (per serving)

Serving size = 1 oz          Servings per container = 12
         Calories             110
         Protein              2 g
         Carbohydrate         24 g
         Fat                  0 g
         Sodium               50 mg

    Percentage of U.S. Recommended Daily Allowance
                   (U.S. RDA)*

         Protein              2
         Thiamine             8
         Niacin               2

NOTE:
   * Contains less than 2 percent of U.S. RDA for vitamin A, vitamin
     C, riboflavin, calcium, and iron
```

Figure 2–1
Example of minimum information that must appear on a nutrition label.

U.S. RDAs are also established for some nutrients, including biotin, pantothenic acid, and copper, for which no RDA is available. The U.S. RDA for children above age 4 and adults is used as the standard for labeling most foods. The others are used for foods and supplements developed especially for the age–sex groups, such as the use on baby foods of the U.S. RDA for infants.

A standard format in content and sequence must be followed when nutrition information is provided on labels. The energy; grams of carbohydrate, protein, and fat; milligrams of sodium; and percentage of the U.S. RDA for protein, five vitamins (A, C, thiamine, riboflavin, and niacin), and two additional minerals (calcium and iron) provided per serving of a food must be listed (Fig. 2–1). Only those nutrients present at a level greater than 2 percent of the U.S. RDA may be listed, and a disclaimer must be included for those contained in insignificant amounts. Sodium content can also be provided on a voluntary basis without necessitating full nutritional labeling.

In addition to these mandatory listings, other nutrients, including fat (as saturated and polyunsaturated fatty acids), cholesterol, and certain other vitamins, may be listed on an optional basis. Reference to any of these optional nutrients must be accompanied by the mandatory listings illustrated in Figure 2–1. When fat and cholesterol content is listed this conditional statement is included: "Information on fat and cholesterol content is provided for individuals who, on the advice of a physician, are modifying their total dietary intake of fat and cholesterol" (Fig. 2–2).

Foods processed for special dietary purposes, such as fat-controlled, sodium-restricted, or low-calorie diets, must follow the mandatory labeling regulations described above. Foods labeled "low-calorie" must have a caloric density of 0.4 kcal or less per gram and contain no more than 40 kcal per serving.

Reduced-calorie foods must be at least one-third lower in kilocalories than a similar food in which the kilocalories have not been reduced and must not be nutritionally inferior to the higher-caloric counterpart. For a food to be labeled "sugar free," "sugarless," or "no sugar," it must also be labeled "low-calorie" or "reduced-calorie" or accompanied by the statement "not a reduced-calorie food."

Five terms may be used on the label to describe sodium content: sodium free (less than 5 mg/serv-

```
               NUTRITION INFORMATION
                    (per serving)

Serving size = 8 oz          Servings per container = 2
         Calories             560
         Protein              23 g
         Carbohydrate         43 g
         Fat                  33 g

    (Percent of calories from fat = 53 percent)

         Polyunsaturated*     22 g
         Saturated*           9 g
         Cholesterol* (18 mg/100 g)   40 g
         Sodium (365 mg/100 g)        810 mg

    Percentage of U.S. Recommended Daily Allowance
                   (U.S. RDA)

    Protein      35      Niacin        25
    Vitamin A    35      Calcium       2
    Vitamin C    10      Iron          25
    Thiamine     15      Vitamin B6    22
    Riboflavin   15      Vitamin B12   15

NOTE:
   * Information on fat and cholesterol content is provided for
     individuals who, on the advice of a physician, are modifying
     their total dietary intake of fat and cholesterol.
```

Figure 2–2
A label may contain optional listings of fats, cholesterol, sodium, and other nutrients.

ing), very low sodium (35 mg or less per serving), low sodium (140 mg or less per serving), reduced sodium (processed so that the usual level of sodium is reduced by 75 percent), and unsalted (processed without added salt, in a product that usually has added salt). Comparative claims may be made when the food contains 25 percent less sodium than the food to which it is being compared. In foods that contain up to 140 mg/serving, sodium content is specified in 5 mg increments whereas in foods that contain more than 140 mg/serving, sodium content is specified in 10 mg increments. Soft drinks and other products that contain 90 percent or more water are temporarily exempt from the sodium regulation.

Encourage clients to use the labels to compare products to determine which product offers the best nutritive value for the money, and for those on modified diets, to use the labels to select those foods appropriate for their needs. Remind them, however, to use the U.S. RDA only as a guideline; on the one hand, the U.S. RDA may overstate their own nutritional requirements and, on the other, not all nutrients needed for health are listed on the labels.

Nutrient Density

The quality of a food is directly related to its nutrient density, and determining the ratio between kilocaloric content and the nutrient composition in a food provides scores that allow nurses and other health professionals to assess the nutritional quality of individual foods and diets. Scores for such foods as fats, sugars, soft drinks, and alcohol are low, indicating a low nutrient density, whereas more nutritious foods, such as turnip greens, give high scores, indicating a high nutrient density. The ratio for each nutrient in a given food or combination of food in a meal can be calculated, and a method using the RDA has been described.[4] Advise clients who have low-calorie requirements because of a sedentary lifestyle to select foods of high nutrient density.

BASIC FOUR FOOD GROUPS

Since the RDA is somewhat too detailed a guide for routine use by much of the general public, the Basic Four Food Groups were designed and have been used for many years in nutrition education to assist people in planning adequate diets that will meet the RDA. In 1979 a new version of the guide was published designating a fifth group. The Basic Four Food Groups are:

1. Milk and cheese group
2. Meat, poultry, fish, and beans group
3. Vegetable–fruit group
4. Bread–cereal group

The fifth group is fats–sweets–alcohol.

Foods of similar nutritive value are classed together in a group and can be substituted one for another within that group. Recommendations are given as to the number and size of servings of foods from each group that should be eaten daily to serve as the foundation of a nutritionally adequate diet. The number and size of servings that one usually sees listed in connection with the Basic Four Food Groups are those for an adult. Adjustments must be made in number and/or size of servings to meet the needs of children and the increased nutrient demands of adolescence, pregnancy, and lactation.[5]

The number of daily servings recommended for adults and the various foods within groups in the Basic Four Food Groups guide are shown in Figure 2–3. The fifth group—fats, sweets, and alcohol—is not shown in Figure 2–3, since there is no recommended daily number of servings for these foods.

Milk and Cheese Group

An 8 oz cup of milk (either whole, skim, low-fat, nonfat, buttermilk, diluted evaporated milk, or yoghurt) or the amount of a food from this group (such as ice cream, ice milk, or cheese) that will provide the same amount of calcium provided by 1 c of milk is considered one serving. Milk used in cooked foods, such as creamed soups, sauces, and puddings, can count toward filling the daily quota from this group. Although foods from the milk and cheese group are good sources of protein of high biologic value and certain vitamins, they are chosen primarily for their calcium content. Equal amounts of milk, cheese, and ice cream are not equal in calcium content, however. The amount of cheese and ice cream necessary to provide the calcium contained in 1 c of milk or plain yoghurt is shown in the diagram below.[6]

AMOUNTS OF FOODS THAT PROVIDE AN EQUAL AMOUNT OF CALCIUM

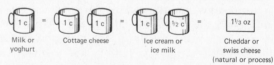

Advise clients that 12 oz (1½ c) of ice cream or ice milk, or 16 oz (2 c) of cottage cheese are required to provide the calcium contained in 1 c of milk. On the other hand 1⅓ oz of cheddar or Swiss cheese has an amount of calcium equal to that contained in 1 c milk.

Meat, Poultry, Fish, and Beans Group

In this group, dry peas or beans, soybeans, lentils, nuts, peanut butter, seeds, and eggs may substitute for meat, poultry, or fish as a source of protein and other nutrients. The amounts of foods that can be used as a protein substitute for 1 oz of meat are shown below.[7]

AMOUNTS OF FOODS THAT PROVIDE AN EQUAL AMOUNT OF PROTEIN

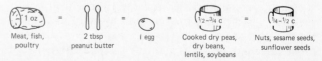

USE THESE FOODS DAILY

MILK AND CHEESE GROUP

Milk or equivalents in cheese, yoghurt, ice cream, or ice milk

Basic servings daily

Children under 9	2–3 c
Children 9–12	3 c
Teenagers	4 c
Adults	2 c
Pregnancy	3 c
Lactation	4 c

MEAT, POULTRY, FISH, AND BEANS GROUP

2 basic servings daily

Meat, fish, poultry, eggs, dry beans or peas, seeds, nuts, peanuts, and peanut butter

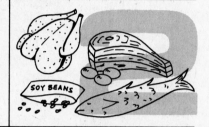

VEGETABLE-FRUIT GROUP

4 basic servings daily

Include a good source of vitamin C daily (such as citrus fruits or tomatoes), and frequently include dark green or deep-yellow vegetables, unpeeled fruits and vegetables and those with edible seeds (such as berries)

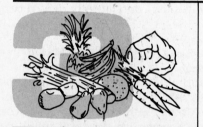

BREAD-CEREAL GROUP

4 basic servings daily

Select only wholegrain and enriched or fortified bread, cereal and pasta (such as macaroni, and noodles) being sure to include some wholegrain bread or cereal daily

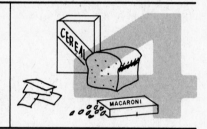

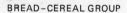

Figure 2–3
A daily food guide. This is the foundation of an adequate diet for all age groups. Additional servings of these foods, as well as other foods, will provide the additional kilocalories needed for growth, activity, and maintenance of desirable body weight. (Source: Lewis CM: Basic and Family Nutrition, A Self-Instructional Approach, ed 2. Philadelphia, FA Davis, 1984, p 67. Adapted from Food. Home and Garden Bulletin No. 228, U.S. Department of Agriculture.)

Two to three ounces of lean cooked meat, poultry, or fish without bone or the amount of eggs, legumes, seeds, nuts, or peanut butter that provides an equal amount of protein is considered one serving from this group for an adult. Therefore, 4 tbsp of peanut butter or 2 eggs or 1 to 1½ c cooked beans would be equal in protein to one 2-oz serving of meat. Legumes, nuts, and seeds are also sources of dietary fiber. While the serving size listed for legumes, nuts, peanut butter, and seeds will provide an equal amount of protein as meat, fish, poultry, or eggs, the biologic value of the protein is not equal; these foods can be combined with animal or grain products to improve protein quality.

Vegetable–Fruit Group

In foods from the vegetable–fruit group, the single serving size for an adult is ½ c or one typical portion (as one medium apple or one medium potato).

Dark green or yellow vegetables, citrus fruit or tomatoes and other foods high in vitamin C content, and unpeeled fruits and vegetables should be in-

cluded. The rationale for this is that the diet should contain a good food source of vitamin C daily and a good source of vitamin A three or four times per week, as well as adequate sources of dietary fiber.

The vegetable–fruit group provides practically all of the vitamin C in the diet and a substantial amount of the vitamin A. The remaining vitamin A comes from whole milk and cheese and fortified skim milk in the milk–cheese group and egg yolk and organ meats, such as liver and kidney, in the meat–fish–poultry–beans group. Butter, fortified margarine, and cream, classified as fats, also contain vitamin A. Vitamin A in the diet is derived from preformed vitamin A (retinol) in foods of animal origin and from provitamin A (the carotenoids) in fruits and vegetables. Fruits and vegetables, particularly those that are unpeeled or contain edible seeds, also provide dietary fiber.

Bread–Cereal Group

The bread–cereal group includes all products made with whole grains or enriched flour or meal (the common breads, cereals, pastas, waffles, pancakes, baked products, flour, and cornmeal). The amounts of one serving of foods from this group for an adult are: 1 slice of bread or 1 oz ready-to-eat cereal or ½ to ¾ c cooked cereal or pasta. Some whole grain bread or cereal should be eaten daily, since these foods provide some vitamins and trace minerals not found in enriched foods. Whole grains and bran are also sources of dietary fiber.

Fats–Sweets–Alcohol Group

With some exceptions, the nutritional contribution provided by this group is limited primarily to kilocalories. For this reason, a basic number of size of servings is not suggested. Included in the group are:

- *Visible fats and oils.* Butter, fortified margarine, cream, cream cheese, vegetable oils and shortenings, mayonnaise, salad dressings, bacon, bacon grease, fatback, fish oils
- *Sweets.* Sugar and foods high in sugar, such as jam, jelly, honey, candy, sweet toppings, soft drinks, and other highly sweetened beverages
- *Alcoholic beverages.* Beer, wine, liquor

Also included in this fifth group because of their low nutrient density are unenriched breads, pastries, and flour products.

Butter, cream, fortified margarine, and fish oils add fat-soluble vitamins, especially vitamins A and D. Vegetable oils are high in vitamin E and in polyunsaturated fatty acids, including linoleic acid, a fatty acid that is essential for growth. Polyunsaturated fatty acids are also valuable for their blood lipid lowering effect. Unrefined dark molasses provides some iron and calcium.

Foods from this group are usually used as ingredients in prepared foods, added to other foods at the table, or used as extras. Advise clients, particularly those gaining unwanted weight, to use these foods in moderate amounts because of their kilocalorie contribution and low nutrient density. Fats provide more than twice the kilocalories per gram than do carbohydrate and protein, and alcohol is a high-caloric food as well as a drug. Few alcoholic beverages are 100 percent alcohol, and the higher the alcohol content, the higher the kilocalories. Moreover, sugar (sucrose) in sticky form, as in cake frosting and sticky candy, may contribute to dental caries.

Nutritional Characteristics of the Basic Four Food Groups

Earlier it was noted that the Basic Four Food Groups serve as the foundation of an adequate diet for all age groups.[8] Each food group is selected for the unique contribution it makes to the total nutritive value of the diet. Figure 2–4 provides a summary

MILK AND CHEESE	MEAT AND ALTERNATIVES
Complete protein Vitamins: A, B (especially riboflavin, B_6, and B_{12}) vitamin D (fortified milk) Minerals: Calcium, phosphorus, magnesium, zinc	Complete protein (legumes, seeds, and nuts are incomplete when used alone) Vitamins: All of the B complex (B_{12} is found only in animal food), A (in egg yolk and liver), E in nuts), D (in egg yolk, liver, salt water fish) Minerals: Iron, phosphorus, magnesium, zinc, calcium (in fish with bones, legumes--especially soybeans, nuts--especially almonds), iodine* (in seafood) Essential fatty acids: Seeds
VEGETABLE–FRUIT	BREAD–CEREAL
Incomplete protein Vitamins: A, C, E (in green leafy vegetables), B complex (especially folic acid, riboflavin, and pyridoxine†) in leafy vegetables) Minerals: Iron and calcium (in leafy vegetables and dried fruits), magnesium (in leafy vegetables and bananas)	Incomplete protein Vitamins: B complex (thiamine, riboflavin, and niacin--all three are added to enriched bread and cereal and are present naturally in whole grains), folic acid and pyridoxine (in whole grain cereal), E (in whole grains and cereal germs)‡ Minerals: Iron and phosphorus (in both whole grain and enriched bread and cereal--iron is added to enriched bread and cereal and is present naturally in whole grains), magnesium and zinc (larger quantities in whole grains than in enriched bread and cereals), calcium (most commercial bread and rolls have dry milk solids added during preparation)

NOTE:
*Iodine is also provided by iodized salt.
†Bananas, potatoes (white and sweet), prunes, raisins, and yeast are also good sources of pyridoxine.
‡Vegetable oils and margarine are also good sources of vitamin E.

Figure 2–4
Major nutrients in the food groups. (Source: Lewis CM: Basic and Family Nutrition, A Self-Instructional Approach, ed 2. Philadelphia, FA Davis, 1984, p 93.)

of the major nutrient contributions of foods from the Basic Four Food Groups. The nutrients included in this summary are those for which a specific RDA is given.[9] For each food group, providing the daily number of servings in the size recommended for each age will provide the RDA for most nutrients and a substantial amount of the energy needs. A diet that provides the recommended basic number and size of servings for adults from the four nutrient-rich groups supplies approximately 1200 kcal. This amount may be sufficient for many sedentary adults who have low energy needs. Active individuals who have higher energy and nutrient requirements can meet these needs by (1) selecting additional or larger servings from the Basic Four or (2) including foods from the kilocalorie-rich fifth group. Inform them, however, that the first choice adds additional nutrients as well as kilocalories. Advise adult clients who wish to avoid gaining weight and overweight clients who wish to reduce that a diet based on the food guide and providing approximately 1200 to 1500 kilocalories may be an excellent starting point. For those gaining unwanted pounds, first cut down on foods from the fats–sweets–alcohol group. Second, cut down on portion sizes from the other groups and select the lower-calorie foods from within each group. For example, fortified low-fat or skim milk products have essentially the same nutrients as whole milk products but fewer kilocalories.

The iron requirements of young children and women during the reproductive period are so high that the additional foods selected for kilocalories by young children and women should be chosen for their iron content as well. Further, the availability of iron from the food supply in relation to the increased iron demand during pregnancy is such that iron supplementation is necessary.[10]

Advise elderly clients that their nutritional needs are basically the same as those of younger adults, with two important exceptions.[10] These are:

1. Elderly adults require fewer kilocalories than younger adults. For this reason, foods chosen in addition to the amounts recommended from the Basic Four Food Groups should be carefully selected so as not to add excessive kilocalories.
2. Iron needs of postmenopausal women decrease to the same level as the recommendation for adult men.

The current nutritional environment—which includes a considerable use of processed foods—necessitates selection of a wide variety of foods from the various food groups to assure that the RDAs for all essential nutrients are met.

FOOD COMPOSITION TABLES

Detailed information is available about the nutrient composition of individual foods.[11] Such data are presented in Appendix 1. However, when considering the nutritive value of specific foods, one should keep in mind that food composition can only be described in terms of representative average values. Because of its biologic nature, food is subject to considerable variations that reflect seasonal, climatic, and genetic influences.

While seasonal and climatic variables are not controllable, considerable progress has been made with genetic maneuvers that have produced improved nutritional strains of some foods, such as cereal grains. Other variables, such as stage of maturity and nutrient losses incurred in food processing, storage, and preparation, also have a bearing on the final nutritive value of the food actually consumed.

Some food processors provide food composition data for their products on request. While some of this information is derived from the traditional food composition tables, other figures may be obtained from a company's own laboratory analysis of its products. A recent innovation is the Nutrient Data Bank, a cooperative effort of the U.S. Department of Agriculture, other governmental agencies, and the food industry. In the future, it is anticipated that this system will provide extensive information about food composition as food research laboratories continually submit food composition data.

DIETARY ANALYSIS

The RDA, Basic Four Food Groups guide, and food composition tables are frequently used in assessing the nutritional quality of a client's diet prior to providing dietary counseling. In some instances, simply comparing food intake with the Basic Four Food Groups guide is adequate. At other times, more precise information is desirable, and it becomes necessary to compare the intake of specific nutrients with the RDA. Both techniques are described below. A 24-hour period is used in the examples, but the methods can be applied to any time period.

Comparison with Basic Four Food Groups

1. Write down the number of servings of all food and beverage intake during the last 24 hours. Estimate the size of servings in the following units:
   a. Milk, ice cream, cottage cheese—cups
      Hard cheese—ounces.
   b. Meat and alternates—ounces or cups (include the ingredients in any mixed dish)
      Peanut butter—tablespoons; eggs—number
   c. Vegetables and fruits—cups or individual portions
   d. Bread and cereal—slices of bread or equivalent in hot bread or rolls;
      Cereal and pasta—cups
   e. Other foods: fats, oils, sugar—teaspoons or tablespoons (3 tsp = 1 tbsp)

Allow approximately 1 tsp of margarine or fat for each serving of cooked vegetables; allow extra fat for fried meats; if breaded and fried, allow extra flour as well

Alcoholic beverages—fluid ounces[12]

2. Convert the amounts listed into servings according to the food group to which it belongs, e.g., 2 eggs = 1 meat serving.
3. Total the number of servings for each of the food groups.
4. For each of the food groups, compare the total servings from the list with the recommended number of servings for that food group. Also, check the food intake list for sources of vitamins A and C and for fiber.

Comparison with RDA

1. Determine the RDA for the person whose diet is being evaluated (Tables 2–1 and 2–2). The RDA is based on a person's age, sex, and recommended body weight. An easy rule of thumb for determining recommended body weight of adults is presented in Figure 2–5, and a method for determining body frame size is given in Table 2–4. To determine kilocalorie needs for an adult, allow 15 kcal per lb per day if body weight is normal (recommended body weight for that person). If overweight, allow 10 kcal per lb per day. If underweight, allow 20 kcal per lb per day. To determine protein needs for an adult, allow 0.8 g of protein per kg (2.2 lb) of recommended body weight. Use Table 2–2 for the RDA for other nutrients.
2. List all food and beverage intake in the last 24 hours (as in Step 1 of dietary analysis using the Basic Four Food Groups).
3. Calculate the nutritive value of each item listed using the food composition tables presented in Appendix 1. Make adjustments as necessary when the amount listed is larger or smaller than the amount given in the food composition table.
4. Total the amounts for each nutrient.
5. Compare the totals for each nutrient with the RDA determined in Step 1. When assess-

---

TABLE 2–4
APPROXIMATION OF FRAME SIZE

Extend your arm and bend the forearm upward at a 90-degree angle. Keep fingers straight and turn the inside of your wrist toward your body. If you have a caliper, use it to measure the space between the two prominent bones on *either* side of your elbow. Without a caliper, place thumb and index finger of your other hand on these two bones. Measure the space between your fingers against a ruler or tape measure. Compare it with these tables that list elbow measurements for *medium-framed* men and women. Measurements lower than those listed indicate you have a small frame. Higher measurements indicate a large frame.

Height in 1-in Heels	Elbow Breadth
Men	
5'2"–5'3"	2½"–2⅞"
5'4"–5'7"	2⅝"–2⅞"
5'8"–5'11"	2¾"–3"
6'0"–6'3"	2¾"–3⅛"
6'4"	2⅞"–3¼"
Women	
4'10"–4'11"	2¼"–2½"
5'0"–5'3"	2¼"–2½"
5'4"–5'7"	2⅜"–2⅝"
5'8"–5'11"	2⅜"–2⅝"
6'0"	2½"–2¾"

(Source: Courtesy of the Metropolitan Life Insurance Company)

---

ing a client's diet in this manner, assume that nutrient intake is acceptable if the average intake for 1 week meets the recommended amount. The recording of a deficient intake on any given day may be insignificant, since the body has some ability to adjust to less than optimum levels of various nutrients. However, habitual intake below the RDA poses a risk of nutritional deficiency.

THE SIX FOOD EXCHANGE LISTS

A simplified method for diet calculation involves the use of the exchange system, which uses food groups similar to, yet somewhat different from, the Basic Four Food Groups. A Food Exchange List is a group of specific amounts of foods such that all the foods in an exchange list are approximately equal in carbohydrate, protein, and fat. Since they are approximately equal in carbohydrate, protein, and fat content, these foods are also equal in kilocaloric content. Thus any food within a given list can be substituted or exchanged for any other food in that list.

The six Food Exchange Lists were developed by the American Dietetic Association, the American Diabetes Association, and the U.S. Public Health Service in 1950 and revised in 1976.[13] Although originally designed for use with diabetic diets, they are also used for calculating other diets that require a controlled amount of kilocalories, carbohydrate, protein, or fat.

WOMEN
Allow base weight of 100 lbs for 5 ft (60 in), ± 5 lbs per in above or below 5 ft

MEN
Allow base weight of 106 lbs for 5 ft (60 in), ± 6 lbs per in above or below 5 ft

NOTE:
Add 10 percent of total for individuals with large frames; subtract 10 percent for small frames. To determine whether large, medium, or small frame, see Table 2-4.

Figure 2–5
Rule of thumb method for determining recommended body weight of individuals of medium body frame.

In the exchange system, most common foods are classified into one of six exchange lists according to their composition. All foods grouped together, in the amount listed, have approximately the same carbohydrate, protein, and fat (and therefore kilocaloric) content. The six exchange groupings are:

- List 1. Milk exchange
- List 2. Vegetable exchange
- List 3. Fruit exchange
- List 4. Bread exchange
- List 5. Meat exchange
- List 6. Fat exchange

In addition, there is a list of free foods that contain no carbohydrate, protein, or fat, which are thus kilocaloric free. The six Food Exchange Lists are presented in Appendix 2. In setting up the lists, a standard was used in determining the amount of each food that would be equivalent to one exchange from each list. In most cases, the standard is low in kilocalories and fat. The standards for the six lists are given in Table 2–5.

In each of the six Food Exchange Lists, the amount of each food listed is equal to 1 exchange. Items to remember when using the exchange system include:

1. Do not confuse servings and exchanges. For example, in using the Basic Four guide, a serving of meat is 2 to 3 oz. However, in the exchange system, 2 to 3 oz of meat is 2 to 3 meat exchanges.
2. In the fruit list, the amount listed as 1 exchange is usually an average-size serving. However, this is not always the case. One exchange of fruits with a high sugar content is a smaller quantity than for fruits with a lesser sugar content.
3. In the vegetable list, those included are relatively low in kilocalories because of their high content of water and nondigestible fiber. Those with a high starch content are listed under bread exchanges. A few salad greens and radishes are kilocalorie free and can be used as desired.
4. The list of kilocalorie-free foods includes several beverages, a number of herbs and spices, and a few vegetables and fruits.

Application of the Food Exchange Lists to meet various dietary needs is presented in Part III of this book.

INTERVENTION

Application of the food guides discussed above in assisting clients to plan adequate diets involves consideration of the many factors that influence food intake. The effect of some of these variables is examined below.*

Family Resources
Family resources that have a bearing on food and nutrient intake include income, equipment, and time.

Income. A number of variables, including (1) number, sex, age, and activities of family members, (2) special dietary needs, and (3) the amount of food produced and preserved at home, influence the cost of providing an adequate diet. In general, the lower the income, the greater the proportion of it must be spent for food in order to obtain a low-cost yet adequate diet. Use guides provided by the U.S. Department of Agriculture to estimate the amounts of food needed to provide an adequate diet for a family at four different cost levels: (1) liberal, (2) moderate, (3) low, and (4) thrifty (see Appendices 3, 4, 5, and 6). The cost of food for the plans is updated periodically by the Department of Agriculture.[14]

When income is low, encourage clients to use these eight guidelines for meal planning and food shopping to improve their nutritional intake at reduced costs:[15]

1. Use a meal pattern as a basis for planning meals; the example below[15] allows for the foods suggested from the Basic Four Food Groups.

---

* Content in this section has been adapted from Lewis CM: Basic and Family Nutrition, A Self-Instructional Approach, ed 2. Philadelphia, FA Davis, 1984, pp 179–197, 221–242.

TABLE 2–5
STANDARDS FOR THE SIX FOOD EXCHANGE LISTS

Standard		Exchange	Carbohydrate (g)	Protein (g)	Fat (g)	Kcal
1 c skim milk	=	1 Milk exchange	12	8	trace	80
½ c vegetable	=	1 Vegetable exchange	5	2	0	25
Average serving of fruit	=	1 Fruit exchange	10	0	0	40
1 slice bread	=	1 Bread exchange	15	2	0	70
1 oz lean meat	=	1 Meat exchange	0	7	3	55
1 tsp margarine	=	1 Fat exchange	0	0	5	45

Breakfast
Fruit or juice
(citrus, melon, or strawberries)
Main dish and/or
cereal with milk
Bread, beverage

Lunch
Main dish
Vegetable or fruit
Bread, beverage

Snack
Fruit or cookies
Beverage

Dinner
Main dish
Two vegetables
(one dark green or deep yellow every
other day)

2. Plan menus based on family preference to avoid waste.
3. Do advance planning of meals and snacks.
4. Use all available resources when planning meals, e.g., the food supply on hand, food stamps, food coupons, advertised specials, and U.S. Department of Agriculture listings of foods in plentiful supply.
5. Keep menus simple.
6. Plan some protein from animal sources at each meal or combine plant proteins at meals to assure that protein of high biologic value is available.
7. Use the less expensive choices from the Basic Four Food Groups (Table 2–6).
8. Use efficient food shopping techniques, e.g., (a) use a supermarket for major food purchases rather than the more expensive neighborhood grocery store unless extra transportation costs would cancel the savings, (b) make cash payments for purchases, (c) avoid impulse buying by shopping with a market list and avoiding shopping when hungry, (d) purchase food in bulk quantity if it is cheaper in bulk, if used frequently by the family, and if adequate storage is available, (e) read labels to determine unit costs, grades, brands, ingredients, nutritive value, and degree of freshness of the product, (f) examine fresh food bargains to be sure they are what the name implies, and (g) select canned foods in which the containers are clean and free of leaks, dents, and bulges.[16]

Equipment and Time. Individuals or families who lack basic food preparation facilities, such as an oven or refrigerator, or those whose time available for food preparation is limited because of employment will need assistance with meal planning to assure an adequate intake. Furthermore, low-income families frequently lack modern conveniences so that

---

TABLE 2–6
GUIDELINES FOR LOW-COST FOODS FROM THE BASIC FOUR FOOD GROUPS

Meat, Fish, Poultry, and Beans
1. Choose meats that yield the most cooked meat per lb for the least cost, e.g., ground beef, liver (pork liver is cheaper than beef or calf liver), frying chicken and whole turkey, canned fish, such as sardines, herring, tuna, and mackerel
2. Choose main dishes made from eggs, dry peas or beans, peanut butter, and cheese in place of meat for some of the main meals during that week
3. Combine a small amount of meat with other ingredients to make soup, stew, or casserole
4. Buy meats in large cuts when possible

Milk and Cheese
1. Use nonfat dry milk or evaporated milk when possible
2. Purchase milk in 1 or ½ gal containers from a supermarket or dairy store

Vegetable–Fruit
1. Do cost comparisons among fresh, frozen, canned, and dehydrated products to determine those that cost least per serving
2. Use fruits and vegetables that are in season and therefore cheaper
3. Use standard grades of canned fruits and vegetables rather than the more expensive fancy grade
4. Freeze or can homegrown fruits and vegetables and those purchased at the peak of their season
5. Purchase fruits and vegetables from bins in the supermarket rather than those that are prepackaged
6. Purchase plain frozen vegetables rather than the boil-in-the-bag type or those frozen in a butter sauce

Bread–Cereal
1. Purchase whole grain bread and cereal or bread, cereal, and pasta with the word "enriched" on the label
2. Select the cheapest cereals from the following scale:
   Uncooked—partially cooked—cooked—sugared
   Least expensive ⟵──────⟶ Most expensive
3. Purchase day-old bread when possible
4. Prepare baked goods at home when possible. When time is a factor, use homemade mixes. Purchase plain bread and rolls rather than sweet or fancy-shaped rolls. The cost of cake and muffin mixes compares favorably with home prepared products

(Source: Adapted from Lewis CM: Basic and Family Nutrition, A Self-Instructional Approach, ed 2. Philadelphia, FA Davis, 1984, pp 233–235, 238–239.)

---

the time and energy involved in taking care of the home is increased. In these situations, encourage the client to plan meals that limit the number of foods served, that require the simplest methods of food preparation, and that include foods requiring little attention during preparation, some foods prepared in advance, and some foods prepared from low-cost convenience foods.[17]

Nutrition Knowledge and Skills
Nurses encounter people of all income and educational levels who lack sufficient knowledge or skills to assemble the essentials of an adequate diet. Assess clients for their knowledge of foods that make up an adequate diet, their ability to plan ahead, and

their ability to purchase, store, and prepare food so that maximum nutritive value is obtained for money spent.[18]

Skill in advance planning of meals provides a framework to assure adequacy of the meals and a basis for efficient food shopping with a list. Encourage clients to plan for 1 week or at least prepare tentative plans for meals and snacks for the next few days. If a local newspaper is available, advertised specials can be used in the plans. In all cases, however, meal plans should be kept flexible so that items on special sale can be used.[18]

The need to plan ahead is especially critical for those individuals or families who encounter periods of inadequate income. Lack of skill in planning is reflected in practices such as splurging on foods and luxuries at the beginning of the pay period and tapering off to a monotonous diet of inexpensive foods as the days go by. When meat is available, it may be used all at once, rather than spread out over a period of time.[18]

Skill in purchasing, storing, and preparing foods for greatest retention of nutritive value is essential for obtaining maximum nutrition for money spent. Those with limited budgets cannot afford the loss of nutrients resulting from poor techniques of food storage or preparation.[18] Nutrients, particularly the water-soluble vitamins, may be lost by exposure to light, air, an alkaline medium, or high cooking temperatures.

For maximum retention of nutritive value, teach clients to use the following guidelines in selection, storage, and preparation of foods:[19]

Selection

1. Purchase fresh fruits and vegetables that are firm in texture and free of blemishes
2. Purchase no more perishables than can be stored adequately

Storage

1. Store potatoes and onions in a cool, dark place
2. Store other perishables in the refrigerator. Allow fresh fruits to fully ripen before refrigeration
3. Keep frozen vegetables frozen until ready to cook, then plunge directly into boiling water
4. Eat frozen fruits as soon as defrosted

Preparation

1. Cook fruits and vegetables in their skins when feasible. If peeling and cutting are necessary, leave in large pieces. If soaking is required, use a small amount of water for a minimum period of time
2. Cook in small amount of boiling water for a short time, until just tender, and cover the container
3. Do not add baking soda to cooking water
4. Roast meats at low temperature (300° to 325°F) to minimize shrinkage. Cook pork, however, at 350°F
5. Use vegetable cooking water and drippings from meat to make gravy and soups. Use all leftovers promptly

---

TABLE 2–7
CHANGING UNDESIRABLE FOOD HABITS

Principle	Application
Obtain knowledge of present food habits	Determine (1) adequacy of resources (income, facilities, and so on), (2) meanings and values attributed to food, (3) specific food choices and preparation techniques
Capitalize on positive aspects of present diet	Reinforce good features of the diet
Choose a specific problem on which to focus	Tackle initially a *small, urgent* problem for which a high rate of success is anticipated
Set realistic goals	A homemaker with limited food preparation skills may feel a real sense of achievement from learning how to prepare a simple dish
Use effective communication skills	Use terminology and visual aids that are geared to the individual's level of understanding
Maintain continuity	Follow-up by the same individual is highly desirable
Evaluate continually	Evaluation may indicate a need for a change in technique, a lack of motivation, or other problems

(Source: Lewis CM: *Basic and Family Nutrition, A Self-Instructional Approach,* ed 2. Philadelphia, FA Davis, 1984, p 197. Adapted from Robinson CH: *Normal and Therapeutic Nutrition,* ed 15. New York, Macmillan, 1977, pp 354–355.)

TABLE 2-8
SUMMARY OF GENERAL DIETARY RECOMMENDATIONS

Agency	Maintain Ideal Body Weight	Reduce Total Fat (%) Calories	Reduce Saturated Fat	Increase Polyunsaturated Fat	Reduce Cholesterol	Reduce Simple Sugar	Increase Complex Carbohydrates	Increase Fiber	Reduce Sodium (g NaCl Equivalent)	Other Recommendations[a]
Senate Select Committee on Nutrition and Human Needs; Dietary Goals, 1977[22]	Yes	Yes (27–33%)	Yes	Yes	Yes (250–350 mg)	Yes	Yes	Yes	Yes (<8 g)	1,7
American Heart Association, 1982,[23] 1983[24]	Yes	Yes (No more than 30–35%)	Yes (<10% of total calories)	Substitute for saturated fat (amount not to exceed 10% of total calories)	Yes (<300 mg)	Yes	Yes	Yes	Yes	5
Surgeon-General's Report, 1979[25]	Yes	Yes	Yes	No	Yes	Yes	Yes	Not discussed	Yes	5,8
American Medical Association, 1979[26]	Yes	For high-risk groups	For high-risk groups	For high-risk groups	For high-risk groups	Moderate	Not discussed	Not discussed	Yes (<12 g)	1,5,8
National Cancer Institute: Prudent Interim Principles, 1979[27]	Yes	Yes	Not discussed	No	Not discussed	Not discussed	Not discussed	Yes	Not discussed	1,5,7
USDA–USDHEW Guidelines, 1979[28]	Yes	Yes	Yes	No	Yes	Yes	Yes	Yes	Yes	1,5,8
Food and Nutrition Board Recommendation, 1980[29]	Yes	Adjust to caloric level	No	No	No	If energy needs are low; for diabetics at risk	For diabetics at risk	As dictated by Basic Four Food Groups	Yes (3–8 g)	1,5,7
National Institutes of Health, Concensus Panel on Lowering Cholesterol, 1984[30]	Yes	Yes (30%)	Yes (<10% of total calories)	Yes (maximum of 10% of total calories)	Yes (250–300 mg)	Not discussed	Not discussed	Not discussed	Not discussed	5

[a] Other recommendations:
1. Moderate/reduce intake of alcohol.
2. Moderate/reduce intake of additives.
3. Moderate/reduce use of processed foods.
4. Associates use of sugar with diabetes.
5. Considers special needs of high-risk groups and special populations.
6. Stresses importance of variety in a well-balanced diet.
7. Encourages exercise.
8. Encourages breastfeeding of infants.
(Source: Adapted from McNutt K: Dietary advice to the public: 1957 to 1980. Nutr Rev 38:353, 1980.)

Established Food Habits

The food habits of an individual family reflect cultural, social, and psychological forces that influence attitudes, feelings, and beliefs about food.[20] Examples of the expression of food habits that are usually strongly entrenched in one's lifestyle are:

1. Meal patterns (time and number of meals per day)
2. Foods chosen for specific meals
3. Food preparation methods
4. Specific food likes and dislikes
5. Value placed on food and eating[21]

People develop food habits when they are young. These habits are an expression of general attitudes developed as a child, and as such, specific foods and methods of preparation may serve as a security blanket when the person is older. The home and family in which a child is reared are predominant influences on specific habits developed.[21] For most persons, a change in food habits often is a very slow process. Cultural food habits are explored in detail in Chapters 19 and 20. Table 2–7 lists important principles and suggestions that nurses can apply when attempting to change a client's undesirable food habits.

GENERAL DIETARY GUIDELINES

In recent years, a number of public and private organizations have recommended dietary guidelines to the public. Most of the guidelines include dietary advice designed to decrease the incidence of the chronic degenerative diseases discussed in Chapter 1 by changing the ratio of the energy-producing nutrients (carbohydrate, protein, and fat) consumed and by reducing the intake of dietary constituents, such as sodium and cholesterol. Table 2–8 provides a summary of the recommendations; note the areas of agreement and disagreement among the recommendations.

Essentially all groups agree on maintenance of desirable body weight and, for middle-aged sedentary persons, a reduction of total fat as a percentage of kilocalories. Likewise, most reports urge a reduction in the consumption of simple sugars as an aid to preventing dental caries. There is not universal agreement on reducing the consumption of sodium and saturated fat or increasing consumption of polyunsaturated fat and fiber, however. Recommendations appearing in the 1980s also tend to stress variety in the diet, moderation in the use of alcohol, and support for breastfeeding of infants.

REVIEW QUESTIONS AND ACTIVITIES

1. Identify the purposes and uses of the Recommended Dietary Allowances, the Basic Four Food Groups, and the six Food Exchange Lists.
2. Compare and contrast the food groups included in the Basic Four Food Groups and the six Food Exchange Lists.
3. Identify the following as they relate to the Basic Four Food Groups:
   a. Numbers and sizes of servings needed daily by adults
   b. Amounts of eggs, peanut butter, cooked beans and peas, nuts and seeds that are equal to 1 oz of meat
   c. Examples of low-cost foods from each group
   d. Guidelines for selecting, storing, and preparing foods from each group for maximum retention of nutritive value
4. Determine your own kilocalorie and protein needs based on desirable body weight.
5. List your Recommended Dietary Allowances for the other nutrients (use Table 2–2).
6. Identify the steps involved in dietary analysis using the Recommended Dietary Allowances as the standard.
7. Compose a list of five adjustments in menu planning that would be appropriate for clients with limited time and limited food preparation facilities.
8. Describe the similarities and differences between the recommendations made by each of the following agencies: (1) Senate Select Committee on Nutrition and Human Needs, (2) the USDA–USDHEW, and (3) Food and Nutrition Board.

REFERENCES

1. Lewis CM: Basic and Family Nutrition, A Self-Instructional Approach, ed 2. Philadelphia, FA Davis, 1984, p 58.
2. Ibid, p 59.
3. National Research Council: Recommended Dietary Allowances, ed 9. Washington, DC, National Academy Press, 1980.
4. Hansen BG, Wyse BW: Expression of nutrient allowances per 1,000 kilocalories. J Am Diet Assoc 76:223, 1980.
5. Lewis CM, op cit, p 66.
6. Ibid, p 68.
7. Ibid, p 69.
8. Ibid, p 78.
9. Ibid, p 92.
10. Ibid, p 79.
11. USDA: Composition of Foods—Raw, Processed, Prepared. USDA Agriculture Handbook No. 8. Washington, DC, U.S. Government Printing Office, 1980.
12. Lewis CM, op cit, p 86.
13. The American Diabetes Association and The American Dietetic Association: Exchange Lists for Meal Planning. New York, 1976.
14. Lewis CM, op cit, pp 180–181.
15. Ibid, pp 222–223.

16. Ibid, p 241–242.
17. Ibid, pp 185, 187.
18. Ibid, p 190.
19. Ibid, pp 191–192.
20. Ibid, p 195.
21. Ibid, p 196.
22. Select Committee on Nutrition and Human Needs: Dietary Goals for the United States, ed 2. Washington, DC, U.S. Government Printing Office, 1977.
23. Grundy SM, Bilheimer D, Blackburn H, et al.: Rationale of the diet–heart statement of the American Heart Association: Report of the Nutrition Committee. Circulation 65:839A, 1982.
24. Task Force Committee of the Nutrition Committee and the Cardiovascular Disease in the Young Council of the American Heart Association: Diet in the healthy child. Circulation 67:1411A, 1983.
25. DHEW: Healthy People: The Surgeon General's Report on Health Promotion and Disease Prevention. DHEW Publication No. 79–55071, Washington, DC, 1979.
26. Council on Scientific Affairs: AMA concepts of nutrition and health. JAMA 242:2335, 1979.
27. Broad WJ: New strength in the diet–disease link? Science 206:666, 1979.
28. USDA and USDHEW: Nutrition and Your Health—Dietary Guidelines for Americans. Washington, DC, Office of Governmental and Public Affairs, 1980.
29. National Academy of Sciences: Toward Healthful Diets. Washington, DC, National Academy Press, 1980.
30. National Institutes of Health Concensus Development Statement: Lowering blood cholesterol. Nutr Today 20:13, 1985.

BIBLIOGRAPHY

Bray GA: Dietary guidelines: The shape of things to come. J Nutr Educ 12:97, 1980.

Greenberg DS: Nutrition: A long wait for a little advice. N Engl J Med. 302:535, 1980.

Guthrie, HA, Scheer JC: Nutritional adequacy of self-selected diets that satisfy the Basic Four. J Nutr Educ 13:46, 1981.

Harper AE: Healthy people: Critique of the nutrition segments of the Surgeon General's Report on Health Promotion and Disease Prevention. Am J Clin Nutr 33:1703, 1980.

Light L, Cronin FJ: Food guides revisited. J Nutr Educ 13:57, 1981.

Mertz W: The new RDAs: Estimated and safe intake of trace elements and calculation of available iron. J Am Diet Assoc 76:128, 1980.

Munro HN: Major gaps in nutrient allowances. J Am Diet Assoc 76:137, 1980.

Nutritive Value of American Foods in Common Units. Agriculture Handbook No. 456. Washington, DC, U.S. Government Printing Office, 1980.

Pennington JAT: Considerations for a new food guide. J Nutr Educ 13:53, 1981.

Pennington, JAT, Church HN: Bowes and Church's Food Values of Portions Commonly Used, ed 14. Philadelphia, JB Lippincott, 1984.

CHAPTER 3

Physiologic and Biochemical Overview of Nutritive Processes

Objectives

After completion of this chapter, the student will be able to:

1. Differentiate among the six major classes of nutrients in relation to (a) chemical nature, (b) need for digestion prior to their use, (c) solubility in water, and (d) functions performed in the body.

2. Teach a client with a digestive disorder the normal process of digestion and absorption.

3. Differentiate among the three major mechanisms of nutrient absorption.

4. Distinguish between the two major processes of cell metabolism.

5. Distinguish among the waste products excreted by the four routes of excretion.

▶ As a physical science, **nutrition** involves the study of the action, interaction, and balance of nutrients contained in food and their relationship to health and disease. It also includes study of the processes by which individuals ingest and digest food and absorb, transport, and metabolize nutrients and excrete the associated waste products. This chapter presents an overview of these nutritive processes to serve as a broad framework for more detailed study of specific nutrients in subsequent chapters.[1]

COMPOSITION OF FOOD

In its natural state, food is made up of three broad categories of organic nutrients: carbohydrates, proteins, and lipids (or fats). Before these complex compounds can be absorbed and used by the body, they must be broken down to their simplest forms during

digestion, namely, simple sugars, amino acids, fatty acids, and glycerol. Three additional categories of nutrients that are also present in foods are vitamins, minerals, and water. These nutrients do not require breakdown to simple forms and can be absorbed and used with little or no change. Note the relationships in Figure 3–1.[2]

Carbohydrates, proteins, lipids, and vitamins
▶ are **organic compounds.** Carbon is a structural component of all organic compounds, but this element is lacking in the inorganic nutrients, water,
▶ and minerals. **Vitamin** is the name given to a group of potent organic compounds (other than carbohydrate, protein, and lipid) that occur in minute quantities in food and are essential for specific body functions. Carbohydrates, proteins, and lipids all contain the elements carbon, hydrogen, and oxygen; proteins are different from carbohydrates and lipids, how-
▶ ever, in that they also contain nitrogen. **Carbohydrates,** better known as sugars and starches, are composed of varying numbers of simple sugars, whereas
▶ **proteins** are composed of many amino acids. In con-
▶ trast, **lipids,** better known as fats, are composed of fatty acids and glycerol.[2]

Content in this chapter has been adapted from Lewis CM: Basic and Family Nutrition, A Self-Instructional Approach, Philadelphia, FA Davis, 1984, pp 3–34.

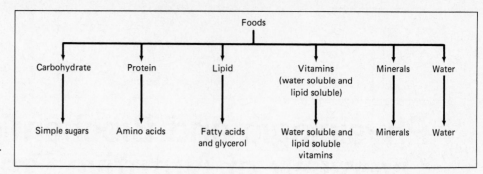

Figure 3–1
Breakdown of food into its nutrient components.

In order for nutrients to be used by the body, they must be soluble, i.e., capable of being dissolved, in the aqueous medium of the body fluids. Most nutrients are readily soluble in water. However, two nutrients, fats and fat-soluble vitamins, are unique in that they are nonwater soluble and require the presence of solution agents for their use (Table 3–1).[3] Bile, a detergentlike secretion from the liver, provides the necessary solubility factor for the digestive breakdown of lipids to fatty acids and glycerol as well as for the passage of fatty acids and lipid-soluble vitamins across the small intestinal wall during absorption. In the intestinal mucosal cells, their solubility is maintained by the formation
▶ of water-soluble lipid–protein complexes called **chylomicrons,** in which the lipids are coated with a layer of protein. As chylomicrons they are transported to the circulatory system for use by the body.

FUNCTIONS OF NUTRIENTS

The major nutrients provided by food are essential for three broad physiologic functions:[4]

1. To supply energy for both voluntary and involuntary body activities
2. To provide structural components for growth and maintenance of body cells
3. To provide components for the formation of regulatory compounds, such as enzymes, coenzymes, hormones, and electrolytes

---

TABLE 3–1
WATER-SOLUBLE AND NONWATER-SOLUBLE NUTRIENTS

Water-soluble Nutrients	Nonwater-soluble Nutrients
Simple sugars	Fats (and fatty acids)
Amino acids	Lipid-soluble vitamins
Glycerol	
Minerals	
Water-soluble vitamins	

(Source: Adapted from Lewis CM: Basic and Family Nutrition, A Self-Instructional Approach, ed 2. Philadelphia, FA Davis, 1980, p 11.)

Carbohydrates, proteins, and lipids are the energy-producing nutrients. Several vitamins and minerals, however, are essential to catalyze, or accelerate, the processes involved in the release of energy. All of the nutrients are involved, either directly or indirectly, in the other two functions.[5] The interrelatedness of the functions of nutrients is illustrated in Figure 3–2.

USE OF FOOD

The use of food for the nourishment of the body requires the coordination of six major physiologic processes. These are schematically represented in the following diagram:[5]

1. Ingestion
2. Digestion
3. Absorption
4. Transport
5. Cell metabolism
6. Excretion

This continuum of ingestion to excretion must be considered as a dynamic unit or working whole. While it may be a very simple matter to trace an individual nutrient through the various physiologic processes, the multitude of events that occur simultaneously in the body must be kept in mind. Each event is affected by other events that preceded it or occur simultaneously with it. The use of each nutrient is interrelated with that of many other nutrients. The maintenance of **homeostasis,** the state of internal balance or equilibrium, by the body is dependent both on an adequate supply of nutrients and on the normal functioning of the various body systems operating within this ingestion–excretion continuum.[5] Thus, if any system is not functioning properly, a breakdown occurs at some point within the continuum.

Ingestion
One of the major factors affecting homeostasis is an adequate supply of nutrients, which ultimately

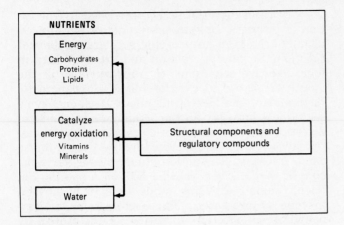

Figure 3-2
Functions of the food nutrients. (Source: Lewis CM: Basic and Family Nutrition, A Self-Instructional Approach, ed 2. Philadelphia, FA Davis, 1984, p 7.)

depends on food intake. All of the nutrients needed by the body are available from food. Many different kinds and combinations of food can provide an adequate supply of nutrients.[6] The following menus, which are characteristic of various ethnic groups, all contain carbohydrates, proteins, lipids, minerals, vitamins, and water.[6]

Swedish
Pickled herring with boiled potatoes
Stuffed cabbage with meat and rice
Rolls with blueberry sauce

Mexican
Lentil–vegetable soup
Tortillas
Refried beans

African
Chicken–peanut stew
Fresh papaya
Cassava meal with eggs, tomatoes, and onions

Greek
Steamed grape leaves with rice and currants
Egg and lemon soup
Baked eggplant, chick pea, and tomato casserole
Flat bread

Some nutrients are present in a wide variety of foods, and, under average conditions of food intake, there is little likelihood of a deficiency occurring. Others are present in less than optimal amounts.[6] Inform clients that if the variety of foods in the diet is limited, deficiencies are likely to occur.

The ingestion of food is controlled by various physiologic, psychologic, and sociocultural factors. None of these controls, however, assures an adequate intake of nutrients.[6] The physiologic factors are the following:

1. The satisfaction of the basic hunger drive.
   Nerve centers or nerve pathways in the brain

are thought to control eating. The neural control system is postulated to respond to various internal and external stimuli that initiate feeding and indicate satiety. Signals that stimulate feeding initiate the search for food; once hunger is relieved, satiety signals take over by inhibiting feeding. In recent years, the liver has been postulated to be involved with monitoring changes in metabolism that signal hunger and satiety.[7]

2. The palatability of specific foods. This is influenced by a combination of sensations produced by stimulation of the taste buds, the olfactory organs, and receptors in the tongue sensitive to temperature and texture variation. Foods palatable to one person may be totally rejected by another.[8]

Attractive, nutritious food can be presented to people, and they may refuse it. The need to satisfy hunger and the psychologic value and sociocultural significance of foods are much likelier determinants of when, how much, and what foods are consumed than is the body's need for nutrients per se. We do not instinctively choose an adequate diet. Foods chosen wisely provide a proper balance of all the nutrients essential for normal body functioning. If they are not properly chosen, however, there may be an excess or deficit of one or more nutrients.[9]

Digestion

► **Digestion,** the second major physiologic process involved in the use of food, is the process by which the complex molecules contained in food are broken down into simpler forms that can be absorbed and used by the body's cells.[9] This involves the breakdown of carbohydrates, proteins, and lipids into simple sugars, amino acids, fatty acids, and glycerol. Vitamins, minerals, and water do not require digestion.

The digestive system consists of a long tube passing through the center of the body with an opening at each end. Until foods are absorbed through the walls of this tube, from a physiologic standpoint they are still outside the body. The main and accessory organs of digestion are listed below and are illustrated in Figure 3-3. The main organs are listed in the sequence in which food passes through them; in Figure 3-3 the accessory organs are starred.

A. Main organs of the digestive tract[10]
   1. Mouth
   2. Pharynx
   3. Esophagus
   4. Stomach
   5. Intestine
      a. Small intestine (approximately 20 ft long and composed of three divisions)
         (1) Duodenum (first 10 in)
         (2) Jejunum (next 7½ ft)
         (3) Ileum (next 12 ft)

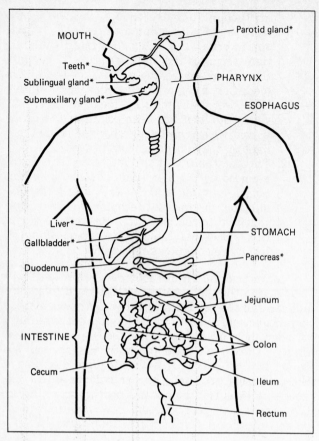

Figure 3–3
*Location of digestive system organs. (*Accessory organs.) (Source: Lewis CM: Basic and Family Nutrition, A Self-Instructional Approach, ed 2. Philadelphia, FA Davis, 1984, p 13.)*

      b. Large intestine (approximately 5 to 6 ft long and composed of three divisions)
         (1) Cecum (first 2 to 3 in)
         (2) Colon (ascending, transverse, descending, and sigmoid)
         (3) Rectum (ends in an opening called the anus)
  B. Accessory organs of the digestive tract
    1. Teeth
    2. Salivary glands
    3. Liver and gallbladder
    4. Pancreas

Digestion of food is accomplished by two main types of processes: mechanical and chemical. Both occur simultaneously as the food moves through the digestive organs. Mechanical digestion involves breaking down the food into smaller pieces so that chemical digestion can take place. As food passes through the digestive tract, the grinding action of the teeth and the contraction and relaxation of the muscular walls of the entire digestive tract accomplish mechanical digestion. The contraction and relaxation of the muscular walls, with the resultant churning action, is known as peristalsis.[11]

Chemical digestion is accomplished by the action of enzymes. **Enzymes** are organic substances, usually protein in nature, that accelerate chemical reactions by catalytic action and are contained in four digestive secretions: (1) salivary juice in the mouth, (2) gastric juice in the stomach, (3) pancreatic juice, and (4) small intestinal juices. Two nonenzyme secretions that play an important role in chemical digestion are (1) hydrochloric acid contained in gastric juice and (2) bile secreted by the liver into the small intestine. The action of enzymes is very specific in that a given enzyme acts on a specific nutrient (Table 3–2). Thus, lipids are split by lipases, protein by proteases, and carbohydrates by carbohydrases.[11] Protein digestion is facilitated by the action of gastric hydrochloric acid, which causes protein molecules to swell and thus be more susceptible to enzyme action. Hydrochloric acid also activates gastric proteases, which are secreted in an inactive form. The action of pancreatic lipase is enhanced by the presence of bile salts contained in bile. The bile salts coat fat droplets in the small intestine, forming soluble complexes called **mixed micelles.**

Through the combined action of the mechanical and chemical processes on foods passing through the main organs of the digestive tract, complex molecules are split into simple ones. Digestion is completed in the small intestine, and the end products are now in a form able to be absorbed across the intestinal wall into the intestinal mucosal cell and finally into the circulatory system.[12]

Absorption
The process of absorption involves the passage of simple forms of nutrients from the intestine to the blood or lymph, where they will be transported to cells. The major organ of absorption is the small intestine. The small intestine is quite a discriminating organ because of its highly developed, specialized tissues.[13] The inner surface of the small intestine contains many folds and is lined with tiny, fingerlike projections called **villi** through which nutrients are absorbed (Fig. 3–4). Nutrients pass from the intestinal lumen, or interior channel, into the mucosa, or interior surface.[13] The walls of the intestine regulate not only the form in which nutrients enter the circulatory system but in some cases also the amount. The intestinal mucosa normally does not allow large molecules, such as intact proteins, to go through. The amount of some of the nutrients absorbed is also regulated by the intestinal mucosa; for example, calcium and iron are absorbed according to the body's need for them.[13]

In the small intestine, most of the nutrients are absorbed from the first and second intestinal segments, the duodenum and jejunum. Nutrients that escape absorption in either of these two sites can be absorbed in the ileum.[13]

The mechanisms by which absorption takes place through the intestinal mucosa are diffusion,

TABLE 3-2
ACTIONS OF ENZYMES IN THE DIGESTIVE PROCESS

Nutrient	Enzyme Action		
	Mouth	Stomach	Small Intestine
Carbohydrate	Starch (amylose and amylopectin) —Salivary amylase (Ptyalin)→ Maltose, maltotriose, and oligosaccharides (Enzyme activity insignificant)	None	*Pancreatic secretions* Starch (amylose and amylopectin) —α-Amylase→ Maltose, maltotriose, and oligosaccharides (α-limit dextrins) *Intestinal secretions* Lactose —Lactase→ Glucose + galactose Sucrose —Sucrase→ Glucose + fructose Maltose —Maltase→ Glucose (2 molecules) α-Limit dextrins —α-Dextrinase (Isomaltase)→ Glucose + maltose
Protein	None	Proteins —HCl Pepsin→ Large polypeptides and amino acids Casein (Milk protein) —Rennin (Present in infants)→ Coagulates milk (paracasein)	*Pancreatic secretions* Proteins and polypeptides —Trypsin Chymotrypsin Carboxypeptidase→ Smaller polypeptides and amino acids *Intestinal secretions* Polypeptides and dipeptides —Aminopeptidase Dipeptidase→ Smaller peptides and amino acids
Fat	None	Tributyrin (butterfat) —Tributyrinase→ Free fatty acids	*Pancreatic secretions* Fat —Lipase (Steapsin)→ Glycerol, monoglycerides, free fatty acids *Intestinal secretions* Fat —Bile (From liver and gallbladder)→ Emulsified fat Monoglycerides —Monoglyceride Lipase→ Glycerol, free fatty acids

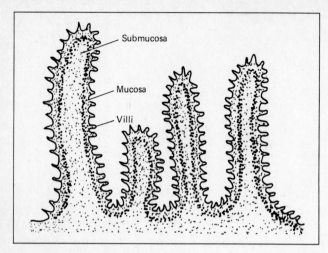

Figure 3–4
Diagram of intestinal villi. (Source: Lewis CM: Basic and Family Nutrition, A Self-Instructional Approach, ed 2. Philadelphia, FA Davis, 1984, p 20.)

carrier-facilitated diffusion, active transport, and oc-
► casionally, pinocytosis.[14] In simple **diffusion,** water, certain electrolytes, and other small water-soluble molecules move freely through pores in the intestinal membranes from the area of higher concentration to the area of lower concentration until equilibrium is established on both sides of the membranes. The large molecular size of most nutrients precludes their transport in this manner. For some of these large molecules, however, diffusion is mediated by
► a carrier; this is called **carrier-facilitated diffusion.** An example is the attachment of the large vitamin B_{12} molecule to a carrier, which ferries the B_{12} across the cell membrane of the intestine into the circulating blood during the process of absorption.

► **Active transport** mechanisms for solute transport can be compared to swimming upstream or walking uphill in that these mechanisms require the expenditure of energy. This energy expenditure allows substances to be transported from an area of lower concentration to an area of higher concentration. Active transport mechanisms appear to be mediated by a carrier molecule that combines with the substances to be transported.

Some substances may be absorbed through the
► process of **pinocytosis.** In this transport technique, the cells of the wall of the small intestine appear to engulf or ingest the substance, move it through the cells, and release it into the circulation. While it is doubtful that this is a significant mechanism for nutrient absorption, on occasion intact proteins may be absorbed in this manner, giving rise to allergic reactions.[14]

Lipids and lipid-soluble vitamins are absorbed as mixed micelles, which diffuse into the intestinal mucosal cell. Once in the cell, the bile salts are released, re-enter the intestinal lumen, and are subse-

quently reabsorbed in the ileum and circulated to the liver for reuse.[14] In a complex series of reactions in the intestinal mucosal cell, fatty acids are resynthesized into complex lipids that, along with the lipid-soluble vitamins, become a part of the chylomicrons, which in turn enter the circulatory system.

While most absorption occurs in the small intestine, a few nutrients are absorbed in the stomach and some from the large intestine as the indigestible parts of food pass through the segments of the colon in preparation for excretion. Water, a small amount of glucose, some minerals, and alcohol, a nonnutrient substance, are absorbed from the stomach. Major nutrients absorbed in the colon are water, some mineral elements, and possibly a few vitamins. The vitamins that may be absorbed in the colon are those that are produced there by the fermentation of intestinal bacteria on undigested food residues. Significant amounts of vitamin K and smaller amounts of the vitamin B complex are produced and absorbed in the colon and possibly the ileum.[15] However, there is uncertainty about how well the vitamins are absorbed from the lower gastrointestinal tract.

Nutrients are absorbed into either the portal vein or the lymph. All water-soluble nutrients readily dissolve in plasma and enter the portal vein

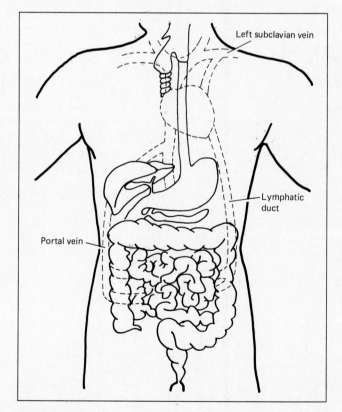

Figure 3–5
Anatomic location of the portal vein and lymphatic duct. (Source: Lewis CM: Basic and Family Nutrition, A Self-Instructional Approach, ed 2. Philadelphia, FA Davis, 1984, p 22.)

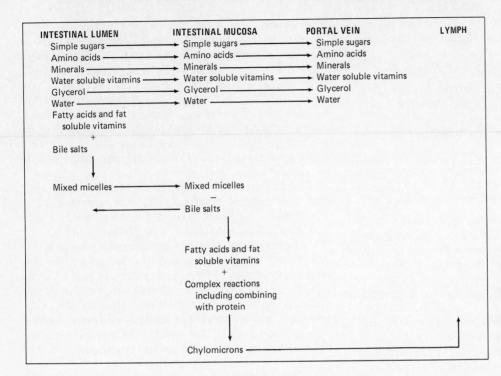

Figure 3–6
A summary of nutrient absorption. (Source: Lewis CM: Basic and Family Nutrition, A Self-Instructional Approach, ed 2. Philadelphia, FA Davis, 1984, p 23.)

and are transported to the liver. Chylomicrons containing the lipids and lipid-soluble vitamins enter the lymphatic system, then the systemic circulation at the left subclavian vein, and are transported, first through the heart and finally to the liver. (See Fig. 3–5 for the anatomic location of the portal vein and lymphatic duct in relation to the digestive tract.) Nutrient absorption is summarized in Figure 3–6.

Nutrient Transport

In the liver, the nutrients undergo further metabolism or are transported directly to the body cells for use or storage. Excesses of some nutrients are stored in the liver. Nutrients are distributed through the arteries and capillaries and finally to the interstitial fluid that surrounds all body cells. As the interstitial fluid bathes the cells, the needed nutrients present in this fluid are transported across each individual cell's membranes to be used by the cell in its metabolic processes. The mechanisms by which the nutrients cross the cell membrane are the same as those mentioned for intestinal absorption: diffusion, carrier-facilitated diffusion, active transport, and pinocytosis. The cell membrane acts as a selective barrier of nutrients into the cell. Figure 3–7 illustrates the passage of nutrients from the capillaries to the interstitial fluid and finally into the cells.[16]

In addition to transporting the nutrients to the cell, the circulatory system also transports oxygen provided by the respiratory system for use in all metabolic processes and transports waste products of cell metabolism from the cell to excretory sites, such as the lungs and kidneys.[17]

Cell Metabolism

The term metabolism is used to describe all of the physical and chemical changes that take place within the cell. Once in the cell, the nutrients are metabolized through numerous physical and/or chemical changes in order to perform the three broad functions of food described earlier in this chapter. Cell metabolism is of two major types: anabolism and catabolism.[18]

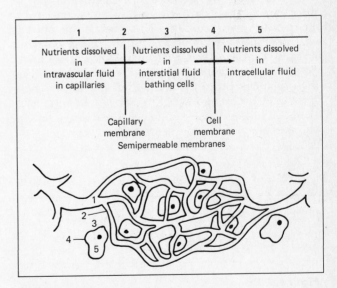

Figure 3–7
Passage of nutrients from capillaries to interstitial fluid and to cells. (Source: Lewis CM: Basic and Family Nutrition, A Self-Instructional Approach, ed 2. Philadelphia, FA Davis, 1984, p 28.)

► **Anabolism** refers to building-up activities, or those processes by which new substances are synthesized from simpler compounds. Examples of anabolism that occur constantly in cells are:[18]

1. Synthesis of body proteins from amino acids
2. Synthesis of body fat from fatty acids and glycerol
3. Synthesis of glycogen from glucose (simple sugar) molecules

► **Catabolism** refers to the breakdown of complex substances to simpler compounds. Three examples of catabolism that occur constantly in cells are:[18]

1. The oxidation of glucose, fatty acids, and fragments of amino acid molecules, with the release of carbon dioxide, water, and energy. The energy is released as adenosine triphosphate (ATP).
2. The breakdown of glycogen to yield glucose (simple sugar).
3. The breakdown of cells due to daily wear and tear. Cellular materials are constantly being catabolized and must be replaced through anabolic processes. The rate of cellular turnover varies with the type of cell and is exceptionally high in the most active cells, such as those of the liver, skin, and the gastrointestinal tract. Even fat cells are constantly being broken down and replaced.

There is a constant interplay between anabolism and catabolism in the cells. Since anabolic processes depend on the energy released from catabolic processes, both proceed simultaneously. In spite of the rapid rate of cell turnover, the body tends to maintain a state of homeostasis.[19]

At any one time there is a metabolic pool of nutrients in the extracellular fluid that constitutes
► the cellular environment. This **metabolic pool** is composed of nutrients from dietary sources as well as those that are salvaged from cellular breakdown. For example, the metabolic pool of amino acids (Fig. 3–8) includes those from the diet as well as those from cellular breakdown. From this metabolic pool, the cell chooses those amino acids necessary to synthesize its specific body proteins.[19]

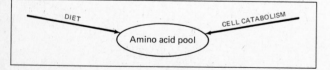

Figure 3–8
The metabolic pool of amino acids includes those obtained from the diet and those obtained from cellular catabolism. (Adapted from Lewis CM: Basic and Family Nutrition, A Self-Instructional Approach, ed 2. Philadelphia, FA Davis, 1984, p 31.)

Excretion

The final physiologic process involved in the use of food is excretion of waste products. The major waste products to be excreted include undigested food residues, metabolic wastes, and dietary excesses. Undigested food residues include foods that are ingested but are not digested or absorbed. In a mixed diet, approximately 98 percent of the carbohydrate, 95 percent of the lipid, and 92 percent of the protein are digested and absorbed. The remaining residue is waste.[20]

Metabolic wastes include carbon dioxide, water, and nitrogenous products of protein metabolism. These waste products are released by the cell into the blood to be transported to their excretory sites.[20]

Dietary excesses that are excreted include excessive water, some mineral elements, and water-soluble vitamins. After absorption, they are transported in the blood to their excretory sites. Excessive carbohydrate, protein, lipid, and lipid-soluble vitamins are not excreted but are stored in the body.[20] Teach clients that the dietary excess of carbohydrate, protein, and lipid can lead to excessive weight gain.

The four routes of excretion are through the large intestine, the lungs, the skin, and the kidneys (Fig. 3–9). The large intestine excretes undigested food residues as well as a small amount of water. The food mass passing from the small to the large intestine is in a liquefied state and contains the nondigestible parts of food. The additional absorption, especially of water, that occurs as the food mass moves through the colon segments produces a semisolid mass that is stored in the lower colon until it is excreted as feces. A small amount of the water contained in the mass is not absorbed but is retained to be excreted with the feces. This water prevents the feces from becoming excessively hard and thus difficult to expel.[21] Teach clients that inadequate fluid intake may lead to constipation.

The excretory function of the lungs includes excretion of the metabolic wastes, carbon dioxide and water. The skin excretes water and some mineral elements, such as sodium, chlorine, and potassium, which are found in sweat. The excretory function of the skin is directly related to regulation of the body's temperature.[22]

The kidneys are an efficient and selective filtering system for the blood, which is constantly circulating through them. The kidneys' primary function is to maintain the normal volume and composition of blood. In order to do this, the kidneys must excrete some metabolic waste products and excesses of nutrients so that there is a relatively constant amount of essential nutrients circulating in the blood at all times. For example, the amount of potassium in the blood must always be in the range of 3.5 to 5.5 milliequivalents (mEq) per liter of blood. If the concentration of potassium in the blood is too high as it circulates through the kidneys, the excess potassium is excreted.[23] The excretory function of the kidneys

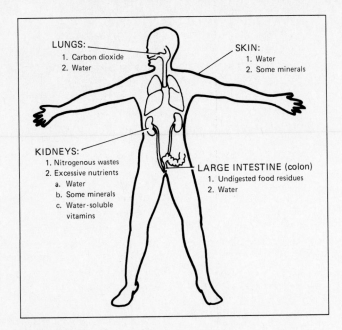

Figure 3–9
The excretion of metabolic wastes by the excretory organs. (Source: Lewis CM: Basic and Family Nutrition, A Self-Instructional Approach, ed 2. Philadelphia, FA Davis, 1984, p 33.)

is under strict hormonal control. The kidneys excrete nitrogenous waste products of protein metabolism, such as urea, uric acid, and creatinine, and excessive nutrients circulating in the blood, including water, some mineral elements, and water-soluble vitamins.[23]

REVIEW QUESTIONS AND ACTIVITIES

1. List the four classes of organic nutrients and the two classes of inorganic nutrients.
2. Identify the chemical element that distinguishes proteins from carbohydrates and lipids.
3. List the three categories of nutrients that do not require digestion prior to absorption.
4. Distinguish between the solubilities of the six categories of nutrients.
5. Identify the three general physiologic functions of nutrients and the functions performed by each nutrient category.
6. List the five major organs and the three accessory organs of the digestive tract.
7. Explain the difference between mechanical and chemical digestion.
8. Explain the difference between the absorption of carbohydrates and lipids and the reason that underlies the difference.
9. Describe the digestion of carbohydrates, proteins, and lipids in relation to sites of digestion and source of enzymes that act on each.
10. Discuss the difference between simple diffusion, carrier-facilitated diffusion, and active transport.
11. List the four routes of excretion and the waste products excreted by each route.

REFERENCES

1. Lewis CM: Basic and Family Nutrition, A Self-Instructional Approach, ed 2. Philadelphia, FA Davis, 1984, p 3.
2. Ibid, pp 3–4.
3. Ibid, p 11.
4. Ibid, p 6.
5. Ibid, p 7.
6. Ibid, p 8.
7. Sawchenko PE, Friedman MI: Sensory functions of the liver—A review. Am J Physiol 236:R5, 1979.
8. Lewis CM, op cit, p 9.
9. Ibid, p 10.
10. Ibid, p 14.
11. Ibid, p 16.
12. Ibid, p 17.
13. Ibid, p 20.
14. Ibid, p 21.
15. Ibid, p 23.
16. Ibid, p 27.
17. Ibid, p 28.
18. Ibid, pp 29–30.
19. Ibid, p 31.
20. Ibid, p 32.
21. Ibid, p 33.
22. Ibid, pp 33–34.
23. Ibid, p 34.

BIBLIOGRAPHY

Davenport HW: Physiology of the Digestive Tract, An Introductory Text. Chicago, Year Book, 1982.
Enloe CF: The pancreas. Nutr Today 17(2):20, 1982.
Friedman HI, Nylund B: Intestinal fat digestion, absorption, and transport: A review. Am J Clin Nutr 33:1108, 1980.
Grossman MI: Neural and hormonal regulation of gastrointestinal function: An overview. Ann Rev Physiol 41:27, 1979.
Guyton AC: Textbook of Medical Physiology, ed. 6. Philadelphia, WB Saunders, 1981.
Makhlouf GM: Function of the gallbladder. Nutr Today 17(1):10, 1982.
Munro HN: Metabolic integration of organs in health and disease. J Parent Ent Nutr 6:271, 1982.
Phillips SF, Stephen A: The structure and function of the large intestine. Nutr Today 16:4, 1981.
Sleisenger MH, Kim YS: Protein digestion and absorption. N Engl J Med 300:659, 1979.

CHAPTER 4

Energy: Sources and Needs

Objectives

After completion of this chapter, the student will be able to:

1. Differentiate between food and body storage forms of potential energy and the form of energy that is used by the body.

2. Distinguish between the priorities given by the body in using food sources of energy.

3. Assess the amount of energy (in kilocalories) that is potentially available from a meal containing a given amount of carbohydrate, protein, and fat, compare (in relative terms) the amount of energy that is potentially available to the amount that is actually available when these substances are oxidized by the cells, and account for the discrepancy.

4. Distinguish between the effects of the major factors affecting total energy requirements.

5. Compare and contrast the effects of the major factors influencing the basal metabolic rate.

6. Teach a client who is in a current state of kilocaloric imbalance how to recognize when kilocalorie intake is adequate for individual needs.

Maintenance of energy balance is a difficult problem for many segments of the population. Overweight and obesity contribute to several chronic diseases, such as diabetes and heart disease, that are now major health problems. In contrast, the inability to maintain desirable weight is a continuing problem for those whose ability to consume or use the appropriate amount of food is impeded by physical or environmental forces. In order to effectively counsel clients to maintain energy balance, a knowledge of the physiologic aspects of energy balance, the energy needs of individuals, and the energy content of foods is essential.

ENERGY SOURCES

Sufficient food to meet the body's energy needs is the first nutritional priority. Energy, in the form

▶ of **adenosine triphosphate** (ATP), is essential for the performance of all body functions. The potential energy in foods must be transformed to ATP before it can be used by the cells. The importance of ATP is shown by the following examples:

1. Sodium ions are constantly diffusing into cells, yet they do not normally accumulate there. Energy, as ATP, is necessary to operate the sodium/potassium pump that ejects the sodium back into the extracellular fluid to maintain normal cellular composition.
2. Amino acids are constantly being linked together to form cell proteins for growth and maintenance. Again, ATP must be available to provide the energy for protein synthesis to occur.
3. Other body functions requiring the use of ATP include the active transport of com-

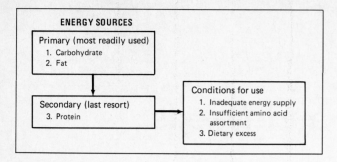

Figure 4–1
Primary and secondary sources of energy.

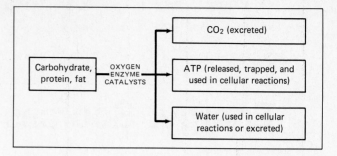

Figure 4–2
Oxidation of substrates for energy with release, trapping, and use of ATP.

pounds across cell and capillary membranes, muscular contraction, nerve impulse conduction, and glandular secretion.

The ultimate source of all the body's energy is the potential energy available from carbohydrate, fat, and protein contained in foods. When times are hard and foods are scarce, carbohydrates, proteins, and fats that have been stored in the body during better days are called on to be oxidized for energy. These body storage forms of potential energy include glycogen, structural protein, and adipose tissue.

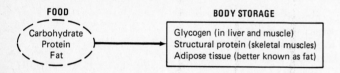

The amount of glycogen stored in the body at any time is very limited. A much larger supply of potential energy is available from adipose tissue and

structural protein, although the supply varies from person to person.

The primary function of carbohydrate and fat in the diet is to provide energy, whereas providing energy is a secondary function of dietary protein. Proteins in foods are necessary to provide the amino acids for the synthesis of structural proteins, hormones, enzymes, and so on in the body. However, there are three conditions in which proteins are oxidized for energy:

1. Inadequate energy supply available from carbohydrate and fat
2. Insufficient assortment of amino acids available in the food protein eaten
3. Dietary excesses of proteins over the amount that the body needs for protein synthesis

Figure 4–1 illustrates primary and secondary sources of energy from the three nutrients.

The digestive end products of food carbohydrates, proteins, and fats or their counterparts derived from the storage form of the nutrients are transported to the cells, where they are oxidized in

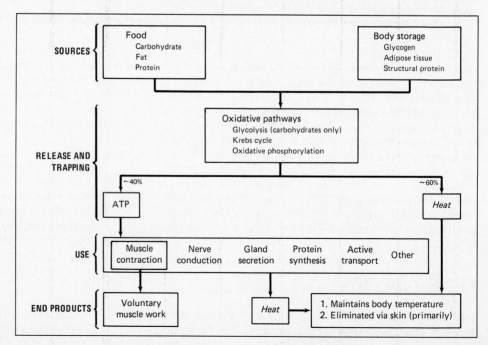

Figure 4–3
The energy cycle.

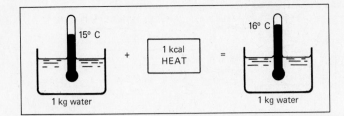

Figure 4-4
Representation of the amount of energy (heat) in 1 kilo-calorie.

a series of biochemical reactions including glycolysis (carbohydrates only), the Krebs cycle, and the electron transport chain. Different metabolites and different end products are involved in each of these pathways. In these oxidations, ATP is released, trapped, and subsequently used by the cells to carry out their metabolic functions (Fig. 4-2).

A few chemical reactions release energy; all others use energy. The most important energy-releasing reaction is the oxidation of carbohydrate, fat, and protein in the pathways mentioned above. Most other cellular reactions use energy as ATP. The two end products produced when ATP is released, trapped, and subsequently used by the body are heat and voluntary muscular work. Figure 4-3 illustrates the points in the energy cycle at which heat and muscular work are produced.

From Figure 4-3, it is evident that heat is produced by both energy-releasing and energy-using reactions. When carbohydrates, proteins, and fats are oxidized to release ATP, much of their potential energy is converted to heat. The energy-trapping system is remarkably inefficient. Theoretically, a molecule of carbohydrate (glucose), when oxidized, will yield 38 molecules of ATP. Actually, only 38 to 40 percent of the potential energy from fat and carbohydrate and 32 to 34 percent of the potential energy from protein are converted to ATP for immediate use or to creatine phosphate for storage in skeletal muscle. The remainder is converted to heat and is, in a sense, wasted.

Once ATP has been used by the cells to perform their functions, it too is converted to heat. The only exception to this occurs when voluntary muscles are used to perform work outside the body, such as walking. In this case, the ATP is converted to work rather than heat.

To summarize, all of the energy that is potentially available when carbohydrates, proteins, and fats (either in food or storage forms) are oxidized to form ATP (release and trapping of energy) is eventually converted to heat or voluntary muscle work. The law of conversion of energy states that energy can be neither created nor destroyed. Just as fossils and prehistoric trees became oil and coal, which are today burned to produce heat energy, likewise food energy is released and conserved as ATP, which is used in the cells to produce heat and work. Heat and the work of voluntary muscles can, therefore, be thought of as end products or by-products of energy metabolism. Heat is essential for maintaining the body's temperature. Amounts produced in excess of this need are excreted primarily through the skin.

MEASUREMENT OF ENERGY

Since heat production is the common denominator of all energy transfers in the body, heat can serve ▶ as a measure of energy; heat is measured in **kilocalories** (kcal). The kilocalorie is used to express the energy needs of the body as well as the energy available from specific foods. The kilocalorie represents the amount of heat required to raise the temperature of 1 kg of water (2.2 lb, or slightly over a quart) 1°C. This is illustrated in Figure 4-4.

▶ In the metric system, the **kilojoule** replaces the kilocalorie as the unit of energy measurement. The U.S. Bureau of Standards adopted the kilojoule as the preferred unit of energy measurement in all branches of science in 1964. It is anticipated that the transition from kilocalories to kilojoules will be effected as soon as the mechanics can be established. With this forthcoming change, an awareness of the use of kilojoules as a unit of measurement is essential. Conversion of kilocalories to kilojoules is shown in Table 4-1; 1 kcal is the equivalent of 4.184 kilojoules.[1] Thus, the conversion factor between kilocalories and kilojoules is 4.184. To change kilocalories to kilojoules, multiply by 4.184. To change kilojoules to kilocalories, divide by 4.184. For example, a dietary allowance of 2500 kilocalories is 10,460 kilojoules.

ENERGY BALANCE

A state of kilocalorie or energy balance exists when the kilocaloric intake from food is equal to the kilocaloric output in the form of heat and work.

Kilocalorie Balance

$$\frac{\text{Kilocaloric intake}}{\text{(food)}} = \frac{\text{Kilocaloric output}}{\text{(heat and work)}}$$

TABLE 4-1
CONVERSION TABLE FOR KILOCALORIES TO KILOJOULES

Nutrient	Kilocalories/g	Kilojoules/g
Carbohydrates	4	17
Protein	4	17
Fat	9	38
Alcohol	7.1	30

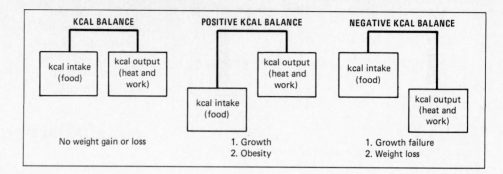

Figure 4–5
Concepts of energy balance.

Clients whose kilocaloric intake is greater than expenditure will be in a state of positive kilocaloric balance; a negative kilocaloric balance exists when kilocaloric intake is less than expenditure. A positive balance is desirable during the growth period to allow for increases in height and weight. After adulthood is reached, however, advise clients to strive for kilocaloric balance to prevent weight gain and pathologic problems frequently associated with obesity. Concepts of energy balance are illustrated in Figure 4–5.

Many adults are able to maintain kilocaloric balance with little effort, and appetite and food intake are geared to energy expenditure. Factors that influence the control of appetite, while many and varied, are still poorly understood. The increasing rate of overweight and obesity in our society is generally considered to result from reduced kilocaloric output rather than from a marked increase in food intake per se, although both may contribute. In treating the condition nurses must manipulate both kilocaloric intake and kilocaloric output so as to create a negative energy balance. This includes advising clients to decrease kilocaloric intake and increase kilocaloric output by doing more muscular work. While the theory behind weight reduction is simple, the practice of it is difficult and the results are frequently discouraging. Prevention of overweight and obesity is the best approach.

KILOCALORIC NEEDS

An individual's energy needs (in kilocalories) are directly related to energy expended as heat or muscular work. Energy expenditure depends on the total metabolic rate:

$$\text{Metabolic rate} = \text{energy expenditure} = \text{kcal needs}$$

Laboratory techniques are available for measuring the total metabolic rate (or rate of heat production) by both direct and indirect methods. These techniques are called **direct** and **indirect calorimetry.** Direct calorimetry involves placing an individual in a special chamber, a calorimeter, and measuring the total amount of heat given off. The metabolic rate can be calculated from the amount of heat given

off. Indirect calorimetry consists of calculating the metabolic rate on the basis of the amounts of oxygen consumed and carbon dioxide excreted in a given period of time. Since the exchange of these gases is directly proportional to the amount of heat being produced, this is a simple method for calculating the metabolic rate. A respiratory device attached to the nose is used to determine the oxygen and carbon dioxide content of inspired and expired air.

The factors contributing to total metabolic rate are shown in Figure 4–6. Of the three factors listed, basal metabolism and muscle activity exert the greatest influence.

Basal Metabolism

► **Basal metabolism** refers to the minimum amount of energy required to maintain life in the resting state, e.g., the energy needed for respiration, circulation, and maintenance of muscle tone and body temperature. This represents the internal work of the body. Voluntary muscle activity, in comparison, represents external work. Factors that determine individual variations in the basal metabolic rate (BMR) are summarized below. Factors that increase basal metabolism result in increased kilocaloric needs; factors that decrease basal metabolism decrease caloric needs.

Size. The effect of body size on basal metabolism is not due to height and weight per se but rather to skin surface area, which is computed from an individual's height and weight. Heat is constantly being lost by radiation from the skin. Since heat loss is proportional to skin surface area, the greater the skin area, the greater the heat loss, and, in turn, the more heat must be produced by the body. Expect

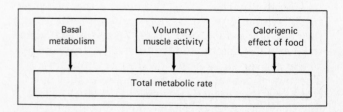

Figure 4–6
Factors contributing to total metabolic rate.

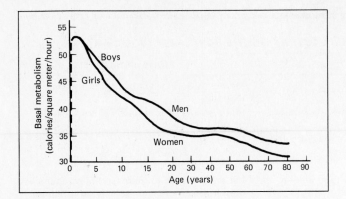

Figure 4–7
Effect of age on basal metabolism. (Source: Mitchell HH: Comparative Nutrition of Man and Domestic Animals. New York, Academic Press, 1962, Vol 1, p 43.)

a tall, thin person to have a greater skin surface area than an individual of the same weight who is short and fat. The tall, thin person will have a higher BMR.

Sex. Men will have a higher BMR than women because of (1) differences in body composition and (2) the effect of the sex hormones. Some tissues are more metabolically active than others, that is, they undergo breakdown and repair more rapidly. Muscle and glandular tissue are more active than bone and adipose tissue. Women characteristically have more fat and less musculature than men, and therefore they tend to have a lower BMR.

Age. Age and growth are responsible for normal variations in basal metabolism. The BMR is highest during the first 2 years of life, decreases in early childhood, increases slightly at puberty, and then declines steadily. These variations are shown in Figure 4–7.

The increased anabolic activities of the cells associated with a rapid growth rate explain the high BMR during the first years of life and the slight increase at puberty. The lessened muscle tone and reduction of muscle mass associated with aging account for the decline in BMR in later life. Advise individuals who fail to adjust kilocaloric intake to the reduced needs that accompany aging to expect a slow and insidious weight gain.

Hormones. The secretions of certain endocrine glands, especially the (1) thyroid, (2) adrenals, and (3) pituitary gland, affect basal metabolism. The thyroid gland, located in the neck, has the most marked effect. Thyroid hormone, secreted by the thyroid gland, regulates the rate of cell metabolism. Any changes in thyroid gland activity will consequently be reflected by changes in the BMR. Excessive secretion of thyroid hormone (hyperthyroidism) may speed up basal metabolism as much as 40 to 60 percent. Advise these clients of a marked increase in

their kilocaloric needs. On the other hand, deficient secretion of thyroid hormone (hypothyroidism) is reflected by a decrease in metabolic rate by as much as 30 to 40 percent. Assist these clients to decrease their kilocalorie intake.

An endocrine secretion with a more transitory effect on BMR is epinephrine, secreted by the adrenal glands located on the kidneys. Expect an increased secretion of epinephrine following intense emotional stimuli, such as fear or anger, to temporarily raise the metabolic rate.

Some of the hormones secreted by the pituitary gland, located at the base of the brain, control the secretions of other endocrine glands, including the thyroid, adrenals, and gonads. Since the pituitary hormones control thyroid gland secretion, clients with abnormalities of pituitary gland secretion will also have altered thyroid gland function and, therefore, altered BMR. Hypersecretion of pituitary hormones may result in an increased BMR; hyposecretion may result in a decreased BMR.

Nutritional State. Persons subjected to prolonged fasting or chronic undernutrition have a lower than normal BMR. The lower BMR may result from a decrease in the mass of active body tissues as well as an adaptive body process that lowers the metabolic rate to conserve energy. The effect of starvation or chronic undernutrition is not a significant factor for most Americans. However, it may explain why chronically undernourished persons from some areas of the world can maintain body weight on kilocaloric intakes lower than predicted needs.

Other Factors. Other factors that influence BMR are listed in Table 4–2. While basal metabolism refers to resting metabolism, excessive muscular activity has an effect on it. The aftereffects of excessive muscular work persist when the work has ceased. For example, the metabolic rate is higher during the night following a day of excessive exercise than following a relatively inactive day.

The many factors that influence the BMR make it difficult to determine the exact number of kilocalories from food needed by an individual to meet basal metabolic needs. However, a general guideline has been established as a result of many research studies on basal metabolism. This guideline suggests approximately 1 kcal per kg of body weight per hour for males and about 0.9 kcal per kg per hour for females (1 kg is 2.2 lb). This represents approximately 1300 to 1700 kcal per day for normal adult females and males. The basal metabolic requirement accounts for the largest proportion of the total energy requirement for most people unless activity is great.

Voluntary Muscle Activity
Voluntary muscle activity is the most variable factor affecting total energy requirements because of differences in activity levels of individuals. Advise

TABLE 4–2
EFFECTS OF VARIOUS FACTORS ON THE BASAL METABOLIC RATE

Factor	Effect on BMR
Pregnancy and lactation	Increases during last trimester and during lactation
Diseases associated with elevated body temperature	Increases (approximately 7% for each 1°F or 13% for each 1°C)
Diseases associated with increased cellular activity, such as cancer	Increases
Sleep	Decreases (approximately 10%)
Intense emotional states (fright, anxiety, suspense, intense mental strain)	Increases (leads to increased hormonal secretion and increased muscle contraction)
Climate and environmental temperature	Increases in extremely cold climates and decreases in extremely hot climates although the effects are not uniform. If heavy work is performed at extremes of high temperature the BMR increases as extra energy is expended to maintain thermal balance. Effects of temperature extremes are often negated through use of appropriate clothing and environmental temperature control. People tend to avoid physical activity at high temperatures, however, and adjustment for this change in activity pattern must be made in determining the total energy allowance.

clients engaged in sedentary activities or occupations, such as teaching or office work, that they require fewer kilocalories than those engaged in more strenuous activities, such as mining, lumbering, or ditch digging. For example, a coal miner (extreme physical activity) may require 5000 kcal per day, while a bank clerk of the same build and age may require only 2500 kcal. (Surprisingly, the intense brain activity involved with studying and taking tests burns up very few kilocalories! Neural activity contributes to the BMR, but intense mental effort uses few kilocalories above the basal expenditure.)

TABLE 4–3
CALORIC EXPENDITURE FOR VARIOUS ACTIVITY LEVELS

	Type of Activity	Kcal Used per Hour
Sedentary	Activities done while sitting that require minimal arm movement, such as reading, writing, eating, watching television or listening to the radio, sewing, playing cards, typing, miscellaneous office work	80–100
Light	Activities done while sitting that are more strenuous, such as rapid typing. Activities done while standing that require some arm movement, such as household duties such as preparing and cooking food, washing dishes, dusting, ironing, walking slowly, personal care, miscellaneous office work	110–160
Moderate	Activities done while sitting that require more vigorous arm movement. Activities done while standing that require moderate arm movement, such as making beds, mopping, sweeping, light polishing and waxing, light gardening or carpentry work, walking moderately fast.	170–240
Vigorous	Activities such as heavy scrubbing and waxing, hanging out clothes, stripping beds, walking fast, bowling, golfing, gardening	250–350
Strenuous	Activities such as swimming, tennis, running, bicycling, dancing, skiing, football	350+

(*Source: Adapted from Page L, Raper N: Food and your weight. Home and Garden Bulletin No. 74, U.S. Department of Agriculture, 1973, p 4.*)

The effect of various activities on energy expenditure has been studied extensively. Although individuals perform tasks with varying degrees of efficiency, some average data on energy expenditure for adults engaged in five levels of activity are given in Table 4–3. A range of the number of kilocalories used is given for each activity level to allow for differences in kilocaloric expenditure for these activities as well as for differences in individual efficiency in performing them. Of the sedentary activities listed, for example, typing requires more kilocalories than reading. The lower limits of the range of figures give a better picture of kilocaloric expenditure for women, while the upper limits give a better picture of kilocaloric expenditure for men. The figures for kilocaloric expenditure include the resting basal metabolism.

Modern living with its many labor-saving devices is conducive to a more sedentary lifestyle and a tendency to gain weight.

Calorigenic Effect of Food

Determination of the BMR requires the subject to be in a postabsorptive state, i.e., fasting for at least 12 hours prior to the administration of a basal metabolism test. The stimulus to metabolism by food intake is not considered a component of basal metabolism. Food intake, however, does increase energy expenditure with subsequent heat production, although the mechanism is poorly understood. This
▶ metabolic stimulus is frequently called the **calori-**
▶ **genic effect** or the **specific dynamic action,** or
▶ more recently, **dietary thermogenesis.** Not all classes of food stimulate metabolism to the same

degree. Protein foods, when eaten alone, have been reported to increase the metabolic rate as much as 30 percent, whereas foods containing carbohydrates and fat produce a much smaller increase in metabolism. A mixed diet, however, contains carbohydrates, fats, and proteins. From such a diet, the average increase in metabolic rate is approximately 6 to 10 percent. Exercise after a meal may increase the calorigenic effect. The popular literature has given considerable emphasis to the high calorigenic effect of protein and, thus, the potential value of a high-protein diet in promoting weight loss. The calorigenic effect of food appears to have more academic than practical application. While the stimulus to metabolism produced by food intake must be considered along with basal metabolic and activity needs in determining total energy requirements, a high-protein diet, in comparison to diets of equal kilocaloric value and varying protein content, produces little practical difference in overall energy use. The characteristic consumption of a heterogeneous diet containing carbohydrate, protein, and fat—and not single food constituents, such as protein—produces less significant results than generally assumed on the basis of experimental results obtained for brief periods with intakes of pure protein, fat, or carbohydrate.

DETERMINING KILOCALORIC NEEDS

Determination of nutrient requirements based on research studies can be applied with a considerable degree of accuracy to groups of people. There is less

---

TABLE 4–4
RECOMMENDED DIETARY ALLOWANCE FOR KILOCALORIES

	Age (years)	Body Weight (kg)	Body Weight (lbs)	Height (cm)	Height (in)	Kcal	Kcal per kg
Infant	0–0.5	6	13	60	24	—	115
	0.5–1.0	9	20	71	28	—	105
Children	1–3	13	29	90	35	1300	100
	4–6	20	44	112	44	1700	85
	7–10	28	62	132	52	2400	86
Males	11–14	45	99	157	62	2700	60
	15–18	66	145	176	69	2800	42
	19–22	70	154	177	70	2900	41
	23–50	70	154	178	70	2700	39
	51–75	70	154	178	70	2400	34
	76+	70	154	178	70	2050	29
Females	11–14	46	101	157	62	2200	48
	15–18	55	120	163	64	2100	38
	19–22	55	120	163	64	2100	38
	23–50	55	120	163	64	2000	36
	51–75	55	120	163	64	1800	32
	75+	55	120	163	64	1600	29
Pregnant						+300	36+
Lactating						+500	

(*Source: Adapted from National Research Council:* Recommended Dietary Allowance, *ed 9. Washington, DC, National Academy Press, 1980.*)

TABLE 4–5
PERCENTAGE OF KILOCALORIES AND
KCAL/G PROVIDED IN THE U.S. DIET BY
KILOCALORIE-CONTAINING SUBSTANCES

Substance	Percentage of Kcal Consumed in the U.S. Diet	Kcal/g
Carbohydrate	46	4
Fat	42	9
Protein	12	4
Alcohol	?	7.1

TABLE 4–6
CARBOHYDRATE, PROTEIN, AND FAT
CONTENT OF SPECIFIC FOODS

Food	Predominant Nutrient(s)		
Whole milk	Carbohydrate	Protein	Fat
Meat		Protein	Fat
Fruit–vegetables	Carbohydrate	Protein[a]	
Bread–cereal	Carbohydrate	Protein[a]	
Butter			Fat

[a] Smaller amounts of protein present in these groups than in milk and meat

accuracy when these determinations are applied to individuals because of individual differences. The method used to estimate total kilocaloric needs depends on the degree of accuracy desired. The most precise determination would require the use of laboratory techniques that measure the amount of heat given off by an individual engaged in various activities. Such methods are usually used for research purposes.

The RDA of the National Research Council gives an allowance for kilocalories that is a useful guide for estimating kilocaloric needs of population groups (Table 4–4). In view of the many factors that influence individual kilocaloric needs, the RDA for kilocalories should not be used to determine individual kilocaloric needs. The RDAs are given for males and females of a stated size and age. Adjustments are necessary for those who differ from the reference standard in size, age, or activity. RDA and other dietary guidelines are discussed in detail in Chapter 2.

While the RDA for kilocalories is a useful estimate of kilocaloric needs of population groups, the

best guide for nurses to use to assess adequacy of kilocaloric intake of individuals is maintenance of the individual's recommended body weight. To prevent insidious and undesirable weight increase, teach clients to weigh themselves at regular intervals and to make adjustments in food intake accordingly. Although kilocaloric excess resulting in overweight is a major health problem in the United States, kilocaloric deficits resulting in underweight and growth retardation in children should be guarded against just as cautiously.

KILOCALORIC CONTENT OF FOODS

Of the kilocalorie-containing nutrients—carbohydrate, protein, and fat—a much greater percentage of total kilocalories is supplied to the diet by carbohydrate and fat than by protein in the typical U.S. diet. Another substance that contributes substantial kilocalories to the diet of many is alcohol. Fat and alcohol are much more concentrated sources of kilocalories than are carbohydrate and protein. Many individuals feel that the current level of fat and alcohol consumption in the American dietary pattern is too high to be consistent with good health. The percentage of kilocalories and kcal per g provided in the diet by the various substances are shown in Table 4–5.

The relationship between grams of nutrients and kilocalories in an 8-oz cup of milk is illustrated in Figure 4–8.

The kilocaloric content of specific foods is directly related to their carbohydrate, protein, and fat content. Most foods contain mixtures of these nutrients. However, one or more of the nutrients predominate in most foods, as shown in the examples in Table 4–6. The kilocaloric content of various foods is included in Appendix 1.

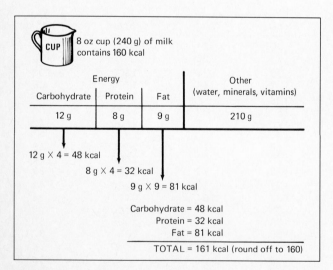

Figure 4–8
Relation between grams of nutrients and kilocalories.

REVIEW QUESTIONS AND ACTIVITIES

1. Identify the two categories of nutrients that are primary sources of energy and one that

is a secondary source and list their body storage counterparts.

2. Describe three conditions in which protein is used for energy.
3. Describe the efficiency of oxidative pathways in trapping the potential energy from energy-yielding substances in a body-usable form.
4. Discuss the role of heat in metabolism.
5. Calculate the kilocalorie value of a meal that contains the following: carbohydrate, 60 g; protein, 20 g; fat, 40 g.
6. Distinguish between kilocalorie balance, positive balance, and negative balance.
7. Discuss the effects of three major factors on total energy expenditure.
8. Explain the effects of four major factors on the BMR.

REFERENCE

1. National Research Council: Recommended Dietary Allowances, ed 9. Washington, DC, National Academy Press, 1980, p 16.

BIBLIOGRAPHY

Acheson KJ, Campbell IT, Edholm EG, et al.: The measurement of daily energy expenditure—An evaluation of some techniques. Am J Clin Nutr 33:1155, 1980.

Beaton GH: Energy in human nutrition. Nutr Today 18(5):6, 1983.

Cunningham JJ: A reanalysis of factors influencing basal metabolism in normal adults. Am J Clin Nutr 33:2372, 1980.

Cunningham JJ: An individualization of dietary requirements for energy in adults. J Am Diet Assoc 80:335, 1982.

Dauncey MJ: Influence of mild cold on 24-hour energy expenditure, resting metabolism, and diet-induced thermogenesis. Br J Nutr 45:257, 1981.

Lewis C: Weight Control. Philadelphia, FA Davis, 1976.

Lord RC: Conversion to the metric system. Sci Am 223:17, 1970.

Mahalko JR, Johnson LK: Accuracy of prediction of long-term energy needs. J Am Diet Assoc 77:557, 1980.

Rothwell NJ, Stock MJ: Regulation of energy balance. Annu Rev Nutr 1:235, 1981.

Sukhatme PV: Autoregulatory homeostatic nature of energy balance. Am J Clin Nutr 35:355, 1982.

Webb P: The measurement of energy exchange in man: An analysis. Am J Clin Nutr 33:1299, 1980.

CHAPTER 5

Carbohydrates

Objectives

After completion of this chapter, the student will be able to:

1. Differentiate between the major classes and subclasses of dietary carbohydrates.

2. Distinguish between the functions of the major food and body carbohydrates.

3. Compare and contrast the carbohydrates contained in foods from the Basic Four Food Groups.

4. Differentiate between the enzymes involved in the digestion of sugars and starch.

5. Distinguish between mechanisms involved in regulating the blood glucose level.

6. Assess a menu to determine its adequacy of carbohydrate content in preventing ketosis.

7. Develop a teaching plan for the prevention of dental caries (as related to carbohydrate consumption) and compare it with a teaching plan for prevention of constipation.

Carbohydrates, a primary source of the body's energy, are also a relatively inexpensive source of many nutrients and provide about 46 percent of the total energy in American diets. Changing patterns of carbohydrate consumption, including an increase in the consumption of highly refined forms, especially sugars, and a decrease in consumption of such complex forms as starch, are provoking nutritional concern. Nurses need to be aware of the major classes of carbohydrate, their food sources, metabolism, and functions in order to work toward preventing and treating disorders related to carbohydrate intake. A knowledge of carbohydrate metabolism is also essential to counteract some types of food misinformation—such as use of the quick weight loss, low-carbohydrate weight reduction diet so frequently advocated.

CLASSIFICATION AND STRUCTURE

Food Carbohydrates

Carbohydrates are composed of a varying number of sugar (or saccharide) units and are classified according to the number of sugar units contained in the molecule. The three major categories of dietary significance are monosaccharides, oligosaccharides, and polysaccharides. **Monosaccharides** consist of a single sugar unit, **oligosaccharides** contain 2 to 10 monosaccharide units, and **polysaccharides** are complex molecules containing more than 10 monosaccharide units. Of the oligosaccharides, the disaccharides consisting of 2 monosaccharides are the most prevalent. Some polysaccharides contain only one type of monosaccharides, whereas others contain several different monosaccharides or monosac-

charide derivatives. Monosaccharides and disaccharides are referred to as **simple carbohydrates;**
▶ polysaccharides are called **complex carbohydrates.**

Monosaccharides. From a nutritional standpoint, glucose, fructose, and galactose are the most important monosaccharides; of these only glucose and fructose are present in significant amounts in foods, such as fruits and vegetables. Galactose does not occur in the free state in foods but is a component of the disaccharide, lactose, present in milk.

Closely related to the monosaccharides is the sugar, D-xylose, and alcohol forms of sugars, such as sorbitol, mannitol, and xylitol. These sugars occur naturally in some foods, and the sugar alcohols are also synthesized commercially and used as sugar substitutes by diabetic clients and others who wish to control their intake of regular sugar. D-Xylose is not used by the body but is excreted in the feces and urine. Nurses use the D-xylose test to detect abnormalities of intestinal absorption in clients with gastrointestinal disorders. The use of the sugar alcohols as sugar substitutes is discussed in Chapter 24.

Disaccharides. The three major disaccharides and their monosaccharide components are:

▶ 1. **Sucrose** or table sugar (1 molecule glucose + 1 molecule fructose)
▶ 2. **Lactose** or milk sugar (1 molecule glucose + 1 molecule galactose)
▶ 3. **Maltose** or malt sugar (2 molecules glucose)

Sucrose is present in certain fruits and vegetables and is used extensively in cooking and commercial food processing. Lactose, found only in milk, is the sole carbohydrate present in any significant amounts in animal foods. Maltose is of little dietary significance except perhaps for the habitual beer drinker; the fermentation of grains, as in the manufacture of beer, produces maltose.

Characteristics of Monosaccharides and Disaccharides. While the kilocaloric values of all the sugars discussed so far are equal, their sweetness and solubilities vary considerably: fructose is the sweetest of the sugars and lactose is the least sweet. All except lactose are very soluble. Because of its sweetness and other properties, fructose is sometimes used as a sugar substitute (see Chap. 24). Be aware that all sugars when used in excessive amounts, are irritating to the gastrointestinal tract, causing an osmotic diarrhea associated with drawing fluid into the gastrointestinal tract. For clients who need to increase their kilocaloric intake, consider adding Polycose (Ross Laboratories) to beverages or foods. This synthetic product has a low sweetness, and consequently relatively large amounts can be used without making the product taste excessively sweet. Because of its low osmolarity, or water-pulling effect, the potential for osmotic diarrhea is minimized.

Polysaccharides. The three major classes of polysaccharides are divided into two groups according to function: those that function in energy storage (in plants and animals) and those that have a structural role (in plants). These are summarized below:

1. Energy storage function
   a. Starch (plants)
   b. Glycogen (animals)
2. Structural function
   a. Dietary fiber
      (1) Cellulose (insoluble plant cell wall polysaccharide)
      (2) Hemicellulose (insoluble plant cell wall polysaccharide)
      (3) Pectin, gums (water-soluble nonstructural polysaccharides)
      (4) Lignin (insoluble noncarbohydrate substance)

▶ **Starch,** the storage form of carbohydrate in plants, is the only digestible polysaccharide of dietary significance. Consisting of many glucose units, starch occurs in two forms in foods: amylose, a straight-chain polysaccharide of glucose, and amylopectin, a branched-chain glucose polysaccharide.

▶ **Glycogen,** the storage form of carbohydrate in animals, is present in small amounts (300 to 350 g) in muscle, where it serves as a quick source of energy for muscle contraction, and in the liver, where it is used to maintain the blood glucose level during periods of fasting. Like starch, glycogen is a polysaccharide of glucose. However, unlike starch, it is present only in a branched-chain form.

Dietary fiber, of which cellulose is the most abundant, includes complex cell wall materials that are nondigestible by humans. Lignin, though classified with dietary fiber, is not a polysaccharide since it does not contain sugar units. Cellulose contains only glucose in a straight-chain form, whereas other fibers contain sugars other than glucose as well as
▶ derivatives of carbohydrate. The term **dietary fiber,** also called bulk or roughage, must be differentiated
▶ from the term **crude fiber.** The latter refers to the insoluble plant material remaining after chemical analysis with weak acid and alkali in nutrient analysis; be aware that this is the form of fiber listed in current food composition tables. Dietary fiber is a more realistic term, since it represents the components actually presented to the digestive tract and may represent a quantity of substances two to five times greater than crude fiber. Figure 5–1 presents a summary of the major classes and subclasses of carbohydrates found in foods.

Body Carbohydrates

Although many types of carbohydrates are ingested in foods, only two, glucose and glycogen, are found in significant amounts in the body. In addition, small amounts of monosaccharides are found in combination with other substances as structural body compounds.

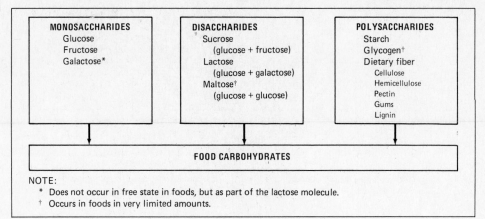

NOTE:
* Does not occur in free state in foods, but as part of the lactose molecule.
† Occurs in foods in very limited amounts.

Figure 5–1
Food carbohydrates.

▶ **Glucose,** also called dextrose or blood sugar, is the simple sugar that is eventually formed in the body when all digestible food carbohydrates are hydrolyzed to their monosaccharide components in the digestive tract and circulated to the liver. Of the three monosaccharides produced by carbohydrate digestion (i.e., glucose, fructose, and galactose), galactose is converted to glucose in the liver, and fructose either is used directly for energy or is indirectly converted to glucose so that the only sugar circulating throughout the body is glucose. There is usually enough glycogen stored in the liver and muscle to supply approximately one-half day's energy needs. Carbohydrate derivatives are sugars, primarily glucose and galactose, in combination with other nutrients, such as protein and lipid, that form structural body compounds. Examples are mucopolysaccharides and glycolipids. The carbohydrates found in the body are summarized in Figure 5–2.

FUNCTION OF CARBOHYDRATES

The primary function of carbohydrates is to provide energy. In addition, individual carbohydrates have regulatory and structural (Fig. 5–2) functions, and carbohydrate-containing foods (except concentrated sweets) are carriers of other essential nutrients, such as minerals, vitamins, and protein. The energy func-

tion and regulatory activities of carbohydrates are discussed in more detail below.

Energy
Protein and fat contribute to the body's energy needs, but carbohydrate plays some specialized roles related to energy production.

1. Glucose is a quick source of energy. Since carbohydrates are digested and absorbed more rapidly than protein or fat, glucose is quickly available for energy.
2. Glucose is the only energy source for the central nervous system under normal conditions. Since these cells do not oxidize fatty acids or amino acids for energy, a decrease in the blood level of glucose to below normal leads to slowing of synaptic activity, followed by shock, coma, and death unless immediately corrected.
3. Glucose exerts a protein-sparing and a fat-sparing action and thus prevents muscle wasting and problems related to excessive oxidation of fats. In order to spare dietary protein for its primary function—protein synthesis—adequate kilocalories (from carbohydrates and fats) must be present. To prevent excessive fat oxidation, some carbohydrate kilocalories must be present.

When dietary carbohydrate is severely restricted, the body oxidizes large amounts of fats and proteins for energy. However, the Krebs cycle (the common oxidative pathway for carbohydrates, proteins, and fats) is not designed to oxidize large amounts of fatty acids in the absence of simultaneous glucose oxidation. The result is that the fatty acids are not completely oxidized, and intermediary

▶ metabolites, called **ketones,** are produced by the liver and accumulate in the blood. Since ketones are strong acids, they cause a type of acidosis called

▶ **ketosis.** Assess for signs of ketosis, including dehydration and loss of body sodium, in clients who follow very low-carbohydrate, high-fat diets for weight reduction. When both glucose and fatty acids are being

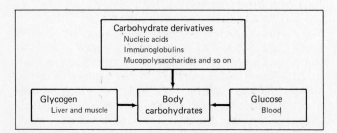

Figure 5–2
Body carbohydrates.

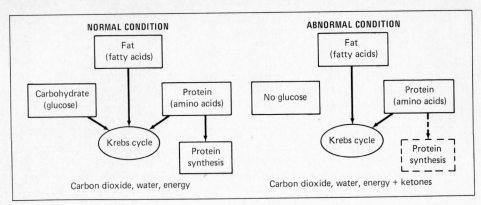

Figure 5–3
Energy oxidation, normal and abnormal.

oxidized simultaneously, only small amounts of ketones are produced by the liver; these are readily oxidized for energy by cells other than those of the liver, such as muscle cells.

Other conditions that cause ketosis due to oxidation of large amounts of fats (fatty acids) for energy in the absence of simultaneous carbohydrate (glucose) oxidation include fasting and insulin deficiency. When insulin is deficient, glucose cannot be transported across certain cell membranes, and energy must be supplied by fats and proteins. Normal and abnormal pathways of energy oxidation are shown in Figure 5–3.

While glucose is the only source of energy for the brain under normal conditions, the brain can adapt to prolonged fasting by using ketones for part of its energy supply. After approximately the third week of fasting, ketones can supply approximately 70 percent of the brain's energy, with the remaining energy being supplied through conversion of body protein to glucose.

Regulatory Function
Carbohydrates that aid in the regulation of gastrointestinal function are lactose and dietary fiber.

Lactose. Some of the lactose in the diet is fermented in the colon to lactic acid. The acid medium thus produced encourages the growth of normal bacterial flora and discourages the growth of undesirable bacterial flora. The normal bacterial flora in the colon synthesize vitamin K and some of the vitamin B complex. When milk sours or is fermented, some of the lactose is converted to lactic acid. Use fermented forms of milk, such as buttermilk, to reestablish the normal bacterial flora in clients whose flora are altered by prolonged use of antibiotics. In making cheese, the lactose-containing fluid part of sour milk (whey) is removed. Hard ripened cheeses made from curds (such as cheddar, Swiss, mozzarella) contain only a trace of lactose. Lactose also enhances the absorption of dietary calcium.

Dietary Fiber. Being nondigestible, dietary fiber may exert a variety of effects in the gastrointestinal tract. These effects are due to four physiologic properties: (1) absorption of water, (2) chelating or binding steroid materials, such as bile acids and cholesterol, as well as certain mineral elements including calcium, iron, magnesium, and zinc, (3) retardation of gastric emptying, and (4) fermentation by intestinal bacteria. Because of these properties, protective effects in prevention and treatment of a variety of abnormal conditions have been proposed. Some are well recognized whereas others remain speculative.

Because of its capacity to absorb water, it is generally well recognized that a high-fiber diet prevents or relieves constipation. Soft, bulky stools are produced that are readily eliminated. Cereal fiber, especially coarse wheat bran, is more effective than fruit or vegetable fiber or fine bran in increasing fecal bulk. The bulk of the food itself may also mechanically stimulate intestinal motility and thus reduce the time for food residues to pass through the gastrointestinal tract (transit time), although there is controversy as to whether this occurs to a significant degree only in clients with decreased motility. Fiber may actually decrease transit time in clients with rapid initial transit time, and adding fiber to the diet has been used successfully in alleviating both constipation and diarrhea in hospitalized clients.[1,2] The cathartic action of fiber may be enhanced by the production of volatile fatty acids secondary to fermentation of fiber by intestinal bacteria. Advise clients who follow a high-fiber diet that this mechanism may not only increase stool volume and alter intestinal transit time but may also lead to an osmotic diarrhea and increased gas production, both undesirable effects. Fiber is also effective in decreasing a high intraluminal pressure in the colon and maintaining the normal size of the colon. Assess the merits for use of a high-fiber diet in treating clients with a high intraluminal colonic pressure, such as those with diverticular disease and irritable bowel syndrome. While a high-fiber diet may be useful in treating these disorders, there is no evidence that they are caused by a low-fiber intake.

The increased volume and velocity of movement of materials in the colon resulting from a high-fiber intake reduce the concentration and exposure time of intestinal tissue to carcinogens produced by bacterial action or those present in food. By this mechanism, a high-fiber intake is thought to be protective against colon cancer. Moreover, there is evidence that bile acids or metabolites of their degradation by bacteria alter colonic structure, although it is not known whether these modifications predispose the colon to the subsequent action of carcinogens.[3] Certain types of fiber bind bile salts, resulting in an increase in their fecal elimination, thereby reducing the bile salt pool available for bacterial degradation. While it is speculated that fiber can modify the intestinal flora that produce harmful substances, it is not known whether fiber can alter bacterial metabolism.

There is also evidence to suggest a potential beneficial effect of a high-fiber diet in protecting against heart disease by lowering the blood cholesterol level. Pectin and guar gum, water-soluble fibers present in fruits, vegetables, and legumes, decrease circulating lipids in both humans and animals.[4] Bile salts are needed for cholesterol absorption; pectin and gums may inhibit cholesterol absorption by binding with bile salts and bile acids. Since the bile salts and acids are excreted in the feces, the liver synthesizes more bile salts from cholesterol, its precursor, to maintain the bile salt pool, thereby possibly lowering blood cholesterol.

Dietary fiber may be important in regulating the blood glucose level and in normal weight maintenance. For instance, pectin and guar gum reduce the after-meal level of blood glucose, insulin, and other hormones[4] and may increase the sensitivity of peripheral insulin receptors. Diets with adequate fiber are now recommended in treating diabetic clients (see Chap. 24). Slowed carbohydrate absorption secondary to a delay in gastric emptying and increased velocity of movement of intestinal contents are possible mechanisms whereby dietary fiber influences glucose metabolism. Delay in gastric emp-

tying may also lead to a feeling of satiety, and high-fiber diets may, therefore, be useful for normal weight maintenance and for weight reduction.

There are possible adverse effects of an excessive intake of dietary fiber. In addition to diarrhea and gas production, a possible decrease in the absorption of nutrients, especially such minerals as calcium, iron, copper, magnesium, and zinc, may precipitate a deficiency of these substances, especially if their intake is minimal. If a wide variety of foods is consumed, however, it is unlikely that the intake of fiber-rich foods will have an adverse effect on nutrient availability. Nonetheless, caution clients against an extreme increase in consumption of fiber-containing foods to avoid the possibility of inducing mineral deficiency. The functions of food and body carbohydrates are summarized in Table 5–1.

FOOD SOURCES OF CARBOHYDRATE

Carbohydrates are found primarily in foods of plant origin. The only significant animal source of carbohydrate is lactose, the sugar in milk. Sources of carbohydrate in the Basic Four Food Groups are summarized below, and Table 5–2 presents the carbohydrate content of various types of foods.

- *Milk and cheese.* Lactose in milk.
- *Meat–fish–poultry–beans.* Dietary fiber and starch in legumes, nuts, seeds.
- *Vegetables and fruits.* Carbohydrate content varies widely. Root and seed vegetables, such as potatoes, carrots, peas, and corn, have a high starch content. On the other hand, leafy vegetables and fruits have a lesser starch content but contain a significant amount of dietary fiber and some sugars, including glucose, fructose, and sucrose. Consequently,

---

TABLE 5–1
FUNCTIONS OF FOOD AND BODY CARBOHYDRATE

Food Carbohydrate	Body Carbohydrate

Is energy source (4 kcal/g)
  Quick glucose source
  Sole energy source for CNS
  Protein- and fat-sparing action
Regulates gastrointestinal function
  Lactic acid production from lactose
  Elimination function of dietary fiber (significance of other properties of dietary fiber in regulatory functions of the body not conclusively known at present)
Provides components for structural carbohydrate derivatives
Carries other nutrients
	Blood glucose: Quick energy source for all cells
	Liver and muscle glycogen: Stored energy
	Carbohydrate derivatives
	  Mucopolysaccharides
	  Glucuronic acid (a detoxifier in the liver)
	  Immunoglobulins
	  Nucleic acids
	  Glycolipids (glucose or galactose plus lipid in nerve tissue)
	  Glycosides (component of steroid hormones)
	  Glucose metabolites (provide carbon residues for nonessential amino acid synthesis)
	Milk production in the lactating mother

TABLE 5–2
AVERAGE CARBOHYDRATE CONTENT OF SOME COMMON FOODS

Food	Amount	Carbohydrate (g)
Milk	1 c	12
Most leafy vegetables	½ c	5
Starchy vegetables	½ c	15
Fruit	1 medium serving	10
Bread	1 slice	15
Meat	1 serving	None
Fat	1 tsp	None
Table sugar	1 tbsp	11

equivalent amounts of these foods are lower in kilocalories than are foods with a high starch content. Foods eaten with peelings, seeds, and seed coverings are particularly high in fiber content.

- *Breads and cereals.* Starch. If whole grain varieties are chosen, dietary fiber is also present in significant amounts. Commercially prepared bran and bran-type cereals are also good sources of fiber.
- *Fats, sweets, and alcohol.* Sucrose in candy, sugar, jam, jelly, syrups, sweet toppings, and other sweets; starch in refined but unenriched breads, pastries, and flour products.

CARBOHYDRATE REQUIREMENTS

Taking into account the nutritive value of carbohydrate-containing foods and the role that glucose plays in controlling excess protein and fat catabolism, the National Research Council recommends that the diet contain 50 to 100 g of digestible carbohydrate daily to offset the undesirable metabolic responses associated with high-fat diets and fasting.[5] However, intakes considerably above this minimal level are desirable (see Chap. 2 for guidelines for carbohydrate consumption). The typical American diet includes 200 to 400 g of carbohydrate daily.

Although dietary fiber is important, it is not now possible to recommend a specific level of intake. Because of the potential for adverse reactions, marked increases in fiber consumption should be avoided. Rather a moderate increase in consumption of fiber should be achieved by increasing consumption of whole grains, legumes, seeds, nuts, fruits, and vegetables. These foods will provide a variety of types of fiber and make a positive contribution to the overall nutritive value of the diet. When a high-fiber diet is indicated, it should contain 13 g of crude fiber daily. A guide for calculating the intake of total dietary fiber has been published.[6]

Fiber-containing foods in descending order of their relative concentration of fiber are bran, nuts, legumes, dried fruits, whole grains, vegetables, and fresh fruits. Caution clients against overcooking fruits and vegetables to preserve their fiber content. Fiber-free foods include animal protein foods (meat, fish, eggs, milk, cheese), fats, sugar, and beverages.

DIGESTION AND ABSORPTION

Of the monosaccharides, disaccharides, and polysaccharides contained in foods, only the disaccharide sugars and starch require digestion. (Monosaccharides are absorbed intact, glycogen occurs in relatively insignificant amounts, and dietary fiber is indigestible.) Disaccharides are hydrolyzed by enzymes called **disaccharidases** secreted by the small intestine. The important disaccharidases are sucrase, maltase, and lactase, which split sucrose, maltose, and lactose, respectively, into their monosaccharide components. Starch is hydrolzyed by amylases secreted by the salivary glands and by the pancreas. Most starch digestion occurs in the small intestine. The end products of carbohydrate digestion—the simple sugars glucose, fructose, and galactose—are absorbed into the portal circulation. As they circulate through the liver, galactose is converted to glucose. Fructose may be used directly for energy or stored as glycogen for eventual conversion to glucose.

METABOLISM

In the body, glucose is the central compound in carbohydrate metabolism. Glucose metabolism is an excellent example of the interrelatedness of nutrient use. Protein and fat metabolism are directly related to glucose metabolism in that protein and fat can be converted to glucose. The glycerol component of the fat molecule (10 percent of the molecule) can be converted to glucose, and 58 percent of amino acid molecules can be converted to glucose. Conversely, glucose metabolites can be converted to glycerol and fatty acids for storage as fat or used for the formation of nonessential amino acids.

There are additional aspects of nutrient interdependence. All nutrients that are oxidized for energy follow a common pathway—the Krebs cycle—that is active in all cells. Furthermore, B vitamins as coenzymes and minerals as enzyme activators are necessary for reactions involved in the nutrient metabolism. The absence of an essential vitamin or mineral will block further metabolism.

Factors Affecting Blood Glucose Level

Although glucose oxidation occurs in all cells, the liver is the major organ for regulating the blood glucose concentration. Hormones from the pancreas, adrenal, thyroid, and pituitary glands exert regulatory effects.

The blood glucose level is the result of a balance

TABLE 5–3
PROCESSES THAT ADD AND REMOVE GLUCOSE
TO AND FROM BLOOD

Processes Adding Blood Glucose	Processes Removing Blood Glucose
Absorption from intestine	Energy oxidation by all cells
Glycogenolysis in liver	Glycogenesis in liver and muscle
Gluconeogenesis from	Lipogenesis and storage in fat deposits
Amino acids (58% of amino acids a potential source of glucose)	Synthesis of carbohydrate derivatives
Glycerol of fat molecules (10% of fat molecule is a potential source of glucose)	Glucosuria (abnormal condition)
Pyruvic and lactic acid (Krebs cycle intermediates of glucose)	

between processes adding glucose to the blood and processes removing glucose from the blood. The regulation is such that blood glucose is in the range of 60 to 120 mg/100 ml of blood in the fasting state under normal conditions. A blood level below 60 mg/100 ml is called **hypoglycemia;** a blood level above 120 mg/100 ml is called **hyperglycemia.** Both hypoglycemia and hyperglycemia are serious conditions that can lead to coma and death if not corrected. These blood sugar levels are summarized below:

- Hypoglycemia: <60 mg/100 ml
- Normal blood glucose: 60–120 mg/100 ml
- Hyperglycemia: >120 mg/100 ml

During the absorption of glucose from the intestine after a meal, the blood glucose level rises to 130 to 140 mg/100 ml of blood. This hyperglycemic state is the stimulus for secretion of the hormone **insulin,** which acts to decrease blood glucose. On the other hand, when an individual is not eating, blood glucose falls to hypoglycemic levels. A number of hormones are thus stimulated to bring about reactions that increase blood glucose. Under normal conditions, the blood glucose level is so well regulated that only insignificant amounts of glucose are excreted in the urine. However, should a client's blood glucose level exceed the kidney's ability to handle it, expect to see glucose excreted in the urine. This abnormal condition, called **glucosuria,** results when the blood glucose level is in the range of 160 to 180 mg/100 ml of blood.

Table 5–3 summarizes processes that add and remove glucose to and from the blood. The list of prefixes and suffixes below may aid in understanding the terminology used in the table.

Prefixes	Suffixes
Glyco-, glycogen	-lysis, destruction
Gluco-, glucose	-genesis, formation of
Neo-, new	or producing
Lipo-, lipid or fat	

Thus, glycogenolysis is glycogen breakdown, glycogenesis is glycogen formation, gluconeogenesis is the formation of new glucose or the formation of glucose from noncarbohydrate substances, and lipogenesis is fat formation.

CARBOHYDRATE IMBALANCE

Problems related to carbohydrate consumption include possible deleterious effects associated with changing food consumption patterns.

Changes in Carbohydrate Consumption Patterns

The changes in food consumption patterns discussed in Chapter 1—a decline in total consumption with a change in the consumption pattern—are thought to have some possible adverse effects on nutritional status. While fewer complex carbohydrates are being consumed, more sugars and syrups are being eaten. Whereas the per capita intake of glucose in the 1700s was less than 5 pounds annually, in 1979 this figure was 90.7 pounds, with an additional per person consumption of 30.1 pounds of sweeteners such as dextrose, corn syrup, and honey.[7] Even when one purposefully refrains from adding sugar to food, it is difficult to avoid a rather large intake since it is added to many processed foods. Advise clients to read food labels to detect unsuspected sources of sugar.

Possible adverse effects related to a high sugar intake include overall nutritional imbalance and a high incidence of dental caries. It is also postulated that a number of degenerative diseases are related to a lack of dietary fiber.

Problems Associated with a High Sugar Intake

Nutrient Imbalance. A high sugar intake provides kilocalories without providing other nutrients. The palatability of foods with a high sugar content may tempt people to consume more of them, reducing the appetite for other foods and resulting in a deficiency of specific nutrients. For example, soft drinks are now the most widely consumed beverage, accounting for approximately 10 percent more of total beverage consumption than does milk. There is little comparison between the nutritive contribution of a glass of milk and a glass of soft drink. Another consideration is the possible contribution of the high sugar intake to obesity. The incidence of obesity is high, and excess weight contributes to the risk of developing such chronic conditions as heart disease, hypertension, diabetes mellitus, and possibly some types of cancer. A final consideration is the possibility of an increased susceptibility to atherosclerosis, a degenerative disease of the arteries that underlies

▶ coronary heart disease. While **hyperlipidemia,** or elevated blood lipid levels, is most closely correlated with increased consumption of fats,[8] some researchers have found that sucrose may be associated with hyperlipidemia, particularly elevated triglycerides and, less consistently, elevated cholesterol.[9] The evidence is far from conclusive, however, that the current high level of sugar consumption is a major factor in the risk of developing heart disease aside from its possible link to obesity, itself a risk factor for heart disease. In contrast, a high fiber intake may be protective of heart disease, although clinical trials with fiber have not been entirely consistent.[4] Some persons are genetically susceptible to an elevated level of blood triglycerides. Advise these clients to restrict their intake of sugar.

Increased Incidence of Dental Caries. Dental caries is an infectious, bacterial disease characterized by demineralization of the dental enamel, dentin, and sometimes the root cementum of teeth. The destructive effects on dental structure occur as a result of the fermentation of carbohydrate by bacteria colonized in dental plaque. By-products of this bacterial activity are (1) sticky, gel-like polysaccharides that adhere tenaciously to the tooth surface and contribute to the further build-up of plaque and (2) organic acids that dissolve the dental enamel. These acids are produced beneath the plaque and are protected from the buffering effect of saliva by plaque.

Dental caries, one of the most prevalent diseases of children, affects over 90 percent of the population. Peak incidence occurs from ages 2 to 8, from adolescence through age 20, and again after age 40. Often classified as a nutrition-related disease, dental caries has a multifactoral etiology that involves an interplay among three factors: the host (a susceptible tooth), the agent (bacterial plaque on the tooth surface), and the environment (local contact between the plaque and fermentable carbohydrate on the tooth surface). Preventive efforts must be directed toward modifying each of these factors.

Although the sugar intake that is typical of the present American diet is thought to be a major contributing factor in the current prevalence of the disease, systemic factors, including genetic, hormonal, immunologic, and nutritional factors during the period of tooth development, may interact to produce a tooth that is susceptible to decay. From a nutritional perspective, the type of diet ingested during all stages of tooth development and maturation and the availability of fluoride during tooth development and maturation can influence the susceptibility or resistance of teeth to decay. Fluoride as a protective factor in tooth decay is discussed in Chapter 9. Other factors found in food that are somewhat caries inhibiting are fat and protein. Fats may be protective by coating the teeth and changing surface activities, by decreasing sugar solubility, or by exerting toxic effects on oral bacteria. Protein may serve a cariostatic function by elevating the level of salivary urea, thus changing plaque pH.

The Role of Carbohydrate in Dental Caries. The local contact of fermentable carbohydrate with the tooth surface is essential to the initiation of the carious process. Although all fermentable carbohydrate foods, including starch, can cause some degree of dental decay, the monosaccharide and disaccharide sugars are the major offenders. Sucrose appears to be the substance most closely related to dental caries, and many investigators believe that this sugar is the most cariogenic of all substances for humans. Concentrated sweet food, such as table sugar, honey, molasses, crude brown sugar, and dried fruits, as well as glucose, fructose, and lactose appear to have a significantly high cariogenic potential. Since saliva contains a starch-digesting enzyme that degrades starch to fermentable products, advise clients that starchy foods may have a potential to produce significant amounts of acid and that, in contrast, fibrous carbohydrate foods that require vigorous chewing (as raw fruits and vegetables) have a protective effect by virtue of their ability to increase salivary flow. The increased volume of saliva helps to buffer plaque acidity and to cleanse the oral cavity of retained food.

The cariogenicity of sugar is related to several factors, including frequency of exposure, exposure at meals vs between meals, and the physical form and length of exposure to the sugar. Since acid formation occurs each time sugar is eaten, the frequency of exposure appears to be more important than the total amount consumed. Thus, small sugar-containing snacks consumed frequently throughout the day may be more damaging than one large daily snack that contains the same amount of sugar. Sugar consumed as part of a meal appears less damaging than the same amount consumed between meals. This presumably results from the clearance of sugar from tooth surfaces by foods and liquids consumed at meals. Sticky, retentive sweets that adhere to the teeth and stay in the mouth longer are more damaging than soluble liquids that are rapidly cleared. For example, a sticky piece of candy may adhere to the teeth for as long as an hour. While liquids are generally less damaging, sugar-sweetened beverages consumed frequently over a prolonged time significantly increase the risk of producing caries, and the acid content of some soft drinks may contribute to erosion of the teeth at the gum line. In teaching clients about diet and dental health, summarize these points: dental caries is most promoted by the frequent, between-meal ingestion of sticky, sweet snacks; the total amount consumed is a secondary consideration.

The sugar alcohols, sorbitol, mannitol, and xylitol, used as natural sugar substitutes have in some instances served to exert a lower caries-producing action than sugar. In fact, xylitol appears to be noncariogenic and in some studies has been shown to have an anticariogenic effect.

Problems Thought to Be Associated with Low Fiber Intake

In recent years epidemiologists have identified a variety of diseases of Western civilization that do not exist in undeveloped countries. The differences in disease patterns are postulated to be due to differences in the fiber consumption of the populations involved. The diseases in question include various conditions or diseases of the gastrointestinal tract (e.g., constipation, diverticular disease of the colon, appendicitis, colonic polyps, cancer of the colon, gallstones, irritable bowel syndrome, hiatus hernia), some vascular disorders (e.g., varicose veins, hemorrhoids, ischemic heart disease, and venous thrombosis), and other diseases (e.g., dental caries, diabetes mellitus, and obesity).

Although dietary fiber has effects that are useful in the treatment of some health problems (e.g., constipation, diverticular diseases of the colon, irritable bowel syndrome, abnormal glucose tolerance), its role in the prevention of the numerous health problems of 20th-century America is much less clear. There are strong statistical relationships between a fiber-depleted diet and the increased incidence of a number of health problems, but there is no direct evidence that lack of dietary fiber causes any of these diseases. Those dietary components that may be increased when fiber is absent, such as sucrose and other refined carbohydrates or fat, also are correlated with some of these health problems.

Many diseases of modern civilization, such as cancer and heart disease, have multiple etiologies that involve aspects of lifestyle and environment other than diet. While research is continuing to try to determine the metabolic properties of the different chemical forms of dietary fiber, avoid coercing clients into thinking that fiber is some type of medicine that should be added in the form of bran (or some other preparation) to an otherwise unrefined diet. Isolated products (such as bran) do not contain the other important elements associated with fiber as it occurs in its natural state in food. It should also be kept in mind that one can never alter the intake of one dietary component without significantly altering the intake of other food components. Thus the question arises: Is the incidence of disease affected by the presence or the absence of a dietary factor?

ABNORMAL CONDITIONS REQUIRING REGULATION OF CARBOHYDRATE INTAKE

Generally, conditions requiring regulation of carbohydrate intake are related to a lack or imbalance of hormones or enzymes necessary for the use of specific carbohydrates. Four examples are given below:

1. A lack of adequate amounts of the metabolically active form of insulin leads to the disease diabetes mellitus, which is associated with a number of metabolic abnormalities including poor glucose transport across cell membranes.
2. A lack of the liver enzyme that converts galactose (a constituent of lactose) to glucose ▶ results in **galactosemia,** the accumulation of galactose in blood and tissues.
3. Lactase deficiency in intestinal secretions leads to intestinal gas, cramps, and diarrhea several hours after the ingestion of milk because of the inability to digest lactose.
4. Hypoglycemia is a condition characterized by an abnormally low blood glucose level. The popular press has suggested that there is a widespread, unrecognized occurrence of the disorder in this country. It has also been suggested that hypoglycemia contributes to other conditions, such as depression, alcoholism, juvenile delinquency, allergies, and so on. Medical evidence does not support these claims. Many individuals with anxiety reactions have symptoms similar to those occurring with hypoglycemia.

Obesity is another condition in which carbohydrate consumption, especially the consumption of simple carbohydrates, must be regulated. While the body can function equally well with a low- or high-carbohydrate intake provided kilocaloric and essential nutrient needs are met, undesirable metabolic responses result when carbohydrate is severely restricted. Some individuals place themselves on popular fad diets for weight reduction that markedly restrict carbohydrates and use large amounts of protein and fat. These so-called ketogenic diets promote a rapid initial weight loss largely as a result of the excretion of water and salt. Persons who follow such diets may experience numerous side effects that are discussed in detail in Chapter 23.

The treatment of diabetes mellitus, galactosemia, lactose intolerance, hypoglycemia, and obesity (including the fad diet approach) are discussed in detail in Part IV.

REVIEW QUESTIONS AND ACTIVITIES

1. Describe the important differences among the three major classes of carbohydrates.

2. Identify the three major monosaccharides, the three major disaccharides, and the three major polysaccharides in terms of their dietary significance and their digestibility.

3. Explain why the term "dietary fiber" is more meaningful than "crude fiber."

4. Identify the two carbohydrates found in significant amounts in the body and the roles of each.

5. Discuss the role of food carbohydrates in providing energy and nutrients and in regulating body metabolism.

6. Explain the rationale for the development of ketosis in clients who markedly restrict their carbohydrate intake.

7. Identify the minimum recommended intake of carbohydrate.

8. Identify the carbohydrate content of foods from the Basic Four Food Groups.

9. Explain the mechanisms whereby dietary fiber is useful in the treatment of constipation.

10. Describe the role of carbohydrates in dental decay and identify dietary recommendations for preventing the disorder.

11. Explain the rationale for abnormal starch digestion in a client with pancreatic dysfunction.

12. Explain the rationale for milk intolerance in clients with abnormal functioning of the small intestine.

13. Identify the amount of carbohydrate contained in the following foods:

Milk, 1 c
Leafy vegetables, ½ c
Starchy vegetables, ½ c
Fruit, 1 average serving
Bread, 1 slice

REFERENCES

1. Stratton JW, MacKiegan JM: Treating constipation. Am Fam Phys 25:139, 1982.

2. Frank HA, Green LC: Successful use of a bulk laxative to control the diarrhea of tube feeding. Scand J Plast Reconstr Surg 13:193, 1979.

3. Vahouny GV: Conclusions and recommendations of the symposium on Dietary Fibers in Health and Disease, Washington, DC, 1981. Am J Clin Nutr 35:152, 1982.

4. Vahouny GV: Dietary fiber, lipid metabolism and atherosclerosis. Fed Proc 41:2801, 1982.

5. National Research Council: Recommended Dietary Allowances, ed 9. Washington, DC, National Academy Press, 1980, p 33.

6. Southgate DAT: A guide to calculating intake of dietary fiber. J Hum Nutr 30:303, 1976.

7. U.S. Department of Agriculture: Sugar and Sweetener Report. SSR, Washington, DC, U.S. Government Printing Office, Vol 4 No. 12, 1979, p 35.

8. Kannel WB: Status of coronary heart disease risk factors. J Nutr Educ 10:10, 1978.

9. Story JA: Dietary carbohydrates and atherosclerosis. Fed Proc 41:2797, 1982.

BIBLIOGRAPHY

Baig MM, Cerdo JJ: Pectin: Its interaction with serum lipoproteins. Am J Clin Nutr 34:50, 1981.

Bohannon NV: Endocrine responses to sugar ingestion in man. J Am Diet Assoc 76:555, 1980.

Burkitt DP: Relationships between diseases and their etiological significance. Am J Clin Nutr 30:262, 1977.

Crapo PA, Olefsky JM: Fructose—Its characteristics, physiology, and metabolism. Nutr Today 15:10, 1980.

Heller SN, Hackler LR, Rivers JM, et al.: Dietary fiber: The effect of particle size of wheat bran on colonic function in young adult men. Am J Clin Nutr 33:1734, 1980.

Jenkins DJA: Dietary fiber, diabetes, and hyperlipidemia. Lancet 1:1287, 1979.

Lewis C: Proteins and Carbohydrates, Lipids. Philadelphia, FA Davis, 1976.

Scheiham A: Sugars and dental decay. Lancet 1:282, 1983.

Spiller GA, Freeman HJ: Recent advances in dietary fiber and colorectal disease. Am J Clin Nutr 34:1145, 1981.

Sreebny LM: Sugar availability, sugar consumptions and dental caries. Comm Dent Oral Epidemiol 10:1, 1982.

Wang Y-M, van Eys J: Nutritional significance of fructose and sugar alcohols. Ann Rev Nutr 1:437, 1981.

CHAPTER 6

Proteins

Objectives

After the completion of this chapter, the student will be able to:

1. Distinguish among simple proteins, conjugated proteins, and derived proteins.
2. Differentiate between the functions of food and body proteins.
3. Compare and contrast the protein content of each of the Basic Four Food Groups in relation to both quantity and quality of protein.
4. Plan a day's menu for an adult client of a given weight that meets the Recommended Dietary Allowance for protein.
5. Distinguish among nitrogen balance, negative nitrogen balance, and positive nitrogen balance and list conditions associated with each.
6. Assess the rationale for development of a negative nitrogen balance in a client on a weight reduction diet that is adequate in both amount and quality of protein.
7. Differentiate between pathologic conditions in which protein intake is increased and those conditions in which protein intake must be restricted.
8. Assess the effects of protein deficiency on body tissues and organs.

Of the approximately 50 nutrients known to be essential for life, protein is one of the most vital, for it is a structural component of all body cells. In addition, many regulatory functions of the body are dependent on an available supply of protein in the form of the amino acid building blocks. The amino acids are also a source of nonprotein nitrogen needed to synthesize important nitrogenous compounds in the body. Thus, protein is essential to the growth, maintenance, and regulatory functions of the body.

Protein provides about 12 percent of the kilocalories in American diets, much of which comes from animal sources. Nutrition surveys indicate that most people consume an adequate amount of protein. However, of increasing concern is the consumption of large amounts of animal protein with its attendant high ratio of animal fat and possible relationships with certain chronic conditions.

STRUCTURE AND CLASSIFICATION OF PROTEINS

Structure

Proteins are organic compounds composed of amino acids. Like carbohydrates and fats, they contain carbon, hydrogen, and oxygen. Unlike carbohydrates and fats, they contain nitrogen, which is their distinguishing feature. Protein is 16 percent nitrogen, and 6.25 g of protein will yield 1 g of nitrogen. Most proteins also contain sulfur and phosphorus, and specialized proteins contain minute amounts of other inorganic elements, such as iron (in hemoglobin) and iodine (in thyroxin).

Proteins consist of amino acids joined to each other by a special linkage, the peptide linkage, to form chains. There are 20 basic amino acids that are included in the structure of most food and body

proteins. Two amino acids joined together form a
▶ **dipeptide,** three a **tripeptide,** and many a **poly-peptide.** Food and body proteins consist of polypeptides. The number of amino acids contained in specific proteins varies considerably. For example, the hormone ACTH contains 23 amino acid units, whereas the blood protein albumin contains over 500 amino acid units.

How can a protein contain such a large number of amino acid units when there are only 20 amino acids? Proteins are made up of combinations of the 20 amino acids, and an amino acid can be repeated many times in a single protein. The specific amino acids included in a protein and the order in which they are arranged in the molecule are specified by the genetic code located in the DNA of cell nuclei and determine the type of protein produced.

Proteins are large molecular weight compounds. In the body they form colloidal solutions that do not diffuse through the body's membranes.

Classification
Proteins may be classified as simple proteins, conjugated (compound) proteins, and derived proteins.

Simple Proteins. Proteins that are made up entirely of amino acids or their derivatives are termed
▶ **simple proteins.** Some examples include:

Albumins and globulins	In body cells and fluids, e.g., serum albumin and serum globulin in the blood, lactalbumin and lactoglobulin in milk
Collagen and elastin	In connective tissue
Keratin	In hair and nails
Zein	In corn
Glutenin	In wheat

Conjugated Proteins. Proteins made up of combinations of polypeptides and nonprotein substances are termed **conjugated (compound) pro-**
▶ **teins.** Some examples include:

Lipoproteins	Polypeptides + lipids
Glycoproteins	Polypeptides + carbohydrates
Phosphoproteins	Polypeptides + phosphoric acid

Derived Proteins. The various stages of breakdown of the protein molecule, such as occurs during digestion of food proteins, result in the formation of
▶ **derived proteins.** A dipeptide is an example.

STRUCTURE AND CLASSIFICATION OF AMINO ACIDS

Structure
All amino acids contain a basic amino group ($-NH_2$) and an acid carboxyl group ($-COOH$). At physiologic pH, these groups are ionized ($-HH_3^+$ and $-COO^-$), which allows them to act either as an acid or base when dissolved in body fluids. This property makes them effective blood buffers. In addition to the amino group and carboxyl group, each of the 20 amino acids has a distinctive side chain, which accounts for the varying properties of the individual amino acids.

Classification
Synthesis of the many proteins needed by the body is dependent upon the simultaneous presence of all 20 amino acids in the amino acid pool. If one amino acid is lacking for a specific protein, no protein synthesis takes place. Instead, all of the amino acids available will be oxidized for energy or converted to glycogen or fat for storage. Some amino acids can be synthesized by the body; others cannot. It is on this basis that amino acids are classified as essential or nonessential.

Essential and Nonessential Amino Acids. In the adult, the cells are equipped with enzymes capable of synthesizing adequate amounts of 12 of the needed amino acids; in infants, this is true of only 11. The amino acids that can be synthesized by the body

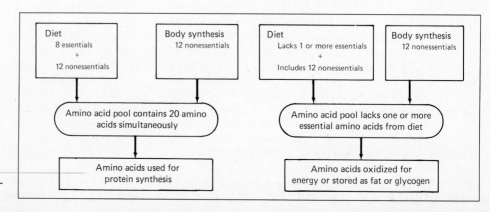

Figure 6–1
Sources and use of amino acids.

TABLE 6–1
ESSENTIAL AND NONESSENTIAL AMINO ACIDS

Essential Amino Acids	Nonessential Amino Acids
Valine	Glycine
Leucine	Alanine
Isoleucine	Serine
Threonine	Cystine
Methionine	Cysteine
Phenylalanine	Tyrosine
Tryptophan	Proline
Lysine	Hydroxyproline
	Histidine (essential for infants)
	Arginine
	Glutamic acid
	Aspartic acid

▶ are called dietary **nonessential amino acids.** Those that cannot be synthesized by the body in adequate amounts or proportions must be supplied by the diet ▶ and are termed dietary **essential amino acids.**

There are two sources of nonessential amino acids: the diet and body synthesis. There is only one source of the essential amino acids: the diet. Since all proteins are made up of both essential and nonessential amino acids, the amino acid pool must contain both types simultaneously in order for protein synthesis to proceed. If the diet is lacking in essential amino acids, the amino acid pool will also be lacking, and no protein synthesis will take place (Fig. 6–1).

The names of the essential and nonessential amino acids are listed in Table 6–1. There is some evidence that histidine may also be an essential amino acid for adults, although this has not been confirmed.

FUNCTIONS

Food Proteins
The primary function of food proteins is to provide the amino acids and nonprotein nitrogen for synthesis of cell proteins, regulatory agents, and nonprotein nitrogenous compounds. Their secondary function is the provision of energy.

Body Proteins
Body proteins have two primary functions: (1) to provide the structural components of all body cells and regulatory compounds and (2) to act in specialized regulatory functions. The provision of energy is a secondary function. The functions of food and body proteins are summarized in Table 6–2.

SOURCES AND QUALITY OF PROTEIN

Most foods, with the exception of pure sugar, fats, and oils, contain some protein. Protein is found in foods of both plant and animal origin. These foods contain mixtures of both essential and nonessential amino acids.

Complete Proteins
Protein foods are rated as to quality relative to their content of the essential amino acids. Thus, a food that contains all eight of the essential amino acids in the correct quantity and ratio for growth and ▶ maintenance is called a **complete protein** food, or ▶ one of **high biologic value.** Except for gelatin, protein foods of animal origin are complete proteins; they contain all eight of the essential amino acids, and they contain some of the nonessential amino acids as well. The protein in human milk has the highest biologic value of all food proteins, followed by egg and cow milk. In addition to being the best quality protein, animal protein foods contain larger amounts of protein than do most foods of plant origin. Teach clients that from the Basic Four Food Groups (see Chap. 2), meat, fish, poultry, eggs, milk, and cheese contain proteins of high biologic value.

Incomplete Proteins
A food that contains only limited amounts or improper proportions of one or more of the essential ▶ amino acids is called an **incomplete protein** food, ▶ or one of **low biologic value.** Protein foods of plant origin, those from the vegetable–fruit group and bread–cereal group from the Basic Four Food Groups, are incomplete proteins. However, two plant protein products whose protein quality approaches that of animal protein are wheat germ and dried yeast. Three additional plant proteins that are commonly substituted for meat are legumes, seeds, and nuts. Even though the protein present in these foods is not as high quality as animal protein, advise clients that these foods provide an amount of protein equivalent to animal protein. Refer to the Basic Four Food Groups in Chapter 2 for the amounts of these foods that provide as much protein as meat. One ounce of meat or an equivalent amount of meat alternates provides approximately 7 g of protein.

Complementary Value
Although plant foods contain incomplete proteins, all plant foods are not lacking in the same amino acid. By combining several plant proteins at the same meal, it is possible to obtain a mixture of amino acids in which all of the essentials are included. For example, cereals such as corn or legumes such as beans are not satisfactory as the sole source of protein at a meal. When combined at the same meal, however, they complement each other, since the missing amino acid in one is supplied by the other. Another way to increase the quality of a plant protein is to consume a small amount of animal food with a larger amount of plant food; macaroni with cheese is an example.

Since animal protein foods are the most expensive components of the diet, plant proteins are used

---

TABLE 6–2
FUNCTIONS OF FOOD AND BODY PROTEINS

Food Protein	Body Protein

Primary function
 To provide amino acids and nonprotein nitrogen for synthesis of cell proteins, regulatory agents, and nonprotein nitrogenous body compounds, such as nucleic acids
 	
 Secondary function
 To supply energy (4 kcal/g)—used for energy when:
 1. Kilocalories from carbohydrate and fat are inadequate
 2. Dietary excesses of protein are present
 3. Amino acid pool is lacking in essential amino acids
	Primary functions
	 1. To provide structural components of all cells and regulatory compounds including hormones and enzymes—as such, provides for:
	   a. Growth
	   b. Continued replacement of normal cells destroyed by wear and tear
	   c. Regulatory processes performed by hormones and enzymes
	 2. To handle specialized tasks
	   a. Regulates water balance (colloidal osmotic pressure of the blood protein albumin draws water from interstitial fluid of cells to maintain blood volume)
	   b. Regulates acid-base balance (proteins are buffers since they can act as acid or base—both cell and blood proteins are part of the body's buffer system)
	   c. Provides resistance to infection (antibodies are proteins)
	   d. Transports nutrients and nutritional substances in the blood (e.g., insoluble lipids are transported as lipoproteins)
	   e. Functions in blood clotting (blood coagulation factors are proteins)
	
	 Secondary function
	 Provides energy—body proteins are catabolized for energy when dietary carbohydrate and fat are insufficient to meet the energy needs of the body

---

extensively by many people. Other individuals choose to eliminate either meat or all animal foods from their diet for sociocultural reasons, as when adopting a vegetarian diet. Remind such clients of these principles of food selection to assure that all amino acids are available in the amino acid pool: (1) choose some complete protein at each meal, and/or (2) choose a varied diet that uses the concept of mutual supplementation of dietary protein.

Let pure vegetarians know that it is possible to obtain a balanced mixture of amino acids without the use of animal protein from meat, eggs, or milk if they eat a variety of (1) whole grain cereals, (2) legumes, (3) nuts, (4) seeds, (5) vegetables and fruits, and (6) dried yeast. Chapter 18 gives a more complete discussion of the supplementary value of various food proteins. Consult other published data[1,2] for further guidelines and recipes.

PROTEIN REQUIREMENTS

While it is convenient to speak of a requirement for protein, the true requirement is not for protein per se but rather for specific amounts and propor-

tions of the essential amino acids and for nonessential amino acid nitrogen.

The amount of protein needed daily to meet this requirement per unit of body weight is highest during the growth periods of infancy and childhood and gradually decreases as adulthood is reached. (The Recommended Dietary Allowance for protein is given in Table 2–2, and the requirement per unit of body weight is given in Table 6–3.)

Table 6–4 gives an estimate of the requirements of essential amino acids. These estimates are based on the assumption that an adequate supply of nitrogen is available for the synthesis of the nonessential amino acids so that the essential amino acids will not be used for this purpose.

DIGESTION AND ABSORPTION

▶ Proteins are split by enzymes called **proteases.** Protein digestion occurs in two organs: (1) the stomach and (2) the small intestine. Three digestive secretions contain proteases: (1) gastric, (2) pancreatic, and (3) small intestinal secretions (see Table 3–2). Secretions from the pancreas are released into the

TABLE 6-3
PROTEIN REQUIREMENT PER KILOGRAM
DESIRABLE BODY WEIGHT

	Age (years)	Protein Requirement g/kg Desirable Body Weight
Infants	0.0–0.5	2.20
	0.5–1.0	2.00
Children	1–3	1.77
	4–6	1.50
	7–10	1.21
Males	11–14	1.00
	15–18	0.85
	19–22	0.80
	22 +	0.80
Females	11–14	1.00
	15–18	0.84
	10–22	0.80
	22 +	0.80
Pregnant		0.80 + 30 g
Lactating		0.80 + 20 g

(Source: Adapted from National Research Council: Recommended Dietary Allowances, ed 9. Washington, DC, National Academy Press, 1980.)

small intestine, where they function in the digestion of foods. An additional substance contained in gastric secretions that is necessary for protein digestion but is not an enzyme is hydrochloric acid. This acid has a catalytic effect by activating proteases contained in gastric secretions and by causing the protein molecules to swell and thus be more accessible for gastric protease action. As dietary protein passes through the stomach and small intestine, the enzymes contained in the three secretions split the large protein molecules into progressively smaller molecules and finally into amino acids, the end product. The enzymes are secreted in an inactive form and activated as they are needed.

Amino acids are absorbed by active transport and diffusion into the portal vein and transported to the liver. The liver removes and degrades dietary excesses of most amino acids to prevent a large build-up in the blood. The remaining amino acids are released to the general circulation for use by the body.

The efficiency of protein digestion and absorption, particularly proteins of plant origin, is less than that of carbohydrate and fat. Whereas 98 percent of the digestible carbohydrates and 95 percent of fats are digested and absorbed, this is true of only 92 percent of dietary proteins. Possible explanations include the presence of digestive enzyme inhibitors in some plant foods that must be inactivated by heating and the presence of dietary fibers that may hinder digestion and absorption.

There is now evidence to suggest that both dipeptides and tripeptides, as well as free amino acids, can be absorbed and that peptide absorption may be more efficient than the absorption of free amino acids.[3] By this mechanism, final hydrolysis to amino acids occurs in the intestinal mucosal cell.

METABOLISM

The metabolism of protein is a composite of anabolic and catabolic processes involving not only the body's structural proteins but all of the nitrogenous substances contained in the body. The processes in the anabolism and catabolism of proteins are summarized in Table 6–5. Like metabolism of carbohydrates

TABLE 6-4
ESTIMATED AMINO ACID REQUIREMENTS OF MAN[a]

Amino Acid	Requirement (mg/kg body weight/day)			Amino Acid Pattern for High-quality Proteins (mg/g of protein)
	Infant (4–6 months)	Child (10–12 years)	Adult	
Histidine	33	?	?	17
Isoleucine	83	28	12	42
Leucine	135	42	16	70
Lysine	99	44	12	51
Total S-containing amino acids (methionine and cystine)	49	22	10	26
Total aromatic amino acids (phenylalanine and tyrosine)	141	22	16	73
Threonine	68	28	8	35
Tryptophan	21	4	3	11
Valine	92	25	14	48

[a] Two grams per kilogram of body weight per day of protein of the quality listed in column 4 would meet the amino acid needs of the infant.
(Source: National Research Council: Recommended Dietary Allowances, ed 9. Washington, DC, National Academy Press, 1980.)

TABLE 6–5
ANABOLISM AND CATABOLISM OF PROTEINS

Anabolic Process	Catabolic Processes

Synthesis of cellular proteins, regulatory substances, and other nitrogenous compounds (such as porphyrines, purine and pyrimidine bases, creatine)	1. Breakdown of cellular protein in response to
	  a. Daily wear and tear
	  b. Inadequate diet, illness, stress, hormonal factors, etc.
	2. Breakdown of amino acids in response to
	  a. Cellular protein breakdown producing amino acids
	  b. Dietary excesses absorbed into circulation
	  c. Amino acid pool lacking essential amino acid

and fats, protein metabolism is under strict hormonal control, and the liver is the major organ of regulation. In addition to effects produced by various hormones, factors that influence anabolism/catabolism are adequacy of the diet and physiologic state of the individual (Table 6–6).

Anabolism

Anabolic processes consist of synthesis of cell proteins, regulatory compounds, and other nitrogen-containing substances. In order for these synthetic activities to occur, the correct amounts and proportion of nitrogen and all 20 amino acids must be present. In addition, the diet must provide adequate energy. When the energy supplied by carbohydrate and fat is not sufficient, protein will be used for this purpose. Assist infants, growing children, and pregnant women with proper food selection to assure that the amount of protein and energy is sufficient to support an increased rate of anabolism during these normal growth periods.

Catabolism

Since an increased rate of cell protein catabolism is characteristic of clients undergoing stresses, such as prolonged immobilization, trauma, and infections, provide these clients with a diet that is high in protein and kilocalories during the rehabilitation process so that tissues can be restored by an increase in the rate of anabolism. When stresses are severe and tissue catabolism is marked, the physician may also consider the ratio of nitrogen to kilocalories provided. Content of the diet can be determined by dividing the protein consumed in grams by 6.25. For example, an egg provides 7 g of protein and 1.12 g of nitrogen.

When cell proteins are broken down not only as a result of illness or inadequate kilocalories or protein intake but also as a result of daily wear and tear, their constituent amino acids are released into the amino acid pool. Some of these can be reused for protein synthesis, but others undergo catabolism. When there are dietary excesses of amino acids, they are also catabolized to prevent an excess build-up in the blood.

The liver withdraws amino acids to be catabolized from the amino acid pool. They are subsequently deaminized and prepared for other uses. ▶ **Deamination** is the removal of the amino ($-NH_2$) group. In deamination, the amino group is split from

TABLE 6–6
EFFECTS OF DIET, HORMONES, AND PHYSIOLOGIC STATE ON THE ANABOLISM/CATABOLISM OF PROTEINS

Increased Cell Protein Anabolism	Increased Cell Protein Catabolism

Occurs during
1. Growth period, including pregnancy
2. Tissue repletion following illness or injury
3. Athletic training for muscle development
4. Secretion of the following hormones
  a. Growth hormone
  b. Androgens
  c. Insulin
  d. Normal level of thyroid hormone
	Occurs during
	1. Periods when diet inadequate in kcal or essential amino acids or both
	2. Immobilization due to illness
	3. Response to trauma, injury, or stress, as from a severe burn
	4. Increased secretion of the following hormones
	  a. Thyroid hormone
	  b. Glucocorticoids

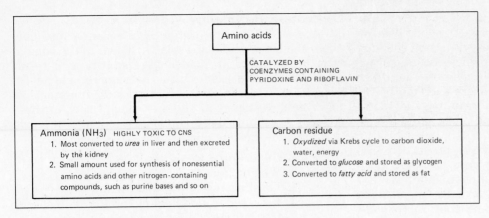

Figure 6–2
Deaminization of amino acids by the liver and further use of ammonia and carbon residue.

the large carbon-containing compound, resulting in the formation of two new compounds: (1) ammonia and (2) carbon residue. Be aware that ammonia is highly toxic to the central nervous system. The liver detoxifies much of the ammonia produced by converting it to the much less toxic compound, urea, which is subsequently excreted in the urine. Suspect ammonia intoxication in clients with severe liver disease in whom protein metabolism is altered. The carbon residue is either oxidized to produce energy or converted to glycogen or fat for storage. Figure 6–2 summarizes deaminization and the further use of ammonia and carbon residue.

Nitrogen Balance

▶ The net result of anabolism and catabolism involving protein substances is termed **nitrogen balance.** Since the presence of nitrogen is the common denominator of both food and body proteins, use an assessment of nitrogen as an index of protein gain or loss in the body. Clients can be in any one of three states relative to nitrogen (and thus protein) gain or loss: (1) nitrogen balance, (2) positive nitrogen balance, or (3) negative nitrogen balance (Table 6–7).

Use an analogy with kilocaloric balance to assist in understanding nitrogen balance. With kilocaloric balance, one is dealing with kilocaloric intake in food and kilocaloric output in heat or work. With nitrogen balance, one is dealing with nitrogen intake in food protein and nitrogen excretion in nitrogenous end products.

Nitrogen balance studies have been performed by measuring nitrogen (and thus protein) intake and excretion over long periods of time in individuals. These studies cover various stages of anabolism and catabolism and permit the classification of given individuals in one of the three categories of nitrogen balance based on their current physiologic state. Expect normal healthy adults to be in a state of nitrogen balance, expect clients with conditions associated with increased protein catabolism to be in negative nitrogen balance, and expect clients with conditions associated with an increased rate of protein anabolism to be in positive nitrogen balance (Table 6–7). Those clients with increased protein catabolism and thus negative nitrogen balance need a high-protein and high-energy diet to reverse the catabolic state into an anabolic situation.

TABLE 6–7
CLASSIFICATION OF NITROGEN BALANCE

Classification	Description and Examples
Nitrogen balance Nitrogen intake = nitrogen excretion → constant body protein content	Tissue build-up equals tissue breakdown, no net protein gain or loss (healthy adults)
Positive nitrogen balance Nitrogen intake exceeds nitrogen excretion → gain in body protein content	Tissue build-up exceeds breakdown; net protein gain (occurs during normal growth cycle including pregnancy, tissue repletion following illness, athletic training for muscular development, effect of hormones that increase protein synthesis)
Negative nitrogen balance Nitrogen excretion exceeds nitrogen intake → loss of body protein content	Tissue breakdown exceeds build-up; net protein loss (inadequate dietary intake, effect of response to trauma and injury, immobilization, debilitating illnesses, effect of hormones that increase protein catabolism)

Excretion of Waste Products

The major waste products of protein metabolism are nitrogen-containing substances, with urea the largest component. Other waste products include carbon dioxide, water, sulfates, and phosphates. The carbon dioxide and some of the water are excreted by the lungs. The remaining wastes, including the nitrogenous compounds, sulfates, and phosphates, are excreted by the kidneys.

The nitrogen-containing waste products of protein metabolism include not only the urea from amino acid breakdown but smaller amounts of other substances produced as end products of metabolism of the other nitrogen-containing body compounds. All of these substances are excreted in the urine ▶ and are collectively called the **nonprotein nitrogen.** The components and sources of nonprotein nitrogen include:

Nonprotein Nitrogen	Source
Urea (largest component)	Waste product of amino acid metabolism
Uric acid	Waste product of purine metabolism
Creatinine	Waste product of muscle creatine phosphate metabolism
Ammonia	Small amount normally excreted
Amino acids	Small amount normally excreted

The normal kidney has no problem in excreting these nitrogenous substances. Clients with advanced kidney disease, however, cannot excrete these wastes. Observe for elevated blood levels of nitrogenous substances, phosphates, and sulfates that contribute to mental confusion and disorientation in these clients.

PROTEIN IMBALANCE

At the international level, the shortage of protein is second only to the shortage of kilocalories in the world's food supply. Protein–calorie malnutrition, with its effects on physical and mental growth and development in infants and young children, is the major nutritional problem in the developing countries of the world. With the continuing growth of the world population, limits on the world's agricultural capacity, and the high cost of animal foods, many are seeking alternatives to animal foods as a source of protein. It is likely that, in the future, greater use will be made of such foods as fish, fish protein concentrates, oilseed meals, algae and microorganisms, textured vegetable proteins, legume and cereal mixtures that have been fortified with amino acids to improve their protein quality, and genetically improved plants, such as hybrid corn with increased lysine content.

Protein Deficiency

While good-quality protein is abundantly available in the United States, a small segment of the population consumes an inadequate quantity as a result of interrelated social, cultural, economic, and health factors. Observe for these signs and symptoms of protein deficiency in high-risk clients, such as those who are chronically ill, elderly clients who live alone, low-income clients, and strict vegetarians:

1. Generalized weakness
2. Weight loss
3. Lowered resistance to infection
4. Retarded wound healing, prolonged recovery from illness
5. Growth failure, brain damage to fetus or early postnatal infant
6. Reduced blood level of albumin leading to edema
7. Anemia in severe deficiency
8. Fatty infiltration of liver

Protein Excess

Protein intake is far in excess of needs for many individuals and for some may account for 15 percent of total kilocaloric intake. At present, there is no compelling evidence that high intakes are either beneficial or harmful,[4] although foods rich in protein, particularly animal protein, are also good sources of other essential nutrients, such as iron, zinc, and B-complex vitamins. Nonetheless, serious toxic effects have been seen in special situations, such as in very small premature infants who consumed diets with 16 percent of the energy as protein.[5]

Moreover, there are now investigations into the possible role of protein excess in the etiology of certain degenerative disorders, such as cancer, heart disease, and hypertension. Evidence from both epidemiologic and laboratory studies suggests that a high protein intake may be associated with an increased risk of cancer at certain sites. Because of the high correlation between fat and protein intake it is not possible to discern from the available data an independent effect of protein. However, the literature on protein is more limited than the literature concerning fats and cancer.[6]

Diets containing animal protein cause high blood cholesterol and atherosclerosis in experimental animals, whereas diets containing vegetable protein do not. Moreover, epidemiologic evidence from several countries shows a correlation between cardiovascular disease and use of animal protein, and replacement of animal protein with soy protein has been found to lower cholesterol in humans.[7] The different effects of animal and plant protein appear to be due to differences in their amino acid content.

Protein intake may also influence blood pressure, although little research has been done in the area. Excessive protein intake is associated with excessive calcium losses through the kidney unless it is counterbalanced by a large intake of calcium. Calcium deficiency has been associated with hypertension (see Chap. 9).

ABNORMAL CONDITIONS REQUIRING REGULATION OF PROTEIN INTAKE

Illnesses, such as advanced liver or kidney disease, are associated with a decreased ability to handle the waste products of protein metabolism, and therefore protein must be restricted in the diet. These disorders are discussed in detail in Part IV.

REVIEW QUESTIONS AND ACTIVITIES

1. Identify the distinguishing chemical element in proteins and the structural units of which proteins are composed.
2. Describe the differences between simple, conjugated, and derived proteins and list an example of each.
3. Distinguish among the roles of carbohydrates, proteins, and fats in providing the body's energy.
4. Distinguish between the structural and regulatory roles of body proteins and identify the six major regulatory functions of body proteins.
5. Explain the difference between essential and nonessential amino acids.
6. Describe the differences between proteins of low biologic value and those of high biologic value with regard to their amino acid content and their food sources.
7. Identify the three major alternates to meat in the diet that provide equivalent amounts of protein to meat, fish, and poultry.
8. Identify the Recommended Dietary Allowance for protein for an adult.
9. Identify the amount of protein contained in an ounce of meat, fish, or poultry.
10. Classify the following clients relative to their state of nitrogen balance:
    a. Normal adult
    b. Normal infant
    c. Normal pregnant woman
    d. Malnourished client who is now consuming a high-protein, high-energy diet
    e. A client on a diet that is low in kilocalories but adequate in protein
    f. A client with major body burns
11. List the three major conditions in which amino acids undergo catabolism.
12. Identify the two compounds that result from the deaminization of amino acids and the fate of each.
13. Identify the seven major waste products of protein metabolism that could be determined by urinalysis.
14. Explain the rationale for dietary protein restriction in clients with advanced liver or advanced kidney disease.
15. Explain the rationale for increasing protein intake in clients with a negative nitrogen balance.
16. Identify the signs and symptoms of protein deficiency.

REFERENCES

1. Robertson L, Flinders C, Godfrey B: Laurel's Kitchen. A Handbook for Vegetarian Cooking and Nutrition. Berkeley, Calif, Nilgiri Press, 1976.
2. Lappe FM: Diet for a Small Planet. New York, Ballentine Books, 1975.
3. Sleisinger WH, Young SK: Protein digestion and absorption. N Engl J Med 300:659, 1979.
4. National Research Council: Recommended Dietary Allowances, ed 9. Washington, DC, National Academy Press, 1980, p 51.
5. Goldman HI, Liebman OB, Frendenthal R, et al.: Late effects of early dietary protein intake on low-birth-weight infants. J Pediatr 85:764, 1974.
6. National Research Council: Diet, Nutrition, and Cancer. Washington, DC, National Academy Press, 1982, pp 6–11.
7. Carrol KK: Hypercholesterolemia and atherosclerosis: Effects of dietary protein. Fed Proc 41:2792, 1982.

BIBLIOGRAPHY

Allen LH, Bartlett RS, Block GD: Reduction of renal calcium reabsorption in man by consumption of dietary protein. J Nutr 109:1345, 1979.
Bessman SP: The justification theory: The essential nature of the non-essential amino acids. Nutr Rev 37:209, 1979.
Cho ES, Anderson HL, Wixom RL, et al.: Long-term effects of low histidine intake on men. J Nutr 114:369, 1984.
Chopra JG, Forbes AL, Habicht JT: Protein in the U.S. diet. J Am Diet Assoc 72:253, 1978.
Hegsted DM: Assessment of nitrogen requirements. Am J Clin Nutr 31:1669, 1978.
Jones AOL, Jacob RM, Fry BE Jr, et al.: Elemental content of predigested liquid protein products. Am J Clin Nutr 33:2545, 1980.
Lewis C: Proteins and Carbohydrates, Lipids. Philadelphia, FA Davis, 1976.
Munro HN: Major gaps in nutrient allowances. The status of the elderly. J Am Diet Assoc 76:137, 1980.
Review: High-protein diets and bone homeostasis. Nutr Rev 38:11, 1981.
Review: Sulfur amino acids and the calciuretic effect of dietary protein. Nutr Rev 39:127, 1981.
Richardson DP, Scrimshaw NS, Young VR: The effect of dietary sucrose on protein utilization in healthy young men. Am J Clin Nutr 33:264, 1980.
Zanni E, Calloway DH, Zezulka AY: Protein requirements of elderly men. J Nutr 109:513, 1979.

CHAPTER 7

Lipids

Objectives

After completion of this chapter, the student will be able to:

1. Differentiate among the three major types of fatty acids in relation to degree of saturation and the need for a dietary source.

2. Differentiate between the functions of food and body lipids and compare and contrast the functions of the major body lipids.

3. Distinguish between the absorption pathways of the end products of lipid digestion.

4. Compare the energy value of lipids with the energy value of protein and carbohydrate.

5. Distinguish between the anabolic and catabolic processes involved in lipid metabolism.

6. Plan a day's menu for a client with an elevated cholesterol level that provides a reasonable balance of fats as specified by the National Academy of Sciences.

7. Plan a day's menu that is low in fat that would be suitable for a client with fat malabsorption.

8. Distinguish between the major sign of essential fatty acid deficiency and the major sign of fat malabsorption and know conditions that may precipitate each.

▶ The term **lipid,** often used interchangeably with fat, is applied to a group of heterogeneous organic compounds related to the fatty acids. This group of compounds includes fats, oils, and fat-related substances that have vital structural and regulatory functions in the body. Oils are fluid at room temperature, whereas fats are solid at room temperature. A common property shared by lipids is their insolubility in water but solubility in organic solvents, such as alcohol, ether, and acetone.

Lipids provide approximately 42 percent of the total energy in U.S. diets. However, there is no physiologic evidence that the human body requires this much fat. Questions are being raised about the relationship of dietary fat to coronary heart disease and

other disorders, and many experts recommend a moderate reduction of fat in the diet. In order to adequately answer clients' questions about fats, nurses need a practical understanding of this category of food nutrients.

STRUCTURE AND CLASSIFICATION

Like carbohydrates and proteins, lipids are composed of carbon, hydrogen, and oxygen, but in different proportions. Because of a lower ratio of oxygen to carbon and hydrogen, lipids are a much more concentrated source of energy than carbohydrates or proteins, providing more than twice as many kcal per g. Some specialized lipids also contain nitrogen and phosphorus as well as carbon, hydrogen, and oxygen.

Just as amino acids and simple sugars are the basic structural units of proteins and carbohydrates, respectively, so are fatty acids and simple alcohols, such as glycerol, or more complex alcohols, such as sphingosine, the basic structural units of lipids.

▶ Like proteins, lipids are classified as simple, compound, and derived lipids. **Simple lipids** are composed only of fatty acids and glycerol, or a more complex alcohol; examples are monoglycerides, diglycerides, and triglycerides containing a molecule of glycerol and one, two, and three fatty acids, re-
▶ spectively. **Compound lipids,** such as phospholipids, lipoproteins, and glycolipids, contain not only glycerol, or sphingosine, and fatty acids but also other substances, such as phosphorus, nitrogen, or
▶ carbohydrate. **Derived lipids** are those substances resulting from breakdown of simple or compound lipids, such as fatty acids and glycerol.

Fatty Acids

▶ **Fatty acids** are organic acids with a methyl ($-CH_3$) group at one end and a carboxyl ($-COOH$) group at the other end of the carbon chain. Most food and body acids contain straight, even-numbered (4,6,8, and so on) carbon chains.

Fatty acids differ from each other in regard to (1) the length of the carbon chain, (2) the state of saturation, (3) the body functions performed, and (4) the need for a dietary source. The nutritional characteristics of food fats—that is, ease of digestibility and therapeutic value in health maintenance and treatment of disease—depend on the type of fatty acids that make them up.

Carbon Chain Length. The carbon chain in fatty acids may be short, medium, or long, containing as few as 4 or as many as 24 carbon atoms.

- Short-chain fatty acids: less than 6 carbons
- Medium-chain fatty acids: 6 to 10 carbons
- Long-chain fatty acids: 12 or more carbons

Most food fats contain predominantly long-chain fatty acids. However, those containing medium-chain and short-chain fatty acids are much easier to digest and absorb.

STEARIC ACID
    $CH_3 (CH_2)_{16} COOH$
      (*no* double bonds, saturated)
OLEIC ACID
    $CH_3 (CH_2)_7 CH = CH (CH_2)_7 COOH$
      (*one* double bond, monounsaturated)
LINOLEIC ACID
    $CH_3 (CH_2)_4 CH = CH - CH_2 - CH = CH (CH_2)_7 COOH$
      (*two* double bonds, polyunsaturated)

Figure 7–1
Examples of saturated, monounsaturated, and polyunsaturated fatty acids.

Degrees of Fatty Acid Saturation. The degree of saturation of a fatty acid depends on the amount of hydrogen bound to the carbons of the carbon chain. With respect to saturation, three types of fatty acids exist: (1) saturated, (2) monounsaturated,
▶ and (3) polyunsaturated. **Saturated fatty acids** contain as many hydrogen atoms as each of the carbons in the chain can hold; they have no double bonds.
▶ **Monounsaturated fatty acids** have one double bond and consequently lack two hydrogen atoms.
▶ **Polyunsaturated fatty acids** have two or more double bonds, lacking four or more hydrogen atoms. Examples of the three types are shown in Figure 7–1.

Essential Fatty Acids. Although all of the fatty acids serve as body energy sources, only three, the polyunsaturated fatty acids linoleic acid, linolenic acid, and arachidonic acid, are known to be essential for growth and metabolism. Since a deficiency of these fatty acids produces specific deficiency signs,
▶ they are called **essential fatty acids.** Of the three,
▶ only **linoleic acid** must be supplied by the diet, and it is, therefore, the only dietary essential fatty acid. Linolenic acid and arachidonic acid can be synthesized in the body from linoleic acid if an adequate supply of the latter is present.

The essential fatty acids perform diverse roles in the body because of their widespread occurrence in the various body lipids (Table 7–1).

Alcohols
Alcohols of varying degrees of complexity are a sec-
▶ ond basic structural unit of lipids. **Glycerol** is the alcohol contained in fats consumed as food and in the body fat stores. The chemical structure of glycerol is similar to that of glucose. When lipids are digested, glycerol is released and used in essentially the same manner as glucose. As such, it contributes to the total available glucose in the diet. Glycerol is also a component of structural lipids in the body, such as certain phospholipids and glycolipids. Other phospholipids and glycolipids contain sphingosine, a more complex alcohol.

FUNCTIONS

Of the major classes of lipids, four of these occur both in foods and in the body. These are:

1. Triglycerides
2. Phospholipids
3. Fatty acids
4. Cholesterol

Two major classes of lipids occur only in the body. These are:

1. Lipoproteins
2. Glycolipids

Triglycerides
The major portion of food fat and body storage fat (adipose tissue) is in triglyceride form. Smaller

---

TABLE 7–1
FUNCTIONS OF LIPIDS

Triglycerides
  Food lipids
  1. Are a major energy source (more concentrated source than carbohydrate or protein—provide 9 kcal/g. All body cells except erythrocytes and cells of the central nervous system oxidize fat for energy
  2. Provide satiety value to meals by delaying gastric emptying
  3. Serve as a carrier of other essential nutrients, i.e., essential fatty acids and the fat-soluble vitamins; also needed for absorption of the fat-soluble vitamins
  4. As an energy source, spare dietary protein for protein synthesis
  Body lipids
  1. Store energy in adipose tissue
  2. Protect body organs from trauma
  3. Act as insulator for body temperature maintenance

Essential Fatty Acids[a]
  1. Are necessary for normal growth and maintenance of tissue
  2. Regulate cholesterol metabolism (transport, formation of metabolites, and excretion)
  3. Maintain the functioning and integrity of body membranes
  4. Are precursors of the prostaglandins—a group of hormone-like compounds that are involved with such body processes as regulation of blood pressure, gastric section, smooth muscle contraction, and the inflammatory response

Phospholipids[a]
  1. Are structural components of cell membranes
  2. Are components of sphingomyelin in the myelin sheath of the brain and nerves
  3. Are components of lipoproteins for transport of water-insoluble lipids in the blood

Cholesterol[a]
  1. Is a structural component of cell membranes
  2. Is a precursor in the formation of body steroids:
    a. Bile acids
    b. Sex hormones
    c. Adrenocortical hormones
    d. Vitamin D (the ultraviolet rays of the sun convert a cholesterol derivative, 7-dehydrocholesterol to vitamin D)

Lipoprotein[a]
  Is the transport form of lipids in the blood

Glycolipids[a]
  Gangliosides and cerebrosides are glycolipids that are structural components of cell membranes; cerebrosides are especially prevalent in nerve tissue.

---

[a] Body lipid(s).

---

amounts of triglycerides also circulate in the blood as a component of the blood lipids. A **triglyceride** is composed of a glycerol base with three attached fatty acids. Derivatives of triglycerides with either one or two fatty acids attached called, respectively, **monoglycerides** and **diglycerides,** are formed during digestion of triglycerides. (The chemical structures of monoglycerides, diglycerides, and triglycerides are shown in Fig. 7–2).

A summary of triglyceride functions is presented in Table 7–1.

Phospholipids

The **phospholipids,** the second major class of lipids, occur to a limited degree in foods but are synthesized primarily by the body (in the small intestine and liver). Like the triglycerides, these lipids contain fatty acids and alcohols, but they are much more specialized in that they contain phosphorus and nitrogen as well.

Phospholipids have many highly specialized functions (Table 7–1), one of which is a role in transporting the water-insoluble lipids in the blood. Phospholipids can mix with both fat and water-soluble substances, making them useful for lipid transport. Triglycerides and cholesterol are first surrounded by phospholipid and are subsequently enveloped by the water-soluble plasma proteins (globulins). The resulting compound, called **lipoprotein,** is water soluble due to its protein content and is the circulating form of lipids in the blood. Lipoprotein components are shown in Figure 7–3.

Fatty Acids

The functions and properties of the fatty acids have been discussed. All of the food and most of the body fatty acids occur not as free acids but as a basic structural unit of other lipids, such as triglycerides and phospholipids. Free fatty acids are released from the triglycerides of adipose tissue as needed to sup-

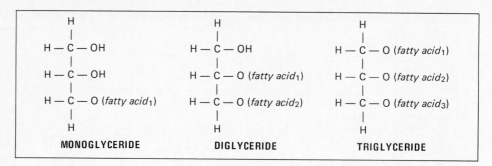

Figure 7–2
*Chemical structure of mono-
glycerides, diglycerides, and
triglycerides.*

ply energy. These free fatty acids are transported in the blood to the cells attached to plasma albumin.

Cholesterol
► **Cholesterol** is a fat-related lipid that is a component of the diet and that is also readily synthesized in the body by the liver and small intestine. Cholesterol metabolism is regulated primarily by the liver, which both synthesizes cholesterol and removes excess cholesterol from the blood by conversion to bile acids and excretion in bile. Linoleic acid also appears to have a role in regulating cholesterol metabolism. Cholesterol has vital structural and regulatory roles in the body (Table 7–1).

Lipoproteins
Lipoproteins are water-soluble complexes containing triglycerides, cholesterol, phospholipids, and protein and are the circulating form of body lipids. Some lipoproteins are synthesized by the intestinal mucosa, others by the liver, and still others are formed directly in the plasma. The intestinal mucosa synthesizes chylomicrons, the lipoprotein class that transports triglycerides absorbed from the intestinal tract to the systemic circulation. Each class of lipoprotein is responsible for transporting a major class of lipid. For example, most of the blood cholesterol is transported as β-lipoprotein, formed in the plasma.

Glycolipids
► **Glycolipids** are a small but important class of body lipids. The name gives a clue to the structure: these

lipids also contain carbohydrate, such as glucose, galactose, or polysaccharides. Glycolipids are an important constituent of nerve tissue (Table 7–1).

FOOD SOURCES

Although some foods are almost pure fat—such as butter and oils—fats in most other foods exist in combination with other nutrients, such as protein and carbohydrate. Major sources of fat include animal foods from the meat–fish–poultry–beans and milk–cheese groups of the Basic Four Food Groups (see Chap. 2) and from vegetable oils, salad dressings, butter, and margarine in the fats–sweets–alcohol group. Most fruits and vegetables are low in fats, although there are some exceptions, such as avocados. Bakery products prepared with the addition of fat, seeds, and nuts are also sources of fat in the diet.

Food fats are composed of mixtures of saturated fat, monounsaturated fat, and polyunsaturated fat. The type of fatty acid that predominates in the food, however, determines its classification.

Food fats of animal origin, such as milk, butter, cheese, eggs, and meat, are composed primarily of
► saturated fatty acids and are called **saturated fats.** Saturated fats of animal origin are also rich in cholesterol, which does not occur in plant foods. Most plant fats contain predominantly polyunsaturated
► fatty acids and are called **polyunsaturated fats.** The best sources of polyunsaturated fats including the essential fatty acids are the vegetable seed oils—soybean, corn, cottonseed, safflower, sesame, and sunflower. Two vegetable oils, peanut and olive, contain predominantly monounsaturated fatty acids
► and are called **monounsaturated fats.**

While nurses can use the plant vs animal classification in helping clients differentiate between saturated and polyunsaturated fat, be aware that there are some exceptions to the rule. Whereas all animal fat contains saturated fat, teach clients that a few plant fats, such as coconut oil, palm oil, and chocolate, are also predominantly saturated fat. The commercial process of hydrogenation (addition of hydrogen to the unsaturated double bonds of a vegetable oil) applied in the production of margarine and solid vegetable shortenings, such as Spry and Crisco, converts a polyunsaturated vegetable oil to a solid

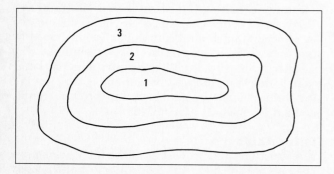

Figure 7–3
Components of a lipoprotein. (1) Triglyceride and cholesterol. (2) Phospholipid. (3) Protein.

TABLE 7–2
FOOD SOURCES OF FAT

Low in Fat	High in Saturated Fat with No Cholesterol (Vegetable Fat)	High in Saturated Fat and Cholesterol (Animal Fat)	High in Unsaturated Fat
Fruits	Regular margarine	Meat fat (beef, lamb, pork, ham higher in saturated fat than poultry, fish, veal; organ meats especially high in cholesterol)	Vegetable oils (safflower, corn, soybean, sunflower, sesame, cottonseed)[a]
Vegetables	Hydrogenated vegetable shortening (Spry, Crisco)		
Legumes	Chocolate	Egg yolks (especially high in cholesterol)	Salad dressings made from above oils (includes many commercial salad dressings)[a]
Cereals	Coconut oil, palm oil	Lard, bacon grease	Soft margarine[a]
Flour	Baked products containing any of the above items	Whole milk, cream (including sour cream)	Peanut oil, olive oil
		Butter	Avocados, olives
		Whole milk cheese, cream cheese	Nuts
		Ice cream, ice milk	
		Baked products containing any of the above items	

[a] High in polyunsaturated fat and essential fatty acids.

saturated fat. Let clients know, however, that soft margarine is produced with a minimum of hydrogenation and retains much of its polyunsaturated fatty acid content.

Table 7–2 summarizes the fat and cholesterol content of foods.

FAT REQUIREMENTS

The amount of fat needed for optimal nutrition is not known, and there is no RDA. Apart from its role in providing energy and serving as a carrier of essential nutrients, including fat-soluble vitamins and essential fatty acids, fat is not a dietary essential.

The National Academy of Sciences states that 3 percent of total energy derived from linoleic acid should be a satisfactory minimum recommended intake of essential fatty acids for those who consume a relatively low-fat diet (i.e., below 25 percent of kilocalories). Assess the client's dietary fat intake, and if the fat intake is high, as is typical of diets currently found in most of the United States, a lower intake may be beneficial.[1] While the National Academy of Sciences does not deem it desirable to make blanket recommendations for dietary changes for the entire U.S. population, use the following guidelines offered by the Academy relative to the amounts and proportions of dietary fat for clients suspected or known to be at high risk for diseases associated with elevated blood lipid levels.[2]

1. Reduce total fat intake (particularly in diets containing below 2000 kcal) so that fat accounts for not more than 35 percent of total kilocalories.

2. Increase the ratio of polyunsaturated to saturated fatty acids; fats containing predominantly saturated fatty acids (i.e., animal fats) should be reduced to a greater extent than fats containing predominantly unsaturated fatty acids (i.e., vegetable fats).

3. An upper limit of 10 percent of kilocalories as polyunsaturated fatty acids is advised.

For those who are overweight and for those who have low energy requirements, the intake of fat, which provides kilocalories but few other essential nutrients, should be reduced.[3]

DIGESTION

► Just as proteases split proteins, **lipases** split lipids. A prerequisite to enzyme hydrolysis of lipids is ► **emulsification,** or the formation of small, uniformly distributed fat globules with a low surface tension. In the emulsified state, a larger surface area with greater ease of penetration is available for enzyme action. A limited amount of natural fats—as in egg yolk—is in a pre-emulsified state. However, most fats require the emulsifying action of bile salts, a digestive agent secreted by the liver and stored in the gallbladder. The bile salts surround the triglycerides and form mixed micelles. In this form lipase activity is accelerated.

The major lipids to be digested are triglycerides, although lesser amounts of dietary cholesterol and phospholipid must also be prepared for absorption. The small intestine is the major organ of lipid digestion. Although a small amount of salivary and gastric lipase are secreted, oral and gastric digestion of lipids is relatively unimportant. Lipase is present in pancreatic and intestinal digestive secretions, although most fats are hydrolyzed by pancreatic lipase.

Through the combined action of bile salts and pancreatic and intestinal lipase, the triglycerides are hydrolyzed in a stepwise fashion to the end products: monoglycerides, free fatty acids, and glycerol (see Table 2–2). Complete breakdown to fatty acids and glycerol does not take place.

ABSORPTION

Of all the nutrients ingested, lipids are the most difficult to absorb. The triglyceride digestive end products presented to the intestinal mucosa for absorption include (1) fatty acids of varying chain lengths (long, medium, short), (2) monoglycerides, and (3) glycerol. However, these products do not follow a common absorption pathway. Monoglycerides and long-chain fatty acids, quantitatively the largest group, follow one pathway, and medium-chain and short-chain fatty acids and glycerol follow another. The difference in absorption pathways is due to (1) the need for a bile as a solution agent for absorption into the intestinal wall, (2) the packaging required inside the intestinal wall to provide continued solubility, and (3) the circulatory route.

Formation of mixed micelles is required to provide solubility for the absorption of monoglycerides and long-chain fatty acids into the intestinal wall. Once the micelles are inside the intestinal wall, the bile salts are released, digestion of monoglycerides is completed, and the lipids require intestinal wall packaging for continued solubility. This packaging consists of a variety of synthetic activities in which triglycerides are reformed and combine with cholesterol, phospholipids, and protein to form chylomicrons, a type of lipoprotein. Chylomicrons are absorbed into the lymphatic system and are the form in which lipids are transported from the intestine to the systemic circulation.

In contrast, short-chain and medium-chain fatty acids and glycerol do not require bile or intestinal wall packaging for solubility and are transported to the systemic circulation via the hepatic portal vein. These differences are summarized in Table 7–3.

METABOLISM

Metabolism of lipids involves the anabolic process
▶ of **lipogenesis,** or fat synthesis, and the catabolic
▶ process of **lipolysis,** or fat breakdown. Both processes are under the hormonal control of the pancreas, pituitary, adrenal, thyroid, and sex glands.

Lipogenesis occurs primarily in three body sites: (1) the intestinal wall, (2) the liver, and (3) adipose tissue. All body tissues, however, are active in synthesizing certain specialized lipids needed for their functioning. The intestinal wall and liver not only synthesize lipoproteins for transport of lipids in the blood, but also are active in the synthesis of other lipids, such as triglycerides, phospholipids, and cholesterol from the products of intermediary metabolism. The lipids synthesized by the liver and intestinal wall are not stored but released to the blood as lipoprotein. In contrast, lipids synthesized by adipose tissue are stored.

Lipolysis also occurs primarily in three body sites: (1) the liver, (2) adipose tissue, and (3) body cells. In addition to synthesizing fat, the liver is also an important organ of lipolysis in that it removes some excess lipids, such as cholesterol, from the blood, with subsequent degradation and/or excretion. When needed, adipose tissue releases its stored triglycerides to the blood as fatty acids and glycerol, and these are subsequently transported to body cells bound to albumin and oxidized for energy. Be aware, however, that blood cells and central nervous system cells oxidize only glucose for energy and do not oxidize fatty acids.

The concentration of lipids in the body, including blood levels and adipose storage, is essentially the end result of the balance between the endogenous (internal) lipogenic and lipolytic activities just described and the exogenous (external) lipids added by the diet. Dietary influences are varied and include (1) consumption of kilocalories, (2) consumption of cholesterol, (3) type of fat consumed (saturated or polyunsaturated), (4) consumption of carbohydrate, and (5) alcohol consumption. With normal metabolic processes and a balanced diet, lipogenesis and lipolysis are also balanced, and body stores and blood concentrations of lipids remain within normal range. If a client's history indicates a dietary imbalance

---

TABLE 7–3
DIFFERENCES IN ABSORPTION FOR GLYCERIDES OF VARYING CHAIN LENGTHS

Glycerides and Long-chain Fatty Acids (Largest Group)	Short-chain and Medium-chain Fatty Acids and Glycerol
Require bile salts as solution agent for transport into the intestinal wall	No bile salts required
Require intestinal wall packaging as chylomicrons	No packaging required
Chylomicrons absorbed into the lymph	Absorbed into portal blood

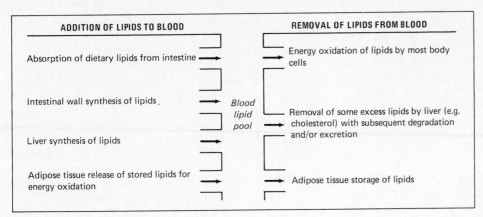

| ADDITION OF LIPIDS TO BLOOD | REMOVAL OF LIPIDS FROM BLOOD |

Absorption of dietary lipids from intestine ⟶

Intestinal wall synthesis of lipids. ⟶

Liver synthesis of lipids ⟶

Adipose tissue release of stored lipids for energy oxidation ⟶

Blood lipid pool

⟶ Energy oxidation of lipids by most body cells

⟶ Removal of some excess lipids by liver (e.g. cholesterol) with subsequent degradation and/or excretion

⟶ Adipose tissue storage of lipids

Figure 7–4
Addition and removal of lipids from the blood lipid pool.

or abnormal metabolic process or both, observe for accumulation of excessive lipids in the blood or adipose tissue. In some conditions, lipids may be stored in the liver. The influences on the blood lipid pool are summarized in Figure 7–4.

DISORDERS INVOLVING LIPIDS

The most common disorders involving lipids include excess body lipids: obesity, fatty infiltration of the liver, and hyperlipidemia. Linoleic acid deficiency has been observed in some instances, and pathologic conditions associated with fat malabsorption are not uncommon. Specific therapies and detailed dietary modifications for these conditions are discussed in Part IV of this book.

Excess Body Lipid Concentrations

Obesity. Excess adipose storage of fat is quite common. According to NHANES I (see Chap. 1) approximately 30 percent of middle-aged women and 15 percent of middle-aged men are obese (weight in excess of 20 percent above desired weight).[4] Major adipose storage sites include subcutaneous tissue, tissue surrounding abdominal organs, and intramuscular connective tissue. Apparently an unlimited amount of fat can be stored when total kilocaloric intake is excessive. Because of its high caloric density (9 kcal/g in comparison with 4 kcal/g for carbohydrate and protein), excess fat intake may be a factor contributing to obesity. However, caution clients that in addition to fat, dietary excesses of carbohydrate and protein also contribute to excess adipose storage of fat and to consider the amount of all the energy-producing nutrients in dietary planning.

Fatty Infiltration and Cirrhosis of the Liver. Recall that unlike adipose tissue, the liver does not normally store lipids but releases the lipids it synthesizes into the blood as lipoprotein, the circulatory form. Fatty liver, or fatty deposits in the liver, is an abnormal condition commonly associated with malnutrition in which the diet is lacking in the pro-

tein and B vitamins needed for lipoprotein formation. If sufficiently severe or long standing, the disorder may be accompanied by necrosis or fibrosis. Although alcohol toxicity is widely accepted as the etiologic agent in Laennec's cirrhosis, also called alcoholic or portal cirrhosis, assess the diet of alcoholic clients since malnutrition may possibly be a contributing factor.

Hyperlipidemia. The condition of elevated blood lipids, called hyperlipidemia, is a common disorder that is thought to be a risk factor in the development of atherosclerosis, a degenerative disease of the arteries, and coronary heart disease. In countries such as the United States whose populations consume large amounts of fat, a sizable proportion of individuals have relatively high blood levels of cholesterol and triglycerides. Although the relative significance of these high blood lipid levels in coronary heart disease is controversial, hypercholesterolemia is generally considered to be one important risk factor among several.[5] Saturated fats tend to elevate and polyunsaturated fat tends to lower blood cholesterol.[6] Monounsaturated fat also tends to lower blood cholesterol but to a lesser degree than polyunsaturated fat.

The average American consumes about 140 g of fat daily, or approximately 42 percent of total kilocaloric intake. Although saturated fat from animal sources contributes the greatest proportion of fat, the increases in fat consumption that have been observed in recent decades are due to increases in consumption of polyunsaturated fats through the use of cooking and salad oils, margarine, and shortening in place of lard and butter.[7] Average cholesterol consumption is 450 mg daily, of which only 10 to 50 percent is absorbed. While dietary modifications are widely used in treating clients with hyperlipidemia, the role of decreasing fat, particularly saturated fat, intake in preventing atherosclerosis and heart disease remains controversial. Refer to Chapter 2 for dietary guidelines regarding fat consumption.

Excessive fat consumption has also been associated with cancer of the colon, breast, and uterus, although the role of fat in the incidence of cancer is even less well understood than its role in heart disease. Diet and cancer are discussed in Chapter 35. Overstimulation of the gallbladder, a condition favoring gallstone formation, may also result from excess fat consumption. Excess fatty acids, particularly saturated fatty acids, favor cholesterol synthesis, leading to supersaturation of the bile with cholesterol, which may precipitate as stones.

Linoleic Acid Deficiency

Poorly nourished individuals may develop linoleic acid deficiency. It is most frequently seen in infants, especially those fed a skim milk formula; in hospitalized clients maintained on prolonged parenteral feedings that do not contain fat; and in clients with persistent fat malabsorption. In clients with a history of the above conditions, observe for signs and symptoms of linoleic acid deficiency, which include:

1. Growth failure (in children)
2. Eczemalike dermatitis
3. Impairment of lipid transport
4. Lowered kilocaloric efficiency
5. Decreased resistance to stress

The most frequently observed symptom is dermatitis. It is interesting to note that in addition to providing a dietary source of linoleic acid as a therapeutic measure, there is also some evidence that the cutaneous application of an oil rich in essential fatty acids, such as sunflower oil, will alleviate the skin rash and biochemical alterations of essential fatty acid deficiency in newborn infants.[8]

Fat Malabsorption

Fat malabsorption resulting in steatorrhea (fat in the stool) occurs as a result of liver or pancreatic disease in which bile or pancreatic lipase deficiency results in impaired fat digestion and absorption. Cholecystitis (gallbladder inflammation) and cholelithiasis (gallstones) are examples of conditions that may result in inadequate bile flow. Cystic fibrosis of the pancreas and chronic pancreatitis may result in pancreatic lipase deficiency. A diminished surface area for absorption, as in intestinal inflammation or resection, also results in malabsorption of fat and other nutrients. Assist clients with any of these conditions to select a nutritionally adequate diet that is low in total fat, both saturated and unsaturated fat content.

REVIEW QUESTIONS AND ACTIVITIES

1. Identify the structural units of lipids.
2. Explain the difference between saturated fat, monounsaturated fat, and polyunsaturated fat.
3. Identify the dietary essential fatty acid in relation to its function, conditions that may

precipitate a deficiency, and major signs of deficiency.
4. Identify foods that are high in total fat content and distinguish between those foods that are high in cholesterol, essential fatty acids, saturated fat, monounsaturated fat, and polyunsaturated fat.
5. Describe the functions of the six major classes of body lipids.
6. Explain the importance of fat as a food nutrient.
7. Calculate the amount of energy provided by 50 g of fat and compare it with the energy provided by 50 g of carbohydrate and 50 g of protein.
8. Explain the importance of bile in lipid digestion and the importance of chylomicrons in lipid transport.
9. Prepare an outline that depicts the digestion, absorption, and metabolic fate of dietary triglycerides.
10. Distinguish between the processes that add lipids to the blood and those that remove lipids from the blood.
11. Discuss the relationship of dietary fats and the blood cholesterol level.
12. Identify the relative amounts and proportions of dietary fats that are appropriate for clients with an elevated blood cholesterol level, as stated by the National Academy of Sciences.
13. Explain the rationale for the development of steatorrhea in a client with fat malabsorption and list foods that must be restricted in the diet because of their high fat content.

REFERENCES

1. National Research Council: Recommended Dietary Allowances, ed 9. Washington, DC, National Academy Press, 1980, p 35.
2. Ibid, pp 35–37.
3. National Research Council: Toward Healthful Diets, Washington, DC, National Academy Press, 1980, p 20.
4. Abraham S, Johnson CL: Overweight Adults in the United States. Vital and Health Statistics of the National Center for Health Statistics, No. 51, 1979.
5. National Research Council: Recommended Dietary Allowances, op cit, p 36.
6. Becker N, Illingsworth DR, Alaupovic P, et al.: Effects of saturated, monounsaturated, and polyunsaturated fatty acids on plasma lipids, lipoproteins, and apoproteins in humans. Am J Clin Nutr 37:355, 1983.
7. Welsh SO, Martson RM: Review of trends in food use in the United States, 1909 to 1980. J Am Diet Assoc 81:120, 1982.
8. Friedman Z, Shochat SJ, Maisels MJ, et al.: Correction of essential fatty acid deficiency in newborn infants by cutaneous application of sunflower seed oil, Pediatrics 58:650, 1976.

BIBLIOGRAPHY

Bach AC, Babayan VK: Medium-chain triglycerides: An update. Am J Clin Nutr 36:950, 1982.

Bliss CM: Fat absorption and malabsorption. Arch Intern Med 141:1213, 1981.

Crawford MA: The role of essential fatty acids and prostaglandins. Postgrad Med 56:557, 1980.

Feigen LP, Hyman AL: Vascular influences of the prostaglandins. Fed Proc 40:1985, 1980.

Glueck, CJ: Appraisal of dietary fat as a causative factor in atherogenesis. Am J Clin Nutr 32:2637, 1979.

Harper AE: Coronary heart disease: An epidemic related to diet. Am J Clin Nutr 37:669, 1983.

Kritchevsky D: Trans fatty acid effects in experimental atherosclerosis. Fed Proc 41:2813, 1982.

Leat WMF: Man's requirement for essential fatty acids. Trends Biochem Sci 6:14, 1981.

Lewis C: Proteins and Carbohydrates, Lipids. Philadelphia, FA Davis, 1976.

McGill HC Jr: Appraisal of cholesterol as a causative factor in atherogenesis. Am J Clin Nutr 32:2632, 1979.

Walker WJ: Changing U.S. lifestyle and declining vascular mortality—A retrospective. N Engl J Med 308:649, 1983.

Vitamins

Objectives

After completion of this chapter, the student will be able to:

1. Compare the properties of water-soluble vitamins and fat-soluble vitamins in relation to their stability in foods, their use by the body, and their potential toxicities.

2. Differentiate between the major functions and results of deficiency of the fat-soluble vitamins.

3. Distinguish among the B-complex vitamins that are involved with release of energy in the body, blood cell formation, and protein metabolism and compare these functions with the major function of vitamin C.

4. Assess the relationship between (a) carotene and vitamin A and (b) polyunsaturated fat and vitamin E.

5. Assess the rationale for administering active metabolites of vitamin D in clients with chronic renal disease.

6. Plan a day's menu for a client that includes at least one good food source of the following vitamins: vitamin A, vitamin E, vitamin K, vitamin C, thiamine, riboflavin, niacin, folic acid, and vitamin B_6.

Vitamins, one of the six major categories of essential food nutrients, can be defined as a group of potent organic compounds needed in minute quantities for cellular metabolic reactions or for the prevention of an associated deficiency disease. Since they cannot be synthesized in sufficient quantities by the body, they must be supplied by the diet.

On the basis of this definition, six major groups of compounds have been classified as vitamins: vitamins A, B, C, D, E, and K. Although a significant amount of vitamin K and some of the B vitamins are synthesized by the body, they are still classified as vitamins. Vitamin D also has some of the characteristics of a hormone. Some vitamins, while classified as a single substance, are actually a group of structurally related compounds that are similar in physiologic activity. Some vitamins are available in foods in their biologically active forms and are called

▶ **preformed vitamins,** and others occur as precursors of vitamins that are transformed in the body
▶ by catalytic action into the **biologically active vitamins.**

CLASSIFICATION AND GENERAL PROPERTIES

Vitamins differ from each other not only in their chemical structure, biochemical function, and distribution in foods but also in their solubility. They are traditionally classified according to their solubility in water or fat and fat solvents. Vitamins A, D, E, and K are fat soluble, and vitamins B and C are water soluble. From a physiologic standpoint, the solubility of vitamins determines their pattern of use, including their absorption, circulation, body

TABLE 8–1
GENERAL PROPERTIES OF THE VITAMINS

Fat-soluble Vitamins (A, D, E, K)	Water-soluble Vitamins (B,C)
1. Soluble in fat and fat solvents, insoluble in water	1. Soluble in water, insoluble in fat
2. Follows absorption and circulation pathway of fats	2. Follows absorption and circulation pathway of water-soluble nutrients
3. Dietary excesses not excreted in urine	3. Dietary excesses excreted in urine
4. Dietary excesses stored in body	4. Minimal storage of dietary excesses
5. Dietary deficiency symptoms develop slowly	5. Dietary deficiency symptoms often develop rapidly
6. Does not dissolve in cooking water; stable with usual cooking methods	6. Dissolves in cooking water; caution necessary to prevent losses in cooking (see Chap. 2)

storage, and excretion (Table 8–1). From a practical standpoint, their solubility determines to a large degree the stability of the vitamin. Fat-soluble vitamins (being insoluble in water) are much more stable with ordinary cooking methods than are the water-soluble vitamins. Heat stability is an additional protective factor for the fat-soluble vitamins; the opposite is true for the water-soluble group. For this reason, caution clients that much of the vitamin B and C content of foods is destroyed by high cooking temperatures and that both fat-soluble and water-soluble vitamins are destroyed by poor food storage techniques that result in wilting and dehydration of fresh food.

METABOLISM

Vitamins contained in foods do not have to be digested. They are absorbed, with little or no change.

Absorption and Circulation
The fat-soluble vitamins A, D, E, and K follow the same absorption and circulation pathway as do fats, since they are absorbed and circulate in combination with fats as components of lipoproteins. In the absence of dietary fat, these vitamins cannot be absorbed. Any factor that decreases fat absorption or circulation will decrease absorption and circulation of fat-soluble vitamins. Examples include:

1. Ingestion of inadequate amounts of dietary fat
2. Inadequate digestion of fat due to bile or pancreatic enzyme deficiency or gastrointestinal hypermotility resulting in diarrhea
3. Inadequate absorption of fat resulting from poor fat digestion, bile deficiency, damage to intestinal mucosa, or hypermotility and diarrhea
4. Inadequate circulation of fat due to impaired lymphatic circulation

The absorption and circulation of the water-soluble vitamins B and C are not dependent on concurrent fat use. Nonetheless, normal digestion, absorption, and circulation processes are necessary for the use of all nutrients. Deficiencies of digestive enzymes, intestinal disease resulting in damage to the mucosal surface, gastrointestinal hypermotility, and inadequate circulation can reduce the cellular supply of all nutrients.

Body Storage and Excretion
Dietary excesses of fat-soluble vitamins are not excreted in the urine but are stored in the body. The major storage site is the liver. However, some of the excesses are stored elsewhere, including adipose tissue, lungs, and kidneys. Excessive intake of these vitamins, with the possible exception of vitamin E, can result in toxic effects. Although vitamin E is generally considered nontoxic to humans, side effects have been observed with excessive ingestion.[1] Toxicity from prolonged excessive ingestion of vitamins A and D is not uncommon. Whereas the natural forms of vitamin K are nontoxic in large doses, excessive doses of synthetic preparations of the vitamin have produced toxic effects. Teach clients that vitamin toxicity can result from indiscriminate self-medication with vitamins and assist them with the correct interpretation of prescription dosages. Failure of physicians to appreciate the potential toxicity of these vitamins can lead to toxic effects. Promiscuous fortification of foods with vitamins may be an additional factor.

In contrast, dietary excesses of the water-soluble group are not stored in the body to any extent but are excreted in the urine, with one exception, vitamin B_{12}. Several years' supply of this vitamin is stored in the liver. A person could eat a diet devoid of vitamin B_{12} for 3 to 5 years without showing evidence of vitamin B_{12} deficiency. Since there is little storage of the other water-soluble vitamins, symptoms resulting from inadequate intake of these vitamins will occur much more rapidly than from inadequate intake of fat-soluble vitamins. Although the evidence of toxicity associated with excessive ingestion of the water-soluble vitamins is less clear-cut than for the fat-soluble vitamins, some adverse reactions have been noted. Vitamin toxicity and adverse reactions are discussed in the section on megavitamin therapy.

VITAMIN AND DRUG INTERACTION

There is a definite relationship between vitamin metabolism and drug metabolism. Certain vitamins influence the absorption and actions of certain drugs, and certain drugs influence the absorption and use of certain vitamins. In addition to the examples presented in the following sections on specific vitamins, a few examples of common vitamin–drug interactions are listed in Figure 8–1.

FUNCTIONS AND IMBALANCES OF VITAMINS

Vitamins are not a source of energy. Generally, they perform regulatory functions, although in a few instances they are constituents of body compounds. Like hormones, vitamins play a catalytic role in metabolic reactions, but a few function in a more general fashion. As catalysts, they function as coenzymes, which combine with specific enzyme proteins to produce the active form of the enzymes; this is particularly true of the B vitamins.

It should be emphasized that vitamin research is continually being conducted, and the knowledge of functions and imbalances is far from complete. The information summarized in this section represents the most widely accepted theories at the present time.

EFFECT OF DRUG ON VITAMIN METABOLISM
1. Oral contraceptives alter the absorption and use of pyridoxine and folic acid and possibly vitamin C, riboflavin, and vitamin B_{12}.
2. Mineral oil taken as a laxative near meal time leaches fat-soluble vitamins. These vitamins are soluble in the mineral oil, which is not absorbed.
3. Administration of an antimetabolite of a vitamin blocks the normal action of the vitamin and produces vitamin deficiency. A common antimetabolite used to block cell division to control malignant tumor growth is methotrexate, a folic acid antagonist. Since a major function of folic acid is to catalyze nucleic acid synthesis, division of normal cells as well as tumor cells decreases. Folic acid deficiency symptoms result.
4. Cigarette smoking may alter the use of vitamin C and result in an increased need for this vitamin.

EFFECT OF VITAMIN ON DRUG METABOLISM
5. Detoxification of drugs by the liver requires enzyme action. Deficiency of such vitamins as vitamin A, vitamin C, vitamin E, or riboflavin results in decreased enzyme levels and diminished drug detoxification.

Figure 8–1
Some examples of common vitamin–drug interactions.

Fat-soluble Vitamins

▶ ***Vitamin A.*** Vitamin A, also called **retinol,** is present in the preformed state in certain animal foods, such as liver, kidney, cream, butter, whole milk and whole milk cheese, egg yolks, and fish liver oils. Margarine, skim milk, and skim milk products are fortified with Vitamin A. Carotenoid pigments present in dark green and deep yellow fruits and vegetables are precursors of vitamin A. They are converted by enzyme action to vitamin A in the intestinal wall during absorption and by the liver, although some may circulate as carotene in the systemic blood.

The functions and signs of deficiency are summarized in Table 8–2. Of the major functions of vitamin A, the most clearly defined relates to its role in vision. It is a constituent of the visual pigments, including rhodopsin (or visual purple) of rod cells necessary for dim light vision. One of the earliest signs of vitamin A deficiency is night blindness, the inability to see well in dim light, especially when going into darkness from bright light, such as when entering a darkened theater. Rhodopsin, being sensitive to light, is broken down on exposure to light. Regeneration of this pigment occurs in the dark only when an adequate supply of vitamin A is available.

Be alert to the possibility of a vitamin A deficiency in clients who follow a very low fat diet and in those with conditions associated with fat malabsorption, such as celiac disease, cystic fibrosis, obstructive jaundice, or infectious hepatitis. Provide a fat-soluble vitamin supplement in a water-miscible form in these cases. Clients with protein energy malnutrition may also be vitamin A deficient, since vitamin A circulates in the blood bound to proteins. With protein deficiency these transport proteins cannot be synthesized.

▶ ***Vitamin D.*** Vitamin D, also called **cholecalciferol** or vitamin D_3, occurs naturally in only a few foods, such as liver, egg yolk, butter, cream, and fish liver oils. Milk and some other foods are fortified with the vitamin. Another source of vitamin D is that which is formed from exposure of a derivative of cholesterol, 7-dehydrocholesterol, in the skin to ultraviolet light. A dietary requirement for vitamin D exists only in the absence of sufficient sunlight exposure.

Vitamin D functions and results of deficiency are summarized in Table 8–3. In the regulation of calcium and phosphorus metabolism, vitamin D is only one factor. Its effects are integrated with the action of two hormones in this regulation: parathyroid hormone (PTH) from the parathyroid glands and calcitonin from the thyroid gland. With normal functioning of vitamin D, PTH, and calcitonin, the blood levels of calcium and phosphate ions are maintained within the range of 9 to 11 mg% and 3.0 to 4.5 mg%, respectively. Further, the ratio of calcium to phosphate ions, the calcium:phosphorus ratio, is also correctly maintained to allow them to func-

---

TABLE 8–2
FUNCTIONS AND SIGNS OF DEFICIENCY OF VITAMIN A

Functions	Results of Deficiency
1. Constituent of visual pigments necessary for normal vision	1. Night blindness, or impairment of visual acuity in dim light
2. Maintenance of epithelial tissues (possibly secondary to role in mucopolysaccharide synthesis)	2. Keratinization of epithelial cells (skin and membranes lining body openings, including the eye, sinus and ear passages, and respiratory, gastrointestinal, and urinary tracts) results in lowered resistance to infection in these areas of the body and can lead to blindness
3. Growth and maintenance of normal bones and teeth (possibly due to role in mucopolysaccharide synthesis or role in stabilizing cell membranes)	3. Growth retardation, abnormal bone growth, and tooth structure
4. Reproduction in experimental animals	4. Reproductive failure in animals
5. Synthesis of steroid hormones	
6. Postulated role in protein synthesis	

---

tion in a variety of catalytic roles. Additionally, calcium and phosphorus are deposited in bone during the mineralization process possibly under the influence of vitamin D, although its specific role is unclear, and this function has not been clearly established.

The recent discovery that vitamin D requires metabolic activation before it can induce physiologic changes has prompted some investigators to regard vitamin D as a prohormone. The activation of vitamin D involves its **hydroxylation** [addition of hydroxyl (OH) groups] by the liver and kidney. One hydroxyl group is added by liver metabolism and a second by the kidney. The hydroxylated forms of vitamin D are more biologically active than the parent compound, and the final hydroxylated form, $1,25\text{-}(OH_2)\ D_3$, or calcitriol, produced by the kidney is the most biologically active form of the vitamin and is now considered a hormone. Synthetic analogs of calcitriol are now available.

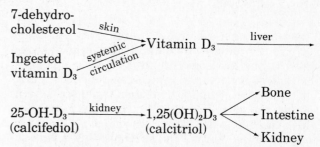

Damage to either the liver or the kidney can reduce the activation of the vitamin and give rise to vitamin D-related bone disorders, even though the intake of the vitamin is adequate. Several disease states, such as bone disease associated with kidney disease (renal osteodystrophy), hypoparathyroidism, neonatal hypocalcemia, certain types of vitamin D-resistant rickets, and osteoporosis, are related to a disturbance in the vitamin D endocrine system, and success is being achieved with use of

---

TABLE 8–3
FUNCTIONS AND SIGNS OF DEFICIENCY OF VITAMIN D

Functions	Results of Deficiency
Regulates calcium and phosphorus metabolism by facilitating:	Hypocalcemia → rickets (in children) or osteomalacia (in adults) in which the mineral content of bone is diminished. May result from deficiency of vitamin D and/or calcium. These disorders may also result from a phosphorus deficiency.
1. Intestinal absorption of calcium and phosphorus.[a]	
2. Mineralization of bone with mineral deposition (least clearly defined function).	
3. Resorption of bone with release of calcium and phosphorus.[a]	
4. Reabsorption of calcium by the kidney.	

[a] Most clearly defined functions.

calcitriol or its analogs in treatment.[2] Administration of calcitriol to osteoporotic postmenopausal women, for example, not only increases calcium absorption but also improves calcium balance, an effect that persists for up to 2 years.

Vitamin D deficiency is most often seen in clients with metabolic disorders associated with poor absorption or impaired activation of the vitamin and in those with inborn errors of vitamin D metabolism. Suspect a deficiency if a client's history includes a malabsorption syndrome, chronic renal failure, or renal tubular defects. The metabolism of vitamin D is also altered in clients receiving corticosteroids and phenytoin (Dilantin). Assess clients who take these drugs on a long-term basis for vitamin D deficiency.

Some ethnic groups follow a practice of shielding children and women from sunlight, making them susceptible to vitamin D deficiency. Dark-skinned people are also susceptible to a deficiency of the vitamin, since melanin pigment retards the formation of vitamin D_3 in the skin. Consider a dietary supplement, particularly for those living in the northern section of the country. Other vulnerable groups include vegetarians and breastfed infants who do not receive a supplement. Milk given to children should be checked to be sure that it is fortified with vitamin D.

Vitamin E. Although vitamin E, also called ▶ **tocopherol,** is a dietary essential, its precise role is still unclear. The vitamin is widely distributed in foods, although wheat germ and vegetable oils (soybean, corn, cottonseed, and safflower) and products made from these are richest sources.

Of the various functions postulated for vitamin E, the only one that has received wide acceptance is its role as a biologic antioxidant. In this role, it traps free radicals generated in the body from normal metabolic processes or from toxic compounds taken into the body. Free radicals induce peroxide formation from polyunsaturated fatty acids, which in turn lead to decomposition of all membrane lipids and cellular damage. Vitamin E thus helps to stabilize cell membranes. The mineral selenium shares a role with vitamin E in preventing peroxidative decomposition of membrane lipids. Vitamin E also protects vitamins A and C from oxidation in the body.

Vitamin E deficiency is very difficult to document. Although generalized instability of cell membranes and cellular degeneration may result from loss of antioxidant properties and subsequent lipid peroxidation, the most easily detected evidence is increased susceptibility of red blood cells to hemolysis. Though various signs of vitamin E deficiency can be observed in experimental animals, it is only in recent years that signs of vitamin E deficiency, including various neurologic and muscle abnormalities, have been observed in humans.

The broad spectrum of deficiency symptoms pro-duced experimentally in animals has prompted many clinicians to give vitamin E a clinical trial in the treatment of numerous conditions. For example, vitamin E has been claimed to be effective in treating a variety of disorders, such as muscular dystrophy, burns, and heart conditions, in improving athletic ability and sexual performance, and in retarding aging, cancer, and cellular damage by air pollutants, such as ozone and nitrogen dioxide. To date, there is no concrete evidence to support claims of this type.

Although vitamin E appears to have low toxicity, some side effects of large doses do occur in both animals and humans, and there are sound reasons to question the safety of ingesting large doses over a prolonged period of time without adequate medical monitoring. In some cases there is a clear need to supplement the diet with vitamin E. High-risk groups for vitamin E deficiency include premature infants and clients with extreme malnutrition, fat malabsorption, or liver disease. Assess the need for vitamin E supplements in these cases. In addition, clients who abruptly terminate a diet that is high in polyunsaturated fats may need to take a vitamin E supplement for an extended period of time following discontinuation of the diet. The need for vitamin E increases in clients who follow a diet high in polyunsaturated fats. The vegetable oils that are high in polyunsaturated fat are also high in vitamin E so that a deficiency in this situation is unlikely. With abrupt termination, however, vitamin E is lost from the tissues faster than the polyunsaturated fat, and a relative state of vitamin E deficiency may develop. Other situations that may necessitate vitamin E supplementation and the side effects of excessive intake that have been reported in isolated cases are discussed in the later section on megavitamin therapy.

Vitamin K. Vitamin K is available naturally from various foods and from bacterial synthesis in the intestinal tract (as vitamin K_1 and K_2). The best dietary sources are green leafy vegetables. Fruits, cereals, dairy products, and meat provide lesser amounts. Approximately one half of the vitamin K comes from intestinal synthesis, and the other half comes from the diet.[3] The synthetic form of ▶ the vitamin (**menadione** or vitamin K_3) has two to three times the biologic activity of the natural forms.

The best known function of vitamin K is to catalyze the liver synthesis of several of the blood-clotting factors, including factor II (prothrombin), factor VII (proconvertin), factor IX (Christmas factor), and factor X (Stuart factor). The role of vitamin K in the synthesis of other plasma proteins that function in bone and kidney metabolism is currently being investigated.

Assess for alterations in blood levels of prothrombin and other clotting factors due to vitamin K deficiency in the following situations:

1. Low blood levels in the newborn because of poor placental transfer and a sterile intestinal tract with no intestinal synthesis of the vitamin. It takes approximately 1 week of milk intake to establish the bacterial flora.
2. Long-term therapy with antibiotics that sterilize the intestinal tract. Use of anticoagulants, such as coumarins (Warfarin, dicumarol), salicylates (aspirin), or large doses of vitamin E (possibly); use of agents that interfere with absorption of the vitamin, such as mineral oil or cholestyramine; or use of agents that increase the turnover of the vitamin in the body (some anticonvulsants, for example).
3. Diseases associated with altered fat digestion and absorption, which may also reduce vitamin K absorption.
4. Liver disease that alters synthesis of blood-clotting factors. In advanced liver disease, vitamin K may not be effective, since the damaged liver may not be able to synthesize clotting factors.

Water-soluble Vitamins

▶ *Vitamin C.* Vitamin C, also called **ascorbic acid,** is currently the subject of much controversy. The questions at issue are the amount of the vitamin needed by healthy persons to maintain health and the effects of taking large doses of the vitamin. Because of the controversy, many people are confused about the amount of the vitamin that they should ingest daily. Most species of animals can synthesize vitamin C from glucose in sufficient amounts to meet their requirements and thus do not require a dietary source. This is not true of humans, however, and a dietary source is required. Vitamin C is present in many fresh fruits and vegetables, especially citrus fruits.

Although vitamin C is important for a variety of biologic functions, its specific mode of action has not been determined. In contrast to most other water-soluble vitamins, no clear-cut coenzyme role has been established. Ascorbic acid is known to function as a reducing agent (giving up hydrogen) in the body. However, this may be a relatively nonspecific effect, although some specific roles for the vitamin have been identified. Its most significant and basic function is to facilitate the formation and maintenance of collagen, a basic structural protein of connective tissue (cartilage, bone, tooth dentin, blood vessel walls, tendon, skin). A deficiency of vitamin C will, therefore, result in faulty collagen formation in connective tissues. Observe for these signs of deficiency when a nutrient analysis reveals that the client's diet lacks vitamin C.

1. Increased permeability of capillaries with bleeding into tissues (easy bruising and hemorrhage)

2. Delayed or incomplete wound healing (scar tissue is connective tissue)
3. Loosened teeth, with gums that bleed easily (gingivitis)
4. Bones that fracture easily

Deficiency symptoms specifically related to other functions of vitamin C (listed below) are more difficult to document. Vitamin C:

1. Facilitates the formation of red blood cells by (a) enhancing the intestinal absorption of iron by reducing ferric iron to ferrous iron, the absorbable form, (b) facilitating the transfer of iron from its transport form in the blood (transferrin) to its storage form (ferritin), and (c) stimulating the conversion of folic acid to its coenzyme form, tetrahydrofolic acid.
2. Plays a role in the synthesis of the neurotransmitters, norepinephrine and serotonin.
3. Plays a role in the synthesis of anti-inflammatory steroids by the adrenal gland. There are high levels of ascorbic acid in the adrenal cortex that disappear during stressful situations when adrenocortical activity is high. Infectious processes, especially those of bacterial origin and with fever, are accompanied by low blood levels of the vitamin.
4. May play a role in lipid metabolism. Its participation in the removal of cholesterol from the tissues to the liver and in the conversion of cholesterol to bile acids has been proposed. Reports on the relationships between vitamin C status and plasma lipid levels are controversial, however, and there is no evidence that large doses of vitamin C are beneficial in clients with normal or high serum cholesterol or triglyceride levels.[4,5]
5. Aids in maintenance of resistance to infection. Although the role is not clear, maintaining optimum tissue saturation levels of the vitamins may be of benefit. At present, however, there is no evidence that resistance to infection is improved with a high intake. For example, there is no evidence available to support the use of megadoses of vitamin C to prevent the common cold.

Therapeutic Value of Vitamin C Supplementation. Consider supplementing the diet with vitamin C for the following clients:

1. Clients with burns or those who have had surgery. The role of vitamin C in wound healing has been recognized for years. Vitamin C apparently migrates to the wound site and stimulates formation of the collagen essential for healing. Postburn skin grafts heal more quickly when vitamin C is present. Many physicians recommend vitamin C supplements in situations associated with trauma.

2. Clients with anemia. Since vitamin C has several indirect roles related to red blood cell formation, its use as adjunct therapy in anemia is warranted. The ingestion of vitamin C-containing foods (such as orange juice) simultaneously with iron supplements or the ingestion of iron supplements that are fortified with vitamin C may promote absorption of the iron.

3. Clients undergoing stressful conditions and those taking certain drugs. Although there is not complete agreement on the relationship between vitamin C and stress, some individuals feel that there is definitely an increased requirement for the vitamin in all forms of stress. In addition to trauma, other stressful situations that increase vitamin C requirements are infections, cigarette smoking, exposure to toxic levels of heavy metals (such as lead, mercury, and cadmium), and frequent ingestion of certain drugs (such as oral contraceptives, phenobarbital, and aspirin).

Vitamin C is also discussed later in this chapter in the section on megavitamin therapy. Because vitamin C is a water-soluble substance, large doses are assumed to be harmless. However, this has not been found to be the case, and further studies are needed to establish the risk:benefit ratio of using large doses of the vitamin in situations for which megadoses are promoted.

B-Complex Vitamins. There are eight B-complex vitamins grouped together because of somewhat similar functions and similar occurrence in foods. These include (1) thiamine (B_1), (2) riboflavin (B_2), (3) niacin, (4) pyridoxine (B_6), (5) pantothenic acid, (6) folic acid, (7) vitamin B_{12} (cyanocobalamin), and (8) biotin. Other substances have some of the properties of vitamins and are sometimes classified with the B-complex group. They are not vitamins, however, since they do not meet the criteria necessary for this classification. Examples include lipoic acid, choline, inositol, coenzyme Q, bioflavinoids, and para-aminobenzoic acid (PABA).

Although the role of the B-complex vitamins in metabolism is not completely understood, all of them function as coenzymes. Some are involved with the release of energy from carbohydrates, proteins, and fats (thiamine, riboflavin, niacin, pantothenic acid, and biotin), others are important in blood cell formation (folic acid and vitamin B_{12}), and pyridoxine performs miscellaneous functions, particularly those involving protein metabolism. All of the B vitamins are involved, either directly or indirectly, in the synthesis of a variety of body compounds. Table 8–4 provides a summary of the functions and sources of specific B vitamins.

Two of the B vitamins, vitamin B_{12} and folic acid, perform vital coenzyme roles in the synthesis of nucleic acids (DNA and RNA), which are present in all cells. Because of this role, they are often referred to as cell-growth and blood-forming factors. These vitamins are interrelated in their functions, although the relationship is not clearly understood. As might be expected, deficiencies of the two vitamins result in abnormal cell division throughout the body, with rapidly dividing cells, such as blood cells and epithelial cells of the gastrointestinal tract, especially affected.

In clients with vitamin B_{12} deficiency, assess for signs and symptoms in the central nervous system, the gastrointestinal tract, and the bone marrow. This deficiency produces (1) degeneration of the spinal cord, (2) inflammation of the gastrointestinal tract, and (3) anemia. Folic acid deficiency also results in gastrointestinal inflammation and anemia but not spinal cord degeneration. Be cautious with giving folic acid supplements. Folic acid supplementation will cure the anemia associated with vitamin B_{12} deficiency, but the neurologic manifestations associated with spinal cord degeneration will not be alleviated. To prevent masking of the potentially lethal neurologic effects of vitamin B_{12} deficiency, federal law prohibits over-the-counter sale of vitamin preparations that contain more than 0.1 mg of folic acid in a daily dosage.

The absorption of vitamin B_{12} (which is also
▶ called the **extrinsic factor**) from the intestine is unique in that it requires the presence of an enzyme.
▶ This enzyme, called the **intrinsic factor,** is a mucoprotein secreted by special gastric glands into the gastric juice. The specific absorption site of vitamin B_{12} is the terminal ileum. If a client's history includes a total gastrectomy or if there is atrophy of the gastric mucosa, be aware that vitamin B_{12} cannot be absorbed. Likewise, absorption will be inhibited with surgical removal of the terminal ileum, the specific absorption site of vitamin B_{12}. However there is significant body storage of vitamin B_{12}, in contrast to other water-soluble vitamins. This storage delays the onset of symptoms of vitamin B_{12} deficiency in those clients who regularly consume animal protein foods, the only significant source of the vitamin. Certain cultural dietary patterns exclude animal foods such as dairy products and/or meats from the diet, however (see Chaps. 19 and 20), and unless suitable alternative sources are chosen, vitamin B_{12} stores may be limited.

Deficiency of the B-Complex Vitamins. Because of the close interrelationship of functions of the B-complex group, deficiency signs or symptoms of single vitamins are seldom seen. For this reason, vitamin supplementation usually involves the entire B group rather than single vitamins. However, four B vitamins, thiamine, folic acid, vitamin B_{12}, and pyridoxine, are sometimes given alone, since situations associated with a deficiency of these vitamins are somewhat easier to differentiate. For example, thiamine, pyridoxine, and folic acid deficiencies are com-

TABLE 8-4
FUNCTIONS AND SOURCES OF B-COMPLEX VITAMINS

Vitamin	Functions	Sources
Energy releasing Thiamine	1. Is a component of the coenzyme thiamine pyrophosphate (TPP) required for (a) the oxidative decarboxylation of alpha-keto acids (pyruvate, alpha-ketoglutarate, and keto analogs of the branded-chain amino acids), (b) the function of transketolase in the hexose monophosphate shunt (thiamine is thus necessary for the release of energy from carbohydrate, protein, and fat and plays an indirect role in the synthesis of nucleic acids and fat). 2. May have a role in neural metabolism that is independent of its coenzyme role.	Pork, organ meats, legumes, nuts, whole or enriched grain products, wheat germ, brewer's yeast
Riboflavin	1. Serves as a coenzyme for a group of enzymes called flavoproteins (FAD, flavin adenine dinucleotide, and FMN, flavin mononucleotide) that exhibit oxidation/reduction activity in the release of energy from carbohydrate, protein, and fat. FMN is also involved in the deamination of amino acids. 2. May also be involved in the synthesis of corticosteroids and the production of red blood cells.	Milk and milk products; organ meats (liver and kidney), egg, green leafy vegetables, whole or enriched grain products
Niacin	1. Is a component of two coenzymes (NAD, nicotinamide adenine dinucleotide, and NADP, nicotinamide adenine dinucleotide phosphate) that are necessary for (a) oxidative release of energy from carbohydrate, protein, and fat, (b) synthesis of fat, cholesterol, and protein, and (3) synthesis of ribose (necessary for nucleic acid synthesis) in the hexose monophosphate shunt.	Preformed—meats, legumes, nuts, peanut butter, whole grain and enriched grains. Precursor (tryptophan)—especially high in animal protein foods
Pantothenic acid	1. Is a constituent of the enzyme coenzyme A (CoA), which (in the activated form—acetyl coenzyme A) catalyzes (a) the oxidative release of energy from carbohydrate, protein, and fat, (b) synthesis of fat, cholesterol, other sterols, porphyrins—constituents of the heme component of hemoglobin—and acetyl choline—a neurotransmitter. 2. Is a constituent of acyl carrier protein (ACP), a compound also needed for fat synthesis.	Liver, kidney, salmon, egg, legumes, nuts (peanuts), whole grains; smaller amounts in fruits, vegetables, milk, molasses, yeast
Biotin	1. Is a coenzyme for carboxylase enzymes that function in the addition of carbon dioxide to organic molecules (called carbon dioxide fixation) as a means of lengthening carbon chains. As a constituent of carboxylases, biotin plays a central role in fat synthesis (as a constituent of the enzyme acetyl-CoA carboxylase) and in carbohydrate metabolism (conversion of pyruvate to oxaloacetate). 2. Other functions of biotin-containing coenzymes in carbohydrate and protein metabolism are less clear, although they may play a role in nucleic acid synthesis, deamination of certain amino acids, gluconeogenesis, formation of antibodies, and synthesis of pancreatic amylase. These suggested roles require further research.	Organ meats, egg yolk, legumes, nuts, mushrooms
Red blood cell formation Folic acid	1. As the coenzyme tetrahydrofolic acid, functions in the transfer of single carbon compounds (e.g., methyl or formyl units) to intermediary compounds. These reactions are important in the synthesis of nucleic acids, some amino acids (e.g., conversion of homocysteine to methionine and histidine to glutamic acid), and heme. Vitamin B_{12} is a cofactor with folic acid in nu-	Green leafy vegetables, liver, peanuts, legumes, whole grains, wheat germ, orange juice

TABLE 8–4 (Continued)

Vitamin	Functions	Sources
	cleic acid synthesis and formation and maturation of blood cells in the bone marrow.	
Vitamin B$_{12}$	1. Functions as a coenzyme (a) in the synthesis of nucleic acids (interrelated with folic acid) and (b) in the conversion of the amino acid homocysteine to methionine. 2. May also be involved in the metabolism of nervous tissue (e.g., in the myelination of neural tissue or in the use of glucose by the brain for energy), although the mechanisms are not clear.	Animal protein foods only (meat, milk, cheeses, fish and shellfish, eggs)
Miscellaneous functions Pyridoxine	1. Functions as a constituent of the enzyme pyridoxyl phosphate (and occasionally pyridoxamine phosphate) in nearly all reactions involved with the metabolism of amino acids and may be involved with the intestinal absorption of amino acids, in the synthesis of heme precursors, and in the conversion of tryptophan to niacin (the relationship of pyridoxine to central nervous system function may in part result from its role in the conversion of amino acids to substances that regulate neurotransmission, e.g., conversion of glutamic acid to gamma-aminobutyric acid and conversion of tryptophan to serotonin). 2. Appears to have an indirect effect on energy production through stabilizing the enzyme phosphorylase, which functions in the release of glucose from liver and muscle glycogen. There is little primary relationship between pyridoxine and fat metabolism, although some roles have been suggested.	Meat (muscle, organ, fish), egg yolk, legumes and nuts, bananas, potatoes (white and sweet), whole grains, wheat germ, legumes, prunes and raisins, yeast

mon in alcoholics. Pyridoxine and folic acid supplements may be necessary for uremic clients undergoing dialysis, and pyridoxine supplements are given to clients taking drugs, such as isoniazid, which alters pyridoxine metabolism.

The general effects of B-complex vitamin deficiency on the various body systems are summarized in Table 8–4. When specific vitamin deficiencies of major significance to the sign or symptom described can be pinpointed, these are indicated. One should keep in mind that the severity of the symptoms is directly related to the severity of the deficiency.

1. Nervous system
   a. Apathy, listlessness, drowsiness, and fatigue result from a slowing of synapses due to lack of energy to the nervous system (deficiency of vitamins, especially thiamine, for energy oxidation. The nervous system normally uses only glucose for energy, and enzyme systems for glucose oxidation are extremely sensitive to thiamine deficiency)
   b. Neuritis and/or neurologic degeneration (thiamine, niacin, vitamin B$_{12}$, pyridoxine deficiency)
   c. Neural hyperactivity → convulsions (pyridoxine deficiency)
2. Gastrointestinal system: Manifestations may be related to lack of any of the B vitamins
   a. Anorexia, weight loss
   b. Indigestion, constipation (thiamine deficiency, especially)
   c. Epithelial changes: red lips and tongue; soreness extending throughout the entire gastrointestinal tract, leading to diarrhea
3. Skin
   a. Dermatitis (greasy or scaly type)
   b. Cracks in skin at corners of mouth and at nasal angles
   c. Poor wound healing
4. Eye: Eyes that are bloodshot, itch, tear, burn, are sensitive to light (riboflavin deficiency, especially)
5. Blood: Anemia (pyridoxine, folic acid, vitamin B$_{12}$ deficiency). Pyridoxine deficiency produces a hypochromic, microcytic anemia, and a macrocytic (megaloblastic) anemia oc-

curs secondary to folic acid or vitamin B_{12} deficiency

6. Heart: Heart failure (severe thiamine deficiency)

VITAMIN REQUIREMENTS

Teach clients that a well-chosen diet will supply adequate vitamins, provided reasonable caution is given to food storage and preparation techniques to preserve nutritive value (see Chap. 2). Normal healthy individuals, except for pregnant women and infants receiving home-prepared formulas (as opposed to commercially prepared premodified formulas), usually do not need vitamin supplements. Folic acid supplements may be required during pregnancy. Neither extra energy nor increased immunity are documented benefits in well-nourished individuals who supplement their diets with multivitamin capsules. The RDAs for selected vitamins are shown in Table 2–1. Estimated safe and adequate intakes of vitamin K, biotin, and pantothenic acid are found in Table 2–3.

VITAMIN SUPPLEMENTATION

In the United States, a vast amount of money is spent annually for unneeded vitamin products. The potency of marketed vitamins varies, and many individuals do not have the knowledge required to compare their own vitamin needs to the vitamin content of supplements. In addition to a waste of resources, there is the potential hazard of vitamin overdosage. One concept should be kept in mind in regard to vitamin supplementation in normal individuals: when used in the amounts listed in the RDAs, vitamins are considered as food. Beyond this point, they should be regarded as drugs. There are no established maximum limits of vitamins and minerals in supplements offered for sale except for children under 12 years of age and for pregnant and lactating women.

There are conditions in which vitamin supplementation is justified and necessary as a part of medical therapy. Refer to Chapter 2 for a discussion of vitamin deficiencies that have been documented in nutrition surveys. However, accompany vitamin supplementation with vigorous efforts to correct the dietary inadequacy. Keep in mind also that various illnesses alter the need for vitamins just as for other nutrients. In many cases, the need for specific vitamins increases far above the RDA (the RDAs meet the needs of healthy persons and do not take into account special needs necessitated by illness). When vitamins are given therapeutically, the dosage may be a maintenance dose (approximately equal to the RDA for the individual) or a therapeutic dose (several times the amount of the RDA to provide for repletion of body stores). Anticipate vitamin supplementation as part of therapy in these situations:

1. Conditions interfering with ingestion
   a. Alcoholism
   b. Diseases associated with chronic anorexia
   c. Mechanical problems (e.g., swallowing)
   d. Mental illness
   e. Diseases requiring a severely restricted diet
   f. Poor eating habits as a result of fads and lack of knowledge, motivation, or resources necessary for the selection and preparation of an adequate diet
2. Diseases associated with digestion and/or absorption problems
   a. Gastrointestinal diseases including pancreatic and liver disease
   b. Malabsorption syndromes
   c. Problems following gastrointestinal surgery
3. Diseases associated with increased metabolic requirements, such as fevers
4. Conditions requiring medications that alter vitamin requirements
5. Periods of rapid growth, such as infancy, pregnancy

MEGAVITAMIN THERAPY

▶ **Megavitamin therapy** is the use of vitamins, at dosage levels at least 10 times the RDA, as pharmacologic agents in the treatment of nonnutritional disorders. As noted earlier, vitamins are organic molecules not synthesized by the body but required in minute amounts from food to sustain metabolic functions. In general, vitamins (particularly the B vitamins) function as catalysts in enzyme systems by serving as coenzymes. Usually, these enzyme systems become saturated with vitamins at levels that approximate the RDA or less. Amounts in excess of that needed to saturate enzyme systems exhibit chemical or druglike effects. Thus, megadoses of vitamins exert chemical, not vitamin, effects, and some of these effects are harmful in varying degrees.

At present, considerable research is being conducted on the pharmacologic use of nutrients in the prevention and treatment of disease. In some instances, beneficial effects have been noted. These include the following:

1. A small number of individuals suffer from vitamin-dependent genetic disease (inborn errors of metabolism) and require supplementation with large doses of the specific vitamin involved. For example, conditions that require large doses of thiamine, niacin, pyridoxine, and vitamin B_{12} have been identified. Megavitamin therapy may also be indicated

in other serious medical illnesses, for example, to counteract the toxicity of an antivitamin.

2. Hemolytic anemia (accompanied by edema and irritability) in premature infants may be relieved by administration of vitamin E. Infants (full-term, premature, or those of low birth weight) may have a relatively low level of vitamin E at birth. This may be due to a lower concentration of blood lipids in newborns or to an inefficient placental transfer of the vitamin. The vitamin E level tends to stabilize at normal within a month after birth, particularly in breastfed babies. However, in some infants—particularly prematures—hemolytic anemia occurs, and a deficiency of vitamin E is considered to be partly responsible. While human milk is a good source of vitamin E, cow's milk contains less. Commercial formulas now contain adequate vitamin E and a favorable ratio of vitamin E to polyunsaturated fatty acids, and formulas designed for prematures contain reduced amounts of iron that can oxidize vitamin E. Consequently, some authorities now conclude that there is no longer a need for the routine administration of a vitamin E supplement to prevent anemia.[6]

3. Intermittent claudication (calf pain when walking) may be relieved in some individuals by prolonged administration of large doses of vitamin E. This condition, however, has a highly subjective component and a variable course. Occasionally there is spontaneous improvement without therapy.

4. Individuals with malabsorption syndromes may require supplements of various vitamins.

While these beneficial effects have been documented, much additional research is needed on the concept of megavitamin therapy in general and of therapy with specific vitamins in particular. There is no evidence that healthy people benefit from megadoses of vitamins or that such doses alleviate symptoms of certain disease conditions. For example, the hypothesis that doses of vitamin C well in excess of that needed for nutritional function are useful for preventing colds or relieving the symptoms associated with colds has not been unequivocally established. Although there is some evidence that megadoses of vitamin C may have a mild antihistaminic effect when a cold is present and give some symptomatic relief in some individuals, the potential risks associated with large doses may outweigh any potential benefit. Whereas some evidence exists for an increased survival time in cancer clients treated with large doses of vitamin C, a recent study showed no benefit for large doses of the vitamin in treating cancer,[7] and the potential exists for harmful effects resulting from excessive use of vitamin C against certain neoplasms.[8]

A committee of the American Psychiatric Association has found no valid support for the hypothesis that large doses of niacin are helpful in the treatment of schizophrenia.[9] Whereas megadoses of niacin may lower serum lipid levels, the benefits of long-term therapy is questionable in view of its side effects and toxicity. Large doses of other nutrients, such as vitamin C, vitamin B_6, riboflavin, pantothenic acid, vitamin B_{12}, and folic acid, used alone or in combination with other therapies are also being recommended to treat various neurologic disorders without well-documented effectiveness.[10] The Committee on Nutrition, American Academy of Pedi atrics, states that megavitamin therapy as a treatment for learning disabilities and psychoses in children is not justified.[11] Some authors also claim that megavitamin therapy may have a role in the treatment of juvenile delinquents and criminals, but this has not been documented.[12] Claims that megadoses of vitamin E are beneficial in treating cardiovascular diseases, such as angina, congestive heart failure, or peripheral vascular disease, or that vitamin E is effective in altering blood cholesterol levels have not been proved.[6] The use of vitamin E in treating retrolental fibroplasia, an eye disease associated with use of oxygen in preterm infants, and bronchopulmonary dysplasia, associated with the respiratory distress syndrome in premature infants, remains controversial, and its use in treating cystic mastitis has not been validated.[6]

Consider the potential toxicity of sufficiently large quantities of any substance, including nutrients and even water. This is especially true for the fetus, infant, and young child. Toxicity associated with the ingestion of the fat-soluble vitamins, especially A and D, is well documented.[10] Although studies of vitamin E toxicity are limited and documentation of toxicity is scant, there is increasing evidence that vitamin E excess may be similar to excesses of other fat-soluble vitamins. Excesses of most water-soluble vitamins are excreted rapidly by the body, but if they are taken in excess of amounts that can be rapidly excreted, they can cause adverse reactions or even be lethal under certain circumstances.

Possible Adverse Effects of Excessive Vitamin Intakes

Fat-soluble Vitamins

Vitamin A

1. Anorexia, diarrhea
2. Scaly dermatitis, hair loss
3. Bone changes (thickening of long bones, bone fragility, bone pain), liver and kidney damage
4. Increased intracranial pressure, headache,

blurred vision, and central nervous system anomalies
5. Teratologic effects in the fetus
6. Optic atrophy and blindness

Regular daily ingestion of supplements of retinol that exceed 3000 retinol equivalents (10,000 IU) by infants and children is recommended only under the direction of a physician. Toxicity in adults is seen with daily intakes of more than 15,000 retinol equivalents (50,000 IU) for long periods. Thus, the Committee on Dietary Allowances of the National Academy of Sciences suggests that regular ingestion of more than 7500 retinol equivalents (25,000 IU) daily is not prudent. In contrast, excessive carotene ingestion is not harmful. Although it may result in yellow coloration of the skin, this disappears when carotene intake is reduced.[13]

Vitamin D

1. Gastrointestinal disturbances (anorexia, nausea, vomiting, weakness, weight loss, constipation, or diarrhea)
2. Polyuria, polydipsia, dehydration
3. Calcification of soft tissues (kidney, lungs, blood vessels, heart)
4. Renal stones
5. Idiopathic hypercalcemia of infancy

The possible long-term effects of dietary intakes that exceed the recommended allowance by severalfold are still unknown, but some evidence suggests that adverse affects may result. In view of the potential toxicity and because of lack of evidence that amounts above the RDA confer health benefits, intakes should closely approximate the RDA for both children and adults.[14]

Vitamin K. Excessive doses of water-soluble, synthetic derivatives given parentally have produced symptoms in infants. Natural forms of vitamin K adminsitered orally in large amounts are not toxic, and vitamin K_1 preparations are recommended for medical use.

1. Hemolytic anemia
2. Hyperbilirubinemia
3. Kernicterus (jaundice of the nuclear masses and ganglia in the medulla oblongata)

Vitamin E. Side effects have been noted in isolated case reports.

1. Fatigue, muscle weakness, and depression
2. Muscle damage and creatinuria
3. Altered vitamin K metabolism leading to prolonged prothrombin time and bleeding tendencies. (This could increase the requirement for vitamin K and be of clinical significance in individuals receiving anticoagulant therapy. These individuals should not take excessive doses of vitamin E.)

4. Various gastrointestinal disturbances, such as diarrhea, cramps, and nausea
5. Increased serum triglycerides and reduced serum thyroid hormone levels
6. Other miscellaneous symptoms, such as headache, dizziness, and blurred vision

While vitamin E is generally considered safe at doses of 300 mg/day or less, caution should be exercised with use of large doses over an extended period of time.[10]

Water-soluble Vitamins. Evidence is limited regarding the possible adverse reactions associated with ingestion of large doses of a number of water-soluble vitamins. However, there is some evidence of adverse reactions associated with ingestion of large doses of vitamin C, niacin, folic acid, and pyridoxine. Presumed allergic reactions have occurred with use of vitamin B_{12}. However, the implications of this have not been clarified.

Vitamin C

1. Promotes renal calculi (associated with the excessive production of oxalate from vitamin C catabolism, elevated uric acid level in the blood, and the excretion of an acid urine that favors the precipitation of uric acid and cystine in those with gout and cystinuria)
2. Elevates blood uric acid and may precipitate gout in susceptible individuals
3. May cause rebound scurvy (following abrupt cessation of the ingestion of large doses of vitamin C)
4. May precipitate hemolytic anemia in individuals with a deficiency of the enzyme glucose-6-phosphate dehydrogenase. (This condition is common in certain ethnic or religious groups, such as American blacks, Jewish people, and Asians.)
5. May alter absorption and metabolism of vitamin B_{12} that may not be overcome by B_{12} supplementation. This effect has been questioned; however, until the clinical significance is clarified, those taking megadoses of vitamin C should have the blood level of vitamin B_{12} monitored
6. Alters the accuracy of certain laboratory tests (e.g., tests for urine sugar and tests for the presence of blood in the stool). Megadoses of vitamin C produce false-negative urine sugar results with the Testape method and false-positive results with the Clinitest method. False-negative test results for blood in the stool are also produced
7. May alter the action of certain drugs (e.g., megadoses of vitamin C reverse the anticoagulant activity of heparin or dicumarol)
8. Induces bleeding in pregnant women, and

may lead to abortion and fetal abnormalities

9. Induces absorption of excess amounts of food iron
10. Produces gastrointestinal disturbances (nausea, abdominal cramps, and diarrhea) especially if large amounts are taken before meals
11. Impairs bactericidal activity of leukocytes
12. Induces high-altitude hypoxia
13. Adversely affects growing bone

While it is not apparent that the ingestion of 1 to 2 g of ascorbic acid is harmful for healthy adults, caution should be exercised when ingesting amounts from 2 to 8 g daily. There is clear evidence that amounts above approximately 8 g per day may be distinctly harmful.

Niacin (Nicotinic Acid)

1. Skin flushing and itching
2. Hepatotoxicity (hyperbilirubinemia and jaundice, elevated serum levels of liver enzymes)
3. Dermatoses
4. Alteration of metabolism of heart muscle with tachycardia and other arrythmias, hypotension, and fainting; may be especially dangerous if taken by an athlete before an event
5. Elevated serum uric acid, which may precipitate gout in susceptible individuals
6. Nausea, vomiting, and diarrhea
7. Peptic ulceration

Folic Acid

1. Antagonizes the protective effect of Dilantin (an anticonvulsant drug) against convulsions in some individuals with epilepsy

Pyridoxine (Vitamin B$_6$). Several case reports[15] have revealed serious neurotoxicity resulting from taking 2 to 6 g (up to 3000 times the RDA) of vitamin B$_6$ for periods ranging from 4 to 40 months. Symptoms included loss of vibration and position sense, leading to difficulty in walking and a diminished ability to perceive touch, temperature, and pain. All of the subjects improved substantially over a period of months following withdrawal of the vitamin, although several years were required for total recovery in several. No symptoms were noticed by the subjects at doses of less than 2 g.

Possible Use of Vitamin Supplements

Although many ideas about nutrition may be ill founded, health professionals must continue to exhibit both open-mindness and healthy skepticism in evaluating research data as they evolve. For those individuals who feel they suffer from a vitamin shortage, the placebo effect of taking a daily capsule

containing amounts of vitamins equivalent to the RDA may be beneficial and should not be harmful. For this purpose, advise clients to choose the cheapest available brand that provides the desired formulation. At the same time, encourage clients to evaluate the adequacy of their food intake, since no dietary supplement can substitute for a balanced diet.

REVIEW QUESTIONS AND ACTIVITIES

1. Identify the four fat-soluble vitamins and the two major classes of water-soluble vitamins.
2. Compare the fat-soluble vitamins and water-soluble vitamins relative to their stability in foods, mechanisms whereby they are used by the body, and body storage.
3. Identify those vitamins that are potentially toxic when excessive amounts are ingested.
4. For each of the following, list major function, major sign of deficiency, and two good dietary sources: vitamin D, vitamin E, vitamin K, and vitamin C.
5. List the eight B-complex vitamins; identify the five that function in energy-releasing reactions, the two that function in blood cell formation, and the one that functions primarily in protein metabolism.
6. Explain the rationale for the following situations:
   a. A client tells you that he becomes temporarily blinded after passing a car while driving at night. You take a nutritional history and discover that he follows a very low-fat diet and rarely eats deep-green or deep-yellow vegetables or fruits.
   b. A client tells you that her physician prescribed a diet high in polyunsaturated fat and also told her to eat foods high in vitamin E.
7. Identify the vitamin that acts as a hormone and list the two body organs that are involved in its activation.
8. Identify the fat-soluble vitamin that exists in both the preformed state and the precursor state and give the name of the precursor.
9. List two good dietary sources of the following B complex vitamins: thiamine, riboflavin, niacin, folic acid, and pyridoxine.

REFERENCES

1. Roberts HJ: Perspectives on vitamin E as therapy. JAMA 246:129, 1981.
2. DeLuca HF: The vitamin D system in the regulation of calcium and phosphorus metabolism. Nutr Rev 37:161, 1979.
3. National Research Council: Recommended Dietary Allowances, ed 9. Washington, DC, National Academy Press, 1980, p 69.

4. Khan AR, Seedarnee FA: Effect of ascorbic acid on plasma lipids and lipoproteins in healthy young women. Atherosclerosis 39:89, 1981.
5. Wahlberg GC, Walldius G: Lack of effect of ascorbic acid on serum lipoprotein concentration in patients with hypertriglyceridemia. Atherosclerosis 43:283, 1982.
6. Bieri JG, Corash L, Hubbard VS: Medical uses of vitamin E. N Engl J Med 308:1063, 1983.
7. Creagen ET, Moertel CG, O'Fallon JR, et al.: Failure of high dose vitamin C (ascorbic acid) therapy to benefit patients with advanced cancer. N Engl J Med 301:687, 1979.
8. Prasad KW: Modulation of the effects of tumor therapeutic agents by vitamin C. Life Sci 27:275, 1980.
9. American Psychiatric Association Task Force on Vitamin Therapy in Psychiatry: Megavitamins and Orthomolecular Therapy in Psychiatry. Washington, DC, American Psychiatric Association, 1973.
10. Dubie MA, Rucker RB: Dietary supplements and health aids—A critical evaluation. Part 1—Vitamins and minerals. J Nutr Educ 15:47, 1983.
11. American Academy of Pediatrics, Committee on Nutrition: Megavitamin therapy for childhood psychoses and learning disabilities. Pediatrics 58:910, 1976.
12. Gray GE, Gray LK: Diet and juvenile delinquency. Nutr Today 18:14, 1983.
13. National Research Council, op cit, p 59.
14. Ibid, p 62.
15. Schaumburg H: Sensory neuropathy from pyridoxine abuse: A new megavitamin syndrome. N Engl J Med 309:445, 1983.

BIBLIOGRAPHY

Bell EF: The role of vitamin E in the nutrition of premature infants. Am J Clin Nutr 34:414, 1981.

DeLuca HF: Some new concepts emanating from a study of the metabolism and function of vitamin D. Nutr Rev 38:169, 1980.

Di Palma JR, McMichael R: Assessing the value of meganutrients in disease. Bull NY Acad Med 58:254, 1983.

Herbert V: The vitamin craze. Arch Intern Med 140:173, 1980.

Herbert V: Toxicity of 25,000 IU vitamin A supplements in "health food" users. Am J Clin Nutr 36:185, 1982.

Kesaniemi MD, Grundy SM: Lack of effect of tocopherol on plasma lipids and lipoproteins in man. Am J Clin Nutr 36:224, 1982.

Konishi F, Harrison SL: Vitamin D for adults. J Nutr Educ 11:120, 1979.

Lewis C: Vitamins and Minerals, Sodium and Potassium. Philadelphia, FA Davis, 1976.

Muller DPR, Lloyd JK, Wolf OH: Vitamin E and neurological function. Lancet 1:225, 1983.

The pathophysiologic basis of vitamin A toxicity. Nutr Rev 40:272, 1982.

Rudman D, Williams PJ: Megadose vitamins: Use and misuse. N Engl J Med 309:488, 1983.

Shearer MJ: Plasma vitamin K in mothers and their newborn babies. Lancet 2:460, 1982.

CHAPTER 9

Minerals

Objectives

After completion of this chapter, the student will be able to:
1. Distinguish between micronutrients and macronutrients.
2. Distinguish between the acid-forming and base-forming properties of foods and their effects on the urinary pH.
3. Compare and contrast the absorption of the macronutrients calcium, phosphorus, sodium, and potassium with the absorption of the micronutrients iron and zinc.
4. Differentiate between skeletal and ionic calcium imbalance.
5. Distinguish among high-risk populations for deficiencies of iron, iodine, fluoride, and zinc.
6. Distinguish between major effects of iodine and fluorine imbalance and techniques designed to prevent imbalances of these two trace elements.
7. Compare and contrast the functions, food sources, and results of deficiency of magnesium, iron, and zinc.
8. Plan a day's menu that meets the Recommended Dietary Allowance for a normal adult female for calcium and iron without the use of milk, cheese, eggs, meat, fish, or poultry.

CLASSIFICATION OF MINERALS

▶ **Mineral elements,** the inorganic class of essential food nutrients, comprise about 4 percent of the total body weight. Approximately 50 mineral elements are found in the human body. Some are present in
▶ relatively large amounts and are called **macronutrients,** whereas others are present in relatively
▶ minute amounts and are called **micronutrients** or
▶ **trace elements.** (The terms micronutrient and trace element are used interchangeably in this chapter.) Essential body functions have been determined for all of the macronutrients and for some of the micronutrients found in the body. Those trace elements (micronutrients) with no known function for either humans or laboratory animals are often referred
▶ to as **trace contaminants.**

At present, a total of 21 mineral elements (7 macronutrients and 14 trace elements) are considered essential or probably essential. While some elements were known to be essential for the health of humans as early as the 17th century (e.g., iron), essentiality for others was proposed as recently as the 1970s. During the last decade several trace elements have been found essential for maintaining the health of certain laboratory animals, and thus the probability that they are essential for humans is receiving active investigation. For some of those thought to be essential for humans—namely, nickel, silicon, tin, and vanadium—many additional years of research are needed to further clarify their practical role in human nutrition. Possible essential roles for other trace elements, such as arsenic and cadmium, are also currently being investigated.

TABLE 9-1
CLASSIFICATION OF MINERAL ELEMENTS

Essential Macronutrients	Essential Micronutrients (Trace Elements)	Probably Essential Micronutrients (Trace Elements)	Trace Contaminants
Calcium	Iron	Nickel	Cadmium[a]
Phosphorus	Copper	Tin	Lead
Sodium	Cobalt	Silicon	Arsenic[a]
Potassium	Zinc	Vanadium	Barium
Magnesium	Manganese		Strontium
Chlorine	Iodine		Mercury
Sulfur	Molybdenum		Boron
	Fluorine		Aluminum
	Selenium		Lithium
	Chromium		Beryllium
			Rubidium
			Others

[a] Preliminary findings suggest a possible essential role.

The macronutrients must be supplied in the diet at levels of 100 mg or more per day, whereas the trace elements must be supplied in the diet at levels of only a few milligrams or less daily. Table 9–1 gives a classification of mineral elements. Many of the trace contaminants are widely distributed in the environment and gain entrance to the body through food, water, and air. There is increasing ecologic concern about environmental exposure to those, such as lead, cadmium, mercury, and arsenic, that are known to be toxic in excess amounts.

GENERAL FUNCTIONS OF MINERALS

The functions of minerals are as varied as the minerals themselves. They are not a source of energy but participate in a variety of structural and regulatory roles. They exert their effects as (1) structural components of essential body compounds and (2) free ions (or ions loosely bound to proteins and other substances) in body fluids. **Ions** are particles carrying an electrical charge; positively charged ions are called **cations,** and negatively charged ions are called **anions.**

Constituents of Essential Body Compounds
Minerals are constituents of such essential body compounds as bone and the mineral-containing molecules of hormones, enzymes, and vitamins. Examples are:

1. *Skeletal minerals.* Calcium and phosphorus (mixed with carbonates of calcium and magnesium) provide skeletal rigidity.
2. *Hemoglobin.* An iron-containing blood protein that transports oxygen and carbon dioxide to and from cells.
3. *Thyroid hormone.* An iodine-containing hormone that regulates the cell metabolic rate.

4. *Vitamin B₁₂.* A cobalt-containing vitamin necessary for nucleic acid synthesis.
5. *Metalloenzymes.* Mineral–enzyme complexes necessary for cell metabolism. Examples include zinc as part of the enzyme carbonic anhydrase and iron and copper as part of the enzyme cytochrome oxidase.

In each instance, mineral deficiency reduces the function of the specific compound involved.

Functions of Ionized Minerals
Free mineral ions or ions loosely bound by proteins and other substances in body fluids are necessary for a variety of body functions. The most important are:

1. Activation of cellular enzyme systems. A number of mineral ions are activators in catabolic and anabolic reactions involving carbohydrates, proteins, and fats. Magnesium ions, for instance, are required for the oxidative release of energy.
2. Maintenance of acid–base balance. Mineral ions, such as sodium, potassium, chlorine, and phosphorus, are essential for maintaining the exact pH of body fluids that is necessary for control of metabolic reactions.
3. Maintenance of osmotic pressure and water balance between intracellular and extracellular fluid. Sodium and potassium ions are especially important for this function.
4. Regulation of permeability of cell membranes. A normal concentration of calcium ions is necessary for this function.
5. Response of nerves and muscles to stimuli. Normal concentrations of sodium, potassium, calcium, and magnesium ions are vital for normal irritability of nerve and muscle fibers.

Like vitamins, minerals are involved in numerous functions in which they catalyze various body reactions. In some instances, they serve as the structural center of an enzyme system (e.g., zinc in carbonic anhydrase), a vitamin (e.g., cobalt in vitamin B_{12}), or a hormone (e.g., iodine in thyroid hormone).

Some mineral elements have been shown to exert a pharmacologic effect. The use of fluoride in the prevention of tooth decay is well known,[1] for example, and lithium salts (lithium is currently classified as a trace contaminant with no essential nutrient function for humans or animals) are used as an antipsychotic drug.

REGULATION OF BODY MINERAL CONTENT

The body's homeostatic mechanisms for maintaining a relatively constant amount of minerals are related primarily to regulating the amount of nutrients (1) absorbed from the intestinal tract and (2) excreted in the urine, bile, feces, and sweat. After absorption into the bloodstream, the mineral elements are transported either as free ions or in combination with plasma proteins or a specific protein carrier.

Effect of Mineral Excretion on Urinary pH

Excretion of excess minerals in the urine is a major method of regulating the total mineral content of the body. Since the minerals are excreted as positively or negatively charged ions, they affect the pH of the urine. Excretion of the negatively charged ions, chlorine, sulfur, and phosphorus, tends to acidify the urine, since these minerals are acid-forming in solution. These acid-forming elements predominate in protein-containing foods, such as meats, eggs, and cereals, although a few fruits and vegetables also tend to acidify the urine (Table 9–2). On the other hand, excretion of the positively charged ions, sodium, potassium, calcium, and magnesium, tends to alkalize the urine, since these minerals produce an alkaline reaction in solution. Akaline elements predominate in fruits, vegetables, and milk. Even such acid-tasting fruits as oranges, grapefruit, and tomatoes produce an excess of alkaline elements when metabolized and will alkalize the urine. Legumes and nuts vary in their effect on the urinary pH. Some foods, such as fats and sugars, have no effect. Generally, mixed diets contain a slight surplus of acid-forming elements, and an acid urine is usually excreted. Expect clients following high-protein diets to excrete a highly acid urine and vegetarians to excrete an alkaline urine.

Proper Mineral Intake

Mineral elements are widely distributed in food and water, and ingesting a varied diet that is balanced with respect to processed and nonprocessed foods is important to avoid the extremes of a deficient or excessive intake. Except for possibly calcium and magnesium, deficiencies of macronutrients are uncommon. Deficiencies of the trace elements iron, fluorine, and possibly iodine are associated with nutritional problems leading to easily recognizable signs in the United States. These problems are discussed in Chapter 1. Moreover, intakes of zinc and chromium are thought to be marginal in some segments of the population. A focus of current concern is on the long-term effects of these marginal intakes.

Since body mechanisms for controlling mineral content are not complete, prolonged excessive intake may produce toxic reactions. As with marginal intake, chronic excessive intake may not be immediately recognizable, and another focus of concern is on long-term effects. A number of people may be prone to mineral imbalance due to consumption of unvaried diets because of economic factors, fads, illness, or because of mineral–drug interactions. Exces-

---

TABLE 9–2
THE ACID–BASE REACTION OF FOODS

Acid-forming Foods	*Alkaline-forming Foods*	*Neutral Foods*
Meat, fish, poultry	Most fruits and vegetables except those listed under acid-forming	Fats: butter, lard, other cooking fats, salad oils
Eggs		Sugar, honey, candy (not chocolate)
Cheese (all types)	Milk, ice cream	
Bread (especially whole grain), crackers, pastries	Nuts: almonds, chestnuts, coconut	Coffee and tea
Cereal (including macaroni, spaghetti, noodles, rice)	Legumes: lima beans, navy beans, dried peas	Cornstarch
Nuts: walnuts, peanuts, filberts, Brazil nuts, peanut butter	Other: molasses, olives, foods prepared with baking powder or baking soda	Tapioca
Legumes: lentils		
Vegetables and fruit: corn, prunes, plums, cranberries and cranberry juice		

sive consumption of refined foods may also be a factor. Trace minerals are lost when grains are refined, and most of these elements are not added back by enrichment.

Current knowledge permits evaluation of daily needs (RDA) for only 6 of the 21 mineral elements that are essential or probably essential for humans (see Table 2–1), and estimated safe and adequate intakes are given for 8 additional ones (see Table 2–3).

MACRONUTRIENTS

Calcium

Functions. Approximately 99 percent of total body calcium is in the skeleton, where it provides rigidity. The remaining 1 percent is in ionic form in extracellular fluid where it functions in (1) the activation of enzymes for blood clotting and muscle contraction, (2) the transmission of nerve impulses, (3) the regulation of cell membrane permeability, (4) maintenance of integrity of intracellular cement substances and of various membranes, and (5) enhancement of myocardial function.

Metabolism. Dietary calcium is incompletely absorbed. Under normal conditions only 20 to 30 percent of that ingested is absorbed, with the remaining 70 to 80 percent being excreted in the feces. The intestinal absorption of calcium is stimulated by the metabolically active form of vitamin D; a low blood level of calcium or of phosphorus stimulates the kidney to produce the metabolically active form of the vitamin. The various factors that influence the efficiency of calcium absorption are summarized in Table 9–3.

The metabolism of calcium (along with that of phosphorus) is regulated by the integrated action of vitamin D, parathyroid hormone, and calcitonin. Respectively, these factors influence calcium blood levels by regulating intestinal absorption, deposition and resorption in bone, and renal excretion. Calcium and phosphorus exhibit a reciprocal relationship in the blood; an increase in the blood level of one causes a decrease in the blood level of the other. The major clinical significance of this is that it serves as a protective mechanism for preventing the products of their concentration (calcium level × phosphorus level) from becoming so high in the extracellular fluid that calcium and phosphorus would react together, with a subsequent calcification of soft tissue, such as the kidneys, lungs, and blood vessels. Calcification and stone formation are not uncommon when the product of the concentrations of calcium and phosphorus is greater than 70. This situation may occur in chronic renal disease in which the kidneys lose their ability to excrete phosphorus and the phosphorus level becomes very high. Normal and abnormal calcium:phosphorus ratios are illustrated in Table 9–4.

The blood calcium level is relatively independent of dietary intake, since the skeleton can take up and release calcium as needed to maintain normal levels. Other homeostatic mechanisms that

---

TABLE 9–3
FACTORS THAT AFFECT THE INTESTINAL ABSORPTION OF CALCIUM

Increased Efficiency of Calcium Absorption	Decreased Efficiency of Calcium Absorption
1. Increased need for calcium (as with a small dietary supply or during growth)	1. Inadequate supply of activated vitamin D (dietary lack or failure of activation mechanisms)
2. Low intestinal pH, which keeps calcium in solution	2. Presence of certain food factors that bind calcium in the intestine:
3. Presence of certain food factors in the intestine:	a. Dietary fiber
a. Vitamin D (activated)	b. Oxalic acid (in foods such as spinach, Swiss chard, beet tops, chocolate, rhubarb)
b. Certain amino acids (e.g., lysine, arginine, serine)	c. Phytic acid (in outer husks of cereal grains)
c. Lactose	d. Excessive fatty acids (which bind calcium as insoluble soaps). Intestinal fatty acid concentration rises secondary to fat maldigestion or malabsorption
	3. Gastrointestinal hypermotility or alkalinity
	4. Antacid and laxative abuse
	5. Aging—the efficiency of calcium absorption is decreased in the elderly

---

TABLE 9–4
NORMAL AND ABNORMAL CALCIUM : PHOSPHORUS RATIOS

Normal Blood Levels	Abnormal Blood Levels (Renal Disease)
Calcium = 10 mg% (average) Phosphorus = 4 mg% (average)	Example: Calcium = 8 mg% Phosphorus = 18 mg%
Ca × P = product 10 × 4 = 40 (calcium and phosphorus are soluble in blood)	Ca × P = product 8 × 18 = 144 (calcium and phosphorus precipitate, causing calcification of soft tissue)

---

serve to maintain a relatively constant calcium blood level include controlled absorption from the intestine and controlled excretion from the urine.

The effect of dietary phosphorus on calcium metabolism and the optimal calcium : phosphorus ratio in the diet is controversial. There is some evidence from experimental animals that excessive phosphorus intake and a low ratio of calcium relative to phosphorus lead to both a decrease in calcium absorption and an increase in bone resorption.[2,3] Because of increasing consumption of phosphorus associated with the use of phosphorus-containing food additives and possibly of certain high-phosphorus soft drinks, these findings may have significance for the development of osteoporosis in humans. The deleterious effects of high phosphorus intakes can apparently be partially offset by increasing calcium intake, however. While soft drinks are not a major contributor to dietary phosphorus intake, should they be substituted for milk, a good source of calcium, the overall effect on calcium–phosphorus metabolism could be substantial.[4]

A high-protein diet, especially in combination with a low intake of dietary calcium, results in an increased renal excretion of calcium. The higher the protein content, the greater the loss of calcium. This urinary loss of calcium can be partially prevented by decreasing the protein intake or increasing the calcium intake.

Sources. Because there is limited distribution of calcium in foods, daily intakes below recommended levels are common. Healthy bone is maintained by a dynamic process of mineralization and resorption that continues throughout life; therefore daily calcium intake is essential. Milk and cheese are the best dietary sources of calcium. Many people do not eat these foods because of personal preference, an acquired allergy, or lactose intolerance. Encourage these people to use other good sources of calcium, such as green leafy vegetables, legumes, nuts, and some types of fish. Table 9–5 lists the calcium content of specific foods.

Imbalance. Calcium imbalance may result from a variety of factors including (1) dietary deficiency of

calcium or vitamin D or both, (2) hormonal imbalance, (3) excessive losses through the kidney or gastrointestinal tract, (4) inflammatory processes or trauma, and (5) conditions associated with rapid bone resorption. Calcium imbalance may be reflected in the skeleton or in the amount of ionic calcium in the extracellular fluid. Specific deficiency symptoms with changes in the amount of total body calcium associated with less than recommended intakes are difficult to document in normal individuals unless the deficiency is severe. In severe deficiency, symptoms are often the result of the combined lack of both calcium and vitamin D. The body compensates for low levels of intake by (1) mobilizing calcium from bone, (2) absorbing a greater percentage of dietary calcium, and (3) excreting less through the urine and feces. These adaptive mechanisms minimize the effects of low calcium intake. Although changes in bone density can be detected by wrist bone x-ray, changes are not evident until as much as one third of bone calcium has been withdrawn. The major causes and effects of the skeletal imbalances are listed in Table 9–6. Osteoporosis, the most common disorder, is a generalized disease of bone characterized by a diminished amount of total bone mass.[5] It apparently results from conditions in which the rate of bone resorption exceeds the rate of new bone formation. The disorder appears to have a multifaceted etiology and occurs secondary to various pathologic conditions. Assess for osteoporosis in clients with prolonged immobilization, hyperparathyroidism, severe protein malnutrition, Cushing's syndrome, prolonged corticosteroid therapy, acromegaly, and hyperthyroidism. While data are not conclusive, there is speculation that a higher incidence of the disorder occurs among individuals with inadequate lifelong calcium intake.

Rickets and osteomalacia, rarely seen in the United States as a result of dietary deficiency, may occur secondary to fat malabsorption or chronic renal disease.

Ionic calcium imbalance, reflected as hypocalcemia or hypercalcemia, is seldom seen as a primary nutritional disorder but most often occurs secondary to pathologic conditions (Table 9–7). **Hypercalcemia** may result in the calcification of soft tissues

TABLE 9–5
CALCIUM CONTENT OF SELECTED FOODS

Food	Serving	Calcium (mg)
Milk products		
Milk (whole)	1 c	288
Yoghurt (made from partially skimmed milk)	1 c	294
Cottage cheese (creamed)	1 c	230
Cheddar cheese	1 oz	213
Ice cream (10% fat)	1 c	194
Legumes–nuts–fish		
Soybeans (cooked)	1 c	54
Almonds (shelled)	½ c	152
Sesame seeds	½ c	82.5
Salmon (canned, red)	3 oz	219
Vegetables		
(Cooked and drained)		
Kale	1 c	206
Collards	1 c	357
Mustard greens	1 c	193
Turnip greens	1 c	267
Dandelion greens	1 c	147
Okra	1 c	147
Broccoli	1 c	136
Spoon cabbage	1 c	252
Rutabagas	1 c	100
Fruits		
Dried apricots (uncooked)	1 c	87
Other		
Blackstrap molasses	1 tbsp	137

(Source: USDA, Agricultural Research Service: Nutritive Value of American Foods in Common Units, Agriculture Handbook No. 456, Washington, DC, 1975.)

and in renal stone formation. Both hypercalcemia and hypocalcemia produce alterations in muscle tone. In hypercalcemia, muscles become hypotonic (decreased muscle tone). Extreme hypercalcemia ▶ may result in cardiac or respiratory failure. In **hy-** **pocalcemia,** muscles become hypertonic (increased ▶ muscle tone) and go into spasm, leading to tetany. **Tetany** is a condition of generalized muscle hypertonicity with tremors and spasmodic muscle contraction due to uncontrolled transmission of nerve im-

TABLE 9–6
SKELETAL CALCIUM IMBALANCE

Imbalance	Causes	Effects

Osteoporosis (most common problem)	1. Excessive bone resorption due to:
	  a. Immobilization
	  b. Hyperparathyroidism
	  c. Other conditions
	2. Diminished hormonal secretion with aging
	3. Long-term inadequate dietary calcium intake
	4. Long-term high-protein intake
		Diminished total bone mass resulting in:
		1. Shortened stature and stooped posture
		2. Fractures
		3. Low back pain

Rickets and osteomalacia	Diminished bone mineralization due to:
	1. Dietary deficiency of calcium and/or vitamin D
	2. Calcium and/or vitamin D deficiency secondary to:
	  a. Fat malabsorption
	  b. Chronic renal disease
	  c. Drug therapy
		Low mineral content in bone resulting in:
		1. Soft, flexible bones and skeletal deformities
		2. Bone pain and generalized weakness
		3. Spontaneous fractures in adults

TABLE 9–7
IONIC CALCIUM IMBALANCE

Imbalance	Causes	Effects

Hypercalcemia	1. Hyperparathyroidism
	2. Rapid build-up of calcium in blood due to:
	   a. Excessive vitamin D
	   b. Immobilization
	   c. Metastatic bone tumors
	3. Milk alkali syndrome
		1. Calcification of soft tissue
		2. Renal stones
		3. Hypotonic muscles → cardiac or respiratory failure

Hypocalcemia	1. Hypoparathyroidism 2. Vitamin D deficiency 3. Low serum protein level 4. Steatorrhea 5. Renal disease 6. Massive cellulitis, peritonitis, burns 7. Use of citrated blood transfusions 8. Temporary dysfunction of parathyroid gland (neonatal tetany) or phosphate overload due to feeding undiluted cow's milk in early infancy	1. Hypertonic muscles → tetany and respiratory failure (must differentiate hypocalcemic tetany from alkalotic tetany due to potassium depletion, vomiting, or hyperventilation)

pulses. Laryngeal muscles are especially sensitive; laryngeal spasm may obstruct respiration, and death may occur unless calcium is administered immediately.

The relationship between calcium intake and blood pressure is now being explored. Animal studies and epidemiologic data show an inverse relationship between calcium intake and blood pressure and that a high calcium intake as well as a high magnesium intake may be protective of hypertension.[6]

Phosphorus

Functions. Phosphorus is closely associated with calcium in relation to its sources, metabolism, and functions. Approximately 80 percent of the total body phosphorus is present as calcium phosphate in bones and teeth. The remaining 20 percent is distributed throughout the other body cells and performs structural functions and many specialized metabolic functions. As an electrolyte, it is the chief intracellular anion. The major functions of phosphorus include:

1. Component of body structures (e.g., skeleton and cell membranes)
2. Regulates the release, transfer, and storage of energy (e.g., phosphorylation of glucose and glycogen to glucose-1-phosphate; component of ATP, ADP, AMP)
3. Necessary for absorption and transport of nutrients (e.g., phosphorylation of glucose and glycerol for intestinal absorption, transport of fat as lipoprotein)
4. Component of essential metabolites (e.g., nucleic acids and B vitamin coenzymes—thiamine, niacin)

5. Regulates acid–base balance (phosphate buffer system)

Absorption. As with calcium, the intestinal absorption of phosphorus is increased by the metabolically active form of vitamin D. Approximately 70 percent of ingested phosphorus is absorbed. The factors that affect the absorption of calcium (Table 9–4) can also be applied to the absorption of phosphorus. Most excess phosphorus is excreted in the urine. The kidneys function in regulating the blood phosphorus level in that the amount excreted is influenced by the blood level. If the blood level of phosphorus is low, phosphorus is reabsorbed from the kidneys and returned to the blood rather than being excreted. Parathyroid hormone leads to an increase in the renal excretion of phosphorus.

Sources. Phosphorus is present in nearly all foods, and a dietary deficiency is extremely unlikely to occur. As with calcium, milk and milk products are excellent sources. Other protein foods, such as meat, poultry, fish, eggs, nuts, and legumes are also good sources of phosphorus (Table 9–8).

Imbalances. Blood levels of phosphorus that are abnormally low or high are usually the result of disease rather than dietary deficiency or excess.

Hypophosphatemia. Low blood levels of phosphorus may result from:

1. Malabsorption (various malabsorption syndromes, prolonged ingestion of phosphate-binding antacids, e.g., aluminum hydroxide)
2. Use of parenteral hyperalimentation formu-

TABLE 9–8
PHOSPHORUS CONTENT OF SELECTED FOODS

Food	Serving	Phosphorus (mg)
Milk (whole)	8 oz glass	227
Milk (skim)	8 oz glass	233
Cheddar cheese	1 oz	136
Chicken, roasted	3⅓ oz	242
Lamb chop, broiled	3⅓ oz	163
Beef hamburger	3 oz	196
Turkey, roasted	3 oz	213
Halibut, broiled in butter or margarine	4½ oz	310
Peanuts with skins, roasted	⅔ c	391

(Source: USDA, Agricultural Research Service: Nutritive Value of American Foods in Common Units, Agricultural Handbook No. 456, Washington, DC, 1975.)

las with inadequate phosphorus supplementation

3. Renal loss of phosphate (vitamin D deficiency; block in vitamin D metabolism due to genetic defect, liver or kidney disease, or use of anticonvulsant drugs; congenital renal tubular disorders; Fanconi syndrome; hyperparathyroidism)
4. Chronic alcoholism
5. Recovery phase of diabetic ketoacidosis and healing phase of severe burns

Symptoms of hypophosphatemia include muscle weakness, anorexia, malaise, failure of bone mineralization, and bone pain.

Hyperphosphatemia. High blood levels of phosphorus may result from renal disease or hypoparathyroidism. Calcification and stone formation may occur when the product of the blood levels of calcium and phosphorus (calcium level × phosphorus level) is greater than 70. In addition, an increased blood level of phosphorus may cause a reciprocal decrease in the blood level of calcium, leading to tetany. A discussion of normal and abnormal calcium:phosphorus ratios (Ca:P) is in the preceding section on calcium.

Magnesium

Functions. Approximately 50 to 60 percent of the total body magnesium is found in bone, where it performs structural functions, and most of the remainder is found within the cells, where it ranks second to potassium as the predominant intracellular cation. Other major functions of magnesium include:

1. Regulation of nerve impulse transmission (must be in proper balance with calcium, sodium, and potassium). At some points, magnesium acts synergistically with calcium and, at other points, antagonistically.
2. Activation of many enzyme systems involved with:

a. Release of energy (e.g., in glycolysis, oxidative phosphorylation, phosphate transfer systems)
b. Protein synthesis (e.g., activation of amino acids)
c. Fatty acid metabolism
d. Bone metabolism

Absorption. The absorption rate of magnesium varies greatly, depending on the amount ingested. Absorption may be as high as 80 percent if the diet is low in magnesium or as low as 25 percent if the diet is high in magnesium. The average absorption is about 30 to 40 percent, with the majority of the excess being excreted in the feces. The absorption of magnesium is not influenced by vitamin D or parathyroid hormone as is the absorption of calcium and phosphorus, but it is diminished by the presence of excess fat, phytate, phosphate, or calcium.

Sources. Magnesium is widely distributed in foods. Especially good sources are dark green leafy vegetables, legumes, nuts, whole grain cereals, and seafood. Refinement of foods is associated with substantial losses of magnesium. Some losses also occur in cooking when cooking waters are discarded. Teach clients to use cooking waters for soups, sauces, and casseroles to conserve mineral content.

Imbalances

Hypomagnesemia. Abnormally low blood levels of magnesium cause symptoms similar to tetany. These include neuromuscular dysfunction (such as hyperexcitability, tremors, convulsions, and mental disorientation) and tachycardia. Deficiency arises from a low dietary intake in conjunction with conditions that decrease absorption or increase excretion. These include:

1. Loss of gastrointestinal fluids (e.g., vomiting or malabsorption)
2. Severe protein–calorie malnutrition
3. Increased renal loss (e.g., diuretics or acute

or chronic renal disease involving tubular dysfunction)
4. Alcoholism
5. Cirrhosis of the liver
6. Prolonged parenteral feeding of magnesium-free solutions
7. Large losses in lactation
8. Hyperparathyroidism
9. Diabetic acidosis

Hypermagnesemia. Abnormally high blood levels of magnesium cause symptoms of extreme thirst, warmth, drowsiness, decrease in neuromuscular irritability, and atrial fibrillation. Hypermagnesemia can result from an unusual increase in absorption (as with the use of antacids containing magnesium) or decreased urinary excretion (as in renal failure).

Sodium, Potassium, and Chlorine

Sodium, potassium, and chloride (the form in which chlorine occurs in the body) are essential macronutrients that are components of body cells and fluids. Sodium is the principal cation in extracellular fluid, potassium is the principal cation in intracellular fluid, and chloride is found in highest concentration in secretions of the gastrointestinal tract and in the cerebrospinal fluid. A detailed discussion of these three minerals is presented in Chapter 10 on fluid and electrolyte balance. A brief overview is presented here. Sodium, potassium, and chloride are very closely interrelated and their major functions in the body involve the regulation and maintenance of:

1. Water balance
2. Osmotic pressure
3. Acid–base balance
4. Neuromuscular excitability (sodium and potassium)
5. Gastric acidity (chloride)

Virtually all of the ingested sodium and chloride and more than 90 percent of ingested potassium are absorbed from the intestine. The kidney provides the major regulatory mechanism for maintaining balance of these ions. Due to the efficient mechanisms regulating their excretion, the body is usually able to function within a wide range of intake. Sodium and potassium are widely distributed in foods, whereas table salt is the major dietary source of chloride. Dietary deficiencies rarely occur. However, deficiencies may result from disease conditions or drug interactions that interfere with the absorption or excretion of these minerals. For example, vomiting, diarrhea, and use of certain diuretics cause loss of these minerals, and Addison's disease causes increased excretion of sodium chloride and retention of potassium. The role of sodium and potassium in the development of hypertension is being investigated (see Chap. 29).

MICRONUTRIENTS

Iron

Functions. The trace mineral iron is a constituent of blood hemoglobin and muscle myoglobin, where it is involved in the transport and storage of oxygen in cells and the removal of carbon dioxide. Iron is also a constituent of heme enzymes, including the cytochromes, catalases, peroxidases, and oxidases. The cytochromes catalyze the oxidative release of energy in the cells.

Classification of Body Iron. Body iron exists as two fractions: the essential or functional component (composed of hemoglobin, myoglobin, the enzymes catalyzed by iron, and the transport form of iron—transferrin, in which the iron is bound to protein) and the storage or reserve component (ferritin and hemosiderin in the bone marrow and reticuloendothelial tissue). The functional component is the larger of the two, comprising slightly less than three fourths of the total body iron. Adult females have a much smaller supply of storage iron than do adult males. It has been noted that at least one third of the adult female population in the United States have little or no reserve iron.

Metabolism. Like calcium and some of the other mineral elements, dietary iron is incompletely absorbed. In contrast to other mineral elements, there is no physiologic regulation of iron metabolism through increased or decreased excretion; the main control of iron status is at the site of intestinal absorption.

A number of factors influence the amount of iron actually absorbed, including the amount and chemical form of the iron ingested, the concurrent presence of various dietary factors that can alter absorption, the condition of the gastrointestinal tract itself, and the body's need for iron. There are ► two categories of iron in foods: (1) **heme iron** (from hemoglobin and myoglobin of meat, liver, fish, poul- ► try) and (2) **nonheme iron** (from plant foods, eggs, dairy products, the nonheme component of meats, and soluble iron supplements). The dietary iron enters the heme and nonheme iron pools in the intestinal lumen. Heme iron, which comprises approximately 40 percent of the iron in meat, liver, poultry, and fish, is much better absorbed (approximately 25 percent) than nonheme iron. Moreover its absorption appears to be affected very little by other dietary components. In contrast, nonheme iron, which comprises the major portion of food iron, is poorly absorbed (5 percent or less). However, its absorption can be markedly altered by components of foods ingested concomitantly: its absorption is increased in the presence of ascorbic acid and a factor present in meat. One milligram of ascorbic acid has about the same enhancing effect as 1 g of meat, fish, or

---

TABLE 9–9
FACTORS THAT AFFECT THE INTESTINAL ABSORPTION OF IRON

Increased Efficiency of Iron Absorption	*Decreased Efficiency of Iron Absorption*

1. Increased need for iron (as during growth or in iron deficiency). Absorption is increased 2–3 times above normal in the iron-depleted individual.
 2. Low intestinal pH. Gastric hydrochloric acid may help to solubilize iron for absorption.
 3. Presence of ascorbic acid (ferric → ferrous state) and meat. These enhance absorption of iron from nonheme sources.
	1. Gastrointestinal hypermotility (e.g., malabsorption syndromes or following gastrointestinal surgery)
	 2. Gastrointestinal alkalinity (as postgastrectomy, use of antacids, and in the elderly)
	 3. Presence of certain food factors that block the intestinal absorption of iron
	    a. EDTA[a]
	    b. Dietary fiber
	    c. Oxalic acid
	    d. Phytic acid
	    e. Calcium phosphate salts (high level)
	    f. Clay (pica)
	    g. Tannic acid
	    h. Coffee and tea
	    i. Phosvitin (of egg yolk)

[a] Ethylenediamine tetraacetic acid—a chelating agent added to certain processed foods (especially carbonated drinks, beer, salad dressings, mayonnaise, sandwich spreads, and sauces) to prevent their oxidation by free metal ions.

---

poultry. Although meat increases the availability of nonheme iron, milk, eggs, and cheese do not increase (and may decrease) iron availability. Conditions that alter iron absorption are summarized in Table 9–9.

Sources. The best food sources of iron are red meats, organ meats, legumes, nuts, green leafy vegetables, dried fruits, whole grain and enriched bread and cereal, molasses, and brewer's yeast. Table 9–10 lists the iron content of certain foods.

The usual American diet provides approximately 6 mg of iron per 1000 kcal of food ingested. When adult females ingest kilocalories at the recommended level (approximately 1800 to 2000 daily), iron intake is approximately 9 to 12 mg, considerably less than the RDA for this age group. To assure that the recommended iron intake is met, teach adult females to include foods in the diet that are known to be high in iron in a well-absorbed form (such as liver and muscle meats) and foods that promote the absorption of iron from other sources (ascorbic acid-containing foods or meat). Provide an iron supplement during pregnancy and for full-term infants by the fourth month (by two months for preterm infants). Iron stores at birth are usually not sufficient to meet needs beyond this age.

Iron imbalance may reflect a deficit or excess of the mineral. Iron deficiency is the most common nutritional deficiency in the United States and a major health problem in other parts of the world. Under some circumstances, however, excessive iron intake or absorption may occur, resulting in signs and symptoms of iron overload.

Iron Deficiency and Iron Deficiency Anemia. Iron status is usually assessed by determining the hemoglobin concentration, and a below-normal hemoglobin level is usually indicative of anemia. The hemoglobin level is an insensitive indicator of iron balance, however, since iron stores and levels of iron-dependent enzymes become depressed before the hemoglobin level drops. Moreover, racial differences

---

TABLE 9–10
IRON CONTENT OF SELECTED FOODS

Food	Serving	Iron (mg)
Beef liver (cooked)	3 oz	7.5
Beef round steak (cooked)	3 oz	3.1
Kidney beans (cooked, drained)	1 c	4.4
Peanuts (shelled and chopped)	1 tbsp	0.2
Peanut butter	1 tbsp	0.3
Turnip greens (cooked, drained)	1 c	1.6
Raisins	1 tbsp	0.3
Apricots (dried)	½ c	2.7
Whole grain bread	1 slice	0.8
White bread (enriched)	1 slice	0.7
Molasses (blackstrap)	1 tbsp	3.2
Baby foods		
Rice cereal (dry, precooked)	1 tbsp	2.2
Beef noodle dinner	1 oz	0.1
Strained veal with vegetables	1 oz	0.2
Strained veal	1 oz	0.5
Egg yolks	1 oz	0.9

(*Source*: USDA, Agricultural Research Service: *Nutritive Value of American Foods in Common Units. Agriculture Handbook No. 456,* Washington, DC, 1975.)

have been observed in hemoglobin concentrations; blacks systematically demonstrate lower levels of hemoglobins than whites,[7] perhaps invalidating the usual criteria for diagnosis of anemia in this group.

Iron deficiency anemia is an extremely common problem, especially in infants, adolescents, and during the female reproductive period, including pregnancy. Factors predisposing to iron deficiency anemia during these periods include the low iron content of milk coupled with the relatively low iron stores of the infant, erratic food habits of the adolescent, menstrual blood loss leading to iron losses of the female during the reproductive cycle, and large fetal iron demands as well as blood loss at childbirth for the pregnant woman. Interestingly, both the NHANES I and the Ten-State Nutrition Survey revealed that the iron status in males is also unsatisfactory (see Chap. 1).

Several studies have shown that iron deficiency is associated with an increase in body lead levels, which in turn exacerbates the iron deficiency.[8] Similar observations have been made with calcium and possibly zinc.[9] Thus there is a possibility of lead toxicity in anemia. Iron intake is frequently inadequate in pregnant women and young children, and both of these groups are quite susceptible to lead poisoning. Given the population's increasing exposure to lead (mainly from leaded gasoline), an adequate iron intake is desirable not only in itself but also to minimize the potential hazards associated with chronic lead exposure.

Although there is no general agreement that iron deficiency in the absence of anemia is a pathologic process, a variety of nonhematologic manifestations have been observed. Various biochemical changes have been observed, and a variety of symptoms, such as fatigue, headache, irritability, cold sensitivity, anorexia, insomnia, depression, and gastrointestinal abnormalities have been noted. Children have been reported to exhibit disturbances, such as hyperactivity, decreased attention span, and perceptual restrictions. In some cases, remediation of these symptoms has occurred too soon after the initiation of iron therapy for augmented hemoglobin levels to be playing a significant role. Some types of pica (see Chap. 19), such as the compulsive eating of ice, have been observed in iron-depleted clients; this is promptly corrected with oral iron therapy.

▶ **Iron Excess.** Iron overload, called **hemosiderosis**
▶ in the absence of associated tissue changes or **hemochromatosis** if there is tissue damage, particularly in the liver and heart has occurred much less frequently than iron deficiency and reflects the body's limited ability to excrete iron. Signs and symptoms of hemochromatosis include a bronze pigmentation of the skin, cirrhosis of the liver, and heart damage. Suspect an excessive accumulation of iron in clients with a history of hemolytic anemia and those who receive repeated blood transfusions for chronic anemia or bleeding disorders. The iron released when red blood cells are broken down is stored. Alcoholics who drink wine with a high iron content and clients with chronic liver disease or chronic pancreatitis may absorb excessive iron.

Be alert to the high prevalence of iron toxicity in infants. Iron-containing medications can be purchased from open shelves at drugstores and supermarkets, and many people are unaware of their danger. The widespread incidence of iron deficiency anemia has resulted in the merchandising of numerous nonprescription iron-containing preparations for the prevention and/or treatment of the anemia. When children have access to medications designed for adults, there is danger of iron toxicity and chronic iron overload.

Iodine and Fluorine

Like iron, iodine and fluorine are two essential trace elements in which documented deficiencies in humans are associated with low concentration of the elements in food and water supplies. Both iodine and fluorine occur in extremely variable amounts in soil and water in various sections of the country. This variability is reflected in their content in foods grown in different geographical locations. Therefore, foods are not dependable sources of either iodine or fluorine.

Iodine

Iodine is present in seafoods and foods grown in seacoast areas. The coastal areas and the southern United States have significant amounts of iodine in both soil and water. Northern and mountainous sections, especially the Great Lakes Region, Pacific Northwest, and Rocky Mountain States, are not as lucky. These areas are often referred to as the "goi-
▶ ter belt." **Goiter** is the enlargement of the thyroid gland.

Fluorine deficiency in soil and water supplies is not as clear-cut. While seafood is a good source of fluorine, local water supplies must be tested to determine fluorine content.

Since everyone does not eat seafood in sufficient quantity to meet the needs for fluorine and iodine and since there is no way of knowing where supermarket foods are grown, other methods must be used to assure an adequate intake of fluorine and iodine. Just as vitamin D is added to milk, vitamin A to vegetable margarines, and iron and some of the B-complex vitamins to white flour, so iodine and fluorine are added to food or water. Iodine is added to common table salt, and fluorine may be added to the water supply in fluorine-deficient areas.

Imbalance. Iodine functions as an integral component of the thyroid hormones, thyroxine and triiodothyronine, which regulate cell metabolism. A defi-
▶ ciency leads to **simple goiter,** also called **nontoxic goiter,** in which the thyroid gland enlarges by increasing in both size and number of epithelial cells.

Thyroid gland enlargement may produce tracheal compression, with respiratory distress.

Clinical studies indicate that iodine nutriture has improved in recent decades. The addition of iodine to table salt has been an effective preventive technique in reducing the incidence of goiter induced by iodine deficiency. It is unlikely that increased iodine intake will reduce the size of goiter once it has developed, however. While goiter still exists in segments of the population, it is not clear at the present time whether it is due to iodine deficiency or other causes. The ingestion of so-called goitrogens (foods that induce goiter by altering the metabolism of iodine) has been implicated in the etiology of goiter in some areas of the world, although it is not known whether this poses a problem in the United States. A number of food substances, including ground nuts, soybeans, and plants of the Brassica genus such as cabbage and rutabagas, are classified as goitrogens. However, cooking the foods inactivates the goitrogenic property. Enlargement of the thyroid gland has been reported in humans who eat soybeans and peanuts.[10]

Iodine excess, like excess of other trace minerals, should be avoided. Iodine excess suppresses the function of the thyroid gland and can cause goiter just as does iodine deficiency. This has been demonstrated in individuals consuming large amounts of seaweed who developed thyrotoxicosis, toxic goiter.[11]

Sources. While the best sources of iodine are seafood and iodized salt, brown algae and seaweed are rich in iodine. However, the latter sources are not prominent in the diet of most Americans. Advise clients that sea salt, which contains chiefly sodium chloride, loses iodine during the drying process.

The Food and Nutrition Board of the National Research Council, which determines the RDA, recommends using only iodized salt in households in all noncoastal regions of the United States.[12] While both iodized and noniodized salt are available, only about one half of the salt presently consumed is iodized, since people have a choice in the type they purchase. Furthermore, salt added to processed foods and salt used by schools and restaurants is unlikely to be iodized. Although the use of iodized salt continues to be an important health measure for those consuming an iodine-deficient diet, the increased availability of iodine in the food supply and environment raises the possibility of goiter being induced by excessive iodine intake in some individuals. Changes in agricultural practices, food technology, use of medications, and environmental pollution may result in an intake of iodine that is considerably in excess of the RDA. The major food items that are responsible for the increased availability of iodine in the food supply are milk and bread. Iodine-containing compounds may be used in feeding dairy cattle (iodized salt blocks or iodine-supplemented feed), in medications used for cattle, and in compounds used to sterilize dairy equipment.

Bread made with iodine-containing dough conditioners is a rich source of iodine, although the practice of using iodate in bread is on the decline. Many therapeutic drugs contain a relatively large amount of iodine. Finally, a significant amount of iodine may be present in air that is polluted by combustion from fossil fuels or organic matter. Although the present iodine intake in the United States can be considered safe, additional increases should be avoided, and iodine-containing compounds used as additives should be replaced with compounds containing less or no iodine when possible.

Fluorine

Fluorine, as the fluoride ion, is a trace element that functions in the formation and maintenance of teeth and bones. It is incorporated into bones and into the dental enamel structure and is required for maximum resistance to dental caries. Fluorine exerts its protective effects against tooth decay by three mechanisms: (1) it stabilizes enamel by converting the enamel mineral, hydroxyapatite, to fluorapatite and the solubility of the mineral in acid is thus reduced, (2) it promotes remineralization of early carious lesions, and (3) it exerts an antibacterial and antienzyme effect on plaque bacteria with a decrease in acid production.

Fluoride exerts both systemic and localized effects on the dental enamel. Systemically, fluoride is deposited within the body of the enamel apatite crystal during mineralization and maturation of the tooth. Topically, fluoride accumulates on the enamel surface. The effect of fluoridated water and oral supplements is primarily systemic, and the effect of topical applications applied by a dentist is primarily local, although there are some of both types of effects associated with each method.

Sources. While fluoride is widely distributed in foods, seafoods and tea are good dietary sources. Drinking water in which fluoride is naturally present in adequate concentration or fluoridated to a level of 1 mg/liter can provide a major source of fluoride. Fluoride is also available in drops and chewable tablets for use as supplements and in tooth pastes, mouthwashes, and tooth gels.

Imbalances. Fluoride deficiency and excess lead to abnormalities in both the teeth and the skeleton. A deficiency is associated with an increased susceptibility of the teeth to decay, whereas excessive fluoride ingestion causes **dental fluorosis,** in which the teeth are mottled in appearance, a condition of cosmetic concern. Adequate fluoride ingestion may provide some protection against bone-related disorders, such as periodontal disease and osteoporosis. Its use has been suggested in conjunction with vitamin D and calcium in the treatment of these disorders. Excessive skeletal deposition of fluoride, however, leads to **osteosclerosis,** an abnormal skeletal density producing symptoms resembling arthritis.

Advise parents that the greatest benefits of fluoride are provided (approximately 50 percent reduction in tooth decay) when it is constantly available in the drinking water from birth throughout life. The major benefits accrue during the pre-eruptive phase of tooth development. There are lesser but still substantial benefits from consuming fluoridated drinking water on a part-time basis (such as in school-fluoridated water systems) or using supplements in the form of chewable tablets, lozenges, or drops. The blood level of fluoride remains relatively constant when drinking fluoridated water, whereas it fluctuates with supplements. Caution parents against adding fluoride drops to milk, since the calcium in milk may reduce the absorption of fluoride. Since the effect of fluoride in preventing dental caries is maximized when used in combination with topical application, encourage clients to see a dentist for fluoride treatments until mineralization and maturation of teeth is completed at approximately 16 years of age. When providing supplements, a dentist adjusts the dosage according to age and the amount of fluoride present in the water supply. Since the amount of fluoride present in infant formulas is negligible, it is safe to provide supplements to infants soon after birth. Provide fluoride supplements for breastfed infants, regardless of the fluoride content of the community water, soon after birth, since little fluoride is transmitted in breast milk.

Since there is little evidence that prenatal supplementation with fluoride has any significant protective effect, the Food and Drug Administration has banned the sale of fluoride preparations designed for use during pregnancy, although this issue is being reexamined.

Zinc

Functions. Zinc is found in all tissues and fluids but is highly concentrated in the eye, skin, hair, nails, testes, bone, liver, and muscle. The major functions of zinc include:

1. Constituent of enzymes involved in many metabolic pathways (e.g., carbonic anhydrase, alkaline phosphatase, carboxypeptidase, lactic dehydrogenase, alcohol dehydrogenase)
2. May have a role in the synthesis and storage of insulin in the pancreas
3. Cofactor for enzymes involved in nucleic acid and protein synthesis
4. Facilitates release of vitamin A stores from the liver to maintain normal concentration of the vitamin in the blood (needed for synthesis of transport protein, retinol-binding protein)
5. May be essential for formation of salivary proteins

Absorption. Approximately 10 to 40 percent of dietary zinc is absorbed, although, like calcium and iron, the amount absorbed probably increases in deficiency states and during pregnancy. Its absorption in the intestinal tract is enhanced by a zinc-binding compound that may be picolinic acid (a product of the vitamin B_6-dependent metabolism of tryptophan that is a component of pancreatic secretions and found in certain foods, such as liver, kidneys, and milk), citric acid, or prostaglandins.[13] Zinc is better absorbed from breast milk than cow's milk. Dietary fiber and phytic acid, present in high concentrations in whole grains, unleavened bread, and legumes, interfere with zinc absorption. Zinc is well absorbed from unleavened bread, however. Other dietary factors that decrease the absorption of zinc are (1) a high ratio of dietary copper to zinc, (2) a high ratio of nonheme iron to zinc, and (3) high doses of EDTA (see section on iron).

Sources. Zinc is present in highest concentration in animal protein foods, with shellfish, particularly Atlantic oysters, being especially good sources. Plant foods contain much less zinc, although legumes, nuts, and whole grains are good sources. Zinc from these sources may not be well absorbed because of the associated phytates and fiber, however. Moderate amounts of zinc are present in eggs, milk, and cheese, although it may not be well absorbed from dairy products.

Imbalance. Zinc deficiency of both a marked and marginal nature have been observed in normal populations as well as those with certain disease conditions. A severe form of zinc deficiency (producing retarded growth, dwarfism, and hypogonadism with retarded sexual development) has been observed in adolescent males in countries of the Middle East where individuals consume a large amount of unrefined cereal and unleavened whole wheat bread that are high in phytate and fiber. Less severe forms of zinc deficiency have been observed in the United States in healthy children from middle-class families[14] as well as in low socioeconomic groups. Conditions that may precipitate a zinc deficiency are as follows:

1. Diminished intake (e.g., in the chronically ill, in individuals who consume a low-protein diet, in prolonged therapy with parenteral formulas that do not contain zinc)
2. Diminished absorption (e.g., the binding of zinc in the intestinal tract by fiber, phytic acid, and the ingestion of clay—geophagia, malabsorption syndromes, inflammatory bowel disease, and protein-losing enteropathy)
3. Increased losses in sweat (e.g., in high environmental temperatures), urine (e.g., renal disease with proteinuria or failure of tubular reabsorption, catabolic states as trauma or infectious processes, alcohol intake, liver diseases, hemolytic anemia as sickle cell dis-

ease, use of some drugs as penicillamine used to treat Wilson's disease), exudates (e.g., burns)

4. Other conditions include:
   a. Pregnancy (possibly associated with rapid placental proliferation during the first trimester)
   b. Use of oral contraceptives
   c. Malignant neoplasms
   d. Acrodermatitis enteropathica (an inborn error of metabolism associated with severe zinc deficiency)

In clients with any of the above conditions, observe for the signs and symptoms of zinc deficiency summarized in Table 9–11.

Groups that are at a particular high risk for zinc deficiency are infants, children, and pregnant women because of their high demands for zinc. The risk is also high for ethnic groups whose traditional diets contain foods high in fiber and phytate, such as black beans and corn tortillas that are staples in the Guatemalan diet, and whole grain and the unleavened bread, Tanok, that are components of the rural Iranian diet. Advise clients following vegetarian diets and clients who eat diets high in protein and phosphorus that their zinc requirements are increased above normal. Zinc intake is inadequate in renal failure clients who follow low-protein diets and those on traditional liquid diets (clear and full liquid).

The toxicity of zinc is relatively low and occurs with the ingestion of 2 g or more. Zinc toxicity may be associated with ingestion of acid foods prepared and stored in galvanized containers, since acid foods dissolve zinc from the container. Another cause of zinc toxicity is the excessive ingestion of zinc supplements, such as zinc sulfate. Assess for vomiting and diarrhea in clients in whom an overdose of zinc is suspected. Excessive zinc intake may also lead to loss of iron and copper, with anemia, and to a lowering of the level of high-density lipoprotein cholesterol[15] (see Chap. 29).

Other Trace Elements

At present, there is much scientific interest in other essential trace elements, including chromium, copper, selenium, cobalt, manganese, and molybdenum. More details on these and other minerals are found in references 1, 16, 17.

TRACE CONTAMINANTS

Many trace elements with no known biologically essential role are present in the body as contaminants. These include aluminum, arsenic, barium, boron, bismuth, bromine, cadmium, germanium, gold, lead, lithium, mercury, rubidium, silver, strontium, titanium, and zirconium. They gain access to the body through ingested food, water, or other substances or through inhaled air, and toxicity is associated with some of these.

Lead poisoning is a common problem, especially in children ages 1 through 6. Caution pregnant women and parents of young children in particular about the dangers of lead poisoning. Lead readily crosses the placenta and the neurologic effects of lead are most severe in the developing nervous system. Moreover, infants and young children apparently absorb more of a given dose of lead than do adults. Excessive amounts of lead can be ingested when children chew on materials that have a lead base paint (e.g., toys, woodwork, or the flaking paint from old homes). The use of dishes with a lead glaze or pewter containers in food preparation and service is an additional source of lead. Lead is also found in a high concentration in plants, soils, and the air in congested traffic areas because of the exhaust from cars using leaded gasoline. A further source of lead ingestion is the burning of refuse containing lead paint or old lead batteries.

Be alert to the fact that lead toxicity is manifest initially by such nonspecific symptoms as pallor, fatigue, and anorexia. However, more severe symptoms, such as convulsions, stupor, and coma, may be evident. Of the children who survive, many may be permanently retarded or have other neurologic handicaps.

An extreme form of cadmium toxicity called Itai-Itai disease, a severe type of osteomalacia, has been noted in Japan as a result of excessive ingestion of cadmium from foods contaminated by industrial wastes. Of the many forms of mercury, methylmercury is the most toxic. Mercury poisoning was reported in Japan from consumption of fish obtained in waters polluted by methylmercury from industrial wastes. Most survivors of this incident were left with permanent neurologic damage.

TABLE 9–11
SIGNS AND SYMPTOMS OF ZINC DEFICIENCY

Nightblindness

Loss of taste acuity (hypogeusia)

Loss of smell acuity (hyposmia)

Anorexia

Delayed wound and burn healing

Mental changes, including lethargy, irritability, emotional disorders, and occasional loss of coordination

Diarrhea, malabsorption, and lactose intolerance

Dermatitis, scaling, and itching particularly around the eyes, nose, mouth, genitalia, rectum, and on the extremities

Hair loss (alopecia)

Delayed growth in children

Delayed sexual development; impotence in adult males

Increased susceptibility to infection

Possible teratogenic effects on the fetus

REVIEW QUESTIONS AND ACTIVITIES

1. Classify mineral elements as macronutrients and micronutrients based on relative amounts contained in the body.
2. List the seven minerals that are classified as essential macronutrients.
3. List seven of the minerals that are essential micronutrients.
4. Differentiate between trace elements and trace contaminants.
5. Identify the two major physiologic mechanisms that regulate mineral content in the body.
6. Identify three foods that contain acid-forming elements, three foods that contain alkaline-forming elements, and three foods that are neutral.
7. Describe the rationale for diminished absorption of calcium and iron in clients with diminished production of gastric hydrochloric acid.
8. Differentiate between the physiologic mechanisms that underlie the absorption of calcium and phosphorus and that of zinc.
9. Explain the differences in absorption of heme and nonheme iron.
10. Discuss the effects of oxalates, phytates, and fiber on the absorption of calcium, iron, and zinc.
11. Explain the difference in the efficiency of absorption of calcium, iron, and zinc in adults under no physiologic stress from the efficiency of absorption of these minerals in pregnant women and in those with a deficiency of the nutrients.
12. Compare the efficiency of absorption of sodium, potassium, and chloride with that of calcium, iron, and zinc.
13. Identify categories of individuals who are at high risk for developing deficiencies of iron, iodine, fluoride, and zinc.
14. Discuss the rationale for fluoridating drinking water and adding iodine to table salt.
15. Identify the two major disorders associated with skeletal calcium imbalance and the two disorders of ionic calcium imbalance.
16. Identify the three major body functions that are regulated by sodium, potassium, and chloride.
17. Identify the following in relation to magnesium, iron, and zinc: two functions, two results of deficiency, and three food sources.
18. Plan a day's menu that includes the RDA for calcium (800 mg) and iron (18 mg) for a 25-year-old client who is following a vegetarian diet that omits all animal foods (use Appendix 1 for your calculations).

REFERENCES

1. National Research Council: Recommended Dietary Allowances, ed 9. Washington, DC, National Academy Press, 1980, p 158.
2. Ibid, pp 126–127.
3. Massey LK, Strang MM: Soft drink consumption, phosphorus intake, and osteoporosis. J Am Diet Assoc 80:581, 1982.
4. Ibid, p 582.
5. Avioli LV: Postmenopausal osteoporosis: Prevention vs cure. Fed Proc 40:2418, 1981.
6. Belizan JM, Villar J, Pinada O, et al.: Reduction of blood pressure with calcium supplementation in young adults. JAMA 249:1161, 1983.
7. Garn SM, Ryan AS, Owen GM, Abraham S: Income-matched black-white hemoglobin differences after correction for low transferrin saturations. Am J Clin Nutr 34:1645, 1981.
8. Ziegler E, Edwards BB, Jensen RL, et al.: Absorption and retention of lead by infants. Pediatr Res 12:29, 1978.
9. Zinc and copper metabolism in $CaNa_2$–EDTA-treated children with plumbism. Pediatr Res 15:635, 1981.
10. Newberne PM: Naturally occurring food-borne toxicants. In Goodhard RS, Shils ME, eds: Modern Nutrition in Health and Disease, ed 6. Philadelphia, Lea & Febiger, 1980, p 473.
11. National Research Council, op cit, p 149.
12. Ibid, pp 149–150.
13. Solomons NW: Factors affecting the bioavailability of zinc. J Am Diet Assoc 80:115, 1982.
14. Hambidge KM, Hambidge C, Jacobs M, Baum JD: Low levels of zinc in hair, anorexia, poor growth, and hypogeusia in children. Pediatr Res 6:868, 1972.
15. Hooper PL, Visconti L, Garry PJ, Johnson GE: Zinc lowers high-density lipoprotein–cholesterol levels. JAMA 244:1960, 1980.
16. Mertz W: The essential trace elements. Science 213:1332, 1981.
17. Mertz W: The significance of trace elements for health. Nutr Today 18(5):26, 1983.

BIBLIOGRAPHY

Allegrini M, Pennington JAT, Tanner JT: Total diet study: Determination of iodine intake by neutron activation analysis. J Am Diet Assoc 83:18, 1983.

Annest JL, Pirkle JL, MacKuc D, et al.: Chronological trend in blood lead levels between 1976 and 1980. N Engl J Med 308:1373, 1983.

Beisel WR: Single nutrients and immunity. Am J Clin Nutr 35 [Suppl]:442, 1982.

Dallman PR, Siimes MA, Stekel A: Iron deficiency in infancy and childhood. Am J Clin Nutr 33:86, 1980.

Leverett DH: Fluorides and the changing prevalence of dental caries. Science 217:26, 1982.

Lewis C: Vitamins and Minerals, Sodium and Potassium. Philadelphia, FA Davis, 1976.

Linkswiler HM: Protein-induced hypercalciuria. Fed Proc 40:2429, 1981.

Monsen ER, Balintfy JL: Calculating dietary iron bioavailability: Refinement and computerization. J Am Diet Assoc 80:307, 1982.

Morek TA, Lynch SR, Cook JD: Inhibition of food iron absorption by coffee. Am J Clin Nutr 37:416, 1983.

Overleas D, Harland BF: Phytate content of foods: Effect on dietary zinc bioavailability. J Am Diet Assoc 79:433, 1981.

Oski FA: The nonhematologic manifestations of iron deficiency. Am J Dis Child 133:315, 1979.

Park YK: Estimation of dietary iodine content of Americans in recent years. J Am Diet Assoc 79:17, 1981.

Prasad AS: Nutritional zinc today. Nutr Today 16:4, 1981.

CHAPTER 10

Fluid and Electrolyte Balance

Objectives

After completion of this chapter, the student will be able to:

1. Compare and contrast the water compartments in the body in terms of (a) relative size and (b) the major cations and anions that comprise the electrolyte composition of each fluid.

2. Compare and contrast the regulatory functions of sodium, potassium, chloride, and phosphate.

3. Differentiate among clinical situations that precipitate imbalances of sodium, chloride, and potassium.

4. Differentiate among the roles of the four major organs involved in regulating fluid and electrolyte balance.

5. Differentiate between the roles of the two major hormones involved with fluid and electrolyte balance.

6. Differentiate between the two major types of acidosis and the two major types of alkalosis in terms of the buffer system alteration involved in each and examples of predisposing causes.

7. Distinguish among the three major types of dehydration and compare dehydration with edema.

8. Assist a client with altered electrolyte status with diet planning that provides for adequate nutrient intake.

Normal life processes depend on the body's ability to maintain a balanced internal environment—or state of homeostasis. This involves the maintenance of an adequate volume, composition, and concentration of body fluids. Water, an inorganic nutrient like the mineral elements, is second only to oxygen in its importance in sustaining life. Water and its dissolved substances are important in regulating body processes: in maintaining normal osmotic pressure relationships, irritability of nerves, contraction of muscles, and acid–base balance and in controlling movement of nutrients into the cells and movement of wastes out of the cells. The constancy of this aqueous environment is maintained within extremely narrow limits by the integration of many physiologic processes.

Illness and trauma can alter the amount and composition of body fluids and may have profound effects unless promptly corrected. In order to provide suitable fluid and electrolyte therapy, nurses need fundamental concepts governing water and electrolytes, which this chapter presents.

BODY FLUIDS: COMPARTMENTS AND COMPOSITION

Body fluids consist chiefly of water and dissolved substances, including electrolytes (substances such as acids, bases, and salts that, in solution, dissociate into electrically charged ions) and nonelectrolytes. Body fluids are distributed within two major com-

▶ partments: the **intracellular fluid** (ICF), or fluid
▶ within the cell, and the **extracellular fluid** (ECF),
or fluid outside the cell. ECF consists of plasma,
lymph, spinal fluid, secretions, and the interstitial
fluid that bathes each cell. ICF comprises approximately two thirds of the total body water (about
40 to 50 percent of the body weight), with the remainder of total body water as ECF. Plasma represents about 5 percent of the body weight and the
interstitial and other fluids about 10 to 20 percent.

There is a constant exchange of water and solutes between the various fluid compartments. These
exchanges occur through a combination of passive
and active transport systems and through pinocytosis (see Chap. 3). The particular type of transport
mechanism involved in the exchange depends on
the type of membrane and the size and concentration of the substances involved.

Water

The total water content of the body varies with age
and body composition (i.e., the amount of lean vs
fat tissue). The percentage of total body weight com-
prised by water is higher in infants than in adults
and higher in lean than in obese persons. Water
accounts for approximately 76 percent of the body
weight of an infant. However, the water content
gradually declines with age to approximately 60 percent in adult males and 50 percent in adult females.
There is a continuing decline as aging progresses.
Very little water is stored in the cell when fat is
deposited. In contrast, approximately 4 g of water
are deposited with 1 g of protein deposited. Therefore, water may account for approximately 50 percent of the body weight of an obese person and 70
percent of the body weight of a lean person.

Electrolytes

▶ **Electrolytes** in the form of cations and anions constitute a major force in regulating fluid balance in
the body. Mineral elements in body fluids occur primarily as salts, which ionize in varying degrees. Substances such as urea and glucose do not ionize in
▶ solution and are thus referred to as **nonelectrolytes.**

The cations of body fluids are sodium, potassium, calcium, and magnesium. The anions include
chloride, bicarbonate, phosphate, sulfate, ions of organic acids (such as lactate and pyruvate), and protein derivatives (proteinates). These electrolytes
must be present in body fluids in a proper balance,
since none operates as a single entity, but, like other

essential substances, they have metabolic actions
that are interrelated.

Because the body fluids contain large numbers
of electrically charged ions, they are referred to as
▶ **electrolytic solutions.** In order for the solutions
to remain stable and thus preserve the integrity
of cells, the solutions must be electrically neutral,
i.e., the number of positively charged particles must
equal the number of negatively charged particles.
The balanced electrolyte composition of the body
fluids is illustrated in Table 10–1. Although many
of the same ions are present in both ECF and ICF,
the numbers of each vary. For example, in the ECF,
sodium is the major cation and chloride the major
anion. In the ICF, potassium is the major cation
and phosphate the major anion. The main difference
between the plasma and the interstitial fluid is the
much greater quantity of protein contained in
plasma. The molecular structure of the plasma proteins is too large to allow their diffusion through
the capillary membrane. With this exception, the
ionic composition of plasma and interstitial fluid is
practically identical.

Sodium. Sodium is the major cation of ECF, representing about 90 percent of the total number of cations.

Regulatory Functions. Sodium plays a major role in
five regulatory functions in the body. In performing
these functions, sodium acts with other ions, such
as potassium, magnesium, and chloride. Because of
the much larger amounts of sodium present, however, it assumes a major role in some of the functions. The regulatory functions of sodium in combination with other electrolytes can be summarized
as follows:

1. Blood osmolality. Since sodium comprises 90
   percent of extracellular cations, it is a major
   force in maintaining the normal osmolality
   of the blood.
2. Fluid balance. Sodium is the major osmotic
   force that maintains the water volume necessary for the cellular environment.
3. Acid–base balance. Sodium is the largest
   component of the total extracellular base
   that buffers acids, such as carbon dioxide and
   ketones.
4. Permeability of cell membranes. The sodium–potassium pump, active in all cell
   membranes, maintains electrolyte differ-

TABLE 10–1			
ELECTROLYTE COMPOSITION OF BODY FLUIDS			
Extracellular Fluid		Intracellular Fluid	
Cations	Anions	Cations	Anions
155 mEq/liter	155 mEq/liter	175 mEq/liter	175 mEq/liter

ences between the intracellular and extracellular fluids.

5. Excitability of nerve and muscle fibers. The diffusion of sodium ions into the cell (and diffusion of potassium ions out of the cell) establishes the membrane potential necessary for the excitability of nerve and muscle fibers.

Sources and Requirements. The main dietary source of sodium is table salt (sodium chloride), which is used in cooking, added to foods at the table, or consumed as a food additive in processed foods. One teaspoon of salt contains approximately 2000 mg of sodium. Sodium is also found naturally in animal protein foods and a few vegetables, such as beets, carrots, celery, and chard. Other vegetables, fruits, cereals, and legumes are low in sodium content unless sodium is added during food processing or food preparation. These food sources of sodium are discussed in detail in Chapter 29. The usual adult diet contains sodium in the range of 2.3 to 6.9 g (100 to 300 mEq) per day.[1]

There is no RDA for sodium. However, the National Academy of Sciences provides an estimated safe and adequate daily dietary intake (see Table 2–3). The physiologic requirements for sodium, while not precisely known, are relatively small. For instance, estimated minimal requirements for infants and young children are approximately 58 mg (2.5 mEq) per day, and healthy adults can maintain sodium balance with an intake of little more than this.[1]

Balance and Imbalance. The normal kidney adjusts to a wide range of sodium intake by excreting more when the intake is large and reabsorbing more when the intake is small. Sodium homeostasis is maintained by the action of the hormone aldosterone on the renal tubules. When sodium intake is nil, an increased secretion of aldosterone rapidly reduces urinary excretion to nearly zero. Conversely, when sodium intake is high, aldosterone secretion decreases and urinary excretion of sodium increases.

Sodium imbalance may be reflected as a decrease or increase in the blood sodium level (hyponatremia or hypernatremia, respectively). An abnormal retention of sodium and water (primarily in the interstitial fluid) occurs with edema. Chronic sodium excess has also been implicated in the etiology of hypertension in genetically susceptible individuals.

▶ **Hyponatremia** results from deficient sodium intake, losses of sodium that exceed water loss, or water intake that exceeds sodium intake, the latter
▶ referred to as **water intoxication.** This syndrome most often develops in clients with conditions associated with loss of both body water and sodium when only the water is adequately replaced. Assess the serum sodium levels and suspect hyponatremia associated with excessive sodium losses in clients whose history includes prolonged use of diuretics, loss of

gastrointestinal fluids from vomiting, diarrhea, or continuous suctioning, nephrotic salt-losing syndrome of the kidneys, adrenal insufficiency, losses associated with trauma, such as burns, or losses associated with visible perspiration.

▶ **Hypernatremia** may occur as a result of excessive sodium intake (salt poisoning). The safety factor between commonly consumed amounts of sodium chloride and toxic levels is low, approximately three to five times the amount commonly eaten by many people. Hypernatremia resulting from salt overload is accompanied by an increase in total body sodium and in the volume of extracellular water. If prolonged, the fluid overload can lead to heart failure. Hypernatremia may also occur as a result of dehydration in which water intake is deficient or water loss exceeds sodium loss. In this case, the concentration of sodium in the blood is increased rather than there being an increase in total body sodium. Clients who are particularly prone to develop hypernatremia associated with dehydration are infants and elderly persons. Assist these clients with consuming adequate amounts of water, particularly when protein intake is high as when high-protein tube feeding formulas are administered. The excretion of the waste products of protein metabolism necessitates an increase in water intake.

Chronic sodium excess, possible in combination with a deficiency of potassium and a high sodium:potassium ratio, has been implicated in the etiology of hypertension in susceptible individuals,[2] although this view is far from unanimous.[3] These relationships are explored in Chapter 29.

Chlorine. Chlorine, which exists in the body almost entirely as chloride, occurs in highest concentration in the ECF closely associated with sodium. However, chloride diffuses freely across cell membranes, and some chloride is found in all body cells, especially red blood cells.

Functions. As the major anion of the ECF, chloride functions with sodium ions in the regulation of acid–base balance and water balance and in normal osmotic pressure relationships. An ion exchange involving chloride and bicarbonate ions occurs in the red blood cells and plasma and assists in maintaining the normal pH of the blood. Chloride also functions in the digestion of food as a component of gastric hydrochloric acid, which provides the acid medium needed for activation of the gastric proteolytic enzymes and for protein digestion.

Sources and Requirements. The major dietary source of chloride is table salt. Although no RDA for chloride has been established, an estimated safe and adequate daily dietary intake is presented in Table 2–3. The amount consumed usually parallels sodium intake and is not deficient under normal conditions.

Balance and Imbalance. The excretion of chloride largely parallels the excretion of sodium in urine, sweat, and via the gastrointestinal tract. In the kidney, the reabsorption of chloride is secondary to the aldosterone-induced reabsorption of sodium. In some situations, however, chloride may be lost independently of sodium or in a greater concentration than sodium. For example, with metabolic acidosis, the kidney may excrete chloride, rather than sodium, in combination with ammonium, in an effort to conserve sodium. Loss of gastric juice, as with vomiting or gastric suctioning, entails a greater loss of chloride than sodium, since gastric juice has a lower concentration of sodium than of chloride. When clients lose excessive chloride, provide chloride replacements to prevent the development of acid–base imbalance. When chloride is lost from body fluids, it is replaced by bicarbonate to maintain electroneutrality. This leads to alkalosis (see below) and has secondary effects on potassium balance.

Potassium. Potassium is the principal cation of the ICF, where approximately 98 percent of the total body potassium is located. Only a small amount of potassium is present in the ECF.

Functions. With other electrolytes, potassium participates in the following regulatory functions:

1. Maintains osmotic pressure of ICF. Just as sodium (the most abundant ion in ECF) maintains the osmotic pressure and thus the volume of ECF, so potassium (the most abundant ion in the ICF) maintains the osmotic pressure and volume of ICF. The shifts of water between ECF and ICF are due primarily to changes in the concentration of sodium and potassium in these compartments.
2. Maintains excitability of nerve and muscle fibers. Although sodium, potassium, calcium, and magnesium all participate in this function, it is primarily the potassium concentration that determines the ease with which nerve and muscle cell membranes can be stimulated and thus transmit nerve impulses.
3. Regulates acid–base balance. Potassium is involved in two aspects of the regulation of acid–base balance: (1) it serves as a cation for excretion of organic acids by the kidney, and (2) it is in secretory competition with hydrogen in the exchange process for sodium reabsorption in the renal distal tubule.
4. Is involved with carbohydrate and protein metabolism. Potassium activates enzymes needed for the oxidation of glucose and is involved with glycogen synthesis. Potassium is stored with the glycogen. Abnormally high blood levels of potassium may be temporarily reduced by administering glucose and insulin, which stimulates entry of glucose into

the cell and stimulates glycogen formation. Potassium is also required for the synthesis of muscle protein from amino acids. A considerable amount of potassium is incorporated into muscle protein as these proteins are synthesized. When muscle protein is broken down, this potassium is released into the ECF from catabolized muscle.

Sources and Requirements. There is no RDA for potassium; however, Table 2–3 provides an estimated safe and adequate daily dietary intake. The mineral is widely distributed in foods. Meat, milk, whole grain cereals, legumes, and many fruits and vegetables are good sources. The usual adult diet contains between 1950 and 5900 mg (50 to 150 mEq). Under ordinary conditions, healthy adults can maintain potassium balance with an intake that approximates 90 mg (2.3 mEq) daily, which also represents the minimal requirements for infants and young children.[4]

Balance and Imbalance. The kidney excretes excess potassium with little difficulty provided renal function is normal, that is (1) renal blood flow is normal, (2) tubular function is normal, and (3) an adequate urine volume is being produced. While excesses are easily excreted, the normal kidney cannot conserve potassium during periods of inadequate intake or increased loss of this nutrient as efficiently as it conserves sodium when intake is low.

▶ Potassium imbalance most commonly results from decreased renal excretion resulting in **hyperkalemia** (elevated blood level of potassium) or from diminished food intake or increased loss of potassium from the body resulting in **hypokalemia** (reduced blood level of potassium).

Determine the blood potassium level and observe for hyperkalemia in clients with any of these conditions:

1. Decreased renal excretion resulting from:
   a. Renal disease with diminished urine volume
   b. Dehydration ⎤ lead to ↓ blood volume →
   ⎟ ↓renal blood flow
   c. Shock ⎦ ∴ ↓ urine volume ∴ ↓ K excretion
   d. Adrenal gland insufficiency with decreased aldosterone production → ↓ Na⁺ reabsorption and ↑ K⁺ reabsorption
   e. Metabolic acidosis
2. Rapid tissue destruction when associated with decreased renal blood flow. Examples include
   a. Severe burns (loss of ECF and proteins; ICF, including K⁺, shifts to ECF)
   b. Crushing injuries (release of K⁺ by damaged cells)
3. Administration of excessive amounts of potassium

In contrast, assess for hypokalemia in clients with these conditions:

1. Decreased intake due to:
   a. Anorexia
   b. Administration of potassium-free IV fluids
2. Increased loss resulting from:
   a. Abnormal loss of gastrointestinal secretions
   b. Increased losses by the kidney, e.g., increased secretion of aldosterone by adrenals, administration of adrenal cortical hormones, administration of diuretics that cause potassium loss, metabolic alkalosis
3. Chronic wasting disease with tissue destruction

Phosphate. Phosphate is the major anion of ICF. Organic phosphates are a part of the structure of all cells and are intimately involved in cellular functions. As a constituent of ATP, it provides the energy needed for all cellular activity. Thus, the ICF contains much more phosphate than does the ECF. Inorganic phosphates (monosodium phosphate and disodium phosphate) function in one of the body's major buffer systems to maintain the acid–base balance. Monosodium phosphate is acid; disodium phosphate is alkaline. Food sources of phosphorus and phosphate imbalance are discussed in Chapter 9.

Measurement of Electrolytes. Laboratory assessments of the amounts of various components of body fluids are reported in one of three units: (1) grams, (2) milligrams, or (3) milliequivalents. Furthermore, these measurements may be per liter of fluid or per 100 ml of fluid. The latter is designated as percent, such as g% or mg%. Ions are measured in terms of milliequivalents per liter (mEq/liter) or as milligrams per 100 ml (mg%). Molecules are measured as milligrams per 100 ml (mg%) or as grams per 100 ml (g%). The following are examples:

Hemoglobin	14–17 g%
Calcium	9.0–11.5 mg% or
	4.5–5.5 mEq/liter
Sodium	135–145 mEq/liter

Grams and milligrams represent weights of ions or molecules, whereas milliequivalents represent numbers of ions. Chemical reactivity (or combining power) is directly related to the number of ions present rather than to the weight of ions present. For example, osmotic pressure is exerted in relation to the number of ions present in solution rather than to the total weight of those ions.

Nonelectrolytes

Compounds of both small and large molecular size constitute the nonelectrolytes of body fluids. Compounds of small molecular size, such as urea, glucose, and amino acids, diffuse freely across the membranes separating fluid compartments and affect water balance only if they occur in the plasma in abnormally large quantities. For example, an exceptionally high level of blood urea or glucose results in the urinary excretion of large quantities of water as the excess urea or glucose is excreted.

Compounds of large molecular size, such as proteins, including the proteins of plasma (albumin and globulins), do not pass readily through the membranes separating the fluid compartments and markedly influence the shift of water between fluid compartments. The proteins exert **colloidal osmotic pressure** (or a water-pulling effect) within the blood vessels and the cells, which protects the volume of fluid in these compartments. For example, the plasma albumin is the principal force that maintains the volume of fluid in the vascular compartment. By exerting a constant pressure that pulls fluid from the interstitial fluid to the plasma, albumin opposes and balances the flow of fluid out of the capillaries as a result of filtration pressure exerted by the force of the blood flowing through the capillaries. When the blood level of albumin falls below normal, the osmotic pressure is reduced and fluid remains in the interstitial fluid—the condition called edema.

REGULATORY CONTROL OF FLUID AND ELECTROLYTE DISTRIBUTION

Many factors control the movement and distribution of water and solutes from one fluid compartment to another. Thus, various abnormalities can affect fluid and electrolyte balance. The two factors that are especially important in maintaining the constant volume, osmolality, and composition of the body fluids are (1) the selective permeability of the cell membrane, which primarily regulates the characteristics of the ICF, and (2) the kidney, which primarily regulates the characteristics of the ECF. The kidney is under hormonal control in regulating fluid and electrolyte balance. The gastrointestinal tract, skin, and lungs also play important regulatory roles.

Membrane Permeability

After nutrients are absorbed from the gastrointestinal tract into the circulatory system, they must pass through two types of membranes before they are available to the cell. These are the capillary and cell membranes.

The capillary membrane is a relatively permeable membrane through which water and nutrients, including ions, diffuse very readily. Since transport across the capillary membrane is relatively easy, the dissolved substances become equilibrated on the two sides of the membrane. For this reason, the concentrations of nutrients and other substances are equal in the blood and interstitial fluid, except for plasma proteins, which, due to their large size, do not diffuse through the capillary membrane.

In contrast to the relative permeability of capillary membranes, cell membranes are highly selective permeability barriers. In order to penetrate the cell membrane, substances must either be small enough to pass through the small membrane pores or else be soluble in its lipoprotein layer. Since many substances needed for cellular reactions do not meet these criteria, transport of many substances across cell membranes is regulated by specialized pumps and gates.

Kidneys

In regulating the characteristics of the ECF, the kidney responds to hormonal stimulation as well as basic renal physiologic processes.

Hormonal Regulation. Hormonal stimulation of the kidney may be induced by changes in the blood volume or the blood osmolality or by stressful situations, such as body injury. In clients with a diminished blood volume, the hormone aldosterone stimulates the kidney to reabsorb sodium—accompanied by water—with a consequent expansion of blood volume. Aldosterone may also be secreted in response to stressful situations. Antidiuretic hormone (ADH) is released in response to an increased osmolality (osmotic pressure) of the blood. For example, in clients who are deficient in water, the osmolality (or tonicity) of the blood is increased due to the high concentration of dissolved solutes, and the release of ADH is thus stimulated. ADH, in turn, stimulates the kidney to reabsorb water, and the client's blood osmolality is restored to normal. The release of ADH is evoked to a lesser extent by a diminished blood volume and by stressful situations, such as surgery. The action of either aldosterone or ADH will diminish the volume of urine excreted because of the increased volume of water reabsorbed.

Physiologic Processes. The four basic physiologic processes involved in the renal regulation of the characteristics of the ECF are (1) glomerular filtration, (2) reabsorption, (3) secretion, and (4) excretion.

As the circulating blood passes through the renal glomeruli, it is filtered through the glomerular capillaries. As this filtrate passes through the tubules, appropriate amounts of the substances needed by the body are reabsorbed through the tubules into the surrounding blood supply and thus are retained. Unneeded substances, including metabolic wastes and ions in excess of body needs, proceed to the collecting tubule to be excreted in the urine. Most of the needed substances are reabsorbed in the proximal portion of the tubules by passive diffusion, that is, from the higher concentration in the proximal tubule to the lower concentration in the surrounding blood supply. Reabsorption in the distal tubule is a more selective process and is under the hormonal influence of aldosterone and ADH.

It is at this point that the secretory function of the renal tubule comes into play. The tubule secretes hydrogen ions or potassium ions to be used in the exchange process with sodium. Secretion in this sense means that hydrogen or potassium ions are removed from the surrounding blood supply by the tubule and transported to the tubular lumen for excretion, in exchange for reabsorbed sodium. When hydrogen ions are more abundant in the blood supply, a hydrogen ion is secreted by the tubules to replace each sodium ion reabsorbed. However, if potassium ions are more abundant than hydrogen ions, a potassium ion is secreted by the tubule and excreted for each sodium ion reabsorbed. This exchange mechanism with sodium not only provides a convenient pathway for excreting ECF excesses of potassium from the diet but also is very important in controlling acid–base balance.

Figure 10–1 illustrates filtration, reabsorption, secretion, and excretion in the kidney.

Gastrointestinal Tract

The fluid and electrolyte components of the gastrointestinal secretions (saliva, gastric juice, bile, pancreatic juice, and intestinal juice) are derived from the blood plasma. They are in a constant state of circulation between the plasma and secretory cells. After functioning in the digestive process, they are reabsorbed and circulated to the plasma for reuse. Approximately 8 to 10 liters of secretions are produced daily by the glands. This volume is greater than the plasma volume itself. Under normal conditions only negligible quantities of these secretions are lost via the gastrointestinal tract. Because of the large volume of fluid and electrolytes contained in the gastrointestinal secretions, serious drains on the body fluids and electrolytes bringing imbalances occur in clients who experience abnormal losses, as with persistent vomiting, diarrhea, gastric, or intestinal suction, or fistula drainage.

Skin and Lungs

With insensible fluid losses (those not noticed by the individual) that occur with evaporation from the skin and expiration from the lungs, expect fluid losses to be moderate and electrolyte losses negligible. However, fluid and electrolyte losses can be excessive in some circumstances. For example, clients with fever, hyperventilation, body trauma, such as burns, or those engaging in vigorous exercise can lose excessive amounts of fluids and electrolytes, causing imbalances unless nurses take corrective action.

ACID–BASE BALANCE

Normal cellular metabolic processes are dependent on the strict regulation of the amounts of acids and bases that are ionized in the body fluids. The symbol pH represents the degree of acidity of body fluids. The acidity or alkalinity of a solution is determined ▶ by its concentration of hydrogen ions. **Acids** are sub-

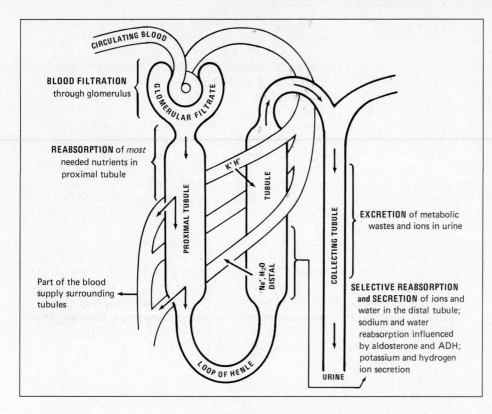

Figure 10–1
Filtration, reabsorption, secretion, and excretion in the kidney. (Source: Adapted from Harper HA, Rodwell VW, Mayes PA: Review of Physiological Chemistry, ed 16. Los Altos, Calif, Lange Medical Publications, 1977, p 613.)

stances that give off hydrogen ions (or protons) in an aqueous solution, whereas **bases** accept or combine with hydrogen ions. Acids and bases are designated as strong or weak depending on the degree to which they ionize in water and yield hydrogen (in the case of acids) or combine with hydrogen (in the case of bases). The greater the hydrogen concentration, the more acid the solution and the lower the pH. The less the hydrogen concentration, the more basic the solution and the higher the pH. A pH of 7 is the point of neutrality between an acid and an alkali.

Although both acids and bases are produced in the body as end products of metabolism, the acid products predominate. In normal conditions, the body fluids are maintained within a narrow range of pH of 7.35 to 7.45. Deficits or excesses of either acids or bases can alter the hydrogen concentration of body fluids and disrupt the cellular environment, with resulting cell death. Extremes of pH of body fluids that are compatible with life are pH 6.8 and 7.8 (Fig. 10–2).

Fluids and electrolytes function through three mechanisms to ensure strict regulation of the normal pH range: (1) dilution, (2) buffering, and (3) direct excretion of metabolites by the lungs and kidneys.

Dilution

Since total body water accounts for approximately two thirds of the body weight, acids and bases are diluted by the water volume.

Buffer Systems

Buffer systems exist in the plasma and/or red blood cells to permit the transport of acidic and basic metabolites from the cell to their excretory sites—the lungs or kidneys—without major changes in pH. A **buffer system** consists of a pair of compounds, a weak acid or base and a salt of this acid or base. The important buffers in the body are mixtures of weak acids and their alkali salts, such as carbonic acid (weak acid) and sodium bicarbonate (alkali salt). Buffers minimize pH changes by reacting with strong acids or bases to form weak acids or bases.

Four major buffer systems are present in the

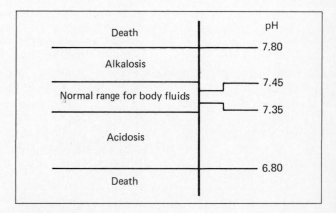

Figure 10–2
Conditions related to various pH levels of body fluids.

body: (1) carbonic acid and sodium bicarbonate, (2) acid and base components of hemoglobin and oxyhemoglobin, (3) monohydrogen and dihydrogen phosphate salts, and (4) the plasma proteins with their alkali salts. The bicarbonate and phosphate systems are important in maintaining the normal pH in both the blood plasma and red blood cells. Proteins are important buffers in the plasma, and hemoglobin and oxyhemoglobin are active buffers in the red blood cells.

Most important of the buffers in maintaining the normal pH of body fluids is the carbonic acid–sodium bicarbonate system. The ratio of these compounds must be maintained at 1:20 (1 part carbonic acid to 20 parts bicarbonate) in order for the blood pH to remain normal. The larger bicarbonate component of this buffer system reflects the body's need to buffer the larger quantities of acids than bases

produced in metabolism, although the system also protects against an excessive amount of base.

Direct Excretion of Metabolites by the Lungs and Kidneys

The lungs and the kidneys are important in maintaining the integrity of the carbonic acid–sodium bicarbonate buffer system and thus maintenance of the normal pH. The lungs ultimately control the supply of carbonic acid in the body fluids, and the kidneys control the supply of sodium and bicarbonate. These organs excrete or conserve carbonic acid and sodium bicarbonate as needed to maintain the 1:20 ratio of carbonic acid to bicarbonate.

Disorders of Acid–Base Balance

Under normal conditions, the processes of dilution, buffering, and direct excretion of metabolites by the

TABLE 10–2
MAJOR ACID–BASE ABNORMALITIES OF THE EXTRACELLULAR FLUID

Acid–Base Abnormality in the ECF	Predisposing Causes	Compensatory Response by Lung/Kidney
Primary bicarbonate deficit (metabolic acidosis)	Excessive production of ketones as in uncontrolled diabetes or in starvation; renal retention of acids (as sulfuric, phosphoric) in renal failure; loss of bicarbonate in renal tubular acidosis; loss of gastrointestinal secretions (as in diarrhea, intestinal suction, or prolonged vomiting); improper use of total parenteral nutrition formulas; hyperkalemia (H^+ and K^+ compete for ion exchange with Na^+)	Hyperventilation; increased renal excretion of H^+ and synthesis of ammonia and decreased excretion of $NaHCO_3$ (renal mechanisms not efficient with renal disease)
Primary carbonic acid excess (respiratory acidosis)	Hypoventilation secondary to respiratory disease (as emphysema, pneumonia), asthma, pulmonary edema, morphine poisoning, asphyxia, and disturbances of respiratory muscles or the regulatory mechanisms in the respiratory center	Increased renal excretion of H^+ and synthesis of ammonia and decreased excretion of $NaHCO_3$; hyperventilation (may be inefficient since lungs directly involved in the cause)
Primary bicarbonate excess (metabolic alkalosis)	Loss of gastric hydrochloric acid in vomiting or gastric suctioning; ingestion of soluble alkalizing salts as sodium bicarbonate; intestinal obstruction (pyloric stenosis); hypokalemia; excessive intake or production of adrenocortical hormones	Depressed respiration; decreased renal excretion of H^+ and synthesis of ammonia and increased excretion of $NaHCO_3$ (concomitant deficit of Na^+ or K^+ may render renal compensation inefficient)
Primary carbonic acid deficit (respiratory alkalosis)	Hyperventilation secondary to acute anxiety, hysteria, salicylate poisoning, high altitude, hot weather, fever, sepsis, peritonitis or other hypermetabolic states, disease of the central nervous system that affects the respiratory center, or hepatic coma	Decreased renal excretion of H^+ and synthesis of ammonia and increased excretion of $NaHCO_3$; depressed respiration (may be inefficient as lungs involved with the cause, though the low level of carbonic acid in the ECF may gradually depress respiration)

lungs and kidneys maintain the 1:20 ratio of carbonic acid:bicarbonate in the body fluid, and the pH of the blood thus remains normal. Any deviation
▶ in this ratio results in **acidosis,** an above-normal
▶ hydrogen ion concentration, or **alkalosis,** a below-normal hydrogen ion concentration (Fig. 10–2). These alterations, which result from excesses or deficits of either carbonic acid or bicarbonate, may be of respiratory or metabolic origin. Respiratory acidosis or alkalosis results from excesses or deficits in the carbonic acid content of the blood, whereas metabolic acidosis or alkalosis results from alterations in the content of bicarbonate in the blood (Table 10–2).

Acidosis may result from an excess of carbonic acid (respiratory) or a deficit of bicarbonate (metabolic). Alkalosis may result from a deficit of carbonic acid (respiratory) or an excess of bicarbonate (metabolic). The lungs and kidneys attempt to compensate for the alteration in the carbonic acid:bicarbonate ratio by altering the excretion of carbonic acid and bicarbonate (Table 10–2).

WATER BALANCE

Regulatory Control

When clients have free access to water, their intake and loss of water are approximately equal, and there exists a state of osmotic equilibrium between the fluid compartments. This equilibrium is normally maintained without conscious effort on the part of the client. The intake of water is regulated by the thirst center in the hypothalamus, and water output is controlled by the kidney—mediated directly by ADH and indirectly by aldosterone.

When clients are depleted of water, their first complaint is thirst. The sensation of thirst is felt when approximately 2 percent of the body weight (as water) has been lost. The rise in blood osmolality associated with the high solute concentration (primarily sodium) or the generalized dehydration of all tissues that accompanies water depletion stimulates the thirst center, and the desire to drink water is initiated. Clients may also be stimulated to drink as a result of drying of the mucous membranes lining the mouth and throat.

The high blood osmolality also stimulates the secretion of ADH, with a resulting increase in the renal reabsorption of water. Depletion of blood volume stimulates secretion of aldosterone, resulting in retention of sodium and water by the kidneys. This hormonal regulation allows the kidneys to adjust water loss to meet varying conditions. For example, when water intake is low or water loss is excessive, as with diarrhea or excessive sweating, the kidneys secrete a smaller volume of more concentrated urine.

Intake and Output

There are two routes of intake and four routes of loss of water in the body. When assessing a client's intake and output, account for all sources of gain and loss. Water is provided by ingestion (as fluids per se and as a component of solid foods) or as an end product of the metabolism of carbohydrate, protein, and fat, so-called **metabolic water.** Water is lost from the skin (as perspiration), the lungs (as water vapor in the expired air), the kidneys (as urine), and the gastrointestinal tract (in feces). The actual intake and output of water depend upon many variables, including the age and food habits of the individual, environmental temperature and humidity, and the presence of pathologic conditions that may alter intake or output.

Water Requirements

Water requirements vary with age; infants and young children have a higher requirement per unit of body weight because they have a less mature renal function and a larger surface area relative to body size than adults. Because of this, be particularly aggressive in replacing fluid losses in these clients to prevent imbalances that can develop quickly. A reasonable water allowance for adults is 1 ml/kcal consumed and for infants 1.5 ml/kcal consumed.[5] Provide additional water to compensate for increased requirements in infants receiving a high-protein formula, in comatose clients, and in clients with fever, polyuria (excessive urination), vomiting, diarrhea, or those taking diuretics or receiving a high-protein diet, and in all clients in a hot environment.

Disorders of Water Balance

Water imbalance, either deficit or excess, leads to acute metabolic difficulties and can result from a deficit or excess of either water or electrolytes or both. A deficit of water in either the ECF or ICF
▶ is called **dehydration,** whereas an excess of water
▶ in the ECF or ICF is called **edema.**

Dehydration. A loss of 10 percent of total body water can lead to symptoms of severe dehydration, while a loss of 20 percent of body water is incompatible with life. Dehydration can result from a deficient intake or excessive losses of fluids and/or electrolytes (primarily sodium) or a combination of the two. Abnormal losses may occur via the gastrointestinal tract, the kidneys, the lungs, the skin, and from tissues damaged by wounds or burns. With dehydration, the electrolyte concentration of body fluids may be normal, increased, or decreased depending on whether the net loss of water is equal to, greater than, or less than the net loss of electrolytes. When net losses of water and electrolytes are approxi-
▶ mately equal, **isotonic dehydration** occurs. Net wa-
▶ ter loss that exceeds electrolyte loss produces **hypertonic dehydration,** and the converse situation (net
▶ electrolyte loss that exceeds water loss) produces **hypotonic dehydration.**

Edema. An increase in body water to 10 percent above the normal volume represents edema. This fluid accumulation is initiated by some defect in the normal circulation of body fluids. Ultimately, it is the accumulation of both sodium and water that leads to the clinical picture of edema. The fluid accumulation may be local or generalized. In clients with edema, determine its basic causes, which may be one of the following: (1) defects in the mechanisms for the removal of fluid from the interstitial tissue spaces, (2) increased renal reabsorption of sodium and water, and (3) decreased renal excretion of sodium and water.

REVIEW QUESTIONS AND ACTIVITIES

1. Identify the two major fluid compartments of the body.
2. Identify the major cation and major anion contained in each of the major fluid compartments.
3. Compare the relative size of the major fluid compartments and subcompartments.
4. Distinguish between electrolytes and non-electrolytes in the body.
5. Describe the unit of measure used to express the number of ions in an electrolytic solution.
6. Describe the role of cell membranes in regulating the fluid and electrolyte characteristics of intracellular fluid.
7. Identify the five regulatory functions of sodium and four regulatory functions of potassium in the body and compare and contrast the regulatory roles of sodium and chloride.
8. Describe the effect on sodium balance in each of the following situations:
   a. A client is losing sodium and water through diarrhea; plain water is being consumed as replacement therapy.
   b. Salt rather than sugar is inadvertently added to an infant formula.
9. Describe clinical situations that precipitate chloride deficiency independent of sodium deficiency.
10. Identify the rationale for each of the following:
    a. Decrease in potassium concentration in the blood when glycogen is stored.
    b. Increase in potassium concentration in the blood when muscle is catabolized.
11. Identify the effect on potassium balance of the following: decreased renal function, loss of gastrointestinal secretions, and severe tissue injury.
12. Explain the roles of the kidney, gastrointestinal tract, skin, and lungs in maintaining fluid and electrolyte balance.
13. Discuss the stimulus for secretion of aldosterone and its effects on sodium, water, and potassium balance.
14. Explain the mechanisms involved in main-taining the pH of the ECF within a range of 7.35 to 7.45.
15. Identify the buffer system imbalance associated with each of the following: metabolic acidosis, metabolic alkalosis, respiratory acidosis, and respiratory alkalosis.
16. Identify the two routes of intake and four routes of loss of body water.
17. Explain the difference between dehydration and edema.
18. *Case study:* A client with a fluid and electrolyte disturbance. Cary is a 6-month-old female infant admitted to the pediatric ward of her local hospital with dehydration and electrolyte disturbances. Medical history, physical examination, and laboratory results are as follows: Diarrhea of 1 week's duration. Parents report feeding the child a high-protein formula prepared from boiled skim milk with no additional fluids. She has lost a total of 10 percent of her body weight, and serum levels of sodium, potassium, and chloride are elevated, and serum bicarbonate is decreased. Her urine volume is low and very concentrated as shown by a high specific gravity.
    a. Describe the type of dehydration that Cary probably has and your rationale for selecting this type over the two other types.
    b. Describe the body's hormonal response to this type of dehydration and its effects on fluid and electrolyte balance and on urine volume.
    c. What type of acid–base imbalance would you anticipate, and what is your rationale for selecting this type over the other three types?
19. *Case study:* Dietary planning for a client with an electrolyte imbalance. Mr. Bradshaw, a 70-year-old black farmer from the rural South has developed chronic renal disease secondary to hypertension. On a recent admission to a university medical center, he was placed on a diet that was restricted in sodium and potassium to control hypertension and hyperkalemia. His diet is to contain 2 g (85 mEq) sodium and 2.5 g (65 mEq) potassium.
    a. Compare the diet order with the usual dietary intake and with the recommended safe and adequate daily dietary intakes of these electrolytes (see Table 2–3).
    b. What information would you like to have about Mr. Bradshaw's eating habits before assisting him with following his diet?
    c. Visit a local supermarket and prepare a list of processed foods that contain added sodium and that may need to be

restricted in the diet. (*Note:* Most canned meats, vegetables, and soups contain added sodium even though it may not be stated on the label.)

d. Refer to Appendix 1 and prepare a list of five fruits that contain 200 mg or more of potassium per ½ c serving and five vegetables that contain 300 mg or more of potassium per ½ c serving and thus must be restricted in the diet.

REFERENCES

1. National Research Council: Recommended Dietary Allowances, ed 9. Washington, DC, National Academy Press, 1980, p 170.
2. MacGregor GA, Markandu ND, Smith SJ, et al.: Moderate potassium supplementation in essential hypertension. Lancet 2:567, 1982.
3. Burstyn P, Hornall D, Watchorn C: Sodium and potassium intake and blood pressure. Br Med J 281:537, 1980.
4. National Research Council, op cit, p 173.
5. Ibid, p 168.

BIBLIOGRAPHY

Attchul AM, Grommet JK: Sodium intake and sodium sensitivity. Nutr Rev 38:393, 1980.

Dahl LK: Salt and hypertension. Am J Clin Nutr 25:231, 1972.

Fregly MJ: Sodium and potassium. Ann Rev Nutr 1:69, 1981.

Lewis C: Vitamins and Minerals, Sodium and Potassium. Philadelphia, FA Davis, 1976.

Patrick J: Interactions between the physiology of sodium, potassium and water and nutrition. J Hum Nutr 32:405, 1978.

Rolls BJ, Wood RJ, Rolls ET, et al.: Thirst following water deprivation in humans. Am J Physiol 239:R476, 1980.

Schachter J, Harper PH, Radin ME, et al.: Comparison of sodium and potassium intake with excretion. Hypertension 2:695, 1980.

Sharer JE: Reviewing acid–base balance. Am J Nurs 75:980, 1976.

Simopoulos AP, Bartley FC: The metabolic consequences of chloride deficiency. Nutr Rev 38:201, 1980.

Stillinger FH: Water revisited. Science 209:451, 1980.

Symposium on fluid, electrolyte, and acid–base balance. Nurs Clin North Am 15:535, 1980.

Tobian L: The relationship of salt to hypertension. Am J Clin Nutr 32:2739, 1979.

PART II

Processes Involved in Providing Nutritional Care

Nurses are confronted daily with clients in both ambulatory and institutional settings who are unable to meet their nutritional needs in a balanced way. In order to deal with the resulting problems, a framework is needed for identifying their nature and providing nutritional care in a systematic manner. Just as nurses use the problem-solving approach—the nursing process—in solving other nursing problems, they can use this same process for dealing with nutritional problems.

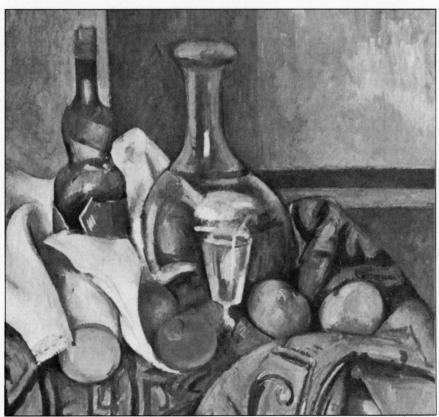

Paul Cézanne *Still Life with Peppermint Bottle*

Much of a nurse's efforts in nutritional care focuses on educating clients to adopt a pattern of eating that meets their individual nutritional requirements. The same problem-solving approach can be used when providing nutrition education.

Part II of this book provides a framework for including nutritional care as a component of total nursing care. The two major topics presented, use of the nursing process in providing nutritional care and concepts of nutrition education and diet counseling, are applicable when providing nutritional care for clients at all stages of the life cycle (discussed in Part III) and for clients with health problems that necessitate nutritional intervention (discussed in Part IV).

CHAPTER 11

The Nutritional Care Process in the Nursing Process

Objectives

After completion of this chapter, the student will be able to apply the four major steps in the nursing process to nutritional needs of clients in the following ways:

1. Assessment
   a. Distinguish between the four major components of nutritional assessment.
   b. Use data from a client's medical history and physical examination to conduct a clinical assessment of nutritional status.
   c. Distinguish between the use of height (or length) and weight and body compositional indices to assess a client's nutritional status.
   d. Evaluate the weight status of an adult of a given height and weight and the growth status of a child of a given height and weight.
   e. Conduct a dietary assessment of a client that includes an evaluation of both nutritional adequacy of foods consumed (using the 24-hour recall method) and a summary of the major factors that affect food intake.
   f. Integrate assessment data into nursing diagnoses, identifying both actual and potential problems.
2. Planning
   a. Determine priority needs.
   b. Identify short- and long-term goals.
   c. Identify outcome criteria by which goals may be measured.
   d. Select from alternative interventions those appropriate for an individual client.
3. Implementation
   a. Recognize how content presented in Parts III and IV may be used as implementation strategies.
   b. Identify barriers that may interfere with effective intervention.
4. Evaluation
   a. Use outcome criteria to evaluate goals.

Because of the complexity of health care, nurses function as part of a health team in delivering client care. Each of the professional members of this team has unique contributions, but there is also an overlap between responsibilities. It is sometimes confusing when working in this gray area. For instance, should the nurse assume any responsibility for dietary concerns when the physician orders the diet and the dietary department prepares and delivers the meal? How does the nurse determine his or her responsibility and that of the registered dietitian? Nursing must identify that aspect of nutritional care that is its major responsibility. This is done through the use of the nursing process. This chapter presents the use of this process in providing nutritional care and concludes with an example of its application. A major emphasis is placed on assessment because interventions related to specific clinical problems are presented in later chapters.

PROCESSES INVOLVED IN PROVIDING NUTRITIONAL CARE

An adaptation of the scientific method, the approach used by scientists in investigating various phenomena, has been successfully used by nursing and other professions that deal with practical problems in providing client care. The adaptation is termed the ▶ **problem-solving method.** However, nursing frequently refers to it as the **nursing process.** This approach involves a four-step process of logical thinking and a pattern of observation that provides the basis for nursing care. The steps in the nursing process are (1) assessment, (2) planning, (3) intervention, and (4) evaluation. Some authors divide the assessment phase into two steps, assessment and nursing diagnosis, thus resulting in a five-step process.

The problem-solving method is as applicable to providing nutritional care as to providing nursing care and can be used by nurses to incorporate nutritional care into the nursing care plan (Table 11–1).

In nutritional care, assessment involves data collection and analysis of those factors that affect the client's nutritional needs and the ability to meet these needs. From this analysis, statements are made about actual or potential problems the client may have that nurses can do something about—the nursing diagnosis. Planning nursing care to deter-

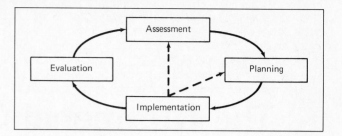

Figure 11–1
The problem-solving approach.

mine possible ways to alleviate the problems is the next logical step, and planning arises from the nursing diagnosis. The implementation phase is the carrying out of the actions identified, and evaluation is an appraisal of the client's response to the actions indicating those problems that have been resolved and those requiring reassessment and alternate plans. In actuality, the steps do not exist in isolation from each other, since nurses continue to collect and analyze data and to plan and evaluate care while implementing a particular care plan. The process is therefore continuous and dynamic, as illustrated in Figure 11–1.

ASSESSMENT

The assessment phase begins with data collection and ends with a diagnosis of the nature and cause of nutritional problems. In general, a nutritional problem exists for any client in whom there is a discrepancy between nutritional needs and nutrient intake and/or use. Relative to intake, the discrepancy may involve excessive, deficient, monotonous, or distorted intake. Because of the multiple influences on food habits, various types of assessment

TABLE 11–1
PROBLEM-SOLVING APPROACH TO NUTRITIONAL CARE

Steps	Description	Components
1. Assessment	Involves data collection, analysis of data, and identification of problems (nursing diagnosis)	Anthropometric data Biochemical data Medical history Physical examination Social history Dietary history Nursing history
2. Planning	Involves setting short- and long-term goals or objectives to correct identified problems, identifying outcome measures, and identifying appropriate actions to achieve goals	Goals must be mutually agreed upon, realistic, and measurable. Appropriate interventions must be specifically stated. Criteria for measuring progress must be defined.
3. Implementation	Involves carrying out the actions identified in the plan	Dietary modifications Client education
4. Evaluation	Involves determination of the degree of success in achieving stated goals or objectives and suggestions for modifications to the plan	Comparison of nutritional status, behaviors and knowledge to goals identified in the plan; analysis to determine reasons for lack of success in achieving goals, if necessary

data must be correlated to determine the cause of existing problems. Factors that are discussed in other sections of the book are not repeated in depth but should be considered when doing the assessment, because they provide clues to the cause of actual or potential nutritional problems. These factors include the following:

1. Level of nutritional knowledge
2. Motivation, feelings, and attitudes about nutrition
3. Cultural, social, physiologic, and psychologic factors
   a. Family resources
   b. Cultural and ethnic influences
   c. Age group influences
   d. Psychologic influences (e.g., use of food for security, punishment, or reward)
   e. Physical conditions that affect food intake or use (e.g., poor teeth, malabsorption, poor vision)
   f. Educational influences

ASSESSMENT OF NUTRITIONAL STATUS

Nutritional status is defined as the state of health of an individual as influenced by intake of the essential food nutrients.[1] Nutritional status, like other aspects of a person's status (e.g., health, financial, social), is the end result of combined interactions between physical and psychosocial forces in the environment. These interactions are illustrated in Figure 11–2. As individuals progress through the stages of the life cycle, various influences interact that may cause a fluctuation on the continuum between adequate nutrition and malnutrition.

In order to provide effective nutritional care for clients in any health care setting, first assess current

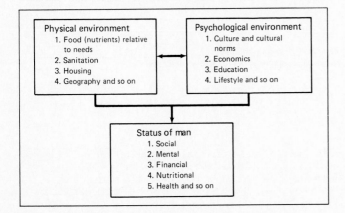

Figure 11–2
An ecologic approach to nutritional assessment. (Source: Adapted from McLaren DS: Nutritional assessment. In McLaren DS, Burman D, eds: Textbook of Paediatric Nutrition, New York. Churchill Livingstone, 1976.)

nutritional status. Use these three major objectives when conducting nutritional assessment: (1) determine the actual and/or potential nutritional status resulting from the intake and use of the essential food nutrients, (2) determine the cause of any actual or potential nutritional problem identified, and (3) provide baseline data for developing a nursing diagnosis and a plan for implementation of ongoing interventions designed to alleviate any nutritional problems. In order to meet objectives 2 and 3, it is important to assess the client's level of knowledge and motivation related to nutrition and the cultural, social, physiologic, and psychologic influences mentioned above.

Assessment Techniques

One can easily spot the grossly overnourished or undernourished client. However, more definitive studies are necessary to identify clients with subclinical imbalances reflecting marginal excesses or deficits in nutrient intake.[2] Attempt to identify clients with marginal imbalances early in order to provide alleviating measures before overt physical signs of disease become apparent. Nutritional imbalances may involve excessive or deficient intake and may be of primary or secondary origin, but the end result is the same. Nonetheless, identification of the cause is essential to effective treatment.

Multiple approaches must be applied to nutritional assessment, since the body uses each of the essential nutrients differently and different standards are used to assess each. Assessment of nutritional status is a complex process that involves correlation of four types of data: (1) clinical, (2) anthropometric (body measurements), (3) biochemical, and (4) dietary. Figure 11–3 includes a summary of the development and evaluation of nutritional disease.

Many of the physical signs of malnutrition may also be related to such nonnutritional factors as inadequate rest or excessive exposure to sunshine. For example, inability to concentrate, irritability, and fatigue may result from a vitamin B-complex deficiency, or the same symptoms may result from inadequate rest. Correct treatment for the situation will depend on correct diagnosis made by correlating data obtained from a physical examination, biochemical analysis, and dietary evaluation.[2]

Clinical Assessment. The nursing history, medical history, and physical examination provide valuable clues for identifying those clients who are at risk of actual or potential malnutrition.

Use the medical history to obtain information about medical and social problems that may place the client at nutritional risk. For example, those clients with a medical problem that interferes with food intake or use or requires medications that interact with specific nutrients may require additional attention from nurses and other members of the health team to meet their nutritional requirements. Use the checklist provided in Figure 11–4 to deter-

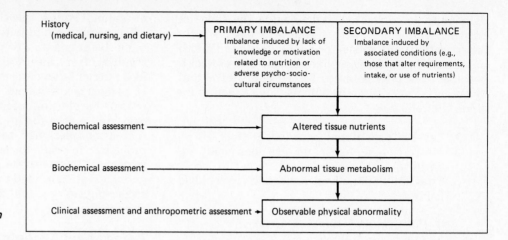

Figure 11–3
Development and evaluation of nutritional disease.

mine the client's degree of risk of developing medical complications unless adequate attention is given to meeting the client's nutritional requirements.

Assess the frequency with which infections occur and adequacy of gastrointestinal function when taking a nursing history. Inadequate nutrition increases susceptibility to infection and predisposes the client to increased severity of infections once they occur. To aid in this assessment, determine how often family members are absent from school or work due to infections. Question the client about appetite and problems related to elimination, such as indigestion, constipation, and diarrhea. Both anorexia and digestive and elimination problems may

	YES	NO
Usual body weight 20 percent above or below desirable?.	____	____
Recent loss or gain of 10 percent of usual body weight?	____	____
Any evidence that income and meals are not adequate for needs?.	____	____
More than half of meals eaten away from home?.	____	____
Does patient live alone and prepare own meals?	____	____
Ill-fitting dentures	____	____
Excessive use of alcohol?	____	____
Frequent use of fad diets, or monotonous diets?	____	____
Any chronic disease of GI tract? (describe)	____	____
Has there been any surgical procedure on GI tract other than appendectomy? (describe)	____	____
Recent major surgery, illness, or injury?	____	____
Recent use of large doses of:		
Catabolic steroids.	____	____
Immunosuppressants	____	____
Antitumor agents.	____	____
Anticonvulsants	____	____
Antibiotics	____	____
Oral contraceptives	____	____
Vitamins	____	____
Other	____	____
Has patient been maintained more than 10 days on IV fluids?	____	____
Any reason to anticipate that patient will be unable to eat for 10 days or longer?	____	____
Is patient known to have:		
Diabetes	____	____
Hypertension	____	____
Hyperlipidemia	____	____
Coronary artery disease	____	____
Malabsorption	____	____
Chronic lung disease.	____	____
Chronic renal disease	____	____
Chronic liver disease.	____	____
Circulatory problem or heart failure.	____	____
Neurologic disorder or paralysis	____	____
Mental retardation	____	____

NOTE:
If all answers to the above items are *No*, the patient may be regarded as a low risk or acceptable risk. The risk increases in direct proportion to the number of *Yes* answers. Patients with more than 3 *Yes* answers should be considered at an increased risk of developing medical complications, unless attention is given to providing their nutritional requirements.

Figure 11–4
Checklist for assessment of nutritional status. (Source: Butterworth CE, Blackburn GL: Hospital Malnutrition. Nutr Today 10(2):9, 1975. Reproduced with permission of Nutrition Today magazine, P.O. Box 1829, Annapolis, MD 21404.)

be either a cause or a result of nutritional deficiency.[3]

The physical examination provides data from observation of specific tissues for physical signs suggesting malnutrition. Parts of the body most commonly exhibiting abnormalities consistent with malnutrition are hair, eyes, skin, teeth and gums, mucous membranes, lips, mouth, tongue, skeleton, nails, muscles, abdomen, lower extremities, and thyroid gland. The signs of good and poor nutrition that can be assessed in these tissues are shown in Table 11-2, and a summary of tissue changes associated with specific nutrient imbalances is found in Table 11-3.

The nervous system may also exhibit signs related to malnutrition. Evaluate the client's general appearance and behavior to gain further clues to relative nutritional status. When looking at or talking to the client, observe whether he or she appears alert and responsive or listless, apathetic, irritable, or not able to concentrate.

In considering the relevance of clinical assessment data to prevention of health problems, be cognizant of the fact that observable lesions occur late in the course of malnutrition. The overt lesions described are easily detected. Much less obvious are the subclinical deficiencies, which are best identified by sensitive biochemical studies in conjunction with the other assessment parameters. Additionally, most clinical signs of nutrient deficiency that nurses are likely to see in community settings are relatively mild and nonspecific.

Anthropometric Assessment

▶ *Commonly Used Techniques.* **Anthropometric assessment** involves body measurements including height, weight, body composition, and, in the case of infants and young children, head circumference. These data are used to assess body fatness, body protein content, and growth in children. As such, anthropometric assessment is an important tool for prevention of health problems. Both obesity and undernutrition, the latter limiting growth in children, are prevalent nutritional problems and are major deterrents to good health. In children, growth failure is one of the earliest responses to undernutrition.

TABLE 11-2
PHYSICAL SIGNS OF GOOD AND POOR NUTRITIONAL STATUS

Tissues	Normal Appearance	Signs Associated with Malnutrition
Eyes	Bright, clear, moist, and shiny with pink membranes; no prominent blood vessels or mound of tissue on sclera	Membranes pale or red; drying of eye, eyelids, cornea; increased vascularization of the cornea (bloodshot eyes); increased sensitivity to bright light, burning, itching, soreness; poor vision in dim light following exposure to bright light (night blindness)
Hair	Shiny, lustrous, and not easily pulled out; healthy scalp	Dull, dry, brittle, thin, depigmented, easily pulled out
Skin	Smooth, slightly moist, good color; no signs of rashes, swellings, dark or light spots	Skin pallor; dermatitis; rough, dry, scaly skin with hardness of papillae at base of hair follicles; sores that fail to heal; petechiae, bruises; depigmentation or hyperpigmentation of the skin
Teeth and gums	Bright, straight teeth without crowding in well-shaped jaw; no evidence of carries (cavities); firm, reddish pink gums with no evidence of swelling or bleeding	Caries present; missing teeth; malposition or abnormal eruption of teeth; worn or mottled tooth surfaces; soft, spongy, bleeding gums
Mucous membranes, mouth, lips, and tongue	Reddish pink color to lips, tongue, mucous membranes; absence of lesions; adequately moist; surface papillae present on tongue	Pale mucous membranes; purplish red to scarlet-red tongue, fissures of the lips and/or corners of mouth; sore mouth and sore, swollen tongue; tongue smooth due to atrophy of surface papillae
Skeleton	Good posture; no malformation present	Poor posture; malformations such as beading of the ribs, bowlegs, or knock-knees
Nails	Firm, pink	Spoon-shaped, brittle, and ridged nails
Muscles	Well-developed, firm	Flaccid, undeveloped, or wasted appearance; tender
Abdomen and lower extremities	Abdomen flat; no tenderness, weaknesses, or swelling of feet and legs	Abdomen swollen; weakness, tenderness, or tingling in feet or legs; edema
Thyroid gland	No enlargement	Enlarged (simple goiter)

(Source: Adapted from Lewis CM: Basic and Family Nutrition, A Self-Instructional Approach, ed 2. Philadelphia, FA Davis, 1984, pp 119, 120, 122.)

TABLE 11-3
TISSUE CHANGES ASSOCIATED WITH SPECIFIC NUTRIENT IMBALANCES

Tissues	Signs Associated with Malnutrition	Nutrient Imbalance
Eyes	1. Nightblindness 2. Drying of eye, eyelids, cornea 3. Increased sensitivity to bright light; burning, itching, soreness 4. Infiltration of cornea by blood vessels	1. Vitamin A deficiency 2. Vitamin A deficiency 3. Vitamin A and/or riboflavin deficiency 4. Riboflavin deficiency
Hair	Dull; dry; brittle; thin; depigmented; easily pulled out	Protein deficiency or protein/calorie deficiency
Skin	1. Skin pallor 2. Dermatitis 3. Rough, dry, scaly skin with hardness of papillae at base of hair follicles 4. Sores that fail to heal	1. Suggestive of anemia from iron, folic acid, or vitamin B_{12} deficiency 2. Vitamin B-complex deficiency (riboflavin, niacin, pyridoxine); linoleic acid deficiency 3. Vitamin A deficiency 4. Protein, vitamin C, or zinc deficiency
Mucous membranes, mouth, lips, tongue, gums	1. Pale mucous membranes 2. Cracks in skin at corner of mouth (cheilosis) 3. Red, cracked lips; purplish red to scarlet-red tongue; tongue smooth due to atrophy of papillae; sore, swollen tongue; sore mouth 4. Soft, spongy, bleeding gums	1. Suggestive of anemia from iron, folic acid, or vitamin B_{12} deficiency 2. Riboflavin deficiency 3. Vitamin B-complex deficiency (riboflavin, niacin, folic acid, pyridoxine, vitamin B_{12}); iron deficiency 4. Vitamin C deficiency
Teeth	1. Dental decay 2. Mottled enamel	1. Calcium, phosphorus, fluoride, vitamins A and D deficiency; possible excess of sucrose in diet 2. Excess fluoride
Skeleton	Bowlegs, knock-knees, chest deformity at diaphragm, beaded ribs, prominent scapulae	Vitamin D, calcium, phosphorus deficiency
Nails	Spoon-shaped, brittle, and ridged	Iron deficiency
Thyroid gland	Simple goiter	Iodine deficiency

(Source: Adapted from Lewis CM: Basic and Family Nutrition, A Self-Instructional Approach, ed 2. Philadelphia, FA Davis, 1984, pp 168–169.)

However, a child's body measurements reflect both genetic and environmental influences. Although nutrition is an important environmental variable, assess for other factors that may compromise health and interact with undernutrition to produce growth retardation, such as recurrent infections or parasitic disease.

The most commonly used anthropometric technique is measurement of height and weight and comparison of these measurements with a height–weight table (for adults) or percentile standards (for children). This technique provides useful screening data for excess or deficient weight.

Height–Weight Table for Adults. Tables of recommended weights have been derived from life insurance statistics that have identified those weights associated with the lowest mortality rates. These statistics indicate that the best weight to maintain throughout the life span is that which is recommended at age 25 for one's height and body frame. Although body weight tends to increase with age, this is not considered biologically desirable. Physical growth is usually completed by approximately age 17 in girls and 21 in boys. Weight subsequently gained is likely to be excess fat. Height and weight of clients over 60 years of age are more difficult to evaluate because of osteoporotic (bone loss) changes, and changes in body composition.

Appendix 7 lists weights of adult males and females ages 25 to 59 years that have been found to best predict longevity, and these figures may be used to determine body weight for adults. Russel notes that these reference weights also appear appropriate for older adults up to age 89.[4] After age 90, however, a weight that represents about 90 percent of the reference weight should be used. Notice in Appendix 7 that height and weight are measured with shoes on and in indoor clothing. When using Appendix 7 to determine body weight, make the appropriate adjustments if the conditions under which the client's weight and height are taken differ from those in the table. Note also that adults are classified on the basis of body frame as small, medium, or large. Refer to Table 2–4 for techniques for approximating body frame size. A range of weights is given for each height and body frame classification. Use the midpoint figure in each case as the recommended weight. Recommended body weight-for-height according to age and sex for individuals 18 to 74 years of age based on NHANES I data have also been published.[5] Many practitioners also use the rule of thumb method described in Chapter 2 for determining recommended body weight.

To correct for limitations inherent in the use of a standard height–weight table, a deviation of 10 percent above or below recommended weight is considered relatively insignificant. Use the following guidelines to classify the weight of adult males and females:[6]

Weight Classification for Adults

Normal weight	Within 10% (±) of recommended weight
Overweight	10 to 20% above recommended weight
Obesity	20% or more above recommended weight
Underweight	10 to 20% below recommended weight
Seriously underweight	20% or more below recommended weight

Growth Charts for Children. Anthropometric assessment is more complex in children than in adults because consideration must be given to the rate of growth and the effects of sexual maturation. Growth spurts and sexual maturation do not occur at the same chronologic age in all children. Height and weight charts for children permit the plotting of a child's height (or length) and weight for age (and for prepubescent children, weight relative to height) from birth to age 18. These charts are reproduced in Appendices 8A through 8D. Growth charts are more useful than height–weight charts for age in determining the growth pattern of individual children over time. By plotting the child's growth at intervals, one can ascertain how his or her growth relates to the pattern of growth of other children of the same age and sex by placing the child in a certain percentile as well as how the child is progressing within his or her own particular pattern. Although growth does not proceed in a smooth curve, most children stay in approximately the same curve during growth. During adolescence, however, many individuals will change in growth percentiles, though they usually return to the original percentile by the time growth is complete. Consider values that fall between the 25th and 75th percentile as normal. Monitor closely those children whose measurements fall consistently above or below these percentiles, since trends toward the upper and lower percentiles may reflect obesity or growth failure, respectively.[7]

In children under 3 years of age, measure the head circumference as well. In infants and young children, the head circumference is related to brain growth, and a small head circumference may reflect a deficiency of protein and/or kilocalories during the prenatal period and the first 2 years of postnatal life. In adolescents, the degree of genital and secondary sexual development is also useful as an index of nutritional status.

Need for Accurate Measurements. To prevent errors in interpretation of anthropometric data, use standard equipment and procedures, and appropriate standards for each index studied. For measuring body weight, use beam balance scales (calibrated two or three times annually with an object of known weight) rather than the spring balance type. Measure recumbent length (vs standing height or stature) during the first 2 years of life. Recumbent length is generally greater than stature by as much as 1 to 2 cm during the early years of life because of the influence of gravity.

Weight and height measurements should be taken at approximately the same time each day. Individuals are lightest in the morning and after vigorous exercise and heaviest after meals. Height also fluctuates during the day. Because of compression of the vertebral discs with daily activity, individuals shrink 1 to 2 cm. Allowances for fluid retention should also be made when measuring weight.

While most references suggest that nude measurements are preferred, this is not often practical. More importantly, correlate measurements with methodology used in developing the reference standards.

Body Compositional Indices. Although height and weight measurements are useful screening tools to detect underweight, overweight, and obesity, neither gives an index of the composition of excess or deficient weight, i.e., fat or protein. With overweight and obesity, the concern is with excessive fat not excess weight per se. For instance, an athlete with well-developed muscles, a muscular child, or a client with edema may be overweight by available standards but not obese. The extra weight is due to muscle bulk or fluid rather than adipose tissue. In contrast, in underweight clients, the concern is with loss of both fat and body protein.

Differentiate between the composition of the gain or loss in clients who are overweight (or obese) or underweight by evaluating skinfold thickness and midarm muscle circumference. Approximately one half of body fat is deposited subcutaneously, and ▶ **skinfold thickness** appears to be a good index of total body fat. Measurement of the thickness of the skinfold (which involves measuring the thickness of a double layer of pinched skin with its attached subcutaneous adipose tissue) can be done with a skinfold caliper at several body sites. The triceps and subscapular sites are most commonly used. However, the triceps fatfold is easier to measure because of its accessibility. This technique is useful not only for detecting a fat (and thus kilocalorie) excess or deficit but also for differentiating between the overweight and overfat client.

▶ The **midarm muscle circumference** indirectly reflects skeletal muscle mass and thus protein stores. When an inadequate consumption of protein or a combined protein–kilocaloric deficit is suspected, evaluate this measurement.

Techniques for measuring skinfold thickness and midarm muscle circumference are given in Appendices 9A and 9B. Percentile standards for these measurements have been published for white individuals 1 to 74 years of age,[8] and race, age, and sex-specific percentiles for triceps skinfold measurements are also available for blacks, ages 6 to 50 years.[9] Upper arm measurements that fall between the 5th and 25th percentiles may indicate moderate nutritional depletion, whereas those that fall below the 5th percentile indicate severe depletion. Conversely, skinfold measurements that fall above the 90th percentile denote probable obesity, and significant obesity may exist when the measurements are above the 95th percentile.

Since no data are available for use as standard for people over age 75 years, the mean triceps skinfold thickness in the 65 to 74.9 years is used as the standard for all people over age 65 years. Because of difficulty in obtaining accurate skinfold measurements in older adults and a great deal of normal variability in the triceps skinfold in older people, Russel suggests that a wide range of skinfold measurements, i.e., 40 to 190 percent of standard, is acceptable before judging a person as having too little or excessive fat stores.[10] A similar situation exists for the midarm muscle circumference measurements. For persons over 65 years, measurements that fall below 20 percent of the standard for persons 65 to 74.9 years may be considered to reflect diminished lean body mass.

Biochemical Assessment. Biochemical assessment uses a variety of biochemical tests to measure levels of nutrients and metabolites in body fluids and/or tissues or to evaluate certain biochemical functions that are dependent on an adequate supply of essential nutrients. In the course of malnutrition, expect most laboratory abnormalities to become evident before physical effects are seen. Because of this, biochemical analysis is a valuable adjunct to other assessment parameters in diagnosing marginal nutritional deficiency states as well as in monitoring the treatment of many common diseases. Should abnormalities be detected, appropriate intervention can then be implemented to prevent overt signs of disease.

As an assessment technique, biochemical analysis is more objective than clinical or dietary methods. If tissue levels of nutrients are normal, it can be assumed that dietary intake is adequate and nutrient use is normal. Because laboratory analysis can detect subclinical deficiency and because of the wide spectrum of nutritional disease and nonspecificity of clinical lesions, a poor correlation often exists between biochemical and clinical findings. Laboratory and dietary intake data are more likely to show a positive correlation than are laboratory and clinical data.

Biochemical studies vary from very simple to quite sophisticated ones. A variety of specimens are available for analysis, including blood, urine, cerebrospinal fluid, tissue biopsy (e.g., liver biopsy), and hair. Ethical considerations preclude extensive use of tissue biopsy. The most common specimens used are blood and urine. These body fluids are analyzed for their content of nutrients and metabolites, though this analysis gives no indication of body nutrient stores. Examples of some of the common blood tests are:

1. Hemoglobin
2. Hematocrit
3. Serum albumin
4. Serum vitamins
5. Serum iron
6. Serum enzymes

Use the results of urine analysis to determine the excretion of those nutrients and metabolites normally excreted in the urine, as well as those not normally excreted. Examples are as follows:[11]

Nutrients normally excreted in urine	Excess water-soluble vitamins
Metabolites normally excreted in urine	Creatinine, urea
Nutrients not normally excreted in urine	Glucose, albumin

The normal laboratory values for various tests of blood and urine are presented in Appendix 10.

The examination of scalp hair as a tool for the biochemical assessment of nutritional status, especially of trace minerals, protein, and calories, is beginning to be explored. Hair is very easily collected, stored, and prepared for analysis. However, there are many variables, such as age, sex, geographic location, and variations within an individual (such as rate of hair growth and distance of the sample from the hair follicle), that must be considered in evaluating and interpreting the data. Some doubts have been expressed regarding the value of hair analysis in determining trace mineral nutriture because of the affinity of the hair to contamination by metallic environmental pollutants. For example, beauty treatments (such as cold waving and bleaching of the hair and use of sprays, conditioners, or tints) have been found to increase the concentration of copper and zinc in the hair. The concentration of these minerals increases with increasing distance of the hair sample from the scalp.

Since the rate of protein synthesis in hair cells is one of the highest in the body, it appears reasonable that any factor that reduces the rate of protein synthesis in the body (such as protein–calorie malnutrition) would be a sensitive indication of the reduction. Visible changes in the hair (thinning, easy

Foods eaten in last 24 hours Kind and amount of food and drink (list main foods in mixed dishes)	NUMBER OF SERVINGS				
	Milk and Cheese	Meat	Vegetable– Fruit	Bread–Cereal	Fats–Sweets– Alcohol[a]
Morning:					
Midmorning:					
Noon:					
Afternoon:					
Evening:					
Before bed:					
Total servings eaten: _____					
Recommended servings: ____ __ ____ ____ ____					
Comparison: ____ __ ____ ____ ____					

NOTE:
   [a] These foods include the following:
      Butter, fortified margarine, cream, bacon, fatback, bacon grease, vegetable oil and shortening, sugar,
      candy, carbonated beverage, alcohol.
      Since these foods provide mainly kilocalories and few nutrients, they should not be used excessively
      in the diet.

Figure 11–5
*Dietary evaluation form.
(Source: Lewis CM: Basic and
Family Nutrition, A Self-In-
structional Approach, ed 2.
Philadelphia, FA Davis, 1984,
pp 135, 172. Adapted from Ex-
tension Service, USDA.)*

pluckability, and hypopigmentation—flag sign) have frequently been noted in children with severe protein–calorie malnutrition. Morphologic changes in the hair, including atrophy of the hair root, are now being investigated as an indicator of protein–calorie deficiency. At present, it appears that hair analysis as an indicator of protein–calorie malnutrition is most useful in those who are severely malnourished rather than suffering from borderline malnutrition. Ease of hair pluckability appears to be related more to protein depletion than to kilocalorie depletion.

Dietary Assessment. Dietary assessment includes (1) an evaluation of the nutrient adequacy of foods consumed and (2) a summary of the major factors affecting food intake. These data are useful for identifying present or potential nutritional problems or pinpointing the cause of nutritional problems that have been identified by other assessment techniques. The data also serve as a useful foundation for any intervention that is necessary to establish and maintain a satisfactory nutrient intake.

While evaluation of the nutrient adequacy of foods consumed is widely used to obtain presumptive evidence of dietary inadequacy or excess, in itself it is not an absolute indicator of adequate nutrition. Use dietary evaluation in conjunction with other assessment techniques to determine nutritional status. In contrast to clinical, anthropometric, and some of the biochemical assessment techniques that reflect long-term nutrient intake, most available techniques for evaluating the adequacy of nutrient intake reflect current intake only.

Dietary Evaluation. Evaluation of the adequacy of nutrient intake has two parts: (1) summary of food intake and (2) comparison with nutrient needs.

Obtain a summary of the client's dietary intake by using either the 24-hour recall technique or a written food intake record. When the 24-hour recall method is used, ask the client to recall from memory the intake of food and fluids for the 24-hour period preceding the interview. This method is simple, requires little technical knowledge, and can be completed within a time span of 15 to 20 minutes. Writing skills on the client's part are not required, and, since it is unannounced, there is no opportunity for the client to modify his/her eating behavior because of an awareness that food intake is being evaluated.

A sample form for recording the data is provided in Figure 11–5. Although a form similar to this may be used for planning the interview, use a conversational and casual approach, being matter-of-fact in vocal tone and facial expression, for the interview itself. Avoid influencing the interaction with verbal or nonverbal behaviors that could portray prejudices, values, assumptions, or perceptions. Be aware of these limitations of the technique in reflecting

SPECIFIC 24-HOUR RECALL		USUAL MEAL PATTERN	
Oatmeal	– 1 c	Cereal	– 1 c cooked
Bread	– 2 slices	Bread	– 2 slices
Margarine	– 2 tsp	Margarine	– 2 tsp
Coffee	– 1 c	Coffee with canned milk	
Canned milk	– ¼ c	and sugar	
Sugar	– 2 heaping tsp		

Figure 11–6
Comparison of 24-hour recall and usual meal pattern.

usual food intake: memory problems, unwillingness to share the information truthfully, and a tendency for the client to overreport small intakes and to underreport large intakes. Moreover, a single day's intake fails to reflect trends in food consumption. To increase the accuracy of the data, guide the client through the activities of the previous 24 hours and determine the times that food was eaten. Avoid labeling meals as "breakfast," "lunch," or "dinner." Ask open-ended questions rather than questions that can be answered with "yes" or "no." Provide models of food and measuring cups and spoons to aid in estimating quantities.[12] Follow up on verbal cues given by the client to get accurate data on adjuvants to the diet, such as sauces and salad dressings. For instance, if the client indicated that salad was consumed, determine what was served with the salad.

To further increase accuracy, repeat the recall randomly over a period of time, combine the recall with the pattern of usual food intake (Fig. 11–6) or the frequency of use of categories of food (Fig. 11–7).

The written food intake record entails having

the client keep a written record of food and beverage intake for a specified period of time. Although the length of time for recording the intake can vary, a 3-day record is frequently chosen. In contrast to the 24-hour recall, the written food record requires writing skills on the part of the client. There may also be the tendency to modify food intake for the period being assessed.[12]

Once the diet summary has been obtained, compare the intake with nutrient requirements, using either the Basic Four or the RDA (see Chap. 2) as the guide to dietary adequacy. While use of the RDA as the standard provides more precise information than does use of the Basic Four Food Groups, either method at best provides only a rough, crude estimate of nutrient intake. The primary value in evaluating the adequacy of food intake is to determine broad areas of dietary weakness.[12]

Assessment of Factors Affecting Intake. Many factors affect food intake and should be assessed for their contribution to actual or potential nutrition problems. Like the data obtained from dietary evaluation, the summary of factors influencing food intake is useful for determining appropriate interventions. Although some of the needed data may be available from the medical record, complete information may be lacking. Table 11–4 summarizes the major data needed.

Use of Nutritional Assessment Data

Once the anthropometric, biochemical, clinical, and dietary data are collected and analyzed, nutritional problems can be identified—and often the cause as well. Some problems are relatively simple and readily amenable to solution, whereas others are more complex and less easily solved.

Not every client will require the in-depth assess-

FOOD ITEM	FREQUENCY OF USE		
	Less than once per week	Not daily but at least once per week	Every day or nearly every day
Milk, cheese, ice cream, yoghurt	____	____	____
Eggs	____	____	____
Meat, fish, poultry	____	____	____
Bread, cereal, pasta and so on	____	____	____
Legumes, nuts, seeds, peanut butter	____	____	____
Fruit or fruit juices	____	____	____
Vegetables	____	____	____
Sugar and desserts	____	____	____
Beverages (coffee, tea, soft drinks, alcohol)	____	____	____
Miscellaneous snack items (chips, candy and so on)	____	____	____
Nutrient supplements (vitamins, minerals)	____	____	____

Figure 11–7
Food frequency checklist.

Table 11–4
FACTORS AFFECTING FOOD INTAKE

The following data related to nutritional intake status should be considered in a dietary assessment:

1. Discrepancy between food intake and nutrient needs (based on 24-hour recall)
2. Client's suggested weight based on body build
   Is client overweight or underweight?
   How does client perceive own weight?
3. Type of diet being followed prior to visit
   If a modified diet is being followed, who gave the diet instruction (physician, dietitian, nurse, self-prescribed, other)?
4. Has there been any change in eating patterns within the last few months?
5. Does the diagnosis or a restricted diet affect eating patterns?
6. Do any of the following factors affect food intake or utilization?

Limited biting, chewing ability	Constipation
Limited swallowing ability	Pica
Limited vision	Alcohol
Limited mobility	Snuff
Limited hand/arm coordination	Laxatives
Nausea	Tobacco
Vomiting	Allergies
Diarrhea	Medications

7. Socioeconomic factors to consider in relation to food intake
   Family size
   Last grade in school
   Income
   Occupation
   Activity level
8. Source of food
   Who purchases food?
   Where (e.g., independent grocery, supermarket)?
   How often?
   Home produced food?
   Food assistance (e.g., food stamps, WIC program, free or reduced priced meals in school or day care center, Meals-on-Wheels, congregate meals)
9. Food preparation and service
   Where are meals and snacks eaten?
   When?
   With whom?
   Who does preparation?
   Cooking and storage facilities
      Stove
      Oven
      Refrigerator
      Freezer
      Dry storage
10. Fluid intake
    Amount and type of fluid consumed with meals
    Amount and type of fluid consumed between meals
11. What relationship does the client see between food intake and health?
12. Do you think the information is reliable?

(*Source: Items 8 and 9 adapted from Lewis CM: Basic and Family Nutrition: A Self-Instructional Approach, ed 2. Philadelphia, FA Davis, 1984, p. 173.*)

ment including the clinical, anthropometric, biochemical, and dietary data discussed above. Reserve the in-depth assessment for those clients who are already at a high risk of malnutrition because of a particular physical, pathophysiologic, or socioeconomic state or those who, on initial screening, appear to require more rigorous assessment.

Selected sources of data have been included to give an overview of what data can be collected and to emphasize the importance of total assessment. However, in many nurse–client situations, the data may be incomplete. For instance, data related to actual intake may be available from the client, but certain anthropometric measures may be missing. Recognition of what data are missing is an important aspect of the assessment process, but identification of problems in such instances should nonetheless be done, based on the available data. Problems may become more severe if interventions are not initiated.

Assessment actually consists of two steps: the process of collecting data and the integration of ▶ these data into a product, the **nursing diagnosis.** Carpenito[13] defines the nursing diagnosis as:

. . . a statement that describes a health state or an actual or potential alteration in one's life processes (physiological, psychological, socio-cultural, developmental, and spiritual). The nurse uses the nursing process to identify and synthesize clinical data and to order nursing interventions to reduce, eliminate, or prevent (health promotion) health alterations which are in the legal and educational domain of nursing.

The formulation of this statement varies from one section of the country to another. However, a national group of nurses has been meeting since 1973 to determine a classification system in order to better clarify nursing diagnoses. This group has identified two accepted nursing diagnoses in nutrition. These are:

- *Nutrition, alterations in:* less than body requirements
- *Definition:* "the state in which an individual experiences or is at risk of experiencing reduced weight related to inadequate intake of nutrients."[14]

- *Nutrition, alterations in:* more than body requirements
- *Definition:* "The state in which the individual experiences or is at risk of experiencing weight gain related to an intake in excess of metabolic requirements."[15]

Although these diagnoses are general in nature, they are made specific to the individual client by combining them with data from the previous step of the assessment phase. These data would provide the etiologic and contributing factors and the manifestations of the problem unique to that individual. For example, a client who was underweight because

of nausea and vomiting related to therapy for cancer, which then caused weakness and fatigue, would have a nursing diagnosis stated as:

- *Alteration in nutrition:* less than body requirements related to nausea and vomiting from cancer therapy resulting in weakness and fatigue.

Examples of etiologic and defining characteristics that were developed by the National Group for Classification of Nursing Diagnosis are found in Tables 11-5, 11-6, and 11-7. Other nursing diagnoses approved by the national conferences that could be related to nutritional status include those concerned with fluid volume deficit or excess, self-care deficit in feeding, disturbance in self-concept—body image related to body size, alteration in bowel elimination, knowledge deficit, and noncompliance.[16]

As can be seen from this discussion, the nursing diagnosis derived from nutritional data should be within the nursing domain, a problem in which a nurse has the legal responsibility and educational preparation to intervene. Problems that demand the attention of a registered dietitian or a physician are not nursing diagnoses. The statement should include the general problem, the related etiology, and the manifestations seen in the individual client. All problems are identified whether they be actual or existing problems or potential ones that might arise as complications.

PLANNING

In planning care, the goal is to develop a course of action to return the client to, or maintain the client

---

TABLE 11–5
NUTRITION, ALTERATIONS IN: LESS THAN BODY REQUIREMENTS

Etiology	Defining Characteristics	
Inability to ingest or digest food or absorb nutrients due to biologic, psychologic, or economic factors	Loss of weight with adequate food intake 20% or more under ideal body weight Reported inadequate food intake less than RDA Weakness of muscles required for swallowing or mastication Reported or evidence of lack of food Lack of interest in food Perceived inability to ingest food Aversion to eating Reported altered taste sensation Satiety immediately after ingesting food	Abdominal pain with or without pathology Sore, inflamed buccal cavity Capillary fragility Abdominal cramping Diarrhea and/or steatorrhea Hyperactive bowel sounds Pale conjunctiva and mucous membranes Poor muscle tone Excessive loss of hair Lack of information, misinformation Misconceptions

(Source: Kim MJ, Moritz DA, eds: Classification of Nursing Diagnoses. Proceedings of the Third and Fourth National Conferences. New York, McGraw-Hill, 1982.)

TABLE 11–6
NUTRITION, ALTERATIONS IN: MORE THAN BODY REQUIREMENTS

Etiology	Defining Characteristics

Excessive intake in relationship to metabolic need	Weight 10% over ideal for height and frame
	Weight 20% over ideal for height and frame[a]
	Triceps skinfold greater than 15 mm in men and 25 mm in women[a]
	Sedentary activity level
	Reported or observed dysfunctional eating patterns
	   Pairing food with other activities
	   Concentrating food intake at end of day
	   Eating in response to external cues, such as time of day, social situation
	   Eating in response to internal cues other than hunger, e.g., anxiety

[a] Critical defining characteristic.
(*Source: Kim MJ, Moritz DA, eds: Classification of Nursing Diagnosis. Proceedings of the Third and Fourth National Conferences. New York, McGraw-Hill, 1982.*)

---

at, the best possible level of health. This phase also contains several steps. First, determine the priority level of each of the problems. Actual problems would take priority over potential ones. In some clinical situations, it might appear that nutritional needs are not high on the priority list, particularly when faced with either a respiratory or circulatory problem. However, an adequate nutritional state is essential for health, and, therefore, nutritional problems should not be ignored. Second, relate the plan directly to the specific problem list and delineate specific goals. Goals follow logically from the problem statement and indicate the status of the client when the problem has been solved. They should be both short term and long term. Recognize, however, that many nutritional problems are not solved over-

night, and, therefore, long-term goals are very important. Goals should meet the following criteria:

1. Mutually defined by and acceptable to the health team and the client
2. Realistic after considering strengths and weaknesses of the client and family and the resources available
3. Reflect the common objectives of the health team but are specific to nursing
4. Least disruptive of lifestyle, yet conducive to health restoration and/or maintenance

Once goals are delineated, identify specific outcome criteria by which progress can be measured. These criteria may be subjective, as measured by the client, or objective, but they must be measurable

---

TABLE 11–7
NUTRITION, ALTERATIONS IN: POTENTIAL FOR MORE THAN BODY REQUIREMENTS

Etiology	Defining Characteristics

Hereditary predisposition
Excessive energy intake during late gestational life, early infancy, and adolescence
Frequent, closely spaced pregnancies
Dysfunctional psychologic conditioning in relationship to food
Membership in lower socioeconomic group
	Reported or observed obesity in one or both parents[a]
	Rapid transition across growth percentiles in infants or children[a]
	Reported use of solid food as major food source before 5 months of age
	Observed use of food as reward or comfort measure
	Reported or observed higher baseline weight at beginning of each pregnancy
	Dysfunctional eating patterns
	   Pairing food with other activities
	   Concentrating food intake at end of day
	   Eating in response to external cues, such as time of day, social situation
	   Eating in response to internal cues other than hunger such as anxiety

[a] Critical defining characteristic.
(*Source: Kim MJ, Moritz DA, eds: Classification of Nursing Diagnoses. Proceedings of the Third and Fourth National Conferences. New York, McGraw-Hill, 1982.*)

and include a time frame in which they are to be accomplished. For example, a criterion related to losing weight should specify the amount of weight to be lost over what period of time.

Since various interventions are available, examine the alternatives and determine which interventions are appropriate for a specific client at a specific point in time. Some interventions may be more acceptable to the client than others, or some may be less costly than others. Consider factors such as these as well as the clinical data in selecting those to be implemented first.

These steps—determining priorities, defining goals, identifying outcome criteria, and selecting interventions—are the essence of the planning phase. The plan should be communicated in writing and coordinated with other health team members so that the plan and the role of each team member in implementing the plan are mutually understood and continuity of care is assured.

Documentation is best done in a standard manner. In many institutions, the nursing care plan is placed on a Kardex, which has appropriate space for the nursing diagnosis, goals and criteria, and suggested interventions written as nursing orders.

IMPLEMENTATION

Implementation involves putting the plan into action. In an institution that is organized through primary nursing, the nurse who is the primary caregiver would be responsible for not only initiating the plan but also for carrying out the specific actions and assuring that the persons who assumed responsibility in his or her absence also followed the plan. In team nursing, the team leader would be responsible for assigning the specific tasks to the appropriate team member. The primary nurse or the team leader would also be responsible for communicating and coordinating the plan with other health team members, such as the dietitian.

Expect numerous barriers to effective intervention when implementing the care plan. Some of the common barriers are:

- For many, motivation to practice preventive aspects of health is lacking. This is one of the most important reasons why good nutritional patterns are difficult to promote. Frequently, motivation to practice good nutritional habits is difficult to establish because the client cannot see the results immediately. Motivation can often be increased by providing rewards that are apparent within a reasonable period of time (such as the loss of 2 lb of weight per week in an obese client).
- Habits and customs are firmly rooted and are usually quite meaningful. This is especially true of food habits among the elderly and various cultural groups.

- Many clients lack knowledge about nutrition and methods of food preparation that are conducive to good nutritional health.
- In the hospital situation, the client is often subjected to malnutrition. For example, food may be withheld because of forthcoming laboratory tests, or the client may be receiving a feeding—such as a liquid diet or an intravenous feeding—that is inadequate to meet nutritional needs.
- In the home situation, the health team member has less control. In contrast to the hospital situation, roles are altered. The nurse or nutritionist is the visitor, though the expert, while the client is the host or hostess who may now feel more like the authority. This may affect the acceptance of suggestions. In addition, in the home situation, there are competing advisors. The influence of storekeepers, druggists, and neighbors may prevent a change in nutritional patterns.

Specific actions related to various clinical problems that will be used as interventions are found in Parts III and IV of this book.

EVALUATION

Like assessment, planning, and intervention, evaluation is part of the continuous process of nutritional care. Base evaluation on the criteria identified when the plan was established. The importance of the rationale for stating criteria in measurable terms is evident in the evaluation phase. A vague criterion, such as "improve dietary habits," is not easily evaluated. A specific criterion, such as "will lose 2 lb per week over the next 4 weeks," can be evaluated by weighing the client at the beginning and end of the 4-week period. Essentially, evaluation consists of again collecting data and comparing those data to the baseline data. Not only should criteria be evaluated but also factors that affect them, such as the acceptability of the intervention to the client. Evaluation indicates those problems that have been solved and those to which the problem-solving approach must be reapplied, e.g., reassessment and identification of continuing or new problems, establishment of new goals, plans of action, implementation, evaluation, reassessment, and so on. Thus the problem-solving approach is a continuous process.

CASE STUDY

Mrs. Jones is a 45-year-old white female who is receiving radiation therapy for cancer. She is 160 cm tall, and her current weight is 40 kg; her weight prior to diagnosis of cancer was 52.3 kg. She has tolerated therapy well but states, "I'm just not hungry," and "I'm tired all of the time." She is on a regular, select diet and eats all of her breakfast but only picks at the food brought to her at lunch and dinner. When questioned, she states, "Nothing tastes good anymore."

Nursing Diagnosis

Alteration in nutrition: less than body requirements related to decreased appetite and decreased taste associated with the effects of cancer and radiation therapy, resulting in weight loss and fatigue.

A. Goals
 1. Increase in kilocalorie and protein intake
 2. Prevention of further weight loss
 3. Decrease in fatigue
B. Criteria
 1. Kilocalorie intake will be 2100 and protein intake will be 100 g per day.
 2. Weight will be maintained at the current level during the period of radiation therapy
 3. Patient will express that she can perform normal activities without feeling tired
C. Interventions
 1. Assess exact kilocalorie and protein intake
 2. Assess level of activity and subjective measure of tiredness
 3. Assess food preference, consistency, and seasonings, and modify diet accordingly; suggest an increase of seasonings and tart flavors; notify dietary department
 4. Keep high-calorie, high-protein liquids available at bedside (milkshakes, eggnogs, or commercial formulas) and maintain cold temperature
 5. Measure liquid intake and maintain at least 2500 ml per 24 hours
 6. Increase amount of food served at breakfast but serve remaining meals in small amounts at more frequent intervals
 7. Provide mouth care before and after eating
 8. Provide a pleasant environment and social interaction at mealtimes to encourage eating
 9. Conserve energy through a balance of activity with scheduled rest periods, particularly after meals
 10. Obtain consultation from dietitian to assist with interventions 1, 3, and 6
D. Evaluation
 After 1 week, Mrs. Jones' weight was 41 kg. Her kilocalorie and protein intake varied on a daily basis but averaged 2000 kcal per day and 80 g protein; fluid intake averaged 2400 ml per 24 hours. She expressed that having small meals, including more seasoning, had made the food more appealing. She took interest in planning her daily schedule and stated that taking frequent rest periods during the day rather than "going until she got tired" helped to eliminate the tired feeling. No change needed in interventions at this time.

REVIEW QUESTIONS AND ACTIVITIES

1. Identify the four steps in the problem-solving approach to nursing care and explain their interrelationships.
2. Describe the characteristics of each of the following four major techniques used to assess nutritional status: (a) clinical, (b) anthropometric, (c) biochemical, and (d) dietary.
3. Identify an adult client in your clinical setting who has been described as being "malnourished."
 a. Use the results of his/her medical and social history and the checklist given in Figure 11-4 to assess the degree of risk of developing medical complications.
 b. List 10 parts of the body that may provide evidence that is suggestive of malnutrition.
 c. Review the results of the physical examination for signs that may be associated with malnutrition in any of the tissues that you listed in b above.
 d. Obtain the client's height and weight and classify his/her weight status, using the height–weight chart given in Appendix 7 to approximate desirable body weight.
4. Use Appendices 8B and 8D and content given in the chapter to evaluate the weight status of a 10-year-old boy who is 130 cm tall and weighs 25 kg and a 12-year-old girl who is 160 cm tall and weighs 55 kg.
5. Describe the use of skinfold and midarm muscle circumference measurements in anthropometric assessment.
6. Identify the two components of dietary assessment.
7. Identify the two components of a dietary evaluation, two methods of performing each, and the advantages and disadvantages of each method.
8. Design a simple form for using the 24-hour recall method of dietary evaluation and that uses the Basic Four Food Groups for evaluating dietary adequacy.
9. Describe three ways for increasing the accuracy of the 24-hour recall method of dietary assessment.
10. Identify additional information regarding factors affecting food intake that should be

obtained when conducting a dietary assessment.

11. Describe the use of nutritional assessment data in arriving at a nursing diagnosis.

12. Your client is an adult female who is 75 lb overweight.
    a. Conduct the appropriate assessment that is needed to establish a nursing diagnosis.
    b. Establish a nursing care plan that meets the four criteria listed in the chapter and that includes specific outcome criteria.
    c. Identify appropriate nursing interventions.
    d. Describe barriers that may impede successful implementation of the nursing care plan.
    e. Describe the evaluation phase of the nursing process relative to the outcome criteria established in b above.

REFERENCES

1. Lewis CM: Basic and Family Nutrition, A Self-Instructional Approach, ed. 2. Philadelphia, FA Davis, 1984, p 117.
2. Ibid, p 118.
3. Ibid, p 123.
4. Russel R: The Problems of Evaluating Nutritional Status of the Elderly. Chapel Hill, NC, Institute of Nutrition, University of North Carolina, 1983, p 7.
5. Jensen TG, Englert DM, Dudrick SJ: Nutritional Assessment, A Manual for Practitioners. E. Norwalk, Conn, Appleton-Century-Crofts, 1983, p 152.
6. Lewis CM, op cit, p 127.
7. Lewis CM, op cit, p 128.
8. Frisancho AR: New norms of upper limb fat and muscle areas for assessment of nutritional status. Am J Clin Nutr, 34:2540, 1981.
9. Cronk CE, Roche AF: Race and sex-specific reference data for triceps and subscapular skinfolds and weight/stature. Am J Clin Nutr 35:347, 1982.
10. Russel R, op cit, p 8.
11. Lewis CM, op cit, p 137.
12. Ibid, p 131.
13. Carpenito LJ: Nursing Diagnosis, Application to Clinical Practice. Philadelphia, JB Lippincott, 1983, p 4.
14. Ibid, p 287.
15. Ibid, p 302.
16. Kim MJ, Moritz DA, eds: Classification of Nursing Diagnosis. Proceedings of the Third and Fourth National Conferences. New York, McGraw-Hill, 1982, pp 279–338.

BIBLIOGRAPHY

Assessment of nutritional status. Am J Clin Nutr 35[Suppl], 1982.

Axelson JM, Csernus MM: Reliability and validity of a food frequency checklist. J Am Diet Assoc 83:152, 1983.

Baker JP, Detsky AS, Wesson DE, et al.: Nutritional assessment: A comparison of clinical judgment and objective measures. N Engl J Med 306:969, 1982.

Campbell C: Nursing Diagnosis and Intervention in Nursing Practice, ed 2. New York, John Wiley & Sons, 1984.

Carter, RL, Sharbaugh CO, Stapell CA: Reliability and validity of the 24-hour recall. J Am Diet Assoc 79:542, 1981.

DuRant RH, Linder CW: An evaluation of five indexes of relative body weight for use with children. J Am Diet Assoc 78:35, 1981.

Gordon M: Nursing Diagnosis, Process and Application. New York, McGraw-Hill, 1982.

Gray GE, Gray LK: Anthropometric measurements and their interpretation: Principles, practices, and problems," J Am Diet Assoc 77:534, 1980.

Hattner JA, Wood P: Assuring quality nutritional care in an acute-care setting. J Am Diet Assoc 77:165, 1980.

Hambridge KM: Hair analysis: Worthless for vitamins, limited for minerals. Am J Clin Nutr 36:943, 1982.

Kim MJ, McFarland GK, McLane, AM, eds: Classification of Nursing Diagnosis. Proceedings of the Fifth National Conference. St. Louis, CV Mosby, 1984.

Krantzler NJ, Mullen BJ, Comstock EM, et al.: Methods of food intake assessment—An annotated bibliography. J Nutr Educ 14(3):108, 1982.

Ometer JL: Documentation of nutritional care. J Am Diet Assoc 76:35, 1980.

St. Jeor ST, Guthrie HA, Jones MB: Variability in nutrient intake in a 28-day period. J Am Diet Assoc 83:155, 1983.

CHAPTER 12

The Nutrition Education Process

Objectives

After completion of this chapter, the student will be able to:
1. Distinguish between the components of planned behavior change and the learning process.
2. Assess the importance of values, attitudes, and beliefs held by the client and nurse in the nutrition education process.
3. Develop a plan for educating a client with a nutritional problem that incorporates (a) concepts of planned behavior change, (b) influence of motivation, values, attitudes, and beliefs held by the client and counselor, (c) major principles of learning, and (d) appropriate teaching techniques.

Opportunities for providing nutrition education present themselves throughout all stages of the life cycle and in various types of health care settings. Interest in nutrition is now at an all-time high, and clients are seeking usable, accurate nutrition information. Bombarded daily by conflicting messages about food and health, they are ready to learn the basic elements of nutrition, even though many are convinced that nutrition information is boring. Clients are also aware of their problems related to food and what works for them within their own lifestyle. These individuals want nutrition information available at the times and places where they are confronted with decisions about food, such as at the points of purchase, preparation, and consumption.

In the past, a considerable quantity of nurses' time has been spent in crisis intervention, e.g., assisting a client who has had a heart attack to adjust to the low-sodium, modified-fat diet component of the therapeutic regimen. However, nutrition plays too great a role in health promotion and maintenance to be relegated to the hit-or-miss, one-shot situation that often occurs in a medical crisis. Efforts must be focused on prevention of nutrition-related health problems, rather than solely on crisis inter-

vention. Within the health care system, a greater emphasis is now being placed on getting clients personally involved in measures that will maintain their health rather than on medical technology to cure disease.

This chapter presents basic principles of nutrition education that should be used when intervening in client situations as presented in Parts III and IV.

NUTRITION EDUCATION AND DIET COUNSELING

Nurses expend considerable effort in providing nutrition education and diet counseling, both of which are important aspects of intervention in the nursing process. Use the problem-solving approach described in Chapter 11 when imparting nutrition information whether it be teaching a pregnant woman in a community setting the principles of the diet or providing reinforcement to the dietitian's teaching about a client's modified diet in a hospital setting. Documentation for the purpose of sharing pertinent information with other team members is also essential.

Nutrition education involves more than disseminating nutrition facts. It is a process, multidisciplinary in nature, that bridges the gap between information and practice. It involves both imparting nutrition information and developing clients' motivation to use the information in their life patterns. Nutrition education continues throughout life and changes in focus as nutritional needs change with maturation (from infancy through old age) and also as research brings out new findings about nutritional needs throughout the life cycle and in wellness/illness management. If the education is effective, the client will put the information into practice as a new habit or as a modification of an old one.

In clinical settings, nutrition education is often provided through counseling. While much informal counsel is given regarding diet—such as that provided by the mass media—**diet counseling** is defined for the professional as the process of providing individualized guidance to assist a person to adjust his daily food consumption to meet his health needs.[1]

Processes Involved in Nutrition Education

Changing a habit of any kind is a difficult and slow process; this is especially true of habits of daily living, such as food habits. Like other behaviors, eating behavior is psychologically motivated, but it is also influenced by biologic, cultural, and situational factors. Any educational program should recognize this interaction. While food habits may change readily if forced by circumstances or if rewards are immediate, change is often impeded by the fact that the immediate reward of _not_ changing often obscures the potential future benefits of the change.

Two of the major processes involved in effective education are planned behavioral change and the learning process itself. The relationship of knowledge to practice, human motivation, and values, attitudes and beliefs are common threads that run through each of these. A client may gain the knowledge needed to change behavior—in this case eating behavior—through diet counseling sessions, but may not actually eat differently because of lack of motivation or because of some deep-seated value or belief about food that impedes the change.

A frequent comment made by nurses is: "Why doesn't Mrs. Jones follow her diet? She has been told repeatedly what she can and cannot eat!" To answer this question, consider these questions, which must be answered before a successful resolution can occur. What is the relationship between Mrs. Jones' knowledge and practice about diet? Is she motivated to follow the diet? What are her values, attitudes, and beliefs related to foods?

Although knowledge is positively correlated to beneficial change, few practices are altered because of knowledge alone. Clients are more likely to transfer knowledge to practice if they are motivated to do so and if the change is consistent with their values. Ethical considerations demand that a delineation be made between the client's and the educator's motivations and values; keep this delineation in perspective.

The key to change in habits is motivation. Consider this question: What is in it for the client? People are motivated by both personal and societal forces, and motivational factors will differ depending on the individual. A motivational force that has particular relevance when providing nutrition teaching is ego involvement. Ego involvement, or self-concern, permeates all actions. For ego involvement to be a positive force in the educational process, tailor the message to the needs and interests of the client, actively involve the client in the process, and recognize the motivational value of praise. Often a nurse's commitment to long-range health goals is not shared by the client; the certain pleasures of the moment may take precedence over the uncertain future gains. Thus, at times the ego involvement of a nurse and client will be in conflict. This must be recognized and kept in focus.

Unless health is clearly threatened, health maintenance alone is usually insufficient as a motivational force. For most, health is not perceived as an end in itself but as a means of achieving life's purposes. While fear of death may be sufficient motivation for the middle-aged man with cardiac insufficiency or chronic renal failure to follow a dietary regimen, it may not suffice for the robust adolescent—for whom death is a remote possibility—to follow a modified-fat dietary regimen as a preventive measure against heart disease. For the adolescent, a more realistic approach would be to discuss how adherence to the particular dietary regimen may help to achieve the goals that the adolescent holds most dear.

Individual values, which are constantly being acquired and shaped through learning, usually reflect those of the culture at large and those of important others in the environment. Be aware that it is very difficult to change food patterns that are deeply rooted in values. When promoting a desired change, avoid creating a communication barrier by failing to perceive the client's values. Weigh questions involving values and consider the benefits of changing vs not changing. Although nurses must be careful not to impose their own values on others, they have both the opportunity and the responsibility to contribute in a positive way to shaping others' values.

Planned Behavioral Change. The elements of planned behavioral change can be used by nurses to improve nutrition through organized intervention. Planned behavioral change is a five-step process: (1) development of awareness of the problem, (2) development of a receptive framework for learning, (3) trial, (4) reinforcement, and (5) adoption.[2]

In the stage of developing awareness of a problem, assist the client to identify specific problems related to food consumption that need to be solved.

This involves outlining facts related to the situation, interpreting the facts, and at times identifying possible courses of action.

To develop a receptive framework for learning, first establish your own credibility. Then become aware of the client's prior perceptions about food and nutrition and identify changes that are needed and feasible. The credible nutrition instructor not only is knowledgeable and enthusiastic about the topic but also has the ability to empathize with the needs and attitudes of the learner—without over-identifying. Prior perception will influence the learning process, and inaccurate facts related to nutrition must first be corrected before new learning can occur. Although certain changes may be needed, they may not always appear feasible to the learner. For example, the retired couple with a reduced income may feel that accepting food stamps is degrading to their integrity and may need considerable encouragement to see this as a feasible option.

The third phase of planned change is trial or experimentation with ideas, techniques, and programs until acceptable ones are found. Strengthen the learning initiated in the trial phase through reinforcement to increase the likelihood that the desired change will be adopted. Learning is reinforced by repetition and by transfer to other similar situations. The reinforcement phase may involve making adjustments whose necessity becomes apparent during the trial. For example, if transportation is identified as a problem for the elderly couple trying to use food stamps, this problem will have to be solved if they are to continue with the program.

The final phase of change is adoption of the desired change into daily habits or practice. Throughout the change process, however, keep in mind that resistance to change is normal. Change takes time and occurs in small steps. If the desired change is complex, approach aspects that are relatively easy and uncomplicated first.

The Learning Process. The processes of teaching and learning are different, though related. According to behaviorist theory, learning, by definition, is behavior change. For example, the client following a sodium-restricted diet who can identify the low-sodium snack foods at a party but who still munches on the salty ones has not learned but has only been informed.

Learning involves an interaction among three aspects of the human personality: cognition ("I know how to do it"), emotion ("I want to do it"), and will ("I will do it").[3] Cognition, or the thought process that leads to formation of concepts and principles, provides the knowledge base for reasoning and analysis. Emotional responses associated with particular items of information or particular situations create tensions that stimulate the client to act. Feeling an unfulfilment, lack, or need, the client wants to do something about it. The will to act to change behavior arises from the conviction that the item of infor-

mation can fill the need and reduce the tensions aroused.

In order to successfully stimulate behavior change, obtain a broad grasp of the client's knowledge, attitudes, and beliefs related to food. This thorough assessment of the total eating pattern reveals not only what problems exist but the why behind them. At the same time, carefully evaluate your own value system related to food and eating and guard against imposing this system on others. Attempt to change only those dietary practices that are harmful. Many dietary practices, although not beneficial, may be harmless and should not be disturbed. For instance, carbonated beverages add little to the nutritive value of the diet but, unless used excessively or contraindicated because of the presence of a particular health problem, do not lead to detrimental effects.

People are never too old to modify a habit or acquire a new skill. While older clients may be resistant to a change in dietary patterns and these changes may be made more slowly, the capacity to learn does not decline with age.

Gear learning experiences to the physical, cognitive, and emotional readiness of the client and present the instruction in terms that the client can understand. Much of the printed nutrition material currently available is geared to middle-class individuals and may not be useful to those with little education. Make a judgment about the amount of details to give; a common mistake is to give too much information at once or too soon. For example, one would not explain the intricacies of the Krebs cycle to someone who simply asked the source of the body's energy. If overwhelmed with information, suggestions, or teaching materials, the client may be unable to distinguish essential from nonessential information. How much one includes is dependent on the level of comprehension and motivation.

Search constantly for techniques to increase motivation to change food habits. Usually, members of various subcultural groups share many common concerns, values, attitudes, and beliefs, and teaching approaches can be directed toward these commonalities. For example, most elderly individuals are concerned about maintaining their independence by living in their own homes. A viable motivational force to accept nutrition teaching may be to correlate nutrition to health maintenance as a means of maintaining independence. However, when using group commonalities as a basis for devising teaching approaches, guard against stereotyping.

When establishing a dietary teaching plan for a client, follow these four learning principles: (1) develop learning objectives, (2) establish contact points for learning, (3) provide for active participation by the learner, and (4) provide feedback and evaluation.

Learning Objectives. Clearly define mutually agreed upon learning goals and objectives in measurable terms of the behavior expected of the client when the content has been mastered. Too often, the focus is placed on the content to be taught rather than on the client's outcome.

Be sure that the objectives are realistic and take into consideration the difficulty of changing lifelong eating patterns. Gear objectives to allow for a series of small steps with rewards established for the successful completion of each step. Even when the motivation is high, small steps are required to permit a feeling of success. The inevitable failure of an immediate massive dietary change often discourages further efforts. For instance, a hypertensive client may be overwhelmed when told that he must immediately restrict all sources of dietary sodium. A better approach for some clients may be to first identify the sodium sources that could be given up most readily, restrict these initially, and then establish a plan for gradual elimination.

Contact Points. Effective learning requires that there be contact or overlap with content or practices that are already familiar. Initiate the teaching at the client's level of information. Change is also easier to make if it is approached within the context of existing practices. Reinforce current positive dietary practices and make every effort to impose as few changes as possible.

Active Participation. Learning is an active process that requires the active participation of the client in planning, selecting teaching methods, and evaluation. A client is more likely to follow a diet if it is planned with him and not for him. For example, a group of elderly clients will be more responsive to topics they helped choose than to abstract or general information that may be irrelevant to their concerns.

Feedback and Evaluation. Frequent and explicit feedback regarding the learner's performance speeds the process of learning by providing motivation—the more immediate the feedback the greater the motivational potential. Include praise as feedback when appropriate and provide reinforcement as necessary for motivation.

Evaluate the learning process constantly in terms of both the client's progress and your effectiveness. At various intervals, assess the learner for changes in attitudes and behavior. This appraisal may take the form of questions that require more than a "yes" or "no" answer, demonstrations by the client, or practice of the change in the client's own life situation.

Two additional aspects of the learning process deserve consideration: (1) the degree to which learning takes place through the human senses and (2) the degree to which information is retained. It has been suggested that 95 percent of learning is initiated by vision and hearing (85 percent through the eyes and 10 percent through the ears), and the remaining 5 percent comes through the tongue, skin, and nose. Retention and learning are also directly related to involvement. As the client becomes more involved by seeing, hearing, and doing, retention increases. Planning tasting parties for young children to introduce them to new foods is a technique that allows for application of these concepts of learning. A child may feel encouraged to eat a different food if he or she participates in a session involving its preparation and eating, with emphasis given to the food's sensory aspects (such as color, texture, sound, smell, and taste).

TECHNIQUES USED IN NUTRITION EDUCATION

A wide variety of techniques can be employed in nutrition education and diet counseling. Since no single technique is adequate for all audiences, use a variety of techniques for individuals or groups with differing needs, interests, and intellectual levels.

Techniques and Tools

Formal and informal techniques are used in teaching individuals, groups, and the population at large. Opportunities for informal teaching constantly arise in conversations with clients in both hospitals and ambulatory care settings. Nurses also provide informal education when serving as role models—"practicing what they preach."

When dealing with problems common to a specific group, such as diabetic clients, a group approach can be successfully used provided the teaching is supplemented with individualized instruction to deal with specific problems. The group approach is beneficial in that clients can share common experiences, such as problems they may be having in following a diabetic diet. Group instruction should be a democratic process in which everyone feels free to participate.

The best results in education and counseling are usually obtained when a nondirective approach is followed. With this approach, guide clients toward seeking solutions to their own particular problems, for example, ask them what they feel they can personally do to solve the problem of failure to adhere to a specific diet.

The usual teaching methods and teaching tools can be used in counseling sessions. The discussion approach, rather than lectures, tends to be more successful in changing food habits. This may be in part because auditory learning alone is only minimally effective for most people. The effectiveness of lectures can be increased, however, when they are accompanied by visual stimulation, such as using the chalkboard, pictures, posters, flip charts, filmstrips, and slides. Demonstrations, when accompanied by return demonstrations, and role playing actively involve the learner and are a definite stimulus to learning.

Other devices can also be used, for example, bulletin, felt, or magnetic boards, opaque or overhead projectors, films, radio, television, or conventional records, printed materials such as pamphlets, flash cards, and programmed instruction, and games, including simulation games.

Printed Materials. Printed materials are by far the most commonly used educational tool with individual clients. The materials used are usually in the form of short printed pamphlets or mimeographed sheets. Assess the reading level of this printed material; its usefulness is diminished if the client's reading ability is limited.

Mass Media. A wide range of formats, including television, radio, and various types of printed materials, are available for providing nutrition education. The potential for providing nutrition education in this manner is tremendous.

Since television station managers are required to accept a certain number of public service announcements, television can be used as a medium for nutrition education. Less expensive than television, radio campaigns can also reach large numbers of people and should not be overlooked as a potentially powerful tool. Radio broadcasts also include public service announcements and special formats, such as talk shows, that allow for more depth in discussing controversial topics.

The mass media also provide several printed formats that can serve as a forum for nutrition education. These include popular magazines, comic books, nutrition books for the lay public, newspapers, and photographs or graphics used in advertising campaigns. Many articles on food and nutrition appear in popular magazines and newspapers. Unfortunately, trained health professionals are not always involved in their preparation, and erroneous or poorly justified recommendations are sometimes made, with a detrimental effect.

Book stores are flooded with books on nutrition designed for the lay public. Some of the popular books are written by individuals presenting sensational ideas about dietary prevention or cures—and thus exploiting the public. A suggested list of reference materials for the lay public has been published by the Society for Nutrition Education,[4] and a similar reference list has been published for professionals.[5]

Audiovisual Materials. Slide–tape presentations, filmstrips, and movies, like television, provide a combination of auditory and visual stimuli to learning. Television has created an audience accustomed to sophisticated audiovisual communication. A listing of audiovisual teaching aids available from various sources is available from the Society for Nutrition Education.[6] This society, in conjunction with the Center for Nutrition Education, has published material to guide the selection and use of nutrition education material and resources.[7]

Games. Games can be a pleasant way to learn. A resource publication contains information for choosing, ordering, and preparing over 100 games for kindergarten through grade 12 in the biologic, physical, earth/space, and general sciences, along with a summary of their rules.[8] The publication includes nutrition-related games. Simulation games, which are imitations of real situations, can also be used.

REVIEW QUESTIONS AND ACTIVITIES

1. Identify five steps involved in planned behavior change and four major learning principles. Give an example of the use of each of these steps and principles in a nutrition education or counseling session with a client of your choice.
2. Discuss the role of the human senses and of personal involvement in the learning process.
3. Describe the influence of motivation, values, attitudes, and beliefs about food and eating held by the client in assisting a client to change nutritional habits. How do the values, attitudes, and beliefs about food and eating held by the nutrition counselor influence the learning process?
4. Visit the patient education center in your clinical setting:
   a. Determine the types of materials that are available for teaching a client with a nutritional problem of your choice.
   b. Evaluate the strengths and weaknesses of each of the available teaching aids.
5. Select a recent popular book about nutrition and assess its appropriateness for use as a teaching aid for the lay public.
6. Prepare a simple teaching aid, either individually or as a group project, that would be useful in teaching clients basic nutrition facts.

REFERENCES

1. American Dietetic Association: Guidelines for developing dietary counseling services in the community. J Am Diet Assoc 55:343, 1969.
2. Gifft HH, Washbon MB, Harrison GG: Nutrition, Behavior, and Change. Englewood Cliffs, NJ, Prentice-Hall, 1972.
3. Williams SR: Nutrition and Diet Therapy, ed. 4. St. Louis, CV Mosby, 1981, pp 298–299.
4. National Nutrition Education Clearinghouse: Nutrition for Everybody. Berkeley, Calif, Society for Nutrition Education, 1981.
5. National Nutrition Education Clearinghouse: Nutrition Information Resources for Professionals. Berkeley, Calif, Society for Nutrition Education, 1978.
6. Society for Nutrition Education: Audiovisuals for Nutrition Education—Education Resource Series No. 9. Berkeley, Calif, 1979.
7. Profiling Nutrition Education Materials, An Instrument with Manual. Oakland, Calif, Society for Nutri-

tion Education and Center for Nutrition Education, 1983.

8. Hounshell PB, Trollinger IR: Games for the Science Classroom. Washington, DC, National Science Teachers Association, 1977.

BIBLIOGRAPHY

Anderson RJ, Kirk LM: Methods of improving patient compliance in chronic disease states. Arch Intern Med 142:1673, 1982.

Christopher C, Shannon B, Sims LS: A multimedia approach to nutrition education. J Nutr Educ 12:8, 1980.

Council on Scientific Affairs, American Medical Association: American Medical Association concepts of nutrition and health. JAMA 242:2335, 1979.

Falck VT: Application of the behavioral sciences to dietary practices. Nutr. Today 16:28, 1981.

Fleming, PL, Brown JE: Using market research approaches in nutrition education. J Nutr Educ 13:4, 1981.

Hertzler AA: Recipes and nutrition education. J Am Diet Assoc 83:466, 1983.

Levy SR, Iverson BK, Walberg HJ: Nutrition education research: An interdisciplinary evaluation and review. Health Educ Q 7:107, 1980.

National Conference on Nutrition Education: Directions for the 1980s. J Nutr Educ 12(2) [Suppl 1], 1980.

Proceeding of the Workshop on Nutrition Education Research: Applying principles from the behavioral sciences. J Nutr Educ 13(1) [Suppl 1], 1981.

Singer EA: Folklore for nutrition education. J Nutr Educ 14(1):12, 1982.

Wardlaw JM: Preparing the nutrition education professional for the 1980s. J Nutr Educ 13:6, 1981.

PART III

Nutrition Throughout the Life Cycle

As a component of comprehensive health care, nutritional care contributes to promotion of wellness, health maintenance, and treatment of disease in all types of health care settings. Indeed, the degree to which clients meet their nutritional needs at the appropriate level is often the decisive factor in health maintenance and restoration.

Nutritional excesses and deficits of differing intensity have been identified in various segments of the population. Both have

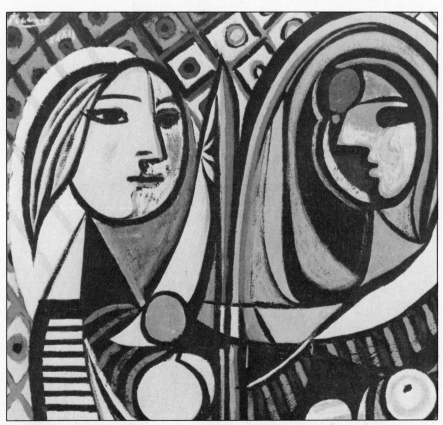

Pablo Picasso *Girl Before a Mirror*

a negative influence on health status. While health problems associated with nutrient deficit are well documented, those associated with excess, except for obesity, are less well defined. The results of several nutritional surveys describing the prevalence of malnutrition were presented in Chapter 1. In these surveys, nutrient adequacy was found to be rather loosely associated with income and educational level. While adequate income or a high level of education is no assurance of an optimum diet, individuals and families with a low income and/or educational level are at a much higher risk of consuming an inadequate diet. The problem of nutritional excess affects all segments of the population.

Throughout the life cycle, food habits and practices must be promoted that will contribute to optimal health and prevent nutrition-related health problems. For instance, nutritional needs of pregnant women must be given special attention to assure the fetus a nutritional environment that promotes optimal growth and development. Part III provides the information needed for nurses to provide nutritional care for clients at all stages of the life cycle. A discussion of alternative dietary practices, including cultural and ethnic dietary patterns, is also included.

CHAPTER 13

Relationship of Nutrition to Growth and Development

Objectives

After completion of this chapter, the student will be able to:
1. Distinguish between the terms "growth" and "development."
2. Compare and contrast the processes involved in the three phases of cellular growth and assess the relationship between nutritional influences on growth of the brain and adipose tissue during each of the three phases.
3. Differentiate between the three phases of physical growth (in height and weight) and assess the relationship between nutritional influences on physical growth during each of the three phases.
4. Assess the overall relationships between hereditary and environmental influences to physiologic and psychosocial growth and development, including the development of food habits in children.

Nutrition is an important environmental influence affecting physiologic and psychosocial growth and development during each phase of the life cycle. Since both nutritional needs and responses to food change as the individual progresses through the life cycle, knowledge of these changes is necessary in order to provide the nutrients required for optimum physiologic and psychosocial development.

Food habits are formed very early in life. In order to foster good eating habits and prevent feeding problems in children, knowledge of the usual response to food at a given stage is as essential as a knowledge of food needs.

Recognition of the relationship between an adequate supply of food and the promotion of growth, development, and health has stimulated governmental agencies to sponsor various programs that provide food and nutrition services to individuals, families, or specific target groups within the family, e.g., pregnant and lactating women and the elderly.

This chapter presents an overview of the fundamental relationship of nutrition to growth and development and the various influences on developing

food patterns. This material provides a framework for study of nutritional needs and responses to food during specific periods of the life cycle, which are presented in subsequent chapters. The governmental food assistance programs are integrated into the appropriate developmental chapters.

GROWTH AND DEVELOPMENT

▶ The term **growth** denotes increase in size as a result
▶ of cell division, and the term **development** refers to increased complexity of function, both physiologic
▶ and psychosocial. The combined term **growth and development** incorporates the complex physiologic and psychosocial changes that occur to transform a helpless infant into a physically and emotionally mature adult.

While growth and development follows an orderly sequence, the timing of each occurrence varies within an age group. For example, babies creep before they walk. However, not all babies begin creeping at the same age. Incisor teeth erupt before the bicuspids, but the age at which the incisor eruption begins varies with individuals. Growth and development are influenced by both hereditary and environmental factors. Environmental influences may be physical (e.g., availability of food) or psychosocial (e.g., exposure to learning stimuli). Nutrition is one of the environmental influences affecting both physiologic and psychosocial growth and development.

In the sections that follow, nutrition is discussed specifically in relation to its effects on (1) physical growth and development and (2) psychosocial growth and development.

RELATIONSHIP OF NUTRITION TO PHYSICAL GROWTH AND DEVELOPMENT

Assessment and Intervention

In order to achieve the maximum genetic potential in physiologic growth and development, food should be adequate in quality and quantity and be consumed at the correct time (developmental stage) to support maximum growth and development of the various organs and tissues. To appreciate the importance of timing of the nutrient supply, a consideration of how growth occurs at the level of both the cell and the body as a whole is necessary.

Cellular Growth. Cellular growth occurs as a result
▶ of **hyperplasia** (cell division with an increase in
▶ cell number) and **hypertrophy** (enlargement in size of existing cells) and occurs in three phases:[1]

- *Phase 1.* Hyperplasia alone or rapid cell division with ↑ DNA; cell size remains constant
- *Phase 2.* Hyperplasia and hypertrophy; cell division with ↑ DNA; cell enlargement with ↑ protein content (hypertrophy)
- *Phase 3.* Hypertrophy alone; cell enlargement with ↑ protein content; cell number remains constant

These three cellular growth phases follow a chronologic schedule for each organ, but the timing of the stages may vary. All body organs grow by hyperplasia in fetal life and for varying periods postnatally.

Phases 1 and 2 are the most critical periods in organ development, since they involve an increase in cell number due to cell division. Malnutrition (either undernutrition or overnutrition) during these phases may affect the ultimate cell number in the organ and has the potential for producing other permanent effects. In contrast, with malnutrition occurring during Phase 3 (hypertrophy alone), the organ may be temporarily smaller or larger, but it returns to normal size when nutritional supplies are present at the optimal level.

Growth in Height and Weight. Physical growth results from an increase in body size as measured by changes in height (stature) and weight. Height

is a better indicator of total body growth than is weight, since growth in height reflects long-term nutritional intake, whereas weight changes reflect recent nutritional experiences.

Although growth is a continuous process from conception to maturity, it does not occur at a uniform rate. Rather, it consists of three growth periods: two periods of rapid growth and one period of slow, uniform growth. Following these periods, growth levels off in the adult plateau and gradually declines with aging. The periods of rapid growth are (1) fetal life through early infancy (first 6 months) and (2) adolescence (ages 10 to 13 in girls and 12 to 15 in boys). The period of late infancy through late childhood (through approximately age 10 in girls and age 12 in boys) is characterized by slow, uniform growth. Since nutritional needs correlate with rate of growth, larger quantities of food relative to body weight are required during growth spurts than during periods of slower growth.

Effects of Malnutrition on Growth. Malnutrition during the growth cycle may alter the growth rate and, consequently, the final size attained. In addition to the effects on the size of the body as a whole, the size of specific organs may be affected. In recent years, cellular development in the brain and adipose tissue (fat tissue) has been intensively studied in relation to nutrient intake, and undernutrition (in the brain) or overnutrition (in adipose tissue) during the critical period of hyperplasia may affect the number of cells in these organs, which, in turn, may have long-lasting effects on their function.

Effect of Malnutrition on Stature. Final height achieved at maturity depends on (1) the rate of growth during and (2) the duration of each growth period. Although nutritional deficiency during any of the growth phases may limit final height attained, pay particular attention to assisting families with children undergoing growth spurts to attain an adequate supply of food, since demands are higher at these times.

The permanence of growth retardation secondary to nutritional deficiency appears to depend on age of onset, duration, and severity of the nutrient lack. Although nutritional rehabilitation results in catch-up growth, the probability of achieving the maximum genetic potential for growth appears to lessen when prolonged, severe malnutrition occurs early in life.

As a result of availability of both good nutrition and good health care in the United States, the height of American children has progressively increased during the past 50 years. However, there are indications that the trend of increasing size in successive generations is diminishing or ceasing, since the growth rate for both boys and girls has leveled off in recent years.

Despite the availability of good nutrition and health care in the United States, growth retardation is a significant nutritional problem. A number of national nutritional surveys have revealed a significant number of children whose heights and weights fall below national standards (see Chap. 1).

Effect of Malnutrition on the Central Nervous System.

Because the brain is the first body to complete its growth, it is the most vulnerable of body organs to undernutrition. The risk of impaired brain development is particularly high if the nutritional deficits occur early in life and are severe and long lasting without treatment. Brain growth occurs by hyperplasia during (1) prenatal life and (2) the first 2 years of postnatal life, with maximum growth occurring 3 months before and 6 months after birth. Following the second year, the brain grows by hypertrophy. By 4 years of age, 80 to 90 percent of adult brain size has been achieved. Undernutrition of significant severity and duration during the hyperplastic growth phase results in structural changes in the brain that are permanent. Because of reduced cell division, the brain contains fewer cells. The smaller brain size is reflected in a below-normal head circumference. Brain functioning is also altered in association with severe malnutrition, and malnourished infants and children exhibit varying degrees of behavioral abnormalities, including impaired learning and intellectual development and, in some cases, mental retardation.

While the irreversible changes in brain structure associated with early malnutrition are easily identifiable, it has not been possible to pinpoint malnutrition as the sole causative factor in the altered brain function that accompanies the malnutrition. Assess other aspects of the environment of malnourished children. Malnutrition is usually associated with a poor social environment in which other factors, such as limited education, poor sanitation, and recurrent infection, interact to produce behavioral changes. The currently accepted theory is that the developmental delays associated with malnutrition are a combined effect of inadequate nutrition and an impoverished social environment.[2] Further, the developmental delays, once thought to be irreversible, can be minimized or reversed with nutrition rehabilitation and environmental enrichment programs. Although one tends to compensate for the other, the best results can be expected when both nutrition and the social environment are improved. Attempt to provide nutritional treatment and rehabilitation for malnourished infants early in the first year if possible, since this improves their chances of recovery of normal or near normal intellectual functioning. With more severe forms of protein-energy malnutrition, the deficits appear to be more long lasting and the potential for rehabilitation less favorable, although recent studies suggest that the potential long-term effects of early, severe malnutrition may be greatly attenuated or, in some instances, virtually eliminated by providing a developmentally supportive environment at a later time.[2]

Effect of Malnutrition (Kilocaloric Excess) on Adipose Cells.

Adipose tissue also grows by hyperplasia and hypertrophy. It has been postulated that the periods of adipose hyperplasia are (1) the third trimester of fetal life, (2) the first and second years of postnatal life, and (3) adolescence (10 to 12 years of age).[3] It has also been hypothesized that adipose cell number becomes fixed during adolescent or early adult life and that kilocaloric excess during periods of adipose hyperplasia can result in a permanent increase in fat cell number with subsequent weight control problems that persist throughout life.[4] Some studies have shown that at all ages obese children have both a greater number and greater size of adipose cells than nonobese children,[4] and the suggestion has been made that the normal person ceases to add fat cells to the body between the ages of 2 and 10 to 12 and then resumes production of new fat cells during puberty. In contrast, the obesity-prone child continues to add fat cells to the body during the first 10 years of life and enters adolescence with an abnormally large number of cells.[5] Other studies have suggested that an increase in fat cell size, but not in fat cell number, occurs in obesity with its onset in adults.[6]

The fat cell hypothesis has been extended further to include a classification of obesity based on the number and size of the fat cells. **Hyperplastic obesity** is associated with an increased number of fat cells, whereas **hypertrophic obesity** is associated with an increase in fat cell size. Thus the more severe form of obesity, with onset early in life, is called hyperplastic–hypertrophic obesity (an increase in both cell number and cell size), and adult-onset obesity, usually a milder form, is termed hypertrophic obesity (increase in cell size only). Weight reduction and maintenance of weight loss are much more difficult in hyperplastic than in hypertrophic types of obesity.

The fat cell hypothesis remains controversial, since data on the development of adipose tissue are far from complete and the notion that fat cell number is fixed in adults can be questioned. Further, the accuracy of the techniques used to measure fat cell numbers has also been questioned, and such studies must be interpreted with great care. In actual practice, there is some overlap in the cellularity and age-of-onset relationships in obesity. Some individuals with early-onset obesity may have a normal number of fat cells, and other individuals with adult-onset obesity may be hypercellular with regard to fat cells. Moreover, the evidence has been reexamined and further studies of adipose tissue have been conducted using tissue from individuals of all ages that show that cell proliferation probably continues into adulthood.[7-9] It has been theorized that there may be a critical size beyond which fat cells cannot increase, and at this point cell proliferation is stimulated. If this scheme operates, both hyperplastic and hypertrophic obesity can exist in adults as well as children. Finally, the results of various experimental studies have not shown clear correlations between the presence of obesity during infancy, a critical period of fat cell division, and obesity in later life. Weight status during later childhood and adolescence tends to be more predictive of weight status in adulthood.

At present it is not clear how important the size and number of adipose cells are in the etiology and treatment of obesity or whether adipose tissue hyperplasia is really irreversible. Although the question, "Does a fat baby become a fat child or a fat adult?" cannot now be answered with certainty, regardless of whether obesity occurs in children or in adults, it is discouragingly refractory to treatment. This is particularly true of obesity with onset early in life. The success rate for maintaining a reduced weight is low regardless of the initial number of cells. Once obesity is established, kilocaloric restriction and weight loss reduce the fat content and size of fat cells but do not change the number. For these reasons, give attention to preventing obesity throughout childhood, taking special care to prevent overfeeding at those stages of development when there is a physiologic deposition of body fat. Begin obesity prevention at the time of the birth of an infant and provide ongoing nutrition counseling regarding feeding techniques during the parents' visits to the clinic or pediatrician.

RELATIONSHIP OF NUTRITION TO PSYCHOSOCIAL GROWTH AND DEVELOPMENT

Assessment and Intervention

To foster maximum psychosocial development, the feeding practices must be adjusted to the level of physiologic and psychosocial development. Dr. Erik Erikson of Harvard University has identified eight stages of growth, with a core psychosocial developmental task at each stage.[10] At each stage, the developmental problem has both a positive ego value and a negative component. These eight growth stages and their correlated developmental tasks (and negative correlate) are listed below.

Infancy	Trust vs mistrust
Toddler	Autonomy vs shame and doubt
Preschooler	Initiative vs guilt
Schoolage child	Industry vs inferiority
Adolescent	Identity vs role confusion
Young adult	Intimacy vs isolation
Middle adult	Generativity vs stagnation
Old age	Ego integrity vs despair

The foods and feeding practices used in nourishing a child should be adjusted to specific behavioral patterns associated with each developmental struggle. Thus, learning and developmental opportunities can be provided through food and its use. This contributes to the achievement of the positive component of the developmental task, as well as to the development of good food habits.

Formation of food habits is a component of growth and development. Formation of these habits is initiated in infancy with the first introduction of food. The process continues throughout childhood, with each year's experience adding to the eating behaviors learned in preceding years. Influences on the developing eating habits and examples as they apply to childhood follow.

Level of Physical Growth and Development

Appetite. The large appetite of the rapidly growing infant whose prime interest is food is in contrast to the small appetite of the slower-growing toddler and preschooler. Recognize the diminished interest in food as a normal process in order to help parents avoid struggles over eating and their negative effects on food habits.

Motor Skill Development. The toddler's development of the gross motor skills involved with walking leads to increased exploratory activity and decreased interest in food. The toddler is also developing the fine motor skills involved in manipulating the utensils needed for self-feeding. In addition, oral skills involved with eating (chewing ability and manipulating the lips and tongue) are being refined. The stage of development of these neuromuscular skills affects the types of foods the child should be served. For example, serve finger foods frequently while manipulative skills are being developed, and change the texture of foods served gradually to allow practice in refining the oral skills involved with eating. This also gives the child practice in using the same oral mechanisms that are necessary for speech.

Level of Psychosocial Development

Broadening Circle of Human Relationships. The food habits of the infant are influenced primarily by the mother or other caretaker. As the child's contacts are broadened (e.g., when the child goes to school), expect food habits of peers and others in the environment to begin to have an influence.

Social Factors. A child learns to use food and eating as a medium of socialization and communication as family meals are shared. Encourage the development of this aspect as a positive experience rather than using mealtime as a time to constantly discipline the child.

Emotional Factors. From birth, food becomes a symbol of love, security, and comfort, and, therefore, food assumes emotional connotations. Food is often used as a reward or punishment (e.g., giving desserts to reward good behavior or withholding them to pun-

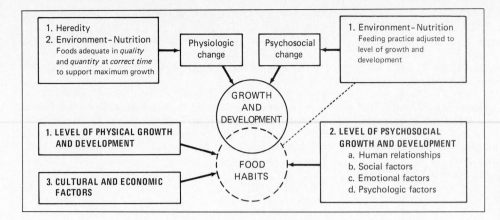

Figure 13–1
Relationship of nutrition to growth and development.

ish inappropriate behavior). Advise parents that foods used in this manner may assume emotional connotations that affect their use in later life.

Psychologic Factors. The inquisitiveness and negativism associated with the development of autonomy in the toddler often involve refusal of food. Again, recognize this as a normal process.

Cultural and Economic Factors. A child becomes acculturated to the foods common to his or her ethnic group or imposed by economic status. As a result of these influences, food and its use assume social, cultural, and emotional significance that is incorporated into developing food habits that may last a lifetime. Infancy and early childhood (toddler and preschool) are the formative years in the development of food habits. To assure the formation of good food habits, assist parents to adjust feeding practices to the child's level of physiologic and psychosocial development.

The overall relationship of nutrition to growth and development is summarized in Figure 13–1. In subsequent chapters of Part III, the eight growth and developmental states as they relate to food and eating will be examined in more detail.

REVIEW QUESTIONS AND ACTIVITIES

1. Explain the terms "growth" and "development."
2. Describe the three phases of cellular growth and the three phases of overall body growth.
3. Identify the pattern of (1) cellular growth in the brain and adipose tissue and (2) overall growth in height and weight in each of the following situations:
   a. An 8-month-old fetus
   b. A 3-month-old infant
   c. A 9-month-old infant
   d. An 18-month-old toddler

   e. A 4-year-old preschooler
   f. An 8-year-old schoolager
   g. A 13-year-old adolescent
4. Explain the relationship among nutrition, growth retardation, and catch-up growth.
5. Discuss the potential for behavioral abnormalities and obesity in association with malnutrition during critical periods of cell division in the brain and adipose tissue.
6. Discuss the effect of nutrition as an environmental influence on psychosocial growth and development and the development of food habits in infants and children and compare these influences with those that affect physiologic growth and development.

REFERENCES

1. Winick M: Malnutrition and Brain Development. New York, Oxford University Press, 1976.
2. Ricciuti HN: Adverse environmental and nutritional influences on mental development: A perspective. J Am Diet Assoc 79:115, 1981.
3. Winick M: Childhood obesity. Nutr Today 9(3):6, 1974.
4. Hirsch J, and Knittle JL: Cellularity of obese and nonobese human adipose tissue. Fed Proc 29:1516, 1970.
5. McKigney JI, Munro HN: Nutrient Requirements of Adolescence. DHEW Publication No. (NIH)76–771 (no date or page numbers given).
6. Sims EA, Horton ES, Salans LB: Inducible metabolic abnormalities during development of obesity. Annu Rev Med 22:235, 1971.
7. Roche AF: The adipocyte-number hypothesis. Child Dev. 52:31, 1981.
8. Chumlea WC, Knittle WC, Roche A, et al.: Size and number of adipocytes and measures of body fat in boys and girls 10 to 18 years of age. Am J Clin Nutr 34:1791, 1981.
9. Chumlea, WC, Knittle WC, Siervogel R, et al.: Adipocytes and adiposity in adults. Am J Clin Nutr 34:1798, 1981.
10. Erikson EH: Childhood and Society, ed 2. New York, WW Norton, 1963, pp 247–274.

BIBLIOGRAPHY

Beardslee WR, Wolff PH, Hurwitz, I, et al.: The effects of infantile malnutrition on behavioral development: A follow-up study. Am J Clin Nutr 35:1437, 1982.

Brozek J: Nutrition, malnutrition, and behavior. Annu Rev Psychol 29:157, 1979

Brozek J, ed: Proceedings of an International Conference on Behavioral Effects of Energy and Protein Deficits. DHEW Publication No (NIH) 79–1906, 1979.

Cravioto J: Nutrition, stimulation, mental development, and learning Nutr Today 16(5):4, 1981.

Falkner F, Tanner JJ, eds: Human Growth. New York, Plenum Press, 1979.

Himes JN: Infant feeding practices and obesity. J Am Diet Assoc 75:122, 1980.

Hurley L: Developmental Nutrition. Englewood Cliffs, NJ, Prentice-Hall, 1980.

Iron deficiency and mental development. Nutr Rev 41:235, 1983.

Oski FA, Honig AS, Howanitz HB: Effect of iron therapy on behavior performance in nonanemic iron-deficient infants. Pediatrics 71:877, 1983.

Pollitt E, Leibel RL, Greenfield D: Brief fasting, stress, and cognition in children. Am J Clin Nutr 34:1526, 1981.

Walter T, Kovalskys J, Stekel A: Effect of mild iron deficiency on infant mental development scores. J Pediatr 102:519, 1983.

CHAPTER 14

Nutrition and the Maternity Cycle

Objectives

After completion of this chapter, the student will be able to:

1. Distinguish among the three phases of pregnancy and the characteristics of each phase.

2. Distinguish between the physiologic and biochemical changes that occur in the major organ systems during pregnancy and the implications of these changes for nursing assessment and intervention.

3. Assess the relationship of nutrition to the outcome of pregnancy from both a generalized and a specific viewpoint.

4. Develop a nursing care plan for the nutritional management of an obese pregnant adult client who develops gestational diabetes during the pregnancy. Adjust the care plan for the periods of labor, delivery, and lactation.

5. Develop a nursing care plan for the nutritional management of an underweight 14-year-old pregnant adolescent who develops toxemia prior to delivery.

6. Distinguish among the effects of smoking, alcohol use, and pica on pregnancy outcome.

7. Differentiate among the three major community nutrition programs that are available for low-income clients.

8. Compare and contrast the characteristics of human and cow's milk.

9. Distinguish between the nutritional implications of the two major types of contraceptive agents.

The course and outcome of pregnancy are influenced by a number of factors that are genetic, biologic, social, psychologic, and nutritional in origin. For each fetus, there is a genetic design that can be fulfilled only in the presence of a favorable environment, including adequate nutrition. Over most of recorded history, special attention has been given to the diets of pregnant women, but there have been vast pendulum swings in the view of prenatal diet as an indicator of the outcome of pregnancy. The influence of nutrition on the course and outcome of pregnancy is currently the subject of considerable interest. Attention is being given not only to the immediate effect of malnutrition on maternal and infant health but also to the long-term effects on the physical and mental development of the child.

This interest has arisen from recognition of the relatively high neonatal and infant morbidity and mortality rates and the relatively high percentage of infants born with a low birth weight. Although the infant mortality rate is declining in the United States, it is still higher than in many other countries. Moreover, the proportion of infants born with a low birth weight (less than 2500 g) also remains high. Infants of low birth weight include those born prematurely (less than 38 weeks gestation) and those who are born after 40 weeks of gestation but are small for gestational age (SGA) because of intrauterine growth retardation. The chance of survival is diminished in low-birth-weight infants; they account for two thirds or more of neonatal deaths. Because of impaired immunologic development, there is also a diminished resistance to infection. Those infants who do survive may require a period of costly medical care and cause continuing concern about their progress in developing normal growth and development patterns. Nutrition is among the factors associated with the incidence of low-birth-weight infants and the related neonatal mortality rates.

The current question with regard to the role of nutrition in pregnancy outcome is not "Does nutrition make any difference?" but rather "What is the magnitude of the effect of diet on pregnancy outcome, and how can these effects be measured?"

New scientific knowledge about the potential benefits of breastfeeding is also becoming available. Until recently, it had been a widely held notion that modern formulas based on cow's milk were biochemically and nutritionally much the same as breast milk. It is now known that the differences between the two milks are more complex and subtle than originally reported.

There is also considerable interest in the nutritional implications of current contraceptive devices, especially sex steroid hormones taken orally and the intrauterine devices (IUDs).

This chapter will focus on nutritional aspects of pregnancy, lactation, and contraceptives.

NUTRITION IN PREGNANCY

Assessment and Intervention

Biologic and Physiologic Changes Associated with Pregnancy. Although pregnancy is a normal physiologic process, it is a period of great physiologic stress, since the pregnant woman synthesizes tissue at a rate greater than at any other period of life. During the course of pregnancy, the woman undergoes a series of physiologic adjustments in order to support fetal growth and development, prepare for lactation, and preserve her own homeostasis. At the same time, there is an exchange of nutrients and waste products between the mother and fetus across the placenta. All of these processes are complex, integrated, and dynamic (i.e., constantly changing throughout the course of the pregnancy). Many aspects of the process are dependent upon the nutrient supply available or have implications for nutrition.

Since the placenta synthesizes several hormones (chorionic gonadotropin, placental lactogen, estrogen, progesterone) that regulate maternal growth and development and control the transfer of substances between the mother and fetus, the development of a healthy placenta is essential to the health of the fetus. Placentas of poorly nourished mothers have been shown to contain fewer and smaller cells, and it has been hypothesized that these placentas are inefficient in nourishing the fe-

tus. However, the effects of maternal malnutrition on the placenta and its function have been studied only to a very limited extent.

The physiologic adjustments that occur are probably under hormonal control, although the precise control mechanisms are poorly understood. During early pregnancy, these physiologic adjustments occur gradually, in response to progressive changes in hormonal function. Many of the needed hormones are synthesized and secreted by the placenta, and the action of some of the placental hormones is similar to the action of the ovarian hormones, estrogen and progesterone.

The stages of pregnancy and the major physiologic and biochemical adjustments are summarized here.

Stages of Pregnancy. Pregnancy is classified into three main stages: implantation, organogenesis, and rapid growth. The period of implantation—in which the fertilized ovum becomes implanted in the uterine wall and development of the placenta begins—occurs during the first 2 weeks following conception. The next 6 weeks (from about 2 to 8 weeks) is the period of organ differentiation (organogenesis), and the beginnings of individual organs and various aspects of skeletal development are established. The final 7 months of pregnancy constitute the period of rapid growth. Fetal organs grow rapidly, and at the same time maternal reserves are being established for labor, the period immediately following labor (the puerperium), and lactation. The greatest growth in length in the fetus occurs during the second trimester, and rapid weight gain takes place during the third trimester.

During the implantation phase, nourishment is provided for the embryo by the outer layers of germ plasm and from secretions of the uterine glands, but during the periods of organogenesis and rapid growth, the external nutrient supply is critical. Evaluate the nutritional intake of pregnant women during these phases in particular, since nutrient deficiency has the potential for contributing to congenital malformations during the period of organ differentiation and for contributing to prematurity or low birth weight during the period of rapid growth. Be aware, however, that medical advice may not be sought during the very early phases of pregnancy, and nausea may be a factor that limits food intake at this time. Thus, those women who are in good nutritional status prior to conception have an advantage over those with poor nutrient intake.

Physiologic and Biochemical Changes in Organ Systems. Major changes occur in various body systems, including the cardiovascular, renal, gastrointestinal, and endocrine systems. Both enzymatic changes and changes in the blood concentration of some substances occur. A major change in body weight also takes place.

Because of the physiologic and biochemical ad-

TABLE 14–1
GUIDELINES FOR EVALUATING SELECTED LABORATORY TESTS IN ADULT PREGNANT WOMEN

Test	Nonpregnant (Normal)	Pregnant (Deficient)
Routine		
Hematocrit (vol %)	36 or above	<33
Hemoglobin (g/100 ml)	12 or above	<11
Serum folic acid (ng/ml)	6 or above	< 3
Other		
Serum albumin (g/100 ml)	3.5–5.0	< 2.5
Total serum protein (g/100 ml)	6.6–8.3	< 5.5
Serum vitamin B_{12} (pg/ml)	200 or above	<80

(*Source: WHO Technical Report Series 405, Geneva, 1968; USDHEW: Ten-State Nutrition Survey, 1968–1970. DHEW Publication No. (HSM) 72–8130, Atlanta, Ga, Centers for Disease Control, 1972; National Academy of Sciences: Laboratory Indices of Nutritional Status in Pregnancy. Washington, DC, National Academy Press, 1978.*)

justments, many features of normal pregnancy resemble those of pathologic disorders (e.g., nutrient loss in the urine, alterations in the blood concentration of such substances as hemoglobin, cholesterol, and albumin, enlargement of the thyroid gland). Biochemical standards for assessing the medical and nutritional status of pregnant women must therefore differ from those used for nonpregnant women (Table 14–1). A recent publication reviews the current state of knowledge regarding laboratory indices reflecting nutritional and metabolic status during normal pregnancy and provides normative data with respect to these indices in healthy pregnant women.[1]

Cardiovascular System. Within the cardiovascular system there is a rise in the volume of plasma (approximately 50 percent) and red cell mass (approximately 20 percent without iron supplements). The disproportionate increase in plasma volume and red cell mass leads to a drop in the hemoglobin concen- ▶ tration, the so-called **physiologic anemia of pregnancy.** The hemoglobin concentration falls from an average of 13 to 14 g/100 ml in a nonpregnant woman to between 11.5 and 12 g/100 ml in late pregnancy. The physiologic anemia can be modified, especially in late pregnancy, by providing supplemental iron.

Other cardiovascular changes include an increase in cardiac output, pulse rate, and venous pressure. High venous pressure in the legs probably contributes to the lower limb edema commonly observed in pregnancy. There is also an increase in the flow of blood to the uterus (the central target for the increased blood flow), the skin, the breasts, and the kidneys. The increased blood flow to the skin and kidneys facilitates waste removal. Some investigators postulate that malnourished women may not be able to adequately expand blood volume and blood flow to the uterus, putting them at risk for complications.

Total body water also increases in pregnancy— not only does maternal blood volume expand but fluid accumulates also in the products of conception and the reproductive organs.

Renal System. To facilitate removal of wastes, there is an increase in renal blood flow, glomerular filtration rate, and renal clearance of substances. Observe the results of laboratory tests. These changes result in the loss of some nutrients in the urine (e.g., glucose, amino acids, iodine, folic acid, sodium, and water). In early pregnancy, urine flow is accelerated, whereas it is diminished in late pregnancy, possibly in association with the pooling of water in the lower limbs.

Gastrointestinal Changes. Question pregnant women who are in their first trimester about appetite and thirst. Increases in both appetite and thirst are often apparent at this time. Morning nausea, though not incongruent with an increased appetite, may temporarily decrease the appetite. Taste preferences may also change, and some women may experience cravings for some foods (such as fruit or highly flavored foods) and aversions to others (such as coffee, tea, ▶ or fried foods). Overt **pica** (an appetite for inappropriate items, such as starch, clay, or chalk) may develop in some women.

Gastrointestinal function is altered. In the stomach, the secretion of gastric acid and pepsin is diminished, as is motility. The hypomotility promotes better digestion but may contribute to nausea. Relaxation of the cardiac sphincter allows some regurgitation of stomach contents into the esophagus, with resulting heartburn. Nutrient absorption is enhanced in the intestine, and hypomotility may result in constipation. Hemorrhoids may develop.

Nausea, vomiting, heartburn, and constipation are all common complaints of pregnant women; manage these with dietary measures when possible. Nausea and vomiting are common in the first trimester of pregnancy, presumably associated with hormonal changes. The symptoms usually subside after 12 weeks. A few women experience pernicious vomiting severe enough to cause weight loss. These clients require hospitalization with intravenous or tube feedings to prevent dehydration and ketosis. Vitamin B_6 may be prescribed for the nausea and vomiting for a limited period of time. A protocol for managing these clients has been published.[2]

Fats are a common cause of gastrointestinal upsets, and the symptoms may also be precipitated by drinking fluid with meals. Control mild nausea and vomiting by advising these dietary adjustments: (1) eat small, frequent, dry meals, (2) drink fluids one-half to 1 hour before or after meals, (3) eat dry foods, such as crackers or dry cereal, before arising in the morning, (4) avoid fried or highly spiced foods and strongly flavored vegetables (e.g., cabbage, turnips, and onions), (5) substitute skim milk for whole milk. Since nausea often subsides by the middle of the day, suggest a larger intake at subsequent meals to compensate for the missed feedings.

Suggest to clients who complain of heartburn that they may be more comfortable if fried foods, highly spiced foods, and strongly flavored vegetables are eliminated from the diet. Encourage them to eat small, frequent meals, to limit the quantity of liquids consumed with meals, and to avoid lying down after meals to reduce reflux.

Constipation is common during the latter half of pregnancy because of such factors as colonic hypomotility, increased uterine pressure on the intestinal tract, limited exercise, or use of iron supplements. Hemorrhoids are aggravated in the presence of constipation. Avoid constipation by providing a diet high in fiber content with a concurrent increase in fluid intake.

Although an increased secretion of saliva is sometimes reported as a complication of pregnancy (particularly in association with nausea), there is little evidence to support this. In contrast to the old wives' tale, "a tooth for every child," dental development is normal during pregnancy, and there is no evidence of demineralization or an increase in the incidence of dental caries. However, gingival edema and gingivitis are not uncommon.

Endocrine Changes. Among the hormonal changes in pregnancy that have nutritional implications are an enlargement of the thyroid gland, an increased uptake of iodine by the thyroid gland, and an increase in the secretion of aldosterone, progesterone, growth hormone, thyroxin, and parathyroid hormone.

Other Changes. The amount and activity of many enzymes (e.g., alkaline phosphatase) are markedly increased. The blood concentration of other substances (such as protein and lipids) is also altered. Check the serum albumin level. This typically falls from about 4 g/100 ml in early pregnancy to between 2.5 and 3.0 g/100 ml. The reason for this change

is not understood. In contrast, the blood level of most lipids rises during pregnancy. For example, blood cholesterol rises from 200 mg/100 ml or less to 250 to 300 mg/100 ml.

Weight Gain. Body mass increases throughout pregnancy in association with fetal growth and deposition of maternal tissues to sustain the pregnancy and prepare for lactation. The actual amount of weight gained by individual women depends on many factors, including age, parity, weight at conception, body frame size, size of the fetus, and the physiologic response to pregnancy (e.g., individual metabolic response to the placental hormones). Total weight gain, the pattern of gain throughout the three trimesters, and the composition of the gain (fat, lean tissue, or fluid) are all important determinants of the outcome of pregnancy; these are discussed in the next section.

Relationship of Nutrition to Pregnancy Outcome. Over the years, various views have been held regarding the relation of nutrition to pregnancy outcome. All too often, these views have been based on gossip, folklore, or superstition. Frequently, the mother has been semistarved (by restriction of kilocalories, sodium, and fluids) in an attempt to prevent ▶ **toxemia**—a complication of pregnancy associated with hypertension, edema, and loss of albumin in the urine—and to produce a small infant that is easy to deliver. Both the parasite theory (the fetus extracts the needed nutrients from the mother's stores, regardless of the quality of her diet) and the maternal instinct theory (the mother instinctively craves and consumes the needed nutrients) have been held from time to time. All of these theories have now been refuted. However, definitive recommendations for the appropriate diet to follow during pregnancy have been difficult to establish because of the sometimes contradictory and conflicting results of research studies.

Widely differing diets have sustained mothers through successful pregnancies, and undernourished mothers may produce healthy children. However, there is evidence that the mother who is in a good nutritional state both before and during pregnancy has a better chance of having an uncomplicated pregnancy and a healthy baby than has a mother with poor nutritional status and poor eating habits.

Because of the many concerns related to maternal nutrition, a special committee was formed by the National Academy of Sciences to study the matter. The report of the committee[3] extensively reviewed existing data on reproductive experiences and concluded that adequate nutrition is one of the most important environmental factors affecting the health of pregnant women and their infants. Data accumulated in both human and animal studies are sufficiently conclusive to indicate that poor nutritional status in the mother is an important factor contributing to maternal complications, fetal and neonatal deaths, prematurity, low birth weight, and neonatal and infant morbidity. This view is supported by results of famine conditions experienced in Holland and Russia during World War II on pregnancy outcome and results of programs in various areas of the world that have provided protein-calorie supplements to pregnant women with poor nutritional status. These studies tend to show an increase in fetal mortality and a downward trend in infant birth weight in association with acute famine conditions and a moderate increase in infant birth weight in association with provision of food supplements during pregnancy. The available data suggest that, in general, maternal malnutrition during the early part of pregnancy affects the physiologic development of the embryo and its ability to survive, whereas maternal nutrition during the latter part of gestation affects final growth of the fetus and, thus, birth weight. The degree of rise in infant birth weight with supplementation appears to depend in part on the nutritional status of the mother. In underweight women who are at risk of delivering a baby of low birth weight, dietary supplementation during pregnancy is effective in increasing birth weight. In contrast, a nutrient supplement is less likely to confer obvious benefits in terms of increased birth weight in adequately nourished women.

The most specific effect of diet on the outcome of pregnancy appears in the relationships of the preconceptional weight of the mother and the amount of her weight gain during pregnancy with the subsequent birth weight of the infant. These two variables rank just behind duration of the pregnancy as the major determinants of infant birth weight, and they act independently of each other. When acting jointly, they become additive in their effects. The mother's prepregnancy weight is an indirect indicator of energy reserves, and weight gain during pregnancy is an indirect indicator of energy intake.

An average weight gain of 24 to 27 lb in women of normal weight is consistent with a better than average course and outcome of pregnancy, although there appears to be considerable individual variation in optimal weight gain during pregnancy. Although the desired amount of weight gain for obese and underweight women has not been established, women who are underweight at conception require a larger gain (30 to 40 lb) to sustain normal fetal growth, and obese women may require a smaller gain. While there is some evidence that 15 to 16 lb is sufficient,[4] most investigators feel that weight gain should not be restricted below the recommended amount for women of normal weight. Although weight gain is currently regarded as the major indicator of dietary adequacy, keep in mind that weight gain per se is a nonspecific and insensitive index of nutrition. It provides little information about nutrient factors other than kilocalories and is only a gross index of fetal development.

Evaluate the pattern of weight gain as well as the total amount. Of the two, the pattern of gain may be of greater importance. A sudden, sharp increase after the twentieth week of pregnancy may indicate water retention and the possible onset of toxemia. The recommended pattern is a minimal gain during the first trimester (1.5 to 3.0 lb), followed by a linear gain of slightly less than a pound (0.8 lb) per week during the last two trimesters. This pattern of gain correlates well with fetal and maternal growth during the pregnancy. There is little maternal or fetal gain in the first trimester, maternal gain is rapid during the second trimester and slows in the third, and most of fetal weight gain occurs during the last trimester. The weight gain grid (Fig. 14–1) illustrates the desired pattern of gain. When weight gain is excessive (7 lb or more per month), distinguish between physiologic fluid retention (normal) and pathologic fluid retention (signaling toxemia).

The lifetime nutritional experiences of the mother are also thought to be important in pregnancy outcome. The nutritional status of the woman entering the childbearing years depends on her lifetime nutritional experiences and reflects the habits, attitudes, and values formed in earlier years. If the mother has always had a diet adequate in all nutrients and is in good health, the likelihood of her delivering a healthy baby is greater than it is for

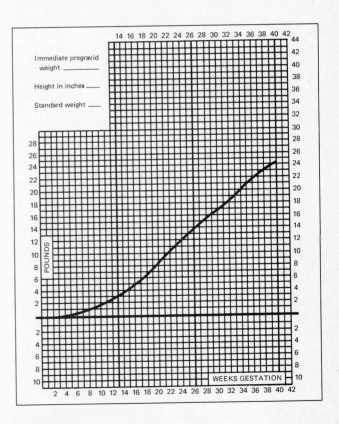

Figure 14–1
Prenatal gain in weight grid. (Source: U.S. Department HEW, Social and Rehabilitation Service, Children's Bureau.)

one who has consistently practiced poor food habits. The capacity to reproduce itself may reflect the adequacy of the diet, since dietary deficiencies may alter fertility and affect the ease of delivery. The size of the pelvis is closely correlated with height. In well-nourished women, the pelvic brim is round. A short stature and the flat pelvis frequently observed in short women may reflect failure to achieve full genetic potential in body structure because of an inadequate diet in childhood. Moreover, pelvic deformities that prevent normal childbearing may be present in women who had rickets in their early years. It is also possible that poor nutrition may produce an intergenerational effect, i.e., be seen in the generation following the one subjected to the nutritional insult, although this question necessitates further research.

Incorporate nutritional assessment, diet counseling, and follow-up into the prenatal care of all women. Even the most affluent and educated women can have nutritional problems in pregnancy. The initial nutritional assessment and counseling should take place preferably during the first prenatal visit, with continuing assessment performed as needed at subsequent visits. This allows for identification of those at high nutritional risk so that appropriate counseling can be provided. The initial assessment should include all four components—anthropometric, biochemical, clinical, and dietary.

Use a table of standard weight for height (see Appendix 7) to arrive at standard weight and plot the client's weight on the weight gain grid with each clinic visit. Visual representation of the pattern in comparison with the normal allows for a quick determination of weight deviations. Give a copy of the grid to the client if she can profit from its use. Of the many biochemical tests, determination of the hemoglobin and hematocrit and urine testing for glucose and ketones are the only ones sufficiently established to be routinely used in evaluating each client. Test the urine routinely. The blood indices are usually evaluated each trimester. Special situations may warrant further evaluation. If the client is following a vegetarian diet (see Chap. 20), a determination of the serum vitamin B_{12} should be made, and measurement of plasma proteins can be useful if protein–kilocalorie malnutrition is suspected. In the latter instance, keep in mind the normal decline of plasma protein levels in pregnancy along with the fact that abnormalities occur only with a severe degree of deficiency.

Evaluate for clinical evidence of nutritional deficiency routinely, remembering that some of the signs may not be evident unless a severe deficiency exists. There may also be confusion in interpreting some of the findings. For example, gingival hypertrophy sometimes occurs normally in pregnancy and may not be a sign of vitamin C deficiency.

The dietary evaluation should consist of a complete nutritional history with an inventory of foods consumed in a 24-hour period (supplemented with a food frequency checklist). The intake of food for a 24-hour period should be evaluated again at subsequent visits if indicated.

In most cases, the prospective mother is anxious to have a normal, healthy baby, and nutritional advice is likely to be better accepted at this time than at other stages of the life cycle. Include the prospective father or other significant family member in diet counseling sessions in order to gain cooperation for following diet recommendations. In this way, the entire family's diet may be improved. If the pregnancy is unwanted, other motivational techniques, such as promoting the mother's own personal well-being, may be necessary.

The need for nutritional information will vary widely and should be determined on an individual basis. The woman having her first baby is likely to require more extensive counseling than one having her second or third child, for whom only a review of the essentials may be necessary.

Nutritional Requirements. Because of the demands of the growing fetus and the physiologic changes that occur in the mother, nutritional requirements in pregnancy (as well as in the subsequent period of lactation) differ from those of the nonpregnant woman. Although the needs for most nutrients known to be essential are increased, the altered requirements do not imply that the mother must "eat for two." Rather, specific recommendations are made in regard to increased need for nutrients.

Nutritional requirements that have been established for normal pregnancy are based on recommendations of the National Academy of Sciences (the Recommended Dietary Allowances,[5] see Chap. 2, and the report of the Committee on Maternal Nutrition[3]). These recommendations are intended to serve as guidelines in determining requirements of individual pregnant women, since needs vary with age, weight, and activity. The nutrient needs of pregnant teenagers are different from those of adults because of the dual growth demand, that of the fetus and that of the teenager herself. Although nutrient needs are greatest during the last trimester of pregnancy, advise clients to increase nutrient intake as soon as the pregnancy is diagnosed in order to build up nutrient stores. Use the food plans given in Tables 14–2 and 14–3 as a guideline for counseling pregnant adults and adolescents regarding their increased nutrient requirements. Except for iron, and in some cases folic acid, vitamin and mineral supplements are not required when foods are selected in the amounts indicated in these food plans.

A limited number of servings of food can supply the additional requirements for energy and nutrients. For instance, the need for the additional 300 kcal, the 30 g of protein, and the increased requirement for vitamin C can be met with the following food combinations:

Food	Protein (g)	Vitamin C (mg)	Kcal
2 c skim milk	16	—	160
2 oz lean meat	14	—	110
1 serving citrus fruit	—	45	40
Total	30	45	310

Energy Needs. Pregnancy imposes additional energy demands to support fetal and maternal tissue growth and to provide for an increase in maternal body mass and metabolism. The actual kilocalorie level varies widely, depending on such factors as age, activity, height, weight at conception, stage of pregnancy, and ambient temperature, and may range from 1800 to 3700 kcal. Energy needs are greatest during the second and third trimesters in association with rapid maternal and fetal growth. However, the larger requirements may be partially offset by a decrease in activity during late pregnancy.

Adjust the kilocalorie level to support the suggested weight gain of approximately 24 to 27 lb. The RDA suggests an additional intake of 300 kcal daily. However, the energy intake should be at least 36 kcal/kg of pregnant body weight for mature women and 40 kcal/kg of pregnant body weight for adolescents to assure adequate use of dietary protein. Use the plotted measurements on the weight gain grid to assess the client's energy status and make adjustments upward or downward as noted by deviations from the normal pattern of weight gain.

Protein Requirement. Additional protein is required for fetal needs and for accessory tissues, blood volume expansion, and growth of the uterus and mammary tissue. The RDA for protein is 30 g above the normal requirement for adults. Very young adolescents require even more, since their own tissues, as well as those of the fetus, are still forming. Use

TABLE 14–2
DAILY FOOD PLAN FOR PREGNANCY AND LACTATION (ADULTS)

Food	Nonpregnant Women	Pregnancy	Lactation
Milk and cheese Includes whole, nonfat, evaporated, reliquefied dry, buttermilk, yoghurt, cheese and foods made with milk or cheese	2 c	3 or more c	4 or more c
Meat–poultry–fish–beans Lean meat, fish, poultry, eggs, legumes, nuts, peanut butter, seeds	2 servings (4–6 oz meat or equivalent amount of meat alternates)	2½ servings (5–7 oz meat or equivalent amount of meat alternates) Encourage use of liver	3 servings (6–9 ounces meat or equivalent amount of meat alternates)
Vegetables and fruit Some raw daily Dark green or deep yellow Vitamin C-rich food Good sources Citrus fruit or juice, green peppers, cantaloupes, fresh strawberries, broccoli Fair sources Other melons, tomatoes, cabbage, potatoes cooked in skins, other green vegetables	1 serving 1 good source or 2 fair sources	1 serving 1 good source and 1 fair or 2 good sources	1–2 servings Same
Other vegetables and fruits	1–2 servings	2 servings	Same
Bread and cereal Enriched or whole grain	3–4 servings	4–5 servings	5 servings
Butter or fortified margarine	Amount as kcal level permits	Same	Same
Additional foods	More of these listed or other foods with amounts adjusted to rate of weight gain		Additional foods as needed to maintain weight
Iron and vitamin supplements	Use according to physician's instructions		Same

---

TABLE 14–3
DAILY FOOD PLAN FOR THE PREGNANT ADOLESCENT

Food	Amount
Milk and cheese Includes whole, nonfat, evaporated, re-liquefied dry, buttermilk, yoghurt, cheese, and foods made with milk or cheese	4 c milk (or 4 servings cheese—1⅓ oz/serving)
Meat–poultry–fish–beans Lean meat, fish, poultry, organ meats, and eggs Legumes, nuts, peanut butter, and seeds	Equivalent of 4 (2–3 oz) servings meat plus 1–2 eggs
Vegetables and fruit Some raw daily Dark green leafy or yellow-orange vegetable/fruit at least every other day 2 good sources (or 1 good source and 1 fair source) vitamin C food daily. See Table 14–2 for classification of good and fair sources	3–4 servings fruit 2–3 servings vegetable (½ c servings fruit and vegetable or ¼ c serving dried fruit)
Bread and cereal Whole grain or enriched	7 servings
Butter, fortified margarine and other fats	Amount as caloric level permits
Additional foods Includes desserts or additional amounts of the above listed foods	As needed to maintain desired rate of weight gain; select nutritious desserts, i.e., pudding, fruit pie, peanut butter or oatmeal cookie
Iron and vitamin supplement	Use according to physician's instruction

(*Source: Adapted from Ritchey SS, Faulkner S: Adolescent Pregnancy, The Influence of Growth, Nutrition and Environment. Cassette-A-Month, American Dietetic Association, Chicago, 1974.*)

---

these guidelines to determine the amount of protein for clients of various ages, based on ideal body weight:

Adult	1.3 g/kg
Age 17–19	1.5 g/kg
Younger adolescents	1.7 g/kg

Minerals and Vitamins. With certain exceptions, routine supplementation of the prenatal diet with minerals and vitamins is unnecessary, since the amounts required can be supplied by an adequate diet. The subject of supplementation is controversial, and the practice has been found neither beneficial nor harmful. Some physicians regard supplementation as an unnecessary expense, whereas others consider the practice as insurance for those clients whose diets are inadequate. In any event, do not allow supplementation to replace diet counseling, which should be provided for all prenatal clients. Consider supplementation on an individual basis; when deemed necessary, the amount of the nutrients given should approximate the RDA. The potential hazards of vitamin supplementation include (1) the possibility of promoting a false sense of security in both the client and the physician and (2) the potential for vitamin toxicity if excessive amounts are administered. Overdosage with certain nutrients (particularly the fat-soluble vitamins) appears to be **teratogenic** (producing fetal malformation) in animals. In humans, some potential exists for fetal toxicity with maternal overdosage with vitamin A, vitamin D, vitamin B_6, vitamin C, and the mineral, iodine.[6] The excessive intake of vitamin A appears to exhibit the most serious consequence for the human embryo and fetus. Urinary tract abnormalities and central nervous system defects have been observed in the newborns of several mothers who ingested large doses of vitamin A at various times throughout their pregnancies. A possible association between maternal vitamin D overdosage and infantile hypercalcemia with attendant facial abnormalities, growth retardation, and aortic stenosis has been suggested, as has the possibility of producing an ascorbic acid and pyridoxine dependency state in the infant with excessive maternal intake of these two vitamins. Finally, congenital goiter may result from a very high intake of iodine. Iodine is a component of expectorants used for treating asthma and other respiratory conditions as well as some prenatal mineral supplements, iodized salt, and kelp tablets. Advise pregnant clients to avoid a large intake of these nutrients as well as others, since they fail to confer any benefit and carry the potential for harming the fetus.

The use of supplements containing vitamins and minerals as a means of preventing neural tube defects (conditions such as spina bifida and anencephaly, which arise due to defective closure of the neural tube in the fetus during the first month of pregnancy) in infants or fetuses of high-risk mothers is being explored. These defects may occur as a result of combined genetic and environmental factors. Poor maternal nutrition is one factor that has been identified.[7] Some preliminary findings showed positive benefits when the nutrient supplement was given to pregnant women who had already borne one or more infants with neural tube defects.[8,9] Although it is not clear which of the nutrients was responsible for the suggested benefits, most attention is being focused on folic acid. The implications of these findings await further study.

Iron. Many women are in a precarious state of iron balance during the reproductive years because the requirement is greater than can be provided by the diet and iron stores (see Chap. 31). Although the efficiency of iron absorption is increased in pregnancy, the added demands on iron requirements (expansion of the red cell mass, transfer of iron to the fetus for storage and to the placenta and umbilical cord, and iron losses incurred at delivery) often exceed the iron supply. For these reasons, advise the client to eat foods high in iron and to take supplemental iron (30 to 60 mg elemental iron daily, which translates to 150 to 300 mg ferrous sulfate) as a prophylactic measure during the second and third trimesters. Supplementation should continue for 2 to 3 months following delivery to replenish iron stores.

▶ **Iron deficiency anemia** is the most common form of anemia in pregnancy. Use the criteria given in Table 14–1 to aid in its diagnosis. Treat anemia by increasing the daily dosage of the iron supplement (500 to 750 mg ferrous sulfate given in three divided doses). Advise the client to consume foods that contain adequate protein, iron, and vitamin C. Teach her that the heme iron that is present in red meat is the best-absorbed form of iron and that the absorption of nonheme iron present in legumes, dried fruits, green vegetables, and grains can be enhanced by consuming a food high in vitamin C, such as orange juice or tomato juice at the meal. Provide a printed handout depicting food sources of iron.

Evaluate the client's compliance with the drug regimen at subsequent visits. Ask her to bring the medication with her, and observe the amount that remains. Question her about the color of her stools; iron supplements create dark stools.

The fetus is an effective parasite in extracting iron from the mother regardless of her state of iron balance. Infants born of anemic mothers will have a normal hemoglobin, although there is some evidence that the iron stores of these infants are low, predisposing them to anemia in late infancy.

Sodium. The sodium requirement is greater in pregnancy because maternal tissue fluid compartments must expand and fetal needs must be met. At the same time, pregnant women lose an increased amount of sodium in the urine secondary to the increased glomerular filtration rate and the salt-losing effect of progesterone produced by the placenta. These losses are compensated for by an increase in the activity of the physiologic mechanisms that promote sodium reabsorption. Thus the old theory that the pregnant woman is a salt retainer is challenged; rather, she is a salt waster.

Edema is one of the cardinal signs of toxemia, since toxemic clients retain sodium abnormally. Be aware that edema in a benign form, either generalized or localized, also occurs late in pregnancy in a large number of otherwise normal women. Although the cause of the generalized edema is not clear, localized edema may be due to factors such as obstruction of the pelvic vein by the enlarged uterus. This edema is not thought to be particularly harmful unless accompanied by hypertension, loss of protein into the urine, or other abnormalities.

The associations among sodium, edema, and toxemia have led to the practice of restricting sodium and prescribing diuretics both to prevent and to treat toxemia. However, there is no evidence that sodium restriction either prevents or alleviates toxemia. Sodium restriction is potentially harmful, since an inadequate intake in the face of excessive loss may lead to diminished blood volume. A sodium-restricted diet may also limit intake of nutritious foods. The sodium intake of women should be at least 2 g per day. Counsel the client to salt food to preferred taste, rather than to either increase or decrease sodium intake. Diuretics are potentially harmful and should not be used.

Calcium. The need for calcium is greatest in late pregnancy to allow for calcification of the fetal skeleton. As with iron, the efficiency of calcium absorption is increased in pregnancy. The RDA for calcium is 1200 to 1600 mg, depending upon age; 1 quart of milk contains approximately 1200 mg of calcium. Other good sources of calcium are fish with edible bones (canned salmon or sardines), clams, oysters, green leafy vegetables, legumes, dried fruits, and soybean curd (tofu), although it is difficult to provide the recommended amount of calcium without milk or other dairy products. With a dietary lack, fetal needs are met by demineralizing the maternal skeleton. This can be especially detrimental to the adolescent whose own skeleton is being mineralized. Tell clients who cannot drink the recommended amounts of milk because of lactose intolerance or other reasons that the amount of calcium contained in an 8 oz cup of milk can be obtained from 1⅓ oz yellow cheese, a carton of yoghurt, or 2 c of cottage cheese. If an adequate calcium intake still remains a problem, consider the use of calcium supplements in the form of calcium carbonate or calcium lactate.

An adequate amount of vitamin D (10 to 15 μg cholecalciferol daily, depending upon age) is needed to promote calcium absorption and bone demineralization. Vitamin D deficiency has been implicated in neonatal tetany.

It has been suggested that a calcium–phosphorus imbalance (high blood phosphorus produces low blood calcium) may lead to leg cramps, but a relationship has not been clearly established. Various treatments for leg cramps have been tried, including milk restriction (because of its high phosphorus content), use of agents that bind phosphorus in the intestine, and supplementation with nonphosphate salts of calcium.

Iodine. The increased metabolism of the thyroid gland results in an increased requirement for iodine. During the second half of pregnancy, the basal metabolic rate may increase up to 23 percent. Since goiter is more likely to develop during pregnancy than at other times, recommend the use of iodized salt for clients who live in areas where the soil and drinking water are deficient in iodine.

Folic Acid. The folic acid requirement is substantially increased in pregnancy in association with increased nucleic acid synthesis and increased formation of red blood cells. The RDA for pregnancy, 800 mg, represents a doubling of the normal amount. ▶ A severe deficiency results in **megaloblastic** (megaloblasts are large, immature red blood cells) **anemia.** The effects of less severe deficiency are not as clear-cut. Several reports have correlated folic acid deficiency with various complications of pregnancy, such as abruptio placentae and other types of prenatal bleeding, spontaneous abortion in early pregnancy, habitual abortion, fetal abnormalities, toxemia, and premature delivery. These reports have not been substantiated, however.

Megaloblastic anemia in pregnancy, though not as common as iron deficiency anemia, is not rare and may accompany iron deficiency. Although routine folic acid supplementation is controversial, consider it as an option in clients who are at an unusually high risk for developing folic acid deficiency, including women with a history of poor dietary intake, frequent or multiple pregnancies, chronic hemolytic anemia, or treatment with anticonvulsant drugs or oral contraceptive agents. If folate supplementation is prescribed, 400 to 800 μg/day is the recommended amount. A prescription is required for a preparation that contains the recommended amount. In addition, assure that the client is receiving adequate dietary sources of folic acid, including leafy green vegetables, legumes, liver, fresh fruits, and whole grains. Treatment of established folic acid deficiency anemia requires a supplement of 1 mg folic acid per day.

Other Vitamins and Minerals. The blood level of most vitamins is decreased in pregnancy, although the significance of this is not known. Supplementation has resulted in normalizing the blood values only in some cases. The low values may represent a deficiency state or a physiologic adjustment. For example, a low blood level of vitamin B_6 (which responds to supplementation) is often noted. Although vitamin B_6 deficiency has been associated with toxemia, this finding has not been confirmed.

While a number of trace minerals (e.g., zinc, chromium, and copper) are essential for normal reproduction in animals, their significance in human reproduction is not known.

Factors Contributing to Nutritional Risk During Pregnancy. Certain conditions related to the client's health status may classify her as high risk during pregnancy. Some of the conditions may already exist at the time of pregnancy, whereas others may develop during the pregnancy itself because of failure to make the needed physiologic adjustments. Many of these conditions, which are physiologic, socioeconomic, and psychologic in origin (Table 14–4), may predispose the client to such complications as prematurity, low infant birth weight, toxemia, and perinatal mortality. Use findings from the medical history and physical examination and

---

TABLE 14–4
SITUATIONS POSING NUTRITIONAL RISKS FOR PREGNANT WOMEN

Medical–obstetric factors
  Weight deviations—obesity, underweight, or abnormal pattern of weight gain
  Multiple pregnancy
  Previous obstetric complications—e.g., toxemia, prematurity, low birth weight, repeated spontaneous abortion, stillbirth and neonatal death, weight deviations
  Addiction—e.g., smoking, alcoholism, drug addiction, pica
  Extremes of age and parity, and short interconceptional period
  Preexisting medical conditions or those that develop during gestation—e.g., infectious diseases such as tuberculosis; preexisting hypertension or renal disease; anemia (especially iron and folic acid deficiency anemia); cardiac disease; gastrointestinal and liver disease; diabetes mellitus (overt or gestational); certain inborn errors of metabolism such as phenylketonuria, cystinuria, and Wilson's disease; and hyperlipidemia—and toxemia

Socioeconomic factors
  Low income or limited food budget
  Inadequate knowledge of nutrition or food resource management—e.g., inaccessibility or lack of knowledge of food assistance programs, limited knowledge or ability to make required dietary changes with ordinary counseling, and lack of budgeting or cooking skills
  Lack of facilities for food preparation and storage
  Ethnic or language barriers—e.g., inability to obtain food of a particular cultural group; inability to read and understand about foods of a particular country
  Alternative dietary patterns—e.g. vegetarian, macrobiotic, or health food diets—and strict regimens for weight loss

Psychologic factors—e.g., depression, anorexia nervosa

other routine screening measures provided in the prenatal health care setting to identify these high-risk clients during the early stage of pregnancy.

Medical–Obstetric Risks

Weight. Weight deviations are common in pregnancy. Use the guidelines given in Table 14–5 to determine if a weight deviation exists. Those who are obese or who gain excessive weight are more susceptible to the development of hypertension or diabetes mellitus. Excessive weight gain in nonobese clients may also predispose them to subsequent obesity. Moreover, excessive prepregnancy weight (up to 180 lb) and excessive weight gain during pregnancy (40 lb or more) result in the birth of larger infants. Newborn infants of obese mothers tend to have a significantly greater amount of subcutaneous fat stores. Infant birth weights above 4500 g are associated with an increased perinatal mortality, and these infants pose mechanical problems in delivery. Keep in mind that many obese people, while ingesting excessive kilocalories, may have an insufficient intake of nutrients.

Those clients who have a low preconceptual weight or who fail to gain an adequate amount of weight during pregnancy have depleted nutrient and energy stores and are at a high risk for delivering a premature infant and/or developing toxemia. Since the fetal period marks the initial stages of brain cell division, prenatal malnutrition increases the potential for retarded brain growth and possible retarded mental development in the child.

Provide intensive diet counseling for clients who are underweight, who gain insufficient weight, or who lose weight in association with vomiting in early pregnancy. The proper management for those who are underweight at conception includes a regimen that allows for the usual gain of pregnancy plus the additional deficit in body weight. A carefully supervised large gain (as much as a total of 40 lb or more) may be indicated for seriously underweight

clients. Assist the client to understand the relationship of weight gain, nutrition, and fetal growth. Set short-term goals for weight gain, such as a gain of 1½ lb for the following week. Suggest a regimen that includes frequent small feedings augmented with high-calorie, high-protein snacks. If the economic situation suggests an inadequate food supply, make a referral to the available food assistance programs (see later). Provide vitamin and iron supplements and monitor weight gain, fetal growth, and fetal status on an ongoing basis.

Although the desired amount of weight gain for obese clients is controversial, less controversial is the issue related to weight reduction during pregnancy or restricting kilocalories to limit the rate of gain during pregnancy for three basic reasons: (1) kilocalorie restriction may result in restricting the supply of nutrients or use of dietary protein for energy rather than for fetal and maternal protein synthesis, (2) severe kilocalorie restriction results in excess fat catabolism and ketosis, and ketosis is hazardous to the neurologic development of the fetus, and (3) inadequate weight gain increases the potential for low infant birth weight and perinatal mortality.

If the client is gaining excessive weight, assist her to adjust the rate of gain to follow the normal pattern—it should not be markedly restricted. Fetal growth is most rapid during the last trimester, and the kilocalorie and nutrient supply at this time is especially critical. At the same time, counsel the client to improve the overall diet quality and correct faulty eating habits that may be contributing to the obesity. Advise her that nonessential foods, such as concentrated sweets and certain fats, can be limited or eliminated without compromising diet quality. Tell the client that weight reduction can safely be initiated at the completion of lactation or, for the nonnursing mother, 2 to 4 weeks postpartum.

Smoking, Alcohol, and Pica. Addictions such as smoking, alcoholism, and pica can also create certain risks. Caution the client who smokes of the potential hazards to both herself and the infant. Prepregnancy weight, weight gain during pregnancy, and long-term weight gain all tend to be lower in smoking women, and these women also tend to experience a greater incidence of complications, such as abruptio placentae and spontaneous abortions. The birth weight of infants of smoking mothers averages 200 g less than that of babies of nonsmoking mothers, with the decrement in birth weight proportional to the number of cigarettes smoked. Higher rates of mortality and morbidity up to 5 years of age have also been observed in children of mothers who smoke during and after pregnancy.[10] Tissue hypoxia induced by carbon monoxide and nicotine is thought to be responsible for the adverse effects, although interaction with other factors, such as inadequate nutrition, may contribute.

Heavy maternal drinking during pregnancy is

TABLE 14–5
GUIDELINES FOR WEIGHT DEVIATIONS IN PREGNANCY

Status	Definition
Underweight	Prepregnancy weight that is less than 85% of standard weight
Inadequate gain	Weight loss during pregnancy or gain of less than 1 kg (about 2 lb) per month during the second or third trimester
Overweight	Prepregnancy weight that is greater than 120% of standard weight
Excessive gain	Gain of more than 3 kg (about 7 lb) per month during the second or third trimester

a widely recognized hazard to the fetus. Many authors have described the teratogenic effects of chronic alcohol ingestion during pregnancy, the features of which have been grouped under the term ▶ **fetal alcohol syndrome.** This syndrome is associated with congenital anomalies, mental deficiencies, and prenatal and postnatal growth retardation. This condition generally exhibits a greater extent of clinical features as maternal alcohol consumption increases, although recent evidence suggests that infants born to 10 percent of women who drink 1 to 2 oz of absolute alcohol per day during the earliest part of pregnancy have some recognizable characteristics of the syndrome.[11] The phase of fetal life most affected by alcohol and the level of alcohol intake that is most harmful have not been determined. Since a safe level of alcohol consumption during pregnancy has not been established, advise the client to avoid alcohol use. For those who do continue to consume alcohol, monitor their nutrient intake closely, since malnutrition may interact with alcohol to produce the adverse effects.

Pica, the ingestion of such nonfood substances as dirt and clay or starch may have detrimental effects through nutrient displacement, interference with nutrient absorption, or ingestion of toxic compounds. Include in the diet history questions to unveil the presence of pica, e.g., do you have a craving for starch? Observe for possible complications, such as iron deficiency anemia, toxemia, and fecal impaction, in pica practitioners. Caution the client who ingests such substances as moth balls or toilet bowl air fresheners of their potentially lethal effects on the fetus (see Chap. 19).

While teratogenic effects have been observed in experimental animals who consumed high levels of caffeine, this has not been confirmed in humans.[12] Nonetheless, it is prudent to advise pregnant women to use caffeine-containing substances, including coffee, tea, cocoa, chocolate, cola and some other soft drinks, and some drugs, in moderation, since a quantitative recommendation regarding caffeine use during pregnancy remains an area of uncertainty.

Age. Consider adolescent girls below age 17 and women above age 35 who become pregnant as high-risk clients. Sexual maturation is achieved about age 12½ or 13, and most girls reach physical maturity at about age 17. Pregnancy after age 17 usually does not present special biologic hazards. However, numerous pregnancy complications are observed in pregnant adolescents, particularly in teenagers 14 years of age and under. The hazards associated with adolescent pregnancy are physiologic, psychologic, and social in nature. It is generally believed that the high incidence of complicated pregnancy in adolescents results from the stresses of pregnancy superimposed on the stresses of adolescence, each with its own nutritional requirements. Many adolescent girls unduly restrict kilocalories to lose weight or have generally poor dietary habits. Assess their di-

etary intake; such nutrients as calcium, iron, B vitamins (especially thiamine, riboflavin, and vitamin B_6), vitamin A, zinc, and copper are often present in marginal amounts in their diets. Approximately 10 to 12 percent of adolescent girls are overweight, while an equal number are underweight. Social and psychologic pressures plague the pregnant adolescent. For instance, social mores are not accepting of the pregnant adolescent, who must leave school.

Provide supplemental folic acid and iron and extensive dietary counseling for the pregnant adolescent client. Follow-up is particularly important for those pregnant teens whose nutritional status is poor, who follow slimming regimens, or whose economic status is poor. Nutrition counseling for pregnant adolescents is further discussed in Chapter 17.

Parity. High parity (e.g., three or more pregnancies during the preceding 2 years) and a short interconceptional period put an additional stress on a current pregnancy. Counsel women to allow sufficient time to replenish nutritional stores following each pregnancy.

Diabetes. Preexisting medical conditions or those that develop during gestation, including diabetes and toxemia, necessitate combining nutritional guidelines for prenatal care with diet therapy for the existing condition. Complications, such as toxemia and perinatal mortality, are especially prevalent in pregnant diabetics. To prevent predelivery and postdelivery complications, pregnancy in a diabetic should be diagnosed as early as possible and a regimen of diet and insulin therapy established to carefully control the blood glucose level. Initiate diet counseling for the client with preexisting diabetes before pregnancy if possible. The pregnant state itself may precipitate the clinical signs of diabetes— ▶ **gestational diabetes**—particularly in obese clients. In pregnancy, the ability to handle a glucose load appears to be impaired. Glucose intolerance with onset in pregnancy is thought to be caused by complex metabolic and hormonal changes that are not completely understood. Insulin resistance may be responsible in part for gestational diabetes. Some women do not adjust as well as others to the altered carbohydrate metabolism and develop diabetes. Although these women regain normal carbohydrate metabolism following pregnancy, observe that the occurrence of gestational diabetes is associated with an increased tendency to develop overt diabetes in later life; 20 to 30 percent of these women develop permanent diabetes within 5 years following the pregnancy if ideal body weight is not attained.

Fetal size is generally larger in pregnant diabetics than in nondiabetics. This is thought to occur as the end result of hypertrophy of the fetal pancreas in response to maternal, and thus fetal, hyperglycemia. The resulting increase in insulin secretion stimulates a greater storage of fat, protein, and glycogen and is also thought to inhibit lung maturation. The larger baby can cause difficulties during labor or necessitate a cesarean section. Evaluate the newborn's blood glucose level, since hypoglycemia may be present during the initial hours after birth.

► Excessive accumulation of amniotic fluid, **hydramnios,** may also occur in pregnant diabetic clients. This fluid accumulation is due to an excessive output of urine by the fetus in excreting the excess glucose. Hydramnios is associated with such complications as premature delivery and toxemia.

Diet and insulin therapy are the cornerstones of treatment for the client who is diabetic at the onset of pregnancy. The client who develops gestational diabetes can usually be managed with diet alone with occasional use of insulin. Assist the client to establish a dietary regimen that allows for strict control of the blood glucose level, absence of ketosis, and adequate weight gain. Kilocalorie and nutrient requirements are the same as for the nondiabetic pregnant woman. Allow a daily kilocalorie intake of 36 to 38 kcal/kg pregnant body weight for the nonobese client and somewhat less, perhaps 30 kcal/kg, if the client is obese. To arrive at a more precise kilocalorie level, document current intake through a diet history or 3-day food record and estimate kilocalorie needs from these data. Use weight gain and the pattern of gain to guide adequacy of the kilocalorie intake. Test the urine for ketones routinely, since their absence can be another guide to kilocalorie adequacy. The carbohydrate, protein, and fat composition of the diet are important. Approximately 45 to 50 percent of the kilocalories should be supplied by complex carbohydrates, 30 to 35 percent by fat, and 15 to 20 percent by protein (about 1.3 to 1.5 g/kg of body weight).

Focus attention on the distribution of both the total kilocalorie intake and its components at various times during the day. To avoid marked fluctuations in blood sugar levels, an even distribution of kilocalories and carbohydrates among meals and snacks is suggested. Establish a meal and snack pattern that includes a minimum of four daily feedings. Six feedings may be necessary for clients who take insulin. Plan a bedtime snack that includes at least 25 g of carbohydrate to protect against early morning hypoglycemia. Educate the client concerning food sources of carbohydrate and the importance of consistent food intake. Review carefully the diet developed early in gestation and make adjustments to accommodate increasing kilocaloric needs and other changes.

Be aware that during the first half of pregnancy, the mother is prone to hypoglycemia, and the blood glucose level after an overnight fast may be 15 to 20 mg/100 ml lower than the level of nonpregnant women. The hypoglycemia, which results from the rapid fetal uptake of glucose, may decrease the requirement for insulin. Nausea, vomiting, and decreased food intake in early pregnancy may inten-
► sify the hypoglycemia and result in **starvation**

ketosis. Differentiate starvation ketosis, which indi-
► cates a need for glucose, from **ketoacidosis,** which indicates a need for insulin. Although ketones are produced excessively in both abnormalities, hyperglycemia is a feature of ketoacidosis and is absent in starvation ketosis. The antagonistic effect of the placental hormones on insulin may result in an increased insulin requirement during the second half of pregnancy. As insulin effectiveness is diminished, the tendency toward ketoacidosis is increased. The secretion of placental hormones reaches maximum levels during the latter stages of pregnancy. Recall that ketosis is hazardous to fetal development.

Toxemia. Toxemia (also called pregnancy-induced hypertension) is a generic term that includes pre-
► eclampsia and eclampsia. **Preeclampsia** is an acute hypertensive disorder that appears after the twentieth week of pregnancy. The hypertension is accom-
► panied by edema of the hands and face and/or **pro-**
► **teinuria** (protein in the urine). **Eclampsia** is the end result of preeclampsia and is further complicated by convulsions and coma. Preeclampsia is characterized by a sharp peak in weight gain due to sodium and fluid retention. The significance of having weight gain follow a gradual, smooth, and progressive curve should be evident.

Toxemia is a major cause of maternal and perinatal mortality. Consider these groups at a high risk for developing the complication: young adolescents, primigravidas, women above the age of 30, women with multiple pregnancies, and low-income women. Epidemiologic studies show a direct relationship between toxemia and per capita income—those states with a low per capita income have a high incidence of toxemia. At present, the incidence of toxemia is declining in the United States as a whole, presumably because of better prenatal care and a better diet.

Toxemia has been called the "disease of theories." Its cause is not known and there are conflicting data on both its etiology and treatment. The belief that such factors as excessive weight gain, high sodium intake, and low protein intake contribute to the disease has led to preventive and therapeutic strategies that restrict kilocalories and sodium or increase the protein content of the diet. Newer evidence suggests, however, that kilocaloric and/or sodium restriction may have deleterious effects, and although the topic is controversial, some investigators feel that a chronic mild nutritional deficiency prior to pregnancy combined with failure to meet the additional protein requirements of pregnancy contribute to the disorder. Others suggest that calcium deficiency may be implicated.[13]

Preeclampsia requires hospitalization, complete bed rest, and medications to lower blood pressure. Provide a diet for the toxemic client that is adequate in kilocalories, protein of high biologic value (1 g/kg dry pregnant weight), and moderate in sodium content and supplement with iron, folic acid, and multivitamins. Delivery cures toxemia, and a cesarean section is necessary in most cases.

Use measures to prevent toxemia: counsel high-risk women regarding their nutritional requirements to assure optimal nutrient intake. Monitor for changes in the weight gain pattern, increases in blood pressure, and presence of protein in the urine. Follow these clients closely throughout pregnancy, see them often, and follow up on missed or cancelled appointments.

Socioeconomic Risks. Low income is the one major factor most often associated with dietary inadequacy. Low income not only limits food purchases but may also limit the availability of food preparation and storage facilities. A pregnant woman with a large family and large financial obligations may neglect her dietary intake.

Guide the low-income client to sources of food assistance, including the Food Stamp Program and the Special Supplemental Food Program for Women, Infants, and Children (WIC program).

Food Stamp Program. The purpose of the Food Stamp Program is to increase the purchasing power of individuals and families who meet the financial criteria for participation in the program. Food stamps or coupons are provided that can be used like money to purchase food. The program is administered by the U.S. Department of Agriculture (USDA) and state and local agencies. At the state level, the program is usually run by the welfare department. Eligibility for the program is based on income and family size. The federal poverty level (defined annually) is used as the cutoff point for determining net income. Once eligibility has been established, a Food Stamp identification card is issued. Subsequently, an Authorization-to-Participate (ATP) card is mailed to the recipient once a month, which notifies the individual of the amount of stamps allotted.

Food stamps are issued by a variety of agencies, which vary with the states and the counties within the states. Some of the most common locations include banks, post offices, county welfare departments, and community action agencies. The individual goes to the location designated to issue stamps in his/her county or city, presents the identification card and ATP card, and receives the stamps. States also have the option of mailing the stamps to the individual. The money value of the coupons received is based on the Thrifty Food Plan (see Chap. 2 and Appendix 6). The money value is determined by subtracting 30 percent of a household's net income from the amount of Thrifty Food Plan allotment for that particular household size. In order to purchase an adequate diet, most households will therefore have to spend cash in addition to the stamps.

Advise clients who receive food stamps that they can spend stamps like money at food stores, supermarkets, or food cooperatives that are registered to accept stamps. Almost all large stores and many small stores are registered. The individual may be asked to show the identification card at the store. Stamps can be used to purchase any food or food product, domestic or imported, for human consumption, as well as plants or seeds to produce food for the household. Advise the client that stamps cannot be used to purchase household supplies, such as soap, paper goods, cleaning supplies, tobacco, alcoholic beverages, and pet food, or to pay bottle deposits.

Program Aides. Since no food assistance program can be effective without concurrent education of families receiving the help, the USDA has funded money for program aides to help meet the goals of the family food assistance programs by providing basic nutrition education for low-income families. The program is administered by the State Agricultural Extension Service. Program aides are selected primarily from the community in which they live and work. They receive intensive training by the County Extension Home Economist on subject matter and techniques for working with the poor. They also receive subsequent training on a continuing basis. The aide's attention is given to working with families not motivated to seek educational assistance. Special efforts are directed toward reaching families with young children. The basic purpose is education in normal nutrition (basic food needs, how to shop and use food stamps wisely). The teaching is done on a one-to-one basis, and the aide comes to the family's home. The aide may take a mother to the grocery store once or twice to show her how to shop wisely. This would not be done on a regular basis, however. A youth component has been added to the program, in which nutrition as a factor influencing growth and development is taught to youth groups.

WIC Program. Programs that provide resources for supplemental foods for needy pregnant and lactating women as well as preschool children are also available. The WIC program, also administered by the U.S. Department of Agriculture is designed to provide supplemental foods to upgrade the nutritional status of individuals who are at a high risk of malnutrition because of inadequate dietary intake and inadequate income during periods of peak growth. The program has the potential for reducing the incidence of certain health problems, such as infant mortality, birth defects, and mental retardation, by providing nutritious foods to supplement the diet of needy individuals.

The WIC program allocates funds to provide food, nutrition education, and certain clinical services to recipients through participating state health departments or comparable state agencies. Indian tribes, bands, or groups recognized by the Department of the Interior and the Indian Health Service may also act as state agencies for purposes of program participation.

Use the following criteria to assess the client's eligibility for the WIC program:

1. Meet these age and status criteria
   a. Pregnant or postpartum (up to 6 months) woman
   b. Lactating woman (up to 1 year)
   c. Infant or preschool child (up to age 5)
2. Reside in a low-income area serviced by an approved health care center that administers the WIC program
3. Are eligible for free or reduced-rate health care at the facility
4. Are considered by a competent health professional on the agency staff (e.g., physician, dietitian, nutritionist, nurse) to be at nutritional risk because of inadequate nutrition or income. This determination is made by medical examination or by nutritional interviews.

Maximum income limits for participation in the program have been established.

While "nutritional risk" is imprecisely defined, criteria usually include the presence of nutritional anemia, inadequate dietary intake, inappropriate growth patterns (e.g., overweight, underweight, or growth stunting in women and obesity or failure to thrive in an infant or child), and, for women, the presence of factors associated with a high risk during pregnancy, such as previous miscarriage, previous delivery of a premature or low-birth-weight infant, high parity, and short interconceptual time.

The supplemental foods provided to program participants are excellent sources of those nutrients known to be lacking in the diets of persons considered to be at nutritional risk: protein of high biologic value, iron, calcium, vitamin A, and vitamin C. The foods provided must meet specified nutritional criteria established by the U.S. Department of Agriculture. For example, cereals and infant formula must contain a specified amount of iron, and fruit or vegetable juice must contain a specified amount of vitamin C. The foods are designed so as not to provide excessive amounts of sugar, salt, and fat. The WIC program has six food package categories with varying amounts and types of food in each package: (1) infants 0 to 3 months, (2) infants 4 to 12 months, (3) children/women with special dietary needs, (4) children 1 to 5 years, (5) pregnant and breastfeeding women, and (6) nonbreastfeeding postpartum women.

Various types of food delivery systems are used by the state agency program to provide the supplemental food to the target population. Systems most frequently used are vouchers, direct distribution, home delivery, or a combination of these. The most commonly used system is the voucher system in which participants are given coupons that are redeemed for food at stores approved to participate.

Project areas must maintain medical records on participants for use in evaluating the effectiveness of the program. The minimal medical data collected are anthropometric measures (height, weight, and, for infants and children, the head circumferences) and blood studies (hemoglobin and hematocrit). Nutrition education is provided for the participants. The effectiveness of the program in terms of reducing the incidence of low-birth-weight infants and other problems has been demonstrated.[14,15]

Those clients with limited nutrition knowledge and limited homemaking skills (e.g., food preparation and budgeting) are also at risk nutritionally. Refer to Chapter 2 for client education guidelines. Additionally, geographic, ethnic, or language barriers may isolate clients from health care facilities or from food assistance programs, such as the Food Stamp Program and WIC. Those unable to obtain the familiar foods of their ethnic background may substitute less nutritious foods from the local markets (such as carbonated beverages for guava juice). Ethnic food patterns are discussed in Chapter 19.

Tailor diet counseling specifically to the needs of those following special regimens, such as vegetarian or health food diets. **Lactoovovegetarians** (those who eat milk and eggs but no meat) will have little difficulty in meeting nutritional needs for pregnancy. However, **vegans** (those who omit all animal foods) may have difficulty consuming adequate kilocalories, protein, vitamin B_{12}, vitamin D, riboflavin, calcium, and iron (see Chap. 20 for a discussion of vegetarian diets). Some fad diets, such as the macrobiotic diet, and strict regimens for weight loss are nutritionally unsound for nonpregnant as well as pregnant women. Advise pregnant women to avoid any type of regimen associated with fasting or ketosis, since ketones can cause fetal damage.

Psychologic Risks. Women with psychologic disorders, such as depression or anorexia nervosa, may not consume adequate kilocalories and nutrients. Limited weight gain, low infant birth weight, and perinatal mortality may result. Provide intensive diet counseling for these clients (see Chap. 17 for a discussion of anorexia nervosa).

DIET DURING LABOR AND FOLLOWING DELIVERY

Assessment and Intervention
During the early stages of labor, limit the diet to carbohydrate-containing foods, such as carbonated beverages, fruit juices, bread, or crackers with jelly, that leave the stomach rapidly. The longer period of time required for gastric emptying of proteins and fats may precipitate vomiting and aspiration if anesthesia is given. During active labor, withhold food to prevent the possibility of vomiting and aspiration. Restrict the first meal following delivery to liquids. Following this, give a normal diet.

Weight loss with delivery and during the first postpartum week averages 18 to 20 lb. Weight is gradually lost over the next several months, and most women return to their prepregnancy weight by about 3 months postpartum if the average amount of weight was gained. Lactating women generally lose the extra weight gained during pregnancy faster than nonnursing women. Since fat is stored during pregnancy as a reserve for lactation, advise nursing mothers not to expect to return to prepregnancy weight until lactation is complete. Assist clients who do not breastfeed to adjust their kilocalorie intake to allow for normalization of weight. If weight reduction is indicated, it can be instituted 2 to 4 weeks postpartum.

NUTRITIONAL CONSIDERATIONS IN LACTATION

Assessment and Intervention

Comparison of Human and Cow's Milk. Although cow's milk can be modified to serve as a suitable food to nourish the infant, there are many differences in the nutritional characteristics of human and cow's milk. Keep in mind, however, that the nutritional composition of breast milk is not constant; it varies with the individual, the stage of lactation, the time of day, the gestational age of the infant, and certain components of the mother's diet.

The stage of lactation greatly influences the nutritional characteristics of human milk. The secretion of the mammary glands undergoes a transitional phase before mature milk is produced. During the first few days after birth, colostrum is produced.
▶ **Colostrum** is a thick, yellowish, transparent fluid that is higher in protein and certain minerals (such as sodium, potassium, and chloride) but lower in fat, carbohydrate, and kilocalories than the milk that follows. Between the third and sixth day, transitional milk (which is still higher in protein) is produced. By the tenth day, the major transition to mature milk has been completed, and by the end of the first month, the milk has assumed the composition and form of mature breast milk. At this time the protein content reaches a consistent level, and as the protein content falls, carbohydrate and fat content rises progressively. Mature milk is composed of a combination of foremilk and hindmilk.
▶ **Foremilk,** a low-fat, low-protein secretion that is continuously secreted into the lactiferous ducts between nursing, accounts for about one third of the milk available to the infant in any nursing period.
▶ The remaining two thirds is **hindmilk,** a secretion higher in protein and fat that is formed and secreted shortly after nursing is initiated. The letdown reflex, a neurohumoral response initiated by the infant's sucking, stimulates the formation of hindmilk.

In human and cow's milk, the water, total solids, total fat, and energy value (20 kcal/oz) are approximately equal. However, the carbohydrate (lactose) content of human milk is about 1.5 times that of cow's milk, and protein and mineral content are only

TABLE 14–6
NUTRIENT CONTENT OF HUMAN MILK AND COW'S MILK

Constituent (per liter)	Human Milk	Cow's Milk
Energy (kcal)	690	660
Protein (g)	9	35
Fat (g)	45	37
Lactose (g)	68	49
Vitamins		
Vitamin A (IU)	1898	1025
Vitamin D (IU)	22	14
Vitamin E (IU)	2	0.4
Vitamin K (μg)	15	60
Thiamine (μg)	160	440
Riboflavin (μg)	360	1750
Niacin (mg)	1.5	0.9
Pyridoxine (μg)	100	640
Folic acid (μg)	52	55
Cobalamin (μg)	0.3	4
Ascorbic acid (mg)	43	11
Minerals		
Calcium (mg)	297	1170
Phosphorus (mg)	150	920
Sodium (mg)	150	506
Potassium (mg)	550	1368
Chlorine (mg)	385	1028
Magnesium (mg)	23	120
Sulfur (mg)	140	300
Iron (mg)[a]	0.56–0.3	0.5
Iodine (mg)	30	47
Manganese (μg)[b]	5.9–4.0	20–40
Copper (μg)	0.6–0.25	0.3
Zinc (mg)[c]	4–0.5	3–5
Selenium (μg)	20	5–50
Fluoride (mg)	0.05	0.03–0.1

[a] Median values at 2 weeks and 5 months of lactation.
[b] Median values at 2 weeks and 5 months of lactation, after which time the manganese content of human milk tends to increase.
[c] Median values at 2 weeks and 37 weeks of lactation.
(*Source:* Pipes PL: Nutrition in Infancy and Childhood, ed 2. St. Louis, CV Mosby, 1981. Adapted from Hambreaus L: Proprietary milk versus human breast milk in infant feeding, a critical approach from the nutritional point of view. Pediatr Clin North Am 24:17, 1977; Siimes MA, Vuori E, Kuitunen P: Breast milk iron—A declining concentration during the course of lactation. Acta Paediatr Scand 68:29, 1979; Vuori E: A longitudinal study of manganese in human milk. Acta Paediatr Scand 68:571, 1979; Vuori E, Kuitunen P: Concentrations of copper and zinc in human milk. Acta Paediatr Scand 68:33, 1978; Nayman R, et al.: Observations on the composition of milk-substitute products for the treatment of inborn errors of amino acid metabolism: Comparisons with human milk. Am J Clin Nutr 32:1279, 1979.)

about one third that of cow's milk. The advantages of these differences in composition are discussed in the next section. Table 14–6 provides a comparison of the nutrient composition of human and cow's milk.

Advantages of Breastfeeding. Human milk has distinct physiologic properties not found in the milk of other species. Thus human milk is the best initial food for the infant. Breastfeeding provides potential benefits for both the mother and baby. The unique characteristics of breast milk provide nutritional and immunologic benefits to the baby. Breast milk is easier for the infant to use than cow's milk formulas, although formulas have been designed to simulate the nutritional characteristics of human milk as nearly as possible. Nonetheless, be supportive of the mother's choice of method—breastfeeding or bottle feeding.

Nutritional Benefits of Breast Milk and Breastfeeding. The ratio of casein to whey proteins (lactalbumin), the major proteins in milk, affects the milk's digestibility. The casein:whey protein ratio in human milk is 40:60. In cow's milk it is 82:18. Casein forms a tough, cheesy curd in the stomach that is difficult to digest. Intestinal obstruction from a bolus of this indigestible mass is possible. Human milk with its lower ratio of casein to whey proteins produces a soft, flocculent, easy-to-digest curd in the stomach. Modification of cow's milk during formula preparation alters the curd and makes it more easily digested by the infant, however. The amino acid pattern of cow's and human milk is also different. For example, human milk contains lesser amounts of methionine and the aromatic amino acids, phenylalanine and tyrosine, and more of the sulfur-containing amino acid, cystine, needed for central nervous system development. Newborns, especially prematures, have a limited capacity to metabolize phenylalanine and tyrosine and to convert methionine to cystine, and they do not synthesize taurine well. Breast milk contains a considerable amount of nitrogen in compounds other than protein. Whether some of the factors in the nonprotein nitrogen of human milk are of nutritional significance to the infant remains to be studied.

The higher lactose content of human milk promotes the growth of microorganisms that produce metabolic acids that lead to a low pH in the gastrointestinal tract. This low pH inhibits the growth of undesirable bacteria and enhances the absorption of certain mineral elements. Infant formula with added lactose tends to have a similar action. Lactose also has a laxative effect. Observe that constipation is not a problem for breastfed babies.

The fatty acids contained in human milk are less saturated than are those in cow's milk. These fats are better absorbed than the fatty acids of cow's milk, which contains larger amounts of the shorter-chain saturated fatty acids. The presence of significant lipolytic activity (lipase enzyme activity) in human milk may also aid fat absorption. Fecal fat loss is less in breastfed babies than in those who are fed cow's milk. However, when they are fed commercial formulas in which the butterfat has been replaced with vegetable oil, the degree of fat absorption is similar to that of breastfed infants. Human milk is a richer source of cholesterol than is cow's milk or infant formulas in which the butterfat is replaced with vegetable oil; these formulas are practically devoid of cholesterol. On the basis of animal experiments, it has been suggested that early expo-

sure to cholesterol stimulates the production of the enzyme systems necessary for cholesterol homeostasis in later life, but conclusive evidence for this is lacking in humans. Moreover, some investigators suggest that exogenous cholesterol may be desirable for synthesis of nerve tissue and bile acids by the infant.

The lesser amounts of protein, sodium, potassium, phosphorus, and chloride of human milk result in a lower renal solute load. The higher renal solute load of cow's milk formulas may predispose infants to dehydration when the environmental temperature is high. However, current commercial formulas provide renal solute loads not greatly in excess of those of breast milk. While the iron content of both cow's and human milk is low, the iron in human milk is better absorbed (about 50 percent vs about 12 percent in unmodified cow's milk), thus protecting the baby against iron deficiency. The lower protein and phosphorus content and higher lactose and vitamin C content of breast milk in comparison to cow's milk are thought to enhance iron absorption, although infant formulas in current use provide most of the advantages of breast milk. Calcium and phosphorus are present in a ratio of 2:1, which allows maximum absorption of both minerals and is protective against hypocalcemic tetany.

Breastfeeding is thought to promote a pattern of weight gain in the infant that protects against infantile obesity and possibly obesity in later life. The protective effect is thought to result from a lesser kilocaloric intake in breastfed babies than in formula-fed babies. Assess the client's feeding pattern. Mothers of breastfed babies usually allow the infant to nurse until satisfied. In contrast, formula-fed babies are often enticed to drink the last drop of formula. Compare the ages at which solid foods are introduced into the diet of breastfed and formula-fed infants. Formula-fed babies are more likely to receive solid foods at a very early age, with an attendant risk of excessive kilocaloric intake and development of poor food habits. Compare the growth patterns of infants fed by the two methods. Formula-fed babies are observed to gain in weight and length more rapidly than breastfed babies, and formula-fed babies generally gain more weight for a specified gain in length than do breastfed babies. The long-term consequences of these differences remain unclear, however, and evidence is lacking in support of the hypothesis that a fat baby becomes a fat child. It is suggested that the change in the composition of breast milk during feeding may satiate the infant or in some may signal a cessation of feeding.

Immunologic Benefits of Breastfeeding. Colostrum and mature milk contain a wide variety of host resistance factors, such as antibodies and white blood cells, that have the potential for providing protection against a range of infections, particularly of the respiratory and gastrointestinal tracts, a property not shared by cow's milk or formula. The protective effect of breastfeeding against respiratory and intestinal infection is particularly evident in countries where sanitary conditions are poor, and there are indications that this is also true in countries with better sanitary conditions.[16] The mechanism of the protective effect is not known, and the effectiveness of breast milk may vary among women as well as within a given woman depending on age and stage of lactation.[17]

Cow's milk protein is a common allergen, but human milk itself does not induce allergic reactions in infants. Intact protein from cow's milk or other allergenic foods is more likely to permeate the gastrointestinal epithelium during the first 6 months of life. Breastfeeding during this time spares the gastrointestinal tract from exposure to food antigens at a time when large molecules may be readily absorbed. If a baby experiences manifestations of allergy while ingesting human milk, examine the mother's dietary intake, since the baby may be allergic to substances in such foods as milk, eggs, or corn that are present in the mother's diet and enter the milk supply. Advise her to eliminate offending foods rather than stop breastfeeding. Although the belief that human milk will prevent a baby from developing allergies or that the overall incidence of allergy is less in breastfed babies has not been proved, breastfeeding for the first 6 months may decrease the child's chances of developing allergic reactions in some cases. However, there is no evidence that it will prevent all allergies.

Contraindications to Breastfeeding.

There are a few circumstances in which breastfeeding is contraindicated or must be terminated. Breastfeeding is impractical if the mother can supply less than half the infant's needs. Situations in which breastfeeding may be contraindicated or should be ended are (1) presence of a chronic illness in the mother (such as cardiac disease, nephritis, severe anemia, tuberculosis, or chronic fevers), (2) return to work by the mother (may require termination), (3) inability of the infant to nurse because of oral anomalies, (4) intolerance to human milk, as in certain inborn errors of metabolism, that necessitates special formulas, and (5) occurrence of another pregnancy. Pregnancy usually does not necessitate immediate cessation of lactation. However, because of the excessively high combined nutrient demands, breastfeeding probably should not continue beyond 20 weeks gestation.

Temporary cessation is usually indicated when the mother acquires an acute infection not yet acquired by the infant. An occasional situation requiring an interruption of breastfeeding is hyperbilirubinemia. This disorder, which causes jaundice of the skin and eyes, results from the build-up of unconjugated bilirubin in the blood. A metabolite of progesterone (pregnanediol) transmitted through the milk inhibits the conjugation (and thus the excretion) of bilirubin. Cessation of nursing for 2 to 3 days allows for sufficient lowering of the serum bilirubin. Breastfeeding can then be safety resumed, and the condition generally does not return when breastfeeding is again instituted. During periods of temporary cessation of breastfeeding, advise the client to manually express her milk to prevent breast engorgement.

Certain drugs and toxins that can harm the infant may be concentrated in human milk. Concern has been expressed about the presence of environmental contaminants, such as polychlorinated biphenyls (PCBs) in breast milk. This lipophilic contaminant tends to accumulate in adipose tissue and can be excreted in breast milk. The presence of environmental pollutants in breast milk has raised questions that have not been resolved in regard to the safety of breastfeeding by all mothers.

Nutritional Requirements of Lactation.

For the woman who chooses to breastfeed, nutrition is particularly important. Many nutrients must be increased above the nonpregnant level, with substantial increases in kilocalories.

Energy Needs.

Additional kilocalories are needed to produce milk. A typical daily milk volume for a lactating woman is 850 ml. The efficiency of conversion of maternal dietary energy to milk energy is 80 percent; therefore, approximately 90 kcal are required to produce 100 ml of milk (or about 800 kcal to produce 850 ml). This additional energy is provided by fat stored during pregnancy (approximately 2 to 4 kg), which may be mobilized to provide 200 to 300 kcal/day for the first 3 months of milk production, and by additional kilocalories from the diet. The RDA of 500 extra kilocalories assumes the use of the stored fat to complete the energy requirement. Tell the client that the kilocalorie requirement should be increased above this level if lactation continues beyond 3 months, if she is nourishing more than one infant, or if she is below the normal weight for her height.

Other Nutrients.

The efficiency of conversion of dietary protein to milk protein is 70 percent. Since 850 ml of milk contains 10 g of protein, the RDA recommends 20 g protein above the nonpregnant allowance to assure an adequate protein intake.

The RDA for calcium remains the same as for pregnancy. The calcium is diverted from calcification of the fetal skeleton to milk production. Even a liberal calcium intake may not be totally successful in counteracting a negative calcium balance.

Although the iron requirement is diminished below the need during pregnancy, remind the client that iron supplementation should continue for several months to replenish iron stores. Supplementation with other nutrients is not required if the diet is adequate (see Table 14–3).

Two to three quarts of fluid are necessary to provide the liquid volume of milk. Contrary to popular opinion, drinking water in amounts larger than that which the mother wishes to drink to quench thirst actually impairs lactation, presumably due to suppression of posterior pituitary secretion. Dehydration reduces milk secretion only when the volume drunk is less than the volume of milk secreted. Counsel the client to use thirst as the guide for fluid intake. Although a high fluid intake does not stimulate milk production, a liberal intake should be maintained to preclude the necessity of forming a highly concentrated urine to compensate for fluid lack.

Effect of Maternal Diet on Lactation. Alterations in the maternal diet can affect the volume of milk produced and the concentration of some components (such as fat and vitamins) of breast milk. In contrast, composition of other nutrients (such as calcium) appears to be largely independent of the mother's nutritional status. With nutritional inadequacy, maternal stores are used to maintain the nutritional value of the milk. Avoid an energy deficit during either pregnancy or lactation that may reduce the volume of milk secreted. Whereas the percentage compositions of carbohydrate, protein, and fat are not affected significantly by the maternal diet, the amount and source of energy may alter the fatty acid pattern. For example, with kilocaloric restriction, the fatty acid composition resembles that of depot fat, indicating mobilization of fat stores. Increased energy intake as carbohydrate results in increased levels of lauric and myristic acids, and a diet high in polyunsaturated fat yields milk that is also high in polyunsaturated fat. There is limited evidence that total fat content may be reduced in malnourished women. While the quantity of protein appears not to be affected by the protein level of the diet, the amounts of two essential amino acids, lysine and methionine, are lower in milk from women consuming a protein-deficient diet. The water-soluble vitamins, vitamin A, and iodine content of breast milk also reflect the dietary levels of these nutrients. This is not the case, however, with the remaining fat-soluble vitamins and minerals, such as calcium, iron, copper, and fluoride. For instance, administration of iron or a fluoride supplement to a nursing mother is not reflected in the milk.

Additional Considerations. There are no foods that require restriction except in individual cases where gastric distress is noted in the infant following ingestion of specific foods. It takes about 4 to 6 hours for food metabolites to get into breast milk; use this period as a guide to determine the offenders.

Most drugs taken by the mother will be excreted in breast milk, and many may depress milk production or have adverse effects on the baby. On the basis of body size, a drug is approximately 12 times more potent in an infant than in the mother. Breast milk is more acidic than plasma, and, therefore, basic drugs (e.g., aminophylline and erythromycin) tend to ionize in this environment and diffuse more readily into the milk. In contrast, weak acids (e.g., penicillins, most diuretics) do the reverse and are less concentrated in breast milk than in plasma. Use the following guidelines for drug therapy for the lactating client:[18]

- *Drugs not to use.* Antimetabolites, most cathartics, radioactive drugs, anticoagulants, tetracycline, iodides, ergot, atropine, metronidazole (Flagyl R), thiouracil, dihydrotachysterol.
- *Drugs to use with supervision.* Lithium carbonate, sulfonamide, reserpine, steroids, diuretics, malidixic acid, barbiturates, phenytoin, narcotics and codeine, chloramphenicol.
- *Drugs not contraindicated.* Occasional aspirin, most antibiotics, antihistamines, antidiarrheals, epinephrine, insulin.

Both alcohol and caffeine are excreted in breast milk; therefore, recommend moderation in their use. In women who smoke 10 to 20 or more cigarettes daily, the milk supply may be reduced, and harmful levels of nicotine will be transmitted to the infant. Alcohol consumption should be limited to the equivalent of two cocktails daily. Oral contraceptives have a deleterious effect on both the quantity and quality of milk produced. If the pills, particularly those with a high content of estrogen, are given soon after delivery, most mothers are unable to continue breastfeeding. For women who select oral contraception, suggest low-dose estrogen or progestogen-only pills or an alternate means of contraception while lactation is in progress.

NUTRITION AND CONTRACEPTION

Assessment and Intervention

The widespread use of contraceptive devices, especially oral contraceptive agents (OCAs or the pill), has prompted active investigation of the nutrition-related effects of various methods of contraception. Attention has been particularly focused on the effects of OCAs and intrauterine devices (IUDs). Investigations with OCA users have revealed alterations in the results of numerous biochemical tests used to assess nutritional status. These findings suggest that requirements for certain nutrients may be altered. However, despite the widespread biochemical and metabolic changes, only a few clinical signs associated with a deficiency of specific nutrients have been observed in OCA users. Many of the changes appear to be reversed when the use of OCAs is discontinued. Considering the large number of OCA users—it is estimated that they are used by one of six women of childbearing age in the United States—more research is needed to identify the specific nutritional and metabolic effects on the user and on her future offspring.

Nutritional Effects of OCAs. OCAs are potent drugs that contain variable amounts of the synthetic hormones, estrogen and progestogens. Since the synthetic forms of the hormones used in OCAs are similar to the natural forms secreted by the placenta during pregnancy, many of the effects noted simulate those observed during pregnancy. For this reason, the norms used for biochemical tests in nonpill users may not apply to pill users. Whereas the physiologic adjustments of OCA use and pregnancy are similar, nutritional requirements are different.

The metabolism of all nutrients studied thus far appears to be altered by the pill, although reports of studies are often contradictory. Body weight tends to increase, various aspects of carbohydrate, protein, and lipid metabolism are changed, and alterations occur in the serum levels of vitamins and minerals. With the latter, the blood concentration of some nutrients is increased, whereas there is a decrease in blood concentration of others. Changes in blood concentration of some nutrients may reflect a redistribution of nutrients among the various body compartments rather than an increase or decrease in use per se. Changes in biochemical test results appear during the first 3 months of pill use and do not usually change further with continued use for several years. Individuals are not equally vulnerable to the changes, and the extent of the changes varies. The variability appears to be related to preexisting hormonal balance and nutritional state, age, hormonal composition of the pill, and duration of pill use. The body may also adapt to the metabolic effects.

Changes in Body Weight and Metabolism of Carbohydrate, Protein, and Lipid. Evaluate the weight status of clients taking OCAs. Many women tend to gain weight at the beginning of pill use. The weight gain occurs secondary to fluid retention and to an increase in lean body tissue.

Most clients on the pill are not as efficient in handling a glucose load as are nonpill users. There is an increase in the frequency of abnormal glucose tolerance tests (GTT), and there may be a slight rise in the fasting blood glucose in healthy women. Caution women with a family history of diabetes mellitus to be especially alert to changes in the handling of glucose that occur with pill use.

Protein synthesis and nitrogen balance are also changed. The hepatic synthesis of certain transport proteins (e.g., transferrin that transports iron, ceruloplasmin that transports copper, and retinol-binding protein that transports vitamin A) is increased. In contrast, the concentration of serum albumin may be decreased, and tryptophan metabolism is altered. Nitrogen retention and an increase in lean body mass contribute to the initial weight gain observed in pill users. This nitrogen retention is not sustained beyond the first few cycles, however, and there is some evidence that nitrogen loss occurs when the pill is discontinued.

Evaluate the blood lipid levels. Plasma triglycerides tend to increase in pill users, but no predictable changes occur in blood cholesterol levels. If the client's history includes familial hypercholesterolemia, she may have an elevation in plasma cholesterol when beginning pill use. Serum triglyceride levels are markedly increased in those with familial hypertriglyceridemia.

Alterations in Vitamin and Mineral Metabolism. The changes in metabolism of various vitamins and minerals that have been correlated with use of the pill are summarized in Table 14–7.

The high serum levels of iron, copper, and vitamin A, which are seen consistently in OCA users, may be linked with an increase in the synthesis of their carrier proteins (i.e., transferrin, ceruloplasmin, and retinol-binding protein). The high vitamin A level may also occur in association with the elevation of serum lipids (vitamin A is fat soluble) or an enhanced synthesis of vitamin A from carotene (carotene levels are found in low concentration in some women). The high vitamin A levels do not imply a decreased requirement, as the high level may reflect a shift of vitamin A from the liver to the serum. It has been suggested that the nutritional requirements for copper and iron are slightly reduced. With regard to iron, OCA use is also associated with a decrease in menstrual blood, and thus iron loss.

Plasma zinc and vitamin B_{12} are usually decreased in OCA users, and some users may also have low levels of vitamin C, vitamin B_6, and folic acid. The availability of thiamine and riboflavin may be reduced by the pill. The low blood concentration of zinc may reflect a shift of this mineral into the erythrocytes to serve as a component of the enzyme, carbonic anhydrase, which increases in concentration with pill use. No explanation is available for the low blood levels of vitamin B_{12} or vitamin C. Interestingly, the tissue levels of B_{12} do not appear to be affected. Like zinc, the altered vitamin C level may reflect a shift in its distribution in the tissues.

Assess routinely the nutritional status of clients taking OCAs and provide diet counseling as a component of routine management. If nutrient inadequacies are detected, evaluate for clinical and biochemical evidence of nutritional deficiencies. Since OCAs tend to alter the body's ability to use certain nutrients, it is imperative that an adequate diet be consumed. Since the interconceptual period is a crucial time for replenishing nutrient stores, it is extremely important to prevent a double inadequacy in clients who have just given birth.

If a marginal diet exists, providing a multivitamin supplement is a reasonable prophylactic measure. As in pregnancy, however, do not allow this practice to substitute for appropriate dietary advice. Much attention has been focused on the relationship between altered vitamin B_6 status and the occasional incidence of depression in some clients, but current evidence does not justify routine supplementation

TABLE 14–7
NUTRITIONAL ABNORMALITIES ASSOCIATED WITH OCAs

Nutrient	Biochemical Defect	Clinical Defect
Iron	Serum level increased; total iron-binding capacity increased	—
Copper	Plasma level increased; ceruloplasmin increased	—
Zinc	Plasma level decreased	—
Vitamin A	Plasma level increased	—
Vitamin B_{12}	Serum level decreased	—
Vitamin B_6	Altered tryptophan metabolism; plasma level decreased	Depression
Folic acid	Serum and erythrocyte levels decreased	Megaloblastic anemia (rare); enlarged cells of cervix
Vitamin C	Plasma, platelet, and leukocyte levels decreased	—
Riboflavin	Erythrocyte level decreased	Glossitis (rare)

(Source: Adapted from Winick M, ed: Nutritional Disorders of American Women. New York, John Wiley & Sons, 1977, p 44.)

with vitamin B_6 or other nutrients.[19] Attempt to correct deficiency states with dietary measures whenever possible.

Intrauterine Devices. The contraceptive action of IUDs involves, in part, the antifertility properties of metabolic copper in the uterine environment. It appears that copper in the IUD is deposited locally in the endometrium of the uterus and is shed during menstruation. It does not spread throughout the general circulation, since no change in circulating copper has been observed.

Although IUD users generally have an increase in menstrual blood loss, the small, copper-containing IUDs cause less blood loss than do other types. Assist clients who use IUDs to maintain a high intake of dietary iron. For those who have excessive menstrual bleeding, supplementation with iron salts may be necessary. Those women with substantial monthly blood loss (more than 50 ml) may need supplemental iron to avoid iron deficiency anemia.

REVIEW QUESTIONS AND ACTIVITIES

1. Identify the three major stages of pregnancy and distinguish between the effects of maternal malnutrition during each stage.
2. Discuss the rationale for the need to use different biochemical indices of nutritional status for pregnant and nonpregnant women.
3. Explain the rationale for the physiologic anemia of pregnancy.
4. Identify the changes that take place in the renal, endocrine, and gastrointestinal systems during pregnancy.
5. Describe the dietary modifications that you would make for pregnant women with the following complaints: (a) nausea and vomiting, (b) heartburn, and (c) constipation.
6. List two maternal characteristics that influence infant birth weight.
7. Identify the appropriate amount and pattern of weight gain during pregnancy.
8. Compare the RDA for energy, protein, vitamins, and minerals for adult pregnant and lactating women. How do these recommendations differ for young pregnant and lactating adolescents?
9. *Case study:* Your client (Mrs. A.) is an obese (150 lb), 25-year-old pregnant female (first trimester) of Spanish-American origin with a limited income.
   a. What hazards does the obesity pose?
   b. Estimate her kilocalorie and protein requirements.
   c. Plan a day's menu that meets her nutritional requirements, using low-cost foods (refer to Chap. 19 for guidelines for ethnic diet patterns and Chap. 2 for low-cost foods).
   d. Describe three community nutrition programs that are available for low-income pregnant women.
   e. What mineral elements need special attention during the pregnancy? What changes occur in the rate of calcium and iron absorption during pregnancy? What

are the hazards of iron deficiency anemia in pregnancy?

f. What would you tell Mrs. A. about her vitamin needs?

g. Why is it necessary to assess for the use of alcohol, tobacco, and the practice of pica in pregnancy?

h. Mrs. A. develops gestational diabetes at the end of the first trimester. Adjust her diet to account for this complication.

i. Describe the dietary adjustments for labor and delivery.

j. Adjust Mrs. A.'s diet pattern for the period of lactation.

10. *Case study:* Fourteen-year-old Alice is in her second trimester of pregnancy. She was underweight at the onset of pregnancy and currently is not gaining an adequate amount of weight.

a. State several reasons why adolescents may have serious nutrition problems during pregnancy.

b. What danger does Alice face due to her underweight condition?

c. Plan a day's menu that meets her nutritional requirements.

During Alice's last checkup, she had an elevated blood pressure and puffiness of the face, hands, and ankles, and her urine analysis revealed the presence of protein.

d. What disorder does Alice likely have?

e. Describe the dietary management of the disorder.

11. Describe the nutritional and immunologic benefits of breast milk.

12. Identify the effects of oral contraceptive use on carbohydrate, protein, and fat metabolism.

13. List three nutrients whose blood levels are increased and six nutrients whose blood levels are decreased secondary to oral contraceptive use.

14. Identify the mineral element for which dietary supplementation may be necessary as a result of use of an intrauterine device.

REFERENCES

1. National Academy of Sciences, Committee on Nutrition of the Mother and Preschool Child: Laboratory Indices of Nutritional Status in Pregnancy. Washington, DC, 1978.
2. Schulman PK: Hyperemesis gravidarum: An approach to the nutritional aspects of care. J Am Diet Assoc 80:577, 1982.
3. Committee on Maternal Nutrition, Food and Nutrition Board, National Research Council: Maternal Nutrition and the Course of Pregnancy. Washington, DC, National Academy Press, 1970.
4. Naeye RL: Weight gain and outcome of pregnancy. Am J Obstet Gynecol 135:3, 1979.
5. National Research Council: Recommended Dietary Allowances, ed 9. Washington, DC, National Academy Press, 1980.
6. Commission on Life Sciences, Food and Nutrition Board, National Research Council: Alternative Dietary Practices and Nutritional Abuses During Pregnancy, Proceedings of a Workshop. Washington, DC, National Academy Press, 1982, pp 21–22.
7. Laurence KM: Neural tube defects: A two-pronged approach to primary prevention. Pediatrics 70:648, 1982.
8. Smithells RW, Nevin NC, Seller MJ, et al.: Further experience of vitamin supplementation for prevention of neural-tube defect recurrences. Lancet 1:1027, 1983.
9. Smithells RW, Sheppard A, Schorah CJ, et al.: Possible prevention of neural-tube defects by periconceptional vitamin supplementation. Lancet 1:339, 1980.
10. Commission on Life Sciences, op cit, p 180.
11. Hanson JW, Streissguth AP, Smith DN: The effects of moderate alcohol consumption during pregnancy on fetal growth and morphogenesis. J Pediatr 92:457, 1978.
12. Linn S, Schoenbaum SC, Monson, RR, et al.: No association between coffee consumption and adverse outcomes of pregnancy. N Engl J Med 306:141, 1982.
13. Belizan JM, Villas J: The relationship between calcium intake and edema- proteinuria- and hypertension-gestosis: An hypothesis. Am J Clin Nutr 33:2202, 1980.
14. Edozien JC, Switzer BR, Bryan RB: Medical evaluation of the special supplemental food program for women, infants, and children. Am J Clin Nutr 32:677, 1979.
15. Hicks LE, Langham RA, Takenaka J: Cognitive and health measures following early nutritional supplementation. Am J Pub Health 72:1110, 1982.
16. Waletzky LR, ed: Symposium on Human Lactation. USDHEW Publication No. (HSA) 79–5107. Washington, DC, U.S. Government Printing Office, 1976, pp 55–56.
17. Whitehead RG: Nutritional aspects of human lactation. Lancet 1:167, 1983.
18. Waletzky LR, ed, op cit, pp 77–89.
19. National Research Council, op cit, pp 101–102.

BIBLIOGRAPHY

Beagle WS: Fetal alcohol syndrome: A review. J Am Diet Assoc 79:274, 1981.
Council on Scientific Affairs: Fetal effects of maternal alcohol use. JAMA 249:2517, 1983.
Kaplan M, Eidelman AI, Aboulafia Y: Fasting and the precipitation of labor. The Yom Kippur effect. JAMA 250:1317, 1983.
Kitzmiller JL: Sweet success: Teaching diabetes and pregnancy management. Diab Educ 9:1 [Suppl] 1983.
Marbury MC, Linn S, Monson R, et al.: The association of alcohol consumption with outcome of pregnancy. Am J Public Health 73:1165, 1983.
McDonald EC, Pollit E, Mueller W, et al.: The Bacon Chow study: Maternal nutritional supplementation and birth weight of offspring. Am J Clin Nutr 34:2133, 1981.
Naeye RL: Influence of maternal cigarette smoking during pregnancy on fetal and childhood growth. Obstet Gynecol 57:18, 1981.

Picone TA, Lindsay HA, Olsen PN, Ferris ME: Pregnancy outcome in North American women. II. Effect of diet, cigarette smoking, stress, and weight gain on placentas and on neonatal physical and behavioral characteristics. Am J Clin Nutr 36:1214, 1982.

Psiaki D, Olson C: Current Knowledge on Breast Feeding: A Review for Medical Practitioners. Ithaca, NY, Division of Nutritional Sciences, Cornell University, 1980.

Ogra PL, Greene HL: Human milk and breast feeding: An update on the state of the art. Pediatr Res 16:266, 1982.

Rosett HL, Weiner L: Prevention of fetal alcohol effects. Pediatrics 69:813, 1982.

Schulman PK: Diabetes in pregnancy: Nutritional aspects of care. J Am Diet Assoc 76:585, 1980.

Stein Z, Kline J: Smoking, alcohol, and reproduction. Am J Public Health 73:1154, 1983.

Thorp VJ: Effect of oral contraceptive agents on vitamin and mineral requirements. J Am Diet Assoc 76:581, 1980.

Weiner L, Rosett HL, Edelin KC, et al.: Alcohol consumption by pregnant women. Obstet Gynecol 61:6, 1983.

CHAPTER 15

Infant Nutrition

Objectives

After completing this chapter, the student will be able to:

1. Assess the major physical and psychologic characteristics of the newborn and infant that have implications for feeding.

2. Develop a teaching plan for managing the diet for the first 6 months of the life of a term infant who is being breastfed, and adjust the teaching plan so that it is appropriate for an infant who is receiving a commercially prepared infant formula.

3. Manage the diet of an infant during the second 6 months of life.

4. Distinguish among regurgitation, vomiting, constipation, diarrhea, and colic in infancy and compare their dietary management.

5. Compare and contrast the nutritional requirements and dietary management of premature and term infants.

Many changes in infant feeding practices have occurred during the twentieth century. Until recently, breastfeeding, an almost universal practice at the turn of the century, was steadily giving way to the convenience of infant formulas. There is now evidence, however, that the trend is slowing or reversing, with a return to breastfeeding. Both the incidence and duration are increasing and this increase has occurred across all levels of income and education.[1] Solid foods are sometimes introduced into the infant's diet at an early age—perhaps during the first few weeks of life—and whole or skim cow's milk may be used as an early replacement for breast milk or formula by some parents.

Infant feeding practices are being carefully evaluated to determine both their short-term and long-term effects. Breastfeeding is encouraged by a number of groups, since breast milk provides the optimum quantity and quality of nutrients to support the infant's growth and development. Breast milk is used as the reference standard for evaluating the adequacy of formulas in supporting growth and

development. For mothers who do not breastfeed, formulas that are modified to simulate human milk as nearly as possible will support adequate growth and development. However, other practices, such as the early use of solid foods, whole milk, or skim milk in the infant's diet, are being discouraged. Knowledge of infant nutrition has not progressed sufficiently to allow the establishment of specific rules or directions in infant feeding, nor are hard and fast rules necessarily desirable. However, nurses should be prepared to help parents establish reasonable feeding practices based on current scientific data.

The infant's growth rate is especially rapid during the first 6 months, and, thus, the food supply is critical during this period. Nutrient imbalances may have lasting effects on growth and development. Concurrent with the rapid growth, there occurs a progressive maturation of motor skills (oral, fine, and gross). During the first year, the infant progresses from a totally dependent feeder to an active participant in the feeding process. Motor control moves from reflexive to voluntary, and the infant who sucks liquids from a nipple at birth gradually learns to chew and swallow solid food and drink from a cup. By 1 year of age, the infant is making an attempt at self-feeding.

ASSESSMENT

Physiologic Aspects of Infancy
Physical characteristics of the infant that affect nutritional needs and the feeding process are (1) a rapid growth rate, (2) limited nutritional stores at birth, (3) a large skin surface area in relation to weight, (4) a skeleton that is not fully calcified, (5) immature digestive capacity, (6) immature kidney function, (7) feeding reflexes present at birth, and (8) feeding position required to prevent infection.

Rapid Growth Rate. The growth rate is especially rapid during the first 6 months, with a weekly gain of 5 to 7 oz. During the second 6 months, the weight gain tapers off somewhat, increasing by only 4 to 5 oz per week. With this rate of weight gain, birth weight is usually doubled by 4 to 6 months and tripled by the end of the first year. Length increases approximately 50 percent by the end of the first year, and the brain weight is 60 percent of that of an adult. A relatively large quantity of food in relation to the baby's size is required to support this rapid rate of growth.

Limited Nutritional Stores. The baby's limited nutritional stores also have implications for nutritional requirements. Note the skimpy look of a newborn; that results from a limited amount of subcutaneous fat. Infants tolerate nutrient deprivation very poorly, even for relatively short periods of time. Although storage of most nutrients is limited, some, such as vitamin A, copper, and iron, are stored in the liver. Iron stores are further augmented after birth from iron added as the initially high hemoglobin level of the newborn gradually drops. In fullterm infants, storage iron is usually sufficient to meet iron needs until birth weight is doubled.

Large Skin Surface Area. The infant's large skin surface area relative to weight leads to large heat and fluid losses from the skin. Since the infant's skin surface area per unit of body weight is approximately double that of an adult, expect the rate of fluid and heat loss to be approximately double that of the adult rate. This contributes to relatively high kilocalorie and fluid needs. Water deprivation is tolerated poorly by the infant because of the high rate of water turnover, the high percentage of the body composed of water, and the limited ability of the immature kidneys to conserve water.

Poorly Calcified Skeleton. At birth, the skeleton is poorly calcified, containing a large percentage of

cartilage and water. Bone mineralization is a process that continues until maturity is reached. The diet must, therefore, contain adequate amounts of such nutrients as calcium, phosphorus, and vitamin D required for bone mineralization.

Immature Digestive Capacity. Observe that the young infant is toothless, and, thus, early feedings must necessarily be liquid or semiliquid. The digestive secretions contain the enzymes necessary for digesting the simple carbohydrates, proteins, and emulsified fats contained in milk. The enzymes that digest starches and other fats gradually develop during the first few months and permit better digestion and absorption. Amylase activity (needed to digest starch) in the small intestine of the young infant is initially very low. Despite this, starch-containing foods (such as cereal, which is usually the first solid food given) do not seem to cause digestive problems. Since the amount eaten is usually very small, gradual enzyme adaptation may occur. Moreover, the young infant's gastrointestinal tract is quite permeable to large molecules, such as intact protein, that can precipitate an allergic response.

Immature Kidney Function. The kidneys do not reach their full functional capacity until the end of the first year. Young infants have a lower glomerular filtration rate and less ability to concentrate the urine than do older infants or children, although by 4 to 6 weeks the ability to concentrate solutes closely approximates the adult level. Greater amounts of some amino acids are excreted (presumably because of low tubular reabsorption), and reabsorption of others is high.

Feeding Reflexes. The reflexes that allow the newborn to actively participate in eating are rooting, sucking, swallowing, gag, extrusion, and satiety. Observe a nursing infant and note that the mouth is reflexively turned toward any object that touches
▶ the cheek. This **rooting reflex** helps to locate the breast or bottle. Stimulation of the lips and tongue
▶ initiates the **sucking reflex.** The fatty sucking pads in the cheeks are an additional aid to sucking. The
▶ **swallowing reflex,** which is stimulated by sucking, is well coordinated with the breathing reflex. The
▶ **gag reflex** comes into play when more food is taken into the mouth than can be swallowed successfully.
▶ In contrast, the **extrusion reflex,** which is strong during the first 9 weeks and begins diminishing at 3½ to 4 months, pushes food that is placed on the tip of the tongue out of the mouth. This reflex provides the thrusting movement of the tongue necessary to extract milk from the nipple. It must diminish in strength before solid food placed on the tip of the tongue can be formed into a ball and carried
▶ to the back of the mouth for swallowing. The **satiety reflex** allows the baby to decide when the feeding is adequate. While breastfed babies are usually allowed to rely on their internal satiety cues, this is

often not the case with the bottle-fed baby, who does not control the feeding situation and who may be encouraged to consume more food than is actually needed. It has been suggested that the changing composition of breast milk that occurs during the process of breastfeeding (notably in fat content) is important in the development of the appetite control mechanism in breastfed babies. The higher fat composition of the hindmilk in comparison with the foremilk may serve as a satiety signal to the infant and gradually motivate the baby to end a feeding. In contrast, the standardized formula given the bottle-fed baby does not allow for the development of self-regulation of food intake.

Feeding Position. Positioning for feeding is vitally important to prevent ear and lung infections. During feeding, the head should be held above the level of the stomach to prevent leakage into the short, straight eustachian tubes and possible otitis media (ear infection). Breastfeeding may help prevent the development of otitis media, since the feeding position at the breast eliminates the possibility for this route of infection. In contrast, if an infant lies on its back while drinking from a propped bottle, milk can enter the eustachian canals.[2] Proper positioning also reduces regurgitation and the possibility of lung infection from aspiration.

Psychosocial Aspects of Infant Feeding

Do not consider the infant's physiologic need for food apart from the psychosocial aspects of development. The infant's developing personality patterns are influenced by the feeding process. At birth, the infant becomes an active participant in the feeding process. Recall that the basic psychosocial need during infancy is to establish a sense of trust in the environment. If needs for food and love are met in the early relationship with the mother or primary caregiver and further broadened by satisfying relationships with other people in the environment, this basic trust is developed. The physical need for food produces discomfort, tension, and crying. The baby's sense of trust begins to develop as he or she consistently experiences pleasurable events, such as relief of hunger by receiving a feeding. Love and affection must be given at this time, as the child can sense a lack of warmth and spontaneity. Feeding time should always be a pleasurable experience for the infant as well as the person feeding. In this type of atmosphere, not only is the sense of trust developed, but also the foundation is laid for agreeable attitudes toward food and the development of sound eating habits.

Nutritional Requirements

Recommended Dietary Allowances. The infant requires the same 50 or so essential food nutrients as do other age groups. The 1980 revision of the RDA lists recommended amounts of nutrients for young (age 0 to 0.5 year) and older (0.5 to 1.0 year) infants (see Chap. 2).

The RDA for infants are derived primarily from the knowledge of nutrients present in human milk, along with a limited amount of experimental data on nutritional requirements. The RDA in turn are used as the basis for evaluating the nutrient composition of commercial formulas. However, given the difficulties inherent in determining the precise nutritional needs of infants, use the RDA only as a rough guide to the nutritional requirements of individual infants.

While infants need the same nutrients as other individuals, a larger quantity is needed per unit of body weight than at other periods of the life cycle. For example, an infant requires 115 kcal/kg of body weight during the first 6 months of life. In contrast, an adult female requires about 36 kcal/kg. Thus, the infant's kilocalorie need per unit of weight is more than three times the adult need. Since nutritional requirements parallel growth, expect the kilocalorie need per unit of weight to undergo a gradual reduction as the infant matures.

INTERVENTION

Meeting Nutritional Needs

For the first 4 to 6 months, the requirement for kilocalories and most nutrients is satisfied by breast milk or an appropriately modified formula consumed in a suitable quantity. Cow's milk is the usual basis for the formula for healthy infants. The differences in nutrient composition of breast and cow's milk were discussed in Chapter 14. Although the kilocalorie value of cow's and human milk is the same, cow's milk contains less carbohydrate and more protein and minerals than does human milk. The fat composition of the two milks is also different. Long-chain unsaturated fatty acids predominate in human milk, whereas saturated fatty acids predominate in cow's milk.

Cow's milk is modified for formula feeding to contain approximately the same nutrient composition as breast milk. The usual modifications include (1) dilution of the high protein and mineral content with water to reduce the renal solute load, (2) addition of a carbohydrate, such as lactose, to approximate breast milk levels and to increase the kilocalories of the diluted formula, (3) removal of butterfat and replacement with a vegetable oil, such as corn oil, to approximate the fatty acid composition of breast milk, (4) addition of nutrients that are lacking in amounts sufficient to meet the RDA, such as vitamin A, vitamin C, vitamin D, vitamin E, iron, and zinc, and (5) treatment with heat to alter the characteristics of the protein and for sanitation purposes. Heat treatment alters the characteristics of the milk protein by producing a softer curd, which is more easily digested, and also significantly improves iron absorption. Heat treatment is especially important for soy-based formulas. The heat processing inactivates the trypsin inhibitor present in raw soybeans and diminishes the goitrogenic effect of soybeans. Commercial formulas are available both with and without the addition of iron (as ferrous sulfate). The specific nutritional content of the brands varies, and changes are made in the content as indicated by research findings. Read the label on individual brands to be sure of the exact nutritive content.

In recent years, some formulas, called "humanized" formulas, have been devised that resemble breast milk even more closely in their content of nutrients, such as protein and minerals. In these milks, demineralized whey is combined with nonfat milk to produce a product in which the ratio of whey proteins to casein is similar to that of human milk (i.e., 60:40). Minerals removed from the whey are added in concentrations similar to those of human milk. Examples of these formulas are SMA (Wyeth) and Similac PM 60/40 (Ross Labs).

Energy and Energy-producing Nutrients. Base the kilocalorie need on needs for basal metabolism, physical activity, and growth. The basal metabolic rate (BMR) in infancy is high, presumably as a result of heat loss from the relatively larger surface area and the larger proportion of metabolic tissue. Assess physical activity on an individual basis. Some infants are quiet and placid and content to interact with the environment primarily with the eyes, whereas others expend considerably more energy crying, kicking, and in other physical movement. Inactive infants may become obese even with a relatively low kilocalorie intake. Excesses or deficits of kilocalories are equally undesirable.

Kilocaloric requirements are met by carbohydrate, protein, and fat. However, the most desirable distribution of these nutrients for infants who are not breastfed is still being investigated. Table 15–1 gives the percentage distribution of carbohydrate, protein, and fat in human milk and in commercial formulas and provides a suggested distribution. Breast milk, cow's milk, and commercial formulas (at normal dilution) provide approximately 20 kcal/ oz (67 kcal/100 ml).

The RDA for protein assumes the use of protein of high biologic value (milk). If vegetable protein is used, as in a vegetarian diet, increase the protein somewhat above the RDA. Excessive protein intake by an infant, as with a formula in which the protein content is greater than 20 percent of total kilocalories, increases the renal solute load. When a high-protein formula is used, provide additional fluids to prevent dehydration.

Lactose is the carbohydrate in human and cow's milk, and it supplies most or all of the carbohydrate in milk-based formulas. Since human milk has a higher lactose content than cow's milk, most commercial formulas add lactose. Other carbohydrates may also be added to formulas—those that modify flavor (e.g., sucrose, dextrose, dextrin, maltose, corn syrup solids) or those that modify consistency (e.g., arrowroot starch, cornstarch, modified cornstarch, and tapioca starch).

Recently, concern has been expressed about the physiologic consequences of feeding infants formulas that are relatively high in polyunsaturated fatty acids, e.g., the linoleic acid content is two to three times the average amount in human milk.

Vitamins, Minerals, and Water. With a few exceptions, the vitamin, mineral, and water content of human milk and commercial formulas is sufficient to meet the RDA for these nutrients. Because the intestinal microflora may not be well established in the newborn, provide an intramuscular injection of vitamin K immediately after birth to prevent any potential for hemorrhage. Some supplementation with vitamin C, vitamin D, iron, and fluoride is also necessary. Specific supplements vary with the age of the infant and the type of feeding, that is, formula or breast milk. With formula, specific supplements depend on whether a commercial formula or one home-prepared from evaporated milk is used. Further, the fluoride content of the water supply affects supplements needed. Use Table 15–2 as a guide for the supplements needed by breastfed and formula-fed babies.

Vitamin C. Vitamin C supplementation is necessary only for the baby receiving an evaporated milk formula. Supplementation should continue until the infant receives a sufficient quantity of vitamin C-containing foods in the diet. After several months, strained diluted orange juice or other vitamin C-containing juice can be gradually introduced. Tell the parents not to heat fruit juices, since heating destroys the vitamin C. When orange juice is introduced, advise parents to observe the infant for allergic reactions, such as a skin rash or gastrointestinal discomfort.

Vitamin D. With rare exceptions, evaporated milk and commercial formulas are fortified with vitamin D, and only breastfed infants require a supplement. An additional source of vitamin D for all infants

TABLE 15–1
CARBOHYDRATE, PROTEIN, AND FAT COMPOSITION OF BREAST MILK AND FORMULA

Nutrient	Human Milk (%)	Most Commercial Formulas (%)	Suggested (%)
Carbohydrate	38	35–46	29–63
Protein	7	9–15	7–16
Fat	55	45–50	30–55

(Source: Based on data in Fomon SJ: Infant Nutrition, ed 2. Philadelphia, WB Saunders, 1974, pp 376, 473.)

TABLE 15–2
SUPPLEMENTS NEEDED BY BREASTFED AND FORMULA-FED BABIES

| | Type of Milk | | | |
	Breast Milk (Well-nourished Mother)	Evaporated Milk Formula	Premodified Formula (No Iron)	Premodified Formula (With Iron)
Newborn	Vitamin D Fluoride[a]	Vitamin C Fluoride	Fluoride	Fluoride
4 months	Iron	Iron	Iron	

[a] If the water supply contains adequate fluoride, a supplement is needed only by the breastfed baby—little fluoride is transmitted in breast milk.

---

is exposure to sunlight. Although some studies have indicated that a water-miscible form of vitamin D is present in human milk and imply that the vitamin D of human milk may be sufficiently high to prevent rickets in the infant, it appears that this is not always the case.[3] Further, some studies fail to support the idea that the forms of vitamin D present in human milk provide significant vitamin D activity,[4] and a supplement is recommended for the breastfed infant, particularly when the mother and infant fail to get adequate exposure to sunlight.

Iron. Since neonatal iron stores are depleted at approximately the time of doubling of the birth weight (4 to 6 months in full-term infants), provide supplemental iron at this time to reduce the risk of iron deficiency and anemia.

The Committee on Nutrition, American Academy of Pediatrics, recommends supplementation with one or more iron sources beginning no later than 4 months of age for full-term infants (4 to 6 months of age for breastfed infants) and no later than 2 months of age for preterm infants.[5] Because of the efficiency of iron absorption from breast milk, an infant who is exclusively breastfed may not need an iron supplement prior to age 6 months, although iron absorption drops significantly when solid foods are added.[6] Although anemia has been observed in breastfed babies, its occurrence is negligible before age 6 months, whereas infants fed a cow's milk formula without added iron may develop anemia by age 4 months. Provide the iron supplement in the form of iron-fortified infant foods (formula or dry infant cereal) or iron-containing drops as an alternative. This supplementation should continue at least through the remainder of the first year. The use of iron-fortified formula from birth may be indicated for some infants, and no ill effects have been associated with this practice.[7] There is evidence to suggest that iron absorption is more efficient during early rapid growth, even though the iron is not immediately used for hemoglobin synthesis.[8]

Fluoride. The fluoride content of all milk is low and must be provided in the water supply, either as natu-

rally occurring or artificially added fluoride or by supplements. Since fluoride is not readily transferred to breast milk, the breastfed baby who is not provided with fluoridated water in addition to breast milk gets little. Supplementation is therefore needed for breastfed infants regardless of the fluoride concentration of the community water. To obtain maximum benefits in preventing dental caries, supplemental fluoride given as drops added to water or juice, tablets, or lozenges should begin soon after birth and continue until the mineralization and maturation of teeth are completed in adolescence. The amount of the supplement is adjusted for the child's age and for the amount in the drinking water. Since calcium can inhibit fluoride absorption, stress to parents that the supplements should not be taken with milk.

Water. The water needs of infants per unit of weight are higher than those of adults. Water turnover in infants is high because of the higher body water content—body water comprises approximately three fourths of their body weight in contrast to two thirds in an adult—the higher skin surface area, and the immaturely functioning kidneys that do not conserve water adequately. The RDA for water is 1.5 ml/kcal of food ingested or approximately 150 ml/kg of body weight.

The water needs of infants are usually satisfied by breast milk and properly prepared commercial formulas. However, caution parents to give the baby additional water to prevent dehydration when environmental temperature is high, when fluid losses are excessive (as in vomiting or diarrhea), when milk intake is inadequate because of illness, or when a high-protein formula is fed. Errors in formula preparation are not infrequent, and feeding an overly concentrated formula to an infant places an extra solute load on the immature kidney, leading to hypernatremia and hypertonic dehydration. A thirsty baby often behaves like a hungry baby. If food is given rather than water, the solute load is further increased and the problem aggravated. When a concentrated form of formula is used, give explicit directions as to its preparation.

Feeding During the First Year

During the first year, the infant's diet is gradually transformed from small, frequent milk feedings supplemented with appropriate vitamins and minerals to a three-meal-a-day plus snack schedule of simply prepared, chopped, table food. Although breast milk or formula and the indicated supplements provide the necessary kilocalories and nutrients for the infant during the first 4 to 6 months, add additional foods to the diet of the older infant to meet nutrient demands, with breast milk or formula continuing to serve as the principal source of kilocalories and nutrients throughout the first year.

Infant Formulas. If the baby is formula fed, give guidance about the types of formulas available and techniques of their preparation and use to avoid contamination. Commercially prepared formulas are available, or they may be prepared at home using evaporated milk as a basis. Commercial formulas are preferred to evaporated milk, since their formulations more closely resemble the nutrient composition of breast milk and iron-fortified forms are readily available. They are available as a liquid concentrate, as a powder, and in a ready-to-use form. Evaporated milk formula is prepared by mixing one can (13 oz) of evaporated milk with 18 oz water and 2 tbsp of corn syrup. This can be made in a quart jar and divided into the desired number of bottles. A single feeding can be prepared by mixing 2 oz milk, 3 oz water, and 2 tsp corn syrup.

The cost of formula is related to its ease of preparation, with the home-prepared formulas the cheapest and the premodified formulas the most expensive. Of the premodified formulas, the liquid concentrate is cheapest, and the ready-to-use form most expensive, with the powdered forms intermediate in cost. The cost of ready-to-use formula is increased by more than half if bought in serving size cans, and it is doubled or tripled if bought in disposable bottles rather than 32-oz cans. Evaluate the merits of the disposable containers in particular situations. Although more expensive, the small cans and bottles may be the only safe source of milk in some home situations, and they are useful when traveling.

Stress to the parents that whole cow's milk, skim milk, generic evaporated milk, filled milk (such as Meadow Fresh or Nutri Whey), and sweetened condensed milk are not suitable for use as a formula. The use of large quantities (1 to 2 liters daily) of fresh pasteurized cow's milk during the first 6 months may contribute to iron deficiency by promoting blood loss through the gastrointestinal tract. Gastrointestinal bleeding is rarely associated with breastfeeding. Its incidence in formula-fed infants is diminished when heat-processed formulas (such as liquid or powdered milk formulas and evaporated milk) are substituted for fresh milk or when the quantity of cow's milk consumed is reduced. Although fresh milk is pasteurized commercially to assure sanitation, the degree of heat used is insufficient to alter the irritating properties of a particular protein fraction that promotes the blood loss. If the infant receives fresh cow's milk after 6 months of age, the American Academy of Pediatrics states that it should not exceed 0.75 quart daily to reduce the risk of blood loss and to encourage the intake of a varied diet that includes iron-fortified cereals.

Skim milk is unsuitable during the first year because of its high renal solute load. Moreover, kilocalorie and fat content are insufficient to permit normal growth. Encourage the parents to continue the use of iron-fortified formula throughout the first year and to limit its volume to a quart daily to make possible the introduction of iron-rich solid foods and to set a pattern for a more varied diet during the second year.[5]

There are a variety of special formulas designed to meet the needs of infants who cannot use standard formulas. For example, infants who are allergic to the protein in cow's milk may be fed meat-based or soybean-based formula preparations. Other conditions may necessitate formulas modified in the type and/or amount of carbohydrate, protein, fat, or electrolytes. Premature infants and low-birth-weight infants also require special formula modifications.

Volume and Frequency of Feedings. Because of the newborn's small stomach capacity, early feedings must consist of a small volume given at frequent intervals, with the volume increased and the time between feeding intervals lengthened as growth takes place. At birth, the stomach holds approximately 2 tbsp. At the end of the first year, the baby can take about 1 c of solids and 8 oz of fluid at a feeding (or approximately one-third to one-half the amount of food an adult can take).

Calculate the approximate amount of formula needed by the baby from the RDA for kilocalories. In the 1980 revision of the RDA, the kilocalorie recommendation for a young infant is 115 kcal/kg of body weight. Thus, a baby who weighs 8 lb (3.6 kg) needs approximately 414 kcal daily. Since conventional formulas provide 20 kcal/oz, the baby needs 21 oz of formula to meet kilocalorie needs. This amount can then be divided into the appropriate number of feedings (approximately six per day during the first month). As the baby grows, adjust the kilocalorie requirement to current weight and kilocalorie requirements per kilogram (which decrease during the second half of the first year). Keep in mind, however, that the RDAs are guidelines only and that adjustments may need to be made for differences in activity level. Use the summary given in Table 15–3 for guiding parents regarding the approximate amount of frequency of feedings during the first year. Assure the mother that if the baby is fed when she or he indicates hunger, a fairly regular schedule of feeding will be established in a relatively short period of time.

TABLE 15–3
SCHEDULE FOR MILK FEEDINGS DURING THE FIRST YEAR

Age	Number of Feedings per 24 Hours	Oz per Feeding	Total Amount per 24 Hours (oz)
1 week	6	2–3	12–15
2–4 weeks	6	3–5	18–30
2–3 months	5	4–6	20–30
4–5 months	5	5–7	25–35
6–7 months	4	7–8	28–32
8–12 months	3	8	24

Solid Food Additions. Prior to 1920, solid foods were seldom fed to infants before 1 year of age. Since that time there has been a gradual reduction in the age recommended for introduction of solids. Today, some infants receive their first solid food within the first month of life. Current concern about the possible association between early introduction of solids and various health problems has prompted many authorities to recommend delay in the introduction of solids until the baby is 4 to 6 months of age.

Nutritional Considerations. Milk cannot adequately supply requirements for energy and some nutrients after 4 to 6 months of age; for example, the kilocaloric requirement exceeds the amount provided by a quart of milk. Since milk is deficient in some nutrients, it is not feasible to meet the increased kilocalorie requirements with milk alone. In infants not receiving iron-fortified formula, birth stores of iron are exhausted by 4 to 6 months.

When solids are introduced, give attention to the quantity consumed, the contribution made to total energy and nutrient intake, and the rate of growth. Caution the parents that replacement of breast milk or formula with foods that are nutritionally inferior can lead to a poor nutritional status. Advise them to introduce food sources of nutrients, such as vitamin C and iron, before these nutrients are eliminated from the diet if a change is made from breast or bottle feedings to plain milk. When solids are introduced, encourage the use of foods high in protein content for the infant who is receiving breast milk or a commercially prepared formula, since these milks are relatively low in protein content. For the infant who may already be taking whole cow's milk that is high in protein content, encourage the use of foods high in carbohydrate content to achieve a better nutrient balance.

Developmental Considerations. Developmentally, the transition from a liquid diet to one that includes foods of a semisolid and solid consistency depends on normal physical development, including maturation of digestive, kidney, and neuromuscular function. Generally, it takes 6 months to a year for the gastrointestinal tract and kidneys to develop fully. Therefore, it is important to provide adequate nutrition without stressing these systems. Development of feeding skills and readiness for changes in food textures depend on the maturation of the central nervous system, which controls the acquisition of fine, gross, and oral motor skills. Although infants can be fed from a spoon during the first month, they are not developmentally ready for semisolid foods until they reach the developmental age of 4 to 6 months. Addition of food of a consistency that the baby is not physiologically ready to handle may lead to frustration of both mother and baby.

The sequence of acquisition of feeding skills, like development in general, follows a predictable pattern. Once readiness for a particular skill has been demonstrated, an opportunity should be given to use the skill. Introduction of solids at 4 to 6 months of age supports the child's neuromuscular development: the extrusion reflex has faded, voluntary swallowing has become established, and the child can sit with support and can communicate satiety by leaning back and turning away.

Discuss with the parents techniques of introducing solid foods that are conducive to the development of sound eating habits. Suggest that new foods can be offered one at a time and at weekly intervals. This allows the infant an opportunity to appreciate their taste and the mother to observe for food sensitivity. The sequence of additions is of little consequence, although iron-fortified infant cereal, mixed with formula or breast milk, is usually the first to be given. Rice cereal is considered to be the least allergenic of the cereals and is usually the first cereal to be introduced. When fruits and vegetables are added, encourage the use of deep green and yellow types to increase the vitamin A level of the diet. Encourage the parents to offer a variety of foods with different shapes and textures and to offer finger foods when teething begins and hand–eye coordination develops and foods that require chewing when the jaw musculature has developed to the point that the infant can bite and chew.

Either commercial or home-prepared foods can be used. While bacteriologically safe, the nutritive

TABLE 15–4
GUIDELINES FOR ADDITION OF SOLID FOODS TO THE INFANT'S DIET DURING THE FIRST YEAR

Age	Food or Supplement and Consistency	Comments
Birth to 4–6 months	Introduce supplements of vitamin C, vitamin D, and fluoride	Nutritional needs are supplied by breast milk or formula and supplements; specific supplements needed depend on the method of feeding and the fluoride content of the water
4–6 months	Introduce commercially prepared dry infant cereal (feed two times daily, morning and evening). If iron-fortified formula or dry infant cereal is not used, a medicinal source of iron should be introduced by 4 months for formula-fed infants and by 4–6 months for breastfed infants	Begin with a single-grain cereal, such as rice, oats, or barley, rather than mixed cereals. Rice cereal is a good first cereal as it is the least allergenic. Wheat cereal or mixed cereal should not be used during the first 6 months because of the potential for allergy
5–7 months	Introduce vegetables, fruits, and their juices, including vitamin C-containing juices, firmer textured foods, and finger foods	Initially, it may be necessary to use commercially prepared strained vegetables or those home-prepared by cooking and straining, pureeing, or blending; fruit may be served raw (ripe, peeled) or canned (use the water-pack type or wash the syrup from syrup-pack type); citrus juices should be diluted for the first few times offered (2 oz of orange juice provides sufficient vitamin C—observe for allergic reactions when introducing orange juice), with tooth eruption, chewing ability and hand-to-mouth movements, finger foods (such as zwieback, hard toast, crackers, or raw peeled apple—avoid foods that splinter in the mouth such as graham crackers), and firmer textured foods (such as mashed or chopped vegetables) are gradually introduced
6–8 months	Introduce protein foods, such as cheese, cooked legumes, meat, fish, chicken, and egg yolk	Depending upon chewing ability, meat should be strained or finely ground and well-moistened and fish mashed; dried beans and peas should be well cooked and sieved (partially cooked legumes or pieces of legumes may cause choking); initially use the commercially prepared egg yolk or prepare at home by hard-cooking and mashing (serve in one-fourth tsp amounts initially)—soft-cooked or poached egg yolk may be added later; the amount of egg yolk may be restricted because of its high cholesterol content
8–12 months	Introduce foods with further variations in texture: potatoes, pasta, and pudding made with a limited amount of sugar; whole egg (toward the end of the year)	Use finely chopped meat that has been boiled, broiled, or baked; coarsely chopped or whole table vegetables and whole fruit (canned fruit or ripe, raw, peeled fruit); iron-fortified, heat-treated formula continues to be appropri-

TABLE 15–4 (Continued)

Age	Food or Supplement and Consistency	Comments
	Continue breast milk or iron fortified formula Wean to a cup	ate throughout the first year to reduce the risk of blood loss and to assure an adequate source of iron; the infant can approximate the lips to the rim of a cup at about 5 months of age, and a true drinking pattern emerges at about 1 year; readiness for weaning is usually apparent by an eagerness to explore the environment and a diminished interest in the breast or bottle; delayed weaning may be a contributing factor in dental caries and iron deficiency anemia

value of the commercially prepared foods varies considerably, and most are either high in carbohydrate and protein or low in fat. The major baby food manufacturers have eliminated salt and most of the sugar from their products. Tell the parents to select plain meat and vegetables rather than prepared mixed dinners and soups, since the dinners and soups are high in water content and contain little meat. Encourage the use of iron-fortified dry infant cereal rather than home-cooked cereal because the infant cereal contains more iron. Commercially prepared egg yolk may be less allergenic than those prepared at home because of the sterilization procedures used.

Provided simple, economic, and nutritious foods are prepared in a sanitary manner, the baby can be fed safely with home-prepared foods, usually at a lower cost than with commercial foods. Tell the parents that foods prepared for family meals can be puréed in a blender or food grinder and used immediately or quick-frozen in small plastic sandwich bags or ice cube trays for later use. Suggest the use of fresh or frozen, unsweetened and unsalted ingredients and to use sugar, salt, and fat sparingly to avoid imprinting a taste preference for these substances. For those not consuming iron-fortified formula or iron-fortified infant cereal, stress the need for a medicinal source of iron, and a fluoride source continues to be important.

By 9 to 11 months of age, the infant is developmentally ready to feed himself or herself and should be allowed the opportunity to develop self-feeding skills. Urge the parents to keep mealtime a pleasant learning experience.

Use Table 15–4 as a guide for assisting parents with the gradual addition of solids during the first year.

Diet of the 1-Year-Old Infant. The gradual addition during the first year of a variety of foods from the Basic Four Food Groups should result in a diet that includes the recommended number of servings from each of the nutrient-rich food groups when the

infant is 1 year old. These include 2 c of milk, two servings of meat or substitute, four servings of vegetables and fruit, and four servings of bread and cereal. While the size of servings will be smaller than for other age groups, the same number of servings should be included. A good practice is to serve small portions and provide seconds, rather than serve large amounts. Infant cereal or other form of iron supplementation may be indicated for vulnerable groups, such as those born prematurely or with a below-average birth weight. In addition, fluoride supplementation should continue for all children who are not receiving fluoridated water.

A suggested meal plan for the end of the first year is given in Table 15–5.

Weaning. Weaning begins when supplemental foods are introduced into the diet and milk no longer serves as the sole source of nourishment. The child is developmentally prepared for weaning during the second half of the first year. At about 5 months of age, the baby can approximate the lips to the rim of a cup, and cup feedings can be gradually introduced after this time.

In many cultures, breastfeeding may continue for periods of 2 to 3 years and is sometimes continued even after the arrival of a new baby. In other cultures, breast milk may be supplemented with semisolid foods within the first few weeks. This situation may lead to less vigorous sucking and diminished milk production, and it usually results in early weaning. Encourage the mother to continue breastfeeding for at least the first 6 months or for as long as it is satisfying to the mother and baby. However some solids should be introduced by 6 months, since protein-rich foods are needed at this time, and by the end of the first year most of the nourishment should be from nonmilk foods. If breastfeeding is terminated before the baby is a year old, advise the mother to substitute an infant formula for the remaining part of the year.

TABLE 15-5
SUGGESTED MEAL PLAN FOR AN INFANT AT THE END OF THE FIRST YEAR

Breakfast	Lunch	Dinner
Fruit or juice	Meat or substitute	Meat or substitute
Cereal	Vegetable	Vegetable
Milk	Enriched bread	Enriched bread
Toast	Fruit	
	Milk	
Fruit juice and finger foods can be offered as snacks		

**Adequacy of Feeding During Infancy.** Assess the adequacy of the kilocalorie and nutrient intake at the time of each check-up by assessing the child's growth, appetite, general appearance and behavior, current nutrient needs, and current dietary intake. Also assess for developmental readiness to make changes in the dietary regimen. Make dietary recommendations based on these assessments.

During early infancy, feedings are probably adequate if the baby is growing satisfactorily, appears satisfied after feeding, and falls asleep promptly and sleeps quietly for several hours following feeding.

Consistent gain in height and weight at a rate characteristic of the infant's age group is one of the best indicators of adequacy of intake. Height and weight measured over a period of time permit calculation of growth, whereas one-time measurements only show size achieved. When a child's height and weight are continuously recorded on a standard growth chart (see Chap. 11), deviations in growth can be easily spotted. Using a home scale daily often gives a false indication of weight gain and may cause unnecessary anxiety. When deviations in growth are observed, such as increments in weight that exceed increments in length or small gains in weight, tell the parents how to make the appropriate adjustment in feeding. For example, if the young infant is gaining excessively, evaluate total food intake. There may be excessive intake of such items as pudding, cereal, or starch-thickened food.

NUTRITION-RELATED PROBLEMS IN INFANCY

Assessment and Intervention
Feeding difficulties in infancy, such as vomiting, diarrhea, constipation, and colic, sometimes occur. The infant who is born with a low birth weight or who fails to thrive requires a specialized type of dietary management. The possible long-term effects of overnutrition or undernutrition in infancy must be considered.

▶ _**Regurgitation, Rumination, and Vomiting.**_ **Regurgitation** or "spitting up" is the return of small amounts of food during or shortly after feeding. In vomiting, on the other hand, the stomach may be
▶ completely emptied. **Rumination** refers to the purposeful regurgitation of food or liquid during or after feeding. Infants who ruminate may also chew or mouth the regurgitant and either swallow it again or spit it out. Rumination usually has a psychologic basis, but consider physical problems, such as esophageal reflux, as a possible etiology. Distinguish among simple regurgitation, rumination, and vomiting, and assess feeding technique and quantity and quality of the feeding to determine the cause and exclude the possibility of serious illness.

Within limits, spitting up is a natural occurrence associated with the immature gastrointestinal tract of young infants. Advise the parents that it usually subsides by 8 to 9 months. The problem may be aggravated, however, by poor feeding technique, such as inadequate burping. Vomiting may be due to feeding problems, such as excess air swallowing, ingestion of too large or too frequent feedings, or ingestion of a formula containing too much fat, which delays gastric emptying. If persistent, suspect a more serious problem, such as allergy, infection, systemic disease, or obstruction, and refer the client to a physician promptly.

Be sure that the volume, concentration, and frequency of the feeding is appropriate and assist the parents to correct improper feeding techniques. Assure that the child is positioned properly during and after the feeding, is burped once or twice during feeding, and that nipples with the openings of the correct size are being used. It may be helpful to have the infant sit upright in an infant seat for a half-hour after feeding before burping.

**Constipation and Diarrhea.** Like vomiting, constipation and diarrhea may be related to feeding or
▶ they may be due to acute or chronic illness. **Constipation** refers to the passage of hard, dry stools that are difficult to expel. Assess the volume of formula consumed by constipated infants. The condition is nearly nonexistent in breastfed babies who get an adequate volume of milk, and it occurs only rarely in babies who get an adequate amount of formula. In formula-fed infants, also assess the amount of water consumed and the carbohydrate content of the formula.

Treat constipation by adjusting the volume of formula, increasing water intake, or adding additional corn syrup to the formula. Use of additional fruits or a solution of equal parts of water and prune juice helps to soften the stool. In an older child, suggest an increase in the bulk constituents of the diet, with a larger intake of whole grain cereal, fruit, and vegetable in addition to increasing the fluid intake.

▶ **Diarrhea** means an increase in frequency, volume, and fluid content of the stools. Acute diarrhea is often the result of bacterial or viral infections, but diarrhea may also be due to feeding an excessive quantity of formula too frequently, use of a formula that is too concentrated, or feeding a contaminated formula. The consequences of acute diarrhea can be severe—dehydration, hypokalemia, acidosis, and decreased lactase enzyme production leading to malabsorption.

Mild to moderate diarrhea of several days' duration can usually be treated at home. Assist the parents with a regime of withholding food for up to 24 hours while maintaining fluid and electrolyte balance with solutions that also contain glucose. Commercial formulas such as Lytren (Mead Johnson Labs) and Pedialyte (Ross Labs) are available for home use. Give the parents precise directions for their use, including recording the amount taken and retained. When the diarrhea subsides, the infant may be given a dilute (10 to 13 kcal/oz) lactose-free formula. Maintain close follow-up, giving the parents explicit directions for gradually increasing the concentration of the formula to standard. Parents may ask about using dilute tea in the nursing bottle. Discourage this practice since it will only overstimulate the already overactive bowel.

Acute diarrhea necessitates hospitalization and repleting fluid and electrolyte losses with glucose–electrolyte solutions. Rehydration may be by the oral route over a period of 4 to 6 hours, with resumption of small frequent feedings as soon as appetite is restored, usually within 6 to 24 hours.

▶ One type of diarrhea, **chronic nonspecific diarrhea,** is a common problem, with onset of symptoms of loose, mucousy stools between 6 and 30 months of age. In contrast to other types of chronic diarrhea, there is no associated malabsorption, and growth and development remain normal. The disorder may persist for as long as 2 years. It has been noted[9] that affected children tend to consume lesser amounts of fat than nonaffected children. Treat this disorder by increasing the fat intake to 4 g/kg body weight. Assist the parents to maintain this diet for approximately 3 weeks and then to taper it down to normal intake. The high fat intake is based on the principle that fat slows gastric emptying time and increases intestinal transit time.

▶ *Colic.* **Colic** is a symptom complex consisting of paroxysmal abdominal pain (presumably of intestinal origin) and severe crying. The symptoms usually subside by 3 to 4 months of age, and the baby appears to grow normally. No single causative factor consistently accounts for colic, and no method of treatment consistently provides relief. Etiologic factors that have been suggested include abdominal distention from air swallowing, gas formed by fermentation of undigested food or overfeeding, hunger, allergy, cold, and emotional conflict. Preventive efforts should be directed toward providing proper feeding techniques (including amounts fed), identifying possible allergies or intolerances, and providing a stable emotional environment. Only occasionally does a change in the diet prevent further attack of colic.

Assist parents of colicky infants to limit the amount of air that the baby swallows while feeding. Advise them to feed the baby at reasonably spaced intervals (3 to 4 hours) and to limit the period of sucking. Suggest two 10-minute sucking intervals, each followed by a 5-minute burping period. Air swallowing increases as the infant becomes tired from prolonged sucking. To assure that air in the stomach does not reach the intestine, stress that the infant be held upright during the feeding. Other therapeutic measures that have been recommended include abdominal massage, distending the rectum with a suppository or greased thermometer, a warm bath, and a small dose of alcohol with warm water and a small amount of sugar.

▶ *Feeding the Low-Birth-Weight Infant.* Low-birth-weight (LBW) infants, those weighing 2500 g or less at birth, may be born prematurely (before the 38th week of gestation), or they may be full-term but small for gestational age (SGA) because of intrauterine growth retardation.

LBW infants are particularly vulnerable to the adverse effects of malnutrition because of greater immaturity of reflexes and of various body systems, more limited nutritional reserves, and greater nutritional requirements than full-term infants. Greater attention must, therefore, be given to the composition, amount, and method of feeding than for full-term infants. Since the full-term SGA infant is not as compromised developmentally as the premature, this infant will require less precaution in introducing early feedings than does the premature. As with prematures, however, nutritional requirements are high because of a greater rate of growth.

Establish as the goal of nutritional care the provision of a level of nutrient intake that will permit the infant to obtain a prompt postnatal resumption of growth to a rate approximating that of the third trimester of intrauterine life (i.e., a gain of approximately 20 to 30 g/day) without imposing stress on the developing metabolic or excretory systems. This is believed to provide the optimum conditions for subsequent normal development. Most LBW infants will achieve a satisfactory growth rate when the kilocaloric intake is in a range of 110 to 150 kcal/kg per day. There are considerable variations in these average values, however, due to both biologic and environmental influences. A protein intake of 2.25 to 5.9 g/kg per day is usually sufficient. Avoid an excessively high protein intake (greater than 6 g/kg per day), however, because such a high intake is associated with increased morbidity and mortality in prematures. There is evidence that the amino acids, cystine, tyrosine, and possibly taurine, are essential for premature infants.

The optimal vitamin and mineral requirements of the LBW infant have not been established. However, proposed recommended intakes for certain vitamins and minerals have been published,[10] and the intake of others is based on recommendations for term infants.[11] Anemia is common in LBW infants, and a daily supplement of 2 mg/day of iron is recommended, beginning at 2 months of age or earlier. The iron may oxidize some of the vitamin E and necessitate larger amounts of this vitamin, particularly when the formula is high in polyunsaturated fat content, to prevent hemolytic anemia. Administer an IM injection of vitamin K at birth and give a daily multivitamin supplement with extra folic acid and possibly vitamin E, depending on the polyunsaturated fat content of the formula. Decreased bone mineralization is a common problem in prematures. Compare the calcium, phosphorus, and vitamin D content of the feeding being used with nutritional requirements to determine if a supplement is needed. Assess the infant's serum sodium level. A large percentage of infants who weigh less than 1200 g at birth may experience hyponatremia during the first weeks of life, possibly associated with high growth requirements and excessive urinary losses. A sodium supplement may be necessary, depending on the amount of sodium in the formula.

The fluid requirement varies with the maturity of renal function and homeostatic mechanisms but is similar to that of the term infant (150 ml/kg per day). The water supplied may not be sufficient in quantity if the formula is highly concentrated or if excess losses are occurring. Monitor daily weight, urine specific gravity, the blood urea nitrogen, and serum levels of creatinine and electrolytes to assess the need for additional water.

Although the subject has been intensively studied during the last several decades, the optimal feeding (i.e., breast milk or a specific type of formula) for the LBW infant has not been precisely defined. The feeding selected should meet nutritional requirements without producing an excessive osmotic load, to avoid diarrhea, excessive renal fluid loss, and acidosis. Human milk offers the properties of a low renal solute load, easily digestible fat, an optimal protein and amino acid pattern, and host resistance factors that may be advantageous to the premature infant. At the same time, the protein, sodium, calcium, and possibly other nutrient levels appear to be inadequate to meet the needs of the growing premature infant. However, new investigations offer intriguing evidence that the composition of milk from mothers who deliver prematurely more closely approximates the infant's nutritional requirements. Preterm milk is higher in protein, sodium, chloride, magnesium, and iron.[12] Preterm milk still lacks sufficient calcium and phosphorus; consider the need for a supplement when it is used. Moreover, use of human milk presents various practical difficulties in obtaining and storing the milk.

Standard formulas based on cow's milk that contain 20 kcal/oz, such as Similac (Ross Labs), Enfamil (Mead Johnson Labs), and SMA (Wyeth) may be used, although there are several formulas that are especially formulated to meet the nutrient needs and nutrient tolerance of the premature infant and thus are more appropriate. These include Enfamil Premature Formula (Mead Johnson Labs), Similac Special Care (Ross Labs), and Preemie SMA (Wyeth). These are available at concentrations of 20 and 24 kcal/oz. Some prematures may require fluid restriction, and in these situations a formula concentration up to 30 kcal/oz may be needed. Carbohydrate or fat supplements can be added to formulas to increase their concentration. Infants whose water balance is threatened (those with infection or diarrhea or those exposed to phototherapy) should not be fed formulas with a kilocalorie density greater than 24 kcal/oz, however.

Restrict the use of soy-based formulas, which are sometimes used during periods of lactose intolerance, to short-term use. The incidence of rickets tends to be greater in LBW infants fed soy-based formula than in those fed milk-based formulas.

Base the feeding regimen for the premature baby on individual evaluation. Feeding methods include nipple feeding, tube feeding, and IV feeding. Evaluate the infant's suck, swallow, and gag reflexes. If these reflexes are coordinated, which is likely in infants at 32 to 34 weeks gestation, and the infant is nonstressed by such medical problems as respiratory distress, nipple feeding can be used. In general, infants less than 32 weeks gestation will require a tube feeding. Intermittent intragastric feeding, continuous intragastric drip, and transpyloric feeding (see Chap. 21) have all been used with some success. If the infant cannot ingest or absorb an adequate amount of kilocalories and nutrients, total parenteral nutrition (see Chap. 21) is indicated.

Initiate feeding as soon as possible for LBW infants. The first feeding should consist of distilled water, followed by glucose feedings to decrease the incidence of hypoglycemia and hyperbilirubinemia, presumed to be physiologic jaundice. Follow the glucose water with a dilute and ultimately full-strength formula concentration.

Monitor nutritional status and provide diet counseling on a continuing basis. Initially, plot the infant's weight daily on a suitable growth chart. Depending on the child's size there should be a daily gain of 10 to 30 g. Measure length weekly. Ideally there should be a weekly increase of 0.8 to 1.0 cm. Additionally, assess for an increase in the head circumference, which should also be 0.8 to 1.0 cm weekly. Weekly determination of skinfold thickness and midarm muscle circumference are useful for determining changes in body fat and muscle size. Evaluate regularly such biochemical indices as serum calcium, phosphorus, alkaline phosphatase, total protein, albumin, blood urea nitrogen, and hematocrit. Keep daily records of intake and output to determine the adequacy of kilocalories and nutrients.

As the child grows, base feeding practices on the infant's corrected age vs chronologic age. To correct for gestational age, subtract the number of weeks that the infant was born prematurely from the chronologic age. Premature infants usually catch up to normal weight by 24 months, length by 36 months, and head circumference by 18 months.

▶ **Failure to Thrive.** **Failure to thrive** is a general term to describe an infant who fails to attain the minimal expected gains in growth and development. Suspect the condition when there is a noticeable decline of growth from an established pattern or when the child's height and/or weight consistently falls below the third percentile for height and weight for age on standard growth charts. Failure to thrive tends to be more severe when both linear growth and head circumference are affected.

Assess for the etiology, which may be either organic or nonorganic in origin. Normal growth and development are dependent on meeting the physical, emotional, and sensory needs of the child. These factors are closely related in the child's development.

In some cases, failure to thrive may result from physical conditions in which the child is unable to ingest or use adequate food. In other cases, failure to thrive may have a psychosocial basis. The child is deprived by his or her caretakers because of ignorance, poor economic status, or deliberate neglect, as in child abuse. Consider all aspects of the child's development, including nutritional, physical, and emotional needs, in developing the nursing care plan.

Nutritional Excesses

Obesity. Excess weight gain in infancy probably reflects an interaction between genetic potential and environmental influences, principally the diet. While the evidence is contradictory, it has been suggested that excessive kilocaloric intake leading to excessive weight gain in infancy may set a pattern for persisting obesity. Use these measures to control weight in an infant so that obesity does not develop:

1. Encourage breastfeeding for at least 3 months.
2. Advise parents to delay the introduction of solid foods until the infant is 4 to 6 months old.
3. Help parents learn how to identify the infant's cues, i.e., when crying is a hunger cry or an expression of another need, such as thirst, or when satiety is expressed as by stopping sucking and pushing the nipple out.
4. Urge parents to allow the infant freedom of body movement, including movement of the extremities.
5. Suggest the use of plain foods (such as vegetables, meat, and fruit) in contrast to higher kilocaloric foods, such as mixed dinners.
6. Tell parents to avoid comparing their infant's food intake with that of friends', relatives', or neighbors' infants.
7. Provide parents with techniques to use when they perceive that the baby is not satisfied with milk alone during the first few months, e.g., a pacifier to provide more sucking and offer water between feedings to satisfy sucking and thirst needs.
8. Advise the parents that the infant may not want that last ½ oz or more of a feeding— do not keep urging the baby to empty the bottle. There are times when extra love and attention may well suffice for the extra food.

Should overweight or obesity occur in an infant, the goal in treatment is not to reduce weight but to slow the rate of gain commensurate with linear growth. Severe dietary restriction may inhibit growth. Suggest that use of foods of high kilocaloric density (such as cereals, fruits, meats, and desserts) be limited and total milk consumption be regulated. Efforts should be made to increase nonfeeding stimulation.

Overuse of Vitamins. Another type of overfeeding is the indiscriminate addition of vitamins to the diet. While there is a need for supplementation with some vitamins when milk is the sole source of nutrients, vitamin supplements become unnecessary as the diet becomes more varied. In actual practice, continued vitamin supplementation is common and poses some risk of vitamin toxicity when the amount consumed from the supplement and from foods—many of which are enriched or fortified with vitamins— is in excess of need. Toxicity of the fat-soluble vitamins, especially vitamins A and D, poses a greater risk than for other vitamins.

Nursing Caries. A common type of dental decay is
▶ called **bottle mouth caries** or **nursing caries.** This refers to rampant caries (occurring shortly after the teeth have erupted but which may not appear until 2 to 3 years of age) that results in destruction of the upper front teeth and sometimes the lower molars by the prolonged pooling of fermentable carbohydrate around the teeth. While sucrose-containing beverages are particularly harmful, any liquid that contains fermentable carbohydrate, including plain milk and breast milk, is an offender. Bedtime bottles are especially destructive as both the swallowing

reflex and flow of saliva are diminished during sleep. This results in the fermentation of undiluted liquid around the teeth. To avoid the incidence of bottle caries, weaning by 1 year of age is recommended. Further, tell parents to avoid sweetened bottles, sweetened pacifiers, and bedtime bottles. If a bedtime bottle is an absolute emotional necessity, suggest that it contain plain water.

Nutrient Deficits. Findings from national nutrition surveys (see Chap. 1) indicate that the overall nutritional status of infants and children in the United States is reasonably good. Although a small percentage of children had clinical findings suggesting deficiency of vitamin A, vitamin D, vitamin C, riboflavin, and niacin, iron deficiency and iron deficiency anemia constituted the major nutritional deficiency disorder among young children and adolescents. Although iron deficiency anemia occurs at all ages and income levels, it is most prevalent between the ages of 6 months and 2 years in the low-income population and in infants of low birth weight. Its high prevalence in low-income groups, however, may be distorted by the greater proportion in those groups of blacks, whose hemoglobin levels are typically lower than whites. A frequent cause is the overuse of milk in the diet, which may limit the intake of iron-containing foods and possibly induce gastrointestinal bleeding, with iron loss. Iron deficiency anemia is less prevalent in breastfed infants than in those receiving a formula. To prevent iron deficiency anemia, recommend the use of iron-fortified formula or iron supplements until the first birthday. No infant under 1 year of age needs more than a quart of formula daily. If this amount is exceeded, assess for milk anemia.

If low income is a factor, suggest the possibility of food stamps and the WIC program (see Chap. 14).

REVIEW QUESTIONS AND ACTIVITIES

1. Identify eight physical characteristics of the newborn and infant that affect nutritional requirements and the feeding process.
2. Discuss the psychologic implications of feeding during the first year.
3. Calculate the kilocaloric requirement of a 7 lb full-term newborn.
4. Calculate the amount of breast milk or formula needed to meet the nutritional requirements of the infant in Question 3. How do these requirements change during the first year?
5. Describe the adjustments that must be made in cow's milk to make it suitable for infant feeding.
6. Compare the nutrient supplements needed by a 6-month-old infant with each of the following types of feedings: breast milk, evaporated milk formula, premodified formula.
7. Discuss the water requirements of infants fed by the methods listed in Question 6.
8. Compare several brands of commercial formulas available for term infants in relation to supplements required and cost.
9. Discuss the hazards associated with use of unmodified whole cow's milk and skim milk during infancy.
10. Compare the volume consumed and frequency of feeding of infants during the first and second 6 months of life.
11. Discuss nutritional and developmental considerations when adding solid foods to the milk diet of an infant.
12. Identify the appropriate age for introducing solid foods into the infant's diet.
13. Describe the dietary advice that you would give to a mother regarding the introduction of solid foods during the first year.
14. Plan a menu for a 12-month-old infant.
15. Discuss the process of weaning of breastfed babies.
16. Discuss dietary approaches for dealing with regurgitation, vomiting, constipation, mild diarrhea, chronic nonspecific diarrhea, and colic in infants.
17. Discuss approaches for preventing obesity, nursing caries, and iron deficiency anemia in infancy.
18. Identify the kilocalorie and protein requirements and the vitamin and mineral supplements that may be required by premature infants.
19. Evaluate the advantages and disadvantages of the use of human milk for premature infants.
20. Identify the three methods for feeding an LBW infant and the indications for use of each method.

REFERENCES

1. Martinez GA, Dodd DA: 1981 milk feeding patterns in the United States during the first 12 months of life. Pediatrics 71:166, 1983.
2. Oseid BJ: Breastfeeding and infant health. Clin Obstet Gynecol 18:149, 1975.
3. Tsang RC: The quandary of vitamin D in the newborn infant. Lancet 1:1370, 1983.
4. Reeve LE: Vitamin D of human milk: Identification of biologically active forms. Am J Clin Nutr 36:122, 1982.
5. Committee on Nutrition, American Academy of Pediatrics: Iron supplements for infants. Pediatrics 58:767, 1976.
6. Oski FA, Landaw SA: Inhibition of iron absorption from human milk by baby food. Am J Dis Child 134:459, 1980.
7. Jelliffee EFP: Infant feeding practices: Associated

iatrogenic and commerciogenic diseases. Pediatr Clin North Am 24(1):49, 1977.

8. Woodruff CW: Iron deficiency in infancy and childhood. Pediatr Clin North Am 24:93, 1977.
9. Cohen SA, Hendricks KN, Mathis RK, et al.: Chronic nonspecific diarrhea: Dietary relationships. Pediatrics 64:402, 1979.
10. Zieglar EE, Biga RL, Fomon SJ: Nutritional requirements of the premature infant. In Suskind RM, ed: Textbook of Pediatric Nutrition. New York, Raven Press, 1981.
11. Committee on Nutrition, American Academy of Pediatrics: Nutritional needs of low-birth-weight infants. Pediatrics 60:519, 1977.
12. Lemons JA, Moye L, Hall D, Simmons M: Differences in the composition of preterm and term human milk during early lactation. Pediatr Res 16:113, 1982.

BIBLIOGRAPHY

Anderson DM, Williams FH, Merkatz RB, et al.: Length of gestation and the composition of human milk. Am J Clin Nutr 37:810, 1983.

Brady MS, Rickard KA, Ernst JA, et al.: Formulas and human milk for premature infants: A review and update. J Am Diet Assoc 81:547, 1982.

Brooke OG: Nutrition in the preterm infants. Lancet 1:514, 1983.

Cone TE Jr: The nursing bottle caries syndrome. JAMA 245:2334, 1981.

Ernst JA, Bull MJ, Rickard KA, et al.: Feeding practices of the very low-birth-weight infant within the first year. J Am Diet Assoc 82:158, 1983.

Ernst JA, Bull MJ, Moye L, et al.: Growth outcome of the very low-birth-weight infant at one year. J Am Diet Assoc 82:44, 1983.

Farris RP, Hyg MS, Frank GC, et al.: Influence of milk source on serum lipids and lipoproteins during the first year of life: Bogalusa Heart Study. Am J Clin Nutr 35:42, 1982.

Gonzalez ER: Study indicates salt is an acquired taste. JAMA 249:2999, 1983.

Gross SJ: Growth and biochemical response of preterm infants fed human milk or modified infant formula. N Engl J Med 308:237, 1983.

Johnson GH, Purvis GA, Wallace RD: What nutrients do our infants really get? Nutr Today 16(4):4, 1981.

Quandt SA: The effect of beikost on the diet of breast-fed infants. J Am Diet Assoc 84:47, 1984.

Roy S III: Perspectives on adverse effects of milk and infant formulas used in infant feeding. J Am Diet Assoc 82:373, 1983.

Williams FH: Human milk banking: Practical concerns for feeding prematures. J Am Diet Assoc 79:565, 1981.

Yeung DL, Pennell MD, Leung M, Hall J: Infant fatness and feeding practices: A longitudinal assessment. J Am Diet Assoc 79:531, 1981.

CHAPTER 16

Nutrition of the Toddler and Preschool Child

Objectives

After completion of this chapter, the student will be able to:

1. Compare the characteristics of physical growth of toddlers and preschoolers.

2. Compare the nutritional requirements relative to body size of toddlers and preschoolers with those of infants and adults.

3. Distinguish between the iron requirements of infants and toddlers.

4. Compare the number and size of servings from each of the Basic Four Food Groups needed by toddlers and preschoolers with those needed by adults.

5. Evaluate the role of snacks in the diet of toddlers and preschoolers.

6. Differentiate between the consistency of foods that are appropriate for toddlers and preschoolers.

7. Develop a teaching plan for the mother of a 3-year-old that is supportive of the child's physiologic and psychosocial development.

The toddler stage begins at 12 to 15 months of age (when the child takes the first steps) and continues until about 3 years of age. The preschool period includes ages 3 through 5. Having progressed from the milk and baby food regimen of infancy, children are not yet settled into family meal patterns. Much of the dissatisfaction expressed by parents about their children's eating habits results from their lack of knowledge of usual food responses at a given stage of development.

Content in this chapter has been adapted from Lewis C: Nutrition of the toddler and preschool child. In Hinton SM, Kerwin DR: Maternal, Infant, and Child Nutrition, Resources for the Professional. The North Carolina Agricultural Extension Service, North Carolina State University, and Nutrition and Dietary Services and Maternal and Child Health Branches, Division of Health Services, Department of Human Resources, State of North Carolina, Raleigh, NC, 1980, pp 1–21.

ASSESSMENT

Characteristics of Physical Growth in Toddler and Preschool Child

In contrast to the rapid and relatively smooth growth rate of the infant, who tripled birth weight (gaining approximately 14 lb) and increased in height by about 50 percent (growing approximately 10 in) during the first year, a slow and sometimes irregular growth rate is characteristic of the toddler and preschool period. Fortunately, the growth rate declines from a gallop in early infancy—if this rate continued, the child would weigh more than 200 tons and be 96 ft tall by the tenth year[1]—to a trot in late infancy, and finally to a fast walk throughout the remainder of childhood until the onset of puberty.

In addition to a leveling off of the growth rate, changes in body composition that affect nutritional

193

TABLE 16-1
GROWTH CHANGES IN THE TODDLER AND PRESCHOOL CHILD

During Second Year	Subsequent Annual Growth until Puberty
~11 to 13 cm increase	~8 to 9 cm increase during the third year
	~7cm increase thereafter
2.5 kg increase	~2.0 kg increase
Progressive increase in muscle mass with disappearance of baby fat	
Calcification of skeleton (bone strength increases more than length) and continued eruption of primary teeth (at age 1, there are usually 6 to 8 teeth; all are usually in by 3 years).	

requirements also occur during this period. The growth pattern of children during this period should approximate the changes shown in Table 16–1.

Nutritional Needs

Recommended Dietary Allowances. The RDAs for the toddler and preschool child are included in the 1980 revision under the 1 to 3 and 4 to 6 age groups (see Chap. 2). Note that from birth to age 6 there is a gradual increase in the quantities of kilocalories and most nutrients needed. This gradual increase in nutrient needs is consistent with the growth pattern characteristics of the period, i.e., slow and progressive growth following the rapid growth spurt of early infancy. The recommendation for vitamin D remains constant throughout the period since 400 IU (or 10 μg cholecalciferol) are required daily during the entire growth cycle. The only nutrient for which the amount recommended decreases during this period is iron. Less iron is required for the preschool child (4 to 6 years) than for the toddler (1 to 3 years). The 15 mg level recommended for the toddler is to aid in replenishing the iron stores used during the rapid growth of infancy.

Whereas the actual amounts of most nutrients needed during the toddler and preschool period show only a small, gradual increase consistent with the gradual increase in body size, keep in mind that nutritional requirements relative to body size are much greater during the entire growth period than during adulthood. Although the nutritional requirements of toddlers and preschoolers relative to body size are less than those of an infant, they are much greater than those of an adult. Two factors account for the greater nutrient requirements relative to body size in childhood than in adulthood. First, kilocalories and nutrients are needed in relatively large amounts to support the anabolic activities that produce growth. Undernutrition may limit growth; for example, a kilocaloric deficit as small as 10 kcal/kg may result in unsatisfactory growth. If a devia-

tion in the growth pattern is observed, suggest that the parents keep a record of food intake for several days; analyze this record for nutritional adequacy. Second, the level of physical activity is usually greater in childhood than in adulthood, although the activity level varies considerably with individual children.

INTERVENTION

Meeting Nutritional Needs

Daily Food Needs. In order to meet the nutritional needs of the toddler and preschool child, use the Daily Food Plan (Table 16–2) as the basis for planning daily meals. The toddler and preschooler should receive the same number of servings of food from each of the nutrient-rich food groups as do adults. Although the number of servings is equivalent to the number needed by adults, note that the size of servings is much smaller to compensate for the smaller amounts of nutrients needed. For example, the appropriate size of fruit and vegetable servings is 1 tbsp per year of age up until approximately 4 years of age.

Children who eat a diet comparable to that shown in Table 16–2 should not require vitamin or mineral supplements, with two possible exceptions, the first being iron. The RDA for iron for the toddler is 15 mg, and an iron supplement may be necessary, since the usual diet consumed by the toddler does not provide this amount. However, the need for a supplement has not been resolved by pediatricians and nutritionists and is not routine at this age. Reduce the potential for iron deficiency by encouraging the continued use of breakfast cereals that are highly fortified with iron, such as dry infant cereals. The labels on cereal boxes indicate the amount of iron present.

The second nutrient that may require continuing supplementation is fluoride. A source of fluoride should be available at least until calcification of the permanent teeth is completed in adolescence. If adequate fluoride is not available from the water supply (either naturally or artificially added), suggest alternate sources including topical application of fluoride by a dentist, fluoride drops added to water or juice, or fluoride lozenges or gels, all provided by prescription.

The appetite of the toddler and preschooler is typically small and is sometimes referred to as ▶ **physiologic anorexia** because of its association with the slow growth rate. Tell the parents to expect a decline in appetite beginning during the latter part of infancy. This decline is often reflected first by a decline in milk intake, usually coinciding with weaning to the cup. Milk consumption may drop to 2 c (or even less) during toddlerhood. In most cases, the appetite tends to improve in the latter

TABLE 16–2
A DAILY FOOD PLAN FOR TODDLERS AND PRESCHOOL CHILDREN

Food	Number of Servings	Size of Servings Toddler (1 through 2 years)	Size of Servings Preschool (3 through 5 years)
Milk and cheese Milk (whole, skim, low-fat, re-liquefied evaporated, soy), yoghurt, ice cream, ice milk, cheese. Calcium equivalent of 1 c milk: 1 c plain yoghurt, 1⅓ oz Swiss or cheddar cheese; 1½ c ice cream or ice milk; 2 c cottage cheese	2 servings (Children who are growing at a faster-than-average rate may need an additional serving)	1 serving = 1 c milk (Milk should be served in child-sized portions, i.e., ½–¾ c)	
Meat–fish–poultry–beans Lean cooked meat, poultry, fish; dry peas, beans, soybeans, lentils, peanut butter, seeds. Protein equivalent of 1 oz meat: 1 egg; ½–¾ c legumes; 2 tbsp peanut butter, ¼–½ c nuts or seeds	2 servings	½–1 oz or 1–2 tbsp	1½–2½ oz or 3–5 tbsp
Vegetables and fruit Dark green or deep yellow fruit or vegetables rich in vitamin A content (e.g., carrots, sweet potatoes, green leafy vegetables, green peppers, cantaloupe, apricots, peaches) Vitamin C-containing foods *Good sources:* citrus fruit or juice, peppers (green and red sweet), cantaloupe, fresh strawberries, broccoli, brussels sprouts *Fair sources:* other melons, tomatoes, cabbage, potatoes cooked in skins, green leafy vegetables, tangerine and lemon, asparagus tips, cauliflower, rutabagas Other vegetables and fruit	4 servings daily to include: 1 serving at least every other day of a food rich in vitamin A 1 serving of a *good* source of vitamin C-containing food or 2 servings of a *fair* source daily 1–3 servings One serving of raw fruit or vegetable should be selected daily	⅓–½ c orange juice or other food high in vitamin C. Size of servings for other foods: 1–2 tbsp or ~⅛ c	⅓–½ c orange juice or other food high in vitamin C; other foods. Size of servings for other foods: 3–5 tbsp or ~¼ c
Bread and cereal Whole grain or enriched	4 servings (If no cereal is eaten, an additional serving of bread or baked goods should be selected)	½ slice bread or ¼–½ oz dry cereal or 1–2 tbsp (~⅛ c) cooked cereal	1 slice bread or ½–1 oz dry cereal or 3–5 tbsp (~¼ c) cooked cereal
Additional foods Butter, margarine, and other fats; desserts and sweets; additional amounts of foods from the four food groups	Amount as needed to meet kcal needs	Some vegetable oil should be included daily. Foods that provide only kcal (e.g., sugar, candy, cake frosting, bottled soft drinks) should be used sparingly as they reduce the appetite for other foods. Select nutritious desserts, such as pudding, fruit, and cookies containing oatmeal or peanut butter	

part of the preschool period, but it may not do so until well into the school-age years for some. A small appetite, especially in toddlers, is of considerable concern to parents accustomed to the voracious appetite of infancy. Tell the parents that, because of the small appetite, food should be served in small, frequent feedings, e.g., three small meals plus two or three small snacks (midmorning, midafternoon, and perhaps bedtime). In relation to snacks, emphasize these three points:

1. Snacks should be carefully spaced to avoid interference with the appetite for meals.
2. Snack choices should contribute to daily food

TABLE 16–3
SUGGESTED MEAL PATTERN FOR THE CHILD 1 TO 6

Breakfast	*A.M. Snack*	*Lunch (or Supper)*	*P.M. Snack*	*Dinner*
Fruit or juice Unsweetened cereal with milk Toast Butter or margarine Milk	Juice (4 oz) or a small cube of cheese or ¼ sandwich	Main dish (such as meat, eggs, fish, poultry, dried peas or beans, cheese, peanut butter) Vegetable or salad Bread Butter or marga- rine Dessert or fruit	Juice (4 oz) or 2 crackers spread with peanut butter or a small ap- ple	Meat, poultry, or fish, or meat alter- nate Vegetable Relish or salad Bread Butter or margarine Fruit or pudding Milk

needs rather than consist of foods supplying primarily kilocalories, such as candy.

3. Snacks should consist of low-sugar foods. Because of the relationship of sugar intake to dental caries, stress that sugar-containing foods should be used sparingly. The current consensus of dentists is that the use of sugar-containing foods should be restricted to meals, and snacks should be limited to non-sweet foods. A suggested meal pattern for the child aged 1 to 6 is given in Table 16–3, and a list of low-sugar snack foods approved by the American Dental Association is given in Table 16–4.

Although frequent feedings are important, overfeeding during this period deserves emphasis. The correlation between obesity in infancy or in childhood and obesity at a later period in life has not been totally clarified, but childhood-onset obesity frequently persists into later life. For this reason, discourage overfeeding.

Consistency of Food Served. The consistency of food served is dependent on chewing ability and development of the manual dexterity required to manipulate utensils involved in self-feeding. Encourage both chewing and self-feeding when the skills necessary to accomplish these tasks are sufficiently developed.

Chewing ability is influenced by the number of teeth. It is initiated with the appearance of up-and-down chewing motions with the mouth and with the beginning eruption of teeth during the fifth to eighth months of infancy. Tooth eruption continues gradually, and at 1 year the child usually has 6 to 8 teeth. All 20 of the primary teeth are usually in at 3 years of age, although there is wide individual variation both in the order of appearance and in the timing of tooth eruption. With tooth eruption, the consistency of the diet should gradually progress from semisolid (baby) food to table foods that are served in mashed, ground, chopped, and sliced forms. Since some meats, such as beef and pork, are hard to chew, it may be necessary to grind them until there are enough teeth to chew them properly. By the time all of the primary teeth are in, suggest that whole table foods can be served with perhaps only the meat cut into bite-sized pieces. Therefore, the toddler eats foods of mashed, ground, chopped or sliced consistency (depending on the number of teeth), whereas the preschool child eats whole table foods requiring no special preparation (other than perhaps cutting meat into bite-sized pieces).

Assess the client's neuromuscular development as it relates to feeding skills. The manual dexterity required for self-feeding is usually developed by the end of the second year, when the child can assume responsibility for his or her own feeding. The transition from drinking from a bottle to using a cup and attempts at finger feeding usually begin toward the

TABLE 16–4
LOW-SUGAR SNACK FOODS

Milk and *Cheese Group*	*Meat–Fish–Poultry–* *Beans Group*	*Vegetable–Fruit* *Group*	*Bread–Cereal* *Group*
Milk, cheese, plain yo- ghurt	Lunch meat and hot dogs (with- out added sugar) Peanut butter Nuts, eggs, chicken, ham, or egg salad	Fresh fruit and vegetables Unsweetened canned fruit Unsweetened fruit or vegetable juices	Toast, plain crackers, such as soda crackers Pizza, hard rolls, snack items such as popcorn, potato chips, pretzels, corn chips

(Source: Adapted from A Snacking Guide, More Or Less. Chicago, American Dental Association, 1975.)

end of the first year, and it takes most of the second year for independence in spoon feeding and cup drinking to be developed. In the interim, advise the parents to expect spilled milk, dropped spoons, and gleeful contrariness from their young toddler as the child explores food and to avoid becoming frustrated by these behaviors. Suggest that during the transition phase finger foods, such as small sandwiches, bits of vegetables, fruit, or cheese, that are easy to manipulate be provided. Finger foods continue to be popular throughout the toddler and preschool period.

Because of the possibility of aspiration, some foods should not be served to toddlers and preschoolers. These include nuts, fruits with large seeds, pits, or tough skins, and gristle around bones. Advise the parents that seeds or pits and fruit peelings should be removed.

Because the gastrointestinal tract of the toddler or preschooler is easily upset, suggest that foods that are very sweet, rich, hard to chew, or fried be used with discretion. Assure that the child receives an adequate amount of fiber to aid normal laxation. Substantial amounts of whole grains, fruits, and vegetables should be provided. Stress to the parents, however, that they avoid a diet that emphasizes high-fiber, low-calorie foods to the exclusion of other common foods.[2]

ASSESSMENT AND INTERVENTION

Psychosocial Development in Toddler and Preschool Child

Individuals exhibit characteristic behavior patterns that are typical of their level of growth and development. Some of these patterns are in response to the level of physiologic maturation, and others are in response to psychosocial developmental struggles.

The psychosocial developmental task of the toddler is to develop the sense of autonomy or the sense of *I* as an independent, self-controlled person who can do things for himself or herself. The toddler uses negativism, dawdling, and ritualism to maintain security while demonstrating the developing autonomy. Constant use of the word "No" reflects the conflict between the child's ego needs and the parents' effort to exert control. Power struggles between parents and child often focus on food and eating. Positive relationships will support the developing sense of autonomy. In contrast, negative relationships may result in feelings of shame and doubt, with the child feeling worthless and incompetent.

The preschool child struggles with the development of initiative (vs feelings of guilt). Initiative is characterized by the enjoyment of energy expended in action, increasing dependability, assertiveness, learning, and the ability to plan. Other developmental tasks of the preschooler are related to this core developmental problem. These include sex identification (the boy imitating the father, and the girl imitating the mother) and development of the superego (the conscience). Given negative relationships, the tension of the conscience results in guilt feelings rather than initiative.

The feeding process provides a mechanism for supporting the positive aspects of these psychosocial struggles and other aspects of psychosocial development. Parents of toddlers and preschoolers welcome help and reassurance regarding perceived eating problems of their children. To foster optimal psychosocial development, help them to adjust feeding practices to (1) correlate with behavior patterns characteristic of a given age and (2) provide learning and developmental opportunities. In so doing, the foundation for the formation of good food habits is laid.

Feeding Practices that Correlate with Behavior Patterns of Toddler and Preschool Child. Typical food responses of toddlers and preschoolers are shown in Figure 16-1.

The small appetite that is common to both toddlers and preschoolers sometimes involves the refusal of food. Thus these periods are sometimes

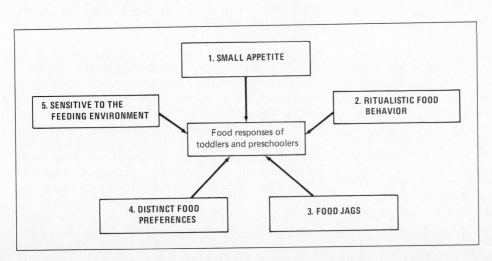

Figure 16–1
Food responses of toddlers and preschoolers.

called the "won't eat" stage. Reasons for the small appetite are:

1. Slow rate of physical growth
2. Increased exploratory activity
3. Short attention span
4. High level of physical activity that may dull the appetite by producing fatigue
5. Susceptibility to illness (such as respiratory infections), which decreases the appetite
6. Negativistic and dawdling behavior (in the toddler) as independence is explored

While the appetite is typically small, tell parents to expect considerable variation from day to day in association with variation in physical activity. Help them to recognize that both toddlers and preschoolers need proportionately fewer kilocalories and that in toddlers the struggle for autonomy often involves food refusal to aid in avoiding conflicts over eating. Let them know that, given appropriate food choices and a pleasant feeding atmosphere, a child will usually eat an adequate quantity of food if he or she feels physically well.

Give them the following suggestions to assure that nutritional needs will be met and that optimal psychosocial development will be fostered during this period of small appetite:

1. Offer a variety of attractive foods in small amounts, in an easy-to-eat form, and at regular intervals. Restrict high-carbohydrate and high-fat snacks that dull the appetite.
2. Allow some choice in food selection.
3. Respect food preferences.
4. Provide a meal environment that is free of distraction. If the child finds it difficult to remain at the table long enough to eat, bring a favorite toy to the table or fix snack foods in a paper bag that can be carried with the child.
5. Allow for a premeal rest period.
6. Provide appropriate substitutes for rejected foods (e.g., if traditional breakfast foods are rejected, serve a hamburger, cheese sandwich, soup, or other favorite food; if vegetables are rejected, replace with fruit).
7. Set reasonable limits that both parents and child can adhere to (for instance, allow a reasonable time for eating. If food is not eaten in this period, casually remove it. The dawdling toddler may need to begin the meal before the rest of the family).

Ritualistic food behavior is characteristic of both toddlers and preschoolers. Such behavior is most common between the ages of 2 and 4 years and reaches a peak at 2½ years. Some examples of food rituals are insisting that the bib be put on the same way, demonstrating a strong preference for certain foods or utensils, eating foods in a certain sequence, insisting that foods not touch each other on the plate, and requesting a specific toy while eating. Since ritualistic behavior provides security, tell parents to respect the need for ritualism to foster optimal psychosocial development.

Food jags are also common in toddlers and preschoolers between 2 and 4 years of age and are characterized by the acceptance of only a limited number of foods for a short period of time. A child, for example, may eat nothing but two or three eggs or several peanut butter sandwiches at every meal and reject all other foods. If treated in a casual manner, children will usually return to a more varied diet after several days. A good plan is to serve other foods in addition to the accepted food, with no issue made if the other foods are rejected. Conflicts over eating may develop if the child is forced to eat.

Toddlers and preschoolers have usually developed distinct food preferences. Children have a more acute sense of taste than adults, and their dislike for certain foods can be very strong. Since parents are the primary socializers of young children, it seems likely that they influence the development of their children's food preferences, although the results of investigations into the relationships between parental food preferences and those of their children are contradictory.[3] A child's food preferences may also be influenced by those of their siblings and peers.[4] Encourage parents to respect their children's food preferences while at the same time continuing to expose them to new foods. When new foods are rejected, they can be offered again at a later time, perhaps prepared differently.

Some studies suggest that vegetables are usually the least well accepted of the food groups, probably because of their strong flavor, with raw vegetables being better accepted than cooked ones. Other studies show, however, that mild-flavored foods are not accepted at a much greater rate than strong-flavored ones and even liver is not a universally disliked food.[5] If strong-flavored vegetables, such as cabbage, onions, cauliflower, and broccoli, are rejected because of their flavor, suggest to the parents that the strong flavor can be diminished by cooking them in an uncovered pot with enough water to extend about ½ in above the vegetables. Some of the strong flavoring substances will escape from the uncovered pan while the vegetables are boiling. Flavor can be gradually intensified as acceptance is established. While this method of cooking may result in the loss of some water-soluble nutrients, it is perhaps reasonable to occasionally sacrifice some of the nutrient content to achieve greater palatability and acceptance. Although acceptance of some foods, such as fruits, is explained by their sweet taste, sweetness does not explain the acceptance of nonsweet foods, such as meat. Toddlers may consume more fruit than vegetables. Help parents to understand that the young child can still get needed nutrients and to assist them to gradually work toward increasing the amount of vegetables eaten.

Like flavor, the form, color, and textures of foods

that are best accepted by young children are the subject of debate.[5] While children are noted to prefer plain foods to mixed dishes, such as casseroles, a decided preference for plain foods has not been documented, and mixed foods, such as pizza, sloppy joes, beef stew, spaghetti, and macaroni with cheese, are often popular. Often toddlers and preschoolers may eat only one food from the plate at a time and may separate a mixture into its component parts and eat them one by one.

Children are also reported to like foods that are colorful, that are soft and fluffy (like mashed potatoes and pudding) rather than sticky, heavy items, and foods that are crisp in texture (like crisp raw vegetables) rather than soggy ones. Again these preference characteristics are difficult to categorize because of local cultural meanings and the variability in perceptions of food qualities.

Children respond to both the quantity of foods served and their temperature. Encourage parents to give small servings initially and allow for seconds. The psychologic effect of an adult-sized serving can overwhelm a small appetite. Also tell parents to serve the child's food at room temperature. It may be necessary to fill the child's plate first, so that it is at room temperature when the meal is served. Young children often appear frightened by hot food. They may stir a food, such as hard ice cream, until it is soupy and less sharply cold.

Young children are sensitive to the environmental situation in which feeding takes place. Given a pleasant feeding environment, the child can master good eating habits and establish a daily routine of eating adequately. Many serious feeding problems develop in early childhood as a result of excessive parental concern and vigilance regarding eating. The attitudes developed in such situations may be carried over into later life. Stress to the parents that the child may try to manipulate them by altering food intake if undue concern is expressed about what is eaten. A casual approach should be taken when food is either accepted or rejected. Give parents these suggestions for creating a feeding environment that is conducive to healthy psychosocial development while at the same time setting reasonable limits on behavior:

1. Establish a regular routine for meals to provide security.
2. Serve meals in a pleasant, relaxed environment that is free of conflict.
3. Provide positive reinforcement for appropriate food behavior.
4. Avoid rigid rules about amounts of food eaten. For instance, a rigid clean-plate rule may lead to unnecessary arguments and may establish a pattern of overeating. Nonetheless, children should learn early in life that they are expected to eat food that is prepared for them.
5. Avoid coaxing ("Just one more bite for Grandpa"), threats ("If you don't eat your supper you're going straight to bed"), bribes ("Clean your plate and you'll get dessert"), or other means of forcing a child to eat. Desserts can be kept in proper perspective by serving those of high-nutrient content, e.g., fruit cup or pudding that can be eaten along with the meal without fear of dulling the appetite. Children frequently respond to coaxing, threats, and bribes by decreasing food intake.

Feeding Practices that Provide Learning and Developmental Opportunities. Food and the way it is used can provide learning situations that foster the psychosocial development of the toddler and preschooler. Food and feeding practices can be used to encourage independence and a sense of achievement, provide a mechanism for socialization, and provide a mechanism for teaching cognitive skills. Make these suggestions for fostering the development of independence and a sense of achievement:

1. Permit the child to eat without being forced.
2. Serve small portions to provide a feeling of success when eating. Fill a glass or cup only half to three-quarters full.
3. Provide foods in an easy-to-eat form (finger foods).
4. Encourage the child to feed himself or herself as soon as he or she is capable.
5. Allow the child to serve his or her own portions.
6. Allow for some choice in food selections.
7. Provide feeding equipment appropriate to ability. The toddler will have fewer accidents when using an unbreakable deep dish and a small glass or cup with a weighted bottom. Spoons and forks should have short, straight handles. A salad fork with blunt tines is suitable for the preschooler. Provide a sturdy chair with a footrest.
8. Give responsibility in food preparation and service according to ability. The preschooler can help plan menus, set the table, wash dishes, and prepare simple foods.

Food and feeding can be a useful socialization medium for the toddler and preschooler. From birth, food becomes a medium of socialization and mode of communication. Being held and fed is the infant's major opportunity to socialize. Sharing food goes hand in hand with communication, since eating together allows for relaxation and conversation. Therefore, toddlers and preschoolers should be provided with group eating experiences (e.g., family meals, nursery school, sharing a meal with a friend) as a means of socialization. In sharing family meals, children should be accepted as family members and included in the conversation. They should not be singled out for constant criticism about table manners. Toddlers and preschoolers are great imitators and follow the examples of others in eating and table manners. Parental example—not criticism—is the best teacher of manners.

Whereas the socializing aspects of sharing family meals are an important consideration for the toddler, food and eating assume greater social significance for the preschooler. Since this is the period for developing sex identification, sharing meals provides an opportunity to imitate the habits of the parent of the same sex. This aids in establishing the child's own sexual identity.

Food may also be used as a mechanism for learning cognitive skills. Food has characteristic properties—color, texture, odor, flavor, temperature—that are a source of stimulation for the child's senses. The young toddler learns textures by touching and squeezing food with the hands. The mouth, too, is a sense organ, and eating foods that vary in texture, odor, and flavor provides the opportunity for learning to differentiate among these sensations.

OTHER CONCERNS

Assessment and Intervention

In recent decades major sociologic changes have occurred that have implications for the nutritional status of toddlers and preschoolers. The large number of working mothers and increasing number of single parents have placed many of these children in day care centers. One or two meals each day may be eaten away from home with peer groups. The types and amounts of foods served and the attitudes of the other children have a great influence on the nutrient intake, and the types of food habits developed may differ greatly from those of the family. Assist parents in selecting a center that serves nutritious food and has a philosophy that reinforces positive food habits. Some day care centers are eligible for assistance with providing food under the Child Care Food Program administered by the U.S. Department of Agriculture. This program provides financial and commodity food assistance for meals served to children 12 years of age and under in licensed or approved child care centers and family and group day care homes. The child care institution can be reimbursed for service of either two meals and one snack or one meal and two snacks per child per day.

Assess the patterns of food use in families with a working mother or with a single parent who works. The pressures of working may increase the frequency with which the family eats at fast-food restaurants and uses convenience foods. Fast foods are often higher in kilocalories, fat, and salt than similar foods prepared at home. Provide guidelines for selecting the items that are lower in fat and sodium. Use of convenience foods may rob children of learning experiences. Children may become confused about the original sources of food, and they may

refuse food, such as vegetables, because they often have to be consumed at the table.

Check how often the child watches television and the types of programs that are watched; some young children may spend a large amount of time at this sedentary activity. Television often gives heavy emphasis to advertising nonnutritious foods. Young children are not able to evaluate claims made about food and may tempt their parents to buy them at the market. Advise parents to monitor the programs viewed by their child. Equally important, caution them about succumbing to the child's pressures to purchase the nonnutritious advertised foods so that they will not be available in the home.

Assess family income. If it is low, the community nutrition programs described in Chapter 14 may be applicable. In addition to the WIC program, the Head Start Program provides services for young children. This federally funded program provides educational enrichment and nutrition services for children aged 3 to 5 from low-income areas. This program is designed to give underprivileged preschool children an opportunity to fulfill their potential in physical and mental development. Nutrition is a significant part of the program, which provides for the service of nutritious meals and snacks, nutrition education for children and their families, and consultation, technical assistance, and training in nutrition for Head Start staff.

Assess for the practice of pica in young children. This practice is not uncommon, particularly between 1½ and 2 years of age, but may persist up to 4 to 6 years of age. Most children begin mouthing objects in the middle of the first year as part of the normal hand-to-mouth stage of development. This type of activity usually subsides in the beginning part of the second year. The activity is considered abnormal when it persists beyond 18 months, especially when it involves a craving for particular nonfood substances, such as dirt, paint chips, and plaster. Lead poisoning may be of particular concern in cities with substandard housing where the child eats paint chips. Determine if anemia is present. The concurrent presence of pica and iron deficiency anemia is not uncommon.

REVIEW QUESTIONS AND ACTIVITIES

1. Identify the characteristics of physical growth in height, weight, and body composition during the toddler and preschool periods.
2. Plan a menu that includes the appropriate number and size of servings from the Basic Four Food Groups for a 2-year-old toddler.
3. Adjust the menu in Question 2 so that it includes the appropriate number and size of servings for a 4-year-old preschooler.
4. Identify the differences in number and size of servings from the Basic Four Food Groups

needed by toddlers, preschoolers, and adults.

5. Calculate the amount of iron contained in the menu in Question 2 and compare the iron content with the RDA for iron for a toddler (use Appendix 1 for your calculations). If the iron content is below the RDA, make the appropriate adjustments in the menu.

6. How do the iron requirements of toddlers and preschoolers differ?

7. List two nutrients for which supplementation may be indicated for toddlers and preschoolers.

8. List three criteria for the appropriate use of snacks in the diet of toddlers and preschoolers.

9. Make a list of several appropriate snack choices from each of the Basic Four Food Groups.

10. Describe the dietary advice about food consistency that you would give to a parent of a 2-year-old toddler. How would this advice differ for a parent of a 4-year-old preschooler?

11. List six factors that may influence the appetite of toddlers and preschoolers.

12. Identify an example of ritualistic food behavior and a food jag. What advice would you give to a parent for handling these food behaviors?

13. List three examples of feeding practices that may increase food acceptance and foster optimal psychosocial development in dealing with each of the following food responses that are typical of toddlers and preschoolers: (a) small appetite, (b) distinct food preferences, and (c) sensitivity to the feeding environment.

14. List three examples of the appropriate use of food to provide learning and developmental opportunities for toddlers and preschoolers.

15. Discuss the potential influences on nutritional status and food habits of young children when the primary caretaker is employed outside the home.

16. List three federal programs that provide nutritional services for toddlers and preschool children.

17. Describe the incidence of pica in children prior to school age.

REFERENCES

1. Beal VA: Nutrition in the Life Span. New York, John Wiley & Sons, 1980, p 265.
2. Committee on Nutrition, American Academy of Pediatrics: Plant fiber intake in the pediatric diet. Pediatrics 67:572, 1981.
3. Birch LL: The relationships between children's food preferences and those of their parents. J Nutr Educ 12:14, 1980.
4. Hertzler AA: Children's food patterns—A review. II. Family and group behavior. J Am Diet Assoc 83:555, 1983.
5. Hertzler AA: Children's food patterns—A review. I. Food preferences and feeding problems. J Am Diet Assoc 83:551, 1983.

BIBLIOGRAPHY

Birch LL: Dimensions of preschool children's food preferences. J Nutr Educ 11:77, 1979.

Birch LL: Effect of peer models' food choices and eating behavior on preschoolers' food preferences. Child Develop 51:489, 1980.

Dallman PR, Siimes MA, Stekel A: Iron deficiency anemia in infancy and childhood. Am J Clin Nutr 33:86, 1980.

National Nutrition Education Clearing House: Preschool Nutrition Education Monograph. Berkeley, Calif, Society for Nutrition Education, 1978.

Phillips BK, Kolasa KK: Vegetable preferences of preschoolers in day care. J Nutr Educ 12:192, 1980.

Phillips MG: Nutrition education for preschoolers: The Head Start experience. Children Today 12:20, 1983.

Pipes PL: Nutrition in Infancy and Childhood, ed 3. St. Louis, CV Mosby, 1985.

Pliner P: Family resemblance in food preference. J Nutr Educ 15:137, 1983.

Schafer RB, Keith PM: Influence on food decisions across the family life cycle. J Am Diet Assoc 78:144, 1981.

Valentine J, Ross CJ, Zigler E: Project Head Start. Children Today 9:22, 1980.

Yperman AM, Vermeersch JA: Factors associated with children's food habits. J Nutr Educ 11:72, 1979.

CHAPTER 17

Nutrition of the School-age Child and Adolescent

Objectives

After completion of this chapter, the student will be able to:

1. Compare the patterns of physical growth and nutritional requirements of school-age children, adolescent males, and adolescent females and relate the nutrient requirements of adolescents to nutrient deficiencies commonly observed in this age group.

2. Use the Basic Four Food Groups to plan menus that meet the nutrient needs of school-age children and adolescents.

3. Compare the psychosocial influences on eating patterns and food choices of school-age children and adolescents.

4. Distinguish among the five school-based nutrition programs.

5. Plan a menu for one day for a school child that conforms to the designated school lunch pattern.

6. Evaluate the potential for reducing the incidence of atherosclerosis by dietary manipulations beginning in childhood.

7. Develop a teaching plan for nutritional management in each of the following situations: (a) a school-age child with dental caries, (b) an obese adolescent female who is pregnant, (c) an adolescent female with anorexia nervosa, (d) an adolescent male who engages in intense physical activity, and (e) an adolescent male with acne.

During the period of late childhood and adolescence, nutrition continues to be an important environmental influence affecting physiologic, psychologic, and sociocultural changes in the individual. In turn, these changes have a great influence on food habits common to these age groups. Perhaps at no other time during the growth cycle do physical and psychosocial changes have so great an impact on food habits as during adolescence.

► The **school-age period** (also called **middle childhood**) refers to children from age 6 to the onset
► of **puberty** (a period characterized by a spurt in physical growth and appearance of the secondary
► sex characteristics), whereas **adolescence** refers to the period from puberty to the completion of physical growth. The end of the school-age period varies widely between the sexes and between individuals of the same sex. In females, the onset of puberty may be as early as 7 to 8 years and as late as 11 to 12 years; for males the ages range from 9 to 10 years to about 14 years.

The mature human body is the end result of a remarkable growth process that requires approximately two decades for completion. The general character of growth is one of decreasing velocity, beginning immediately after birth and changing significantly only during adolescence, when the velocity of growth seems to increase suddenly. At the end of this growth period (approximately age 17 in girls and 21 in boys), adult stature is largely attained, although there is some evidence that growth in stature can continue for another decade.

203

Growth occurs by increases in height and weight. Gains in height reflect bone growth in three body compartments: (1) the head, (2) the trunk (i.e., the spinal column), and (3) the legs. Because of differences in the rate of growth in these three compartments at different stages of the growth cycle, the body has a characteristic appearance at different ages. In contrast to gains in height, gains in weight reflect a composite of growth in all body tissues—bone, muscle, fat, organs, and fluids.

Over the past century an increase in the size of children in successive generations has been evident in industrialized societies. Each generation of children has grown taller and heavier and matured earlier sexually than the previous generations. For example, the gain in height in successive generations has averaged 1 inch every 30 years or so. There are indications, however, that the maximum genetic capacity for adult stature has been reached in the United States, although adult weight attained is still

▶ increasing. The age of **menarche** (onset of menstruation in females) has changed from an average age of 17 years to the current average age of 13. This trend is thought to be related to improvements in medical care, especially improved nutritional status.

ASSESSMENT

Physical Changes

School-Age Children. In marked contrast to the dramatic, rapid rate of growth that occurs during the prenatal and early postnatal period, observe that growth is relatively slow and steady during the early years of middle childhood. The period is sometimes

▶ called the **latent period** because it is significantly more serene and poses fewer overall problems, including feeding problems, than do the periods of early childhood and adolescence. The end of the period, however, overlaps with the onset of adolescence, and there begins a spurt in physical growth. The prepubescent growth spurt is characterized by an increase in body size that occurs at a rate matched or exceeded only by the rate of the developing fetus and the infant in early postnatal life.

There is little difference between the sexes in yearly gains in height and weight until the approximate age of 9 to 9½ years, although males tend to be slightly taller and heavier than females. However, note that females from about the age of 9 to 13½ years of age tend to be taller and heavier than males because the growth spurt begins about 2 years earlier in females than in males. After this age, the situation is reversed. Physical characteristics of the school-age period that have implications (either direct or indirect) for nutritional needs are summarized in Table 17–1.

Adolescents. Adolescence is a period characterized by rapid, recognizable changes in the individual's

makeup. The period has no specified age-defined beginning or end. It is a period not only of physical maturation but of social, psychologic, and cognitive maturation as well. After the relatively uniform growth of childhood, physical growth during adolescence increases in velocity, and reproductive development takes place. Within 4 years after the onset of puberty, adult sexual maturity with the ability to procreate is reached. Do not confuse sexual maturity with maturity in other parameters, however. For instance, social, psychologic, and cognitive maturation do not occur until the later years of adolescence.

The most rapid phase of adolescent growth is

▶ known as the **growth spurt,** and its highest point is called its peak. The growth spurt begins in females at an average age of 10 years, reaching a peak rate at approximately age 12. In males the spurt in growth begins 2 years later, peaking at about 14 years. Thereafter, growth continues but at a slower rate. The peak velocity of increase in stature and weight precedes menarche in females and sperm production in males. The weight increment curve in both boys and girls has a lower peak and lasts longer than the height curve. Recognize that the growth spurt relative to the rate of growth and duration is more intense and prolonged in males than in females and that differences in body composition between the sexes become apparent. Males deposit proportionately more lean body tissue and skeletal muscle mass while concurrently decreasing total body fat, and females deposit proportionately more fat during adolescent growth. The fact that males on the average are taller and heavier than females at maturity may be explained by the males' later and more prolonged growth period, and by their larger growth potential. The growth spurt represents the only time in extrauterine life when growth velocity actually increases. Table 17–2 provides a summary of the major physical changes that have an influence on nutrition for the adolescent.

Recommended Dietary Allowances

While biologic age provides more accurate data for determining nutritional needs, most authorities use the more convenient method of stating needs according to chronologic age. Note that the RDA (see Chap. 2) for school-age children and adolescents make no distinction between the sexes in nutrient requirements until after the age of 10. At this point, separate allowances are given for males and females in three age categories (11 to 14, 15 to 18, and 19 to 22). The specific allowances given, which for the most part reflect extrapolations from data on infants and adults, reflect the larger male requirement for kilocalories and a number of nutrients and the difference in maturation patterns between males and females. For example, energy requirements reach a maximum for females in the 7 to 10 age range (2400 kcal) and for males in the 19 to 22 age range (2900 kcal).

TABLE 17–1
PHYSICAL CHANGES IN THE SCHOOL-AGE CHILD

Physical Characteristics	Comments
Slow growth rate: average annual weight gain of 2.2–3.9 kg with increasing age in males and 2.3–4.4 kg with increasing age in females; average annual height increment of 5.2–5.8 cm in males and 5.8–6.5 cm in females	Growth characterized by spurts and plateaus with a pronounced spurt toward the end of the period; weight gain is generally more rapid in fall and winter; appetite tends to parallel growth rate; body type is confirmed, i.e., short children tend to remain short, tall children tend to remain tall during this period
Vigorous physical activity	Wide individual variations in activity level, however
Loss of deciduous teeth and eruption and maturation of permanent teeth (first molars erupt at about age 7; most permanent teeth, except for second and third molars, have erupted by age 12)	Continued need for nutritional support to foster the development and maintenance of healthy teeth (e.g., control of the frequency of sucrose ingestion, provision of a source of fluoride, provision of adequate calcium, phosphorus, and vitamin D)
Nutrients stored in preparation for adolescence	For example, the greatest retention of calcium and phosphorus in the skeleton precedes the growth spurt by 2 or more years.
Brain size approximates that of adult brain	Growth in head circumference slows (circumference increases from about 20 to 21 in. between the ages of 5 and 12)
Lymphoid tissue reaches peak of development and generally exceeds amount of this type of tissue present in normal adult	Enlarged tonsils and adenoids may be surgically removed if they are foci of infection.
High incidence of respiratory infection during the early school years but resistance gradually increases	Response to infection is similar to adult response
Declining activity of lactose enzyme in susceptible populations	Assess for milk tolerance

TABLE 17–2
PHYSICAL CHANGES IN THE ADOLESCENT

Physical Characteristics	Comments
Rapid increase in height and weight	Increase in both cell number and cell size; growth spurt contributes about 50% to adult body weight and about 15% to final adult height
Development of secondary sexual characteristics	*Girls:* development of the breasts, appearance and elaboration of pubic and axillary hair, menarche, differential deposition of adipose tissue on hips, thighs, buttocks, enlargement of pelvis *Boys:* growth in size of penis and testes, appearance and elaboration of pubic, axillary, body, and facial hair, increase in the size of the larynx, broadening of the shoulder girdle, increase in lean body mass (muscle and skeletal tissue)
Appear to be able to resist infectious diseases	Incidence of respiratory infections is lower than during early childhood; most prevalent infections are infectious mononucleosis, serum hepatitis, and venereal disease
Completion of tooth eruption and maturation	Eruption and maturation of all 32 permanent teeth complete by age 21 (the second molars usually erupt by age 13 or 14 and the third molars may erupt as late as early 20s)
Increased activity of sebaceous glands	Acne may be a consequence of changing hormonal secretions

Pattern of Nutrient Requirements

School-Age Children. A decline in nutrient requirements relative to body size is characteristic of late childhood, during which time the rate of growth is slow and steady. Be aware that this is an important period from a nutritional standpoint, however, because nutrients are being stored in preparation for the increased demands that occur with rapid growth during the latter part of the period. During this period, kilocaloric and nutrient requirements increase gradually. Although the elementary schoolchild needs somewhat more kilocalories and nutrients, the changes are not startling. Throughout childhood and until the growth spurt, daily kilocaloric requirements increase by approximately 100 kcal each year. A useful rule of thumb for approximating daily kilocaloric needs is to allow 1000 kcal for the 1-year-old and add 100 kcal for each additional year of age.

Adolescents. The sharp rise in nutrient requirements per unit of body weight during adolescent growth results in an increased need for all essential nutrients. Kilocalories and certain nutrients, e.g., protein, B vitamins, iron, zinc, calcium, phosphorus, iodine, and fluoride, require special consideration because of their particular role in growth and development. Due to the greater increase in lean tissue and skeletal mass that occurs in males during the growth spurt, there is a greater dietary demand for protein, iron, and zinc than is required for the growth spurt in girls. Kilocaloric requirements (and the need for the B vitamins necessary for energy metabolism) increase as the basal metabolic rate (BMR) increases to support growth. The BMR is higher in males than in females because of their higher muscle and lower fat content. Energy requirements are also affected by the level of physical activity, which varies. Males are generally more physically active than females.

Protein requirements are increased since nitrogen is stored—a positive nitrogen balance occurs during growth. A kilocaloric deficit, even with an adequate protein intake, can compromise protein synthesis and deposition of lean body mass during growth periods. The folic acid requirement is considerably increased, since this B vitamin is needed for the increased rate of cell division.

In females, iron requirements increase to replace the iron lost in menstrual blood. In males, the increased muscle mass and rise in red blood cell production bring higher iron requirements. The number of red blood cells rises considerably in pubescent males, probably as a result of increased androgen production, whereas the red cell mass remains constant in females. When growth is rapid, males require more iron than do menstruating females. The high iron requirement continues until the menopause for females, but the need for iron decreases for males after the cessation of growth.

The need for calcium and phosphorus increase concomitantly with the increase in size of the skeleton and progressive bone mineralization. It is during the growth spurt that approximately 45 percent of adult skeletal mass is formed.[1] Research studies indicate that emotional stress may adversely affect calcium retention in the body. Since teenagers are subject to considerable emotional stress, this finding has particular significance for this age group. There is some evidence that a low dietary intake of calcium may result in a decrease in bone density, which may be a predisposing factor to osteoporosis in later life (see Chap. 37). If calcium intake is inadequate during peak adolescent growth, bone growth may be limited in some individuals.[1] A generous body storage of calcium also provides extra protection for the adolescent who becomes pregnant soon after the peak of height velocity. Zinc is needed for growth and sexual maturation, and iodine requirements increase in association with the increased need for thyroid hormones to support growth. A source of fluoride continues to be important until the calcification and maturation of teeth are complete.

Assess for the presence of special situations not uncommon in adolescence, such as the use of drugs, alcohol, cigarettes, contraceptive devices by the female, or the occurrence of pregnancy, that have a direct or indirect effect on nutrient needs and nutritional status. Drugs, alcohol, and cigarettes may pose a nutritional risk either directly—by altering nutrient metabolism—or indirectly—by affecting appetite. Pregnancy increases nutrient requirements.

INTERVENTION

The nutrient requirements of school-age children and adolescents are translated into a daily food plan in Table 17–3. Base specific dietary recommendations on the stage of physical maturation rather than chronologic age. Nutrient needs are greatest during the growth spurt and gradually decrease as the individual achieves physical maturity.

Use the client's appetite for judging the approximate amount of food needed. Appetite tends to parallel the growth rate. The appetite of normal healthy children naturally increases to provide for the increased amounts of food needed for growth. While the small appetite that is characteristic of toddlers and preschoolers may continue into the school years in some children, usually by 8 to 10 years of age, the appetite is very good and corresponds to the slow, steady growth rate. With the onset of the growth spurt, the appetite becomes voracious—adolescents are constantly hungry. However, females require fewer kilocalories than males because of their smaller physical size and usually lower levels of physical activity. Assist female teenage clients to select foods of high nutrient density in order to meet all of the nutrient needs without exceeding the energy allowance.

TABLE 17–3
FOODS TO MEET NUTRITIONAL REQUIREMENTS OF ELEMENTARY SCHOOL CHILDREN AND TEENAGERS

Food	7–10 Years		10–Teen Years	
Milk and cheese (whole, dry, skim, reliquified evaporated, soy milk, buttermilk, and other dairy products)	6–9 years: 9–10 years:	2–3 c 3 or more c	10–12 years: 12–16 years: Pregnant teens:	3–4 c 4 c 5–6 c

Calcium equivalent of 1 c milk:
    1 c plain yoghurt
    2 c cottage cheese
    1½ c ice cream
    1⅓ oz cheddar or Swiss cheese
    (natural or process)				

Meat–fish–poultry–beans
  Substitutes for protein for 1 oz meat:
    1 egg
    ½–¾ c cooked dry beans, dry peas,
    soybeans, lentils
    ¼–½ c nuts or seeds
    2 tbsp peanut butter
	2 servings (1½–2 oz/serving)		2 servings (2–3 oz/serving)	

Vegetables and fruit
  Eat one vitamin C source daily (e.g., citrus fruit, melon, strawberries, broccoli, tomatoes, raw cabbage)
  Eat one vitamin A source at least every other day (e.g., deep yellow-orange or very dark green vegetable or fruit)
  Use unpeeled fruits and vegetables and those with edible seeds frequently
	4 or more servings
	(⅓ c each)
			4 or more servings
			(½ c each)	

Bread and cereal (whole grain or enriched bread, cereal, rice, or pasta). One serving is:
  1 slice bread
  1 roll, muffin, or biscuit
  ½–¾ c cooked cereal, rice, or pasta
  1 oz dry cereal
	4 servings or more (very active children need more for energy)		4 servings or more
			Teenage boys: 6 or more servings (very active teens and athletes need more for energy)	

Additional foods Fats and oils, such as butter, margarine, mayonnaise, and vegetable oils; sweets and desserts; a source of vitamin D	As needed to meet kilocaloric needs; sweets should be consumed in moderation and with meals rather than as snacks, to reduce potential for dental caries; a source of vitamin D (such as vitamin D-fortified milk) is recommended throughout the growth period; nutritious snacks include milk, fruits, vegetables, juices, cheese, cold meat cubes, peanut butter on bread or crackers, custard, yoghurt, and nonsugared cereal			

Kilocaloric need	2400 (7–10 years)		*Girls:*
			  11–14 years:
			  15–22 years:
			Boys:
			  11–14 years:
			  15–18 years:
			  19–22 years:
				2200
				2100
				
				2700
				2800
				2900

Rehabilitation of the drug- or alcohol-dependent client requires nutritional therapy, and nutrient supplementation may be necessary for the adolescent female using contraceptives. Alcoholism is discussed in Chapter 36, contraceptive use in Chapter 14, and adolescent pregnancy later in this chapter.

ASSESSMENT AND INTERVENTION

Psychosocial Influences on Food Choice and Eating Patterns

Two major influences on the continuing development of food habits in the school-age child and adolescent are (1) the basic developmental tasks for the two age groups (as described in Chap. 13) and (2) the decline in family influence on food choice as children mature.

School-Age Children. The school-age years are characterized as the period during which children are faced with the challenge of developing a sense of industry (vs feelings of inferiority). The major thrust of this period of psychosocial development is determination on the part of the child to master the activities in which he or she is involved. Great efforts are placed on producing—and the child applies himself or herself to skills and tasks that go beyond playful expression. The child learns to cooperate in group activities, and considerable energy is expended in organized sports and games. There is increasing cognitive–intellectual development, and the child learns to solve problems. The sense of adequacy develops as horizons widen with new school experiences and challenging learning opportunities. There is movement away from dependence on parental standards and toward peer standards. It is a period of gangs, cliques, and hero worship. During this period, the child must also adjust to the changing body image and self-concept involved in coming to terms with the masculine or feminine social role. The period is thus characterized by considerable emotional stress; for example, the child must not only learn to get along with other children but also respond to pressures generated for self-control of the changing body. The child's fear of inferiority—feeling inadequate, defeated, unable to learn, to compete, to compromise, or to cooperate—is based on the knowledge that he or she is still a child who lacks the abilities to compete successfully in the adult-oriented world. Educate parents as to how they can contribute to the development of the sense of industry and avoid the feelings of inferiority by having realistic expectations of the child, encouraging peer activities as well as home responsibilities, and giving recognition to accomplished tasks.

The food behavior of the school-age child reflects these developmental changes. For instance, a wide variety of activities may take priority over food, and it may be difficult for the child to be punctual for meals. There is less parental supervision, more independent choice of food, and more peer influence on what and where the child eats. This may result in poor dietary habits, particularly if less nutrient-dense foods replace foods of high nutrient density. For some children, peer pressure leads to acceptance of previously rejected foods, whereas for others it may lead to excessive intake of such foods as soft drinks and candy. Conflicts may arise because of unrealistic parental expectations, which may include food-related behavior, such as adult table manners.

By the school-age period, dietary intake is usually smooth and regular, with gradual acceptance of a wider variety of foods and increase in appetite. Food patterns acquired at this age are likely to become lifelong practices. Stress to parents or other caretakers that the child needs supervision and supportive guidance in selecting nutritious foods so that growth is not compromised. Moreover, if the child goes into adolescence with a good nutritional status, he or she is better equipped to cope with the associated stresses.

In some cases, children may be left to their own devices in preparing breakfasts, and inadequate supervision may be available for the after-school hours. The consequences may be inadequate or skipped breakfast and foraging for snacks in the afternoon to satisfy the appetite. Snacking is common in this age group, especially after school, since for many children this may be the hungriest time of the day. Emphasize the importance of an adequate breakfast; skipping breakfast may impair the child's late morning problem-solving performance.[2,3] Stress that nutritious snacks, such as fruit or vegetables cut in bite-size pieces, juices, and milk, should be available in the home, and stress the desirability of knowing what foods are consumed during the day.

During late childhood, children want to grow normally and be like their peers. They are ready to learn about the relationship of food to the body. Assist the child to eat wisely by emphasizing that what is eaten does indeed make a difference in the way he or she grows. Inquire about the child's food patterns; school-age children like to share experiences with others. Give guidance about how to evaluate nutrition information, such as that provided by the mass media. Encourage them to share in responsibilities, such as meal planning, marketing, food preparation, and gardening, and to become involved in nutrition-related projects in the school and community. Urge participation in the school breakfast and/or school lunch program and give them information as to how to make nutritious choices.

Adolescents. The developmental task of the adolescent is identity formation and the assertion of independence. He or she asks: Who am I? What am I? How do I feel? Tasks center largely around the adolescent-related sexual development and preparation for an adult role in a complex society. The period produces numerous psychologic, emotional, and social conflicts, and the adolescent is characterized by vacillating moods and extremes of behavior. Changes in body image occur in association with sexual development. Males and females share an overriding concern for body image and peer group identification. While the period of rapid growth lasts only 2 to 3 years, the attendant social, psychologic, and cognitive maturation continues over a much longer period. The conflicts of adolescence may have many nutritional consequences.

Because of growing independence and a schedule that demands spending more time outside the home, many of the food choices of the adolescent are made independently. Away from home, a casual style of eating is often adopted, and meals may often be consumed at fast-food outlets. Irregular eating patterns, meal skipping, and increased snacking are often characteristic of the period. Breakfast and lunch are the meals most frequently skipped, and girls tend to skip breakfast more often than do boys. Adolescents snack frequently, and snacks may account for 12 to 17 percent of the RDA for energy and nutrients in their diets.[4] Snacking tends to be beneficial in meeting nutritional needs (except for the obese, because of the added kilocalories), since those who eat more frequently are more likely to ingest an adequate diet.

The peer group is the setter of adolescent norms in dress, food, and other areas. The peer influence may extend beyond the immediate group and include others, such as national idols or respected adults. Food practices may change because of the influence of others rather than for health reasons. Out of a desire to be accepted, new eating patterns may evolve, some of which are faddish, grossly restricted, or eccentric. Adoption of nontraditional diets, such as vegetarian, health food, fruitarian, or macrobiotic diets, is not uncommon in this age group. Food choices are often made on the basis of status, enjoyment, or sociability. Frequently diet is used to try to influence physical appearance, and nutritional health may be compromised by attempts to conform to cultural ideals. Adolescent girls are under constant pressures to diet. Society's idolization of slimness, the difference in the timing of the growth spurt in boys and girls that results in girls being taller than boys from about age 9 to 13½, and the more pronounced physiologic fat deposition in girls during adolescence all contribute to these pressures. Males are especially interested in physical fitness and competitive sports, and they may adopt a special type of diet (such as one that includes a larger amount of steak and eggs) as part of a muscle-building regimen. Both sexes may use diet in an attempt to control acne.

Assess physical activity on an individual basis. It may be high in adolescents who participate in competitive sports and low in those with sedentary pursuits.

Take into account the social and attitudinal characteristics and the timing and rates of growth when counseling adolescent clients. Encourage the development of good food patterns, since they may become the more stable food habits of the adult. Accept the fact that the traditional patterns of eating at home may not apply, and focus dietary advice on food selections at any time of day to meet total nutritional needs.

Since adolescents are totally absorbed in the growing-up process and are interested in using foods to achieve the things they want, relate nutrition information to these concepts. Discuss the relationship of nutrient intake to the skeletal and body compositional changes that are occurring and explain how adolescents can use food to improve appearance, vitality, and popularity. Because many adolescents are concerned about weight, this can often provide the basis for effective nutrition education. Some teenagers are also interested in ecologic issues, and these concerns can be incorporated into nutrition education. Provide information within the framework of the current pattern, such as how to provide an adequate vegetarian diet, rather than try to change the pattern. Mere repetition of the amounts and types of food needed from the Basic Four Food Groups may appear boring. Group sessions that focus on nutrition topics, such as food facts and fads, are an effective educational method. Colorful leaflets and pamphlets are available from such sources as the National Dairy Council. Use a positive approach that reinforces desirable habits and that involves

adolescents in arriving at solutions to their own problems.

Caution against kilocaloric restriction without medical supervision, since this practice may compromise growth. If for any reason the diet is restricted either in total quantity or in specific food groups, evaluate customary intake to detect deficiencies and to provide a basis for counseling.

Child Nutrition Programs

School-based nutrition programs for children include the School Lunch Program, School Breakfast Program, Special Milk Program, and the Summer Food Service Program for Children. The Child Care Food Program is discussed in Chapter 16. These programs are all administered by the U.S. Department of Agriculture and, at the local level, by state educational agencies. For participating schools, the federal government offers cash and food assistance to the states.

National School Lunch Program. Since 1946, the National School Lunch Program has provided nutritious lunches daily in schools throughout the nation. In order to qualify under the program, participating schools must (1) operate the program on a nonprofit basis for all children, (2) serve meals that meet nutritional guidelines established by the USDA, (3) provide lunches free or at a reduced price for children who are unable to pay full price, and (4) insure that children receiving free or reduced-price meals are not overtly identified. All public and nonprofit private schools of high school grade and under, as well as public and licensed nonprofit private residential child care institutions, may participate in the program. Public and licensed nonprofit private residential childcare institutions include homes for the mentally retarded, orphanages, temporary shelters for abused or runaway children, juvenile detention centers, homes for unwed mothers and their infants, and hospitals for chronically ill children.

To meet nutritional standards established by the USDA, participating schools must conform to a school lunch pattern that provides approximately one third of the RDA for nutrients on an average over a period of time. The pattern consists of four components (with a total of five food items):

1. Protein-rich food (i.e., meat or a meat alternate, such as cheese, eggs, legumes, or peanut butter)
2. Milk (includes low-fat, skim, buttermilk, whole, and flavored milk—the milk choices must include an unflavored milk with reduced fat content)
3. Fruit and/or vegetable (2 servings)
4. Bread or bread alternate (i.e., enriched bread, muffins, cornbread, biscuit, or rolls made of enriched or whole grain flour or cornmeal, enriched or whole grain rice, macaroni, or noodle products)

The USDA recommends that serving sizes be adjusted to the needs of the various age groups (from 1 year through high school age). Minimum portions of food to be served to children for each of four age groups have been identified, and maximum quantities have been specified for a fifth group (12 years and older). However, these children would be able to select smaller portion sizes if desired. Service of two small meals (which together meet the lunch pattern requirements) is recommended for children ages 1 through 5 in child care institutions, to conform with their smaller appetites.

In order to reduce plate waste, senior high school students are offered all five items comprising the lunch pattern (priced as a unit) but are required to select a minimum of three of the items in order for the lunch to be eligible for federal reimbursement. This practice is optional for students below the senior high level. The sale of foods that provide minimal nutritional value is restricted until the end of the last school lunch period each day in schools participating in the School Lunch and School Breakfast Programs. The sale of these items (which include carbonated beverages, water ices, chewing gum, and some candies) is thought to contribute to a decline in the consumption of nutritious foods in school and to reduce participation in the school meals program.

Children who receive free or reduced-price lunches are issued the same color lunch tickets as other children. Eligibility to receive free or reduced price lunches is based on the USDA family size/family minimum income criteria announced annually by the Secretary of Agriculture.

Schools must promote activities, involving students and parents, aimed at improving acceptability of the program.

School Breakfast Program. Similar to the School Lunch Program, the School Breakfast Program provides meals to students on a full-price, reduced-price, or free basis depending on the size and income of the student's family. The breakfast program plays an important role in improving the diets of needy children. Regulations require that the breakfast consist of one-half pint milk, one-half c fruit or vegetable or both or full-strength fruit or vegetable juice, and one serving of bread or an equivalent grain product. A serving of a protein-rich food should be included as often as possible.

Special Milk Program. Under this program, children attending a school or institution that does not participate in any other federally subsidized meal program may purchase milk at a reduced price or, if needy, receive it free.

Summer Food Service Program for Children. This program spans the gap in the school food programs by providing meals to children (age 18 or below) during extended vacation periods. It operates during the summer or during any school vacation of more than 3 weeks for schools that have a continuous school year calendar.

The program may be sponsored by any public or nonprofit private, nonresidential institution or residential summer camp in areas where at least one half of the children are eligible for free or reduced-price school meals. Children may be served breakfast, lunch, and snacks, all free. Meals and snacks served must meet specific criteria established by the USDA.

In addition to the above program, the USDA also distributes commodity foods (surplus food) to schools and provides funds for nutrition education. The Nutrition Education and Training Program (or NET) provides funds for nutrition education for schools participating in the breakfast and lunch programs. The NET program is coordinated at the state level and provides training for children, teachers, and school food service personnel that emphasizes the relationship of food, nutrition, and health.

For many school-age children, the school lunch provides the first introduction to group feeding, and it may offer the most balanced and well-planned meal of the day for some. Learning experiences are provided by the school lunch itself—exposure to new foods and methods of food preparation—and teachers may integrate nutrition education into the classroom experience as part of the curriculum. An effective program of nutrition education will integrate the learning potential of the school lunch with the classroom activities. However, the hurry and confusion of the average school cafeteria may make this setting less than desirable for eating, enjoying, and learning about food.

Since it is not mandatory that all lunch items served at school be selected, be sure that adequate counseling and guidance are given to assure that a nutritional lunch is chosen.

NUTRITION-RELATED HEALTH PROBLEMS

There are no definitive studies of the current nutritional status of children during late childhood and adolescence. Despite claims that adolescents have the poorest dietary intake of the population, their nutritional health is generally good. Although nutritional deficiency may be seen in all ethnic and income groups, it tends to be greatest in minority groups who are economically disadvantaged. Nutritional imbalances, both excess and deficiency, seen in late childhood and adolescence generally reflect problems that exist in the rest of the population, such as dietary deficiencies of calcium and iron, overweight and obesity, and dental decay. Hyperlipidemia is also of concern in children and adolescents. Anorexia nervosa and bulimia, eating disorders that develop in some young people, have nutritional ramifications, and diet is often mentioned as a factor in acne vulgaris. Diet is an important consideration in adolescent pregnancy and athletic performance.

Nutrient Deficiency

Assessment and Intervention. Although nutrition surveys have revealed scattered evidence of nutrient deficiency in the school-age population, more evidence of deficiency has been noted in adolescence. Among the various age groups surveyed in the Ten-State Nutrition Survey, adolescents between the ages of 10 and 16 had the highest prevalence of unsatisfactory nutritional status, with male adolescents exhibiting more evidence of malnutrition than females.[5] Before the survey, the adolescent male was largely overlooked in deference to the female.

The stress of growth, in combination with the psychologic stress of growing up, make the adolescent period extremely vulnerable to malnutrition. The practice of meal skipping, the use of fad diets, and the restriction of certain foods for various reasons may all contribute to nutrient inadequacy. Because adolescence is the last major period of growth, the kinds and amounts of food teenagers eat can have an impact on their final development.

Nutrients most often consumed in inadequate amounts in teenage diets are iron, calcium, riboflavin, and vitamin A. If nutritional deficiency is suspected, assess the client's dietary pattern; those who skip meals, eat few snacks, and consume smaller quantities of foods at meals have the poorest diets. Since snacks comprise a large part of the diet of children and adolescents, encourage snacking as an integral part of the total eating pattern. Monitor the kinds of snacks available, however, and discourage the practice if it constitutes overeating.

Iron Deficiency Anemia. Iron deficiency anemia has been a common finding in all of the national nutrition surveys regardless of age, socioeconomic status, ethnic group, or sex. The incidence is greater during the two periods of rapid growth—infancy–early childhood and adolescence—although the NHANES survey provided some dietary and biochemical evidence of iron deficiency in black school-age children (6 to 11 years). The greater prevalence in blacks may be due to lack of appropriate standards, as there is evidence that blacks of all ages have slightly lower hemoglobin levels than whites.

Both adolescent males and females are susceptible to anemia. The demand for iron is increased in both sexes, and few adolescents consume the recommended amount of 18 mg of iron daily in their diets. Since the need for iron as a component of growth is closely related to deposition of lean body mass, the risk of anemia in the male is highest when growth is most rapid. In females, the risk is highest in those with large menstrual losses. The Ten-State Nutrition Survey, which studied low-income groups primarily, showed that anemia occurs more frequently in pubescent males than in females.

Although iron deficiency is rather easily corrected with iron medication, do not neglect efforts to change dietary habits through counseling to avoid recurrence of the problem at a later date (see Chap. 12).

Calcium Deficiency. The tendency of some adolescents, particularly females, to decrease milk intake decreases their consumption of calcium and riboflavin. Calcium consumption of males tends to more closely approximate the RDA of 1200 mg. Assess soft drink consumption, since there is concern about the replacement of milk (high in calcium) with soft drinks (high in phosphorus). The resulting calcium:phosphorus ratio may deviate from the normal (1:1) and lead to abnormal calcium absorption at a time when calcium needs are high for bone mineralization.

While low intakes of vitamin A are frequently cited, there is little evidence of a clinical deficiency in teenagers.

Dental Caries. Dental caries is a universal finding in nutrition surveys and occurs in children regardless of socioeconomic status. The development of dental caries in childhood and adolescence may be associated with frequent ingestion of between-meal snacks composed of sticky, refined sucrose-containing foods, such as sugary confections and baked goods. In the Ten-State Nutrition Survey, the caries index in adolescents rose progressively as the proportion of these components rose in the diet.

Since few children and adolescents consume food in a three-meal-a-day pattern, advise them about the proper use of sucrose-containing foods and the continuing need for fluoride to reduce the tendency for tooth decay. At the same time, stress other aspects of oral hygiene, such as brushing and flossing the teeth. Adolescents may be motivated to improve dental health if they are fully informed about the effect of poor dental hygiene on their appearance.

Nutrient Excess: Obesity

Assessment and Intervention. Obesity that has its onset in childhood or adolescence is a particular problem because it tends to persist into adulthood and becomes especially refractory to treatment. The incidence of the disorder in childhood and adolescence is difficult to assess, particularly in view of the normal body compositional changes that occur during adolescence. Differentiate between the early transient fatness that is typical of pubescent growth and a permanent acquisition of excess fat that may not be recognized until after it has occurred. Observe that obese children tend to mature earlier and achieve greater skeletal growth than their counterparts of average weight.

Obesity with onset prior to adulthood carries some of the risks that are similar to those of obese adults, but for the adolescent, the psychologic and social consequences may be profound. Assess the obese adolescent client's psychologic status, since obesity at this time may lead to altered body image and poor self-concept and other disturbed personality traits.

The major goal in treatment is weight maintenance, not weight reduction, which allows the child to grow up to his or her weight. Avoid stringent dietary restriction until after the pubertal growth spurt has occurred. Low kilocalorie intake may result in protein catabolism, thus interfering with normal growth and development. Kilocalorie restriction just prior to the growth spurt may jeopardize the growth in height that would automatically rectify the problem. If weight reduction is indicated, carefully monitor growth in stature and skeletal maturation. If treatment is initiated after growth is complete or nearly complete, use the techniques described for adults in Chapter 23. Combine the dietary regimen with a program of increased physical activity to increase energy output and provide diversion.

Promote measures directed toward preventing obesity throughout the growth cycle. Encourage children of all ages to participate in activities that can be performed on an individual basis and continued throughout life, such as hiking and swimming. Suggest to parents that toys and games that require movement on the part of the child will increase energy expenditure, and encourage family outings that include exercise. In particular, aid the adolescent to establish realistic goals for weight maintenance.

Hyperlipidemia

Assessment and Intervention. Hyperlipidemia, especially elevated blood cholesterol, is clearly a risk factor for atherosclerosis in adults and may contribute to atherogenesis in children. There is some evidence to suggest that atherosclerotic lesions may have their origin in infancy and progress throughout the life span. Fatty streaks and fibrous plaques have been identified in the arteries at a very early age, and although the relationship of these lesions to fibrotic plaques in the adult is the subject of controversy, some authorities suggest that they are the precursors of the end-stage atherosclerotic lesions.[6] Advanced atherosclerotic lesions may be present in young adults. Some young soldiers who died of battle trauma in World War II and in the Korean and Vietnam Wars were afflicted with severe coronary disease.[7,8]

Because of the relationships of diet, blood cholesterol, and coronary artery disease and the evidence that atherosclerosis may begin in early life, some authorities suggest that diet modifications should be instituted in healthy children over the age of 2 years as a measure to prevent coronary arterial disease.[6] Although the efficacy of a fat-controlled diet in healthy children in altering the incidence of coronary heart disease in later life has not been directly demonstrated, experience with fat-modified food patterns demonstrates that they are nutritionally adequate.

Moreover, a major benefit is the possibility that dietary habits learned in childhood will persist into adulthood. Assess the dietary fat and cholesterol intake of children and adolescents. If intake of these factors is excessive, suggest moderate reductions. Identify children with more specific risk factors, such as a family history of coronary heart disease, obesity, or diabetes mellitus, and provide dietary counseling of a more specific nature for such clients (see Chap. 29). Although it is generally agreed that children with elevated blood lipids should be placed on an appropriate diet to reduce their health risks, it would seem advantageous also for children and adolescents with normal blood lipid levels to adhere to a fat-controlled diet.

Anorexia Nervosa and Bulimia

Assessment. While anorexia leading to reduced food intake is characteristic of a number of psychologic disorders, such as hysteria, depression, and schizophrenia, the term **anorexia nervosa** is used to describe a specific syndrome of food refusal that appears in some adolescents. The disorder has its origin usually during puberty or later in adolescence. Less commonly, it appears after 20 years of age. It occurs 10 times more frequently in females than in males. A spectrum of the disorder occurs that ranges from very mild symptoms that require little or no intervention to very severe forms that necessitate hospitalization.[9] Anorexia nervosa is observed more frequently in affluent societies than in undeveloped countries, and the victims are more often members of upper- and middle-class families than lower-class families. While reliable data on prevalence are not available, it is widely held that the incidence of the condition is increasing.

Anorexia nervosa manifests itself as self-induced starvation in the absence of any initial organic disease and can lead to death if untreated. The term "anorexia" as applied to the disease is actually a misnomer, since the appetite is not lost—the client simply refuses to eat. A preoccupation with food and body weight, induced by a morbid fear of being unable to control eating and consequently becoming obese, is a characteristic manifestation of the disease. In the pursuit of thinness, the anorexic client engages in extreme dieting and frantic exercise programs leading to severe weight loss in the absence of organic disease.

In the anorexic client there is confusion between the awareness of hunger and the feeling of having no control over eating. Whereas true loss of appetite may occur in advanced stages of malnutrition, anorexic clients do experience hunger. Actually, the condition is characterized by alternating periods of starvation and binge eating. If anorexic clients give in to hunger, they may eat a large quantity of any type food or fluid that is available—this binge may then be followed by induced vomiting or use of laxatives or diuretics. Anorexics may be very knowledgeable about food, be expert calorie counters, and be very manipulative about energy intake and expenditure. Hyperactivity, exercising to the point of exhaustion with denial of fatigue, and a drive for intellectual excellence are typical.

The bizarre eating and exercise patterns lead to serious biologic, metabolic, neuroendocrine, and psychologic problems. These are followed by severe social isolation. The physical signs are essentially those of a healthy person subjected to protein–calorie malnutrition and starvation. There may be severe wasting of muscle and fat. The client's weight may be only 10 to 50 percent of previous weight, and a body weight of 70 lb is not uncommon. Other physiologic manifestations may include cessation of menses, dry scaly skin, dry stringy hair or lanugo hair (fine, downy) over the body, cold intolerance, lowered basal metabolism, hypotension, bradycardia, abnormal glucose tolerance, diminished sweating, constipation, abdominal pain, erosion of the tooth enamel secondary to induced vomiting, and electrolyte imbalance. If untreated, malnutrition and electrolyte imbalance may lead to death.

Severe psychologic problems may also develop, although there are marked differences in the manifestations. The effects on the psyche of the underlying disorder may be intensified by the severe malnutrition. Insomnia is a common manifestation; some may sleep no more than 3 to 4 hours a night. The body image is distorted—the body may be seen not as a part of self but as something extraneous. The client takes pride in the weight loss and does not perceive the body as ugly. The size of others tends to be overestimated. Other psychologic problems are psychotic-like thinking, splitting of the ego, and regression to earlier levels of mental functioning. Hyperactivity gives way to weakness, apathy, and depression.

▶ Differentiate anorexia nervosa from **bulimia,** a disorder affecting young people, particularly women 18 years of age and older and a much lower percentage of males. Bulimia shares some of the characteristics of anorexia nervosa but is considered by some health professionals as a separate disorder. Bulimia is characterized by the sudden ingestion of large amounts of food in a short period of time (as much as 4000 to 5000 kcal or more), followed by fasting, vomiting, or purging, particularly with laxatives or enemas. The behavior is by conscious choice with regard to vomiting and purging and is usually secretive. The prevalence of the disorder can only be speculated upon at present, but it affects as many as one half of the clients with anorexia nervosa.

Little data are available at present about the bulimia syndrome. It is not known whether the behavior represents a sequel to or a distinct subgroup of anorexia nervosa. The victims are primarily from the middle and upper socioeconomic classes, and college students, actresses, and models are particularly vulnerable. Over half of the affected clients are of normal weight, and the disorder occurs in fewer than 5 percent of obese clients. Bulimic clients have an exaggerated fear of becoming fat, and in many cases the symptoms begin at the conclusion of a weight reduction diet.

Indulging in food binges alone can lead to obesity, and when followed by fasting, vomiting, or purging, it may lead to dehydration, electrolyte imbalance, and malnutrition. Frequent vomiting can lead to esophageal irritation and extensive dental erosion and decay. Endocrine and metabolic disorders, including menstrual disturbances, have occurred, particularly with radical practices, and salivary gland enlargement is common.

Intervention. The goal of treatment of anorexia nervosa is to assist the client with the development of a positive and secure self-image and a change in attitude toward food. In the absence of these changes, weight gain alone may represent a continuation of the pathologic desire to gain approval. Nutritional rehabilitation is dependent upon the resolution of any negative perceptions held.

For clients who have a mild form of the disorder, provide counseling about adolescent growth, normal nutrition, and the serious consequences of malnutrition. If the disorder is complicated by stresses, such as family problems or depression, shift the focus of concern away from eating by dealing with the particular stress. Once the focus of conflict is removed, the normal hunger drive may take over. With more severe forms of illness, various combinations of psychologic and diet counseling are necessary for a prolonged period of time.[9] Hospitalization may be necessary for clients with severe illness for correction of severe weight and fluid and electrolyte imbalances and for dealing with strong resistance to treatment. Other clients may be treated on an outpatient basis.

Design a plan of dietary treatment that initially allows for maintenance of current body weight, followed by gradual improvement of nutritional status while a low weight is being maintained, and finally, a gradual weight increase through normal self-feeding. Take a detailed dietary history to form the basis for the dietary management. Estimate current kilocalorie and protein intake and determine current eating patterns, family eating patterns, and food preferences and aversions. Differentiate between true aversions and those that resulted from dietary manipulations. Determine eating patterns prior to the onset of illness and the progression that was followed to reach current practices.[10]

Involve the client with the plan of nutritional care and explain its rationale. Establish a realistic weight gain goal that will reestablish normal physiologic function. Initially, it may be necessary to select a lower goal, with reevaluation as the goal is achieved. Explain the nutritional needs for growth, development, and maintenance of tissues and how these needs are met by food. Describe the energy needs for weight control, both to reach and to maintain an appropriate body weight.

Since the body's kilocalorie needs are diminished in the emaciated state, the kilocalorie level of the normal teenage diet cannot be tolerated initially. Design a diet that at first includes kilocalories sufficient to meet the basal energy requirement, with adjustments slightly upward or downward to conform with current intake. Make weekly increments of approximately 200 kcal during the early stages of treatment, with greater increases made as eating becomes more comfortable.[11] Include foods from each of the Basic Four Food Groups, with portion sizes increased as kilocalorie increases are made. Include three meals, with or without snacks, depending on the client's choices. Instill confidence in the client to eat the recommended amounts of food by involving him or her in the process of determining the kilocaloric level and explaining the rationale for the level to be used. Alert the client to the possibility of rapid weight gain initially due to fluid retention secondary to expansion of the extracellular compartments, electrolyte retention, and repletion of glycogen stores.[11] There may also be some gastric distention with each addition to the diet, but the contracted stomach adjusts relatively rapidly to the increased volume of food. Emphasize to the client that additional foods can be eaten as long as the prescribed diet is consumed. Ask the client to keep a record of foods consumed in the early stages of treatment and review these records for a general trend of foods consumed. When the client reaches the weight gain goal, readjust the diet plan to allow for weight maintenance.

Provide diet counseling for bulimic clients that focuses on the appropriate quantities of food needed for weight maintenance. Providing a set of dietary guidelines may give them a feeling of control and assurance of adequate nutrition and help them to structure and regulate their daily schedule without weight gain. Encourage regularity in dietary habits to assure weight stability and minimize the likelihood of eating binges or long periods of fasting. Assist clients with time management that may help to avoid extremes in overactivity and boredom, which may contribute to the eating problem.

Adolescent Pregnancy

Assessment and Intervention. Despite a decline in the birth rate in the general population, births to teenagers have risen and now comprise a large proportion of all births. A large percentage of teenagers who give birth become pregnant again within a year, bringing a strong likelihood of subsequent pregnancies at short-term intervals while the mother is still in her teens.

Pregnancy in the adolescent does not appear to result in competition between the mother and child for nutrients. Growth and pregnancy appear to compete only in those rare instances when fertilization takes place before or very soon after the menarche. Pregnancy in girls with adequate nutritional reserves and in whom the pregnancy occurs at least 2 years after menarche does not appear to affect the health of the mother or the baby. In girls, growth in lean body mass is nearly complete by the age of fertility. Some growth potential remains, however, and the needs for this growth must be considered when planning the diet.

Since one of the most significant influences on the size of the newborn (and hence its well-being) is maternal weight gain during pregnancy, encourage pregnant teenagers to eat a well-balanced diet that allows for the normal gain of her own body as well as for the fetus and products of conception. Young teenagers will need to gain about 4 kg (8.8 lb) more than older teenagers or adults during pregnancy in order to meet their own growth needs and the needs of the fetus.[12]

The RDA for pregnancy and a diet plan for pregnant adolescents are discussed in Chapter 14. As with adult pregnant women, use weight gain as the indicator for adequacy of energy intake in the pregnant adolescent. Assess the nutrient content of the client's diet, particularly those that are often low in teenage diets, including iron and calcium. The RDA for calcium increases to 1600 mg to meet the needs of the growing adolescent and to allow for mineralization of the fetal skeleton and deciduous teeth. Be sure that a prenatal vitamin supplement with added folic acid and an iron supplement are prescribed. Caution the client against dieting to minimize the obligatory gain in weight and stress that this practice could lead to ketosis, a condition that is ill-tolerated by the fetal nervous system.

Follow a nonauthoritarian approach when counseling the client. Determine what is important for the individual and gear the instruction toward these values. Stage demonstrations, such as allowing the client to observe a mother breastfeeding her baby to dispel some of the mystique about breastfeeding. Be sure that she knows how the baby is fed during intrauterine life, and propose the notion that if such foods as soda pop and candy are inappropriate for a newborn, they are just as inappropriate for feeding the baby in the uterus.

Nutrition in Athletic Performance

Assessment. Nutritional requirements of adolescents actively engaged in sports are beginning to receive serious consideration. The high school athlete is particularly interested in diet, and programs to both gain and lose weight are undertaken to achieve a desired ratio of muscle strength to body weight. A particular mystique is associated with the athlete's diet. In spite of sound nutritional principles that constantly evolve from nutritional research, dietary practices that are unsound, faddish in nature, and sometimes dangerous continue to appear. Some of these practices are evident in current theories related to diet and athletic performance. Although nutritional needs for athletic performance are based on relatively straightforward principles and are not dissimilar from the usual nutritional demands, the competitive atmosphere of sports often makes the amateur athlete the recipient of faddish notions. For example, protein supplements are claimed to be needed for muscle building and honey is claimed to enhance physical performance. Super or wonder foods or drugs do not substitute for adequate nutrition for the athlete.

The athlete, like the nonathlete, requires a diet that provides suitable proportions of carbohydrates, protein, fats, minerals, vitamins, and water. Because of the specific demands of exercise, certain nutrient factors require special attention. The most significant of these are kilocalories (and the balance of carbohydrates, protein, and fat providing the kilocalories), water, electrolytes (especially sodium and potassium), and iron. While deficits of any nutrient can impair athletic performance, provision of adequate kilocalories and proper replacement of fluid and electrolytes are of prime importance.

Nutritional Requirements. Kilocaloric needs increase with exercise, and athletes may need 3000 to 6000 kcal daily to maintain weight. Contrary to popular opinion, protein does not increase muscle mass—proper training and exercise do. While the protein requirement does not increase with exercise per se, the requirement does increase slightly for the development of the increased muscle mass that accompanies exercise, for restoration of tissue loss through trauma and loss of protein, hemoglobin, and myoglobin in the urine, and for restoring losses of nitrogen through the skin due to heavy sweating. Moreover, protein does supply some glucose via gluconeogenesis during prolonged exercise. If protein from a variety of sources provides from 10 to 15 percent of the total kilocalorie intake, it will be sufficient to meet all of the above needs relative to athletic training and competition. The need for certain B-complex vitamins, especially thiamine, riboflavin, and niacin, increases as the kilocalorie requirement increases. Large fluid losses may occur in those who participate in heavy exercise in hot weather and will necessitate replacement. Electrolyte losses, particularly of sodium, potassium, chloride, and magnesium, accompany the sweat losses, although the losses are small due to renal conservation of minerals. Assess the client's iron status. Teenage males and females of childbearing age are susceptible to low iron stores. Iron deficiency anemia adversely effects athletic performance. A condition called ▶ **sports anemia** is sometimes seen during the early stages of strenuous training. At present, its cause and significance are unknown.

Energy Sources. Body stores of carbohydrate and fate are the major energy sources for muscular activity, although body protein may contribute as much as 10 percent of the energy expended when exhaustive exercise is performed and glycogen stores are low. The relative contribution of carbohydrate and fat depends on the duration and intensity of the activity and the adequacy of the oxygen supply. These two nutrients supply an approximately equal proportion of energy during light-to-moderate activity of limited duration. During prolonged exercise at less than full effort, the percentage of energy provided by fat increases to approximately 75 percent. As the duration and intensity of the exercise increase, the oxygen supply to muscles becomes increasingly inadequate and the body's metabolism shifts to the use of carbohydrate (glycogen) without the use of oxygen (anaerobic metabolism). The ability to sustain prolonged vigorous exercise is directly related to initial glycogen stores. A high initial level enables the individual to maintain an optimal pace throughout the duration of the activity.

This knowledge has led to the practice of supersaturating the muscles with glycogen in a dietary ▶ manipulation called **glycogen loading** to improve performance in endurance-type athletic events lasting 60 minutes or longer. The procedure is of no value for short or intermittent strenuous events, such as football. The technique begins 7 days prior to competition. Initially, the muscle glycogen stores are depleted by strenuous exercise while consuming a low-carbohydrate (100 g), high-protein, high-fat diet. Three days before the competition, a high-carbohydrate (250 to 525 g), moderate-protein, low-fat diet is consumed. Exhaustive exercise is not recommended since it depletes glycogen stores. With this technique, the stores of muscle glycogen are approximately double the usual reserve capacity of trained athletes. A less rigorous approach (modified carbohydrate loading) is also used. Glycogen loading may also serve to conserve body protein reserves during exercise.

The rate of fat metabolism may be increased by ingesting caffeine prior to and during endurance activities. Since caffeine spares glycogen, one can exercise longer without feeling exhausted.

Intervention. To meet the increased kilocalorie demands, advise the client to increase food intake in a balanced way rather than to focus on a particular category, such as protein. In so doing the demands for other nutrients, including protein and vitamins, will be met automatically. The percentage distribution of carbohydrate, protein, and fat is 50 to 55, 10 to 20, and 30 to 35, respectively. Emphasize the use of complex carbohydrates. High-protein diets, protein supplements, and a pregame meal high in protein have been widely advocated for athletes, probably because of the association between protein and muscle tissue and the association between animal protein and strength and power. Athletes' customary preference for diets high in animal protein reflects a psychologic rather than a physiologic preference. A high protein intake can theoretically inhibit athletic performance by contributing to acidosis and dehydration. A larger amount of fluid is needed to excrete the nitrogenous wastes and fixed acids produced by protein metabolism. Hyperuricemia with a threat of gout is a further complication. A high-protein diet deprives the body of more efficient fuel sources.

There is no conclusive evidence that the intake of specific vitamins, such as vitamin C, above the level that normally occurs in an adequate diet enhances athletic performance. In view of the potential side effects associated with excessive vitamin consumption, do not advocate supplementation. While the daily use of a multivitamin supplement is generally considered safe, megavitamin therapy can be abused.

Stress the importance of adequate water intake before, during, and after exercise to prevent dehydration, organ damage, heat stroke, and death. Individuals seldom voluntarily drink as much water as is lost in the sweat. In order to determine the amount of fluid that needs to be replaced, athletes should weigh themselves before and after an event. In replacing fluids, keep in mind that maximum fluid intake should not exceed the limit of gastric emptying time (about a liter per hour) and that cold beverages leave the stomach more rapidly than warm drinks. Drinking small amounts of beverages at short intervals (i.e., 100 to 200 ml at 10- to 15-minute intervals) is preferable to drinking large amounts every hour or so. Athletes involved in endurance competition should consume approximately 600 ml of fluid about 2 hours before the competition and approximately 400 to 500 ml 10 to 15 minutes before the event. After the event, the athlete should drink water until the lost weight has been regained. For weight losses of 4.0 to 7.5 percent, as much as 24 to 36 hours may be needed for rehydration.

Athletes need not replace salt losses hour by hour but can usually correct the losses following the event. Recommend that extra salt be added to foods consumed and foods with high salt content be eaten. A liberal fluid intake should accompany the sodium replacement to avoid dehydration that may accompany an excess salt load on the kidney. Advise against the use of salt tablets, which may lead to nausea, vomiting, gastrointestinal distress, and accelerated water loss. Unless an athlete is sweating excessively (e.g., losing more than 5 lb a day) salt tablets are not necessary. By including potassium-rich foods in the diet, all except excessively large potassium losses are likely to be replaced. Electrolyte supplements should be used only on the advice of a physician. Replacement solutions should be of optimal osmolarity to avoid delayed gastric emptying, gastric fullness and distress, and dehydration associated with the administration of hypertonic solutions. Solutions that contain up to 2.5 percent glucose, less than 10 mEq sodium/liter, and less than 5 mEq potassium/liter are recommended.

Many commercially available electrolyte-containing beverages have osmolarities that can result in fluid retention and gastrointestinal distress. Iron needs can be met by including more iron-rich foods in the diet or by iron supplements for clients who are clinically diagnosed as being iron deficient.

While glycogen loading may be beneficial for some individuals participating in endurance events, there are some possible negative effects. The water retention that accompanies glycogen storage may lead to muscle heaviness, stiffness, and sluggishness, and there may be fluid and electrolyte imbalances, although the long-term effect of glycogen loading on muscles is unknown. Athletes with active diabetes mellitus or elevated serum triglycerides should seek medical advice before engaging in carbohydrate loading, and the atherogenic potential of a diet high in fat and protein requires consideration. Since carbohydrate loading does add to the demands of the muscles, it should be used only for endurance events and used sparingly. Do not recommend the technique for children and adolescents.

Although there is some evidence that use of caffeine may enhance physical capacity by sparing muscle glycogen, weigh the potential benefits against the potential risks. Caffeine may be associated with a variety of side effects, since it is a central nervous system stimulant.

Advise that the pregame meal should be eaten about 3 hours in advance of the event to allow for digestion and absorption and thus prevent competition for the blood supply between the digestive system and muscles. Suggest that the meal be modest in size (approximately 500 kcal) and consist of foods high in complex carbohydrate and contain some protein and a minimal amount of fat. Abundant fluids should be provided, and foods that are gas forming or high in fiber or salt should be restricted. The meal may consist of lean meat, vegetables, fruit, bread, and skim milk. Recommend that concentrated sweets not be eaten less than 2 hours before the event, since this may produce a transient hypoglycemia early in the event and lead to premature exhaustion of glycogen stores in endurance performers.

Weight Control for the Athlete. Athletes may be tempted to either lose or gain weight, depending on the type of sport involved. In sports events that match competitors on the basis of weight, such as wrestling, athletes are tempted to achieve the lowest possible weight and frequently attempt a large weight reduction in a short period of time. Fluid restriction, use of sweat baths, and crash dieting are all practiced. The harmful effects of each are evident. However, the immediate physiologic effects of dehydration are more drastic than those of semi-starvation. Caution against these practices, particularly in growing adolescents whose health and well-being may be adversely affected. When weight loss is indicated for adult athletes, a reduction in body fat, not in protein or water, is desired, and this should be achieved at a rate no greater than 1 kg per week, with a moderate decrease in food intake and moderate increase in exercise. Water deprivation limits work capacity and may be responsible for collapse and even death of athletes during the stress of the game. Estimate the amount of body fat and project the desired amount of fat loss. Advise the client to add an hour of exercise daily while modestly decreasing kilocalorie intake by 500 to 750 daily to achieve a total daily deficit of 1000. Involuntary weight loss representing a negative energy balance is common in athletes. Monitor regularly the adequacy of total energy intake by scheduled recording of body weight, and make estimates of body fat with skinfold calipers.

Others participating in contact sports, such as football, frequently want to increase body weight in order to maximize their performance. Regimens to gain weight should result in an increase in muscle mass, not fat. Excessive body fat reduces speed and limits endurance. Help the athlete to understand that only muscle exercise will increase muscle mass and that specific increases in protein or vitamins in the diet are not indicated. Suggest the addition of 1000 kcal to the daily diet to attain a gain of approximately 2 lb per week. Use of drugs, such as anabolic–androgenic steroids, are not recommended, since these drugs may disrupt the normal growth pattern in an adolescent.

Kilocaloric balance becomes an especially important consideration when activity diminishes during off-seasons and in postcompetitive years. Many develop a weight problem at these times because they fail to recognize the diminished kilocaloric demand.

Acne Vulgaris

▶ *Assessment and intervention.* Acne vulgaris is a skin disorder characterized by inflammation of the sebaceous glands, primarily on the face, chest, and back where the glands are more numerous. Many adolescents experience complexion problems associated with acne, and the disorder is believed to be related to changes in hormonal secretion. There is some evidence that acne may involve some interrelated deficiency of zinc and vitamin A, since reduced blood levels of zinc and retinol-binding protein (a vitamin A transport protein whose synthesis probably requires zinc) have been found in subjects with acne.[13]

The treatment of teenage acne is subject to many fads and fallacies, and the relationship of dietary factors to acne has been the subject of controversy for many years. A popular belief is that certain foods cause or aggravate the condition. The foods most frequently incriminated are chocolate, nuts, milk and dairy products, cola drinks, iodized salt, and foods high in sucrose or fat. Controlled studies have failed to consistently demonstrate that limita-

tion of these foods is beneficial. Although iodides may be a factor in triggering acne, it is doubtful that they are a significant factor in the pathogenesis.

Assist the client with acne to trace his or her food history to determine if there are foods that seem to aggravate the condition on an individual basis, and any identified foods should be limited in the diet. Advise adolescents to eat a variety of foods to maintain healthy skin and that the acne will resolve with age. Discourage self-treatment with systemic or topical nutrient supplements. Large doses of vitamin A have not been shown to have a consistent or long-lasting effect and can produce serious,
▶ even fatal illness. **Retinoic acid,** the acid form of vitamin A, applied topically is effective therapy for clients with mild to moderate acne, and recently, the synthetic derivative of vitamin A, 13-*cis*-retinoic acid has been approved for oral use for treating severe cystic acne. Clients who receive this drug should be monitored closely for side effects, which may include transient elevation of blood lipids and other symptoms. Reducing the dosage is indicated for clients who experience side effects. Since retinoids in general also appear to be teratogenic, advise clients of childbearing age to use contraceptive measures during and 3 to 6 months following treatment.

REVIEW QUESTIONS AND ACTIVITIES

1. Discuss the following aspects of growth during the school-age period: (a) pattern of physical growth, (b) difference in growth pattern at the beginning and end of the period, and (c) implications of the pattern of growth for nutritional requirements.
2. Explain the rationale for use of biologic age rather than chronologic age for assessing the nutritional requirements of adolescents.
3. Compare the characteristics of growth in male and female adolescents and relate the growth pattern to nutritional requirements during the period.
4. Identify the differences in changes in body composition that occur in males and females during adolescence.
5. Identify two minerals whose deficiency is common in association with high requirements during adolescence.
6. Plan a menu for one day that includes the appropriate number of servings of food from the Basic Four Food Groups for an elementary school child and adapt the menu so that it is appropriate for a high school student.
7. List two major influences on the food habits of school-age children and adolescents.
8. List two examples of the effects on food habits of the psychosocial developmental tasks of school-age children and adolescents.
9. Identify the characteristics of each of the following child nutrition programs: (a)

School Lunch Program, (b) School Breakfast Program, (c) Special Milk Program, and (d) Summer Food Service Program for Children.

10. Identify the components of the School Lunch Program and describe how it may be modified to reduce food waste.

11. Explain the rationale for a high degree of susceptibility of school-age children and adolescents to dental caries.

12. Describe the dietary advice that you would give to a pregnant adolescent who is obese. What additional factor must be accounted for in establishing the desired amount of weight gain in pregnant adolescents?

13. Explain the rationale for categorizing atherosclerosis as a pediatric problem and for implementing a fat-controlled diet in childhood.

14. Identify the manifestations of anorexia nervosa and discuss its dietary management.

15. Differentiate between anorexia nervosa and bulimia.

16. Discuss the need for the following nutrient factors in the diet for athletes: (a) kilocalories, (b) protein, (c) vitamins, (d) water, (e) electrolytes, and (f) iron.

17. Discuss the appropriate replacement of fluids and electrolytes during athletic performance.

18. Describe the potential hazards of the following practices sometimes followed by athletes: (a) glycogen loading, (b) high protein intake, and (c) extreme measures for weight loss.

19. Describe the dietary advice that you would give to a client with acne.

REFERENCES

1. Greenwood CT, Richardson DP: Nutrition during adolescence, World Rev Nutr Diet 33:1, 1979.
2. Pollit E, Lewis NL: Fasting and cognitive function. Psychiatric Research 17:169, 1982/83.
3. Pollitt E, Leibel RL, Greenfield D: Brief fasting, stress, and cognition in children Am J Clin Nutr 34:1526, 1981.
4. Brown PT, Bergan JG, Murgo CF: Current trends in food habits and dietary intakes of home economics students in three junior high schools in Rhode Island. J Home Econ Res 7:324, 1979.
5. USDHEW, Health Services and Mental Health Administration: Highlights, Ten-State Nutrition Survey, 1968–1970. DHEW Publication No. (HMS) 72–8134, Atlanta (no date), p 10.
6. Task Force Committee of the Nutrition Committee and the Cardiovascular Disease in the Young, Council

of the American Heart Association: Diet in the healthy child. Circulation 67:1411A, 1983.
7. Enos, WF, Beyer, JC, Holms R: Pathogenesis of coronary disease in American soldiers killed in Korea. JAMA 158:912, 1955.
8. Inter-Society Commission of Heart Disease Resources, Atherosclerosis Study Group and Epidemiology Study Group: Primary prevention of the atherosclerotic diseases. In Wright IS, Fredrickson DT, eds: Cardiovascular Diseases. Guidelines for Prevention and Care. Washington, DC, U.S. Government Printing Office, 1974, p 15.
9. Huse DM, Lucas AR: Dietary treatment of anorexia nervosa. J Am Diet Assoc 83:687, 1983.
10. Ibid, p 688.
11. Ibid, p 689.
12. Frisancho AR, Matos J, Fiegel P: Maternal nutritional status and adolescent pregnancy outcome. Am J Clin Nutr 38:739, 1983.
13. Michaelsson GL, Vahlquist LJ, Juhnlin L: Serum zinc and retinol-binding protein in acne. Br J Dermatol 96:283, 1977.

BIBLIOGRAPHY

Crawford PB, Clark MJ, Pearson DL, Huenemann RL: Serum cholesterol of 6-year-olds in relation to environmental factors. J Am Diet Assoc 78:41, 1981.

Gam SM, Levelle M: Reproductive histories of low weight girls and women. Am J Clin Nutr 37:862, 1983.

Garfinkel PE, Garner DM: Anorexia Nervosa: A Multidimensional Perspective. New York, Brunner/Mazel, 1982.

Garn SM, Hopkins PJ, Ryan AS: Differential fatness gain of low income boys and girls. Am J Clin Nutr 34:1465, 1981.

Harper JM, Mackin SD, Sjogren DO, Jansen GR: Alternate school lunch patterns in high schools. II. Student and foodstaff reactions. J Am Diet Assoc 77:282, 1980.

Mahan LK, Rees JM: Nutrition in Adolescence. St. Louis, Mosby, 1984.

Mallick MJ: Health hazards of obesity and weight control in children. A review of the literature. Am J Public Health 72:78, 1982.

Nutrition and physical fitness. J Am Diet Assoc. 76:437, 1980.

Neuman P, Halvorson P: Anorexia Nervosa and Bulimia: A Handbook for Counselors and Therapists. New York, Van Nostrand Reinhold, 1983

Peterson DS, Barkmeier WW: Oral signs of frequent vomiting in anorexia. Am Fam Phys 27:199, 1983.

Sherman W, Costill D: The marathon: Dietary manipulation to optimize performance. Am J Sports Med 12:44, 1984.

St. Pierre RG, Rezmovic V: An overview of the National Nutrition Education and Training Program evaluation. J Nutr Educ 14(2):61, 1982.

The enigma of anorexia nervosa. Nutr Rev 41:121, 1983.

Winnick M, ed: Adolescent Nutrition: Current Concepts in Nutrition. New York, John Wiley & Sons, 1982, Vol 11.

CHAPTER 18

Nutrition for Adults and Elderly Persons

Objectives

After completion of this chapter, the student will be able to:

1. Differentiate among the three age periods encompassed by the period of adulthood and the psychosocial developmental task for each period.

2. Distinguish between the type of dietary advice that would be given to young and middle-age adults in meeting their nutritional needs.

3. Assess the effects of two major categories of physiologic determinants and five major categories of psychosocial determinants of nutritional status/needs of elderly persons.

4. Compare and contrast the nutritional requirements of elderly adults with those of young and middle-age adults.

5. Distinguish between the community nutrition programs that are designed for physically handicapped persons and those that are designed for individuals who are socially isolated.

6. Develop a nursing care plan for the nutritional management of elderly clients who have each of the following problems: (a) lack of teeth, (b) difficulty swallowing due to lack of saliva, (c) diminished taste and smell acuity, (d) vague complaints of gastrointestinal distress, (e) constipation, (f) diminished renal function, (g) limited income and cooking facilities, (h) living and eating alone, and (i) belief that nutrient supplements will prolong life and relieve complaints of chronic illness.

The adult years are commonly divided into three age periods or stages: young, middle, and elderly (or **senescence**). Chronologically, early adulthood covers roughly ages 18 to 40, middle adulthood, ages 40 to 60 or 65 years, and elderly adulthood, ages 60 or 65 years and older. In recent years, other age classifications of older adults have been recognized including the young old (ages 60 or 65 to 75) and the old old (ages 75 plus). It is difficult to pinpoint stages of adult development based on chronologic age alone, since no specific birthday separates the various stages. In terms of chronologic age, for example, some persons may be considered old who, in reality, are young in appearance and attitudes.

The process of aging is continuous, beginning with conception and ending with death. From conception throughout the growth cycle, anabolic processes exceed catabolic processes. Once physical growth ceases during early adulthood, the situation is reversed, and catabolism exceeds anabolism (except for pregnant and lactating women). The end result is a gradual net decrease in the number of cells in the body, which may impair organ functioning to some degree. The effects associated with decreased renewal of cells and tissues do not become obvious for many years. However, the progression of aging varies widely among individuals; be cautious in making generalizations. Whereas physical growth is generally complete and metabolism begins to slow down in early adulthood, the body's cells and tissues remain in a dynamic state and metabolism continues.

As with other age groups in the life cycle, the adult of all ages is subject to various physiologic and psychologic influences. From a physiologic perspective, differences in heredity, environment, and availability and use of health care facilities account for the variability seen between individuals of the same age in overall physiologic and health status. Although the role of nutrition in the aging process has not been precisely determined, nutrition does influence the development and progression of certain chronic diseases that accompany aging. The likelihood of developing chronic illnesses is increased in the older age groups, although these illnesses may become apparent during the middle-age period. The active period of life may be extended by the application of good health practices, including sound nutritional practices, throughout life. If these practices have not been established previously, appropriate changes should be made during the early and middle years.

NUTRITION OF YOUNG AND MIDDLE-AGE ADULTS

Assessment and Intervention

The years between the 20s and the 60s are usually the most productive years of life, during which the individual makes significant contributions to society. Although health status is usually relatively good during this period, certain practices, such as the use of alcohol in excess, cigarette smoking, stressful employment, too little exercise, and consumption of a diet containing excessive amounts of kilocalories, fat, sugar, and sodium and too little fiber, may be factors contributing to the development of such chronic disorders as obesity, cardiovascular disease, diabetes mellitus, gastrointestinal disorders, and dental problems. The hectic schedule followed by many may lead them to feel that they do not have the time to attend to their health. Motivation is needed in order to help them realize that neglect of health is detrimental. Middle-age people are more likely to be able to afford the necessary food and medical care needed for preventive health care. Economics and inconvenience of health care facilities may be deterrents to preventive care for younger adults.

With the cessation of physical growth, requirements for kilocalories and specific nutrients decline to maintenance levels for adults. A gradual decline in the kilocalorie requirement accompanies the slowly declining metabolic rate that is characteristic as aging progresses. Nutritional requirements remain relatively stable during the adult years, except that iron needs decrease for females at menopause, which occurs in the middle-age period (see the RDA in Chap. 2).

Although physical growth ceases during early adulthood, psychosocial development continues during the period. Erikson describes the developmental task during the period as that of establishing intimate relationships. In reaching for adult intimacy, young people seek a source of emotional fulfillment to replace the nuclear family. Failing to achieve this task, the young adult becomes increasingly isolated from others. Other developmental events that may occur during young adulthood include becoming established in one's own home and a career, marriage, and parenthood. The young adult, however, may adopt any one of a number of lifestyles, and the ages of career decisions, marriage, and parenthood vary widely.

Direct educational efforts toward assisting young adults to develop a healthy lifestyle in order to prevent or delay the onset of chronic diseases. For clients in this age group, advice about dietary intake to meet nutritional needs is very simple. Assist them with the prudent selection of foods from the Basic Four Food Groups (see Chap. 2), with attention given to avoidance of excessive kilocalories, fat, sugar, and sodium and to ingesting a moderate amount of fiber. In this way, their RDA will be met and a good nutritional status will be maintained for the continuing life cycle.

Assist them to establish regular exercise patterns that can be maintained throughout the remainder of life in order to control weight during the period. Without regular exercise, weight may gradually increase. Determine the amount and type of physical activity by the degree of physical fitness and tolerance. Stress that regular dental care should be continued during this period to reduce the potential for tooth loss and other dental problems.

In the young adult, establishing independence by moving away from home and assuming responsibility for providing food is facilitated if learning food management skills has been a part of the home and school educational process. For the inexperienced cook and those with busy schedules, use of some convenience foods of high nutritional value or eating at a restaurant or cafeteria that offers a varied menu may be helpful initially.

Diet and nutrition become of major importance with pregnancy and parenthood. Provide guidance for following a diet adequate to meet the demands of pregnancy and for establishing family patterns of eating that will foster optimal physical and psychosocial growth and development of the infant and child. Parents may be particularly motivated to follow good nutritional practices during the childbearing years and be interested in feeding their children a nutritious diet and teaching them good food habits. A special concern for women during this period is the effect of contraceptive agents on nutritional status (see Chap. 14). Women who use contraceptive agents may be at risk of developing deficiencies of particular nutrients; continue to monitor their nutritional status.

During the middle years, the so-called generation in the middle, adults are striving to seek a sense of generativity. This is achieved by reaching beyond the few intimate relationships established in young adulthood with spouses or close friends and becoming concerned with the next generation and even with humanity in a broad sense. Middle-age people act as a bridge between the younger and older generations. Should generativity not be achieved, there occurs a sense of stagnation or self-absorption.

It is during this period that chronic disorders, such as hypertension, atherosclerosis, obesity, and periodontal disease, may become manifest, and it is necessary to individualize the diet counseling to meet specific needs. Counseling must include the role of diet modifications in management of the disorders (see Part IV). It is also during this period that health-related concerns may be manifest by an interest in changing certain lifestyle habits related to exercise, diet, and smoking in order to prevent these disorders. Should smoking be discontinued, assist with the control of food intake so that the individual can avoid gaining weight.

NUTRITION OF ELDERLY ADULTS

Assessment
Advances in medical care, environmental sanitation, and nutrition have produced an environment in which much of the population is living beyond retirement years. Not only are people living longer, but in many cases there is greater freedom from disease for longer periods of time. The stereotyped thinking of the past, which tends to perceive all older adults as incapacitated and impoverished, no longer holds true. An increasing number of older adults are healthy, physically active, and financially comfortable.

The percentage of the population 65 years and older is rising annually, and the average age of individuals in that group is also increasing. At present, approximately 11 percent of the population is 65 years or older. In particular, the population of those 75 years and older is increasing more rapidly than the population of the elderly as a whole. It is estimated that 20 percent will be 65 and older by the year 2030. The number of elderly females is proportionately larger than males because of the longer life expectancy for women. Mortality rates among the elderly have been declining during the past several years. The average life expectancy in 1982 reached an all time high of 74.5 years (72 years for males and 77 years for females).

Although many elderly persons are essentially well and independent, others are chronically ill, institutionalized, or homebound. Approximately 5 to 6 percent of the elderly live in institutions, and the rest live in the community with a spouse, relatives, friends, or alone. Elderly women are more likely to live alone than men because of their longer life expectancy and fewer opportunities for remarriage. A larger percentage of the elderly live in urban areas than in rural areas.

Although the elderly currently constitute only 11 percent of the total population, they use 30 percent of the nation's health care services, and much attention is now being focused on their general well-being and special needs, including nutritional needs.

Determinants of the Nutritional Status and Nutritional Needs of the Elderly. The nutritional status of the elderly reflects current dietary practices, which are influenced by a variety of physiologic and psychosocial parameters. In turn, the physiologic parameters are influenced by both heredity and environment, with lifetime eating habits acting as an important environmental influence. A model illustrating the interrelationships between physiologic and psychologic parameters that influence the nutritional status of the elderly is given in Figure 18–1. The effects of physiologic parameters, such as chronic disease, often coexist in the elderly with psychosocial factors, such as inadequate income or social isolation. There is a strong interplay between physiologic and psychosocial influences as they affect food intake and nutritional status.

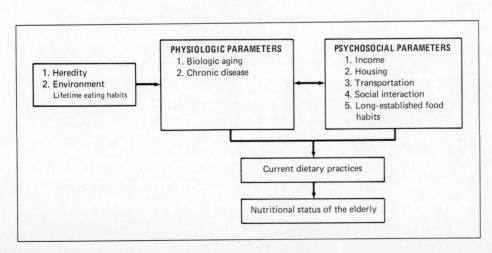

Figure 18–1
Parameters influencing the nutritional status of the elderly.

Be aware that today's elderly represent a particularly heterogeneous group that varies widely in chronologic age (65 to 115 years), income level, educational level, lifestyle, dietary habits, and health status. The only commonality binding the group is chronologic age, which is a poor index of either biologic age or health status. Some individuals, for example, are healthy and active at over 90 years of age, whereas others are hampered at an earlier age by conditions, such as impaired vision and mobility or chronic diseases, that necessitate dietary modifications.

Physiologic Determinants. The physiologic parameters that influence current dietary practices, and thus nutritional status, include the effects on the intake and use of food of (1) biologic aging and (2) chronic disease. The onset and progression of biologic aging, as well as the development of some chronic diseases, are influenced by both heredity and environmental factors, including lifetime eating habits.

Biologic Aging. Aging is not a process that begins late in life—it begins with conception and continues throughout life. Biologic aging is attributed to decreased organ function as a result of cell loss, diminished cellular efficiency, and altered metabolism, possibly in association with a decline in the rate of activity of enzymes and hormones. As a result, the body loses reserve capacities, adaptability, and the capacity to function well under stress. The changes may vary considerably between individuals of the same age group. In addition, variations occur within the same individual, since age does not uniformly affect all body organs. For instance, a 70-year-old man may have the cardiac output of a 60-year-old and the renal function of an 80-year-old. Although the genetic component of aging is evident, environmental factors play a large role in both the timing and the rate of aging changes. Such factors as environmental stress, physical activity, intake of food and drugs, and psychologic experiences that are unique to each individual bring marked differences in body function and status. The role of nutrition in modulating the aging process per se is unknown. Animal feeding experiments that restricted food or energy without concurrent undernutrition have shown a delay in aging and increased longevity, but comparable findings have not been demonstrated in humans.

Age-related changes occur in practically every part of the body, and changes in the body organs involved with food intake and use may negatively affect nutritional status (Fig. 18–2). In spite of the large number of changes that occur during aging, most functions are affected to only a moderate degree, particularly in the resting state. When stressed, changes may be evident, however. Moreover, there is confusion between changes related to aging and those due to disease, since many older people experience chronic diseases in their later years, and the existence of concurrent disease has not always been controlled for in studies of aging people. Much of the available data have been attained through cross-sectional studies, using different subjects with each group, creating doubt whether the changes are indeed real.

FOOD INGESTION. Assess the elderly client's dental status, swallowing ability, and sense of taste and smell. Decreased ability to bite and chew results from tooth loss, failure to replace lost teeth with dentures, or use of ill-fitting dentures. By age 65, 50 percent of

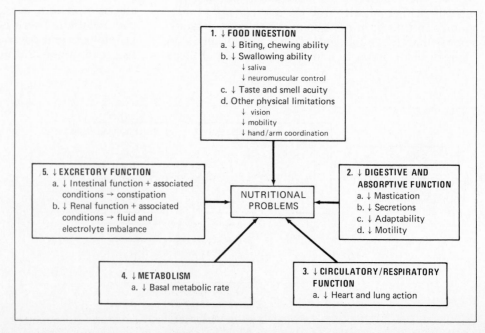

Figure 18–2
Physiologic factors contributing to nutritional problems in the elderly.

Americans have lost all of their teeth, with the percentage increasing with increasing age. Despite being edentulous, elderly clients still prefer the variety and consistency of foods they enjoyed when younger, and ground or pureed foods are often unpopular. Many older people manage to masticate food well with gums calloused by use over the years or to maintain good nutritional status when foods that require little biting or chewing are served. On the other hand, clients with ill-fitting dentures tend to avoid foods that are hard, sticky, or irritating when they become lodged in pockets or cracks in the mouth.

Decreased swallowing ability may result from decreased secretion of saliva or diminished neuromuscular control of swallowing. Each of these occurs with aging or may be associated with various chronic diseases or their treatment. Inspect under the tongue for moisture to denote the presence (or absence) of saliva. Clues to diminished neuromuscular control include drooling, inability to close the lips tightly, and a tendency to pull the tongue slightly to one side on protrusion.

The senses of taste and smell and the ability to discriminate between odors decline with increasing age. Although many specialists in geriatrics accept the concept that this is part of the aging process, others disagree.[1] Sensory decline may be due to other factors, such as smoking and disease. The sense of smell is most frequently the first sensory system to show a decline with age. The decline begins to occur as early as the late 30s or early 40s, whereas the decline for taste generally appears a little later. These declines are associated with a decline in numbers of papillae, numbers of taste buds per papilla, and degeneration of the olfactory cortex of the brain, which is very vulnerable to degenerative changes of aging. Loss of taste initially affects the taste buds located anteriorly on the tongue and then progresses posteriorly. The taste buds lost first are those that detect a sweet or salty taste, leaving those that detect the bitter or sour, and, thus, the bitter and sour tastes become more pronounced. Salt is often used to compensate for the losses of taste and smell acuity, which poses a problem for those on sodium-restricted diets. Some observations suggest that sensitivity to sugars increases from early childhood through adolescence, plateaus in adulthood, and finally decreases in later life. Somewhat similarly, sensitivity to the salty taste decreases in later life, but the decrease is greater in men than in women. The ability to discriminate among odors also changes, and older persons can best discriminate fruits from other foods. Be aware also that some diminution of the sour and bitter taste sensation occurs initially when wearing dentures because the palate is covered, but perception frequently improves with the passage of time.

Determine if other physical limitations, such as diminished hand and arm coordination, mobility limitations, or diminished vision, are present. These may limit the client's ability to shop for, prepare, and eat food. Neuromuscular coordination and the ability to maintain fine discriminating movements in the hands decrease with age, resulting in loss of manual dexterity, with subsequent problems in manipulating utensils, preparing foods, and so on. This problem may be compounded by the presence of neurologic or arthritic disease that may, in addition, limit mobility. Diminished vision interferes with reading food labels, package directions, and recipes.

DIGESTION AND ABSORPTION. Decreased digestive and absorptive function may occur with aging, although the magnitude of the decline has not been fully established. Much of the literature on secretory and motor function in the elderly presents conflicting ideas. The large reserve capacity of the gastrointestinal organs may partially compensate for diminished function. The gastric secretion of hydrochloric acid is less efficient, but effects of the relative achlorhydria on digestion and absorption have not been clearly demonstrated. Lack of gastric acid and a decrease in intrinsic factor may account for the greater prevalence of vitamin B_{12} deficiency in the elderly, and there is some evidence that protein digestion may become less efficient, with reduced proteolytic enzyme secretion. Ptyalin secretion is also reduced. The absorption of calcium is decreased in older people, and the intestine loses some of its physiologic adaptability. This may account for its decreased ability to adapt to a low-calcium intake in later years, although this may be due to changes in the kidney with failure to activate vitamin D rather than from changes in the intestine itself.[2]

Nonetheless, the gastrointestinal tract is a frequent cause of chronic distress in the elderly. Symptoms, such as heartburn, gas, and abdominal distention, are common but may be related to such factors as poor eating and bowel habits, a preoccupation with food, and emotional tension.

CIRCULATION AND RESPIRATION. Evaluate the client's cardiac and respiratory function. The diminished circulatory and respiratory function that occurs with age may negatively affect nutritional status. The reduced pumping action of the heart, reduced lung capacity, and diminished blood supply result in a lessened ability to nourish the cells and remove wastes.

BASAL METABOLISM. Basal metabolism declines with age, dropping about 16 percent from age 30 to age 70. It is generally held that the change in metabolism with age is related to changes in the ratio of lean to fat tissue mass in the body—the proportion of adipose tissue increases at the expense of the lean body mass. As muscle cells disappear, they are replaced by fat and fibrous connective tissue.

EXCRETION. Excretory function, both intestinal function and renal function, declines with age. There occurs a thinning of the muscle layers, and motility is probably decreased in some people, contributing to constipation, a common problem in the elderly. If constipation is among the client's problems, determine if associated conditions that can precipitate constipation are also present. These include (1) ingestion of an unbalanced diet (e.g., irregular meal times, inadequate fluids and fiber), (2) ingestion of calcium-containing antacids (e.g., calcium carbonate), (3) psychologic stress (e.g., anxiety or depression), and (4) decreased physical activity.

Renal function is reduced by the aging process. There is a decline in the number of nephrons and a decrease in renal blood flow, glomerular filtration, and the ability to concentrate or dilute the urine. Because of the diminished renal function, the elderly are particularly prone to fluid and electrolyte imbalances in stressful situations.

Chronic Diseases. In their later years, many people experience one or more chronic diseases that may be related to the biologic changes associated with aging, to heredity, and to other factors including current or past nutritional practices. Although over three fourths of the noninstitutionalized elderly have one or more chronic illnesses, only about one fourth of the elderly population are severely impaired and unable to carry on major activities. Most noninstitutionalized elderly persons think that they are in fairly good health, and their chronic conditions can usually be controlled sufficiently so that they can lead fairly normal, active lives.

Be aware that the existence of chronic disease may affect food intake or use—and thus nutritional status—in four ways. First, a modified diet that may be unappetizing or nutritionally inadequate may be necessary. A common example is the sodium-restricted diet required for cardiovascular problems. Second, nutrient/drug interactions that are secondary to necessary drug therapy may alter nutritional needs. For instance, anticonvulsant drugs (such as phenytoin) increase the need for folic acid and vitamin D. Use of psychotropic drugs (such as the phenothiazines) may result in obesity due to increased appetite. Third, physical conditions that limit mobility (such as arthritis), vision (such as glaucoma), or neuromuscular coordination (such as stroke) may limit the ability to secure or ingest food. Finally, altered nutrient use associated with the disease itself (such as malabsorption secondary to gastric or pancreatic insufficiency) may result in malnutrition.

The incidence of disease and disability that leads to alterations of dietary intake, absorption, and metabolism of nutrients increases after age 75. Common disorders include obesity, diabetes mellitus, cardiovascular disease, hypertension, gastrointestinal disorders, degenerative bone and joint diseases, and anemias.

OBESITY. Obesity is especially prevalent in older females. In relation to obesity, note that there is a tendency to increase both body weight and the percentage of fat with age. Beginning with the teenage period, there is a progressive increase in body fat. This increase in fat deposition reaches a peak in later life, followed by a decline. The phenomenon is observed in both men and women, although the pattern is different for the sexes. For example, data from cross-sectional studies show that in males the gradual increase in weight throughout adult life reaches a peak in the middle years (about age 40 or 50) and is then followed by a decline. In females, the peak and decline of the weight increment are observed approximately a decade later. Since these data were derived from cross-sectional rather than longitudinal studies, it is not known whether the pattern is a phenomenon of aging per se or whether it reflects a higher mortality rate for the fattest individuals. The changes in adiposity that occur with age may be an important factor in the increased susceptibility of the elderly population to diabetes mellitus, cardiovascular disease, and other disorders that increase mortality. Furthermore, even a moderate degree of overweight (about 20 percent above desirable weight) has been shown to carry a risk of elevated mortality.[3] This is contrary to the widely held view that moderate overweight carries no increased risk.

DIABETES MELLITUS. Assess the blood glucose level of elderly clients. With increasing age, there is an impaired ability to use glucose. This age-dependent decrease in carbohydrate tolerance may lead to the diagnosis of diabetes mellitus even though true diabetes mellitus may be absent. Although there is no way to distinguish the effects of aging per se on insulin secretion from the effects of a genetic tendency to develop diabetes, glucose intolerance in the elderly may well be related to dietary factors. For example, excessive adipose tissue is associated with a resistance to the action of insulin. The pancreas responds to the insulin resistance by increasing insulin secretion. Over a period of time, the stress on the insulin secretory mechanism may unmask those with a genetic trait for diabetes. The presence of diabetes accelerates the process of atherosclerosis and thus increases the risk of developing cardiovascular disease.

CARDIOVASCULAR DISEASE AND HYPERTENSION. The highest incidence of cardiovascular disease occurs in clients over 45 years of age. Elevation of blood cholesterol and, to a lesser extent, elevation of blood triglyceride are associated with an increased risk of developing coronary heart disease. An increase in both blood cholesterol and blood triglyceride occurs with age in both males and females. Data from national nutrition surveys show that in males the blood cholesterol rises rapidly up to the age of 35 to 44 years, reaches a peak in the 55- to 64-year age group, and declines slightly after this period. In females, blood cholesterol increases less rapidly than for males in the age groups 25 to 34 and 35 to 44 years, but after age 45, the increase is much more rapid than in males. The level declines after age 55 to 64 in males, but the levels for women continue to rise.[4] Other studies have shown that serum triglyceride levels gradually increase with age in both males and females. In males, the triglyceride level reaches a peak at age 45 to 50, followed by a decline. The peak is reached a decade later in females (age 55 to 60).[5] There have been attempts to correlate the increase in blood lipids with body weight increments with age.[6] The similarity of the peaks in body weight and serum lipids suggests that increasing adiposity with age may be in some way responsible for the changes in serum lipids observed with age. It has been noted that neither serum lipids nor glucose increases with age in populations in which the people remain thin throughout adulthood.

Mean blood pressure tends to increase with age, with the sharpest increase in both sexes occurring after age 45. Observe that pressure elevations are most frequently seen in obese clients.

GASTROINTESTINAL DISORDERS. Gastrointestinal disorders commonly observed in the elderly are esophageal reflux (heartburn), hiatal hernia, irritable colon, diverticular disease of the colon, and cancer of the colon. The incidence of gallstones also increases with age. The presence of these disorders may alter the client's ability to maintain a good nutritional status.

DEGENERATIVE BONE DISEASE. The prevalence of degenerative bone diseases, including osteoporosis and periodontal disease, increases in the elderly population. Osteoporosis is very common in women after the age of 50 and in men after the age of 60. Bone loss is a general phenomenon of aging, beginning in both sexes during the third or fourth decade of life but progressing more rapidly in women (and especially postmenopausal women) and in Caucasians. The disorder is estimated to affect as many as 25 percent of aging women.[7] In addition to a low level of physical activity and the hormonal effects of the onset of menopause, a number of nutritional factors have been implicated in its etiology. These include long-term low calcium intake, a low level of vitamin D, diminished calcium absorption with age, an inappropriate ratio of dietary calcium to phosphorus, alcoholism, and a high protein intake (see Chap. 39). Periodontal disease is the major cause of tooth loss after age 40. In addition to bone disorders, many elderly persons have chronic conditions, such as arthritis and the aftereffects of stroke, that may limit mobility.

ANEMIA. The incidence of anemia significantly increases with age and although no difference has been found between young adults and active older adults in their ability to absorb iron administered as ferrous sulfate,[8] the fall in hemoglobin concentration

in older people may be at least partially related to the aging process. Postulated mechanisms include the decline in lean body mass, which decreases the oxygen requirement (and thus the need for hemoglobin), a decline in testosterone secretion or testosterone sensitivity in males (and thus a decrease in the stimulation of red blood cell production), and shortened red blood cell survival time. If the client is anemic, assess the dietary iron intake, since anemia in the elderly is frequently due to inadequate iron intake. For instance, the RDA for iron in those above age 50 years is 10 mg daily, and approximately 10 to 12 mg of iron is contained in 2000 kilocalories. Since many elderly people consume 1500 kcal or less daily, iron deficiency may exist. If iron intake appears sufficient, probe for other possible causes, such as chronic blood loss or infection. Deficiencies of folic acid or vitamin B_{12} may also contribute to anemia.

Psychosocial Determinants. The final crisis of adult psychosocial development, according to Erikson, is integrity vs despair. Those older adults who can look back in retrospect and feel satisfied that their lives had meaning will feel a sense of integrity. In contrast, if life is seen as a succession of wrong turns, missed opportunities, or futile efforts, a feeling of despair results. Achievement of this developmental task may have a bearing on the client's nutritional status. Psychosocial deterrents to good nutritional status that may affect some elderly people are shown in Figure 18–3. Assess for the effects of these factors that may affect the availability or acceptance of food. Inadequacies in any of these areas may negatively affect nutritional status.

Income, Housing, and Transportation. Inadequate income, housing, and transportation often accompany retirement, decrease in earning capacity, and loss of economic leverage. Although the percentage of the population age 65 and older living below the poverty level has declined in recent years, poverty is still more concentrated in the over-65 group than in the population at large. Programs, such as Medicare and Medicaid, have provided some measure of economic security to older adults. In a study by the USDA, it was found that households headed by senior citizens had an average income of less than half that of households headed by people under 65 years during the 1972–1973 study period and that senior citizens spent an average of 22 percent of their before-tax income on food, compared with 17 percent for those under 65. Senior citizens also spend more money on food at home, and less on food away from home, than other age groups and allocate more money for the purchase of fresh fruits and vegetables and less to red meats, dairy products, beverages, and prepared foods.[9] Food intake of many elderly individuals is below desirable levels, and economic factors are largely responsible for the nutritional deficiencies.

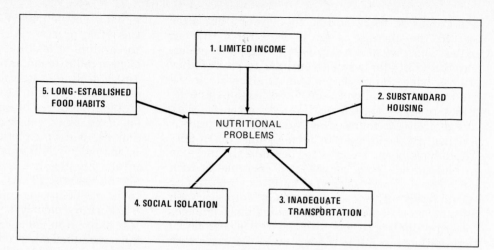

Figure 18–3
Psychosocial deterrents to good nutritional status in the elderly.

Some elderly live in substandard housing characterized by a lack of adequate food preparation and storage facilities, refrigeration, space, and other essentials. These limitations narrow the range of foods purchased and prepared and may necessitate the use of high-cost convenience foods. Inadequate transportation limits the procurement of food. Fear for personal safety may inhibit venturing to shop. The more accessible neighborhood store, where costs are higher, may be chosen over the less expensive but less accessible supermarket.

Social Interaction. Behaviorally, eating and food intake are closely intertwined with emotions and moods. Loss of appetite may result from feelings of isolation, depression, or the need to attract attention. In contrast, others may respond to these same feelings by overeating and becoming obese. Sweets may become a major source of emotional satisfaction. For others, food may serve as a sedative, making them less aware of their unpleasant situation. Food and eating serve as a mode of communication and socialization. Food eaten by oneself lacks the social aspects of eating in another's presence. Socially isolated persons have a decreased incentive to prepare and eat food and may rely on quickly prepared foods that are high in simple carbohydrate content.

Established Food Habits. By middle age and late maturity, eating patterns become relatively fixed, and change in patterns is difficult except with alterations in food tolerance. Familiar food patterns serve as a security blanket and coping device for dealing with life. The eating habits of today's elderly population were formed in an environment totally different from today's environment. The elderly may become confused at the vast array of food choices available in today's supermarket, as their habits were formed at a time of limited food choice. Food selection for some may, therefore, be limited to long-accustomed foods. Moreover, today's elderly received no formal nutrition education, since at the time of their youth,

nutrition as a science was also in its youth. While many elderly have positive attitudes toward health, food, and eating and food habits and beliefs free of food faddism, lack of nutrition knowledge may subject many others to faddist notions that promise extended life and relief from chronic disorders, and they may be unable to differentiate between reliable and nonreliable data. Consider also the food habits that stem from a particular cultural or ethnic group.

Nutritional Requirements. Although nutritional requirements of the elderly are different from those during other periods in the life cycle, recommendations of nutrient intake to promote optimal health cannot be made with certainty, and little distinction is made between the nutrient needs of younger and older adults in the 1980 RDA (see Chap. 2). Note that the nutrient values are designated to cover the age span of 51 years and above, since it is not now possible to make estimates of nutrient requirements for specific age categories in the older age group. Also note that the kilocalorie requirements are given for two age categories in the older age group: 51 to 75 years and 76 years and above. This represents the most significant differences in nutritional requirements between older and younger adults that are reflected in the RDA—kilocalorie requirements decline with increasing age in both males and females. A decrease in basal metabolism associated with an apparent loss in lean body mass (the RDA allows for a 2 percent reduction in the BMR per decade for the two older age groups) and a decrease in physical activity with age account for the decrease in kilocalorie requirements. Assess kilocalorie requirements individually, however, and base them on the level of physical activity maintained by specific clients. Activity level is quite variable in older adults, and some remain very active physically. The cessation of iron loss in menstrual blood accounts for the decline in iron requirements of postmenopausal women. A decrease in the requirements of the B vitamins (thiamine, riboflavin, and niacin) needed for energy metabolism is reflected in the requirements for older males but not older females.

Some controversy surrounds the RDA for several nutrients, particularly protein, calcium, and vitamin D. The protein requirements of older adults have recently been reexamined by several groups of investigators, with conflicting results. Whereas some studies suggest that the protein requirement may be increased in older people, other studies do not support this finding and suggest that the protein need does not change or may even decrease. In view of the declining energy requirement with age (not accompanied by a decline in the protein requirement) and the increasing incidence of recurring episodes of chronic disease in older people that may increase protein needs, the National Academy of Sciences notes that it appears prudent to ensure that the elderly receive 12 percent or more of their total kilocalorie intake in the form of protein,[10] or at least 0.8 g/kg body weight. A recent study showed this amount to be insufficient to maintain nitrogen balance in a majority of the subjects, all of whom were over 70 years of age and consuming adequate energy.[11]

The absorption of calcium is diminished in older adults, and chronic calcium deficiency may exist. Much controversy surrounds the RDA for calcium and the relationship between dietary factors in the etiology and treatment of osteoporosis and periodontal disease. According to some investigators, the RDA of 800 mg daily is insufficient and it should be increased to 1000 to 1500 mg to achieve calcium balance and optimal skeletal health, especially in postmenopausal women.

Although there is little information about the requirement for vitamin D, there are indications that it may be higher than for younger adults, and some investigators recommend that elderly persons consume 15 to 20 μg daily,[12] which is considerably in excess of the RDA of 5 μg.

Intervention

Use the daily diet plan given in Table 18–1, which lists the recommended number and size of servings of foods from the Basic Four Food Groups, to serve as the foundation for planning an adequate diet for the elderly client. Appropriate exchanges within the food groups are also listed in Table 18–1. Since nutrient requirements are the same (except for those mentioned above), older adults need the same number and size of servings of food from the Basic Four as do younger adults.

The fact that kilocalorie needs diminish with age without a proportionate decrease in need for most nutrients may predispose the elderly to obesity and/or nutrient deficiency. Weight increase with age is not desirable; encourage elderly clients to maintain the weight throughout life that was correct for them at age 25. To assure nutritional adequacy and prevent weight gain, stress that the client should select foods of high nutrient density rather than cutting down proportionately on all foods. For example, low-fat forms of milk and cheese and lean meat should be used, and fat seasonings for vegetables and nonessential foods, such as sugar and alcohol, should be reduced.

There is no evidence that nutrient supplements, such as vitamins and minerals, are needed by elderly individuals who eat an adequate diet. Gradually diminishing tissue reserves of some nutrients indicate the need for a constant adequate supply, however. It is difficult to meet the RDA when the diet supplies less than 1200 to 1400 kcal daily. Therefore, it may be necessary to provide vitamin/mineral supplements if it is necessary to markedly restrict kilocalorie intake because of obesity. Older women who are sedentary and small in body size may normally require only 1300 to 1400 kcal and may need supplements. When supplements are indicated, use individual needs as well as the standards presented in the RDA to guide the amounts. Occasionally, megavitamin therapy has been suggested for the treatment of symptoms commonly associated with senility. This type of therapy uses supplements of the water-soluble vitamins and minerals in quantities 20 to 200 times the RDA, with claims that such treatment gives benefits above those obtained with the usual practice of medicine. Controlled studies made by several groups of psychiatrists and psychologists have not validated these claims.

Symptoms often associated with senility, such as malaise, apathy, confusion, and anorexia, will respond to nutritional therapy if they are a result of nutritional deficiency. Those symptoms due to biologic aging or a chronic disease do not respond to nutrient supplementation.

Although the RDA describes nutritional requirements for healthy aged individuals, each client has his or her own unique nutritional requirements dictated by current health status. These individual needs are affected by both the physiologic and psychosocial parameters described earlier. Consider the added stresses of injury or disease in the overall assessment of needs, using the RDA as the guideline for maintaining nutrition in health. Individualize diet counseling according to the specific problems identified.

Tables 18–2, 18–3, and 18–4 provide a summary of suggested nursing interventions to prevent negative nutritional effects in clients who have difficulty ingesting an adequate amount of food because of dental problems, diminished swallowing ability, and diminished acuity of taste and smell.

Use these interventions for clients whose vision, mobility, and hand/arm coordination are limited because of aging or disease:

1. Provide foods, utensils, and assistance with feeding appropriate to ability, for example, finger foods, lightweight dinnerware and mugs with room for all fingers to grasp the handle, a moistened towel or sponge placed under trays and glasses to prevent slippage,

TABLE 18–1
A DAILY DIET PLAN FOR THE ELDERLY

Food	Amount	Size of Servings and Substitutions
Milk and cheese (Includes whole, nonfat, reliquified evaporated, and reliquefied dry milk, buttermilk, yoghurt, fortified soy milk, cheese, and foods made with milk)	2 c	Calcium equivalent of 1 c milk: 1½ c ice cream; 2 c cottage cheese; 1⅓ oz American cheese; 1 c plain yoghurt
Meat–poultry–fish–beans	2 servings	1 serving = 2–3 oz cooked lean meat, fish, poultry. Protein equivalent of 1 oz meat: 1 egg; ½–¾ c cooked legumes; ¼–½ c nuts or seeds
Vegetable–fruit	4 servings daily to include:	1 serving =
Dark green or deep yellow fruits or vegetables for vitamin A (carrots, sweet potatoes, green leafy vegetables, green peppers, yellow or orange fruit)	1 serving at least every other day	1 c raw leafy vegetable; ½ c cooked vegetable or fruit; 1 medium size fruit such as an apple or peach
Vitamin C-containing foods *Good sources:* citrus fruit or juice, peppers (green and red sweet), cantaloupe, fresh strawberries, broccoli, brussels sprouts *Fair sources:* other melons, tomatoes, cabbage, potatoes cooked in skins, green leafy vegetables, tangerines and lemons, asparagus tips, cauliflower, rutabagas	1 good source or 2 fair sources	
Other vegetables and fruits, use unpeeled vegetables and fruits and those with edible seeds frequently	1–3 servings	
Bread–cereal (Whole grain or enriched)	4 servings (If no cereal is eaten, eat an additional serving of bread or baked goods)	1 serving = 1 slice of bread; ¾ c cold cereal; ½ c cooked cereal, macaroni, spaghetti; 5 saltines; 1 small biscuit or muffin; 2 graham crackers
Butter–fortified margarine–other fats	Amount as kcal level permits	Select foods from this group carefully because of their high kcal content; many fats have little nutritional value
Additional foods (Desserts, alcohol, additional amounts of above listed foods)	Amount as kcal level permits	Select nutritious desserts, such as fruit and pudding, and cut down on strictly calorie-containing foods, such as sugar and alcohol

TABLE 18–2
POTENTIAL NUTRITIONAL PROBLEMS AND SUGGESTED INTERVENTIONS FOR LACK OF TEETH

Nutritional Problem	Interventions
Decreased biting and chewing ability result in: Decreased emotional pleasure from eating ∴ anorexia. Selection of soft carbohydrate foods (cereal, bread, jam, mashed potatoes) ∴ nutritional deficiency (protein, vitamins, minerals). Decreased digestive enzyme flow ∴ maldigestion and malabsorption.	Include easy-to-chew foods on menu frequently (e.g., fish, cheese dishes, peanut butter, eggs, legumes, some prepackaged dinners, canned fruit and vegetables). Serve hard-to-chew foods (e.g., whole meat, fresh fruit and vegetables) in minced, chopped or cubed form; cubed meat may be served in a soup, casserole, or stew. Fortify foods with dry skim milk powder to increase protein content (e.g., cooked cereal, cream soup, puddings)

TABLE 18–3
POTENTIAL NUTRITIONAL PROBLEMS AND SUGGESTED INTERVENTIONS FOR LACK OF SALIVA AND DECREASED NEUROMUSCULAR CONTROL OF SWALLOWING

Nutritional Problems	Interventions
Decreased saliva results in: ↓ Moisture and lubrication → difficulty swallowing ∴ nutritional deficiency ↓ Cleansing of the teeth → dental caries Altered taste sensation → anorexia ↓ Digestive enzyme (ptyalin) → possible ↓ starch digestion Decreased neuromuscular control → Difficulty swallowing ∴ nutritional deficiency	Increase moisture in the diet by increasing fluid intake and serving moist foods (e.g., meat with broth or gravy, vegetables and potatoes with cream sauce, salad dressing) Provide sips of water with solids Assume position for eating with the head well up to aid in swallowing

arm support (pillows or armchair) while eating.

2. Assist with a suitable arrangement of kitchen equipment and utensils (consult an occupational therapist).
3. Provide cookbooks with large print.
4. Investigate the feasibility of home meal delivery or homemaker services. Additional suggestions are available in a manual designed for the aging and for people with disabilities.[13]

The Meals-on-Wheels program is designed for elderly or slightly handicapped individuals who can remain in their own homes provided some provision is made for their meals. Frequently, private groups, such as women's clubs, family service organizations, or church groups, organize the program. Food may be purchased from a local hospital or other food service establishment and delivered by volunteers. Some programs make no charge for the meals, while others charge according to ability to pay. Food stamps may be used in payment, or the Welfare Department may pay in some cases.

A program may provide for the delivery of one, two, or three meals at one time daily (or 5 days per week). A three-meal plan would provide a hot lunch (to be eaten when received), a cold meal for the evening, and a cold breakfast for the next morning. A three-meal service requires refrigeration in the home. Home-delivered meals may also be provided as a component of the Congregate Meals Program (see below). This program provides meals at least once a day for 5 or more days to participants.

Homemaker services are sponsored by public or voluntary agencies, such as the Welfare Department and family service organizations. Individuals are trained to fulfill homemaker functions for families in which there is no one to perform this role. Some of the terms used to designate this individual are homemaker, home health aide, housekeeper, and visiting homemaker. Nutrition services provided may include meal planning, marketing, food preparation, and food service.

To improve digestion and absorption and diminish gastrointestinal distress, stress the proper chewing of food or eating food in a finely divided state. The ingestion of small frequent meals should also

TABLE 18–4
POTENTIAL NUTRITIONAL PROBLEMS AND INTERVENTIONS FOR DIMINISHED TASTE AND SMELL ACUITY

Nutritional Problem	Interventions
Decreased taste and smell acuity result in: Anorexia ↓ Digestive enzyme flow ↓ Emotional pleasure from eating	Increase food flavors by: Using herbs and spices high on the flavor scale; e.g., mustard, horseradish, onion Serve foods at the optimal temperature for taste perceptions; e.g., hot or warm foods may enhance aromas and compensate somewhat for decreased taste Amplify food odors with artificial flavors (e.g., add simulated odors, such as simulated green bean odor to green beans) Chew foods well to release more molecules to come into contact with taste and smell receptors Switch around from food to food while eating (to counteract sensory adaptation) Use different food textures (to partially compensate for losses in taste and smell acuity)

be encouraged. Small, frequent meals reduce the work load of the heart and lungs and provide better nutrition. Assist the client to identify individual food intolerances, e.g., fatty foods or the so-called gas formers. Many foods are said to produce gas, but controlled studies to date have confirmed only gas production resulting from bacterial fermentation of nonabsorbed carbohydrates in the colon (including sugars and the complex carbohydrates found in beans, such as navy and pinto beans).

Discourage the habitual use of laxatives in controlling constipation. Many older clients use mineral oil as a laxative. Its use is not recommended since the fat-soluble vitamins may not be absorbed, and it may lead to pulmonary problems (see Chap. 34). Rather, encourage the client to eat meals at regular times, increase fluid intake (especially prune juice), and increase fibrous food intake. Although fiber has traditionally been avoided by elderly persons, it appears appropriate for them to consume a moderate but not excessive amount for its laxative properties. Raw vegetables may be better accepted when served in a shredded form, and fresh fruits may be more readily eaten when peeled, sliced, or cubed. Stress the need to increase fluid intake when fiber is increased and to increase fiber consumption gradually.

To compensate for the declining renal function, advise the client to increase total fluid intake and to space fluid intake throughout the day and evening to decrease the osmotic work of the kidney. Enough liquid should be consumed to allow for the excretion of at least 1500 ml of urine daily. Usually 2 liters of fluid is sufficient, but an additional 1 to 2 liters should be added when fluid loss is excessive. Some elderly patients may reject water; alternate fluids, such as juice, soup, milk, carbonated beverages, diet beverages, coffee, tea, and jello, may be substituted. Give consideration to the nutritive value of fluids that are recommended.

If the client's income is limited, give information about low-cost nutritious foods and money-saving shopping techniques (see Chap. 2). Discuss with them their eligibility for food stamps, and if they are eligible, encourage them to use the stamps. Some elderly persons refuse to use stamps because they feel they do not want to accept charity. Investigate other possible resources, such as food buying cooperatives and group feeding centers. Shopping buses and reduced bus fares for the elderly are useful for those clients without transportation. Suggest the use of one-dish meals, a hot plate, double boiler cooking, and canned foods when facilities are limited (see Chap. 2).

To overcome a feeling of indifference toward food preparation and eating when clients live alone, encourage them to create a social environment by using techniques to increase meal interest when eating alone and by eating with others when possible. Assist them with planning meals on a structured basis and to plan other kinds of company, such as music, a magazine, or eating by a window with a view. Suggest that they invite a friend or neighbor to share one meal a day, to form a community eating group or club, or to participate in an established community nutrition program.

The Congregate Meals Program for the Elderly, conducted by the Administration on Aging and operated by state and local agencies, provides a nutritious meal to older citizens in a congregate setting to bring them out of isolation. The program specifies that at least one hot or other appropriate meal meeting at least one third of the RDA must be served daily for 5 or more days per week. The components of the meal and amounts to be served are listed below:

1. Milk (fortified whole, skim, low-fat, flavored, buttermilk, yoghurt, cheese): ½ pint
2. Meat, fish, poultry, eggs, cheese: 3 oz (such meat alternates as legumes, nuts, and peanut butter may be used occasionally)
3. Vegetables and fruits: 2 (½ c) servings
4. Bread or bread alternates: 1 serving
5. Butter or fortified margarine: 1 tsp
6. Dessert: 1 (½ c) serving. Includes fruit, fruit juices, pudding, gelatin dessert, ice cream, ice milk, sherbert, cakes, pies, cookies, and similar foods
7. Beverages: Coffee, tea, decaffeinated beverages, soft drinks, and fruit-flavored drinks may be used but cannot substitute for the milk requirement

Where feasible and appropriate, menus must be provided that meet the particular dietary needs arising from the health requirements, religious requirements, or ethnic backgrounds of eligible individuals. The program is designed to serve individuals over 60 years of age who do not eat properly because of income, social isolation, or lack of mobility and skill to shop and prepare foods. Spouses (regardless of age) are also served. Meals may be home-delivered for those who are homebound by reasons of illness, disability, or extreme transportation problems. The spouse of the homebound individual, regardless of age or condition, may also receive a home-delivered meal.

Supportive services that must be available to participants are outreach and nutrition education. The nutrition service providers are expected to cooperate with other community agencies to assure that participants receive other needed social services, such as health and welfare counseling, health services, shopping assistance, escort services, and transportation. Volunteer participation in the program, particularly by older persons, is strongly emphasized in order to maximize available resources.

The project sites are located where there is a large concentration of eligible individuals including the low-income and other target groups. The centers are located as near as possible to where the individuals live. Often they are in churches, community centers, housing projects, or senior citizen centers. The food may be prepared at the project, or it may be contracted to a school or restaurant and transported to the center.

Project participants are given the opportunity to pay all or part of the cost of the meal. The participants themselves determine if they will pay and how much. This is kept in strict confidence. Each project develops its own fee schedule regarding the cost of the meal, and food stamps may be used in payment.

The participants are given a voice in decision making regarding the project—in such matters as the type of meal, when it will be served, the cost, and the environment in which it is served.

Use the following interventions to decrease nutritional problems associated with long-established food habits:

1. Provide foods consistent with established habits. This entails knowledge of diet history and food preferences.
2. Approach change cautiously by building on positive habits rather than suggesting radical change. The elderly can change if sufficient time is given and suggested changes are presented slowly and repetitiously, with consideration given to socioeconomic, cultural, religious, and educational background.
3. Capitalize on nutrition interest by channeling it toward sound understanding of factual data. Education techniques that actively involve the elderly in planning are more effective than formal lectures.
4. Evaluate the meaning and possible consequences of faddist beliefs to the client. Whereas the potential danger of health quackery should not be ignored, following a faddist notion may sometimes serve as a coping device and may improve nutritional intake.

REVIEW QUESTIONS AND ACTIVITIES

1. Identify the three adult age periods, the approximate ages associated with each period, and the psychosocial developmental task associated with each period.
2. Describe the pattern of nutritional requirements during the period covered by years 18 to 50 and identify the further changes in nutritional requirements that occur as aging progresses.
3. What dietary advice would you give to a young adult married couple that would be consistent with both their physiologic and psychosocial needs? How would the dietary advice differ for the middle-age parents of this young couple?
4. List two physiologic factors that may influence nutritional status in older adults.
5. List four factors that may lead to a decrease in food ingestion in older adults and plan

interventions to modify the possible negative effects on nutritional status of each of these factors.
6. What changes occur with age that may modify the digestion and absorption of food?
7. Discuss the controversy related to the current RDA for protein and calcium.
8. Fractured bones heal slowly in some older women. Why?
9. Describe the dietary advice that you would give to an elderly client who frequently complains of symptoms of heartburn, gas, and abdominal distention in the absence of organic disease.
10. In what way must food selection differ between older adults and young adults in order to meet nutritional needs while at the same time avoiding excess weight gain?
11. Discuss age-related changes that may occur in intestinal and renal function, and plan nursing interventions for coping with these changes.
12. Identify four factors associated with chronic disease that may affect food intake and/or use in the elderly.
13. For an elderly couple, plan a low-cost menu for 1 day that could be prepared on a single burner hot plate.
14. Identify the community nutrition programs that are available in your area for elderly clients in each of the following circumstances: (a) low-income, (b) moderately physically handicapped, and (c) living alone.
15. Under what circumstances may nutrient supplements be justified for elderly clients?
16. Your elderly client is purchasing supplements from a health food store in the belief that they will provide extra energy. What advice would you give this client?

REFERENCES

1. Kamath SK: Taste acuity and aging. Am J Clin Nutr 36 [Suppl]:766, 1982.
2. Bowman BB, Rosenberg IH: Digestive function and aging. Human Nutr Clin Nutr 37C:75, 1983.
3. Garrison RJ, Feinleib M, Castelli WP, McNamara PM: Cigarette smoking as a confounder of the relationship between relative weight and long-term mortality: The Framingham Study. JAMA 249:2199, 1983.
4. Abraham S, Johnson CL, Carroll MD: Advance data from Vital and Health Statistics of the National Center for Health Statistics. Washington, DC, U.S. DHEW, Feb 1977.
5. Bierman EL: Obesity, carbohydrate, and lipid interactions in the elderly. In Winick M, ed: Nutrition and Aging. New York, John Wiley & Sons, 1976, p 172.
6. Ibid, p 174.
7. Young EA: Nutrition, aging, and the aged. Med Clin North Am 67:295, 1983.
8. Nordstrom JW: Trace mineral nutrition in the elderly. Am J Clin Nutr 36[Suppl]:788, 1983.

9. Gallo AE, Salathe LE, Boehm WT: Senior Citizens: Food Expenditure Patterns and Assistance. USDA, Agricultural Economic Report No. 426, Washington, DC, 1979.
10. National Research Council: Recommended Dietary Allowances, ed 9. Washington, DC, National Academy Press, 1980, p 50.
11. Gersovitz M, Motil K, Munro H, et al.: Human protein requirements: Assessment of the adequacy of the current Recommended Dietary Allowance for dietary protein in elderly men and women. Am J Clin Nutr 35:6, 1982.
12. Parfitt AM, Chir B, Gallagher JC, et al.: Vitamin D and bone health in the elderly. Am J Clin Nutr 36 [Suppl]:1014, 1982.
13. Klinger JL (with the Institute of Rehabilitation Medicine, New York Medical Center and Campbell Soup Co.): Mealtime Manual for People with Disabilities and the Aging, ed 2. Camden, NJ, Campbell Soup Co., 1978.

BIBLIOGRAPHY

Bolinder J, Ostman J, Arner P: Influence of aging on insulin receptor binding and metabolic effects of insulin on human adipose tissue. Diabetes 32:959, 1983.

Fieldman EB, ed: Nutrition in the Middle and Later Years, Boston, John Wright–PSG Inc, 1983.
Lewis C: Nutritional Considerations for the Elderly. Philadelphia, FA Davis, 1976.
Morrison SD: Nutrition and longevity. Nutr Rev 41:133, 1983.
Natow AB, Heslin JA: Geriatric Nutrition. Boston, CBI Publishing, 1980.
Posner BM: Nutrition education for older Americans: National policy recommendations. J Am Diet Assoc 80:455, 1982.
Raskind M: Nutrition and cognitive functioning in the elderly. JAMA 249:2939, 1983.
Rivlin RS: Nutrition and the health of the elderly: A growing concern for all ages. Arch Intern Med 143:1200, 1983.
Roe DA: Geriatric Nutrition. Englewood Cliffs, NJ, Prentice-Hall, 1983.
Schiffman SS: Taste and smell in disease. N Engl J Med 308:1337, 1983.
Symposium on evidence relating selected vitamins and minerals to health and disease in the elderly population in the United States. Am J Clin Nutr 36[Suppl]:977, 1982.
Symposium on nutrition and aging. Am J Clin Nutr 36[Suppl]:735, 1983.
Weimer JP: The nutritional status of the elderly. J Nutr Elderly 2:17, 1983.

CHAPTER 19

Cultural Influences on Dietary Practices

Objectives

After completion of this chapter, the student will be able to:

1. Compare and contrast traditional Asian dietary patterns with regard to the following aspects: (a) staple food, (b) positive nutritional aspects, (c) potential negative nutritional aspects, and (d) techniques for improving the nutritional quality.

2. Develop a teaching plan for assisting a black American client who follows the traditional southern dietary pattern to improve the nutritional quality of the diet, and adjust the teaching plan for a Mexican-American client.

3. Distinguish between the traditional dietary practices of Italians and Middle and Near Easterners.

4. Distinguish between the traditional dietary practices of the two major categories of Native Americans.

5. Differentiate between the dietary practices of the following three religions: (a) Judaism (Orthodox), (b) Islam, and (c) Seventh-Day Adventist.

6. Plan a day's menu for an ethnic group that is prevalent in your area and adjust the menu so that it is appropriate for both an adult and a child.

Nurses need an understanding of the cultural basis of food habits, since often the diets that are prescribed by the health team or the foods that are served to clients who are hospitalized because of illness violate the clients' fundamental beliefs about food and its relationship to their health and well-being. The United States is a nation of immigrants.[1] Native Americans, Aleuts, and Eskimos migrated here thousands of years before the Europeans and may be considered the only natives.[2] The men, women, and children who have come to this country brought with them their own unique food habits and nutritional beliefs and practices. There are at least 106 ethnic groups and more than 170 Native American groups in the United States,[2] and the members of these groups often maintain the dietary practices unique to their group.

This chapter explores various cultural, that is, ethnic and religious, nutritional beliefs and dietary practices. The foods that are commonly eaten or avoided by members of several specific ethnic groups will be listed. Religious beliefs that affect nutrition will be described.

ETHNIC DIETARY PRACTICES

The food practices of America's ethnic groups are extraordinarily diverse. As these ethnic groups immigrate to the United States they typically strive to retain their ethnic dietary practices, and a complex web of factors determines the pace and scope of dietary change. These factors include prevalence of the ethnic group within a geographical area, ac-

233

ceptability of American food choices, and value placed on ethnic preservation or acculturation. Other factors, such as socioeconomic status, availability of transportation, and food meanings and beliefs, may also significantly affect dietary change. The following sections describe a variety of ethnic groups and their dietary practices.

Asian

Chinese, Japanese, and Filipino

Assessment. Although food patterns of the Chinese, Japanese, and Filipinos are different in many respects, there are also numerous similarities, and for this reason they are considered here as a group. The type of diet followed by individuals from these countries who now live in the United States is influenced by the length of residence in this country but may also reflect the geographical area from which they migrated and certain traditional beliefs about food. Tables 19–1, 19–2, and 19–3 list specific foods commonly found in Chinese, Japanese, and Filipino diets.

First-generation Japanese (referred to as "Isei") and recent arrivals from Japan follow the ancestral food pattern, whereas the children of these immigrants (called "Nisei") have developed a more westernized type of diet. For them, the practice of eating a typical Japanese meal is infrequent, perhaps once a week to once a month, or reserved for a dinner out. Recent immigrants from the Philippines tend to follow their typical meal pattern of a heavy breakfast, lunch, a light afternoon meal, and dinner. The light afternoon meal tends to be eliminated after several years in the United States or when the person is employed full time. On the other hand, the meal pattern of Chinese and Japanese immigrants is based on three meals, usually described as breakfast, lunch, and dinner.

Chinese food is characterized by four distinct diet styles reflecting different geographic regions. The Mandarin cooking popular in northern China uses both delicately seasoned and pungent sweet–sour dishes. Freshwater fish, seafood, and dishes made with thickened sauces, sugar, and dark red soy sauce highlight Shanghai cooking, popular in the coastal area. The third region is inland China where Szechwan cooking is best known for its unusual pepper seasoning. Finally, the Cantonese cooking of the southern region is the least greasy of all types and has subtle flavors. Rice is the staple food of the southern and central regions, with wheat predominating in the north.

The eating habits of the Chinese are further influenced by the belief that for health maintenance there must be a balance in hot and cold foods consumed. Hot and cold refers to the reaction of the food in the body rather than to temperature or seasoning and reflects traditional Chinese beliefs about

food and disease. Foods and disease are categorized as either hot or cold. To restore balance, diseases classified as hot must be treated with cold foods and vice versa. The hot–cold food theory is discussed in more detail with Hispanic dietary practices later in this chapter.

Food choices in the Asian diet tend to be varied, including a wide variety of meat (such as poultry and seafood), eggs, legumes, fruits, and vegetables. The latter include many plants, weeds (as seaweed, radish leaves, and shepherd's purse), and sprouts (as bamboo and bean). Although other cereals are used in varying degrees, polished white rice is the staple in most areas and plays a role similar to bread in the American diet. Noodles are popular in some areas. Seafood is the main animal protein source in the Japanese diet. Except for the bones and hair, all parts of the carcass, such as spinal cord, skin, blood, and brains, are often used. Fish and shellfish are sold alive in China because dead fish are considered unfit for eating. A variety of meats is used, but the total quantity consumed is small, and milk and cheese are not used extensively. The limited use of these animal foods is influenced by agricultural necessity as well as the Buddhist tradition of eating no meat. Often milk is not used beyond infancy, due to lactase deficiency (see Chap. 5), but may be given to the sick. A white cheese resembling farmer's cheese is eaten in some areas, and cheese is used to some extent in the Philippines.

Although meat and milk are used in limited amounts, other protein-containing foods, such as eggs and legumes, are used extensively. Eggs of chicken, pigeon, or duck are added to soups and vegetable dishes. Fermented and other types of preserved eggs are eaten in a manner similar to sweets in this country. Abundant use is made of legumes and nuts, which may be substituted for meat. The soybean is widely used in China and Japan, where dozens of products, such as soybean milk (used in infant feeding), soybean curd (tofu), and soybean paste (miso), are prepared from it.

Vegetable oils (such as peanut, sesame, and soybean) and lard are used in cooking. Soy sauce is a frequent ingredient and contributes to the high salt intake of the diet. The wide use of soy sauce may present a problem to clients if a sodium-restricted diet is indicated. Although tea is the traditional beverage, coffee is now popular also. Few desserts are eaten.

Because of a shortage of fuel, such quick-cooking techniques as sauteeing or stir-frying in a small amount of hot oil or fat and steaming or boiling for short periods are used in food preparation. The cooking water is usually served with the food. Quick-cooking and use of the cooking liquid result in a significant retention of nutrients in food. Meats may be served separately or in combination with vegetables. Ovens are not used in China. Although the cooking time itself is brief, much preparation is generally required. In keeping with the philosophy of

TABLE 19–1
CHARACTERISTIC CHINESE FOOD CHOICES

Milk and Alternates	Meat and Substitutes	Vegetable– Fruit	Bread– Cereal	Other
Flavored milk	Meat	Vegetable	Rice	Soy sauce
Milk (cooking)	Pork	Bamboo shoots	Noodles: fried,	Sweet and sour
Ice cream	Beef	Beans: green, yel-	white, and clear	sauce
	Organ meats	low	White bread	Mustard sauce
	Lamb	Bean sprouts	Barley	Ginger
	Goat	Bok choy (cab-	Millet	Plum sauce
	Poultry	bage)		Red bean paste
	Chicken	Broccoli		Tea
	Duck	Carrots		Coffee
	Fish	Celery		Soybean oil
	Whitefish	Corn		Peanut oil
	Carp	Cucumbers		lard
	Shrimp	Eggplant		
	Lobster	Greens: collard,		
	Oyster	Chinese broccoli,		
	Sardines	mustard, kale,		
	Eggs	spinach, radish		
	Legumes	leaves		
	Soybeans	Leeks		
	Soybean curd (tofu)	Lettuce		
	Black beans	Mushrooms		
	Peanuts	Peppers		
	Nuts	Potatoes: white		
	Almonds	and sweet		
	Cashews	Scallions		
		Shepherd's purse		
		Snow peas		
		Taro		
		Tomatoes		
		Water chestnuts		
		White radishes		
		White turnips		
		Fruit		
		Apples		
		Bananas		
		Dates		
		Figs		
		Grapes		
		Kumquats		
		Litchee nuts		
		Loquats		
		Mangoes		
		Oranges		
		Papayas		
		Peaches		
		Pears		
		Persimmons		
		Pineapples		
		Plums		
		Tangerines		
		Winter melons		

(*Source: Adapted from Nutrition During Pregnancy and Lactation. Sacramento, California Department of Health, 1975, p 82.*)

Confucius, foods are chopped or cut into small pieces before they can be eaten. The practice of washing rice prior to cooking results in loss of the water-soluble nutrients it contains.

Raw foods are popular in Japan, including vegetables, eggs, and fish, often served with a pungent green mustard. The Japanese also consume smoked, canned, and dried fish. Marinating is popular with both the Japanese and Filipinos, and marinades may be applied to meats prior to their roasting or broil-

ing. In the Philippines, fresh vegetables are sometimes marinated for salads. Deep frying (tempura) is used by both groups in preparing meats, fish, and some vegetables. Japanese eating habits have undergone extensive changes since World War II as the culture has become considerably westernized. There is a trend toward greater consumption of wheat products, protein foods such as milk, cheese, and meat, and convenience foods.

Nutritional deficiencies likely to be noted in the

TABLE 19–2
CHARACTERISTIC JAPANESE FOOD CHOICES

Milk and Alternates	Meat and Substitutes	Vegetable–Fruit	Bread–Cereal	Other

Milk
Cheese
Ice cream
	Meat
	  Beef
	  Pork
	Poultry
	  Chicken
	  Turkey
	Fish
	  Crab
	  Tuna
	  Carp
	  Mackerel
	  Sardines (dried
	  form, called
	  mezashi)
	  Salmon
	  Sea bass
	  Globefish (puffer)
	  Shrimp
	  Abalone
	  Eels
	  Squid
	  Octopus
	  Fish sausage
	Eggs
	Legumes
	  Soybean curd
	  (tofu)
	  Soybean paste
	  (miso)
	  Soybeans
	  Red beans (azuki)
	  Lima beans
	Nuts
	  Chestnuts (kuri)
		Vegetable
		  Bamboo shoots
		  Bok choy (cabbage)
		  Broccoli
		  Burdock root
		  Carrots
		  Cauliflower
		  Celery
		  Cucumbers
		  Eggplant
		  Green beans
		  Groud (kampyo)
		  Mushrooms
		  Mustard greens
		  Napa cabbage
		  Peas
		  Peppers
		  Radishes (white rad-
		  ish, called daikon;
		  pickled white rad-
		  ish, called takawan)
		  Seaweed
		  Snow peas
		  Spinach
		  Squash
		  Sweet potatoes
		  Taro (Japanese
		  sweet potatoes)
		  Tomatoes
		  Turnips
		  Water chestnuts
		  Yams
		Fruit
		  Apples
		  Apricots
		  Bananas
		  Cherries
		  Grapefruit
		  Grapes
		  Lemons
		  Limes
		  Melons
		  Oranges
		  Peaches
		  Pears
		  Persimmons
		  Pineapples
		  Pomegranates
		  Plums (dried pick-
		  led plums, called
		  umeboshi)
		  Strawberries
		  Tangerines
			Rice
			Rice crackers
			Noodles (whole
			wheat noodle,
			called soba)
			White bread
			Oatmeal
			Dry cereals
				Soy sauce
				Nori paste (used to
				season rice)
				Bean thread
				(konyaku)
				Ginger (shoga,
				dried form, called
				denishoga)
				Tea
				Coffee
				Pickled vegetables
				Soybean oil
				Suet
				Saki (rice liquor)

(Source: Adapted from Nutrition During Pregnancy and Lactation. Sacramento, California Department of Health, 1975, p 84.)

traditional diet of Asians are associated with the limited consumption of milk, cheese, and meat. For this reason, the diet may be inadequate in kilocalories, protein, calcium, and riboflavin.

Intervention. Since adults may be intolerant of milk as a result of lactase deficiency, the same techniques described in the next section for black Americans are also relevant for Asians. To increase kilocalorie, protein, calcium, and riboflavin intake, encourage an increase in the consumption of tofu or beans. Six ounces of tofu contains an amount of calcium equivalent to 1 c of milk if calcium salts are used to precipitate the curd. Discourage the washing of rice before preparation and the ingestion of raw eggs, which may be contaminated with *Salmonella.*

TABLE 19-3
CHARACTERISTIC FILIPINO FOOD CHOICES

Milk and Alternates	Meat and Substitutes	Vegetable– Fruit	Bread– Cereal	Other

Milk: flavored and evaporated
 	
Cheese: gouda, cheddar
	Meat
	  Pork
	  Beef
	  Goat
	  Deer
	  Rabbit
	  Variety meats
	Poultry
	  Chicken
	Fish
	  Sole
	  Bonito
	  Herring
	  Tuna
	  Mackerel
	  Crab
	  Mussels
	  Shrimp
	  Squid
	Eggs
	Legumes
	  Black beans
	  Chick peas
	  Blackeyed peas
	  Lentils
	  Mung beans
	  Lima beans
	  White kidney
	  beans
	Nuts
	  Cashews
	  Peanuts
	  Pili nuts
		Vegetable
		  Bamboo shoots
		  Beets
		  Cabbage
		  Carrots
		  Cauliflower
		  Chinese celery
		  Eggplant
		  Endive
		  Green beans
		  Leeks
		  Lettuce
		  Mushrooms
		  Okra
		  Onions
		  Peppers
		  Potatoes: white
		  and sweet
		  Pumpkin
		  Snow peas
		  Spinach
		  Squash
		  Tomatoes
		  Water chestnuts
		  Watercress
		  Yams
		Fruit
		  Apples
		  Bananas
		  Grapes
		  Guava
		  Lemons
		  Limes
		  Mangoes
		  Melons
		  Oranges
		  Papayas
		  Pears
		  Pineapples
		  Plums
		  Pomegranates
		  Rhubarb
		  Strawberries
		  Tangerines
			Rice
			Cooked cereal: farina, oatmeal
			Dry cereals
			Noodles (rice and wheat)
			Spaghetti
				Soy sauce
				Coffee
				Tea

(Source: Adapted from Nutrition During Pregnancy and Lactation. Sacramento, California Department of Health, 1975, p 86.)

Vietnamese

Assessment. The food preferences of Vietnamese immigrating to the United States are similar to those of other South Asian groups. Milk and milk products are not typically part of the Vietnamese diet, although infants and small children often consume evaporated milk. Tea is the principal beverage. Fish, seafood, pork (including heart, tongue, liver, stomach, intestines, and coagulated blood), chicken, peanuts, soybeans, and Chinese sausage are acceptable high-protein choices. Bananas, mangoes, melons, oranges, papayas, and pineapples are favored fruits. Vietnamese vegetables that are typically available in the United States include bamboo shoots, bean sprouts, bok choy, carrots, cabbage, cauliflower, greens, green pepper, snow peas, eggplant, mushrooms, and water chestnuts.

Rice is the primary cereal grain, although other grain products, such as bean thread, noodles, and French bread, are also frequently eaten. Lard is used for frying, and sweets are made from rice gluten flour, fruit, or seeds.

The daily food pattern often begins with a breakfast of strong coffee with a great deal of cream and sugar, and sometimes leftover foods. Lunch and dinner stress rice with soups containing meat, fish, and vegetables or a main course of meat or seafood cooked with salt or fish sauce.

Intervention. Encourage the use of vegetables,

fruits, and milk products, and discourage the excessive washing of rice. Other changes in the typical diet of immigrant Vietnamese that would improve the nutritional quality include less emphasis on candy, sodas, and sweets.

Black American

Assessment. The dietary practices of black Americans reflect the food patterns of the regions where they live. Consequently, southern blacks generally have the same pattern as other southerners, while blacks who are natives of the north may identify very little with this regional food pattern, although they may adopt some of these habits.

Historically, poverty has been extreme among blacks, and this has been reflected in their diet. The traditional foods used include many found commonly throughout the south (Table 19–4). Pork, chicken, and fish are favored meats. Various dried legumes and small wild game are also used as protein sources. Milk and cheese are not used extensively, and buttermilk, ice cream, and evaporated milk are the preferred items from this group. A large majority of adult black Americans may not be able to tolerate large amounts of milk because of lactase deficiency, although milk is generally well tolerated until late childhood. Wide use is made of hot breads, rice, grits, and vegetables, including the green leafy types. The long-cooking technique using salted fat seasoning is popular, with the pot liquor being consumed as well as the vegetables. Fruits in season, such as oranges, melons, grapes, and peaches, are often eaten as a snack. Salads are not common. Sweets, particularly molasses, other syrups, pies, cakes, cookies, and carbonated drinks, play a prominent role in the diet, and carbonated drinks often displace fruit juice or milk as a beverage. Frying, stewing, and barbecuing are favorite cooking methods, even when an oven is available for roasting or baking. The diet contains considerable fat, since pork fat is often used for frying, and fatty meats, such as pig's feet, pig's ears, and spareribs, which contain large amounts of bone, fat, and connective tissue relative to lean protein tissue, are a part of the diet.

The word "soul," often used in relation to black culture, relates to various cultural aspects, such as music and food, that originated from a feeling of kinship that is recognizable but difficult to define. The specific foods that have been designated as soul foods are those that give a sense of well-being and pleasure and give rise to particular sentiments or feelings. Such foods had their origins in the socioeconomic climate of the pre-Civil War south as the slaves attempted to make the most of the low-status foods discarded by the plantation owners. Vestiges of American Indian foods as well as those of the African black culture can be identified. Typical soul foods include blackeyed peas (often cooked with rice and called "Hoppin' John"), boiled greens with fat-

back, pot liquor, sweet potatoes (often served in a pie or candied), pork products such as chitterlings, hog maw, hog jowl, pig's feet, tails, ears, and snout (sometimes made into souse meat or scrapple), neck bones, corn bread, fried chicken, fried fish, especially catfish and porgies, and game, such as opossum, squirrel, racoon, and rabbit. Blacks who migrate from the south tend initially to retain many of their favorite southern dishes. With time, their diet blends with the foods typical of the new area.

The ethnic food pattern of black Americans tends to lack variety and be excessive in sodium and saturated fat. The kilocaloric level may be high, with a large consumption of fried foods, fatty meats, and refined carbohydrate foods, such as bread, rice, and high-calorie desserts. Obesity is a major problem within this group, especially among women, and there is a high incidence of hypertension. Positive aspects of the black American diet include the wide use of leafy green vegetables and other vegetables and plant sources of protein, such as blackeyed peas and lima beans.

Intervention. Assist black American clients who follow a dietary pattern similar to that described above to improve the overall nutritional quality of the diet by substituting vegetable fat for pork fat, decreasing sodium intake, and increasing intake of milk products. Even with lactase deficiency, a nutritionally significant amount of milk can be tolerated, especially if taken with other foods. Moreover, cheese and fermented milk are often well tolerated, and calcium can be obtained from leafy greens. Suggest alternatives to salt and saturated fat for seasoning, and assess the diet for adequacy of protein and iron, since these nutrients may be lacking in the diet. If the expense of animal protein foods is a factor, use the concept of protein complementation discussed in Chapter 20 to assure protein of adequate quality from plant sources. When assessing the iron status of black clients, recall that they tend to have slightly lower hemoglobin readings even though they may not be nutritionally deficient in iron.

Hispanic

The Hispanic population of the United States is composed of many ethnic groups. The dietary practices of Mexican-Americans, Puerto Ricans, and Cubans are explored in this section.

Mexican-American

Assessment. The dietary practices of people of Mexican heritage who live in the United States, chiefly in the southwest, reflect a blend of Spanish and Native American influences. Because of limited availability and the high cost of animal protein foods, the traditional diet is based largely on plant foods (Table 19–5). Chili peppers, corn, and dried beans are the staples, although corn is being gradually replaced by wheat.

TABLE 19-4
CHARACTERISTIC SOUTHERN BLACK AMERICAN FOOD CHOICES

Milk and Alternates	Meat and Substitutes	Vegetable– Fruit	Bread– Cereal	Other
Homogenized milk (as available)	**Meat**	**Vegetable**	Refined cereals: white rice, hominy grits, and refined dry cereals	Lard
Evaporated milk	Pork and ham (most popular) including such pork products as country cured ham, hog jowls, ham hocks, hog maw (stomach), fatback (streak of lean), bacon, sausage, heart, lungs, kidneys, brains, liver, pig's feet, tails, ears, and snout, neck bones, spareribs, chitterlings	Broccoli		Butter
Dry milk		Cabbage		Gravy
Cheddar and processed cheese		Carrots	Hot breads: biscuits, cornbread, muffins, hush puppies, spoon bread hoe cakes[a]	Molasses
Cottage cheese		Corn		Cane syrup
Ice cream		Cucumber		Jams and jellies
		Greens: collard, kale, mustard, spinach, turnip tops		Carbonated beverages
		Green beans	Commercial white bread	Fruit drinks and fruit-flavored beverages, as Kool-Aid
		Green pepper	Macaroni	
		Lima beans	Spaghetti	
	Beef (including cured tongue)	Okra	Crackers	
	Poultry	Onions	Baked desserts: cakes, pies, cookies, other sweet breads	
	Chicken	Peas		
	Turkey	Potatoes: white and sweet		
	Small wild game and birds	Pumpkin		
	Squirrel, rabbit, opossum, dove, quail	Summer squash		
		Tomatoes		
	Fish	Yams		
	Catfish	**Fruit**		
	White buffalo fish	Apples		
	Mullet	Bananas		
	Spots	Grapes		
	Croakers	Grapefruit		
	Perch	Melons: watermelon and cantaloupe		
	Butterfish	Oranges		
	Trout	Peaches		
	Red snapper	Plums		
	Salted fish, as herring	Tangerines		
	Canned fish, as tuna, salmon, sardines			
	Shrimp			
	Scallops			
	Oysters			
	Crabs			
	Clams			
	Crayfish			
	Eggs			
	Legumes			
	Dried blackeyed peas			
	Kidney and pinto beans			
	Nuts			
	Peanuts, and peanut butter especially			

[a] Originally baked on a hoe over an open fire.

For the Mexican, the chili plant is indispensable, since good health is believed to accompany its liberal use. A variety of green and red chili peppers is eaten fresh or dried; these peppers are rich sources of vitamins A and C. Corn is used in numerous ways and may be eaten fresh in the form of a type of hominy (pasole) or steamed and dried on the cob (chicos). A dough (masa) made from dried corn is used in the preparation of the popular tortilla, and cornmeal is used to prepare a gruel (atole). The prac-

TABLE 19–5
CHARACTERISTIC MEXICAN-AMERICAN FOOD CHOICES

Milk and Alternates	Meat and Substitutes	Vegetable– Fruit	Bread– Cereal	Other
Evaporated milk (for infants)	Meat	Vegetable	Tortillas: corn and wheat flour	Salt pork
Custard (flan)	Beef	Corn: fresh, pasole, chicos	Rice	Bacon
Puddings (e.g., rice pudding—arroz con leche)	Pork and pork intestine	Carrots	Oatmeal	Coffee
Cheese (small amounts)	Cold cuts	Chili peppers	Dry cereals: corn-flakes and sugar coated	Tequila
Champarrado (milk with chocolate and cinnamon)	Goat	Tomatoes		Beer
	Lamb	Potatoes: white and sweet	Noodles	Fruit drinks
	Tripe	Beets	Spaghetti	Kool-Aid
	Sausage (chorizo)	Cabbage	Macaroni	Carbonated beverages
	Poultry	Greens: tropical and wild, spinach	White bread	Popsicles
	Chicken	Peas	Sweet bread (pan dulce)	Lard (manteca)
	Eggs	Pumpkin	Atole (cornmeal gruel)	Pork cracklings
	Legumes	Squash: zucchini and other	Polvillo (gruel)	Guacamole
	Pinto beans	Green beans	Sopaipilla (fried biscuit)	Chili sauce
	Calico beans	Turnips		Chili powder
	Pink beans	Lettuce		Salsa (tomato, pepper, onion relish)
	Garbonzo beans	Onion		Salt
	Lentils	Prickly pear cactus leaf (nopales)		Sugar
	Refried beans (frijoles)	Fruit		Garlic
	Peanuts	Apples		Oregano
	Peanut butter	Bananas		Coriander (cilantro)
		Prickly pear cactus fruit (tuna)		Cumin (comino)
		Oranges		Saffron
		Melons		
		Peaches		
		Canned fruit cocktail		
		Apricots		
		Zapote (or sapote)		
		Avocado		

tice of soaking the corn used in making hominy and dough in lime water adds a significant amount of calcium to the diet. The trend toward using wheat rather than corn in dough preparation may consequently reduce calcium consumption. Although corn is the basic cereal, some rice and wheat are used, and rice may be cooked with milk as a dessert. Sugar-coated, prepared breakfast cereals, oatmeal, and wheat rolls are popular.

Beans of various types, such as pinto and calico beans, are eaten at nearly every meal. Usually they are cooked, mashed, and refried with lard until they absorb all of the fat in the pan (frijoles refritos). They may be used in soups (sopas) or in combination with meat (chili con carne) or cereal (topopo, corn tortillas filled with refried beans, shredded lettuce, and olives). The variety of vegetables used is not as great as with some other ethnic groups, and potatoes, chili peppers, and tomatoes are the most popular items. The use of fruits, often considered a dessert or snack, depends on cost and availability, and they are usually eaten fresh and sometimes canned.

The consumption of milk and cheese is largely limited to the use of evaporated milk in infant feeding. However, some milk may be used in the preparation of cereals and puddings. When cheese is used, the Mexican varieties are preferred.

Meat consumption is small, and meat typically appears in combination with other foods. Beef and chicken are well liked, whereas fish is used infrequently. Characteristic combination dishes that use varying amounts of meat, cheese, legumes, cereals, and vegetables include tacos (tortillas filled with seasoned ground meat or cheese served with lettuce and chili sauce), burritos (a combination of a large tortilla, green or red chili peppers, and diced, cooked meat or refried beans), enchiladas (small tortillas filled with shredded meat, cheese, and vegetables served with chili sauce), tamale (seasoned ground meat placed on masa, wrapped in corn husks, steamed, and served with chili sauce), and chili con carne (meat and beans with chili peppers and garlic seasoning). A vegetable mixture used for making gravy and sauces (mole poblano, a mixture of wheat flour, peanut butter, sugar, cocoa or bitter chocolate, cottonseed oil, and spices) is said to contribute a significant amount of protein to the diet.[3]

The Mexican-American food pattern emphasizes sugar and other sweets. Foods are highly seasoned. Ground chili peppers, onion, cumin, and garlic are used most frequently, although other herbs, such as oregano and coriander, are sometimes used. Lard is the basic fat, and such foods as meat, eggs, beans, macaroni, and potatoes are often fried. Vegetables and some meats may be prepared by boiling. A large quantity of coffee is used, and it is sometimes given to children.

American influences can be identified in the evolving Mexican food pattern: there is increasing use of such foods as wheat, oatmeal, ready-to-eat cereal, soft drinks, popsicles, and fruit drinks. The practice of including a merienda (a later afternoon snack) is less common among those who have lived in this country for some time.

Assess for the presence of nutrient inadequacies associated with the limited use of milk and vegetables, especially the dark green and yellow varieties. Overcooking of vegetables contributes to potential deficiencies. Although several nutrient inadequacies have been documented in surveys, vitamin A deficiency appears to be the most significant problem.[4]

Intervention. To increase the amount of vitamin A in the diet, counsel the client to increase the use of foods such as carrots. Stress that vegetables should be cooked in small amounts of water for shorter periods of time. Encourage the use of various forms of dairy products in the diet, particularly if the indigenous practice of lime-soaking techniques is abandoned. Simple dishes, such as melted cheese on tortillas (quesadillas) and tortillas made with nonfat dry milk can be prepared. Be aware of the high incidence of lactose intolerance in older children and adults when seeking methods to increase intake of calcium, however. Since the incidence of obesity is high among Mexican-Americans, examine the nutrient:kilocalorie ratio of the diet. The high use of foods, such as pastries and carbonated beverages, and the frequent use of lard or oil to fry foods contributes excessive kilocalories. Encourage the client to limit the intake of sweets and nonessential fats.

Puerto Rican

Assessment. Although most Puerto Ricans living on the mainland were born here, many follow the traditional food habits of their parents who came from the island. Staple foods common to most Puerto Rican diets include rice, legumes, viandas (starchy root vegetables and fruits indigenous to the area, such as yams, cassava, green bananas, and plantains), dry salted codfish, lard, sugar, and coffee (Table 19–6). Sofrito, or refrito (a combination of tomatoes, peppers, onions, garlic, salt pork, and seasoning) is a basic sauce used in the preparation of rice, legumes, and other foods. Because of their high cost, other fruits and vegetables, milk, and meat may be consumed in small quantities.

The majority of families eat a breakfast composed of a coffee–milk mixture (cafe con leche) with or without bread, a lunch of viandas with codfish and oil, and a dinner of rice, beans, and viandas or bread. Urban dwellers may eat rice and beans twice a day, and between-meal eating is common. Oatmeal and eggs may be added to breakfast and other meats and fruits to daily meals when possible.

Rice is consumed in large quantities, approximately 7 oz daily per person, and contributes a large portion of the kilocalories in the diet. It may be boiled and dressed with lard (arroz blanco or white rice), stewed with beans and sofrito (arroz con habichuelas), cooked with chicken, sofrito, and seasonings (arroz con pollo), or made into a chicken-rice soup (asopao). Chopped sausages or codfish may also be prepared with the rice. Arroz con dulce is a dessert made with sweetened rice.

Viandas, high in starch content, contain a fair amount of iron, B vitamins, and vitamin C. They often replace bread in the diet and may be used much like potatoes with fish or meat. A popular one-dish meal in rural areas is serenata, hot boiled viandas served with oil, vinegar, and codfish, with sliced onion, avocado, and hard-cooked egg sometimes added. Sancocho is a soup of meat and vianda. In the United States, white and sweet potatoes may be substituted for the tropical viandas.

Legumes are usually boiled until tender and combined with sofrito or stewed with rice. Although codfish is a primary protein source, consumption of various types of beef, pork, and chicken rises with increased income. Pork intestines are well liked and are eaten fried (cuchifritos) or stewed with native vegetables (salcocho) or with chick peas.

The amount of milk consumed varies, but it is used primarily for infant feeding and for flavoring strong Spanish coffee and very sweet cocoa and chocolate drinks. Milk is usually boiled before use. A cup of cafe con leche may contain 2 to 5 oz of milk. Cooked cereals are often prepared with milk rather than water. Although locally grown fruits and vegetables are abundant, and some are relatively inexpensive, very few are consumed, and imported canned fruits are often preferred. A native fruit, the acerole, or West Indian cherry, is the richest known natural source of vitamin C.

Desserts are not always served, but fruits cooked in syrup are a frequent dietary item. A favorite beverage is black malt beer (malta). This high-calorie, nonalcoholic beverage is believed to be very nourishing and is combined with beaten egg and served to convalescents, the aged, and pregnant women. It contributes some protein, iron, and B vitamins to the diet.

TABLE 19–6
CHARACTERISTIC PUERTO RICAN FOOD CHOICES

Milk and Alternates	Meat and Substitutes	Vegetable–Fruit	Bread–Cereal	Other

Cafe con leche (coffee and boiled milk)	Meat
	  Beef
	  Pork and pork intestine
	  Sausages
		Vegetable
		  Sofrito
		  Viandas
		    Green banana (piche verde)
		    Green plantain (plantano verde)
		    Ripe plantain (plantano maduro)
		    White sweet potatoes (batata blanca)
		    Yellow sweet potatoes (batata amarillo)
		    White yams (ñame blanco)
		    Breadfruit (panapen)
		    Tanier (yautia)
		    Cassava (yuca)
		  Beets
		  Eggplant (chayote)
		  Onions
		  Carrots
		  Green beans
		  Okra
		  Tomatoes
		  Spinach
		  Chard
		  Yellow squash (calabaza)
		  Lettuce
		  Cabbage
		  Green peppers
		  Onions
		  Pumpkin
		Fruit
		  West Indian cherry (acerola)
		  Papayas
		  Mangoes
		  Guava
		  Oranges
		  Grapefruit
		  Pineapples
		  Imported canned fruits (fruit cocktail, peaches, pears, apples)
		  Bananas
		  Fruit nectars
		  Fruit paste (guava, bitter orange, pineapple, mango)
		  Cashew nut fruit
		  Boiled papaya preserves
			Rice (arroz)
			Wheat bread
			Noodles
			Cornmeal and cornmeal mush
			Oatmeal
			Cream of wheat
			Cakes
			Pies
			Arroz con dulce (rice, sugar, spices)
				Lard
				Olive oil
				Butter
				Salt pork
				Ham butt
				Annato (yellow coloring)
				Sugar molasses
				Coffee (mocha)
				Carbonated beverages
				Garlic
				Black malt beer (malta)

Sweetened cocoa and chocolate drinks	Fish
	  Dry salted codfish (bacalao)
	  Fresh fish (coastal areas)			

Cereals cooked with milk	Poultry Chicken			
Native white cheese (queso blanco)	Eggs			

Ice cream	Legumes (granos)
	  Chick peas
	  Pigeon peas
	  Navy beans
	  Red kidney beans
	  Dry peas			

Fresh cow's milk				

Intervention. Assist Puerto Rican clients to improve their diets by supplementing the staple foods with milk, meat, egg, green and yellow vegetables, and native fruits. For those living in this country, stress the use of less expensive foods from each food group and give some help in substituting local foods for the similar but more expensive imported foods. The use of nonfat milk, cheaper cuts of meat, margarine instead of butter, and replacements for out-of-season fruits and vegetables would provide better nutrition for less cost. Since rice and beans offer a combination of high nutritive quality, encourage their use. When served at the same meal, the essential amino acid patterns are complementary. Nonfat dry milk is well accepted, but the client must be taught how to use it. Encourage the use of whole grain cereals.

Assess for the presence of obesity, which may be a problem because of the large amount of sugar and fat used.

Cuban

Assessment. In recent years there has been a large influx of Cuban refugees into Florida and other southern states. Cuban dietary practices are similar to those of other West Indian groups, with the Spanish influence predominating. Rice is a staple food and is served with dinner and supper. Breakfast tends to be inadequate and often includes sweetened coffee and bread or crackers. Both carbonated beverages and coffee are popular. Protein sources in the traditional diet include meat, fish, poultry, eggs, legumes, milk, and cheese. Black beans are a favorite and are often mixed with rice. Fruits and vegetables, including plantains, are used liberally, and native fruits and vegetables are preferred. Fruits serve as the basis for sweets, but flan, a custardlike dessert, is also popular. Meats are usually fried, preferably with lard. Characteristic cuban food choices are summarized in Table 19–7.

Intervention. To improve the nutritive quality of the diet, encourage the practice of combining black beans and rice to attain a high-quality amino acid mixture and increasing the consumption of calcium-rich vegetables, such as spinach and broccoli. The addition of cheese to the breakfast meal would improve the adequacy of this meal and increase the calcium intake. Advise the client to decrease the

---

TABLE 19–7
CHARACTERISTIC CUBAN FOOD CHOICES

Milk and Alternates	Meat and Substitutes	Vegetable–Fruit	Bread–Cereal	Other
Milk: whole, skimmed, condensed, dry	Meat Beef Pork Lamb Veal Sausages	Vegetable Beans: green and yellow Berenjena Boniato (white yams)	Rice Cornmeal Cornstarch Imported cereals (as oatmeal, corn flakes)	Sour cream Lard Olive oil Peanut oil Soy oil
Goat's milk (usually given to the sick)	Poultry Chicken	Carrots Chayote Lettuce	Plantain	Butter Margarine
Cheese: Gouda, cream, and native cheese (queso de mano)	Fish Fresh, salted, smoked, canned	Onions Peppers, green Potatoes	Desserts: cakes, pies, guava, prune, and mango pastes, moron cookies, ter-	Shortening Coffee
Ice cream	Eggs	Tubers, native: yuca, ñame, ma-	rejas, boniatillo, bu-	Tea
Custard (flour)	Legumes Black beans Red beans Kidney beans Navy beans Lima beans Split peas	langa (white and yellow) Tomatoes Fruit Anon Bananas Caimito Chirimoya Coconut Grapefruit Guanabana Mamey Mangoes Maranon Oranges (sweet and sour) Papayas Zapote	nuelos, cafiroletas	Beer Wines Carbonated beverages Seasonings: vinegar, cumin, oregano, bijol, salt, pepper, garlic

(*Source:* Adapted from Krause MV, Hunscher MA: *Food, Nutrition and Diet Therapy*, ed 5. Philadelphia, WB Saunders, 1972, p 195.)

consumption of carbonated beverages and to substitute vegetable oils for lard.

Beliefs Concerning Hot and Cold

Assessment and Intervention. Assess the food beliefs of Hispanic clients. As do the traditional Chinese, many members of the Hispanic community believe that food, in the proper combinations, plays a vital role in the prevention of illness and the restoration of health, and they ascribe to a hot and cold food theory. While the hot–cold classification system may vary from person to person, essentially there are certain foods that are classified as hot and others classified as cold. If these foods are eaten in the proper amounts and combination, the body is maintained in the correct balance. Examples of cold foods are avocado, bananas, chicken, fruits, honey, and lima beans, and examples of hot foods are chocolate, coffee, cornmeal, garlic, kidney beans, onions, and peas. Illness occurs if these foods are eaten in improper combinations or amounts. For example, fridad del estomago, "cold stomach," is caused by eating too many cold-classified foods. A pregnant woman may avoid hot-classified foods, an infant who has a formula that is classified as hot may be fed whole milk, classified as cold, and a woman who is menstruating or post partum may avoid cold foods. Illness is treated by restoring the body's balance. When an illness is classified as hot, it must be treated by the ingestion of a cold food. The postpartum condition is classified as cold, and, therefore, chicken is avoided since it is a cold food.[5]

Italian

Assessment. Pasta of various kinds and bread are staples of the Italian diet, although there are some regional variations in food customs. Northern Italians use more meat, dairy products, and root vegetables, whereas the diet of southern Italians includes more fish, olive oil, and highly seasoned foods. Few Italian-Americans were born in Italy.[6] They have adopted many of the food customs of the United States, although bread and pasta continue to be an important part of the diet pattern.

Daily meals, which are usually eaten at a leisurely pace, consist of a light breakfast, a large main meal, and an additional light meal. The main meal may be eaten in the middle of the day or at night. Breakfast may consist of a beverage (coffee for adults and milk for children) and bread served without butter. Soups, such as minestrone (made with vegetables, chick peas, and pasta) and pasta e fagioli (made with dried legumes), are often served as the main food for light meals. Bread and cheese with coffee or wine may also serve as a light meal.

Milk is used in limited amounts, and goat's milk is more popular than cow's milk. Although the total amount of meat consumed is smaller than for some other groups, a wide variety or meats, fish, and meat substitutes is used. Characteristic meat dishes include cacciatora (chicken browned in oil and simmered in a wine–tomato sauce), scallopine (thin, floured veal strips browned in oil and simmered in a wine–herb sauce), spaghetti with meat balls, and baccala (dried, salted codfish, soaked for several days, browned in oil, and simmered in a tomato–herb sauce). Combinations of various meat mixtures and pastas are used to prepare lasagne, manicotti, ravioli, tortellini, and canneloni.

Fruits and vegetables are popular, and raw fruit is often served for dessert. Salads are a part of most meals, and insalata, a salad prepared with a combination of greens and served with a dressing of oil, vinegar, salt, pepper, and garlic, is a frequent accompaniment. Bread is served at every Italian meal. White crusty bread is now more popular than dark bread, which was formerly the bread of choice. Pasta, in a variety of shapes and enhanced with many different sauces, may be served several times per week. Pasta prepared with meatless sauces or with fish is traditionally served during Lent and Advent. Polenta, a thick cornmeal mush, may be eaten plain or in a casserole with sausage, tomato sauce, and cheese.

Olive oil is widely used for cooking and seasoning. Many main dishes are prepared by sautéing the seasonings and meat in oil, covering with a liquid, and simmering on low heat for several hours. Vegetables are frequently boiled and then sautéed in oil. Herbs and spices, including garlic and tomato puree, are used generously in many dishes. Wine flavors many foods and is typically served as a beverage with meals. Lavish cakes, pastries, and frozen delicacies are served on festive occasions. Characteristic foods are summarized in Table 19–8.

Intervention. Since the typical Italian-American diet provides a wide variety of foods, nutritional needs are likely to be met. Additional meat and milk, especially for young children, will further improve nutrient intake. Suggest the use of nonfat dry milk or evaporated milk, domestic cheese, and cheese bought in wedges for economy. Encourage cooking methods other than frying, and discuss methods of cooking vegetables that require a shorter cooking time and less oil.

Middle and Near Eastern

Assessment. Many food habits are shared by inhabitants of the countries of the Middle and Near East. Much of the food supply is home-produced, since many of these people are farmers and herdsmen. Bread is the staff of life, and cereal grains contribute a large percentage of the energy value of the diet. Bread is served at every meal, and for the Greek, each bite of food is accompanied by bread. A popular staple is bulgur, a product prepared from wheat that is boiled, dried, and cracked.

Milk from the goat, sheep, and cow is used fre-

TABLE 19–8
CHARACTERISTIC ITALIAN FOOD CHOICES

Milk and Alternates	Meat and Substitutes	Vegetable– Fruit	Bread– Cereal	Other
Milk (in coffee, often half milk and half coffee)	Meat Beef Veal	Vegetable Broccoli Escarole and	Bread: wheat, crusty white Italian Rice	Salad dressing: oil, vinegar, salt, pepper, garlic
Cheese: parmesan, mozzarella, provolone, ricotta, casicavallo, romano, gorgonzola, locatelli	Sausage Organ Meats Cold cuts: salami, mortadella (bologna-type sausage), coppa (peppered sausage), prosciutto (cured ham)	other salad greens Beans: green and fava Zucchini Other kinds of squash	Polenta (corn meal) Pasta: macaroni, spaghetti, egg noodles Pastasciutta (pasta with gravy or sauce)	Olive oil Herbs and spices; oregano, rosemary, basil, saffron, parsley, nutmeg, garlic
Ice cream Custard	Lamb Pork Poultry Chicken	Celery Asparagus Eggplant Artichokes	Pizza Facacci (whole wheat bread) Cakes and filled pastries	Salt pork Lard Butter Dry wines
	Fish Fresh, canned (tuna, sardines, anchovies), dried (codfish), shellfish (shrimp, lobster, clams, mussels) Octopus Squid Snails	Peppers Tomatoes Spinach Swiss chard Mustard greens Dandelion greens Mushrooms Fennel Onions Cauliflower Radishes		Liqueurs Coffee Espresso
	Eggs Legumes Kidney beans Lentils Chick peas Split peas	Fruit Grapes Oranges Tangerines Figs Persimmons		
	Nuts Almonds Chestnuts Hazelnuts Pistachios Walnuts	Pomegranates Olives Pears Plums Melons Quinces Cherries Dates Apricots Apples Raisins		

quently in soured and fermented forms (e.g., yoghurt) and as soft and hard cheese. Sweet milk is seldom used. Adults consume little milk, although it is often served hot and sweetened to children. Meat, fish, and poultry are all consumed, with lamb the favorite meat. Pork is often restricted by religious customs, and beef may be too expensive. Although meat prepared on hickory skewers is popular, it is more often served with varying combinations of vegetables and/or cereal grains. Examples include shashlik (marinated mutton or lamb roasted on a skewer with slices of tomato and onion), keib (a combination dish of lamb and ground wheat), breast of lamb stuffed with rice and currants, vegetables (such as grape leaves, cabbage leaves, and squash) stuffed with chopped meat, rice, or bulgur and seasonings, and stews with cereal grains and

vegetables. Dishes of eggs, legumes, and nuts combined with starchy foods and vegetables often replace meat dishes. Cold boiled beans seasoned with oil and vinegar may be used for breakfast.

Vegetables, cooked with olive oil or meat fat, may be served hot or cold. They are also used in stews, stuffed with wheat, beans, nuts or meat, or served as salads with olive oil and vinegar. Seasonal fruits are used for desserts and are eaten raw or in compotes. Dates, olives, and figs are well known in this region of the world.

Bread is baked on griddles in round, flat loaves. In addition to serving as the staple starchy food at meals, cereals such as rice and bulgur are combined with meat, nuts, or legumes as main dishes. The preferred beverage of these countries is black, heavily sweetened coffee that retains the pulverized bean. Rose water is often used in sweets and each country has its own distinctive herbs and spices. Note that the diet is rich in fat. Olive oil, sesame oil, and meat fats are used extensively in meat and vegetable dishes. Characteristic food choices are listed in Table 19–9.

Intervention. Discourage the excessive use of saturated fats and assure that dietary sources of calcium are adequate. Evaluate the protein content of the diet, particularly for the meals when meat is not served, to be sure that the supply of essential amino acids is adequate.

Native American

Assessment. Native Americans include American Indians and Eskimos. Typical American Indian food habits are difficult to describe because of the large number of tribes represented in the population, the

lack of information about the specific food habits of each tribe, and the fact that some Indians are integrated into the general population, whereas others live on reservations. Traditionally, each tribe had its own unique dietary practices based on one or more staple food items. These staple foods were determined primarily by geographical location—the tribes subsisted either by hunting, fishing, and herding animals, such as sheep and goats, or by cultivating the land. Foods were often prepared over an open fire, and soups and stews composed of wild game and vegetables were commonly served. The food situation was often one of feast or famine, since food storage and preservation techniques were limited.

Some of the traditional foods eaten by American Indians include acorn bread, fried bread (sopapillas), smoked salmon and smoked salmon eggs, venison, and berries. Native dishes include wasna, a combination of powdered dried meat, dried berries, sugar,

TABLE 19–9
CHARACTERISTIC MIDDLE AND NEAR EASTERN FOOD CHOICES

Milk and Alternates	Meat and Substitutes	Vegetable– Fruit	Bread– Cereal	Other

Milk: soured and fermented forms of cow's, goat's, or sheep's milk (yoghurt, leben, matzoon)
Cheese: soft and hard
	Meat
	  Lamb
	  Mutton
	  Goat
	  Camel
	  Some beef and pork
	Poultry
	  Chicken
	  Duck
	  Goose
	Fish
	  Fresh, salted and smoked octopus, squid, shellfish, roe
	Eggs
	Legumes
	  Lentils
	  Chick peas
	  Peanuts
	  Soybeans
	Seeds and Nuts
	  Chestnuts
	  Hazelnuts
	  Pignolias
	  Pistachios
	  Seeds of caraway, pumpkin, sesame
		Vegetable
		  Onions
		  Tomatoes
		  Squash
		  Okra
		  Peppers
		  Broccoli
		  Spinach
		  Peas
		  Green beans
		  Dandelions
		  Cucumbers
		  Eggplant
		  Grape leaves
		  Artichokes
		  Cabbage
		  Cauliflower
		  Potatoes
		  Salad greens
		  Leeks
		Fruit
		  Olives
		  Melons
		  Dates
		  Figs
		  Grapes
		  Cherries
		  Quinces
		  Oranges
		  Raisins
		  Apricots
		  Lemons
		  Pears
		  Plums
		  Currants
		  Peaches
			Wheat: whole and cracked (bulgur)
			White and dark breads
			Rice
			Barley
			Corn (polenta)
			Baklava (pastry with nuts and honey)
				Sheep's fat and other meat fats
				Olive oil
				Seed oils
				Sour cream
				Turkish coffee (Giaour)
				Honey
				Sugar
				Apricot candy
				Turkish paste
				Wine
				Hickory embers, for broiling
				Coffee
				Lemon juice

and fat, and wajupi, a fruit pudding of berries, cornstarch, and sugar. They also consumed a variety of wild fruits, game, fish and shellfish, herbs, and maple sugar, as well as sheep and goats. Soups or stews made with game or other meat and vegetables were commonly consumed.

Much cultural blending of food patterns occurred between the European settlers and the American Indians. An excellent example of the melding of foods is found in the southwestern United States, where the food patterns reflect Anglo, American Indian, Mexican, and Spanish influences. Many of the plant foods widely eaten today, such as corn, potatoes, peppers, squash, pumpkin, beans, cranberries, and wild rice, originated with the American Indians. Popcorn was an American Indian creation.

It is not possible to identify a typical food pattern today because of extensive acculturation in much the same way that other ethnic food patterns have become assimilated. The current living situation has interfered with the ability to consume traditional foods. Food choices are dependent on income and food availability as well as place of residence (i.e., reservation, rural, or urban). Although traditional eating patterns are preferred, they are often not followed, even on reservations, because of the unavailability of familiar foods. A blend of American and traditional foods can usually be identified in everyday meals, consisting of breakfast, lunch, and dinner. Traditional meals that incorporate foods with religious or ceremonial significance are served primarily on special occasions.

Today there is increased interest in understanding the American Indian cultural heritage and reviving traditional foods and methods of preparation. There also appear to be distinct nutritional advantages for American Indians in reviving some of their food customs, many of which are nutritionally superior to those adopted in recent times.

Nutrition surveys of various tribes reveal nutrient deficiencies that may be mild to marked, and the growth of children tends to be below the norm for North American children.[7] The infant mortality rate is higher than that of the general population, and the incidence of such chronic diseases as tuberculosis is still high.[8]

The traditional diet of Eskimos, which consisted almost entirely of frozen, dried, or fresh game and fish, supplemented seasonally with berries, roots, leafy greens, and seaweed, has also suffered from American acculturation. The adaptation of food habits that include such foods as sugar, candy, and soft drinks has been associated with the incidence of health problems, such as dental decay, that were nonexistent in earlier times.

Intervention. Emphasize the need to ingest adequate kilocalories, protein foods, vegetables, fruits, and milk products while avoiding excessive sweets. Be aware that the incidence of lactose intolerance is high in both Indians and Eskimos, however. Support the practice of breastfeeding and the use of weaning foods that are low in sugar, fat, and salt.

RELIGIOUS DIETARY PRACTICES

Many associations have developed between religion and food. The earliest religious practices made use of food as an offering to the gods. Most religious teachings include proscriptions or prescriptions regarding foods and eating practices that have deep significance and must be considered when providing nursing care. Although the reasons for the religious food practices are often obscure, in many cases they symbolize major events in the history of the religion, or they may be used an as affirmation of faith. For example, foods are used in many Jewish feasts and holy days to symbolize past events. The Jewish practice of serving kosher foods, requiring considerable labor and self-discipline, is clearly a demonstration of faith and belief. In Christian churches, Holy Communion symbolizes a past event and demonstrates faith.

At present, rituals within several religions are practiced in varying degrees. While religious prescriptions may not be followed in daily meals, they may be observed on religious holidays and feasts. The abolition of certain laws by some religious groups in recent years has changed customary dietary habits. Dietary restrictions and fast days for Roman Catholics have been liberalized by the Vatican, beginning in the mid-1960s. However, customs vary with locality. A somewhat more liberal interpretation is being given to the dietary laws of the Greek Orthodox Church. However, Greek Orthodox regulations still include the restriction of animal foods on Fridays, certain Wednesdays, and during the first and last weeks of Lent. The Church of Jesus Christ of Latter-Day Saints (Mormons) continues to prohibit the use of alcohol, tobacco, tea, and coffee for its members.

In the United States there are several religious bodies that strongly influence dietary habits. Of these, Jewish, Islamic, and vegetarian groups, such as the Seventh-Day Adventists and Zen Buddhists, will be discussed here.

Judaism

Assessment. Judaism has traditionally used food in its religious feasts and ceremonies and has observed dietary laws based on Biblical and rabbinical regulations. The body of laws regulating food intake, known as the rules of kashruth, defines those foods that are **kosher,** or fit. Although self-purification and service to God form the basis of the laws, hygienic or ethical considerations probably also contributed.

At present, Jewish families differ in food practices according to their particular group affiliation and country of origin. Orthodox Jews observe the laws under all conditions and place a great value on traditional and ceremonial practice of the religion. In contrast, Reform Jews may minimize the significance of the laws, which are considered purely ceremonial. In between are Conservative Jews, who adhere nominally to the laws and sometimes make a distinction between observing the rules inside and outside the home. For the majority of Jewish people, foods typical of their country of origin are used to the extent that they are consistent with dietary laws.

The rules of kashruth regulate the selection, preparation, and service of food and classify foods into four types:

1. Foods that are inherently kosher (pareve) and may be eaten in their natural state. These include fruits, vegetables, vegetable fats, cereal products, eggs that are free of blood, fish that have fins and scales (e.g., halibut, sole, cod, tuna, salmon), coffee, and tea.
2. Foods that require some processing in order to be kosher. The allowed meats and poultry are included in this category. Acceptable animals must be declared healthy and quickly and painlessly slaughtered by an ordained shochet (ritual slaughterer). The meat is then koshered (cleansed of blood) by one of two methods: (1) soaking in cold water for half an hour, salting with coarse salt, draining for 1 hour to remove the blood, washing thoroughly under cold running water, and draining again, or (2) quick searing. Meats with a high blood content, such as liver, are rinsed, drained well, and broiled on a grill. They may then be fried, chopped, or combined with other foods. The permitted fish and eggs do not have to undergo this process. Meats must come from a specific type of animal: cloven-hoofed creatures that graze and chew their cud, such as cows, sheep, goats, and deer. Only the forequarter segments (the rib cage forward) and organs are permitted. The hindquarter can be eaten only if the hip sinew of the thigh vein is removed.
3. Foods that are prohibited. These include pork, blood in any form (including eggs with blood spots, and fish without fins and scales (shellfish and eels).
4. Foods that cannot be combined at the same meal. These are meat (fleishig) and milk or milk products (milchig). Usually two meals contain dairy products and one contains meat and its products. Whereas milk or dairy products may be eaten just prior to a meat meal, 6 hours must elapse after the meal before they are again permitted. At meat meals, butter may not be used even on bread or for seasoning vegetables, nor may cream be added to coffee. Separate utensils and dishes

must be used to prepare and serve meat and milk meals. This necessitates two separate sets of utensils and dishes, one for meat and one for milk meals. Vegetables cooked in a milk pot must be considered a milk dish. Foods that are inherently kosher, such as cereals, fruits, vegetables, eggs from permitted birds, and permitted fish, are considered neutral and may be eaten at either milk or meat meals.

Kosher products are so certified by a reliable rabbinical authority. Either the rabbi's name or the copyrighted symbol of the Union of Orthodox Jewish Congregations of America (U) appears on the sealed package. It is necessary to check the listing of ingredients on many packaged foods for the inclusion of meat, lard, or other animal fat, and milk. For example, many breads and margarines have milk added and cookies and crackers may be prepared with lard. A kosher food package should be presented to the user with the seal unbroken. It should be opened by the user, in his presence, or by one authorized by the religious authorities to do so. Because rabbis vary in their kosher interpretation of some foods, such as gelatin, Jewish clients should consult their rabbi regarding use of questionable items.

Many of the traditional Jewish foods are related to the different festivals and to special dishes prepared for the Sabbath. Some examples are gefilte fish (a stuffed fish often served as an appetizer), tzimmes (any combination of meat, vegetables, or fruit, such as brisket, carrot, sweet potato, and brown sugar), cholent (a casserole of beef, potato, and dried beans), challah (white bread baked as a twist or coil), and kugel (a sweet pudding of noodles or potatoes, almonds, raisins, and spices). Other representative foods are found in Table 19–10.

The Jewish diet contains a considerable amount of pastries filled with fruit and nuts, cakes, preserves, fatty foods, and the like. Bread, cereal, legumes, fish, and dairy products are used abundantly. Legumes and vegetables may be combined with meat in casseroles or served in soups, which are especially popular and may be served at every meal. Root vegetables and potatoes are used extensively, and cereals, such as barley, are frequently served as a vegetable or in soup. Many foods are highly salted, although unsalted butter is preferred. Pickles and relishes that contain a large amount of salt are widely used. Soft drinks may be served at meat meals when milk beverages are not permitted.

The food regulations associated with religious festivals are usually observed by more liberal groups as well as the orthodox. The major ones are summarized below.

1. *Sabbath.* No food is cooked or heated on the Sabbath, which begins at sundown Friday and ends with the first visible star on Saturday evening. Sabbath foods are prepared on Friday and kept warm or served cold. Some

TABLE 19-10
CHARACTERISTIC JEWISH FOOD CHOICES

Milk and Alternates	Meat and Substitutes	Vegetable– Fruit	Bread– Cereal	Other

Milk: fresh, butter-milk
Cheese: cottage, pot, American, Muenster, Swiss
	Meat
	  Beef } Koshered forequarters and organs
	  Lamb
	Poultry
	  Chicken
	  Turkey
	  Goose
	  Pheasant
	  Duck
	  Dove
	  Pigeon
	  Squab
	Fish
	  Trout
	  Cod
	  Tuna
	  Haddock
	  Carp
	  Flounder
	  Salmon
	  Whitefish
	  Halibut
	  Sturgeon
	  Smoked and salted fish (herring, salmon, sturgeon)
	  Gefilte fish (stuffed fish)
	  Caviar
	Eggs (without blood spots)
	Legumes
	  Chick peas (nahit)
	  Lentils
	  Dried beans
		Vegetable
		All vegetables may be used without restriction; especially popular are:
		  Onions
		  Spinach
		  Sorrel leaves
		  Radishes
		  Broccoli
		  Cucumbers
		  Carrots
		  Chicory
		  Potatoes: white and sweet
		  Green peppers
		  Tomatoes
		  Cabbage
		  Beets
		  Turnips
		Borscht (a meatless soup containing meat stock, beets and other vegetables, and sour cream; or with meat, beets and other vegetables, and sour cream)
		Schav (a soup containing spinach or sorrel leaves)
		Latkes (potato pancakes)
		Fruit
		All fruits may be used without restriction; especially popular are:
		  Oranges
		  Grapefruit
		  Apples
		  Peaches
		  Pears
		  Apricots
		  Dried fruits
			Brown rice
			Oatmeal
			Barley
			Millet
			Egg noodles
			Crusty rolls
			Rye bread
			Pumpernickel bread
			White seed rolls
			Challah (braided egg bread)
			Matzo (flat unleavened bread)
			Bulke (light yeast roll)
			Farfel (grated noodle dough)
			Kasha (buckwheat groats)
			Kloese (dumplings)
			Bagels (doughnut-shaped hard yeast rolls)
			Blintzes (thin, filled, and rolled pancakes)
			Cakes and pastries:
			  Leckach
			  Strudel
			  Teiglach
			  Kuchen
			  Bubke
			  Sponge cake
			  Cheesecake
			  Macaroons
			  Hamantashen
			Lukshen (noodles)
				Butter (unsalted preferred)
				Sour cream
				Cream cheese
				Beef and chicken fat
				Vegetable oil and shortening
				Preserves
				Pickles and relishes
				Soft drinks
				Wine (sabbath and holidays)
				Coffee
				Tea

special Sabbath dishes were mentioned previously.

2. *Passover.* During the 8-day ceremonial festival held in the spring, the use of leavened bread is prohibited. Rather, an unleavened bread, matzo, is eaten and all baked products are prepared from a flour of ground matzo (matzo meal) or potato starch leavened with egg white. Observance of Passover necessitates an additional two sets of dishes, since those that have had contact with leavened foods cannot be used. Consequently, an Orthodox Jewish family needs four sets of dishes, one each for meat and milk meals during Passover and one each for these meals at other times.

3. *Fasting days.* Yom Kippur (the Day of Atonement), occurring 10 days after the Jewish New Year in September, is a day of fasting. No food or drink is consumed for 25 to 26 hours (depending on sunset). The Fast of Esther, usually observed by only the very pious, is another holy day.

Intervention. Because of the restriction on combining meat and milk, the consumption of milk by children of Jewish families that rigidly observe the dietary laws may be inadequate. Encourage its use at breakfast and the dairy meal, keeping in mind, however, that the incidence of lactose intolerance is high among the Jewish population. Explain that cream cheese is not a milk substitute and discuss the use of other cheeses that are high in protein and calcium content. Since all kosher meat is expensive, suggest the use of the less expensive cuts and use of other sources of protein, such as fish and cheese. Discourage the excessive use of delicatessen-type meats, such as corned beef, pastrami, and salami, because of their high sodium and fat content. Stress the need to increase the variety of vegetables consumed, including more green leafy and yellow vegetables. Deemphasize the use of rich pastries and provide ideas for substitute desserts, such as milk puddings and ice cream or ice milk for dairy meals and fruit for meat meals. Fruit juice can also serve as a beverage for meat meals rather than soft drinks.

Islam

Assessment. The Islamic religion prohibits the consumption of these foods:

1. Pork, animal shortening, blood, and gelatin
2. Other animal meats unless slaughtered according to a prescribed ritual. Many Muslims will eat the kosher meat and poultry slaughtered by the Jewish ritual. Freshwater fish are exempted from the slaughtering ritual and are allowed in the diet.
3. Alcoholic beverages and alcohol-containing products, including flavoring extracts. The drinking of stimulants, such as coffee and tea, is also discouraged.

Vegetarian

Assessment. A lacto-ovo-vegetarian diet (milk, eggs, and plant foods) is recommended for Seventh-Day Adventists, who are committed to a philosophy of healthful living. Other religious groups who practice vegetarianism include adherents of Hinduism, Brahmanism, Buddhism, and Jainism, whose basic tenets involve the preservation of animal life because of a belief in transmigration of souls. Some Roman Catholic religious communities, such as the Trappists and Carthusians, follow a simple agriculturally based lifestyle that excludes the consumption of meat.

The Zen macrobiotic diet is an outgrowth of the interpretation of Zen Buddhism and was introduced into the United States and Europe by the late Japanese writer, George Ohsawa. The goals of this rigid nutritional system are largely spiritual, seeking to balance Yin (centrifugal forces) and Yang (centripetal forces) in all aspects of life, including diet. Ohsawa maintained that by following his principle, one could ward off all human illnesses. Self-treatment of disease is common among his followers, and medical consultation is discouraged.

Vegetarian diets are discussed in detail in Chapter 20.

Intervention. Be knowledgeable of the characteristic food habits and the beliefs and value systems that support cultural or religious beliefs. Place emphasis on the desirable features of the established food pattern and on methods of food preparation that preserve maximum food values. Attempt to change only those that are not compatible with good nutrition and good health.

REVIEW QUESTIONS AND ACTIVITIES

1. Identify six factors that may influence the degree to which immigrants to the United States retain their traditional dietary practices.
2. Identify the staple food of most Asian countries.
3. Compare the use of cereal grains and animal protein foods among the different countries of Europe and Asia.
4. Identify the ethnic groups in which lactose intolerance is a common problem, and describe the dietary advice that you would give for dealing with this problem.
5. Describe the dietary advice that you would give to assure adequacy of essential amino acids for clients whose dietary pattern includes little animal protein.
6. Identify the two food groups of the Basic Four Food Groups from which there is limited consumption in the traditional Asian diet.
7. Describe the food preparation methods used by Asians and the implications of these methods for the nutritional value of food.
8. What changes would you recommend in the regional diets of the south and southwest with regard to characteristic food choices and methods of food preparation?
9. What problems in dietary adjustment would you anticipate for a Puerto Rican family who just came to the United States? A Cuban family?
10. Identify the ethnic groups that ascribe to the hot–cold theory of foods and disease, and discuss the significance of this belief for nursing intervention.
11. How do the traditional diets of Italians and Middle and Near Easterners compare with regard to foods used and methods of food preparation?
12. Describe the basic foods consumed in the traditional diets of American Indians and Eskimos. Discuss the influence of the use of foods common to the typical American diet on the nutritional health of these two groups.

13. Discuss the role of kosher foods in relation to Orthodox Jewish dietary practices, including foods that are inherently kosher, foods that require special processing in order to be kosher, foods that are forbidden, and foods that must not be combined at the same meal.

14. How do the dietary practices of Muslims and Seventh-Day Adventists differ from those of Orthodox Jews?

15. Select the ethnic group that is most prevalent in your area:
    a. Plan a day's menu that meets the criteria of the Basic Four Food Groups for an adult.
    b. Adjust the menu so that it is appropriate for a child.

16. Interview a client from one of the ethnic groups described and compare the actual food practices of the client with those described.

17. Survey the food markets in your community and identify those that offer ethnic foods.

REFERENCES

1. McLemore SD: Racial and Ethnic Relations in America. Boston, Allyn and Bacon, 1980.
2. Thernstrom S, ed: Harvard Encyclopedia of American Ethnic Groups. Cambridge, Mass, Harvard University Press, 1980.
3. Knight MA: Nutrition influences of Mexican-American foods in Arizona. J Am Diet Assoc 55:557, 1969.
4. Larson LB, Dodds JM, Massoth DM, et al.: Nutritional status of children of Mexican-American migrant families. J Am Diet Assoc 64:29, 1974.
5. Harwood A: The hot–cold theory of disease: Implications for treatment of Puerto Rican patients. JAMA 216:1153, 1971.
6. Anderson O, Dibble MV, Turkki PR, et al.: Nutrition in Health and Disease, ed 17. Philadelphia, JB Lippincott, 1982, p 262.
7. Moore WM, Silverberg MM, Read MS: Nutrition, Growth, and Development of North American Indian Children. Washington, DC, DHEW Publication No. (NIH) 72–26, 1972.
8. Bass MA, Wakefield LM: Nutrient intake and food patterns of Indians on Standing Rock Reservation. J Am Diet Assoc 64:36, 1974.

BIBLIOGRAPHY

Crane NT, Green NR: Food habits and food preferences of Vietnamese refugees living in northern Florida. J Am Diet Assoc 76:591, 1980.

Day M-L, Lentner M, Jaquez S: Food acceptance patterns of Spanish-speaking new Mexicans. J Nutr Educ 10:121, 1978.

Feitelson M, Fiedler K: Kosher dietary laws and children's food preferences: Guide to a camp menu plan. J Am Diet Assoc 81:453, 1982.

Fidanza F: Changing patterns of food consumption in Italy. J Am Diet Assoc 77:133, 1980.

Fitzgerald TK: Southern folks' eating habits ain't what they used to be—If they ever were. Nutr Today 14(4):16, 1979.

Grivetti LE, Paquette MB: Nontraditional ethnic food choices among first generation Chinese in California. J Nutr Educ 10:109, 1978.

Hertzler AA, Wenkam W, Standal B: Classifying cultural food habits and meanings. J Am Diet Assoc 80:421, 1983.

Jerome W, Kandel R, Pelto G: Nutritional anthropology: Contemporary approaches to diet and culture. Pleasantville, NY, Redgrave Pub. 1980.

Kuhnlein HV, Calloway DH, Harland BF: Composition of traditional Hopi foods. J Am Diet Assoc 75:37, 1979.

Nalbandian A, Bergan JG, Brown PT: Three generations of Americans: Food habits and dietary status. J Am Diet Assoc 79:694, 1981.

Smith LK: Mexican-American views of Anglo medical and dietetic practice. J Am Diet Assoc 74:463, 1979.

Toma RB, Curry ML: North Dakota Indians' traditional foods. J Am Diet Assoc 76:589, 1980.

Whang J: Chinese traditional food therapy. J Am Diet Assoc 78:55, 1981.

Wilson CS: Food customs and nurture: An annotated bibliography on sociocultural and biocultural aspects of nutrition. J Nutr Educ 11(4) [Suppl] 1979.

CHAPTER 20

Alternative Dietary Practices

Objectives

After completion of this chapter, the student will be able to:

1. Distinguish among the overall dietary patterns of the five major categories of vegetarians.

2. Design a teaching plan for assisting an adult lacto-ovo-vegetarian to select a nutritionally adequate diet, and adapt the teaching plan so that it is appropriate for an adult vegan and an infant vegan.

3. Differentiate among natural, organic, and health foods.

4. Evaluate common claims or fallacies related to each of the following topics: (a) nutrient content of the food supply, (b) need for dietary supplements, (c) natural vs synthetic vitamins and minerals, (d) organic vs chemical fertilizers, (e) curative powers of specific foods, and (f) detrimental nature of food chemicals.

5. Develop a nursing care plan for the nutritional management of a client who practices pica (specifically clay eating).

A number of current diets and food practices are sometimes used as alternatives to those considered traditional or typical of most Americans. In recent years both vegetarian and health food diets have gained popularity. It is estimated that there are 6 million vegetarians in the United States, and the number is growing. The upsurge of interest in the practice cannot be attributed to any one specific cause but rather to a blend of religious, ethical, health-related, ecologic, and economic influences. In some cases, adoption of these patterns may reflect misguided and potentially dangerous faddism. The new vegetarians are not a homogeneous group in their motivations, nor are they homogeneous in the type of diet they adopt. The patterns vary from those that are nutritionally adequate to those that are totally inadequate. Many but not all vegetarians use health foods as well. The rise in interest in health foods stems largely from concerns related to pollution of the environment and contamination of the food supply associated with the use of pesticides, chemical fertilizers, and food additives. Pica is another nontraditional practice, although not new. Vegetarian diets, health food diets, and the practice of pica are explored in this chapter.

Content related to health foods and vegetarian diets in this chapter was adapted from Lewis CM: Food Fads and Vegetarian Diets (self-instructional packages prepared pursuant to contract 223–76–8200 with the Food and Drug Administration, DHEW, and distributed through the Health Sciences Consortium, University of North Carolina, Chapel Hill, NC).

VEGETARIAN DIETS

Assessment

▶ The term **vegetarian** refers to the elimination of animal foods (meat, dairy products, and eggs) from the diet and the use of plant foods, including vegeta-

---

TABLE 20–1
CATEGORIES OF VEGETARIAN DIETS

Classification	Foods Allowed	Foods Eliminated
No red meat vegetarian	Fish, poultry, dairy products, eggs, plant foods	Beef, veal, pork, lamb
Lacto-ovo-vegetarian	Dairy products, eggs, plant foods	All meat
Lacto-vegetarian	Dairy products, plant foods	Meat and eggs
Ovo-vegetarian	Eggs, plant foods	Meat and dairy products
Vegan (strict or pure vegetarian)	Plant foods only	All animal foods (meat, dairy products, eggs)

---

bles, fruits, whole grain or enriched bread and cereal, legumes (dry peas, beans, lentils), yeast, nuts and nutlike seeds, vegetable and nut oils, sugars, and syrups. Determine the specific dietary practice in clients who tell you they are vegetarians, since in actual practice, vegetarianism reflects a variety of diet categories. For example, the elimination of animal foods varies from the avoidance of red meat only to total elimination of animal foods. Some diets classified as vegetarian restrict all meat but allow dairy products and eggs. The three most common types of vegetarian diets are summarized in descending order of degree of restriction in Table 20–1.

Two additional categories that depict extreme forms of vegetarianism are the fruitarian, who consumes largely fruits, and the Zen macrobiotic (see Chap. 19), who may follow any one of ten diet levels, with the highest level containing only cereals and tea. Assess the diet of these clients carefully, since dietary inadequacy can be severe.

Potential Health Benefits of Vegetarian Diets.
There is some evidence to suggest that reliance on plant dietaries may, over a period of time, significantly reduce the incidence of several nutrition-related disorders: obesity, heart disease, hypertension, cancer, osteoporosis, and some gastrointestinal disorders. Since much of the supporting data are epidemiologic in nature and contradictory data exist in some areas, further studies are needed to clarify these relationships.

Since plant foods are low in kilocalories and high in fiber, the vegetarian diet (particularly the vegan diet) tends to be low in kilocalories and rather bulky. In order to maintain body weight, the vegetarian must consume larger quantities of food than if consuming kilocalories in a more concentrated form, as in animal foods. Some studies show that vegetarians tend to be leaner than nonvegetarians, and those who adopt a vegetarian diet usually lose weight rather than gain weight.[1,2] Although there may be an increase in energy output associated with

the altered lifestyle, no data on this relationship are currently available. Other studies have found no difference between the weights of vegetarians and nonvegetarians, however.[3]

Seventh-Day Adventists, who have traditionally practiced a lacto-ovo or vegan diet, have a lower mortality rate from heart disease than has the general population, according to some studies.[4] Although their longer life may be partially due to abstinence from smoking, the eating pattern may also be a factor. The blood cholesterol level (a major indicator of coronary risk) tends to be lower in vegetarians than in nonvegetarians,[5] and the serum cholesterol level tends to be lower in pure vegetarians than in lacto-ovo-vegetarians. The blood cholesterol level in the vegetarian may be related to two characteristics of the diet: (1) the modified fat intake (i.e., intake of less total fat, saturated fat, and cholesterol and use of polyunsaturated fat) and (2) the high fiber intake. Other studies have suggested that vegetarians tend to have lower blood pressures than those eating a conventional diet.[6-8] The intake of foods from animal sources appears to be significantly associated with an increase in blood pressure.

There are data to suggest that death rates from most cancers are lower in Seventh-Day Adventists than in the general population.[4,9] Although abstinence from alcohol and tobacco may be related to this finding, the vegetarian diet pattern may also be important. The diet pattern of vegetarians (low in kilocalories, fat, and refined foods and high in fiber) should theoretically provide a protective effect. For example, some studies have shown positive correlations in the etiology of cancer at certain sites, especially the breast and colon, with diets high in kilocalories (leading to obesity), fat, and refined foods and low in fiber.

Other research suggests that vegetarians are less prone to osteoporosis than are those consuming meat, since studies have shown greater bone densities in vegetarians than in nonvegetarians. A recent study showed that lacto-ovo-vegetarians have about half the bone loss after age 60 years experienced by those who consume meat.[10] One hypothesis given for this finding is that vegetarians (who eat predominantly an alkaline ash diet) require less dissolution of bone to provide the alkaline components (e.g., calcium) needed to buffer acids associated with eating an acid ash diet. Meat is the primary dietary source of acid ash. Another possibility is the potential for negative calcium balance and probable bone loss in association with a long-term high protein intake.[11]

Epidemiologic evidence suggests that a high-fiber diet (characteristic of a vegetarian diet) may be effective in the prevention of certain gastrointestinal disorders, such as hiatal hernia, gallstones, diverticular disease, hemorrhoids, polyps, and appendicitis.[12] These relationships remain to be substantiated.

Potential Health Hazards of Vegetarian Diets.
The major potential health hazard associated with vegetarian diets is nutritional deficiency associated with an inadequate consumption of kilocalories and essential nutrients. In addition to kilocalories, nutrients that may be only marginally present (or totally absent) in vegetarian diets are protein (both in quality and quantity), vitamins (especially vitamin B_{12}, vitamin D, and riboflavin), and minerals (especially calcium, iron, and zinc). The relative content of these nutrient factors in animal and plant foods is summarized in Table 20–2.

Kilocalories.
Assess the kilocalorie level of the vegetarian client's diet. Since many plant foods are low in kilocalories and high in fiber, a relatively bulky diet results, especially with a vegan diet. Consequently, the volume of food required to meet kilocalorie needs can become a problem unless the selection is well planned. Assess also the client's protein status. A major health hazard associated with inadequate kilocalorie consumption is the body's preferential use of dietary protein for energy rather than for growth or maintenance, leading to protein–calorie malnutrition. Recent concern has been expressed about the increased incidence of protein–calorie

malnutrition among vegetarian children, particularly children of the new vegetarians. Some studies report anthropometric data in some of the children that are below standards.[13]

Protein.
Both the quantity and quality of protein can be of concern, especially for the strict vegetarian, unless a variety of foods is selected. With respect to protein quantity, the RDA for adults is 0.8 g/kg of body weight (or 56 g for a 70-kg man and 46 g for a 58-kg woman). This allowance, based on the average protein requirements for adults with corrections made for individual variation and efficiency of protein utilization, assumes that protein will be provided by a mixture of plant and animal sources. However, when foods of plant origin supply all of the dietary protein, the client must consume a larger quantity to compensate for the less efficient digestion of many plant products. No figures have been published as to the exact amount.

Plant foods are less concentrated sources of protein than are animal foods, and the largest quantity is found in legumes (dry peas, beans, lentils), nuts, and nutlike seeds. Lesser amounts are present in cereal grains, vegetables, and fruit. Although soybean milk is also a good protein source, the quality of the protein contained in some brands is not equivalent to that in cow's milk. An adult vegetarian should have no problems consuming an adequate amount, but be aware that pregnant women, infants, and small children, whose requirements relative to body weight are greater, may get an insufficient quantity from a vegan diet.

Protein quality is determined by the content of essential amino acids in a food. Animal protein foods supply all of the essential amino acids in optimal amounts for body needs and are said to be of high biologic value. In contrast, plant protein foods are of low biologic value because they contain insufficient quantities of one or more essential amino acids. However, the protein from some legumes (particularly soybeans and chick peas) is almost equivalent in quality to animal protein. Plant foods vary in the specific amino acids available in limited quantity

---

TABLE 20–2
NUTRITIVE CONTENT OF ANIMAL FOODS RELATIVE TO PLANT FOODS

Nutrient Factor	Content in Animal Foods Relative to Plant Foods
Kilocalories	More concentrated in animal than plant foods
Protein (*quantity* and *quality*)	Greater *quantity* of protein and higher *quality* protein in animal than in plant foods
Vitamins Vitamin B_{12} Vitamin D Riboflavin	Animal foods are the *only* source of vitamin B_{12} and of the natural form of vitamin D (egg yolk, butter, liver, some fish); animal foods provide significant amounts of riboflavin, with dairy products and organ meats the best source
Minerals Zinc Iron Calcium	More concentrated in animal than plant foods: all animal foods are good sources of *zinc;* meat and eggs are the best sources of *iron;* dairy products are the best sources of *calcium*

TABLE 20–3
LIMITING AMINO ACIDS IN PLANT FOODS

Essential Amino Acids	Generally Limited	Limiting Amino Acids in Specific Foods
Leucine	Lysine	Cereal grains: lysine
Isoleucine	Methionine	
Lysine	Tryptophan	Legumes (except peanuts): methionine (and occasionally tryptophan)
Threonine		
Methionine		
Tryptophan		Nuts and seeds: lysine (and occasionally tryptophan)
Phenylalanine		
Valine		
Histidine[a]		Leafy vegetables: methionine

[a] Essential for children; *may* be essential for adults.

▶ (referred to as **limiting amino acids**). A summary of the essential amino acids, those generally limited in plant foods, and limiting amino acids in specific plant foods is found in Table 20–3.

Vitamins. Evaluate the client's vitamin B_{12} status. Animal foods contain the only practical source of vitamin B_{12}, and this vitamin may be totally lacking in vegan diets. Vitamin B_{12} is required for cell division (including blood cells) and for normal nerve function. A deficiency is manifest as anemia (macrocytic) and the more serious condition, spinal cord degeneration. Deficiency may be a problem in clients following a vegan diet for a prolonged period. Since dietary excesses of vitamin B_{12} are stored, an adult who has ingested animal foods for a lifetime will have sufficient liver storage to last for a number of years. The body's conservation of the vitamin via enterohepatic circulation may explain the extended period of time prior to manifestations of symptomology in some clients. In other cases, the high folic acid content of vegetarian diets may mask the anemia, resulting in a failure to diagnose the deficiency until irreversible nerve damage has occurred. A recent study documented low blood levels of vitamin B_{12} in vegetarians who did not take a supplement.[14]

Vitamin D, necessary for the use of calcium and phosphorus, is another nutrient not contained in plant foods and normally obtained from two major sources: (1) vitamin D-fortified milk, and (2) conversion of a derivative of cholesterol in the skin to the vitamin. Assess the client's sunlight exposure. Unless there is daily exposure, vitamin D deficiency may be a problem for the vegan. There are several reports of vitamin D-deficiency rickets in vegetarian children.[15] Milk products are the most significant source of riboflavin for many people, and vegans may be susceptible to deficiency of this vitamin.

Minerals. Although calcium, iron, and zinc are present in significant amounts in some plant foods, recall that they are absorbed less well from plant sources than from animal foods. Whole grains and some leafy vegetables contain phytates and/or oxalates that may combine with the minerals to form insoluble compounds that are not absorbed. Large amounts of plant fiber may also decrease mineral absorption. At present, however, there is no evidence to indicate that there is an increased incidence of mineral deficiencies associated with diminished absorption, nor is information available about possible long-term effects. A recent report suggests that some vegetarians may be marginally deficient in zinc,[16] and there is evidence of low iron stores in vegetarian young women.[17]

Intervention
Advise the client to increase the amounts of foods consumed from each of the major food groups to assure kilocalorie adequacy and to apply the concept of protein complementation to assure protein quality.

Since plant foods vary in the specific limiting amino acids, foods with complementary amino acids can be combined at the same meal to produce a balanced mixture with an amino acid pattern equivalent to animal protein. Note the following example of protein complementation:

Cereal grains: ↓ Lysine and ↑ methionine (and contain adequate amounts of other essential amino acids)

Legumes: ↑ Lysine and ↓ methionine (and contain adequate amounts of other essential amino acids)

Cereal grains + legumes = amino acid pattern of ↑ biologic value

The foods do not have to be combined as a mixed dish, only eaten at the same meal.

Both lacto-ovo-vegetarians and vegans can use protein complementation to assure adequate protein quality. Lacto-ovo-vegetarians can eat milk or eggs at each meal to supply the amino acids missing in plant foods, or, like vegans, they can combine plant foods with complementary amino acid patterns (Table 20–4). Lappe offers a more complete guide to complementary protein patterns.[18] To safeguard protein quality, tell the vegan client to eat a variety of plant sources at each meal, selecting from cereal grains, legumes, nuts, seeds, vegetables, and fruits.

TABLE 20–4
COMPLEMENTARY PROTEIN PATTERNS

Food Combinations	Examples
Grains + legumes (*Note:* a blend of soybean flour and cereal malts in suitable proportions is almost equal in nutritive value to milk protein for children)	Beans and rice, beans and corn, blackeyed peas and rice, baked beans and brown bread, wheat bread and peanuts
Seeds and nuts + legumes	Sesame seeds and soybeans and sesame seeds and chick peas
Grains and milk products	Cereal and milk

Meat analogs can serve as an alternate source of protein for vegetarians. Meat analogs are plant protein products (legumes, nuts, seeds, or grains) that have been texturized, flavored, and fortified with nutrients to resemble meat, such as beef, ham, chicken, fish, sausage, bacon, or frankfurters. The soybean is the most common plant source because of the relatively high biologic value of its protein. Analogs are available in an increasing number of markets in frozen, dehydrated, or canned forms. Some are designed as meat extenders (e.g., to add to ground beef), whereas others are total meat replacements. Although not essential to a well-planned vegetarian diet, they can facilitate meal planning and preparation. However, some contain egg white or nonfat dry milk (to improve quality) and would not be suitable for vegan diets. The ingredient label lists the contents. The availability of analogs allows those individuals who find it difficult to give up meat to follow a degree of vegetarianism.

Plant protein products can be formulated to meet whatever standards are specified and thus can be made to provide the known nutrients in animal protein sources. The labels should be checked for nutritional adequacy since, at present, vitamin and mineral content may differ from the meats they simulate. A potential advantage of analogs is their lower content of fat and kilocalories in comparison to their animal counterparts. Disadvantages are their relatively high cost (less than meat but greater than conventional plant foods) and their high sodium content, which often precludes their use by individuals who must restrict dietary sodium.

Recommend the use of foods that contain adequate amounts of other nutrients that are likely to be deficient or else advise that a supplement be taken (Table 20–5). Vitamin D supplementation is especially important for children and pregnant and lactating women, and the same criteria for iron supplementation described in Chapters 14 and 15 apply. Counsel vegetarians not only to consume good food sources of iron but also to include a good food source of ascorbic acid to enhance iron absorption. Children and pregnant and lactating women may also require

a calcium supplement. Although soybean milk or nut-based milks are alternative calcium sources for the vegan, the calcium content is not equivalent to that of cow's milk unless it is fortified with calcium. Commercially prepared soy- or sesame seed-based milk are usually, but not always, fortified with calcium, vitamins A and D, and vitamin B_{12}. Homemade milk substitutes, usually prepared from soy, are rarely fortified with vitamins or minerals.

Suggested Vegetarian Diet. Use the traditional Basic Four Food Groups to serve as a foundation for an adequate diet for vegetarians. The major difference in application to the vegetarian diet is in relation to the meat–poultry–fish–beans and milk and cheese groups. Suggest these four general changes for vegetarians (lacto-ovo-vegetarian *or* vegan):

1. Increase the total amounts of food eaten from all food groups to supply adequate kilocalories and other nutrients
2. Reduce substantially the intake of foods of low nutrient density (the fats–sweets–alcohol group)
3. Substitute whole grain cereals for refined types
4. Select a wide variety of foods chosen from legumes, nuts, seeds, meat analogs, whole grains, vegetables, and fruits

Refer to Table 20–6 for specific adjustments in the Basic Four Food Groups for a lacto-ovo-vegetarian diet and the additional changes necessary for a vegan diet. Smith[19] gives a guide for the specific number of servings of food from the food groups for various age groups for the lacto-ovo-vegetarian. A sample 1-day menu for a vegan, with possible modifications for a lacto-ovo-vegetarian, is given in Table 20–7.

A well chosen lacto-ovo-vegetarian diet is adequate to meet the nutritional needs of all age groups. Vegan diets are not recommended during periods of growth. Recognize, however, that nurses may well encounter vegetarian families in which the infants and children are also following a strict vegetarian regimen. Follow the general guidelines outlined below for feeding an infant.

Although breastfeeding is the method of choice, a properly fortified soy formula can promote satisfactory growth and development. The formula must contain adequate amounts of kilocalories and critical nutrients, such as protein, calcium, iron, riboflavin, and vitamins B_{12}, A, and D. No supplements are needed until the child is 4 to 6 months of age. The infant should be gradually introduced to a variety of strained legumes, cereals, vegetables, and fruit, later moving to mashed and chopped foods when the teeth erupt. Foods should be selected for their nutritional value, giving special attention to foods that provide iron, protein, and vitamins A, B, and C. If not included in the formula, iron supple-

TABLE 20–5
ALTERNATIVE NUTRIENT SOURCES FOR THE VEGETARIAN DIET

Nutrient Factors	Food Groups[a]				
	Meat Alternates	Milk and Cheese	Vegetable–Fruit	Bread–Cereal	Other
	[Legumes (dry peas, beans, and lentils), nuts and nutlike seeds, peanut butter, meat analogs, eggs]	[Regular milk, cheese, soybean milk]	[Fresh, canned, frozen, or dried fruits and vegetables]	[Enriched or whole grain bread and cereal]	
Kilocalories	V:[b] Omit eggs	V: Omit regular milk and cheese			
Protein (quantity and quality)	V: Omit eggs and use mutual complementation for protein quality	V: Omit regular milk and cheese			
Vitamin B_{12}	L-O-V:[b] Eggs V: Meat analogs fortified with vitamin B_{12}	L-O-V: Regular milk and cheese V: Soybean milk fortified with B_{12}		V: Cereals fortified with vitamin B_{12}	V: Medicinal supplement; nutritional yeast grown on vitamin B_{12}-enriched media; seaweed, algae, and fermented soy products (tempeh, miso, and soy sauce are not considered reliable sources)
Vitamin D		L-O-V: Regular milk and cheese V: Fortified soybean milk		Some cereals fortified with vitamin D	Margarine fortified with vitamin D; exposure to sunlight; medicinal supplement; cod liver oil
Riboflavin	All meat alternates V: Omit eggs	L-O-V: Regular milk and cheese V: Soybean milk	Green leafy vegetables, asparagus, broccoli, brussels sprouts, okra, winter squash, avocado	Whole grain or enriched bread and cereal	Yeast; wheat germ
Calcium	V: Legumes (especially navy beans and soybeans), nuts and nutlike seeds (especially almonds, filberts, sesame, and sunflower seeds), calcium-precipitated tofu	L-O-V: Regular milk and cheese V: Fortified soybean milk	Largest amount in green leafy vegetables (especially kale, collards, mustard, turnip, and dandelion greens); moderate amounts in other vegetables (especially okra, broccoli, spoon cabbage, rutabagas); most dried fruits		V: Medicinal supplement
Iron	All meat alternates V: Omit eggs		Green leafy vegetables; dried fruits	Whole grain or enriched bread/cereal	Medicinal supplement; brewer's yeast
Zinc	All meat alternates V: Omit eggs	L-O-V: Regular milk and cheese		Whole grain bread and cereal	
Iodine					Iodized salt in low iodine areas (Great Lakes region, Ohio Valley, Texas, western mountain areas), seaweed

[a] Increase intake of foods from all groups except fats–sweets–alcohol as needed to maintain weight.
[b] L-O-V, lacto-ovo-vegetarian; V, vegan.

TABLE 20–6
VEGETARIAN DIET BASED ON THE BASIC FOUR FOOD GROUPS

Conventional Basic Four	Lacto-ovo-vegetarian Diet	Vegan Diet
Meat–poultry–fish–beans group Foods included: Meat (i.e., red meat, fish, poultry), eggs, legumes, nuts, peanut butter, and seeds Number of servings: 2 (one additional serving for pregnant and lactating women) Size of servings: Cooked meat, 2–3 oz.; eggs, 2–3; cooked legumes, 1–2¼ c; nuts and seeds, ½–1½ c; peanut butter, ¼–⅓ c (smaller servings for children)	Meat and alternates group *Delete* meat, fish, poultry *Increase* consumption of meat alternates including legumes (especially soybeans), nuts (especially peanuts, almonds, and cashews), seeds, eggs *Add* meat analogs if desired	Meat and alternates group *Delete* meat, fish, poultry, and eggs *Increase further* the consumption of meat alternates (especially soybeans), nuts (especially peanuts, almonds, and cashews), and seeds *Add* meat analogs if desired *Use* the concept of *protein complementation* by using a variety of legumes and whole grains, with some seeds or nuts in meals each day
Milk and cheese group Foods included: Whole, skim, nonfat, low-fat, evaporated; cheese; ice cream; yoghurt Number of servings: Adults, 2 c; children 10 years and under, 2–3 c; pre-adolescents and adolescents, 4 c; pregnant women, 3 c; lactating women, 4 c; pregnant adolescents, 5–6 c Calcium equivalent of 1 c milk: Yoghurt, 1 c; cottage cheese, 2 c; ice-cream, 1½ c; cheddar or Swiss cheese, 1⅓ oz	Milk and cheese group *Increase* consumption of milk and cheese, giving special emphasis to low-fat forms as needed to maintain weight	Milk and cheese group *Delete* milk and cheese *Add* soybean milk that has been fortified with vitamin B_{12}, calcium, vitamin A, and vitamin D (take a vitamin B_{12} supplement if no foods are used that are fortified with the vitamin)
Vegetable–fruit Foods included: All fresh, canned, frozen, or dried fruits and vegetables, to include a daily source of vitamin C (e.g., citrus fruit, melon, strawberries, tomato), and a source of vitamin A every other day (e.g., deep yellow-orange or very dark green fruits and vegetables) Number of servings: 4 Size of servings: ½ c or one medium portion (e.g., 1 orange) for adults with smaller servings (¼–⅓ c) for children	Vegetable–fruit *Use a variety* of fruits and vegetables *Include* a food high in ascorbic acid content at each meal to enhance iron absorption	Vegetable–fruit *Increase* consumption of vegetables and fruits giving emphasis to variety, increased use of green leafy vegetables, and increased use of dried fruits) *Include* a food high in ascorbic acid content at each meal to enhance iron absorption
Bread–cereal Foods included: Whole grain or enriched bread, cereals, and pastas Number of servings: 4 Size of servings: 1 slice bread; 1 oz cold cereal; ½ c cooked cereal, with smaller servings for children	Bread–cereal *Increase* consumption of breads and cereals giving special emphasis to whole grains as needed to maintain weight	Bread–cereal Same as lacto-ovo-vegetarian
Other foods Foods included: Additional servings of foods from the above groups, sugar, fats, oils, and alcohol Number of servings: As needed to maintain weight	Other foods *Reduce consumption* of empty calorie foods from fats–sweets–alcohol group	Other foods Same as lacto-ovo-vegetarian

mentation should begin at 4 months of age with iron-fortified infant cereal or a medicinal source. Calcium and vitamin D supplements should also be given, since their intake drops as milk intake declines with the introduction of solid foods.

At weaning, the soybean formula or a properly fortified soybean milk should be given by cup. In addition to the soybean milk, combinations of legumes and cereals should be fed at each meal for their complementary amino acid patterns, since either food alone will supply inadequate protein. The child's limited stomach capacity presents a major problem at weaning. Since the infant's and young child's need for kilocalories and other nutrients are much greater in relation to body weight than are the needs of the adult, relatively large quantities of food are necessary to support a satisfactory rate of growth. Monitor carefully the rate of growth of children in a vegan family to assure that adequate nutrients are being consumed. Using unprocessed foods to meet energy needs of infants and young children is a challenge, even for the professional.

TABLE 20–7
SAMPLE MENU FOR 1 DAY FOR VEGAN, WITH POSSIBLE MODIFICATIONS FOR A LACTO-OVO-VEGETARIAN

Meal	Vegan Diet	Lacto-ovo-vegetarian Modification
Breakfast	½ grapefruit	(same)
	Cooked whole wheat cereal with honey or molasses	(same)
	Fortified soybean milk	Cow's milk
		Egg
	Toasted wheat–soy bread	(same)
	Margarine	(same)
	Beverage[a]	(same)
Snack[b]		
Lunch	Navy bean soup	(same)
	Peanut butter sandwich on whole wheat bread	(same)
	Dried apricots	(same)
	Beverage	(same)
Snack		
Dinner	Pinto bean and rice casserole	Macaroni and cheese
	Cooked turnip greens	(same)
	Carrot–raisin salad	(same)
	Oatmeal bread	(same)
	Margarine	(same)
	Fresh peach	(same)
	Beverage	(same)

[a] Beverages could include coffee, tea, vegetable or fruit juice, vegetable broth, or milk (soybean milk for the vegan and cow's milk for the lacto-ovo-vegetarian).
[b] Snacks could include milk, fresh or dried fruit, nuts, or raw vegetables.

It is difficult to get young children to eat a sufficient volume of bulky foods, such as legumes, whole grains, seeds, and nuts in forms they can easily digest and to eat foods in precise proportional relationships. An increase in consumption of bulky plant foods is not considered advisable, and the inclusion of fortified soybean milk or cow's milk is recommended.

HEALTH FOOD DIETS

Assessment

Definitions. There are no traditional or official standards or definitions for health food, but the term generally includes organic and natural foods as well as some other types. These terms may be defined as follows:

▶ **Natural foods** are marketed as those foods that contain no added preservatives, emulsifiers, or artificial ingredients and that have not been processed or refined.

▶ **Organic foods** are those that are allegedly grown without agricultural chemicals (pesticides or fertilizers) and processed without chemicals or additives.

▶ **Health food** is a more inclusive term that includes organic or natural foods as well as dietetic, vegetarian, and other foods (some of which contain artificial chemicals). The connotation is that the foods are invested with special health-giving properties. The term includes conventional foods that have been subjected to less processing than usual (such as unhydrogenated nut butters and whole grain flours) and less conventional foods, such as brewer's yeast, pumpkin seed, wheat germ, and herb teas.

Health Food Fallacies and Facts. In recent years, the American food supply has often been characterized by misleading terminology. Foods that are considered "natural," "organic," and "health foods" are in some way perceived as safer, more nutritious, and somehow better for you than foods characterized as "processed" or "synthetic," or that contain "chemicals" and "additives." There has been a rapid rise in the health food industry and the health food diet pattern, sometimes predicated on misinformation about exaggerated claims of the virtues or hazards of a given food or diet. Many of the concerns expressed are legitimate and require continuing surveillance by existing regulatory bodies.

Three broad categories of fallacies provide the framework for the natural, organic, and health food diets. These fallacies are: (1) the food supply is nutritionally depleted, (2) some foods or nutrients are virtually miracle foods because of their curative powers, and (3) the food supply is poisoned with chemicals (food additives).[20] These are described below, along with facts related to each.

1. Fallacy. "The food supply is so nutritionally depleted (due to soil depletion and nutrient losses in food processing, transportation, storage, and cooking) that ordinary foods cannot supply an adequate amount of nutrients. Consequently, the population is suffering from widespread, subclinical nutritional deficiency, requiring daily supplementation with vitamins, minerals, and other dietary supplements. Natural forms of vitamins are superior in quality to synthetic forms. Additionally, organic fertilizers produce foods of superior nutritional quality."

Facts. There is no scientific evidence to support any of these claims. Let us look at each aspect of the first fallacy ("The food supply is nutritionally depleted") in more detail.

Nutrient Content of the Food Supply. Be aware that nutritional losses indeed occur in food handling, whether it is processed commercially or at home or stored in an unprocessed state. Although these losses occur with commercial food processing, transportation, and storage, modern technology minimizes nutrient losses, is safe, and is well standardized. Some nutrients lost in processing are replaced by enrichment (such as adding B vitamins and iron to white bread). However, there is some concern related to the low levels of some of the trace mineral elements (such as zinc and chromium) in highly processed foods. The rigid commercial processes applied in the freezing and canning of fruits and vegetables at their peak nutrient quality may result in foods that are nutritionally superior to similar foods prepared at home. Improper home processing and cooking techniques can seriously deplete nutritional values.

Need for Dietary Supplements. A varied diet selected from the Basic Four Food Groups will provide optimal nutrition for all age groups, with a few exceptions. Pregnant women require supplements of iron and possibly folic acid, infants also require a supplemental source of iron, and women during the child-bearing years as well as young children may need an iron supplement.

Natural vs Synthetic Vitamins and Minerals. Both natural and synthetic vitamins react similarly in the body. Further, all minerals are natural, since the same chemical elements are present in foods and in the earth. Interestingly, some products labeled "natural" are not necessarily so. Some natural or organic vitamins contain added synthetic compounds because natural extracts are too bulky for a pill or capsule. Moreover, organic and natural foods contain pesticide residues as do conventional foods, but the residues in both cases are within established levels.

Organic vs Chemical Fertilizers. There is no significant difference in the nutritional value of foods grown with organic fertilizers (animal manures, humus) and chemical fertilizers. The principal advantage of organic fertilizers is that they improve the physical properties of the soil. Since plants use only inorganic nutrients, organic fertilizers must be converted to inorganic compounds by soil bacteria before use. Fertilization affects quantity of yield, not quality. The nutritional properties of a plant are determined by genetic makeup—a plant will not grow in a nutrient-deficient soil. Except for mineral elements, the plant synthesizes its own nutrients rather than absorbing them from the soil in a preformed state. Some regional soil patterns do reflect deficiencies of some trace minerals not required by plants but essential for animals (e.g., iodine, fluorine). Should the plants absorb these nutrients, they serve as a suitable vehicle for entry into the food chain of animals that need the nutrients. These deficiencies are not due to soil depletion and are corrected by adding the lacking mineral to chemical fertilizers or to food or water (e.g., iodine to salt, fluorine to water). Organic fertilizers can only return to the soil those elements yielded in producing animal feed, which is then recycled through the animal to produce organic fertilizer.

Since there are no industry standards for natural, organic, and health foods, some foods sold as such are not as they are promoted. However, efforts are being made at the federal level to control the advertising of these foods.

Although the excessive use of chemical fertilizers has contributed to ecologic problems and the precepts underlying organic farming are useful, large-scale organic farming is impractical at the present time.

The nutritional superiority of whole grain breads and cereals over their refined counterparts is well recognized. However this superiority is in no way related to the type of fertilizer used. Rather, it is related to current regulatory systems that provide for addition of certain B vitamins and iron to refined products but not for the addition of the other nutrients lost in the refining process, such as trace minerals and vitamin E.

2. Fallacy. "Some foods or nutrients are virtually miracle foods because of their curative powers. A number of foods (e.g., whole grains, fertile eggs, granola cereal) and nutrients (especially vitamins A, C, and E) fall into this category."

Facts. While many of the foods are very nutritious, they do not have curative powers. For example, there is no scientific evidence that organically grown Chicosan rice is a treatment for cancer or that blackstrap molasses increases longevity.

The claims that massive doses of vitamin C will prevent or cure the common cold, that large doses of vitamin A over a prolonged period are beneficial in the treatment of acne vulgaris, and that vitamin E cures or prevents a variety of conditions (e.g., sterility, miscarriage, cancer) have not been substantiated by well-controlled clinical trials.

3. Fallacy. "The food supply is poisoned with chemicals (food additives)."

Facts. While there are valid concerns about the safety of the large numbers of additives present in the food supply, the issue is sometimes exaggerated or distorted. The inability to predict with certainty the absolute safety of any chemical (including food chemicals) creates doubt, fear, and anxiety. When chemicals once considered safe (such as cyclamates) are removed from the market based on new data, anxiety mounts further. Let us look at what is known about food additives.

Chemical Nature of Food. All foods in their natural state are mixtures of chemicals. Some of these chemicals are nutrients (carbohydrate, protein, fat, minerals, vitamins, and water). Others are nonnutrient substances, such as colors, flavors, emulsifiers, antioxidants, and chelating agents.

In addition to the naturally occurring chemicals, foods also contain additives, which are of two types. Intentional additives are those added to perform a specific function, such as to prevent spoilage or oxidation or improve nutritive value. In contrast, incidental additives are those that become part of the food secondary to their use in food production or processing and serve no functional purpose in the final food product. Potential sources are pesticides, fertilizers, adjuvants to animal feed, and packaging materials, such as polyvinyl chloride, that migrate from the wrapping to the food.

All food chemicals (those naturally occurring or added) are potentially toxic (i.e., capable of producing injury) but hazardous (i.e., with some probability that injury will result from their use) only in sufficiently large quantities. There are safe and unsafe doses of all chemicals, both natural and synthetic. Even naturally occurring chemicals in some foods are toxic if consumed in sufficiently large quantities. For example, arsenic is present in fish, goitrogenic substances are found in rutabagas and some other vegetables, solanine (a toxic alkaloid) is present in potatoes. Common table salt is toxic in doses three to five times the normal usage. Actually, more is known about the relative safety of food additives than about naturally occurring toxicants.[21]

Purposes of Additives. Although a large number of additives are used in food processing, they comprise only a small portion of the weight of food consumed. Many of the food additives are derived from natural sources (such as spices, natural flavoring and coloring compounds, or nutrients) or are closely related to chemical substances that occur in natural foodstuffs. About three fifths of food additives are artificial flavors and colors, emulsifiers, stabilizers, and thickeners whose main purpose is to make food more attractive. Other additives are used as preservatives, antioxidants, or as leavening, anti-staling, or mold-retarding agents. Table 20–8 provides a summary of the functions, purposes, and examples of food additives.

Regulatory Control of Food Additives. The use of additives in food is regulated by the Food and Drug Administration, which defines criteria and tolerance levels for additives and continually monitors their use.

Criteria to Be Met by Additives. All additives in food, including new ones proposed for use as well as those currently in use, must meet the following four criteria. The additive must be (1) of benefit to the consumer directly or indirectly, (2) used in the smallest amount needed to achieve the desired effect, (3) safe for intended use (i.e., with virtual certainty that no injury will result), and (4) free of carcinogenic properties. This latter criterion results from a specific government regulation (the Delaney clause) that bans the use of any additives found to be carcinogenic to test animals, even in massive quantities fed under extreme circumstances. The banning of cyclamates resulted from the application of this regulation. Each additive undergoes extensive testing with laboratory animals to meet criteria 3 and 4.

Tolerance Levels for Additives. Tolerance levels for additives (both intentional and incidental) that are considered safe are set by the Food and Drug Administration. The level refers to the amount of the chemical that can be present in a food. These minimal tolerance levels are set after extensive testing with laboratory animals and usually provide for a 100-fold margin of safety above the amount that proved harmless in test animals. In actual practice, the margin of safety may be more or less than 100, depending on the nature of the deleterious effects observed in test animals fed high doses of the substance, the scope of the toxicologic data available, and a judgment regarding the reliability of the available data.

Monitoring. Monitoring for the continued safety of additives is done continually to observe for deleterious effects that may emerge through experience with prolonged and varying conditions of use. Safety in the use of additives is also reappraised as warranted by advances in knowledge, increased sophistication of toxicity test procedures, and use of certain substances well beyond their anticipated exposure patterns. This continuous monitoring has resulted in changes in the use of some additives in recent years. Cyclamates and the colorants red dye #2 and #4 and carbon black have been removed from use because of hazardous effects in animals, even though there have been no observable effects in humans. Other additives are permitted in foods only under specified conditions and with limited levels of use.

TABLE 20-8
FUNCTIONS, PURPOSES, AND EXAMPLES OF INTENTIONAL FOOD ADDITIVES

Function	Purpose	Examples of Additives Used	Examples of Foods in Which Additive Is Used
To improve nutritive value	Restores nutrient values lost in processing or increases nutrient values above those naturally present	Potassium iodide, fluorine, vitamin D, thiamine, riboflavin, niacin, iron, vitamin A, vitamin C	Salt, water, milk, bread, cereal, margarine, fruit drinks
To enhance flavor	Increases taste appeal (and possibly food acceptance)—a variety of natural flavors and spices, and artificial flavors are used	Amylacetate, benzaldehyde, methylsalicylate, monosodium glutamate, citrus oils, spices (such as pepper, cloves, ginger), vanillin, and artificial flavors (mainly fruit flavors)	Soft drinks, bakery goods, ice cream, candy, sausage, fruit-flavored toppings, and gelatin
To maintain appearance, palatability and wholesomeness	Delays food spoilage due to microbial action and delays oxidation, which causes rancidity in fats and browning of fruits when cut and exposed to air	Sodium chloride, sodium benzoate, propionic acid and its calcium and sodium salts, potassium sorbate, chlorotetracycline, butylated hydroxyanisole (BHA), butylated hydroxytoluene (BHT), tocopherols (vitamin E), citric acid, ascorbic acid, sulfur dioxide	Pickles, salted meats, maraschino cherries, bread, cheese, antibiotic dip for fish and dressed poultry, vegetable oils and shortenings, potato chips, pudding and pie filling mixes, whipped topping mix, fruit (canned, frozen, dried)
To impart and maintain a desired consistency	Provides homogeneous consistency and texture (emulsifiers) and maintains smooth, uniform textures	Mono- and diglycerides, lecithin, vegetable gums (such as carob bean, guar, and carrageenin), gum arabic, agar-agar, methyl cellulose, pectin, gelatin, sodium alginate, dextrin	Salad dressings, margarine, butter, chocolate milk, evaporated milk, ice cream, cream cheese, jam and jelly, mixes (cake, pudding, pie filling, whipped topping), candy, frozen desserts, frozen whipped topping, baked goods (cakes, cookies, quick breads, crackers), processed cheese and cheese spreads, chocolate, soft drinks, beer
To control pH (acidity or alkalinity)	Reduces or increases the acidity or sourness of a food (buffers, acids, alkalis, neutralizing agents); substances are useful as leavening agents in baked goods, in controlling the texture of candy, in neutralizing sour cream to make butter, and in making fruits easier to peel for canning	Tartaric acid, potassium acid tartrate, sodium bicarbonate, citric acid, adipic acid, lactic acid	Baking powder, baked goods, gelatin desserts, soft drink mixes, fruit sherbets, processed cheese, and cheese spreads
To impart a desired and characteristic color	Increases attractiveness (and possibly food acceptance)—both natural and synthetic food colors are used; most colors used today are FD & C (a list of approved coal-tar derivatives) synthetic derivatives, since sufficient natural colors are not available	FD & C colors, beta-carotene, annatto, powders of chlorophyll, tomato, or beet	Butter, margarine, baked goods, soft drinks and soft drink mixes, candy, jam and jelly, fruit-flavored gelatin, cheese, ice cream, pudding and pie filling mixes, frankfurters
To serve as maturing and bleaching agents in milling and baking	Alters color of certain foods (e.g., certain cheeses and wheat flour—changes yellow pigment of wheat flour to white) and modifies gluten characteristics of wheat flour to improve baking results	Chlorine dioxide, nitrosyl chloride, chlorine, potassium bromate, potassium iodate	Certain cheeses, wheat flour
To perform other miscellaneous functions	Anticaking agents (to keep salts and powders free-flowing), flavor enhancers (to increase the effect of certain other kinds of flavors), humectants (to help retain moisture in certain foods), firming agents (to produce desirable crispiness or texture), curing agents (to give flavor and color to certain meats), sequestrants (to combine chemically with traces of metals naturally present in foods), and nonnutritive sweeteners	Calcium stearate, sodium silico aluminate, monosodium glutamate, sorbitol, glycerine, propylene glycol, alum, sodium nitrate and nitrite, sodium citrate, saccharin	Table salt, garlic salt, coconut, pickles, frankfurters and other sausages, dairy products, dietetic foods

Benefits vs Risks of Additives. The use of additives contributes to the quantity, quality, and safety of the food supply. Without their use, the scope of the food supply would be limited, and many aesthetic and convenience qualities would be lost. For example, baked goods would go stale overnight, canned fruits and vegetables would be mushy and discolored, table salt would harden.

Present evaluation and regulatory procedures provide practical assurance of the safety of additives. There is no available evidence to indicate that consumption of additives has endangered human health. However, present evaluation techniques do not insure absolute protection from injury. They do not totally eliminate the possibility of long-term effects of additives or synergistic relationships between themselves and other food chemicals. Limitations in testing procedures as well as the heterogeneity of the population (including individuals of all age groups and different physiologic states and food habits) preclude predictions of absolute safety under all conditions of use.

Although decisions about the use of additives must be based on assurance that their use will be safe (i.e., with virtual certainty that no injury will result), at times reasoned judgement must be applied, based on comparison of benefits and risks. Few human decisions are based on absolutes. At the same time, many individuals (scientists and nonscientists alike) think that there are too many additives in the food supply. Their very number (over 2000 intentional additives) increases the difficulty of identifying the potentially unsafe ones. Benefit–risk comparisons suggest that those with the fewest benefits relative to risks be eliminated and those with the greatest benefits relative to risks retained, at least until a virtually safe substitute can be found.

Intervention

Inform clients who ask about the relative merits of natural, organic, and health foods that they are neither more nor less nutritious than similar foods available at the supermarket. Let them know that practically any varied, well-selected diet (including the health food diet) that excludes excessive amounts of highly processed foods can be nutritionally adequate. By the same token, the health food diet is not essential to health, just as no one specific diet pattern is necessary for such benefits. In view of the high cost of health foods,[22] encourage health food users to optimize their purchases, just as when shopping at any other food store. Advise them to shop at the largest and best established stores and to insist on getting the quality of products for which they pay.

Encourage proper cooking techniques to preserve nutrient values (see Chap. 2) and discourage supplementation with massive doses of vitamins, which can be dangerous. Because of the known toxicity of excessive amounts of vitamin A and the possible toxicity of prolonged excessive supplementation with others, such as vitamins C and E, unrestricted use of these vitamins is not recommended.

Influence the decision-making processes about the quantity, quality, and safety of the food supply by the choices you make at food markets (health food or conventional) and by being informed and communicating with decision makers (i.e., government agencies and food manufacturers).

PICA

Assessment

The term pica refers to the compulsive ingestion of nonfood substances. The list of items ingested by its adherents is extensive, but those who engage in the habit usually show a preference for a specific item. A variety of substances have been reported to be eaten, including dirt, clay, laundry starch, paint and plaster chips, pieces of clay pots, ashes, fireplace soot, charcoal, match ends, paper, chalk, coffee grounds, bean clods, paraffin, mothballs, toilet bowl air freshener, antacids, baking soda, and milk of magnesia. In some cases an excessive intake of a particular type of food, such as ice, celery, potato chips, carrots, pickles, chewing gum, and pretzels, can be considered as pica. The ingestion of clay or ► dirt is called **geophagia,** of laundry starch, **amylo-**
► **phagia,** and of excessive ice, **pagophagia.** The practice of pica is not dissimilar from other compulsions or cravings for, e.g., alcohol, tobacco, coffee, or a favorite food.

Incidence. Pica has been practiced for centuries, and its incidence in pregnant women has been frequently noted. It is not limited to any one geographic area, race, creed, sex, or cultural status, but be aware that the practice is not uncommon among pregnant women, particularly low-income black women of southern rural heritage.[23] During pregnancy, pica often occurs in the form of clay or laundry starch eating. Boxes of clay may be brought to obstetric clients as gifts and are sometimes sold in farmer's markets. Starch eating (especially Argo laundry starch) may replace the clay when people move from the rural south to the urban north. Nonetheless, clay eating has moved to the cities, where the clay can sometimes be purchased in supermarkets or is received by mail from relatives.

Pica may also occur in children, chiefly toddlers and preschoolers (see Chap. 16). It generally does not occur in persons past 6 years of age except in brain-damaged or mentally ill children, pregnant women, and women of some subcultural groups. Whereas mouthing objects is a part of normal infant development, pica involves a further step—the development of a craving for a particular substance, such as dirt, starch, flakes of paint or plaster, paper, and the like. Mothers of many children with pica also engage in this practice, particularly during pregnancy, and eating of dirt in childhood may be related to subsequent pica during pregnancy.

Etiology. There appears to be no single motive for the practice of pica. It may be related to physiologic, sociocultural, or psychologic factors or any combination of these. The diversity of practices of various ages and races precludes defining a single etiology, and group similarities and differences must be considered; for example, clay ingestion may be etiologically distinct from that of ice or any other substance. Pica in a 2-year-old white male may have little in common with that of a 35-year-old black woman. Pregnancy appears to be an especially important variable, since the incidence is highest at this time.

Discuss with the client who practices pica the underlying reason. From a physiologic standpoint, hunger has been said to motivate the eating of clay and starch as a replacement for inaccessible foods. The filling of the stomach associated with their ingestion may lead to a feeling of satiety, and starch does provide kilocalories. Also hypothesized is the notion that certain substances will relieve the sensation of nausea and increased salivation sometimes experienced in pregnancy. Still others have suggested that pica represents an instinctive effort on the part of the practitioner to compensate for nutrient deficiencies, such as trace mineral lack. While the instinctive aspect has no basis in proven fact, a strong and persistent link between pica and iron deficiency has been demonstrated, although the exact relationship between the two is unclear. Anemia that is sometimes responsive to iron therapy often occurs in pica practitioners. Some suggest that iron deficiency is the cause of the pica, whereas others say iron deficiency is its result. There are data to support both contentions. To date, pagophagia is possibly the closest to being explained as a result of iron lack.[23]

From a sociocultural perspective, pica may have a basis in culture and tradition. This may be especially true of the consumption of clay and starch in the south, which may be perpetuated by tradition as women pass the habit to their children.

Pica has sometimes been explained on a psychologic basis, as, for some, it appears to meet various individual needs providing mental relaxation, sensory pleasure, and social approval. Many like the odor, taste, and pleasure associated with chewing the various substances. In some communities, the behavior is socially acceptable. Pica has qualities of compulsive behavior, since the craving must be satisfied with a specific substance. Many women have unusual food cravings or aversions associated with the stress of pregnancy, which are usually transient and not explainable on a physiologic basis, though they are sometimes described as an attention-getting device. A predisposition to oral fixation has been suggested as the basis for pica that occurs in childhood and later adult life.

Detrimental Effects. If the client is a pica practitioner, determine the specific type and amount of the substance being consumed and the duration of the practice. The detrimental effects of pica are generally related to the specific type of practice, the amount of the substance consumed, and the length of time the substance has been eaten. Determine if nutritional deficiencies are present that may occur as a result of displacement of nutritious foods in the diet or through interference with absorption. While the cause–effect relationship between anemia and pica has not been completely determined, both nutrient displacement and interference with nutrient absorption are thought to contribute. Clay is thought to chelate (bind) iron as well as other minerals in the intestinal tract, thus inhibiting their absorption.

The ingestion of substances that provide kilocalories, such as starch, could contribute to obesity if ingested in excessive quantities. Pica practitioners are subject to the potential toxicity of some of the substances consumed and to quantities of nutrients not tolerated in disease states. A prime example is lead poisoning, which occurs in children who chew on toys, furniture, or the paint flakes from lead-based paint. Congenital lead poisoning has resulted from maternal lead poisoning secondary to pica for wall plaster. The eating of mothballs and toilet bowl air freshener during pregnancy has led to transplacental poisoning, with resulting hemolytic anemia in the newborn. Clients who practice geophagia are predisposed to intestinal parasites and fecal impaction. In some cases, maternal complications, such as toxemia and hypertension, have been linked to pica, and the potassium contained in clay has produced life-threatening hyperkalemia in some clients with chronic renal disease. Wearing of the dental enamel occurs in clients who eat large amounts of hard substances, such as ice.

Intervention

Treat any associated complications, correct nutritional deficiencies, and provide iron supplements if anemia is present. In view of the cause–effect relationships noted between iron deficiency and pica, maintenance of an adequate hemoglobin level cannot be overemphasized. A therapeutic trial with iron supplements, even in the absence of anemia (as demonstrated by a low hemoglobin level), may be indicated in pica practitioners.

Since pica is potentially harmful if excessive amounts of the substances craved are eaten regularly, direct efforts toward control of pica. Because the habit may be rooted in cultural values and meet emotional needs, it may be difficult to alter. For instance, how many people have broken similar habits (such as smoking and drinking) as a result of threatening lectures about health dangers? For this reason, ultimate control of the practice rests with primary prevention.

Since the etiology of pica appears to be multifaceted, use a multidisciplinary team approach in its prevention. Nurses play a valuable role in both case finding and referral to other health team members, since they are often the first to interview clients in health care settings. Identify pica-prone clients before the development of symptoms so that corrective approaches can be applied. Pica may not be detected by the usual assessment techniques. Elicit information by asking questions that are both open-ended (Do you crave anything in particular?) and straightforward (Do you eat ice, laundry starch, coffee grounds?). Once pica is detected, direct efforts toward providing information about harmful effects; provide nutrition education and refer the client to agencies that can enhance the client's social welfare. During this process, guide the client toward a self-directed solution, which for many may simply be a limitation in daily consumption.

Current laws forbid the sale of lead-based interior paint, but advise clients who live in older buildings that it may be present. Caution clients to use lead-free paint for home projects, such as repainting and constructing furniture and toys.

REVIEW QUESTIONS AND ACTIVITIES

1. Identify the foods allowed in the diet in each of five categories of vegetarian diets.
2. Discuss the potential health benefits of following a vegetarian diet.
3. Explain the relationship between the adequacy of kilocaloric and protein intake in a vegan diet.
4. Compare the total quantity of protein needed by a vegan with that needed by a nonvegetarian of the same age and sex.
5. Explain the concept of protein complementation as a technique for obtaining adequate protein quality in a vegan diet, including examples of appropriate combinations.
6. Describe the role of meat analogs in vegetarian diets.
7. List three vitamins and three minerals that may be present in marginal quantities in an ill-planned vegetarian diet, and identify alternate food sources for these nutrients.
8. Identify the most serious pathologic manifestation of vitamin B_{12} deficiency.
9. Plan a nutritionally adequate menu for 1 day for a lacto-ovo-vegetarian client.
10. What adjustments must be made in the menu in Question 9 so that it is appropriate for a vegan client?
11. Design a lesson plan for teaching the following clients the principles of a nutritionally adequate diet: (a) an adult lacto-ovo-vegetarian, (b) an adult vegan, and (c) the mother of an infant who is being fed a vegan diet.
12. Explain the differences between natural, organic, and health foods.
13. Discuss the nutrient content of the current food supply and the need for dietary supplements by the population at large.
14. Compare the effects of natural and synthetic vitamins and minerals in the body.
15. Compare the effects of organic and synthetic fertilizers.
16. What dietary advice would you give to a client who is taking large doses of vitamin E for preventing cancer?
17. List two major categories of chemicals contained in food, and discuss two major types of food additives used in food production and food processing.
18. Identify the postulated etiology of pica and the groups associated with its highest incidence.
19. Your client has eaten a substantial quantity of clay for several years.
    a. Identify the potential medical complication for which you would assess.
    b. Why is iron deficiency a potential problem?
    c. Describe the nursing interventions that are appropriate in this situation.

REFERENCES

1. Committee on Nutritional Misinformation, Food and Nutrition Board, National Research Council: Vegetarian diets. J Am Diet Assoc 65:121, 1974.
2. Sanders TA, Ellis FR, Dickerson JW: Studies of vegans: The fatty acid composition of plasma choline phosphoglycerides, erythrocytes, adipose tissue, and breast milk and some indicators of susceptibility to ischemic heart disease in vegans and omnivore controls. Am J Clin Nutr 31:805, 1978.
3. Taber LAL, Cook RA: Dietary and anthropometric assessment of adult omnivores, fish-eaters, and lacto-ovo vegetarians. J Am Diet Assoc 76:21, 1980.
4. Phillips RL, Kuzma JW, Beeson WL, Lotz T: Influence of selection versus lifestyle on risk of fatal cancer and cardiovascular disease among Seventh-Day Adventists. Am J Epidemiol 112:296, 1980.
5. Sacks FM, Donner A, Castelli WP, et al.: Effect of ingestion of meat on plasma cholesterol of vegetarians. JAMA 246:640, 1981.
6. Sacks FM, Rosner B, Kass EH: Blood pressure in vegetarians. Am J Epidemiol 100:390, 1974.
7. Armstrong B, Van Merwyk AJ, Coates H: Blood pressure in Seventh-Day Adventist vegetarians. Am J Epidemiol 105:444, 1977.
8. Rouse IL, Beilin LJ, Armstrong BK, Vandongen R: Blood pressure-lowering effect of a vegetarian diet: Controlled trial in normotensive subjects. Lancet 1:5, 1983.
9. Phillips RL: Role of life-style and dietary habits in risk of cancer among Seventh-Day Adventists. Cancer Res 35:3513, 1975.
10. Marsh AG, Sanchez TV, Midkelsen O, et al.: Cortical bone density of adult lacto-ovo-vegetarian and omnivorous women. J Am Diet Assoc 76:148, 1980.

11. Allen LH, Oddoye EA, Margen S: Protein-induced hypercalciuria: A longer-term study. Am J Clin Nutr 32:741, 1979.

12. Burkitt DP, Walker ARP, Painter NS: Effect of dietary fibre on stools and transit-times and its role in the causation of disease. Lancet 2:1408, 1972.

13. Dywer JT, Andrew EM, Berkey C, et al.: Growth in "new" vegetarian children using the Jenss–Bayley curve fitting technique. Am J Clin Nutr 37:815, 1983.

14. Dong A: Serum vitamin B_{12} and blood cell values in vegetarians. Ann Nutr Metab 26:209, 1982.

15. Curtis JA, Kooh SW, Fraser D, Greenberg ML: Nutritional rickets in vegetarian children. Can Med Assoc J 128:150, 1983.

16. Freeland–Graves JH, Bodzy PW, Eppright MA: Zinc-status in the vegetarian. J Am Diet Assoc 77:655, 1980.

17. McEndree LS, Kies CV, Fox HM: Iron intake and iron nutritional status of lacto-ovo-vegetarians and omnivore students eating in a lacto-ovo-vegetarian food service. Nutr Rep Int 27:199, 1983.

18. Lappe FM: Diet for a Small Planet. New York, Ballantine Books, 1975.

19. Smith EB: A guide to good eating the vegetarian way. J Nutr Educ 7:111, 1975.

20. Margolius S: Health Foods: Facts and Fakes. New York, Public Affairs Pamphlet No. 498, 1973.

21. Coon JM: Natural food toxicants—A perspective. In Present Knowledge in Nutrition, ed 4. New York, The Nutrition Foundation, 1976, p 545.

22. Gourdine SP, Traiger WW, Cohen DS: Health food stores investigation. J Am Diet Assoc 83:285, 1983.

23. Committee on Nutrition of the Mother and Preschool Child, National Research Council: Alternative Dietary Practices and Nutritional Abuses in Pregnancy, Proceedings of a Workshop. Washington, DC, National Academy Press, 1982, pp 44–96.

BIBLIOGRAPHY

American Dietetic Association: Position paper on the vegetarian approach to eating. J Am Diet Assoc 77:61, 1980.

Bergen JC, Brown PT: Nutritional status of new vegetarians. J Am Diet Assoc 76:151, 1980.

Bowerman SJ, Harrill I: Nutrient consumption of individuals taking or not taking nutrient supplements. J Am Diet Assoc 83:298, 1983.

Dubrick MA: Dietary supplements and health aids—A critical evaluation. Part 3—Natural and miscellaneous products. J Nutr Educ 15:123, 1983.

Freeland-Graves JH, Greninger SA, Vickers J, et al.: Nutrition knowledge of vegetarians and nonvegetarians. J Nutr Educ 14(1):21, 1982.

Fulton JR, Hutton CW, Stitt KR: Preschool vegetarian children: Dietary and anthropometric data. J Am Diet Assoc 76:360, 1980.

Gibson RS, Anderson BM, Sabry JH: The trace metal status of a group of post-menopausal vegetarians. J Am Diet Assoc 82:246, 1983.

Hartbarger JC, Hartbarger NJ: Eating for the Eighties: A Complete Guide to Vegetarian Nutrition. Philadelphia, WB Saunders, 1981.

Read MH, Thomas DC: Nutrient and food supplement practices of lacto-ovo-vegetarians. J Am Diet Assoc 82:401, 1983.

Robertson L, Flinders C, Godfrey B: Laurel's Kitchen. New York, Bantam Books, 1978.

Schultz TD, Leklem JE: Dietary status of Seventh-Day Adventists and nonvegetarians. J Am Diet Assoc 83:27, 1983.

Strobl CM, Groll L: Professional knowledge and attitudes on vegetarianism: Implications for practice. J Am Diet Assoc 79:568, 1981.

Truesdale DD, Whitney EN, Acosta PB: Nutrients in vegetarian foods. J Am Diet Assoc 84:28, 1984.

PART IV

Nutrition in Secondary Health Care

The preceding parts of this book focused on the use of food in a manner conducive to the prevention of nutrition-related health problems.

Adequate nutrition, important for maintaining optimal health at all ages and in all normal physiologic conditions, is equally important for restoration of health during periods of disease and other physiologic and psychosocial stress. Part IV describes those disease conditions that are treated, controlled, or otherwise

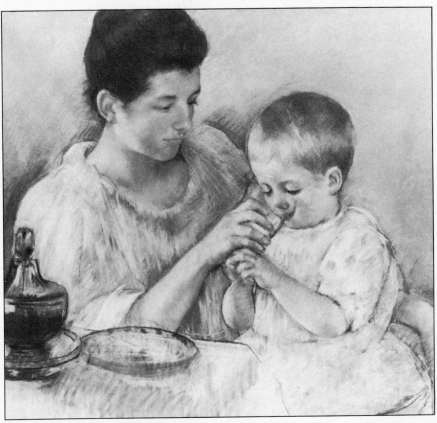

Mary Cassatt *Mother Feeding Her Child*

supported by diet modifications and discusses the specific diet modifications that are necessary. Not all disease states require a modified diet. In these situations dietary evaluation and counseling may be necessary to assure an adequate intake and thus prevent the complicating effects of poor nutritional status. In some instances, a modified diet is the primary mode of therapy—an example is the use of a diet restricted in kilocalories to treat uncomplicated obesity. In other cases, a modified diet and insulin are used to treat insulin-dependent diabetes. Finally, diet therapy may be used to support other treatment regimens—an example is the progression from a liquid to a regular diet following surgery.

For hospitalized clients, aggressive nutritional care may well reduce the length of hospitalization. Nutritional care is especially important for acutely ill hospitalized clients. However, it is equally important in the long-term care of the chronically ill. Hospitalized infants, elderly persons, and those who are acutely ill are especially likely to exhibit dramatic changes from day to day in their physical or mental status. Nutritional care is also a component of the follow-up care provided for clients upon discharge from a hospital. Although they are prepared during hospitalization for the return to home and community, many clients may be unable to cope with lifestyle changes necessitated by diet modifications or other aspects of treatment. Therefore, referral for follow-up and support through an outpatient clinic, physician's office, or other community agency is an important aspect of the nursing care plan. For some outpatients, effective nutritional care may delay or even eliminate the need for further hospitalizations.

The nursing care plan should include nutritional care and be developed in an individualized, organized, and coordinated manner. There is no typical client, since most clients present a variety of conditions or problems that affect nutritional requirements, appetite, or enjoyment of food. Treat the client as a whole person and give consideration to the effect of various physiologic, psychologic, socioeconomic, and cultural factors on present nutritional needs and on plans for continuing care. No one standard of care will suffice for all clients with a particular medical problem. Rather, develop an individualized plan for each client, using input from the client as well as from members of the health care team. The plan should have built-in flexibility to allow for changes as conditions change.

Meeting the nutritional needs of hospitalized clients requires an interdisciplinary team effort. Because several team members are involved, roles may overlap. For example, both dietitians/ nutritionists and nurses are involved in supervising meal service and observing and reporting food intake. Since staffing patterns and thus responsibilities vary within hospital settings, specific roles should be clarified for each setting to permit an integrated approach to nutritional care. Because of their unique expertise, dietitians and nutritionists should provide the leadership in promoting nutritional care. To assure coordination of nutritional care, communication among team members is essential. While verbal communication is informative, at best it is sporadic and does not replace documentation, which can be shared by all team members.

CHAPTER 21

Nutritional Care of the Hospitalized Client

Objectives

After completion of this chapter, the student will be able to:

1. Evaluate the nutritional adequacy of standard hospital diets.

2. Compare and contrast the seven major characteristics of each of the three major categories of liquid formulas used for enteral feeding.

3. Distinguish between the nutrient composition and nutritional adequacy of two types of peripherally infused nutrient solutions and nutrient solutions infused via a central vein.

4. Differentiate between the complications associated with tube feeding and total parenteral nutrition.

5. Develop a nursing care plan for the nutritional management of a client with a severe systemic infection, and adjust the plan to be appropriate for a severely burned client.

6. Distinguish between the effects of drug therapy on nutritional status and the effect of food, substances consumed with food, and nutritional status on drug therapy.

7. Develop a nursing care plan for an elderly client whose diagnosis includes protein–calorie malnutrition complicated by a chronic disease and surgery.

Disease conditions are accompanied by numerous physiologic and psychologic stresses that may predispose the affected individual to malnutrition. Should hospitalization become necessary, the psychologic and physical effects of hospitalization itself may further compound the effect of the disease on nutritional status. Some acute situations (such as body trauma from surgical injury, severe burns, fractures, and severe infection) have a profound effect on nutritional status because they produce a catabolic state with secondary negative nutrient balance and exceptionally high nutrient demands. Any illness associated with bedrest and immobilization also leads to negative nutrient balance, especially of nitrogen and calcium. Malnutrition may occur secondary to the treatment used for disease. For example, the adverse effects of various drugs on the nutritional status is a topic much investigated at present. Because of certain practices that do not support optimal nutrition for hospitalized clients, considerable attention has been given recently to ▶ **iatrogenic malnutrition** (malnutrition produced inadvertently as a result of treatment by the medical team) in the hospital setting. At the same time, research has unveiled new methods for providing nutritional support for those clients at greatest risk of malnutrition as a result of excessively large nutrient demands or inability to ingest or use an appropriate amount of food.

This chapter, which focuses on (1) the effect of illness and hospitalization on nutritional status, (2) hospital malnutrition, (3) methods for providing nutritional support in the hospital, (4) nutrition in physiologic stress (surgery, burns, infections), (5) nu-

271

trient–drug interactions, and (6) techniques for assessing hospital malnutrition, is designed to assist nurses with assessment and integration of nutritional care into the total nursing care plan. In order to arrive at a correct nursing diagnosis and plan effective intervention, nurses must be aware of the effects of illness, hospitalization, and treatment on the client's nutritional status. Moreover, the client's nutritional status may change frequently throughout the hospital stay, and nurses can be aware of this by including nutritional assessment as part of their nursing histories. Of particular importance are obtaining baseline assessment data (see Chap. 11) at the time of admission and continuous monitoring of nutritional status during the hospital stay. Diet counseling may be a component of the interventions provided by nurses for hospitalized clients who may require ongoing care. Refer to Chapter 12 for nutrition education guidelines that need to be considered as a basis for planning diet counseling.

EFFECT OF ILLNESS AND HOSPITALIZATION ON NUTRITIONAL STATUS

Assessment

Physiologic Aspects. Disease processes or the treatments used, such as drug, radiation, or diet therapy, may alter (1) food intake, (2) nutrient requirements, or (3) nutrient use. Observe for diminished food intake in clients with disease conditions accompanied by anorexia (loss of appetite), alteration in the sense of taste, or mechanical problems that limit intake, such as obstruction in the gastrointestinal tract. In some situations the client may simply be too weak to eat. Although diminished food intake is a more common problem, assess for excessive food intake in clients with certain psychologic or endocrine disorders.

Evaluate for the presence of disease conditions that alter nutrient requirements. Requirements for kilocalories or certain nutrients can either increase or decrease because of changes in metabolism or excessive losses. Expect metabolic changes with concomitant large energy and nutrient demands to accompany fever, infection, and body trauma, since these conditions produce a catabolic state and consequent negative energy and nutrient balance. In particular, severely burned clients may have such large nutrient demands that it is not possible to consume sufficient food by the oral route, and other methods of nutritional support must be provided. Evaluate for metabolic changes that lead to negative nutrient balance, especially negative protein and calcium balance, in immobilized clients. Interestingly, these effects of immobilization can occur even when one is immobilized in the absence of illness, for example, in the case of an astronaut confined to a space capsule.

In certain metabolic disorders or diseases, there is an inability to use specific nutrients. For example, the amino acid phenylalanine cannot be metabolized in clients with phenylketonuria, and tolerance for glucose is impaired in clients with diabetes mellitus. Some modes of treatment, such as drugs and radiation therapy, may adversely affect nutritional status. Diet modifications that are (1) excessively restrictive, (2) bland-tasting or otherwise unflavorful, or (3) planned without regard for the client's usual food habits may be either nutritionally inadequate or rejected by the client.

Psychosocial Aspects. Illness may be accompanied by psychologic stresses that have the potential for altering food intake. It has been suggested that psychologic stresses may be sufficiently severe to bring hormonal changes, which in turn lead to negative nutrient balance, such as negative nitrogen and calcium balance. The client who is sick may be anxious and fearful about the outcome of the illness and its economic ramifications and may express either verbally or nonverbally fear of loss of independence and the need to depend on others. With hospitalization, anxiety may be accentuated as the client is faced with loneliness, interruptions of routines, and loss of privacy and individual control. Meals must frequently be eaten alone, at a time when the comfort and companionship of others are most needed. If the meal must be consumed in bed, there may be difficulty in managing the tray and utensils. Assess for these additional factors that may decrease food intake: (1) meals may be served at unaccustomed hours, (2) the diet may consist of unfamiliar foods, (3) the freedom of movement may be restricted, and (4) there may be frequent interruptions in the day's routine to perform laboratory tests, interviews, physical examinations, treatments, and (5) the environment may be poor (such as the presence of bedpans). Moreover, the client is expected to interact with a wide variety of unfamiliar people, such as the physician, nurse, dietitian, technicians, and perhaps has to share a room with a stranger. All of these stresses may produce psychologic responses, and mood swings involving such mechanisms as withdrawal, anger, denial, bargaining, regression, and depression are common.

Evaluate food acceptance and food intake in clients who experience these mood swings. For example, rejection of a modified diet may be one way of maintaining some personal control over the unpleasant situation, or registering complaints about the food served may be perceived as a safe way to express unhappiness. The client may also use diet as a means of getting attention from the family or hospital personnel by requiring excessive attention to minor details or displaying loss of appetite.

Hospital Malnutrition. In recent years, there has been much concern about the high prevalence of malnutrition, especially protein–calorie malnutrition (PCM), in hospitalized clients, and continuing research is aimed at assessing its nature and frequency.[1-3] Many clients may enter the hospital with borderline PCM as a result of long-term or debilitating illness, and the pattern may continue in the hospital if the client does not eat the food that is served or receives nutritionally inadequate nutritional support measures. Use the data summarized in Table 21–1 to determine the presence of undesirable hospital practices that may have adverse effects on the nutritional status of clients; more desirable alternatives are also summarized in Table 21–1.

Consequences of Hospital Malnutrition. In the malnourished state, a self-perpetuating phenomenon becomes manifest that results in symptoms of progressive starvation. As the client eats little and stays in bed, he or she becomes progressively weaker. As weakness increases, the client becomes even more apathetic and food intake decreases further, the period of hospitalization is prolonged, and morbidity and mortality rates increase. Observe for these adverse effects of malnutrition: (1) increased suscepti-

bility to infection, (2) impaired wound healing, (3) increased incidence of complications associated with a prolonged period of debilitation and bedrest, and (4) alteration in the body's use of medications.

The increased susceptibility to infectious disease results from the impairment in cell-mediated immunity that is associated with malnutrition. Protein deficiency and iron deficiency, in particular, depress cell-mediated immunity. Wound healing is impaired in the malnourished state. The nutrients particularly important in wound healing are protein, vitamin C, vitamin A, zinc, copper, and iron.

An increased incidence of complications associated with prolonged debilitation and bedrest usually accompany malnutrition. These complications include pneumonia, decubiti, thromboembolism, fecal impaction, and stress ulcers. For example, with progressive muscle weakness, the strength of the cough reflex is diminished, and pneumonia may ensue. There is deterioration in the respiratory-regulating reflexes with malnutrition—the sensitivity of the respiratory center to the normal levels of blood oxygen and carbon dioxide decreases. Decubiti may accom-

---

TABLE 21–1
UNDESIRABLE AND DESIRABLE HOSPITAL PRACTICES AS RELATED TO NUTRITIONAL STATUS

Undesirable Hospital Practices that May Adversely Affect Nutritional Status[a]	Practices that May Improve Nutritional Status[b]
Failure to record height and weight on admission and at regular intervals thereafter	Record weight and height routinely on admission and at regular intervals subsequently
Rotation of staff at frequent intervals; continuity for patient care is lacking	Maintain continuity of client care by adequate observation and recording of significant data
Diffusion of responsibility for patient care among health team members; lack of communication among team members	Develop a plan that clearly delineates the role of the various team members (i.e., the physician, nurse, and dietitian) in nutritional care
Prolonged use of intravenous feedings consisting primarily of glucose and saline	Provide nutritional supplements when the use of glucose and saline feedings is prolonged
Failure to observe and record patient's food intake	Observe and record food intake in a manner that can be evaluated in relation to quality and quantity
Withholding of meals because of diagnostic procedures	Provide replacements for missed meals
Use of tube feeding of uncertain composition, in inadequate amounts, and under unsanitary conditions	Specify the nutrient composition of tube feeding, feed the required amount, and maintain sanitary conditions
Inadequate knowledge of the nutrient composition of nutrient supplements, e.g., vitamin mixtures	Administer nutritional supplements of known composition that are appropriate to meet the specific needs of the client
Failure to recognize the increased nutrient demands of injury or illness	Provide nutritional support with recognition of the specific requirements of the client (e.g., increased requirements associated with injury or illness)
Failure to provide optimal nutritional support for the surgical client (e.g., failure to assure an optimal nutritional status before surgery and failure to provide adequate nutritional support during the postsurgical period)	Provide optimal nutritional support for the surgical client (e.g., prepare the client nutritionally in cases of elective surgery and provide adequate nutritional support in the postoperative period)
Failure to recognize the role of nutrition in providing resistance to infection and in recovery from infection; undue reliance on antibiotics	Include nutritional therapy in the regimen for prevention and treatment of infection; avoid sole reliance on antibiotics
Failure to provide nutritional support until the client is in an advanced state of depletion—which may be irreversible	Avoid nutritional depletion by providing ongoing nutritional support that begins with admission
Limited availability of laboratory tests, or failure to use those available, in assessing nutritional status	Use available laboratory tests in assessing nutritional status

[a] (*Source: Adapted from Butterworth CE: The skeleton in the hospital closet. Nutr Today 9:8, 1974.*)
[b] (*Source: Adapted from Butterworth CE: Hospital malnutrition. Cassette-A-Month, American Dietetic Association, Chicago, 1976.*)

pany the loss of subcutaneous fat and skin integrity.

The body's use of medications is altered in the malnourished state. There are alterations in the intestinal absorption of drugs, in the body's response to drugs, and in the detoxification of drugs. For example, with protein or vitamin C deficiency, detoxification of drugs is diminished, and the response of a client with cancer to therapy (with drugs or radiation, for example) depends on the nutritional state.

METHODS OF NUTRITIONAL SUPPORT IN HOSPITAL SETTINGS

Intervention

As the relationship between nutrition and health becomes more clear, the medical community is becoming increasingly concerned about the quality of nutritional care provided to hospitalized clients. In some hospitals, nutritional support teams composed of physicians, dietitians, nurses, and pharmacists have been organized to assure that the client receives the proper nutrients by the most appropriate method. The variety of foods and food preparation methods, as well as products and procedures, currently available for both enteral and parenteral feeding makes it possible to meet the total nutritional needs of most hospitalized clients. Although the major responsibility for providing nutritious food in hospitals rests with its dietetic service, the actual provision of nutritional care is a shared responsibility of the health team members. To adequately nourish the client, cooperate with other health team members to assure that (1) the diet order prescribed by the physician is formulated to meet the nutritional needs of the client as closely as possible, (2) the food that is delivered to the client by the food service department is attractive, palatable, and nutritious, and (3) the client receives the assistance and encouragement necessary to assure that the food is eaten.

Standard Hospital Diets. Most hospitals have prepared or adopted a diet manual that compiles the routine, modified, and test diets used in the institution. The manual can serve as a guideline for ordering diets by the physician as well as a tool for communication among the health team members.

TABLE 21–2
DESCRIPTION OF STANDARD HOSPITAL DIETS

Diet	Indications for Use	Comment
Regular	Used for clients requiring no particular modification	Based on the RDA and Basic Four Food groups; foods that may cause digestive disturbances are omitted; can be increased in kcal and protein content by the addition of extra amounts of milk, meat, or high-protein supplements. Some hospitals may offer a prudent regular diet as a health-promoting measure (a prudent diet offers foods low in saturated fat and cholesterol with substitution of polyunsaturated fat)
Soft		
Traditional	May be used during the transition phase in the progression from a liquid to a regular diet; in the convalescent phase of acute infections; mild gastrointestinal disturbances	Based on the RDA and Basic Four Food Groups; modified in texture so as to include foods that are low in fiber and thus easy to chew and foods that are simply prepared, mild in flavor, and easily digested; texture modifications for clients with chewing problems should be evaluated on an individual basis
Mechanical or dental soft	May be used by clients who have chewing problems because of lack of teeth or suitable dentures	
Liquid		
Full	May be used before and after surgery, in infectious diseases, in situations where chewing and swallowing problems are present, and with gastrointestinal problems	Allows use of foods that are liquid at room or body temperature and low in fiber and easily digested and absorbed; may contain adequate kcal but is low in iron and other nutrients; can increase the kcal and nutritive value by addition of cream to milk, nonfat milk to beverages and soups, strained meat to soups, and sugar or Polycose to beverages; provide at least 6 feedings daily
Clear	May be used before and after surgery or when illness is acute—nausea, vomiting, distention, diarrhea, anorexia, and so on	Allows fluids that are transparent and consist primarily of carbohydrates that leave little residue after digestion; is nutritionally inadequate and should be used as the sole source of nutrition for no more than 24–48 hours; provide at least 6 feedings daily

Nurses use the manual to obtain the rationale for use of specific diets, a list of foods allowed and avoided on each diet, a sample menu, and nutritive evaluations. The manual also serves as a teaching tool and reference document for physicians, nurses, and other professionals.

The most commonly used diets in hospitals are the regular diets (also called general, full, or house diets) for infants, children, and adults and diets that are modified in consistency (i.e., liquid—clear and full liquid—and soft diets). Some hospitals provide a light (or convalescent) diet, but others omit this classification and use the soft diet as a substitute. The modifications in consistency are sometimes re-
► ferred to as **progressive hospital diets** and are used when the client's physical, neurologic, or psychologic condition necessitates a modification in texture or consistency. The objective of the progressive dietary regimen is to provide nutritional support

as the client progresses stepwise (i.e., from clear liquids to full liquids to soft foods to regular diet). A description of standard hospital diets is given in Table 21–2, and a general listing of foods allowed on each type of diet is summarized in Table 21–3. Although regular and soft diets are planned to meet the RDA for kilocalories and nutrients, it is difficult to meet the RDA when a liquid diet is used. With careful planning, the nutritional value of a full liquid diet can be adequate, except for fiber content, although a clear liquid diet is totally inadequate nutritionally. A comparison of the kilocalorie, protein, fat, and carbohydrate content of a full and clear liquid diet is shown in Table 21–4. Commercial products are available for supplementing both clear and full liquid diets.

Enteral Feedings. Hospitalized clients may be nourished via the enteral route (using the gastroin-

TABLE 21–3
FOODS ALLOWED ON ROUTINE HOSPITAL DIETS

Food Grouping	Clear Liquid	Full Liquid	Soft	Regular
Soup	Fat-free broth, bouillon	Same, plus strained soups	Same	All
Bread and cereal		Refined or strained whole grain cereal gruels	White or fine-grain bread and cereal, macaroni, spaghetti and noodles, soda crackers, melba toast, zwieback	All
Protein foods		Milk, milk drinks as eggnog, milkshakes, cocoa, milk-based commercial supplements	Same plus: tender, minced or ground meat, poultry, fish, sweetbreads, liver (cook by stewing, baking, broiling, creaming); mild cheeses (as cottage, cheddar, Swiss); eggs (except fried)	All
Vegetables		Juices	Cooked, milk-flavored low-fiber vegetables (no fried and greasy vegetables, gas-forming or raw vegetables; potato without skin	All
Fruit	Pulp-free fruit juice as apple and grape	Juices	Same plus: cooked or canned fruit without seeds or skins (as apples, peaches, apricots, pears, plums, ripe banana, fruit cocktail, Royal Anne cherries); citrus fruit sections without membranes; and ripe avocado	All
Desserts	Plain gelatin, water ices	Plain gelatin, plain ice cream, sherbet, junket, custard, and plain puddings, water ices	Same plus: plain cake and cookies with or without plain frosting, fruit whip, and any other smooth desserts	All
Miscellaneous	Tea, coffee or coffee substitute, sugar, lemon, carbonated beverages, fruit-flavored powders, plain stick candy, ice chips	Same as for clear liquid plus: Fats: cream, butter or margarine Sweets: honey and plain syrups Spices: salt and pepper in moderation Other: cocoa or chocolate for flavoring	Same as for clear liquid plus: Fats: crisp bacon, cream cheese Sweets: Jelly, candy (without fruit or nuts), honey, molasses, sugar, syrups Spices: In moderation, including vinegar for seasoning Other: Gravy, cream sauces	All

TABLE 21-4
NUTRITIVE VALUE OF CLEAR AND FULL LIQUID DIETS

	Clear Liquid	Full Liquid
Kilocalories	600–900	2000[a]
Protein (g)	5–15[b]	70
Fat (g)	0	80
Carbohydrate (g)	100–130	250

[a] The kilocalorie and nutritive value can be increased by adding pureed meat and vegetables to cream soups, incorporating nonfat dry milk into beverages and soups, adding glucose (or Polycose, Ross Laboratories) to beverages, and adding butter or margarine to cereal gruels and soups.
[b] Primarily from gelatin, a source of incomplete protein.

testinal tract) or the parenteral route (through infusion of nutrients into a vein). If the client can ingest, digest, and absorb an adequate amount of food and nutrients, use either of two categories of enteral feeding: (1) oral feeding, using the appropriate standard hospital diet, or (2) tube feeding. Be aware, however, of the nutritional inadequacies of standard liquid regimens, particularly clear liquids. Many commercial products are available for oral supplementation or to provide nutritionally complete oral or tube feeding.

Three basic categories of commercially prepared and pasteurized formulas are available:

1. Milk-based formulas
2. Blenderized diet feedings
3. Defined formulas diets (predigested formulas)

All of these have the characteristics of convenience and ease of preparation, consistency in nutrient content for a given brand, and freedom from bacterial contaminants prior to opening the container. At full strength, these preparations all provide approximately 1 kcal/ml and can meet total nutritional requirements when given in adequate volume. The blenderized diets and milk-based formulas are reasonably well balanced with regard to the percentage of kilocalories supplied by carbohydrate, protein, and fat, although some of the milk-based products have a relatively high protein content. In contrast, most of the defined formula diets, which are designed to meet special metabolic requirements, are very high in carbohydrate content, moderate in protein content, and moderate to low in fat content. Other characteristics also vary among the categories (Table 21–5). Use the physical condition of each client, including digestive/absorptive capacity and tolerance for specific nutrients, to make the best formula choice. For example, a client who is intolerant of lactose in milk should receive a lactose-free formula, and defined formula diets are suitable for clients with gastrointestinal disorders associated with a diminished ability to digest or absorb food/nutrients.

In addition to the above types of formulas, specialty formulas of three additional types are available:

1. Formulas designed for clients who have failure of specific organs, such as the kidneys or liver, or who are unable to tolerate conventional fats

TABLE 21-5
CHARACTERISTICS OF THE MAJOR TYPES OF COMMERCIAL FORMULAS USED FOR ENTERAL (ORAL OR TUBE) FEEDING

Characteristic	Type of Formula		
	Blended	Milk Based	Defined Formula
Nutritional adequacy	Provides approximately 1 kcal/ml at full strength; can meet nutritional requirements of most patients when given in adequate volume	Provides approximately 1 kcal/ml at full strength; can meet nutritional requirements of most patients when given in adequate volume	Provides approximately 1 kcal/ml at full strength; can meet nutritional requirements of most patients when given in adequate volume
Consistency (viscosity)	Most viscid (must use large tube when used as tube feeding)	Moderately viscid (can use small tube when used as tube feeding)	Least viscid (can use small tube when used as tube feeding)
Degree of digestion required	Complex forms of carbohydrate, protein, and fat that require complete digestion before absorption	Complex forms of carbohydrate, protein, and fat that require complete digestion before absorption	Predigested forms of carbohydrate, protein, and fat that require minimal or no digestion, leading to rapid absorption
Lactose content	Large amounts	Large amounts[a]	Lactose free
Osmolality	Hypertonic	Hypertonic[b]	Hypertonic
Residue	Moderate	Low	Minimal
Cost	Moderate	Moderate	Expensive

[a] Brands in this category have been developed that are lactose free.
[b] Brands in this category have been developed that are essentially isotonic.

2. Formulas designed for clients who have increased metabolic needs due to such factors as severe infections or burns
3. Feeding modules that supply single nutrients (carbohydrate, protein, or fat) or a combination of two or more

Formulas designed for clients with liver and kidney failure are altered in their content of specific amino acids. Be aware that many of these products are nutritionally incomplete and thus cannot serve as the sole method of nutritional support. For clients who cannot use conventional fats, consider the use of a nutritionally complete formula that substitutes medium-chain triglycerides (MCT) for long-chain fats. An MCT oil is available that can be used as cooking oil in food preparation. Use feeding modules (such as Polycose) to supplement oral or tube feedings. Feeding modules can also be combined to yield a unique formula for specific client needs.

Tube Feedings. Oral feeding is preferred to tube feeding, but there are many situations in which clients cannot ingest an adequate amount of food, yet have a functioning gastrointestinal tract. For these clients, tube feeding is an alternate method of ingesting food. In recent years, improved formulas (discussed in the previous section) and improved feeding techniques (including the availability of small flexible feeding tubes and food pumps) have enhanced client acceptance and overall success of tube feeding. Depending upon the client's condition and tolerance for food, tube feeding may serve as the method of total nutritional support for long periods of time or as an adjunct to oral food intake. With adequate instruction, many clients can maintain themselves with tube feeding at home.

Tube feedings may be administered into the stomach (via a tube inserted through the nose or mouth or by a surgical opening into the esophagus or the stomach), the duodenum (via a tube inserted through the nose), or the jejunum (via a tube inserted through the nose or a surgical opening into the jejunum). A feeding catheter can be inserted into the jejunum at the time of abdominal surgery.

Consider the use of tube feeding for clients whose oral intake may be inadequate because of any of the following conditions:

1. Oral or phargyngeal lesions or following oral or pharyngeal surgery
2. Loss of reflex ability (e.g., clients with a stroke or those who are unconscious or semicomatose)
3. Mechanical obstruction in the gastrointestinal tract (peristalsis must be present and the gastrointestinal tract must be patent below the level at which the feeding is administered)
4. Malnutrition secondary to disease conditions (e.g., mental retardation, psychologic disorders involving food refusal, severe infections,

cancer, hyperthyroidism, and conditions associated with extreme anorexia)
5. Severe burns
6. Metabolic disorders, such as liver and kidney diseases (use special formulas designed for these conditions)
7. Gastrointestinal diseases, such as inflammatory bowel disorders and pancreatic disorders (use defined formula diets that require minimal digestion and are rapidly absorbed)

To aid in the client's acceptance of tube feeding, explain the rationale for the feeding and its nutritional content and openly discuss all of the client's questions. If oral intake is possible (many clients can eat with the tube in place), provide favorite foods. Unless contraindicated, add favorite fluids, such as coffee, through the tube. Encourage the client to chew and savor the taste of food without swallowing it. Encourage ambulation when possible, not only to improve morale but also to promote protein synthesis.

Weigh the client daily and keep accurate records of intake and output to guide adequacy of energy and nutrient intake. Provided an adequate volume of formula is taken, formulas that supply 1 kcal/ml given at full strength will meet the nutrient requirements of most clients. The nutrient composition varies widely among the various formulas, however. Use the nutrient composition given on the can of formula to evaluate the nutrient adequacy on an individual basis. For most clients, a total volume of 3000 ml of full-strength formula containing 1 kcal/ml is adequate to permit weight maintenance or weight gain. Formulas are also available that have a kilocalorie density greater than 1 kcal/ml for clients who have large kilocaloric needs. Observe for the complications of tube feeding, which can include drying of the oral cavity, irritation of the nares, dehydration, diarrhea, constipation, nausea, gastric retention, aspiration, and dumping syndrome. Provide adequate nasal care and oral hygiene to prevent nasal and oral problems. Avoid dehydration by providing additional water by tube. Most formulas contain about 80 percent water, which may not be a sufficient amount for some clients. To prevent such problems as diarrhea, nausea, and gastric retention, avoid giving concentrated formulas too rapidly. Intolerance for lactose or bacterial contamination of the formula can also lead to diarrhea. Aspiration can be a particular problem in clients who receive gastric feedings, and the dumping syndrome (see Chap. 26) is not uncommon in clients receiving duodenal and jejunal feedings. Correct administration technique[4] can diminish the risk of these complications. Defined formula diets produce little residue. Advise clients receiving this type of formula to expect a bowel movement about every 5 days. The low residue content of other formulas may lead to constipation in some clients, which may necessitate the use of medication for relief.

Parenteral Feedings. In many situations, it is impossible to supply nutrients by mouth or tube feeding because of conditions that require total rest for the gastrointestinal tract for varying periods of time. The period of rest needed may be short (such as the first several days after gastrointestinal surgery) or relatively long term (such as in severe malabsorption syndromes). In these cases, use **parenteral nutrition**—a term generally synonymous with **intravenous feeding**—as the method of nutritional support. Fluids containing varying quantities of glucose, amino acids, fat, mineral salts, and vitamins can be infused into either a peripheral or a central vein. Differentiate between peripherally infused solutions and centrally infused solutions. A peripherally infused solution is the conventional method of nutritional support; infusion into a central vein (i.e., vena cava) is a recent innovation. Formulas infused into a central vein are more nutritionally adequate than are nutrients infused peripherally.

Adequate water, mineral salts, and vitamins can be given by either route. The ability to provide adequate kilocalories and protein in a volume of fluid that does not produce circulatory overload or other side effects is the factor limiting the nutritional adequacy of peripherally infused solutions. Expect clients who are maintained for long periods of time on standard intravenous therapy to be in negative nitrogen balance and show characteristics of debilitation and emaciation.

The ability to provide complete nutritional support, including adequate kilocalories and protein, by using a central vein as the site of infusion (called **total parenteral nutrition** or TPN) is a medical achievement of the past decade. The use of TPN solutions has enabled the health team to avert nutritional deficiency in critically ill clients—many with accelerated requirements—who cannot otherwise obtain adequate nutrients for long periods of time. This mode of therapy is not without the risk of complications, however, and to avoid or minimize side effects a team approach is necessary. Members of the team must be knowledgeable concerning those aspects of nutrition and metabolism involved and also must be proficient in the technical skills needed for administration.

Standard Intravenous Therapy. Provide short-term nutritional support by delivery of nutrients into a peripheral vein. Since none of the available solutions provide all of the needed nutrients, encourage a rapid return to regular eating. If this is impossible, the use of TPN solutions may be indicated. The major objectives in the use of conventional intravenous fluids are first, to provide water and mineral salts to maintain or restore fluid and electrolyte balance and, second, to provide a source of kilocalories to minimize tissue catabolism and prevent ketosis. While sodium chloride and potassium salts are the major mineral salts provided, others such as magnesium, phosphate, and calcium can be provided as needed. Glucose (5 percent, D_5, or 10 percent, D_{10}) is generally used as the source of kilocalories. The amount of kilocalories provided by conventional intravenous therapy is limited by the concentration of glucose that can be used without irritating the veins and by the volume of fluid that can be given without causing fluid overload. Ten percent glucose in water ($D_{10}W$) is the highest concentration of glucose that can be infused into a peripheral vein without causing phlebitis or thrombosis. One liter of D_5W provides 200 kcal, and 1 liter of $D_{10}W$ provides 400 kcal. Provided renal function is normal and there are no abnormal fluid losses (as from vomiting or diarrhea), fluid tolerance in an adult is approximately 35 to 50 ml/kg of body weight, or a total of about 3 to 3.5 liters per day. Thus, the use of glucose as the sole energy source limits the kilocalorie intake to approximately 600 to 1200 daily, an amount that is grossly inadequate for hypermetabolic states, such as traumatic conditions (e.g., surgery, burns, fractures). Kilocalorie intake can be more nutritionally adequate when amino acids and fat are added.

The combined use of glucose, amino acids, and fat as energy sources (with amino acids also supplying nitrogen) represents a modification of TPN, although a peripheral rather than a central vein is the infusion site. Be aware, however, that limitations still preclude providing sufficient kilocalories to meet the requirements for many conditions; a daily maximum is approximately 2000 kcal.

Replacement of fluid and electrolytes is usually accomplished by the intravenous infusion of D_5W (isotonic glucose) in saline (sodium chloride) solutions, with potassium and other salts added as needed. Balanced electrolyte solutions—those that contain salts of sodium, potassium, magnesium, chloride, phosphate, and lactate in a ratio resembling the proportion of these cations and anions in normal plasma—are also available commercially and are used in certain conditions. The rate and amount of the infusion should not exceed the body's ability to use the nutrients. Use urine volume as the guide to adequacy of fluid replacement; the daily production of approximately 1000 ml of urine in an adult is a desired amount. Administer potassium-containing solutions slowly, and assure that renal function is adequate to prevent hyperkalemia and untoward effects on muscle function.

Use specialized types of replacement solutions in certain disorders, such as acid–base imbalances, renal failure, and adrenal insufficiency. To prevent and treat shock, use fluids containing substances that exert colloidal osmotic pressure, such as whole blood, plasma, albumin, or dextran. These tend to maintain the circulating blood volume and also compensate for the blood volume lost in hemorrhage and replace fluid that has left the circulating compartment because of increased capillary permeability.

Total Parenteral Nutrition. TPN, formerly referred
▶ to as **hyperalimentation,** is a useful way to provide
complete nutritional support for extended periods
to clients whose energy and protein requirements
are large and for whom conventional intravenous
therapy, oral feeding, or tube feeding is inadequate
or contraindicated. Appearing first in the late 1960s,
the techniques of administration and solutions available for use have become sufficiently refined that
even home administration is now possible, and there
is now an increased use of TPN in home settings.

The technique involves infusion of a hypertonic
nutrient solution into a vein of large diameter, the
superior vena cava, via the subclavian vein (in
adults) and the internal or external jugular vein
(in children) (Fig. 21-1). The concentrated nutrient
solution is thus rapidly diluted by the high blood
flow of the central vein. The occurrence of phlebitis
or thrombosis is minimized since nutrients are sent
to the periphery in isotonic concentration. This technique can provide sufficient kilocalories and nutrients to support positive nitrogen balance and
weight gain in malnourished infants and adults, although it is not known whether nutrients taken
through a vein are used in the same way as those
taken by mouth.

Components of the Nutrient Solutions. TPN solutions
are formulated according to individual client needs
—there is no standard TPN formula. The major components are sources of kilocalories, nitrogen, minerals, vitamins, essential fatty acids, and water. The
solution is extremely hypertonic (1800 to 2400
mOsm/liter) to provide sufficient kilocalories and
nutrients in an allowable volume of water. A general
guide to kilocaloric and nitrogen composition of TPN

TABLE 21-6
RECOMMENDED ENERGY AND PROTEIN CONTENT OF TPN FORMULAS

	Kcal/kg Body Weight	G Nitrogen/kg Body Weight[a]
Adults	30–50	0.2–0.3
Infants	125–130	0.6–0.74

[a] 1 g nitrogen = 6.25 g protein.

formulas for adults and infants is given in Table
21-6.

The energy needs of a sedentary adult client
without preexisting deficits or a hypermetabolic
state can be met by approximately 30 kcal/kg of
weight per day, but in cases of extreme stress, infection, or body trauma, the need for kilocalories may
double or even triple. An important consideration
in TPN formulas is the kilocalorie:nitrogen ratio.
Although the optimum ratio has not been determined, a ratio of 150:1 has been suggested as a safe
guide. Clients undergoing severe stress secondary
to burns, severe infection, or major trauma may
need lower ratios, and clients with only normal
maintenance requirements may do well with higher
ratios. Protein losses increase more rapidly than
does the metabolic rate in severely stressed clients.[5]
A kilocaloric intake of 45 kcal/kg per day and a
protein intake of 1.8 g/kg per day provide a kilocalo-
rie:nitrogen ratio of approximately 150:1.

A hypertonic glucose solution (20 to 50 percent
concentration) is the major kilocalorie source in
TPN solutions. The high concentrations are necessary in order to supply the daily kilocaloric need
without using fat. A synthetic crystalline L-amino
acid solution is the usual nitrogen source. These
amino acids are better used than protein hydrolysates, which contain peptides that are lost in the
urine in large quantities. Specialized amino acid solutions are available for clients with deranged amino
acid metabolism, including those with renal and
liver dysfunction and clients who are severely trau-
matized or infected. Electrolytes, trace minerals,
and vitamins are added directly to the base solution
of glucose and amino acids in amounts approximating known or estimated daily requirements.[6,7] Vitamin K and iron are not routinely added to the TPN
solution. Monitor the prothrombin time and red
blood cell indices and administer vitamin K and iron
as needed. Acetate is routinely added to the TPN
solution to prevent acid–base imbalances, and heparin is added to prevent clotting in the catheter. Albumin and insulin can be added to the solution if
needed. Avoid adding other medications since in-
compatibilities with the nutrient solution can occur.
Infuse a fat emulsion about twice weekly to provide
essential fatty acids; the fat emulsion also adds additional kilocalories.

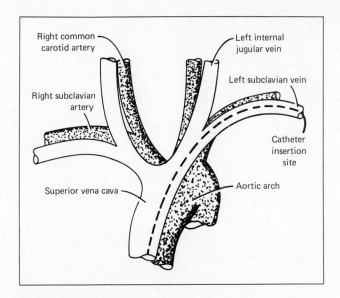

Figure 21-1
*The site of catheter insertion for TPN. The right subcla-
vian, innominate, or jugular vein may also be used as
the site of catheter insertion.*

The nutrient composition of a typical liter of TPN solution is as follows:

Glucose (20%)	200 g
Amino acids (4.5%)	42.5 g
Sodium	50 mEq
Potassium	35 mEq
Calcium	10 mEq
Phosphate	10 mM
Magnesium	8 mEq
Zinc	1.0 mg
Copper	0.4 mg
Manganese	0.1 mg
Chromium	4 μg
Vitamins	(see Reference 6)

Two to four liters of this solution is usually given daily.

Assess baseline vital signs and record body weight at the beginning of TPN therapy and monitor these indices regularly to aid in detecting complications (Table 21–7). A weight gain in excess of ½ lb daily suggests fluid retention. It is necessary to record intake and output, to monitor the results of laboratory tests, to test the urine for glucose and acetone, and to observe for edema and dehydration on a regular basis. Provide good oral hygiene to prevent oral inflammation and infection.

Since the client is lacking the pleasure associated with eating, provide emotional support on a continuing basis. Hallucinations can occur in clients for whom eating is especially pleasurable. Advise the client to expect a weight gain and also to expect smaller, fewer stools. Explain that TPN often suppresses the appetite.

When TPN is to be discontinued, avoid doing so abruptly. Rather, provide a period of transition that uses two overlapping feeding methods to assist the client in maintaining nutritional status. Some clients can be started directly on oral feedings of high-calorie high-protein foods while maintaining TPN in gradually decreasing amounts as oral intake increases. Other clients may require a period of tube feeding in combination with TPN before initiating oral intake. For clients who have not eaten for a long period of time, the transition to oral feeding may be difficult. In these cases, first, assure that the client can swallow properly and, second, try liquids, and later give soft or pureed foods. Restrict lactose and fat initially, since these may be difficult to digest and absorb. Management of TPN in adults and children is discussed is greater detail elsewhere.[8,9]

NUTRITION AND PHYSIOLOGIC STRESS

Assessment
Stress evokes a predictable series of neuroendocrine responses. The magnitude of the response corresponds to the severity of the stress and may range from very mild to very severe. Examples of physiologic situations that induce the stress response,

---

TABLE 21–7
COMPLICATIONS OF TPN THERAPY

Infection and Sepsis	Mechanical Complications	Metabolic Complications
Contamination of entrance site during catheter insertion	Puncture or laceration of subclavian artery	Hyperglycemia leading to glycosuria, osmotic diuresis, hyperosmolar non-ketotic dehydration, and coma
Long-term catheter placement	Air embolism	Ketoacidosis in diabetic clients
Seeding of catheter with blood-borne organisms or organisms from a distant site of infection	Pneumothorax	Postinfusion hypoglycemia
Contamination of infusate	Hemothorax	Electrolyte disturbances
	Hydrothorax	Hypo- and hyperkalemia
	Brachial plexus injury	Hypo- and hypernatremia
	Mediastinal hematoma	Hypo- and hypercalcemia
	Thoracic duct injury	Hypophosphatemia
	Pericardial tamponade	Hypomagnesemia
	Central venous thrombophlebitis	Hypo- and hypervitaminosis A and D
	Intrahepatic abscess	Essential fatty acid deficiency
	Endocarditis	Trace element deficiency
		Abnormal plasma aminograms
		Prerenal azotemia
		Liver function abnormalities and cirrhosis
		Cholelithiasis and acalculus cholecystitis
		Congestive heart failure and pulmonary edema
		Anemia
		Bleeding

listed in increasing magnitude of the response elicited, are elective surgery (uncomplicated), trauma (as from multiple injuries sustained in a vehicle accident), severe infection (as peritonitis), and major burns. At times, stressful stimuli may be combined in the same client; for example, infection may be a complication of surgery, trauma, or burns.

In response to stressful stimuli, the body directs its physiologic efforts toward adaptations for survival. The stress reaction is characterized by a catabolic, hypermetabolic state as the body's neural and hormonal mechanisms convert to metabolic pathways that provide glucose and energy to cells and preserve an adequate blood volume. The hormones involved are (1) those that influence the balance between anabolism and catabolism in the body and (2) those that influence water balance. The stress response favors a high catabolic:anabolic hormone ratio that produces a negative nitrogen balance in order to provide nutrient substances for survival. Amino acids are catabolized for energy via gluconeogenesis, and there is an increase in fat catabolism, bringing ketosis. Observe for weight loss and hyperglycemia in stressed clients. Be aware, however, that weight loss may be masked due to retention of sodium and water. Potassium losses are also incurred.

The period of hypermetabolism and catabolism is usually accompanied by a period of low kilocalorie and protein intake. The duration of the catabolic phase (with concomitant nitrogen loss) varies with the severity of the stress. As the stress becomes resolved, the processes described above are reversed as the client enters into an anabolic phase of metabolism, with positive nitrogen balance and slow weight gain.

Surgery. Surgical procedures are a form of planned trauma, and the metabolic response to stress discussed above is applicable here. Assess the nutritional status of all clients for whom surgery is contemplated, since both obesity and undernutrition add to the client's surgical risk. Unless the surgery is urgent, consider the postponement of the surgery until a realistic weight status has been achieved.

Preoperative Nutrition Intervention. During the preoperative phase of surgery, provide nutritional repletion as necessary for clients who are underweight. It may be necessary to use a combination of oral intake, tube feeding, and TPN to reduce their operative risks. Repletion by the enteral route may be the best method, since there is limited evidence to suggest that better resistance to infection is provided by enteral nutrition than by nutrients given intravenously. Assist obese clients with weight reduction (see Chap. 23).

In the immediate preoperative preparation, clear the gastrointestinal tract of partially digested food to prevent vomiting, aspiration, and other side effects during anesthesia or recovery from anesthesia. The presence of food may also increase the possibility of postoperative gastric retention and dilatation. If the surgery involves the gastrointestinal tract, food may interfere with the surgical procedure itself. The client is NPO (nothing by mouth) for at least 8 hours before surgery. For surgery scheduled in the morning, food and fluids are generally allowed until midnight on the day preceding the surgery. A light breakfast may be given when the operation is scheduled for the afternoon and local anesthesia is to be used. For gastrointestinal surgery, provide a low-residue diet for 2 to 3 days before the operation to clear the operative site of residue. An often ignored aspect of preoperative care is the additional malnutrition that may occur when surgery is cancelled and the client may not be fed for another 24 hours or longer. Give interim feedings in these cases to prevent dehydration and further energy and protein depletion.

Postoperative Nutritional Management. Nutritional management during the postoperative period involves two phases: (1) a period of parenteral infusion and (2) a period of progression to normal food intake. In either phase, the extra nutritional needs of the previously malnourished client must be added to the routine support measures used. In some cases, the surgical procedure may necessitate temporary or permanent use of a modified diet.

Until gastrointestinal peristalsis returns (measured by the return of bowel sounds), use parenteral therapy for nutritional support. The goals of management during this period are, first, to maintain fluid and electrolyte balance and prevent dehydration and shock and, second, to provide kilocalories to minimize tissue catabolism, prevent ketosis, and provide energy for the brain. The amount of parenteral fluids given during the period reflects the total amount of fluid, sodium, potassium, and glucose needed to (1) meet baseline requirements (Table 21–8), (2) replace abnormal losses (as in wound drainage, vomiting, or fever), and (3) replace deficits existing at the time of treatment.

Initiate oral feeding as soon as possible after the return of gastrointestinal peristalsis in order to stimulate normal gastrointestinal function and an early return to a full diet. In this way, severe energy and protein deficits can be averted. The period of delay in oral intake depends on the type of surgery. Encourage ambulation as soon as possible to increase the appetite and prevent losses of protein and calcium. If dressing changes and treatments are involved, time those that might bring anorexia as far away from mealtime as possible. Encourage clients to eat and drink slowly to prevent air swallowing, which contributes to gas formation in the gastrointestinal tract. According to individual tolerance, the client progresses from water to clear liquids to full liquids to a soft and finally to a regular diet.

TABLE 21–8
BASELINE REQUIREMENTS FOR FLUID, ELECTROLYTES, AND GLUCOSE IN THE ADULT SURGICAL CLIENT

Nutrient	Amount	Comment
Water	1250–3000	Specific amount depends on age, sex, and body cell mass; renal efficiency may be abnormal in surgical clients, and there is an increased renal solute load secondary to catabolism of body cell mass; baseline requirements are increased with fever, sweating, and increased metabolism; unless there is serious impairment of renal function, a daily urine volume of 1200–1500 ml is desirable in the average adult following surgery
Sodium	76 mEq	There is sodium retention immediately after surgery secondary to the increased secretion of aldosterone (sodium diuresis occurs 5–7 days after surgery); the sodium requirement is increased by abnormal losses (as from intestinal secretions) and decreased by excesses (as with an overexpansion of the extracellular fluid)
Potassium	40 mEq	Potassium chloride should not be administered in concentrations in excess of 40 mEq/liter of fluid; the baseline requirement should be dissolved in at least 1000 ml of otherwise isotonic fluid
Glucose	100–125 g	This amount of glucose will prevent approximately one-half the nitrogen loss resulting from catabolism of the lean body mass and will also prevent ketosis; amounts in excess of this (even up to 400 g/day) will not completely prevent the breakdown of the body cell mass

Nutrition and Wound Healing

Assessment and Intervention. Synthesis of collagen, which is the end product of wound healing, is dependent on an adequate supply of energy and nutrients needed to stimulate the inflammatory response and to form fibroblasts—cells that form collagen—and new blood vessels in the area of the wound. In addition to sources of glucose for energy, protein, and oxygen, several vitamins and trace minerals are needed for the wound to heal.

Vitamin C is needed for collagen synthesis; provide 2 to 4 g daily for clients whose wounds are substantial, as with a severe burn. Vitamin C deficiency not only retards wound healing but may also lead to disruption of old wounds. Although the exact mechanism whereby vitamin A is needed for wound healing is not known, a deficiency results in a decrease in the inflammatory response needed for the early phases of healing as well as a decrease in the subsequent phases. Provide a maximum amount of 1000 to 25,000 IU daily for clients with severe wounds. Avoid excesses, however, which can lead to adverse effects. Although vitamin E has been promoted for its beneficial effects, this vitamin actually acts as an anti-inflammatory agent and can halt the inflammatory phase of healing. Zinc and iron are also needed for collagen synthesis, and copper must

be present in adequate amounts for the healing process to occur. An excessive amount of zinc is no more beneficial than an adequate amount. Iron is important not only for its role in collagen synthesis but also as a component of hemoglobin needed to provide the oxygen necessary for collagen synthesis. Assess for anemia; if the hematocrit falls below 24 percent, wound healing is likely to be adversely affected due to a lack of oxygen.

Assess for the presence of other conditions that can lead to wound infection and retarded wound healing. These include (1) preoperative malnutrition with a prolonged convalescence, (2) presence of obesity, and (3) poorly controlled diabetes mellitus. Malnutrition and weight loss lead to a decreased resistance to infection. Since the wound is a relatively good scavenger of energy and substrates, the malnutrition and weight loss must be significant before wounds fail to heal. Obesity causes added stress on the wound, presents a mechanical barrier to the arrival of healing cells to the wound area, and may have an adverse effect on pulmonary function and thus the oxygen supply. Moreover, obesity may be associated with insulin resistance—insulin is needed for the early phases of collagen synthesis. Because of the role of insulin in wound healing, be alert to the need for strict control in diabetic clients during the crucial early inflammatory phases of healing.

Burns

Assessment and Intervention. The metabolic stress of a burn injury varies from the simple mechanisms involved with wound healing to an all-out effort by the body to overcome profound shock, extensive loss of body tissue, and persistent bacterial invasion. Assess for altered capillary dynamics, hypermetabolism, negative nitrogen balance, and weight loss, which characterize the post-traumatic metabolic response to a major burn. These changes drastically increase the nutritional requirements. The kilocalorie need frequently exceeds that of any other condition. However, in a given client, precise nutritional requirements are dependent on the extent of the burn, age, previous nutritional state, and presence of complicating metabolic disorders. If the kilocalorie need is not satisfied, weight loss occurs in proportion to the extent of the burn. Diminished peristaltic and absorptive function and anorexia also accompany severe burns.

During the immediate postburn phase, reestablish fluid and electrolyte balance and prevent shock by administering an appropriate intravenous formula. Maintain a urinary output of at least 15 ml/hour for an infant, 25 ml/hour for a child, and 30 ml/hour for an adult. After the client has become stabilized, consider the enteral infusion of a defined formula diet (such as Vivonex HN, Eaton Labs) to prevent ulceration and bleeding of the gastric mucosa. Some investigators have found this treatment superior to both antacids and cimetidine in preventing ulceration and bleeding.[10] Provide a high-kilocalorie, high-protein diet to minimize weight loss (at least) or to fully meet energy nutrient requirements (at best). Use the formula given in the last part of this chapter (assessing hospital malnutrition) to determine the kilocalorie and protein requirement. As much as 3000 to 6000 kcal and 150 to 200 g of protein or more may be needed daily. Provide multivitamin supplements, including 2 to 4 g of vitamin C and 1500 to 2500 IU of vitamin A. Assess the need for providing supplements of zinc, iron, and copper.

The sheer volume of food required often makes it difficult to achieve nutritional balance, and spontaneous food intake may account for no more than 60 percent of need. Provide small frequent feedings to promote acceptance of the high-kilocalorie, high-protein intake and record the amount of feeding consumed. Avoid constipation by including foods high in fiber content. The judicious use of fats not only adds kilocalories in a concentrated form but also may lessen the tendency for constipation. Raw vegetables served as finger foods may increase vegetable consumption in children. Educate the client about the importance of an adequate dietary intake and allow the client some control in planning the diet. Encourage the family to prepare favorite dishes as occasional treats. Dressings should not be changed in close proximity to mealtimes, and do not permit meals to be interrupted by other aspects of care.

Supplement oral feeding with tube feeding or TPN as needed to achieve the desired level of intake. A defined formula diet such as Vivonex HN can provide as much as 8000 to 9000 kcal when given by continuous infusion over a 24-hour period.

Provide good oral hygiene to prevent oral complications and to relieve thirst, which may be a problem in the early postburn period. When possible, encourage ambulation to improve the appetite and reduce the calcium and protein losses associated with immobilization. Encourage an adequate fluid intake to prevent renal calculi, which also complicates immobilization.

Once the burn is covered with skin (by grafting or healing) the catabolic phase is reversed, since protein loss from the wound ceases, the metabolic rate returns to normal, and there begins the phase of tissue repair or anabolism. With wound closure, observe that the appetite and food intake improve in association with improved morale and increased exercise. During this phase, there is a continuing need to supply food in adequate quality and quantity to restore the body mass. At the end of the anabolic stage, control kilocalorie intake to prevent post-traumatic obesity, however.

Infections

Assessment and Intervention. A generalized infectious illness causes widespread metabolic and biochemical changes that become evident within hours after the onset of the infectious process. A systemic infection can lead to overt nutritional deficiency by increasing nutrient requirements, by decreasing nutrient intake, absorption, or use, or by increasing nutrient excretion. Be aware that any acute infection triggers the stress response, with accompanying hypermetabolism and negative balances of nitrogen, potassium, phosphorus, magnesium, and sulfur, and a consequent weight loss. Typically, there is a decrease in protein synthesis, an increase in protein catabolism, and alteration in the amino acid profile. There is a redistribution of iron and zinc. The plasma levels of these minerals fall as they accumulate in the liver. In contrast, plasma levels of copper rise.

Fever may be present, bringing further increases in catabolism and losses of heat and nutrients in sweat. The catabolic response persists into convalescence, and the magnitude of the loss is proportional to the severity and duration of fever. Observe for a decrease in food intake because of generalized malaise, pain, discomfort, and anorexia. In respiratory infections, coughing, dyspnea (shortness of breath), nasal obstruction, and mouth breathing may further limit food intake, and if the gastrointestinal tract is involved, nausea, vomiting, and diarrhea may contribute to decreased intake or malabsorption. Prior to the onset of fever, there is an increased renal excretion of sodium chloride, although retention of sodium and water occurs during the febrile phase of an acute infection. This excess is usually lost during postfebrile diuresis. Evaluate for the presence of dehydration, electrolyte depletion, and acid–base imbalances if there is severe diarrhea, vomiting, sweating, or hyperventilation. Should metabolic acidosis occur, intracellular sodium concentration increases, and the problem is overload, not dehydration. Before resolution of the infection and repletion of nutritional deficits, resistance to infection is lowered, and the client may be predisposed to secondary infections.

The nutritional requirements during infection are related to the severity and duration of the infection. Direct management toward controlling fever and provide a diet with sufficient energy and key nutrients to prevent or minimize the concomitant nutrient depletion. Correct fluid and electrolyte imbalances by the intravenous route to permit return of the hematocrit and protein concentration to normal. Differentiate between a sodium deficit and an overload; appropriate therapy may include fluid and sodium restriction rather than the administration of saline solutions, which could precipitate cardiac failure or cerebral edema.

If the client's infection is severe, increase the protein content of the diet by 50 percent. Kilocaloric requirements may be increased by 200 to 300 percent over basal needs. Supplement with vitamins and minerals at a dosage level that is double the normal amount. Be cautious in increasing the iron intake, however, since this may be harmful to host defense against the infectious disease. The nutrient losses associated with an acute infection of short duration can usually be replenished within several weeks if the client was well nourished previously. However, it may be necessary to provide tube feeding or TPN if the illness is life threatening and the client is losing substantial weight.

NUTRIENT–DRUG INTERACTIONS

Assessment and Intervention

Nutrients and drugs interact in a twofold manner: (1) drugs may alter food intake or the absorption, use, and excretion of nutrients, and (2) foods and nutrients may alter the use of drugs or, in a few instances, exert a direct pharmacologic action. The interactive process may involve prescription and nonprescription medications and a wide variety of nutrients. Both nutritional balance and drug response may be affected, resulting in either overt clinical changes or in changes that are both subtle and hard to detect.

Effects of Drugs on Nutrition. The mechanisms responsible for drug-induced alterations in nutrient balance are (1) alteration in food intake and (2) phar-

macokinetic influences whereby absorption, metabolism, or excretion of nutrients is affected.

Nutritional status may be indirectly affected by drugs that either decrease or increase food intake or produce gastrointestinal irritation. Anorexia is a side effect of many drugs. Observe for other side effects that can lead to a decrease in appetite, including nausea and vomiting, altered taste acuity, change in taste sensations, or dry mouth. Expect, for example, a client who has received an excessive amount of digitalis to be anorectic and nauseated, a client who takes griseofulvin (an antifungal agent) to have a decrease in taste acuity, and a client who takes an anticholinergic drug to experience a dry mouth. Antineoplastic drugs produce several side effects, including anorexia, altered taste, nausea, vomiting, and oral ulceration, all of which lead to a reduction in food intake. On the other hand, assess for excessive food intake and overweight in clients who take drugs that increase the appetite, such as corticosteroids and psychotropic agents, including the phenothiazine tranquilizers and tricyclic antidepressants. Note, however, that some drugs may have different effects on appetite at different times or under different circumstances. For example, the tricyclic antidepressants may cause either weight gain or loss. The appetite often improves as depression lessens. However, the drug may cause nausea, vomiting, gastrointestinal distress, altered taste, and anorexia. While small doses of alcohol may increase the appetite, large doses serve as an appetite depressant.

Malabsorption may be induced by drugs that increase intestinal motility, including laxatives, or by those that damage the intestinal mucosa, such as neomycin and colchicine. Moreover, many nutrients require energy for transport across the gastrointestinal membranes, i.e., they are actively transported, and malabsorption can result from inhibition of the active transport mechanism by drugs. An example is the calcium malabsorption that occurs secondary to the use of such drugs as phenobarbital, primidone, phenytoin, and glutethimide. These drugs accelerate the catabolism of vitamin D and its metabolites, which are needed for the intestinal transport of calcium.

Nutrient imbalance can result secondary to a drug's effect on nutrient metabolism or use. Many nutrients must be converted to a metabolically active form before they can perform a nutrient function. These biologic transformations usually occur in the liver, although other organs, such as the kidney or intestine, may be involved. An example is pyridoxine. The various forms of this vitamin must be converted to the metabolically active coenzyme, pyridoxal phosphate. Several drugs, namely, isoniazid, hydralazine, and levodopa, form complexes with pyridoxal phosphate; thus the coenzyme is inactivated. Observe for symptoms of pyridoxine deficiency secondary to the use of these drugs.

Other examples of altered metabolism of nutrients by drugs involve (1) the need for nutrients to metabolize drugs and (2) common metabolic pathways shared by certain nutrients and drugs. For example, the metabolism of phenytoin and other anticonvulsants requires folic acid as a coenzyme. Expect an increase in the use of folic acid and a relative depletion of folate following administration of these anticonvulsant agents. Hepatic enzymes that metabolize the anticonvulsants, such as phenytoin and phenobarbital, also metabolically inactivate vitamin D. Chronic administration of the anticonvulsants induces the formation of increased amounts of the enzymes responsible for their degradative metabolism. The subsequent decreased activity of vitamin D produces hypocalcemia and bone changes, in particular, osteomalacia.

Evaluate the need for supplemental vitamin D and folic acid in clients who receive anticonvulsant therapy on a long-term basis. Be cautious, however, in providing a large folic acid supplement—rather, administer small supplements. Folic acid may interfere with the metabolism (or possibly absorption) of the drug and lead to decreased blood levels of the drug. A similar metabolic interaction occurs between pyridoxine and levodopa. Clients who take this drug should avoid an excessive intake of pyridoxine to prevent reversal of the therapeutic effects of the drug because of metabolic interactions.

Under certain conditions, the desired therapeutic effect of a drug is achieved through its deliberate interference with the body's use of a particular nutrient. Examples are methotrexate, used in cancer chemotherapy, and anticoagulants, used in the prevention and treatment of thrombophlebitis. Methotrexate is antagonistic to the action of folic acid, whereas the anticoagulants have anti-vitamin K properties.

Some drugs increase the fecal or urinary loss of nutrients. Excessive use of antacids containing aluminum hydroxide can lead to phosphate depletion and bone demineralization (rickets or osteomalacia). The aluminum hydroxide combines with phosphate in the gastrointestinal tract, and the resulting aluminum phosphate is excreted in the feces. Aspirin increases the urinary loss of vitamin C, and the renal excretion of electrolytes is affected to a significant extent by the administration of diuretics. Assess for urinary loss of potassium, calcium, magnesium, and zinc in clients who are being treated with diuretics. Table 21–9 provides a summary of the effects of selected drugs on nutrient balance.

Prevent drug-induced malnutrition by identifying those at greatest risk and providing dietary changes or nutrient supplements for these groups. Expect drug-induced malnutrition to occur most frequently in clients who are long-term users of multiple drugs and who are already at nutritional risk because of a marginal diet, chronic disease, drug abuse, or physiologic stress, i.e., the fetus, growing child, and the elderly. In particular, assess for the effects in hospitalized clients and in elderly persons living in institutionalized settings who are taking several drugs. In the elderly, risk factors often interact together, since many older clients take one or more drugs on a chronic basis, consume marginal diets, and suffer from chronic diseases that can lead to nutritional deficiency. Moreover, the aging process itself, associated with such factors as diminished gastrointestinal absorption and diminished ability to detoxify drugs, alters the use of both drugs and nutrients. In this situation, the added stress imposed on nutritional status by drugs may be sufficient to produce clinical symptoms.

Use all four parameters of nutritional assessment discussed in Chapter 11. Exert caution, however, in interpreting the results of laboratory indices with concomitant use of drugs, since some drugs can influence assays for certain nutrients. Avoid administration of medications that contain disallowed nutrients for clients with certain conditions, such as a cough syrup containing sugar for a diabetic or a medication that contains sodium for a client on a sodium-restricted diet.

Effect of Foods and Nutrients on Drug Therapy. Just as drugs may alter a client's nutritional state, various dietary components or dietary patterns may alter the effectiveness of drug therapy either by altering the absorption, metabolism, or excretion of a drug or by altering the response to the drug. Some of the mechanisms resemble those whereby drug therapy influences nutritional status. The interactions have both positive and negative effects on drug response. In some cases, the effectiveness of the drug is increased or the side effects are decreased when the drug is administered simultaneously with food. In other cases, the effectiveness of the drug is diminished or side effects become evident when the drug is given in close proximity to eating or when certain types of foods are consumed simultaneously.

Alterations in Drug Absorption. The most widely reported effect of foods on drug therapy involves alterations in drug absorption when the drugs are taken simultaneously with food. Both the rate and the total amount of a drug absorbed may be increased or decreased when taken with food. Although simultaneously food intake increases the absorption of drugs in some instances, as a general rule drugs are absorbed more slowly when taken with food, and in some cases the total amount of the drug absorbed is reduced (see Table 21–10 for examples). This effect is generally attributed to such factors as the delaying effect of food on gastric emptying, changes in gastrointestinal pH induced by food, chelation of drugs by food constituents, or competition between drugs and nutrients for absorption.

The presence of food in the stomach slows the rate of gastric emptying, thereby delaying the delivery of some drugs to the intestine for absorption. Meals that are high in fat or large in size have the greatest effect. Since drugs are better absorbed in

TABLE 21–9
EFFECTS OF SELECTED DRUGS ON NUTRIENT BALANCE

Drug	*Effect*
Abused drugs	
Alcohol	↓ or sporadic food intake; ↓ fat digestion (pancreatitis); ↓ absorption of D-xylose, glucose, fat, vitamin B_{12}, folic acid, thiamin; ↑ urinary excretion of zinc, magnesium, and calcium
Narcotics (e.g., heroin, codeine)	General malnutrition
Anti-inflammatory agents	
Colchicine	↓ absorption of fat, cholesterol, carotene, sodium, potassium, vitamin B_{12}, lactose, nitrogen
Corticosteroids	↑ appetite; ↓ glucose tolerance; ↓ muscle protein and negative nitrogen balance; ↑ serum lipids and liver fat; ↓ renal sodium loss → edema; ↓ calcium and phosphorus absorption; gastric inflammation → ulcer; ↑ catabolism of vitamin D; osteoporosis; ↑ urinary excretion of calcium, magnesium, zinc, potassium, vitamin C ↑ conversion of tryptophan → niacin (↑ need for vitamin B_6); poor wound healing
Nonsteroidal anti-inflammatory drugs	Gastrointestinal bleeding (aspirin, indomethacin, phenylbutazone); ↑ thiamine and vitamin C excretion (aspirin); folic acid responsive megaloblastic anemia (chronic use of phenylbutazone); inhibition of vitamin C metabolism (aspirin); ↓ iron absorption (aspirin)
Anorexics	Appetite suppression; possible growth retardation in hyperkinetic children with use of dextroamphetamine and methylphenidate—catch-up growth occurs when drug discontinued
Antacids	Systemic alkalosis → inactivation of thiamine; ↓ iron absorption (carbonate antacids and magnesium trisilicate); ↓ phosphate absorption (aluminum and magnesium antacids); ↓ vitamin A absorption (aluminum hydroxide); steatorrhea (calcium carbonate); some contain excessive sodium → edema in susceptible individuals; when combined with excessive milk intake → hypercalcemia
Anticholinergic drugs	Slow gastric emptying and ↓ intestinal motility; ↑ absorption of riboflavin (propantheline); xerostomia
Anticonvulsants and sedatives (hydantoins and barbiturates)	Deficiency of folic acid and vitamin D (supplements should be provided—the dose of supplemental folate should be small, since large doses tend to decrease the blood level of the anticonvulsant and precipitate seizures); ↑ catabolism of vitamin K (can cause vitamin K deficiency in newborns of mothers taking anticonvulsants); ↓ absorption of vitamin B_{12} and xylose; ↓ serum levels of calcium, magnesium, and vitamin B_6; ↑ serum copper; ↑ blood glucose (Dilantin); gingival hyperplasia (Dilantin)
Antidepressants	Stimulation of the appetite → weight gain (gastrointestinal side effects may → weight loss); monamine oxidase inhibitors react with tyramine-containing foods to produce headache and hypertensive crisis; avoid concomitant use with alcohol to avoid further depression of the central nervous system
Antimicrobials	Appetite suppression; change in intestinal flora → diarrhea; ↓ intestinal synthesis of B vitamins and vitamin K (broad-spectrum antibiotics, such as chloramphenicol, tetracycline, penicillins, sulfonamides); colitis (clindamycin, lincomycin, ampicillin, tetracycline, chloramphenicol); ↓ in protein synthesis, altered hemoglobin synthesis, and aplastic or hypoplastic anemia (chloramphenicol); damage to intestinal mucosa, inhibition of mucosal enzymes, precipitation of bile acids, fat, and cholesterol → steatorrhea, diminished pancreatic lipase activity and malabsorption of medium-chain triglycerides, nitrogen, disaccharides, carotene, vitamins A, B_{12}, and K, iron, calcium, sodium, and potassium (neomycin and to a lesser extent, polymyxin, kanamycin, and bacitracin); unpleasant aftertaste (oral penicillins); high content of sodium and/or potassium (IV penicillin G); mucosal block in folate uptake (salicylazo-sulfapyridine—Azulfidine); chelates minerals such as calcium, magnesium, iron, zinc—coadministration with antacids, milk, or iron preparations decrease absorption of both the drug and the minerals, ↑ blood urea nitrogen (tetracycline); binds pyridoxine and produces peripheral neuropathy (isoniazide—daily pyridoxine supplement necessary); ↓ absorption of vitamin B_{12}, folate, carotene, xylose, iron, fat, and cholesterol (para-aminosalicylic acid)
Cytotoxic agents	Negative protein balance (inhibits protein synthesis); ↓ in food intake secondary to nausea, vomiting, anorexia, stomatitis, buccal ulceration, glossitis, gingivitis, pharyngitis; and altered taste (nitrogen mustard produces a metallic taste); ↓ nutrient absorption secondary to inflammation of the gastrointestinal tract; anemia
Chelating agents	Chelation of metals → ↓ absorption; ↑ urinary excretion of vitamin B_6, zinc, copper (penicillamine); ↓ taste acuity and aftertaste → suppression of the appetite (penicillamine)
Diuretics	↑ renal loss of sodium, water, potassium, calcium, magnesium, and zinc; most diuretics are capable of producing hypokalemia (except spironolactone and triamterene), hypomagnesemia, ↓ carbohydrate tolerance, and water and electrolyte imbalance; sodium depletion (with concurrent severe dietary sodium restriction); hypokalemia (poses a risk of digitalis toxicity in those taking digitalis glycosides); hyperkalemia (with the use of triamterine and spironolactone); hyperuricemia and precipitation of gout in susceptible individuals (thiazides, furosemide, ethacrynic acid); hyperglycemia, especially in pregnant women,

TABLE 21–9 (Continued)

Drug	Effect
	hypertensives, and those with latent diabetes (thiazides, furosemide, ethacrynic acid); hypocalcemia (furosemide, ethacrynic acid, mercurials, spironolactone, and triamterine); hypercalcemia in clients prone to the disorder (thiazides); hypomagnesemia (thiazides, furosemide, ethacrynic acid, mercurials, spironolactone, triamterene—?, poses a risk of digitalis toxicity in those taking digitalis glycosides); zinc depletion (thiazides, furosemide, ethacrynic acid, mercurials—?); hypomagnesemia and hypocalcemia may be aggravated by the concurrent use of digitalis glycosides that also ↑ the renal loss of these nutrients; ↓ serum folate (furosemide—this diuretic is antagonistic to the action of folate)
Hypocholesterolemics	Cholestyramine: steatorrhea; malabsorption of cholesterol, vitamins A, D, K, B₁₂, folate, calcium, iron, monosaccharides; ↑ renal excretion of calcium; osteomalacia; hyperchloremic acidosis Clofibrate: ↑ fecal excretion of sterols; inhibits intestinal mucosal enzymes involved in carbohydrate digestion; ↓ absorption of vitamin B₁₂, xylose, and sugar, carotene, medium-chain triglycerides, iron, and electrolytes; ↓ blood level of vitamin K; unpleasant or altered taste sensation → suppression of appetite Neomycin: see antimicrobials
Hypoglycemics	↓ absorption of glucose, xylose, amino acids, fat, calcium, water, electrolytes, and vitamin B₁₂ (biguanides); ↓ absorption of glucose (sulfonylureas, e.g., tolbutamide); altered taste sensations (e.g., phenformin, sulfonylureas); need to restrict alcohol use to avoid side effects, such as flushing, nausea, shortness of breath, palpitations (tolbutamide), and lactic acidosis (the biguanide, DBI)
Laxatives	↑ gastric motility; ↓ intestinal uptake of glucose; steatorrhea; fecal loss of calcium, phosphate, and electrolytes—especially bicarbonate, sodium, and potassium; excessive use may result in hypokalemia, hyponatremia, osteomalacia, dehydration, and hypoalbuminemia; mineral oil may cause malabsorption of carotene and fat-soluble vitamins; excessive use of milk of magnesia may cause mild steatorrhea and loss of phosphate; excessive use of phenolphthalein, colocynth, jalop, podophyllin, and bisacodyl may cause protein-losing enteropathy; excessive use of phenolphthalein may cause decreased absorption of vitamin D and calcium
Oral contraceptives	↓ serum levels of folate, riboflavin, vitamin C, vitamin B₁₂, pyridoxine, and zinc, ↑ serum levels of vitamin A, iron, and copper
Surfactants (stool softeners)	Alters fat dispersion and permeability of mucosal cell membrane and may ↑ absorption of fat, cholesterol, and vitamin A (e.g., Tween 80, polysorbate 80, and dioctyl sodium sulfosuccinate)
Tranquilizers	Stimulation of the appetite → weight gain (gastrointestinal side effects may → weight loss); hyperglycemia, glucosuria, hypercholesterolemia (phenothiazines). Avoid concurrent use of alcohol to diminish the risk of further central nervous system depression
Miscellaneous Anticoagulants	Excessive use of anticoagulants (e.g., coumarin derivatives) may produce vitamin K deficiency. Other drugs that may enhance the anticoagulant response are chloral hydrate, clofibrate, phenylbutazone, indomethacin, salicylates, certain acid sulfonamides, quinidine, quinine, cinchophen, ethanol, and possibly anabolic steroids and dextrothyroxine. In contrast, excessive ingestion of vitamin K-rich foods (such as green leafy vegetables) may result in decreased effectiveness of the anticoagulant
Ferrous sulfate	Nausea, vomiting; inhibits absorption of tetracycline and its derivatives: a time interval of 3 hours should be allowed between oral ingestion of the two drugs to avoid interactions; ascorbic acid ↑ absorption
Hypotensive drugs Digitalis glycosides	↓ glucose absorption; ↑ urinary excretion of calcium and magnesium; toxicity (producing nausea, vomiting, anorexia, and diarrhea) may be induced by hypokalemia, hypomagnesemia, or hypercalcemia
Guanethidine	Diarrhea, nausea, vomiting, dry mouth, weight gain
Hydralazine	Pyridoxine deficiency; ↑ magnesium excretion; anorexia, nausea, vomiting, and diarrhea
Methyldopa	May ↑ need for folate and vitamin B₁₂; dry mouth, gastrointestinal distention, constipation, or diarrhea
Reserpine	↑ gastric motility and secretion; can cause nausea, vomiting, anorexia, diarrhea, and weight gain
Potassium chloride	↓ absorption of vitamin B₁₂
Levodopa	May induce pyridoxine deficiency (especially in those with high requirements, such as the malnourished and alcoholics); however, pyridoxine supplements diminish the effectiveness of the drug; ↑ urinary loss of sodium and potassium; may ↑ requirement for folate and vitamin B₁₂; effectiveness of the drug ↓ by a high-protein diet—amino acids and the drug compete for absorption; the daily protein intake should be approximately 0.5 g/k/day, and the medication should not be taken concurrently with high-protein foods (such as milk and cheese)

TABLE 21–10
EFFECT ON ABSORPTION OF SELECTED DRUGS WHEN CONSUMED WITH FOOD

↓ Rate of Absorption	↓ Extent of Absorption	Absorption Promoted by Food Intake
Acetaminophen	Antipyrene	Carbamazepine
Aspirin	Aspirin	Dicumerol
Amoxicillin	Ampicillin	Griseofulvin
Cimetidine	Cephalexen	Erythromycin estolate and
Capuride	Erythromycin stearate	erythromycin ethylsuccinate
Cefaclor	Fluorouracil	Hydralazine
Digoxin	Indomethacin	Hydrochlorothiazide
Furosemide	Isoniazid	Lithium salts
Metronidazole	Levodopa	Metoprolol
Sulfonamides	Lincomycin	Nitrofurantoin
	Methacycline	Propranolol
	Nafcillin	Propoxyphene
	Penicillins G and V	Riboflavin
	Phenacetin	Spironolactone
	Phenobarbital	
	Propantheline	
	Propylthiouracil	
	Rifampicin	
	Solatol	
	Tetracycline	
	Theophylline	

the nonionized, more fat-soluble state, the pH of gastric and intestinal fluids also affects absorption. The presence of food in the stomach raises gastric pH, which generally affects the dissolution of drugs taken in a tablet or capsule form more than absorption per se. For instance, the rise in gastric pH following food consumption may destroy the enteric coating on time-release drugs, leading to higher blood levels in a shorter period of time than is desired. Consumption of acidic fluids, such as colas, lemon juice, or cranberry juice—all with a pH below 2.5—may aid the dissolution and thus the absorption of weakly basic and even some weakly acidic drugs. Be aware, however, that acid-labile drugs, such as penicillin G, may be impaired by mixing the drug with acidic beverages to mask the disagreeable taste.

Drugs may directly interact with food substances, such as metal ions or nonabsorbed polysaccharides found in high-fiber foods, in the gastrointestinal tract by chelating with these substances. Tetracycline, a broad-spectrum antibiotic, may combine with such metals as calcium, iron, and aluminum, leading to failure of absorption of both the nutrient and the drug. A similar type of chelating reaction may occur with the simultaneous ingestion of oral zinc or iron salts and foods containing phosphates (as milk) and phytates found in high-fiber foods.

A high dietary intake of protein decreases the therapeutic effect of levodopa, a drug used to treat Parkinson's disease. Amino acids compete with levodopa for absorption. In other situations, the simultaneous ingestion of food may have a beneficial effect by either increasing the absorption of the drug or

decreasing the gastrointestinal irritation associated with the drug. For instance, the absorption of drugs that have poor dissolution properties or that are fat soluble is enhanced when consumed with food. Griseofulvin, an oral antifungal agent that is highly fat-soluble, is better absorbed when taken in conjunction with a high-fat meal. Some drugs are intrinsically irritating to the gastrointestinal tract, and such side effects as nausea and vomiting are common, and the presence of food in the stomach may counteract the direct irritation of the drug. Table 21–11 provides a list of drugs to be taken with or

TABLE 21–11
DRUGS REPORTED TO IRRITATE THE GASTROINTESTINAL TRACT

Aminophylline	Nalidixic acid
Aminosalicyclic acid	Nitrofurantoin
Ammonium chloride	Pancreatin
Aspirin	Phenformin
Aspirin–phenacetin–caffeine (APC)	Phenylbutazone
Chloral hydrate	Potassium salts
Chlorpromazine	Prednisolone
Chlorpropamide	Prednisone
Phenytoin	Probenecid
Ferrous salts (fumerate, gluconate, lactate, sulfate)	Procyclidine
	Reserpine
Griseofulvin	Sulfinpyrazone
Hydrochlorothiazide	Tolbutamide
Hydrocortisone	Triamterene
Indomethacin	Trihexyhemidyl
Isoniazide	Trimeprazine
Metronidazole	

immediately after meals or snacks or with an antacid to buffer the irritating effects. Although propantheline, an anticholinergic drug used to decrease gastric secretion and motility in clients with gastric ulcer, has irritating effects, it may lose some of its pharmacologic effects when given before meals.

Time the administration of drugs appropriately in relation to food intake and assist the client to develop a meal and drug schedule consistent with both nutrient and drug needs. If food is to be avoided because of possible interference with drug absorption, stress to the client that the drug should not be taken in the time period of 1 hour before to 2 hours after a meal. Advise clients taking tetracycline to separate the ingestion of tetracycline and dairy products. Moreover, the simultaneous ingestion of baking soda or antacids, sometimes used to reduce the secondary gastrointestinal distress, also reduces tetracycline absorption. Assist the client to detect hidden sources of metal ions, including the cooking of acidic foods in aluminum or iron cookware. It may be prudent to advise that drugs not be taken simultaneously with a high-fiber diet. Advise clients for whom griseofulvin is prescribed to take the drug in conjunction with high-fat meals. Assist clients who are being treated with levodopa to plan a protein-restricted diet (0.5 g/kg per day), with the protein distributed in meals throughout the day. Unless contraindicated because of a fluid restriction, advise the client to consume a full glass of water with the drug to aid in its dissolution and absorption.

Alterations in Drug Metabolism. Nutrients or nonnutrient substances consumed with food can alter the rate of metabolism, that is, the rate of inactivation or degradation, of drugs or other chemicals. Exposure to foreign substances, such as drugs, leads to an increase in the synthesis of enzymes involved

▶ with their metabolism, a phenomenum called **enzyme induction.** The production of drug-metabolizing enzymes occurs primarily in the liver, but these enzymes are located also in other body sites, such as the intestine and kidney. Enzyme induction leads to an accelerated rate of drug clearance. Assess for the concurrent presence of other substances consumed with food that can also induce drug-metabolizing enzymes, increase the rate of drug clearance, and alter drug response. These include alcohol consumed habitually (and without concurrent cirrhosis of the liver), theophylline contained in chocolate and tea, curry powder, food additives such as BHA and BHT, polycyclic hydrocarbons contained in mineral oil, tobacco smoke, and charcoal-broiled meat, caffeine consumed in small amounts, and chemicals, such as endoles, that are present in such foods as cabbage, turnips, brussels sprouts, cauliflower, spinach, dill, and alfalfa. Although individually the changes in drug metabolism induced by these substances are small, the effects are additive. Assess total exposure to these enzyme inducers to determine their potential effect on drug clearance and drug response. In particular, advise clients to avoid alcohol ingestion concurrently with drugs.

Failure of enzyme induction prolongs drug response, leading to drug toxicity. Malnutrition, particularly a deficiency of protein (both quality and quantity), vitamin C, niacin, riboflavin, and zinc, decreases enzyme activity and the rate of drug metabolism. Assess the nutritional status of clients who experience unexplained drug toxicity. During the assessment, determine the blood albumin concentration, which is likely to be low in malnourished clients. Many drugs are transported in the blood partially complexed with plasma proteins, particularly albumin. Drug toxicity may be potentiated by a low blood albumin level, since more drug is directly available to the target tissue. In addition to causing drug toxicity, malnutrition may lead to a poor response to drug therapy.

Also assess for other dietary practices that may lead to drug toxicity in association with release of excessive amounts of drug from body storage sites, particularly adipose tissue. Fat-soluble drugs may be concentrated in adipose tissue. Erratic dietary practices, such as rapid weight loss, skipping meals, and use of low-carbohydrate diets can release an excessive quantity of drugs into the bloodstream. Of particular concern is drugs taken on a long-term basis, such as antipsychotics and anticonvulsants.

Certain drugs consumed with specific foods may inhibit drug-metabolizing enzymes. For instance, the enzyme monoamine oxidase metabolizes the potent vasopressor tyramine, found naturally in a number of foods (Table 21–12) in the intestinal mucosa and liver. Advise clients who take monoamine oxidase inhibitors, such as procarbazine, to avoid consuming tryamine-containing food to prevent severe side effects, including hypertensive crisis or even death. In contrast, other nonnutritive substances consumed with food may inhibit drug metabolism. Methylxanthines present in coffee, tea, and chocolate inhibit not only their own metabolism but also that of other methylxanthines, when taken in excessive amounts.

Alterations in Drug Excretion. Renal excretion is the primary route for drug elimination, although some drugs are excreted in the bile. The effect of foods on drug excretion is related to the capacity of certain foods to alter the urinary pH and, thus, the degree of ionization of drugs that are acidic or basic in reaction. Drugs in a nonionized form are not readily excreted in the urine—rather, they diffuse more readily from the urine into the blood. Generally, basic drugs are more readily excreted in acidic urine, and the converse is true for acidic drugs.

Be aware that acid ash and alkaline ash diets, used for therapeutic purposes in some situations, can change urinary pH sufficiently to alter drug excretion, although extreme shifts below pH 5.0 or above 8.0 are not easily achieved by diet alone. Toxic

TABLE 21–12
FOODS HIGH IN TYRAMINE CONTENT

Ripened cheese and foods containing ripened cheese (such as pizza and macaroni and cheese)	Pickles
Yoghurt	Baked potato
Fermented meats (bologna, salami, pepperoni, summer sausage)	Yeast and yeast extracts
Beef and chicken liver	Wine (chianti, sherry, some red wines)
Pickled and kippered herring	Some beers
Lox (smoked salmon)	Patés
Snails	Chocolate
Overripe bananas	Licorice
Canned figs	Soy sauce (contains dopa)
Avocados	Sour cream
Broad (fava) beans (contain dopa)	Coffee and colas (containing caffeine)
Raisins, dates	Meat extracts (such as marmite)
Pineapple	Papaya products (including meat tenderizers)
Sauerkraut	Nuts
	Soups (canned or packaged)

manifestations are also possible. Toxic symptoms and changes in electrocardiogram tracings have been reported in clients taking quinidine (an antiarrhythmic agent, basic in reaction) simultaneously with antacids and an alkaline ash diet. Use urine acidifiers, such as methionine, or urine alkalizers, such as sodium citrate or sodium bicarbonate, to promote the desired urinary pH for excretion of a specific drug. Vitamin C is sometimes used as a urine acidifier, although it is doubtful that vitamin C alone can acidify the urine to a significant extent.

ASSESSING HOSPITAL MALNUTRITION

In hospital settings, the implication is often made that weight loss is to be expected in clients with certain types of illness. However, aggressive nutritional support at the time of admission can prevent the development of malnutrition, and aggressive nutritional support can improve the ability of malnourished clients to withstand the stress of a disease or of a surgical procedure.

Providing adequate kilocalories and protein for critically ill clients is a major challenge. The kilocalorie level must be sufficient to meet the basal energy expenditure (BEE), with additional amounts to compensate for hypermetabolism, weight loss, and physical activity. Use the guidelines below for determining kilocalorie and protein requirements:

Males: BEE = 66 + (13.7 × weight in kg) + (5 × height in cm) − (6.8 × age)

Females: BEE = 655 + (9.6 × weight in kg) + (1.7 × height in cm) − (4.7 × age)

Suggested kilocalorie intakes for clients with various conditions are:

- Well-nourished, unstressed client, light hospital activity: 1.2 × BEE

- Stressed or undernourished client on tube feeding: 1.5 × BEE
- Stressed or undernourished client on TPN: 1.75 × BEE
- Severely burned clients: 2.0 × BEE

Sufficient protein should be provided to allow for a positive nitrogen balance and weight gain. General guidelines for clients with normal renal and hepatic function are:

- Nonstressed clients: 1.0 g/kg
- Moderately stressed clients: 1.5–3 g/kg
- Severely depleted or severely stressed clients: 3–4 g/kg

Starvation alone does not cause a high mortality rate until a 40 percent weight loss has occurred. In contrast the risk of mortality is high after only a 25 percent weight loss when the starvation is combined with illness or injury.

Use the nutritional assessment techniques described in Chapter 11 to aid in determining the nutritional status and degree of risk of hospitalized clients. Additional dietary, biochemical, and anthropometric techniques that are useful in assessing protein–calorie malnutrition and progress with nutritional therapy are discussed below.

Dietary Assessment

A useful dietary technique is to calculate the actual amount of kilocalories and protein consumed periodically and enter this information in the client's medical record. This information is usually provided by the dietitian–nutritionist. Compare actual intake with the client's estimated energy and protein requirements.

Biochemical Assessment

Use the results of the laboratory tests summarized in Table 21–13 to assess hematologic and visceral protein status, muscle mass, and immunocompe-

TABLE 21–13
BIOCHEMICAL ASSESSMENT OF PROTEIN–CALORIE MALNUTRITION

Assessment Parameter	Laboratory Test	Comments
Hematologic status	Hemoglobin and hematocrit	Evaluates for anemia
Visceral protein (i.e., liver, heart, kidney) status	Transport proteins, such as total serum protein, albumin, transferrin, retinol-binding protein and thyroxine-binding prealbumin (serum transferrin can be determined from the total iron-binding capacity—TIBC)	Evaluates synthetic activities of the liver and indirectly reflects visceral protein status
Lean body mass	Creatinine height index (CHI); (3-methyl-histidine—3-MeHis—an amino acid present almost exclusively in muscle is being investigated as a way of measuring muscle mass)	Determined from a 24-hour urine collection; creatinine excretion is related to the muscle mass and is constant for a given individual regardless of dietary intake and indirectly reflects lean body mass
Nitrogen balance	Urinary urea nitrogen	Determined from a 24-hour urine collection; when combined with an accurate record of protein consumed, the state of nitrogen balance can be approximated
Host defense and immune function	Total lymphocyte count (white blood count and differential to determine the percentage of lymphocytes present)	Evaluates cell-mediated immunity
	Reactivity to skin test antigens	Evaluates cell-mediated immunity

tence in hospitalized clients. These indices are useful not only for detecting protein–calorie malnutrition but also for assessing the effectiveness of nutritional therapy. Keep in mind, however, that these are primarily indirect measures of the parameters being assessed and that sensitivity and specificity of the tests vary widely and can be influenced by such factors as the concurrent presence of physiologic stresses, metabolic disorders, or drug therapy.

Anthropometric Assessment. In order to assess the client's weight status, first, assure that height and actual weight are recorded as part of the initial screening process. Second, compare actual weight with both recommended body weight (see Chap. 11) and usual body weight. If these are not comparable, evaluate the percentage of weight change by using this formula:

$$\text{Percent weight change} = \frac{\text{Usual weight} - \text{actual weight}}{\text{Usual weight}} \times 100$$

Standards for determining whether this weight change over a period of 1 week to 6 months is either significant or severe are published elsewhere.[11]

In the presence of weight loss, determine the composition of the loss, i.e., fat or muscle, by observing arm circumference, triceps skinfold, and arm muscle circumference measurements. Evaluate the results according to standards given in Chapter 11. Procedures for determining these measurements in a supine position have been published,[12] along with a detailed discussion of a variety of nutritional assessment techniques in current use.

REVIEW QUESTIONS AND ACTIVITIES

1. Identify the nutritional manifestations of physiologic stress and state three examples of acute conditions that elicit this response.
2. *Case study:* Your client is a 70-year-old male, Mr. A., who has been readmitted to the hospital following a weight loss of 20 lb during the past several months secondary to gastrointestinal cancer. He has been receiving chemotherapy and radiation therapy on an outpatient basis, and during this hospitalization surgical removal of the tumor is planned. His tolerance for solid food of normal consistency is poor.
   a. List signs and symptoms that may indicate that protein–calorie malnutrition is a possible diagnosis in Mr. A.'s case.
   b. Identify anthropometric and biochemical tests that could be used to assess for protein–calorie malnutrition.
   c. As you care for Mr. A. in the clinical setting, use Table 21–1 to identify undesirable practices that should be guarded against to prevent further deterioration in Mr. A.'s nutritional status.
   d. Identify two categories of enteral feedings and three categories of parenteral feedings that could be used to meet Mr. A.'s nutritional needs and compare the potential for meeting his nutritional requirements with each of these feeding methods.
   e. Consult the hospital dietitian and discuss the various brands of commercial formu-

las that are available for oral or tube feeding in the following categories: (1) milk-based, (2) blenderized diet feedings, and (3) defined formula diets.

f. With the assistance of the dietitian and your clinical instructor, identify a formula that would be suitable as an oral supplement for Mr. A., using criteria of (1) nutritional adequacy, (2) degree of digestion required, (3) lactose content, (4) osmolality, (5) residue content, and (6) cost.

g. What additional characteristic would be of concern should Mr. A. receive the formula as a tube feeding?

Additional information: In preparation for surgery next week, Mr. A. has been placed on a combination of oral food intake as tolerated and tube feeding given by the nasogastric route.

h. What advantages does this feeding regimen have over other types of feeding regimens in reducing Mr. A.'s operative risk, including postoperative wound infection?

i. List complications of tube feeding that you would observe for and compare these complications with the metabolic complications of a client receiving total parenteral nutrition.

j. Describe the appropriate diet regimen during the immediate preoperative and postoperative periods.

k. List nutrient supplements that should be given to promote proper wound healing and reduce other nutritional risks during the postoperative period.

Additional information: Following surgery, Mr. A.'s chemotherapy and radiation therapy are reinstated.

l. Identify the potential effects of the chemotherapy on Mr. A.'s nutritional status.

3. Explain the alterations in requirements for kilocalories, protein, minerals, vitamins, fluids, and electrolytes that occur in infectious diseases and burns and the appropriate nutritional therapy in each case.

4. Discuss the effects of drugs on (a) food intake, (b) absorption of nutrients, (c) metabolism of nutrients, and (d) excretion of nutrients.

5. List an example of a drug that affects each of the nutritive processes stated in Question 4.

6. Explain the effects of food or substances contained in food on absorption, metabolism, and excretion of drugs.

7. Describe the rationale for the development of drug toxicity in malnourished clients or those who follow erratic eating patterns.

8. Describe the twofold interaction that occurs (a) between tetracycline and metals such as calcium and iron, (b) between anticonvulsants and folic acid, and (c) between pyridoxine and levodopa.

REFERENCES

1. Bienia R, Ratcliff S, Barbour GL, Kummer M: Malnutrition in the hospitalized geriatric patient. J Am Geriatr Soc 30:433, 1982.
2. Jensen JE, Jensen TG, Smith TK, et al.: Nutrition in orthopaedic surgery. J Bone Joint Surg 64-A:1263, 1982.
3. Chandra RK, Joshi P, Au B, et al.: Nutrition and immunocompetence of the elderly: Effect of short-term nutritional supplementation on cell-mediated immunity and lymphocyte subsets. Nutr Res 2:223, 1982.
4. Konstantinides NN, Shronts E: Tube feeding. Am J Nurs 83(9):1312, 1983.
5. American Dietetic Association: Handbook of Clinical Dietetics. New Haven, Yale University Press, 1981, p B-56.
6. AMA Department of Foods and Nutrition: Nutrition advisory group statement on multivitamin preparations for parenteral use. J Parent Enter Nutr 3:258, 1979.
7. AMA Expert Panel: Guidelines for essential trace element preparations for parenteral use. JAMA 241:2051, 1979.
8. Shils ME: Parenteral nutrition. In RS Goodhart, ME Shils, eds: Modern Nutrition in Health and Disease. Philadelphia, Lea & Febiger, 1980, p 1125.
9. Reimer LL, Michener WM, Steiger E: Nutritional support of the critically ill child. Pediatr Clin North Am 27:647, 1980.
10. Mabogunje OA, Andrassy RJ, Isaacs HJ, Mahour GH: The role of a defined formula diet in the prevention of stress-induced gastric mucosal injury in the rat. J Pediatr Surg 16:1036, 1981.
11. American Dietetic Association, op cit, p A-27.
12. Jensen TG, Englert DM, Dudrick SJ: Nutritional Assessment, A Manual for Practitioners. Norwalk, Conn, Appleton-Century-Crofts, 1983, p 74.

BIBLIOGRAPHY

Adams MM: Guidelines for planning home enteral feeding. J Am Diet Assoc 84:68, 1984.

Beisel WR: Effects of infection on nutritional status and immunity. Fed Proc 39:3105, 1980.

Bushman L, Russel R, Warfield L, et al.: Malnutrition among patients in an acute-care veterans facility. J Am Diet Assoc 77:462, 1980.

Byrne, WJ, Burke M, Fonkalsrud EW, Ament ME: Home parenteral nutrition: An alternative approach to the management of complicated gastrointestinal fistulas not responding to conventional medical or surgical therapy. J Parent Enter Nutr 3:555, 1979.

Chernoff R: Nutritional support: Formulas and delivery of enteral feeding. I. Enteral formulas. II. Delivery systems. J Am Diet Assoc 79:426, 430, 1981.

Jensen TJ, Dudrick SJ: Implementation of a multidisciplinary nutritional assessment program. J Am Diet Assoc 79:258, 1981.

Jensen TG, Englert DM, Dudrick SJ, Johnston DA: Delayed hypersensitivity skin testing: Response rates in a surgical population. J Am Diet Assoc 82:49, 1983.

Klein GL: Aluminum loading during total parenteral nutrition. Am J Clin Nutr 35:1425, 1982.

Maillet JO: Calculating parenteral feedings: A programmed instruction. J Am Diet Assoc 84:1312, 1984.

Michel L, Serrano A, Malt RA: Current concepts: Nutritional support of hospitalized patients. N Engl J Med 304:1147, 1981.

Morath MA, Miller SF, Finley RK: Nutritional implications of post-burn bacteremic sepsis. J Parent Enter Nutr 5:488, 1981.

Parrish G, Gibney A: Total parenteral nutrition—An update. Nutr Support Serv 2:9, 1982.

Pollack MM, Wiley JS, Kanter R, Holbrook PR: Malnutrition in critically ill infants and children. J Parent Enter Nutr 6:20, 1982.

Robinson LA: Vitamin regimens in parenteral nutrition: A dilemma. J Parent Enter Nutr 6:76, 1982.

Roe DA: Handbook: Interactions of Selected Drugs and Nutrients in Patients, ed 3. Chicago, American Dietetic Association, 1982.

CHAPTER 22

Nutrition and Pediatric Disorders:
Congenital Anomalies and Metabolic Disorders

Objectives

After completion of this chapter, the student will be able to:

1. Plan a day's menu for a 3-year-old hospitalized child that is adequate in kilocalories and protein.

2. Develop a nursing care plan for the nutritional management of a child with a combined cleft lip and palate during the presurgical and postsurgical phases of management, and adjust the plan to be appropriate for an infant with a mild form of pyloric stenosis who is receiving medical management only.

3. Compare and contrast the metabolic defect and clinical manifestations of the classic forms of the following inborn errors of metabolism: (a) galactosemia, (b) phenylketonuria, (c) maple syrup urine disease, (d) familial hypercholesterolemia, and (e) Wilson's disease.

4. Plan an appropriate dietary regimen for a 1-month-old infant with each of the following disorders and adjust the plan for that same child at the age of 6 years: (a) galactosemia, (b) phenylketonuria, and (c) maple syrup urine disease.

5. Distinguish between the dietary management of familial hypercholesterolemia and Wilson's disease.

In many instances, congenital anomalies and inborn errors of metabolism are manifested at birth or shortly thereafter and pose immediate problems in nutritional management. In other cases, the congenital anomaly or hereditary disorder may not become manifest until later in life. Do not view the terms **congenital** and **hereditary** as synonymous. An abnormality may be congenital, i.e., present at birth, but not genetically determined. Conversely, a genetically determined abnormality may, in some instances, manifest itself for the first time after an individual reaches adulthood.

This chapter focuses on the following aspects of nutritional therapy for pediatric disorders:

1. Feeding the ill child
2. Congenital abnormalities of the gastrointestinal tract
3. Inborn errors of metabolism that are most frequently encountered

FEEDING THE ILL CHILD

Assessment and Intervention

Just as with ill adults, maintenance of optimal nutrition in sick children plays an important role in the control and rate of recovery from acute and chronic illnesses. In planning diets for sick children, keep in mind the nutritional requirements of normal children relative to age, size, rate of growth, and degree of physical activity and modify the kinds and amounts of foods served according to the needs imposed by illness and the child's ability to eat. Assess the nutritional requirements of ill children. These requirements are at least the same as and often greater than those of well children of the same age and stage of development. Superimposed on the normal nutritional requirements for growth are those created by illness. These special needs are most prominent in chronic illnesses and illness characterized by hypermetabolism or impaired use of nutrients. Some clinical signs associated with illness may actually be due to nutritional deficiency rather than an inherent component of the disease process.

Consider the emotional response of the child and parents to an illness that necessitates hospitalization before devising a plan for nutritional care, especially if the plan needs to be followed on a long-term basis after discharge. Illness of a child brings emotional tensions in both the child and the parents or caretakers. If hospitalization is necessary, expect the child to experience anxieties associated with separation from the family and fears regarding the illness. When the hospitalized child is removed from the familiar setting of the home and placed in the care of adults who do not know him or her, the child is subjected to many new environmental factors that require adjustment. Questions such as "Where will I sleep?" or "What will I get for supper?" may be paramount.

When they become ill, children may also regress to an earlier developmental stage, and well-established feeding schedules may be completely disrupted by the illness and transfer to a strange environment. For instance, the baby who has made good progress toward accepting solids and toward cup drinking may refuse everything but the nursing bottle, or a toddler who can feed himself or herself well may now desire to be fed. If understanding care is given, this type of behavior may be only temporary.

Illness and hospitalization may also bring undesirable changes in eating behavior, and hospitalized children often present more than the usual number of feeding problems. The trauma of medical or surgical treatments and separation from home and family may cause a child's interest in food to decrease. Often the types and amounts of food the child will accept are limited. There may be wide fluctuations and capriciousness of appetite. This is often true not only from day to day but from meal to meal or even from the beginning to the end of the meal. Not all the feeding problems of sick children are associated with lack of appetite, however. Some children with long-term illnesses may seek in food a partial compensation for lack of emotional satisfaction and may become obese. These children need help in developing other outlets for their frustrations. Explain to parents of children who experience emotion-related changes in eating behavior the underlying rationale, and remind the parents how their own response to the child's illness and medical regimen may affect the child's eating behavior. It is imperative, therefore, to bridge the gap between the known and the unknown and link past and pres-

ent experiences to make the transition from home to hospital less disruptive. Since food has particular meanings for a child and represents part of the home life, the regular appearance of food in an acceptable form may be one aspect of reassuring the child that the new surroundings are stable and someone stands ready to meet his or her needs. As soon as possible after admission, take a dietary history to identify usual eating patterns and to serve as a basis for planning the child's meals.

Present food in a manner and form that is acceptable; include some familiar food at meals and serve the food in the manner to which the child is accustomed. Alteration of eating habits or acquisition of new feeding skills is difficult during hospitalization. The child's preferences should be catered to insofar as possible, particularly in acute, short-term illnesses, such as an acute gastrointestinal or respiratory infection, although food intake may become a more serious problem in the child with a long-term illness.

If a modified diet is a part of the medical regimen, plan the diet within the framework of the child's usual diet as well, giving consideration to ethnic food patterns. Make an effort to establish a plan that does not make a child appear different from his or her peers in the types of foods allowed when this is possible. Being like their peers is important to children, who do not like to be viewed as different.

In situations necessitating a modified diet to be followed after discharge from the hospital, explain the rationale for the feeding program and conduct diet counseling sessions jointly with the child and parents as a component of the total educational process directed toward teaching the family to live with the disease process. Initiate these counseling sessions in the hospital and continue them on an ongoing basis during follow-up sessions in the home, outpatient clinic, or periods of rehospitalization. The child should have a clear understanding of what is expected of him or her and how to assume responsibility for implementing the diet commensurate with age and capabilities.

Involve the child and parents in activities that will allow them to identify foods suitable for the diet, such as identifying foods served on the food tray, preparing foods suitable for the diet, using games to identify foods or concepts, using movies, slide–tape presentations, and other visual aids available in the hospital or clinic education center, planning menus suitable for the diet, and keeping records of foods consumed and comparing the records with the diet plan. Use group teaching sessions when possible to allow the child and parents to interact with others experiencing the same problem. Also provide information about available resources, such as financial aid or community support groups. Periodic changes in the diet to meet the increased nutritional requirements associated with growth will also require an explanation.

CONGENITAL ANOMALIES OF THE GASTROINTESTINAL TRACT

Assessment and Intervention

Numerous congenital anomalies of the gastrointestinal tract have the potential for altering nutritional status. In some instances, failure to thrive results from such factors as gastric dumping, intestinal malabsorption, gastrointestinal obstruction, or vomiting. Examples of these conditions, which in some cases necessitate immediate surgical repair, are omphalocele, pyloric stenosis, small bowel obstruction, intestinal atresia, meconium ileus, necrotizing enterocolitis, Hirschsprung's disease, and imperforate anus. In other congenital anomalies, such as cleft lip and palate, surgery is delayed for a period of time, and specialized feeding techniques are necessary until the surgery, which is done in phases, is complete.

In those defects necessitating immediate surgery, expect nutrient demands to increase as a result of the increased nutrient losses sustained by the malabsorption, vomiting, and so on, as well as the metabolic trauma of surgery. Provide total parenteral nutrition for those clients and progress to oral feeding as soon as the gastrointestinal tract has recuperated from the surgery.

Consult a pediatric textbook for a full discussion of the conditions mentioned and their treatment. Only pyloric stenosis and cleft lip and palate are discussed below.

Pyloric Stenosis. Pyloric stenosis is a serious disorder that is not uncommon in infants and that carries a high rate of mortality unless diagnosed and treated in the early stages. The pylorus is the opening from the stomach to the duodenum. In pyloric stenosis the pylorus is elongated, thickened, and almost cartilaginous in consistency. Hypertrophy of the circular muscular layer leads to severe narrowing of the lumen. The disorder usually becomes manifest during the second or third week of life. Onset is rare prior to 1 week of age and is seldom delayed until the second or third month. Suspect the disorder in infants who vomit during or shortly after feeding, although in some instances the vomiting may be delayed for several hours. In the beginning stages, observe for a pattern of regurgitation or occasional nonprojectile vomiting, although the vomiting becomes projectile usually within a week after onset. In some clients, the vomiting is intermittent, whereas in others, vomiting occurs after every feeding. Gastric peristaltic waves, which progress from the left upper quadrant toward the pylorus, are visible immediately after feeding or just before vomiting. Assess for dehydration, weight loss, and acid–base imbalances, particularly hypochloremic alkalosis, which occurs secondary to the vomiting.

Surgical correction is the treatment of choice; if the condition is mild and medical rather than surgical management is selected, use the following feeding regimen:

1. Provide continuous gastric suction or frequent lavage and give formula or breast milk between aspiration (some formula-fed infants show improvement when given breast milk)
2. Give small frequent (e.g., every 4 hours) milk feedings (frequent feedings thickened with cereal may be better tolerated by formula-fed infants)
3. Maintain the infant in a semi-upright position for an hour or so after feeding
4. Refeed if vomiting occurs and a large volume of the feeding is lost; refeedings are often retained
5. Use total parenteral nutrition as necessary to correct dehydration, acid–base abnormalities, and malnutrition

Instruct the parents in the proper feeding technique and follow the child's progress with the feeding regimen. If no improvement occurs, surgery is advised.

Cleft Lip and Palate. Cleft lip and cleft palate are developmental defects occurring in the first trimester of pregnancy. The exact pathogenesis of the defect is unknown, but most researchers feel that a number of factors, both genetic and environmental, are involved in the etiology. Nutritional deficiencies, infections, and various drugs have all been implicated.

Cleft lip and cleft palate may occur singly or together in affected clients, and the clefts may vary in severity. In severe forms of cleft lip, there is complete lip separation extending into the floor of the nose. Assess the client's dental status; the alveolar ridge may also be involved and defective, or absent teeth may be additional anomalies. Palatal defects may involve both the soft and hard palate, and there may be a cleft in one or both sides of the upper gums. Since normal sucking and swallowing ability is dependent upon lip and tongue control and properly formed palates, expect feeding problems to arise in affected clients (Table 22–1). Muscular movement of the soft palate is essential for speech, and speech may be affected.

Rehabilitation of the child with cleft lip or palate may require several years to complete, and it requires medical, surgical, dental, speech, and nutritional therapy. The timing for surgical correction depends upon the degree of deformity and individual patterns of development and facial growth. Thus the timing of surgical and orthodontic procedures is an individual matter. The initial surgical repair of a cleft lip is usually done when the infant is 1 to 2 months of age and is gaining weight satisfactorily. The initial surgical repair may be revised at 4 to 5 years of age. Palatal repair may be carried out between the ages of 6 to 9 months and 4 to 5 years. Growth increases the size of the palate and thus

TABLE 22–1
POTENTIAL FEEDING PROBLEMS AND POSSIBLE ALTERNATIVE FEEDING TECHNIQUES IN CHILDREN WITH CLEFTS

Feeding Problem	Suggested Alterations in Feeding Technique
1. Difficulty in sucking milk from the nipple, usually due to a lack of suction caused by the cleft	1. a. Use a large, soft nipple (boil new nipples to soften) with an enlarged opening (enlarge the opening with a heated needle or ice pick or turn nipple inside out and cut an X with a razor and revert the nipple to normal position—nipple opening should not be so large that when the bottle is upturned, the milk runs out too rapidly, however); infants learn to use chewing motions to get milk through the nipple b. Use alternate feeding devices, such as a medicine dropper, asepto syringe, or special feeders, such as the Brecht feeder (a bulb-type syringe with a rubber or plastic tip on the end) or Beniflex feeder (a soft plastic bag with a horizontal cross-cut nipple attached: Mead Johnson Labs): *Note:* special feeders that necessitate little effort to suck or chew should be discontinued as soon as possible in order to promote development of musculature needed for speech c. Encourage breast feeding if the mother is enthusiastic about this feeding method and is knowledgeable about the inherent problems, and if the infant has sufficient strength; mother manually extends the nipple by placing the index finger on the top edge, and the middle finger on the bottom edge, of the nipple areola. The infant can use the jaws, tongue, cheeks, and gums to press or milk rather than suck the milk from the breast.
2. Excessive air swallowing, bringing distention and discomfort due to improper feeding position or the increased time and effort involved in getting milk from the nipple	2. a. Hold the infant's body in an upright position (and tilted slightly backward) while feeding; experiment with varying degrees of tilting to find the position that best suits the infant b. Burp often during feeding and burp after feeding; to burp, set the infant upright at a 45-degree angle to allow air to be expelled—putting baby over the shoulder and patting the back may bring excessive belching and vomiting c. Feed the infant rapidly enough to prevent becoming overtired but not so rapidly that it induces choking
3. Reflux of fluid and food through the nose as a result of their being forced through the cleft by the normal action of the tongue	3. a. Maintain upright position while feeding (reflux of fluids and food through the nose sometimes occurs regardless of the feeding procedure used) b. Encourage the child to eat solid foods slowly and take small bites c. In rare instances, a plastic appliance may be placed over the cleft to keep fluid or food from entering the nose d. Surgical repair practically eliminates food coming out of the nose
4. Episodes of choking due to feeding excessive quantities of food, feeding too rapidly, allowing milk to strike the back of the throat directly, feeding foods of a consistency that cannot be handled, or possible transfer of the parent's fear of the child's choking to the infant	4. a. Aim milk so that it hits the side of the cheek rather than the back of the throat b. Decrease the quantity and rate of feeding (i.e., provide small amounts of liquids or smaller bites of food during feeding and allow adequate time for swallowing) c. Experiment with the consistency of semisolids to determine the consistency the child can best handle; some infants can eat strained foods that have been thinned with milk, fruit juice, or broth whereas others tolerate strained foods thickened with graham cracker crumbs or other substances (strained foods should not be fed from a bottle unless spoon-feeding is difficult) d. Maintain a calm approach while feeding to avoid transmitting fears to the infant
5. Prolonged feeding process, causing fatigue in child and person feeding	5. a. Feed as rapidly as is feasible without inducing choking b. Provide small frequent meals (e.g., 5–6 small meals) for the older child c. Be patient during the feeding process
6. Irritation of the mouth and nose by acid or spicy foods	6. a. Avoid very acid and spicy foods and use alternates of equal nutritive value b. Mix acid or spicy foods with bland foods to cause less irritation

TABLE 22-1 *(Continued)*

Feeding Problem	*Suggested Alterations in Feeding Technique*
7. Certain types of foods getting stuck in opening of palate in some children	7. a. Dislodge food by rinsing with milk or water or swabbing (some children can suck the food down) b. Avoid gooey or pasty foods that tend to cling to the roof of the mouth, or prepare them in such a manner that they do not cling (common offenders are nuts, peanut butter, cooked cheese dishes, leafy vegetables, fruit peelings, and creamed dishes)
8. Difficulty in chewing, often due to dental caries and malocclusion	8. a. Encourage proper dental care and oral hygiene (e.g., follow feedings with water to remove excess food from the mouth) b. Provide chewy foods, such as bread crusts, when infant is teething to aid in development of jaw muscles and better tooth alignment c. Provide foods in a form that is easy to chew (e.g., ground or chopped meat)

aids in the closure of the cleft. Like lip surgery, palatal surgery is often not completed for several years. Occasionally, a child may be treated by a temporary or permanent dental appliance instead of surgery.

Prior to surgical intervention, use the feeding techniques outlined in Table 22-1 to establish a suitable feeding regimen for the child. Give the parents detailed information about the child's day-to-day care and treatment, including positioning for feeding and use of special feeding devices that may be indicated. Provide them with support in ventilating their feelings about giving birth to a deformed child and in promoting the development of a healthy parent–child relationship that is essential to a positive feeding experience. Stress an approach that calls attention to other attributes of the child and emphasizes normal interactions, such as holding and cuddling the child.

Tell the parents to expect their child to undergo the same developmental processes as other children and describe to them the usual food responses of children of comparable age. Since early feedings are likely to be tiring and lengthy, encourage the parents to provide rest periods during feeding and to burp the child frequently to expel inspired air. Introduce solid foods into the child's diet at the usual age and give instructions to the parents regarding any special preparation techniques that may be necessary and outline to them those foods that may produce problems.

Prior to surgery, assess the child's nutritional status to assure that there are sufficient reserves to withstand the stress of surgery and to promote normal wound healing. In preparation for palatal surgery, introduce the child to the postsurgical routine (spoon feeding, cup drinking, and use of a variety of liquids, such as fruit and vegetable juices, broth, bouillon, and flat carbonated beverages) so that the child becomes accustomed to this routine in advance.

Following cleft lip surgery, give the infant clear liquids for the first couple of feedings. After this,

initiate formula feeding. At the discretion of the surgeon, the feeding device may be a medicine dropper, syringe, or whatever feeding device the child is accustomed to using. To prevent contamination of the sutures and infection, provide a small amount of water to follow the feeding and cleanse the suture line thoroughly after each feeding. Special feeding devices may be used for a month or more following surgery.

Palatal surgery necessitates the use of a liquid diet for approximately 2 weeks (clear fluids for the first 5 days and full liquids the next 10 days). A soft diet is then given for about 10 days, after which the child may receive a normal diet. Tell the child and parents to avoid hard foods, such as hard candy, for a period of 1 to 2 months or longer postoperatively. Feed the child solids from the side of a spoon, being careful not to insert the spoon into the mouth where it may damage the suture line. Give fluids from a cup and avoid the use of a nipple or straw for a period of time. While straw drinking is not permissible during the postoperative period, after the palate is completely healed, drinking liquids through a straw aids in the development of muscles needed for speech.

INBORN ERRORS OF METABOLISM

Assessment
The more common metabolic diseases determined in part by genetic factors—diabetes mellitus (Chap. 24), obesity (Chap. 23), gout (Chap. 37), and familial hyperlipoproteinemia (Chap. 29)—are discussed in other chapters of the book. Only those relatively rare metabolic disorders (inborn errors of metabolism) whose onset is in early infancy and that respond to dietary management are included here.

▶ The term **inborn errors of metabolism** refers to a number of relatively rare, hereditary, molecular disorders resulting from a biochemical defect in the structure or function of a protein. Inborn errors of
▶ metabolism result from gene mutations (a **mutation**

is a slight change in the chemical composition of a gene) that cause abnormal protein molecules, such as hemoglobin and enzymes, to be produced. Genes control not only such physical characteristics as sex and hair and eye color but also metabolism, by controlling the synthesis of enzymes that catalyze metabolic reactions. If the genes are not coded correctly (i.e., mutant), an enzyme may be missing or abnormal, bringing an inborn error of metabolism. All of the biochemical and clinical abnormalities associated with an inborn error of metabolism are caused by an abnormality of a single gene that is responsible for a single specific step in metabolism. Mutations may result from physical or chemical factors, such as extremes of high temperature or pH, exposure to x-rays, ultraviolet rays, or cosmic rays, radioactive materials, LSD, or mustard gas compounds. In some cases, the effect may not be observable, whereas in others, the effect may be quite obvious.

Assess for the mechanism by which an improperly synthesized enzyme can influence cellular reactions in affected clients:

1. Defects in membrane transport in which a substrate cannot enter the cell (e.g., in glucose–galactose malabsorption, glucose and galactose cannot be absorbed from the intestine or the proximal kidney tubule)
2. Defects in the metabolism of specific substrates bringing:
   a. Failure to synthesize adequate amounts of essential products (e.g., the albino lacks melanin pigment due to inactivity of the enzyme, tyrosinase, needed to metabolize tyrosine to melanin)
   b. Accumulation of the precursor substrates or metabolites that may have toxic effects on certain body tissues; e.g., in hereditary galactokinase deficiency, galactose cannot be converted to galactose-1-phosphate, and the galactose accumulates and results in cataracts; in Tay-Sachs disease, a lipid substance (ganglioside) accumulates in the neuronal cells of the brain, bringing blindness, mental retardation, paralysis, and death, usually before the age of 4 years; in Gaucher's disease, a lipid substance (glucocerebroside) accumulates in the reticuloendothelial cells of the liver, spleen, lymph nodes, and bone marrow, and the accumulation of this compound in the neurons is responsible for brain damage in the infantile form
3. Development of alternate pathways and metabolites for disposal of precursor substances, e.g., in phenylketonuria, the conversion of phenylalanine to tyrosine is blocked. Phenylalanine is metabolized to other compounds, which can be detected in the urine in affected individuals

Over 300 different inborn errors of metabolism have been identified, and in many of these the actual enzyme defect has been pinpointed. A number are represented by a single case. With improved methods of diagnosis and the development of large-scale screening programs, the number of cases being identified is increasing. Moreover, medical advances have made it possible to treat many of the disorders, and children who once died in infancy now survive to adulthood and have children themselves. Thus, the population of individuals with inborn errors of metabolism is also increasing.

The clinical expressions of the effect of the gene mutation vary widely; some are asymptomatic, whereas in others the effects of the mutant gene are minimal in infancy, although some effects are observed in later life. Still others are so severe that death occurs in utero or in early life. An example is Tay-Sachs disease (an abnormality of glycosphingolipid metabolism), which is incompatible with life and in which death occurs by early childhood. Several mutations, including phenylketonuria, galactosemia, and branched-chain ketoaciduria, lead to severe mental retardation unless the disorder is detected and treated early. Since the brain grows rapidly in infancy and early childhood, expect the effects of certain inborn errors of metabolism to be especially detrimental to this organ. Interference with brain growth cannot be rectified at a later time.

Inborn errors of metabolism are classified in different ways by different authors. However, they are most commonly classified according to the particular metabolic pathway that is disturbed, i.e., carbohydrate, amino acid, lipid, vitamin, mineral, and so on. Galactosemia (an inborn error of carbohydrate metabolism), phenylketonuria, and maple syrup urine disease (inborn errors of protein metabolism), hyperlipoproteinemia (an inborn error of lipid metabolism), and Wilson's disease (an inborn error of mineral metabolism) are discussed in the remaining sections of this chapter.

Inborn Errors of Carbohydrate Metabolism: Galactosemia

Assessment. Enzyme deficiencies or diminished enzyme activity may give rise to a number of disorders of carbohydrate metabolism, affecting either the monosaccharides (pentoses, fructose, glucose, and galactose), the disaccharides (sucrose, isomaltose, and lactose), or the polysaccharides (glycogen and starch). Depending on the nature of the disorder, these inborn errors of carbohydrate metabolism may be relatively harmless, or they may bring intestinal malabsorption or severe pathologic conditions associated with the accumulation of metabolites in amounts that are toxic.

Galactosemia is a group of inherited disorders characterized by an increase in levels of the monosaccharide galactose or its metabolites in cells, blood, and urine resulting from an inability to convert galactose to glucose. Galactose is derived from the enzymatic hydrolysis of lactose (milk sugar) in the intestinal tract, and most galactose is metabolized by the liver. The disease is seen in approximately 1 of every 65,000 live births in the general population. Galactosemia may present itself in its classic form, characterized by an increase in the blood and urinary levels of galactose and the accumulation of its metabolite, galactose-1-phosphate, in red blood cells, liver, spleen, kidney, heart, cerebral cortex, and the lens of the eye due to a defect in the enzyme, galactose-1-phosphate uridyl transferase. The more rare variant form leads to the accumulation of galactose as a result of a deficiency of the enzyme, galactokinase.

The classic form of the disease may be mild or severe in symptomology. In severe cases, clinical manifestations become evident shortly after birth when the affected infant ingests milk. Observe for the following complications: vomiting, diarrhea, anorexia, hypoglycemia, manifestations of liver involvement, such as jaundice, and enlargement of the liver and spleen, polyuria (excessive urination), manifestations of damage to the renal tubules, including proteinuria, generalized amino aciduria, and phosphaturia (urinary excretion of protein, amino acids, and phosphorus), and unless treated early, brain damage with cerebral edema and severe intellectual impairment. Because the lens of the eye can convert galactose to the sugar alcohol, galactitol, cataracts also develop; cataracts may develop in utero. Most untreated children who survive beyond infancy show progressive mental and growth retardation.

In the variant form of galactosemia characterized by galactokinase deficiency, the toxic effects of exposure to galactose are milder and are manifest primarily as cataract formation, abnormal galactose tolerance, and elevated levels of galactose in the blood and urine. There are no gastrointestinal disturbances, and mental development is normal. In this disorder, galactose-1-phosphate does not accumulate, and the damage results from the high concentration of galactose itself. The disorder may not be diagnosed until cataracts are identified in later infancy and childhood, since for the most part the condition is asymptomatic in the newborn period except for a transient increase in intracranial pressure that has been identified in some affected infants.

Detect the presence of galactosemia by assessing the galactose level in blood and urine and galactokinase and galactose-1-phosphate uridyl transferase activity from assays of erythrocytes or cultured skin fibroblasts. Prenatal diagnosis may be made by determining enzyme activity in cultured amniotic fluid cells.

Intervention. Initiate treatment of the disorder in the first few weeks of life by removal of all sources of galactose from the diet in order to prevent mental retardation, cirrhosis of the liver, renal damage, cataracts, and growth failure. With treatment, progression of cataracts can be halted, and there is some evidence that cataracts may improve if treatment is initiated early. Results are not satisfactory if the cataracts have become dense.

Dietary galactose is derived primarily from the consumption of the disaccharide, lactose, that is present in mammalian milks. Provide a lactose-free formula for infants, and use foods that are free of lactose and galactose when solid foods are added. Examples of alternate formulas for infants that replace lactose with sucrose, maltose, or glucose as the sole carbohydrate source are included in the food list for a galactose-free diet given in Table 22–2. Because of the lactose content of breast milk, breast-feeding is contraindicated. Advise the parents to continue the use of the milk substitute as a beverage or use it in food preparation after weaning, since it is difficult to provide recommended intakes of such nutrients as calcium and riboflavin without the use of these milk substitutes.

Since galactose is a component of lactose, all types of milk, milk products, and foods prepared with milk must be omitted. Advise the parents to scrutinize food labels carefully since lactose or milk products are added to many foods. Caution them to omit products that list such items as milk, butter, cream, cheese, nonfat dry milk solids, whey, whey solids, curds, or casein as ingredients on the label. In contrast, lactate, lactic acid, and lactalbumin do not contain lactose and are safe to use. The lactose content of drugs, especially tablets that may contain lactose as a filler or sweetening agent, must also be considered.

Although there is no consensus as to when, if ever, dietary control can be relaxed, some authorities suggest that diet regulation can be somewhat relaxed during later childhood (ages 12 to 13 years) to make the diet more socially acceptable. A conservative approach is to restrict milk and dairy products throughout life but to allow prepared foods that contain small amounts of milk, such as sauces and baked goods, at the time the child enters school. Continue careful biochemical monitoring for brain and liver damage and cataracts, however. Many affected clients will voluntarily limit galactose intake throughout adult life because of habit or due to discomfort associated with the ingestion of significant amounts of galactose-containing foods.

Recommend galactose restriction during pregnancy for females who are at risk of having an offspring affected with galactosemia, since there is evidence that damage can occur in utero.

Provided the diagnosis is made and treatment is instituted before irreversible organ damage has occurred, affected children may have normal physical development and near normal intellectual functioning.

Inborn Errors of Amino Acid Metabolism

There are over 100 inherited disorders of amino acid metabolism. Some of these are harmless, but others cause profound illness or intellectual impairment early in life. In many of these disorders, enzyme deficiencies give rise to clinical problems because

TABLE 22–2
FOOD LIST FOR A GALACTOSE-FREE DIET

Foods Allowed	Foods Not Allowed
Milk substitutes Casein hydrolysate Nutramigen (Mead Johnson Labs) Soybean-based formula Isomil (Ross Labs) Neomullsoy (Syntex Labs) Prosobee (Mead Johnson Labs) Soyalac (Loma) Meat-based formula Meat Base (Gerber Products)	Breast milk, all animal milks, imitation or filled milk; cream; cottage, and hard cheese; yoghurt; ice cream, ice milk, milk sherbet; custard and pudding made with milk
Meat and substitutes Plain beef, lamb, veal, pork, ham, fowl, fish Kosher frankfurters Eggs (prepared without milk, cream, butter, margarine) Nut butters (peanut butter) Nuts	Creamed, buttered, or breaded meat, fish, eggs, poultry; frankfurters, cold cuts, and liver sausage containing milk, lactose, or galactose; organ meats (liver, brains, sweetbreads, kidneys, pancreas, heart)
Fruits and vegetables All fresh, frozen, canned, or dried fruit except those listed as Not Allowed All fresh, frozen, canned, or dried vegetables except those listed as Not Allowed	All forms of fruit (including dietetic fruits) processed with lactose or galactose; vegetables seasoned with butter or margarine; creamed or breaded vegetables, vegetables processed with milk or lactose; instant mashed potatoes or commercially packaged fried potatoes containing lactose or other galactose-containing substances
Breads and cereals Cooked and dry cereals, bread or crackers without added lactose (e.g., saltines, graham crackers, hard rolls—contact local bakery if not sure); macaroni, spaghetti, noodles, rice; tortilla	Cereals, bread, or crackers that have milk, milk products, or lactose added; dry cereals; cream of wheat or rice; pancakes, waffles, and French toast; zwieback; crackers made with butter or margarine; prepared muffin or biscuit mixes
Fats All vegetable oils All shortening, lard, kosher-type margarines; bacon; mayonnaise; olives; salad dressings made without milk products or lactose	Butter; cream; cream cheese; margarine with added lactose; salad dressing containing butter, milk, or lactose
Miscellaneous Clear soups, vegetable soups made with allowed vegetables, homemade cream soups made with milk substitutes; water-based gravies; angel food cake, baked desserts, and puddings made from milk substitutes, water, or vegetable oils; water and fruit ices; gelatin made with water; cocoa powder; carbonated beverages; fruit drinks and punch base without lactose; sugar-free and regular chewing gum with safe ingredients; plain sugar or rock candies, marshmallows without lactose; sugar (brown and granulated white); molasses, honey, and corn syrup; carob powder; lactose-free jam, jelly, and marmalade; chocolate (unsweetened, bittersweet, and semisweet); artificial sweeteners made with allowed ingredients; catsup, mustard, pickles; pure spices and seasonings; instant coffee without lactose; nondairy creamers like Cremora or mocha mix (in limited quantities); unbuttered popcorn, plain corn chips and potato chips; plain alcoholic beverages; beer; wine	Soups, sauces, and gravies made with milk, cream, butter or margarine; commercially prepared desserts made with nonallowed ingredients; chocolate drinks; cocoa mix; Ovaltine; malt or malted milk mix; powdered soft drinks; candy (butterscotch, caramels, milk chocolate, peppermint, toffee); milk chocolate and chocolate syrup made with unallowed ingredients; artificial sweeteners containing lactose; dietetic and diabetic preparations; nondairy creamers containing lactose; snack foods made with nonallowed ingredients; dried, shredded coconut; party dips; food colors, powdered foods, spice blends, and syrups containing lactose; cordials and liquers; premixed alcoholic drink mixes containing unallowed ingredients

See Chapter 27 for additional information on low-lactose diet.
(*Source: Adapted from California Department of Health, Maternal and Child Health Branch: Parents' Guide to the Galactose-Restricted Diet, Sacramento, 1976.*)

toxic amounts of some metabolites accumulate, whereas others are present in insufficient quantities. Transient disorders of amino acid metabolism may be present in early infancy, though their clinical significance is unclear. The offspring of mothers with amino acid disorders are exposed to (and may be damaged by) the biochemical abnormality in utero.

This phenomenon has been documented for phenylketonuria,[1] and there is suggestive evidence that similar (although probably less severe) effects may be present in other severe amino acid disturbances.

The inborn error of amino acid metabolism that has received most attention is phenylketonuria. The response of this disease to dietary management has been extensively evaluated and has, in many ways, served as a model for the study of other amino acid disturbances.

Phenylketonuria

Assessment. Phenylketonuria (PKU) represents a group of inherited disorders, occurring with a frequency of approximately 7 of every 100,000 live births in the United States, that may appear in the classic form or in a number of variant forms. The classic form of PKU is characterized by the absence or inactivity of the hepatic enzyme, phenylalanine hydroxylase, needed to catalyze the hydroxylation of the essential amino acid, phenylalanine, to the nonessential amino acid, tyrosine. This situation leads to the accumulation in plasma and cells of
▶ phenylalanine and metabolites called **phenylketones** that arise from alternate pathways of phenylalanine metabolism and the excretion of large amounts of these substances in the urine. Tyrosine levels are low or normal. Suspect PKU in an infant on a normal diet whose phenylalanine blood level is 30 to 60 mg/100 ml after the third day of life. Normal values range from 1 to 2 mg/100 ml. There are at least six defined mutations of the enzyme complex that lead to varying degrees of impairment.

Observe for these complications and manifestations in untreated clients: (1) mental retardation and a diminished IQ level, (2) decreased life expectancy (approximately three fourths die by the age of 30 years), (3) hyperactive behavior and convulsive disorders, (4) reduced pigmentation of the hair, skin, and iris of the eye, (5) eczema, and (6) a musty odor to the urine and sweat. The exact cause of the mental retardation is not known, although it is theorized that either the elevated plasma phenylalanine concentration, the accumulation of the catabolic byproducts of phenylalanine, or a deficiency of tyrosine[2] leading to depressed protein synthesis produces central nervous system damage during critical periods of central nervous development. In PKU, there is incomplete myelination, and it has been suggested that there may be decreased myelin synthesis. The lack of melanin pigment probably accounts for the lesser pigmentation than is usual for family and climate. Tyrosine is the precursor of melanin.

A delay of only a few weeks in initiating treatment may lead to a reduction in the IQ level, and a marked reduction may be evident by 6 to 9 months of age. Although many of the symptoms, including certain behavioral characteristics, improve with treatment at any age, mental retardation, once established, is not reversible with diet control.

While all clients with PKU have hyperphenylalaninemia, not all with hyperphenylalaninemia have classic PKU. Approximately one third of infants who have a positive screening test for PKU do not have the classic form of the disease. These cases may represent benign variants, presumably

with no risk of brain damage. Several variant forms associated with progressive neurologic damage have been reported, however. They are unresponsive to diet therapy alone. These forms are rare and are associated with altered biopterin (a folacinlike cofactor needed for phenylalanine hydroxylase activity) metabolism.

Despite the fact that the fetus may have active phenylalanine hydroxylase, maternal elevations of blood phenylalanine may lead to fetal malformations or intrauterine brain damage. There is some evidence that diet control during pregnancy can partially reduce these risks, and successful attempts with diet therapy have been described.[3]

Mass screening of newborns for PKU is required by law in most states. If a newborn is suspected of having PKU from this screening test, use results of blood and urine tests to confirm the diagnosis and to differentiate classic PKU from benign forms of hyperphenylalaninemia.

Intervention. Follow these objectives of dietary management: (1) restrict dietary phenylalanine intake to an amount that allows for maintenance of the desired range of phenylalanine blood level and (2) provide all nutrients (including phenylalanine, tyrosine, other amino acids, vitamins, minerals, and water) and energy in an amount sufficient to promote normal growth and development. The specific amount of phenylalanine allowed varies according to the needs for growth, the severity of the disease, and the clinical response. In classic phenylketonuria, the tolerance for phenylalanine varies between 250 and 500 mg/day, whereas in the mild variant forms, an amount greater than 500 mg/day can usually be handled. At present, there is no consensus on need for diet therapy in clients whose blood phenylalanine levels range between 5 and 20 mg/100 ml. In clients whose blood levels are not excessively high or if only minimal diet restrictions are necessary to control the disorder, test the possibility of safely discontinuing the diet every few months. Use the results of laboratory tests, such as the blood levels of phenylalanine and tyrosine and urinary levels of phenylketones, to aid in this assessment. Since tyrosine becomes an essential amino acid during phenylalanine restriction, it is included in special formulas designed for clients with PKU. Initiate treatment in affected infants during the early weeks of life to allow the child to reach his or her developmental potential. For women at risk, the phenylalanine-restricted diet should be initiated before conception and continued throughout the pregnancy.

Since natural protein foods contain approximately 5 percent phenylalanine, the diet is based on synthetic or partially synthetic preparations that are low in phenylalanine or phenylalanine-free. The most commonly used preparation in the United States is Lofenalac (Mead Johnson), a casein hydrolysate to which carbohydrate, fat, vitamins, and minerals are added. This product contains a low

TABLE 22–3
APPROXIMATE NUTRITIVE COMPOSITION OF SPECIAL DIETARY PRODUCTS PER 100 G POWDER

Nutrient	Lofen-alac (MJ)[a]	PKU-Aid (MS)[b]	Low-methio-nine Isomil (RL)[c]	Phenyl-Free (MJ)	3200-AB (MJ)	MSUD-Aid (MS)	MSUD Diet Powder (MJ)	Methio-naid (MS)	3200-K (MJ)	Histi-naid (MS)	80056 (MJ)
Calories	460	240	516	406	460	248	476	242	518	240	445
Protein (g)	15	60	12.5	20.3	15	64.4	8.2	63.1	15.8	61.2	0
Fat (g)	18	0	28.1	6.8	18	0	20.1	0	28	0	20.4
CHO (g)	60	0	57.0	66	60	0	63.7	0	51.1	0	65.3
L-Amino Acids (g)											
Essential											
Isoleucine	0.75	2.6	0.56	1.10	0.86	0	0	2.4	0.76	2.5	0
Leucine	1.41	6.1	1.02	1.73	1.76	0	0	32	1.31	3.8	0
Lysine	1.57	6.1	0.77	1.89	1.91	7.1	0.8	6.0	0.98	5.8	0
Methionine	0.45	1.5	0.14	0.63	0.56	1.9	0.25	0.2	0.18	1.6	0
Phenylalanine	0.08	<0.07	0.6	0	0.08	3.8	0.55	4.3	0.86	2.2	0
Threonine	0.77	4.8	0.51	0.94	0.65	3.3	0.55	3.2	0.59	3.1	0
Tryptophan	0.19	0.9	0.12	0.28	0.20	1.2	0.20	0.9	0.18	1.1	0
Valine	1.20	4.6	0.52	1.26	1.38	0	0	3.2	0.80	3.1	0
Histidine	0.39	1.8	0.28	0.47	0.40	2.7	0.25	2.8	0.38	0	0
Nonessential											
Arginine	0.34	3.1	0.83	0.69	0.39	5.1	0.50	4.4	1.08	4.6	0
Alanine	0.64	4.1	0.53	NL	0.76	7.1	0.45	5.6	0.68	5.9	0
Aspartate	1.34	8.1	1.29	5.20	1.60	12.1	1.14	9.5	1.94	10.6	0
Cystine	0.025	1.5	0.15	0.35	0.042	2.1	0.25	3.7	0.107	1.8	0
Glutamate	3.78	9.3	2.48	1.88	4.31	13.3	2.09	11.0	3.12	12.3	0
Glycine	0.35	3.1	0.52	3.35	0.40	3.9	0.60	4.3	0.67	5.9	0
Proline	1.13	3.6	0.6	NL	1.13	2.3	0.90	1.6	0.77	1.9	0
Serine	1.02	4.8	0.68	NL	1.09	2.4	0.60	1.7	0.81	1.9	0
Tryosine	0.81	6.0	0.40	0.93	<0.04	3.8	0.65	4.3	0.55	4.5	0
Glutamine	NL[d]	NL	NL	4.75	NL	NL	NL	NL	NL	NL	0
Vitamins											
Vitamin A (IU)	1151	0	2200	2030	1151	0	1190	0	1296	0	1308
Vitamin D (IU)	288	0	340	406	288	0	297	0	324	0	327
Vitamin E (IU)	7.2	0	12	10	7.2	0	7	0	8.0	0	8
Vitamin C (mg)	37	0	60	53	37	0	39	0	42	0	41
Thiamine (μg)	360	2000	0.5	609	360	2000	370	2000	360	2000	409
Riboflavin (μg)	430	2000	0.6	1015	430	2000	450	2000	490	2000	491
Vitamin B_6 (μg)	290	2000	0.5	508	290	2000	300	2000	290	2000	327
Vitamin B_{12} (μg)	1.4	20	35	2.5	1.4	20	1.5	20	1.6	20	16.4
Niacin (μg)	5800	25,000	9	8122	5800	25,000	5900	25,000	6500	25,000	6545
Folic acid (μg)	72	400	0.12	102	72	400	74	400	81	400	82
Pantothenic acid (μg)	2200	20,000	7	3046	2200	20,000	2200	20,000	2400	20,000	2454
Choline (mg)	61	0	94	86	61	0	63	0	69	0	69
Biotin (μg)	36	600	0.13	30	36	600	40	600	36	600	41
Vitamin K (μg)	72	0	0.12	102	72	0	74	0	81	0	82
Inositol (mg)	22	0	0	30	22	250	22	100	24	100	25
Minerals											
Calcium (mg)	432	2500	650	609	432	2500	491	2500	486	700	491
Phosphorus (mg)	324	1500	440	457	324	1500	268	1500	324	1500	270
Magnesium (mg)	51	300	40	71	50	300	52	300	49	80	57
Iron (mg)	8.6	25	10	12	8.6	50	9	50	10	4	10
Iodine (μg)	32	150	120	46	32	150	33	150	36	60	37
Copper (μg)	430	2500	500	609	430	2500	400	2500	500	500	491
Manganese (mg)	0.7	3.5	0	1	0.7	3.5	0.7	3.5	0.8	0.5	0.8
Zinc (mg)	2.9	15	4	4.1	2.9	15	3	15	4	0.9	3.3
Sodium (mEq)	9	61	10.4	11	9	61	9.7	61	9	34	2.8
Potassium (mEq)	12	66	10.4	18	12	66	8.6	66	11.4	19	7.9
Chloride (mEq)	9	80	12.7	14	9	80	10.5	80	9	NL	3.5

In these formulas, protein = nitrogen in g × 6.25.
[a] MJ, Mead Johnson Company.
[b] MS, Milner Scientific.
[c] RL, Ross Laboratories.
[d] NL, not listed.
(*Source: Pediatric Nutrition Handbook. American Academy of Pediatrics, 1979, pp 224–225, Table 26. Copyright American Academy of Pediatrics.*)

(0.08 g/100 g) but significant amount of phenylalanine. Initially, Lofenalac should provide 85 to 90 percent of the protein requirement, since most protein-containing foods contain an excessive amount of phenylalanine. Since Lofenalac may not provide sufficient phenylalanine to support growth, it must usually be supplemented with natural protein sources. Standard infant formula or evaporated milk is the usual supplement for an infant, and other natural foods (such as fruits, vegetables, and cereals) are added as the child begins to take solid food. Breast milk of mothers with phenylketonuria contains a high concentration of phenylalanine, and these mothers should not breastfeed.

Another product available for use by PKU clients is Phenyl-Free (Mead Johnson), which is composed of synthetic L-amino acids, is free of phenylalanine, and is higher in protein content than Lofenalac. Because Phenyl-Free does not contain phenylalanine, more natural foods can be incorporated into the diet and less diet supplement consumed, thereby facilitating clinical management in children over 2 years of age. Additional kilocalories and the required phenylalanine can be provided by conventional foods given in prescribed amounts. (The nutrient composition of Lofenalac and Phenyl-Free is found in Table 22–3.)

Use data provided in Table 22–4 to determine the phenylalanine, protein, and energy requirements of the child and the composition of the formula needed (i.e., the amount of Lofenalac and supplemental milk, if any) for each client. The amount of water to be used is determined by fluid requirements for the child's age, preference for fluids, and taste for Lofenalac. Fluid (130 to 200 ml/kg) must be provided in an amount sufficient to prevent dehydration, and some may be offered between formula feedings. Older children, according to individual tolerance, will demand extra fluid. Because Lofenalac is frequently given in a concentrated form (i.e., 1 measure of Lofenalac to 1 oz water or 45 kcal/oz) infants and children using the formula tend to be more thirsty than those taking regular formula or milk. The protein, phenylalanine, and energy not provided by the Lofenalac formula are given as regular foods. Solid foods should be introduced at the appropriate age as for any child. The amount to give is determined by subtracting the phenylalanine, protein, and energy supplied by the Lofenalac–milk mixture from the total phenylalanine, protein, and energy requirement. The serving lists for the phenylalanine-restricted diet (Appendices 11 and 12) are then used to determine the kinds and amounts of food to select. The serving lists are stated as phenylalanine equivalents. Foods of similar phenylalanine content are grouped together and can be exchanged for one another within a given list. This system of exchanges provides for variety in the diet. Frequent adjustment in the diet prescription may be necessary, particularly during the first 6 months, based on growth and development, degree of hunger, and laboratory analysis of serum phenylalanine levels.

Even with solid food additions, Lofenalac re-

TABLE 22–4
RECOMMENDED INTAKE AND PRESCRIBED SOURCES OF PHENYLALANINE, PROTEIN, AND ENERGY FOR PKU INFANTS AND PRESCHOOLERS

Age (months)	Suggested Phenylalanine	Suggested Protein[a]	Suggested Energy[b]	Percent Protein from Lofenalac	Amount of Lofenalac	Evaporated Milk[c]
	(mg/kg/day)	(g/kg/day)	(kcal/kg/day)		(ms[d]/kg)	(oz)
0–3	58 ± 18[e]	4.4	120	85	2½–3	1–3
4–6	40 ± 10[e]	3.3	115	85	2–2½	½–2
7–9	32 ± 9[e]	2.5	110	90	1½–2	½–1½
10–12	30 ± 8[e]	2.5	105	90	1½–2	½–1
		(total g/day)[b]	(kcal/day)		(total ms/day)	
13–24	25[f]	25.0	1300	90	16	0–1
25–36	24 ± 8[e]	25.0	1300	90	16	None
37–48	20[f]	30.0	1300	90	19	None
49–72	18[f]	30.0	1800	90	19	None

[a] Considerable controversy exists over protein need of both normal and PKU infants, particularly when it is provided by a casein hydrolysate. Because of this, recommended protein intake during infancy is the amount found by the Collaborative Study to promote normal growth (Acosta PB, Wenz E, Williamson M: Nutrient intake of treated infants with phenylketonuria (PKU). Am J Clin Nutr 30:198, 1977).
[b] From Joint FAO/WHO Ad Hoc Expert Committee: Energy and Protein Requirements, FAO Nutrition Meetings Report Series No. 52, Rome, Food and Agriculture Organization, 1971, p 33.
[c] 1 oz evaporated milk contains 106 mg phenylalanine, 2.2 g protein, and 44 kcal.
[d] A measure of Lofenalac = 10 g or 1 tbsp.
[e] See reference a.
[f] From Acosta PB, Wenz E: Nutrition in phenylketonuria. In H Bickel, FP Husdon, LI Woolf, eds: Phenylketonuria and Some Other Inborn Errors of Amino Acid Metabolism. Stuttgart, George Thieme Verlag, 1971, pp 181–196.
(*Source:* Acosta PB, Wenz E: Diet Management of PKU for Infants and Preschool Children. DHEW Publication No. (HSA) 78–5209, Rockville, Md, 1978, p 14.)

mains the major source of dietary protein and supplies part of the energy need. With weaning, the PKU child—just as non-PKU children—tends to decrease the total quantity of formula ingested. At this stage, part of the Lofenalac can be reconstituted for drinking and part may be incorporated into prepared products, such as cookies, bread, pastries, puddings, and sauces. Bread made from low-protein flour can be home-prepared or purchased commercially. While the taste of Lofenalac may be unpleasant for older children and adults, it is usually well accepted by young infants.

Since the child is usually receiving only a special modified formula during early infancy, implementation of the diet is relatively easy. The diet becomes more difficult to follow when other foods are added, however. It is essential that the diet be adequate in energy from nonprotein sources to prevent rises in the blood phenylalanine secondary to endogenous protein catabolism due to inadequate energy. Inadequate phenylalanine intake, febrile illness, and infection also lead to increased protein catabolism. A number of low-protein products are available commercially for increasing nonprotein energy intake (Table 22–5). Refer to Appendix 12 for a list of foods free of phenylalanine.

Educate the parents by interpreting the meaning of the diagnosis and its treatment, assisting with planning and implementing the diet plan, and aiding in their adjustment to the tensions—physical, emotional, and financial—associated with coping with the disease. Give the parents a copy of the calculated diet pattern and demonstrate the techniques of formula preparation, with a return demonstration given by the parents, at the beginning of treatment and with each change in diet. Teach the parents how to calculate the diet themselves. Provide a form on which to record the child's daily intake, and with each clinic visit, compare this record with the diet prescription. When solid foods are introduced, provide a copy of the exchange lists (see Appendix 12) and assist the parents with their use in planning daily menus. Advise parents to anticipate problems with acceptance of the formula, because of its taste, particularly as the child grows older and if other family members indicate a dislike for it. Since the formula remains the major protein source, provide recipes for incorporating it into prepared foods. When the child can comprehend, explain the reason for the diet modifications at a level that he or she can understand. Caution all individuals in contact with the child against offering the child foods that are not part of the diet. When the child goes to school, make teachers aware of the restrictions.

Parents may express many concerns, such as feelings of guilt and anxiety and of frustrations associated with having to constantly monitor and record food intake, the cost of the diet, and other aspects of the child's care. Encourage them to voice these concerns but at the same time to understand the absolute necessity of following the diet carefully and to aid the child to develop normally by coping with the normal developmental stages without major dietary indiscretions. Provide the parents with practical suggestions for organizing their daily schedules to allow both the child with PKU and other family members to receive proper attention. Since Lofenalac and Phenyl-Free are expensive, direct families to sources of financial assistance if necessary.

Frequent home visits by a public health nurse or nutritionist are necessary to provide continuing guidance or support. Establish a communication network between visits, either by telephone or written correspondence.

TABLE 22–5
COMMERCIALLY AVAILABLE LOW-PROTEIN PRODUCTS

Product	Source
Cellu Wheat Starch	Chicago Dietetic Supply, Inc.
Lo Pro Pastas	405 East Shawnut Ave.
Low Protein Baking Mix and Bread	La Grange, IL 60525
Controlyte	D. M. Doyle Pharmaceutical Co.
	Highway 100 at West Twenty-Third St.
	Minneapolis, MN 55416
Low Protein Bread and Mix	Ener-G Foods, Inc.
Potato Mix	1526 Utah Ave., South
Egg Replacer	Seattle, WA 98134
Aproten Low Protein Pastas, Rusks, Porridge	General Mills Chemicals, Inc.
	4620 W. 77th St.
Cal-Power Beverages	Minneapolis, MN 55440
Dietetic Paygel Baking Mix	
Dietetic Paygel Wheat Starch	
Low Protein Canned Bread	
Prono Imitation Jello	

(Source: Acosta PB, Wenz E: Diet Management of PKU for Infants and Preschool Children. DHEW Publication No. (HSA) 78-5209, Rockville, Md, 1978, p 25.)

Careful monitoring of treatment is essential throughout the period of dietary management. Monitor serum phenylalanine levels and the child's growth closely to detect both excesses and deficiencies of phenylalanine. Adjust the diet in accordance with phenylalanine blood levels and growth pattern. The goal is to maintain a serum phenylalanine level of 2 to 10 mg/100 ml. The allowed range of serum phenylalanine is above the normal level to avoid the possibility of phenylalanine deficiency and to allow for a wider choice of normal foods. Phenylalanine deficiency brings growth failure, anemia, hypoproteinemia, generalized amino aciduria, dermatitis, and frequent infections. Teach parents how to take blood samples for monitoring purposes.

To monitor growth, assess height, weight, and head circumference on a regular basis to aid in determining the adequacy of the diet and make dietary adjustments accordingly. Because of the severe restriction of protein intake, evaluate hemoglobin levels at frequent intervals. Intake of other nutrients, such as magnesium and zinc, may also be low when the primary protein source is synthetic or semisynthetic diets, and supplements may be necessary. Criteria for monitoring the nutritional status in pregnant women and infants of these women during the first year have been published.[3]

Controversy exists as to how long rigid dietary control should continue. Some authorities take the view that diet control can be relaxed by age 4 or 5 years, since the danger of brain damage is greatest during the first few years of life. Results of discontinuing the diet at this age are variable, although significant drops in IQ have been noted with diet discontinuation. At present the practice of liberalizing the diet at an early age is being questioned. The need to provide diet control for pregnant PKU women is related to considerations given to discontinuing diet control. Since the diet must be controlled during pregnancy, this may be facilitated by maintaining some degree of control in female clients.

Disorders of Branched-chain Amino Acid Metabolism: Maple Syrup Urine Disease (Branched-chain Ketoacidemia)

Assessment. There are numerous disorders involving defects in the degradation of the branched-chain amino acids (BCAA), valine, leucine, and isoleucine, which lead to the accumulation in plasma and urine of one or more of the BCAA or small molecular ▶ weight organic acids (**keto acids**).

In normal metabolism, amino acids are catabolized by reactions involving transamination and oxidative decarboxylation to metabolites that enter metabolic pathways of carbohydrate or fat. In transamination, the amino group is removed from the individual amino acids and subsequently converted to urea, leaving the keto acid derivative of the individual amino acid (Fig. 22–1). The keto acids are further degraded by oxidative decarboxylation (removal of carbon dioxide) to simple acids. Oxidative decarboxylation is a complex reaction involving at least two (and probably three) different enzymes and several cofactors that contain B vitamins. Some of the disorders of BCAA are due to defects in the transamination of the amino acid(s), leading to elevated plasma and urinary levels of the amino acid involved, whereas others are due to defects in decarboxylation, leading not only to an elevation of the involved amino acids in the plasma and urine but also to elevations of their keto acid derivatives.

Several variants have been described for each defect, and the onset may be within a few days of birth or may be delayed until late infancy or childhood. The most severe forms lead to severe ketoacidosis, neurologic defects, and other abnormalities that may cause death within a few days. Alternatively, there may be mental retardation or recurring episodes of ketoacidosis, often precipitated by an infection or a sudden increase in protein intake.

Some of the variants are responsive to large doses of certain B vitamins, since several of the enzymes involved require specific vitamin-containing

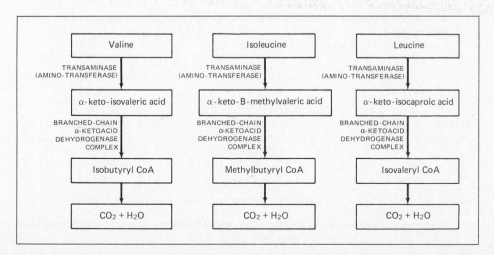

Figure 22–1
Metabolism of valine, isoleucine, and leucine (BCAA).

cofactors. In those disorders that do not respond to pharmacologic doses of vitamins, the use of a protein-restricted diet or of a diet restricting the offending amino acid(s) is necessary.

Maple syrup urine disease (MSUD), which is characterized by the accumulation in body fluids of both BCAA and their keto acid derivatives (BCKA), is discussed in more detail below. MSUD, also called branched-chain ketoaciduria, is a complex disorder of metabolism of the BCAA that has a very rare incidence—1 in 50,000 to 200,000 live births. Suspect a diagnosis of MSUD in newborns whose urine, sweat, and ear wax have an odor of maple syrup. The name of the disorder is derived from this characteristic odor.

In this disease, there is impairment of branched-chain alpha-keto acid dehydrogenase (see Fig. 22–1), a multienzyme complex involved with the second step in the degradation of the BCAA, and the keto acids cannot undergo oxidative decarboxylation with production of metabolites that are oxidized for energy. A defect in several enzymes may be responsible for the disease. Assess for the accumulation of BCAA and BCKA in the blood and other body fluids (including the cerebrospinal fluid) and for their excretion in large amounts in the urine. Urinary excretion of the BCKA leads to metabolic acidosis. Blood levels of the amino acid, alanine, are decreased, and that of alloisoleucine, a metabolite of isoleucine, is increased. This last compound occurs only in clients with MSUD and is a specific marker for the disorder.[4]

Like PKU, the disorder appears in a classic form and several variants—intermittent (late manifesting), mild, and a form responsive to thiamine. It may be difficult to distinguish between the intermittent and mild forms, and the relationship between enzymatic and environmental factors in these two disorders is not completely understood.

In the classic form of the disease, the affected infant may appear normal at birth, but observe for symptoms of progressive neurologic dysfunction and fragrant urine during the first week. Neurologic impairment is manifest as poor sucking, irregular respirations, lethargy, alternating muscle rigidity and flaccidity, and convulsions. The baby may also have a high-pitched cry. Untreated clients with a severe form of the disease usually die within the first few weeks of life from severe neurologic damage. Should the untreated client survive beyond infancy, expect retarded physical and mental development.

Differentiate between the classic and the intermittent form of MSUD. The latter form is episodic in nature and may not be detected until late infancy or early childhood. Be aware that clinical symptoms, including severe metabolic acidosis, may be triggered by a specific stimulus, such as an infection, surgery, or a high-protein load. Affected children may have normal plasma levels of BCAA between episodes of illness. During attacks, however, which may be so severe as to bring death, plasma levels are increased (Table 22–6).

A few cases of a mild form of the classic variant have been reported, and a thiamine-responsive type has been identified. Thiamine (as thiamine pyrophosphate) serves as a coenzyme for the decarboxylation reaction of the BCKA. Affected children may improve when given a 10 g/day thiamine supplement. The mechanism of action of the thiamine may involve stabilization of the decarboxylase enzyme and prolongation of its biologic half-life.

Base the diagnosis of MSUD on suggestive evidence provided by the sweet, maple syrup odor of the urine, and confirm it by assessing the plasma levels of BCAA and decarboxylase enzyme activity (see Table 22–6).

Intervention. Initiate a diet that restricts (but not excludes) the BCAA immediately after diagnosis of the classic form of the disorder to prevent death or permanent neurologic damage. The treatment of the disorder from early infancy (initiation of the diet within the first week is essential) may permit normal growth and development. Like phenylala-

TABLE 22–6
PLASMA CONCENTRATION OF BCAA AND ENZYME ACTIVITY IN MSUD

MSUD Variant	Plasma Concentration of BCAA	Keto Acid Decarboxylase Enzyme Activity
Classic	10 × normal	<5% of normal
Intermittent	>10 × normal during attacks	10–20% of normal during attacks
Mild	5–15 × normal	~25% of normal
Thiamine-responsive	3 × normal	<40% of normal

(Source: Short SH: A review of selected inborn errors of metabolism. Cassette-A-Month, American Dietetic Association, Chicago, 1974.)

nine, valine, leucine, and isoleucine are essential amino acids; thus the diet must supply the anabolic requirements while not providing excessive amounts. MSUD is more difficult to control than PKU, since three amino acids have to be adjusted individually, and clients are more sensitive to small changes in dietary intake.

Use a semisynthetic diet (i.e., synthetic amino acids plus natural food supplements to maintain growth) to treat the severe form of the disease. A formula that consists of a mixture of crystalline L-amino acids devoid of the BCAA and that contains appropriate amounts of carbohydrate, fat, vitamins, and minerals (e.g., MSUD Diet Powder, see Table 22–3) and additional protein to provide the needed amounts of the essential BCAA is used. For infants, add a small amount of milk or milk-based infant formula to the formula to supply the needed protein. Older children can eat an appropriately balanced mixture of natural foods of known composition to meet nutritional requirements and enhance variety. The formula remains the basis of the diet for older children, however. In addition to MSUD Diet Powder, other commercial products devoid of the BCAA are available that require varying degrees of supplementation, e.g., MSUD-Aid (see Table 22–3), that must be supplemented with fat-soluble vitamins, carbohydrate, and fat as well as additional protein to serve as a minimal source of the BCAA.

Several food equivalent systems similar to the exchange system used for diabetes mellitus and PKU have been published.[5-8] Tabulated food lists for the equivalency system listed in reference 8 are available from Nutrition Division, Clinical Investigation Unit, the Hospital for Sick Children, 555 University Avenue, Toronto, Ontario, Canada, M5G, 1X8.

A low-protein diet may be appropriate in managing the intermittent and mild forms of the disease, and sometimes those clients with a mild form of MSUD do well with no diet restrictions. During episodes of acute disease, however, a strict diet is needed.

Use the same educational strategies described for PKU to assist parents of the MSUD child with dietary management. Stress that rigid dietary control measures are necessary, since small fluctuations in intake produce wide fluctuations in the serum concentration. Diet control must be maintained throughout life. Be aggressive with management in the presence of infections, which bring tissue catabolism and increases in the serum levels of BCAA. Encourage the intake of sweetened, low-protein fruit juice when infection is present to reduce tissue catabolism. Peritoneal dialysis (see Chap. 30) may be necessary at these times to wash the amino acids from the body pools to avoid brain damage.

Monitor the effectiveness of dietary control on a continuing basis by frequent blood testing, use of diet records, and anthropometric measurements.

Inborn Errors of Lipid Metabolism: Familial Hypercholesterolemia

Assessment and Intervention. Genetic abnormalities of lipid metabolism may bring (1) altered vascular transport of lipids as lipoproteins from the intestine to the tissues secondary to hyperlipoproteinemia or hypolipoproteinemia (elevated and depressed levels of lipoproteins, respectively) and (2) accumulation of complex structural lipids in body tissues, such as the brain, liver, and kidney (lipoidoses).

The hyperlipoproteinemias have assumed considerable significance in the health problems of contemporary society because of their association with such problems as atherosclerosis, coronary heart disease, diabetes mellitus, and obesity. The familial forms of hyperlipoproteinemias are included in the discussion of this topic in Chapter 29. Of the six major types of primary hyperlipoproteinemia, only familial hyperchylomicronemia (type I hyperliproteinemia) and familial hypercholesterolemia (type II hyperlipoproteinemia) are likely to be encountered in the pediatric population. Familial hypercholesterolemia is discussed in more detail below.

Most of the blood cholesterol is incorporated into lipoproteins, with the majority circulating in the blood in the low-density lipoprotein fraction (LDL). Hypercholesterolemia occurs in a number of metabolic disorders, including familial hypercholesterolemia. In familial hypercholesterolemia, there is an abnormality in the cell membrane receptors for cholesterol, leading to faulty feedback inhibition of cholesterol synthesis by the liver, and both the blood cholesterol and LDL levels are increased. This disorder is classified as type II hyperlipoproteinemia and affects 1 in 300 to 500 persons in the population. Assess the blood cholesterol level in children of affected parents; plasma levels may range from 300 to 600 mg/100 ml in moderate forms of the disease to as much as 650 to 1000 mg/100 ml in more severe forms. Affected clients face a major risk of developing premature atherosclerosis and coronary heart disease and even myocardial infarction as a child in the more severe forms. Observe also for cholesterol deposits (**xanthomas**) on tendons in hypercholesterolemic clients.

Treat moderate degrees of hypercholesterolemia with a diet low in fat, with an increased ratio of polyunsaturated fat to saturated fat, and limited in kilocalories. This regimen will lower blood cholesterol and has no known harmful side effects, although pediatricians have expressed concern about manipulating the diet during the period of infancy. For older children and adults, restrict cholesterol to less than 300 mg/day as well. In families including both parents and children with familial hypercholesterolemia, encourage the entire family to share the same dietary regimen.

Use a combination of diet and drug therapy for

more severe forms of hypercholesterolemia. Cholestyramine and nicotinic acid are sometimes used. Both medical and surgical management are necessary in clients with extreme forms of hypercholesterolemia who face serious risks of myocardial infarction as a child. Refer to Chapter 29 for a complete discussion of diets altered in fat and cholesterol.

Inborn Errors of Mineral Metabolism: Wilson's Disease

Assessment and Intervention. Inborn errors in the metabolism of several trace minerals, including zinc, copper, and iron, have been identified, and the clinical manifestations of these disorders resemble those either of a deficiency state or of chronic toxicity. These disorders are as follows:

Zinc	Acrodermatitis enteropathica
Copper	Menkes' kinky hair syndrome
	Wilson's disease
Iron	Hemochromatosis

The specific defect leading to these abnormalities is unconfirmed at present, although several, including a defect in a specific mineral-binding protein, increased absorption, and maldistribution of a specific mineral, have been proposed. Only two of these disorders, acrodermatitis enteropathica and Wilson's disease, respond to diet therapy. The skin rash, diarrhea, and abnormal unsaturated fatty acid metabolism associated with acrodermatitis enteropathica respond to zinc supplements and dietary copper restriction in a component of the treatment of Wilson's disease (discussed below).

In Wilson's disease, copper accumulates in such tissues as the brain, liver, kidney, and the cornea of the eye probably due to a defect in the copper-binding protein, ceruloplasmin. The insidious accumulation of copper in these tissues leads to irreversible damage as the client ages. Prompt diagnosis is difficult because of the variable features of the disease and the wide range in age of onset of symptoms. The onset of symptoms correlates with the time required for the copper accumulation to become damaging, and some of the manifestations may not occur until the teenage years or young adulthood. Assess for these clinical manifestations in affected clients: (1) acute or chronic liver disease, (2) hemolytic anemia, (3) damage to the basal ganglia of the brain, leading to disorders of movement, (4) change in the higher brain centers, leading to psychologic disorders and other neurologic manifestations, (5) copper-stained rings in the cornea, and (6) renal damage with proteinuria, amino aciduria, glucosuria, phosphaturia, and uricosuria (excretion of uric acid in the urine). The serum copper concentration is usually depressed, and urinary excretion is markedly increased. With acute or chronic liver damage, copper may be released suddenly, bringing a transient hemolytic anemia. Alternately, the liver copper may be released slowly to be distributed to other tissues.

Effective treatment can arrest the progress of the disease in symptomatic clients and prevent the tissue abnormalities if the diagnosis is made in the presymptomatic stage. Test the siblings of affected clients in order to detect the disorder in the early stages. Use a combination of diet and drug therapy to treat Wilson's disease, since neither suffices when used alone. Promote an increase in the renal excretion of copper by administering chelating agents, such as D-penicillamine, and restrict dietary copper intake to 1.0 mg/day. This combined therapy leads to a negative copper balance and removal of excess tissue copper.

The usual dietary copper intake ranges from 3 to 6 mg/day, of which approximately one half is absorbed. Restriction of the dietary intake to less than 1 mg/day necessitates an unappetizing regimen making reduction of dietary copper intake alone an ineffective treatment. Advise the client to avoid the following high-copper foods: shellfish, organ meats, coffee, chocolate, cocoa, tea, mushrooms, nuts, dried fruits, dried legumes, and poultry. The copper content of foods has been published.[9] Check the copper content of the client's water supply and suggest the use of distilled water if necessary. Advise the client to avoid the use of copper cookware in food preparation. Be alert that siblings of affected clients are susceptible to the disease, and evaluate these siblings for the presence of the disorder so that treatment can be initiated in the early stages.

REVIEW QUESTIONS AND ACTIVITIES

1. Discuss common psychologic responses of hospitalized children and nursing implications for intervention.
2. Describe nursing interventions that could be used to assist school-age children adjust to a prolonged modified diet.
3. Plan a day's menu that is adequate in kilocalories and protein for a 3-year-old child who is hospitalized and receiving a regular diet. [Use the RDA charts given in Chapter 2 (see Tables 2–1 and 2–2) and Appendix 1 to determine kilocalorie and protein needs and to calculate the kilocalorie and protein values.]
4. Discuss appropriate feeding techniques for the medical management of infants with a mild form of pyloric stenosis.
5. Differentiate between a cleft lip and a cleft palate.
6. Compare the presurgical and postsurgical dietary regimens for cleft lip and cleft palate.
7. Identify the rationale for the necessity of initiating prompt diet therapy in infants with galactosemia, phenylketonuria, maple syrup urine disease, and Wilson's disease.

8. **a.** Prepare a chart that lists the biochemical defects and metabolic consequences that may occur in untreated cases of each of the following inborn errors of metabolism: (1) galactosemia, (2) PKU, (3) MSUD, (4) familial hypercholesterolemia, and (5) Wilson's disease.

   b. List those problems that are common to all of the disorders and those that are different.

9. Discuss the recommended duration of dietary control for galactosemia, PKU, and MSUD and the implications of these disorders for affected clients who are pregnant.

10. **a.** Outline the essential points to be covered in counseling parents of infants who are diagnosed with each of the following disorders: (1) galactosemia, (2) PKU, and (3) MSUD.

    b. Visit a supermarket and identify lactose-containing packaged foods that must be eliminated on a galactose-free diet.

    c. Consult a pharmacist to determine lactose-containing medications that cannot be used by galactosemic clients.

    d. Consult the hospital dietitian to determine the special formulas available for treating galactosemia, PKU, and MSUD. Assess their nutritive content and identify what supplements, if any, are needed by 6-month-old infants using these formulas.

11. Identify adjustments that should be made in the diet of infants with PKU and MSUD when solid foods are added to the diet.

12. Develop a teaching plan for parents of 6-month-old infants with PKU and MSUD.

13. Compare and contrast the management of moderate and severe forms of familial hypercholesterolemia.

14. Identify foods that must be eliminated from the diet in clients with Wilson's disease.

15. *Case study:* Your client today is 8-day-old Jimmy, who has just been diagnosed with phenylketonuria and is receiving Lofenalac formula. His weight is 4.7 kg and his height is 56.1 cm. Jimmy's parents are overwhelmed with the diagnosis; they have another young child who is unaffected by the disorder.

    a. Why is breastfeeding contraindicated for clients with phenylketonuria?

    b. What is Lofenalac?

    c. Describe the rationale for adding a source of phenylalanine to the Lofenalac formula. What food sources may be used for infants? for older children?

    d. Why is it necessary to use Lofenalac to provide a large percentage of the protein requirement?

    e. How are the requirements for phenylalanine, protein, energy, and fluid determined? Why is the energy level important?

    f. What teaching tools would you use in instructing the parents on formula preparation?

    g. Discuss ways of relieving Jimmy's parents of their anxiety regarding the diagnosis.

    h. List some of the problems that the family may encounter in maintaining Jimmy on a phenylalanine-restricted diet as he grows older.

    i. What is Phenyl-Free, and how can it be used in Jimmy's diet?

    j. Discuss the use of the food exchange system for phenylalanine-restricted diets in planning Jimmy's diet when solid foods are added.

    k. Discuss ways of incorporating Lofenalac into the diet after Jimmy is weaned.

    l. Should Jimmy develop an infection with fever, how will this affect the control of the disease?

    m. How would you monitor the effectiveness of treatment?

REFERENCES

1. Lenke RL, Levy HL: Maternal phenylketonuria and hyperphenylalaninemia. An internal survey of the outcome of untreated and treated pregnancies. N Engl J Med 303:1202, 1980.
2. Bessman SP, Williamson ML, Koch R: Diet, genetics, and mental retardation. Interaction between phenylketonuric heterozygous mother and fetus to produce nonspecific diminution of IQ: Evidence in support of the justification hypothesis. Proc Natl Acad Sci USA 75:1562, 1978.
3. Acosta PB, Blaskovics M, Cloud H, et al.: Nutrition in pregnancy of women with hyperphenylalaninemia. J Am Diet Assoc 80:443, 1982.
4. DiGeorge AM, Rezvani I, Garibaldi LR, Schwartz M: Prospective study of maple syrup urine disease for the first four days of life. N Engl J Med 307:1492, 1982.
5. Smith BA, Waisman HA: Leucine equivalency system in managing branched-chain ketoacidemia. J Am Diet Assoc 59:342, 1971.
6. Noel MB, Stanley PB, Girz JC, et al.: Dietary treatment of maple syrup urine disease (branched-chain ketoacidemia). J Am Diet Assoc 69:62, 1976.
7. Acosta PB, Elsas LJ: Dietary Management of Inherited Metabolic Disease: Phenylketonuria, Galactosemia, Tyrosinemia, Homocystinuria, Maple Syrup Urine Disease. Avondale Estates, Ga, ACELMU Publishers, 1976, pp 72–75.
8. Bell L, Chao E, Milne J: Dietary management of maple syrup urine disease: Extension of equivalency systems. J Am Diet Assoc 74:357, 1979.
9. Pennington JT, Calloway DH: Copper content of foods. J Am Diet Assoc 63:143, 1973.

BIBLIOGRAPHY

Acosta P, Bell L: A Parent's Guide to the Child with MSUD. Tallahassee, Florida State University Center for Family Services, 1982.

Acosta PB, Fernoff PM, Warshaw HS, et al.: Zinc and copper status of treated children with phenylketonuria. J Parent Enter Nutr 5:406, 1981.

Bell L, Acosta PB, Chan L: Amino acid content of low-protein recipes. J Am Diet Assoc 80:579, 1982.

Bondy PK, Rosenberg LE, eds: Metabolic Control and Disease, ed 8. Philadelphia, WB Saunders, 1980.

Daeschel I, Kramish MJ, Coleman RA: Diet and growth of children with glycogen storage disease types I and III. J Am Diet Assoc 83:135, 1983.

Fischler K, Koch R, Donnell GN, Wenz E: Developmental aspects of galactosemia from infancy to childhood. Clin Pediatr 19:38, 1980.

Glorieux FH, Marie PJ, Pettifor JM, et al.: Bone response to phosphate salts, ergocalciferol, and calcitriol in hypo-phosphatemic vitamin D-resistant rickets. N Engl J Med 303:1023, 1980.

Hostetter MK, Levy HL, Winter HS, et al.: Evidence for liver disease preceding amino abnormalities in hereditary tyrosinemia. N Engl J Med 308:1265, 1983.

Mark-Savage CL, Keen CL, Hurley LS: Reduction by copper supplementation of teratogenic effects of D-penicillamine. J Nutr 113:501, 1983.

Queen PM, Fernoff PM, Acosta PB: Protein and essential amino acid requirements in a child with propionic acidemia. J Am Diet Assoc 79:562, 1981.

Tenbrinck MS, Stroud HW: Normal infant born to a mother with phenylketonuria. JAMA 247:2139, 1982.

The dietary treatment of phenylketonuria. Nutr Rev 41:11, 1983.

Williamson ML, Koch R, Azen C, Chang C: Correlates of intelligence test results in treated phenylketonuric children. Pediatrics 69:161, 1981.

Wolf BW, Hsia YE, Sweetman L, et al.: Propionic acidemia: A clinical update. J Pediatr 99:835, 1981.

CHAPTER 23

Body Weight Imbalance

Objectives

After completion of this chapter, the student will be able to:

1. Differentiate between the etiologic factors and complications of obesity and underweight.

2. Develop a teaching plan for an adult obese client using a balanced, kilocalorie-controlled diet, increased physical activity, and techniques of behavior modification.

3. Distinguish between the potential health hazards associated with fasting (prolonged and supplemented), low-carbohydrate, ketogenic diets, and drug therapy used for weight reduction.

4. Develop a nursing care plan for all stages of the dietary management of a client following gastric bypass surgery for morbid obesity.

5. Manage the diet for an underweight client.

Obesity and underweight are both common conditions. However, obesity is by far the most prevalent weight imbalance in the United States. The attention given to the management of obesity practically eclipses the efforts directed toward the smaller group who need to gain weight. Yet, the health hazards are as great for underweight as for obesity, and the conditions merit equal medical attention. The definition, diagnosis, classification, incidence, causes, complications, treatment, and prevention of obesity and underweight are discussed in this chapter. Obesity in children and adolescents and anorexia nervosa (a cause of serious underweight in some adolescents) are discussed in Chapter 17.

OBESITY

Assessment

Definition and Diagnosis. Although the terms obesity and overweight are often used interchangeably, ▶ **obesity** is best defined as an accumulation of excessive adipose tissue in the body. In contrast, **overweight** denotes no specific reference to body composition but refers to a body weight that exceeds given weight standards, such as available height–weight tables. Overweight may or may not be due to excessive body fat accumulation; obese people are usually overweight but not all overweight people are obese.

Body fat development follows an age- and sex-specific developmental pattern, and at all ages females have higher levels of body fat than males. The development of fat begins in late prenatal life, increases rapidly in infancy, and shows a slow, steady increase during childhood. There is an increase in fat deposition during adolescence, and the pattern differs for males and females. In males, a mild increase in fat deposition occurs before the growth spurt, followed by a decline, whereas females show a steady increase in subcutaneous fat deposition throughout adolescence, tapering off after age 16 or 17. The percentage of body weight composed of fat in young adult males is approximately 15 to

20 percent; in females, fat comprises 20 to 25 percent of body weight. During later adult life total body fat increases in both sexes, although actual body weight changes little as lean body mass decreases at a proportional rate. Obesity in males and females may be defined as a body fat content greater than 25 and 30 percent, respectively. With marked obesity, 40 to 50 percent or more of total body weight may consist of fat.

Diagnostic tools for measuring body fat involve sophisticated techniques, including the use of ultrasound and measurement of body density by underwater weighing, that are usually reserved for research purposes, and diagnosis of obesity is generally based on anthropometric measures (discussed in Chap. 11), such as determination of height and weight and skinfold thickness.

Overweight and obesity in adults are defined in relation to tables of recommended weight (see Chapter 11 and Appendix 7) that are derived from life insurance statistics or the body mass index, also called the quetelet index (weight in kg divided by height in meters squared—wt/ht²). With the use of life insurance company tables, weight is expressed as relative weight (the ratio or percentage of actual to recommended weight). Consider adults whose body weight is 10 to 20 percent above recommended weight as overweight and those with a body weight greater than 20 percent above the recommended body weight as obese. The normal limits for body mass index in adults are 20 to 25 for men and 19 to 24 for women. A body mass index that falls between the top acceptable value for either sex and 30 is considered overweight whereas a body mass index greater than 30 in either sex represents obesity. A state of morbid obesity exists in clients whose weight is more than twice the recommended body weight for height listed in the life insurance company tables or whose body mass index is 45 or more. A nomograph based on the body mass index has been developed for assessing body weight.[1] Use the

standards given in Table 23–1 for evaluating excess weight in children.

Assessment of height and weight do not give any real index of fatness. In contrast, assessment of skinfold thickness is helpful in quantifying the amount of fat and differentiating between overweight and overfat. Use skinfold measurements as a screening tool, but be aware that these measurements may be of little value for assessing obesity in clients whose fatfolds are greater than the calipers can accommodate, for example, those with body weight in excess of 150 percent of recommended weight. In adults, skinfold values greater than 18 mm in males and 25 mm in females indicate obesity.[2] Percentiles for triceps skinfolds for adults and children, based on data obtained from NHANES I, have been published.[3,4]

Classification. Obese individuals may be broadly classified into two groups: those with developmental obesity and those with reactive obesity. **Developmental obesity** manifests itself gradually over a period of time, possibly from infancy. In contrast, suspect **reactive obesity** in clients whose weight gain follows a stressful situation, such as the death of a loved one, separation, or hospitalization.

In childhood and adolescence, assess for two additional types of obesity. The first type is associated with an increase in adrenal androgens and clients will demonstrate these characteristics: (1) an increase in lean body mass and fat, (2) advanced sexual and skeletal maturation, a tendency toward tallness, and early menarche in the female, and (3) long-standing obesity with onset in infancy or early childhood. Because of earlier maturity, the client may attain a somewhat shorter stature as an adult. In clients with the second type of obesity, height and bone age are normal, there is no increase in lean body mass, but there is a history of weight gain in middle or late childhood.

TABLE 23–1
STANDARDS AND EVALUATION OF WEIGHT FOR AGE AND WEIGHT FOR STATURE, FROM BIRTH TO AGE 18

Age	Standards	Evaluation
Birth–36 months	National Center for Health Statistics Growth Charts (see Appendices 8A and C); plot weight for age and weight for length	Probable excess weight: 85–95th percentile on either graph Significant excess weight; >95th percentile on either graph
3 years–18 years	National Center for Health Statistics Growth Charts (see Appendices 8B and D); age 3–18, plot weight for age; age 3–10 in girls and 3–11½ in boys, plot weight for stature*a*	

a Body compositional changes with the pubertal growth spurt render plotting weight for stature invalid.

Incidence. The incidence of obesity is difficult to define precisely because of different methodologies and poor standardization of techniques used in its assessment. According to NHANES I data, approximately 30 percent of middle-age women and 15 percent of middle-age men are obese (i.e., they weigh more than 120 percent of recommended weight).[5] Observe that the prevalence is greater in black adult females than in white females. This trend is reversed in males—obesity is more common among white than black men. For both black and white men, a lower income level is associated with a lower level of obesity. In younger women, obesity is more prevalent in the lower-income groups. In older women, both black and white, lower income is associated with a lower prevalence of obesity.[6]

Etiology. Whereas obesity results from an imbalance between energy intake and energy expenditure, its etiology is complex and no one theory of causation provides a total explanation. Its etiology may reflect a combination of genetic, physiologic, environmental and social, and emotional factors.

Genetic Factors. Although obesity as an inherited trait has been observed in experimental animals, human genetic obesity (i.e., individuals with specific enzyme defects) has not been detected. The mixed racial heritage of the U.S. population and the interaction of many environmental factors known to contribute to obesity are difficult to control in studies. Regardless of whether obesity is due to genetic factors, environmental determinants, or genetic–environmental interaction, the familial incidence is strikingly high. Observe that obese parents tend to have obese children. Family studies demonstrate that if one parent is obese, 20 to 40 percent of the children will develop obesity, and the proportion rises to 40 to 80 percent if both parents are obese. This is in contrast to an incidence of less than 10 percent in children of parents of average weight.

A genetic basis for obesity is supported by studies with twins, both identical and fraternal, reared in similar and different environments. Note that identical twins, even when reared in different homes, tend to show more similar weights than do fraternal twins, even when the latter are reared together in the same environment. However, skinfold thicknesses of both natural and adoptive children correlate well with those of their parents, suggesting an influence of social factors and shared environment. Length of living together also appears to be related to the degree of similarity in fatness observed in spouses.[7]

The importance of a genetic determinant or predisposition to obesity is further illustrated by the high correlation between inherited body type and the likelihood of developing obesity. The lean, tall
▶ **ectomorph** is much less likely to become obese than
▶ the round, soft **endomorph**, whose abdominal area tends to be larger than the chest. There may be a

genetic basis for obesity, but it is likely that genetic and environmental interactions influence the development of obesity. Observe for lifestyle, attitudes, and habits toward food and exercise that may combine with genetic tendencies to produce the observed familial pattern.

Physiologic Factors. Physiologic factors that may influence the development of obesity are metabolic abnormalities, excessive kilocaloric consumption during periods of adipose cell division, and use of certain drugs.

Metabolic Abnormalities. Metabolic abnormalities that may be associated with the development of obesity include alteration in the physiologic control of hunger and satiety, defective heat production, and imbalances of certain hormones.

Although regulatory mechanisms that control hunger and satiety and thus food intake are ill-defined, it is hypothesized that failure of these mechanisms may be a factor leading to obesity. In spite of wide fluctuations in food intake, many people maintain a balance between food intake and energy expenditure that keeps their weight comparatively stable over a period of years. Obese persons, however, may be unable to adjust food intake to physiologic need. There are some indications that in the obese, hunger and eating behavior become dissociated, and eating is not initiated or terminated appropriately with food consumption. For example, it has been suggested that obese subjects tend to respond to external cues associated with eating—sight, smell, taste of food, the time of day that meals are eaten—rather than to feelings of hunger per se.[8] Assist parents of infants and children to respond to the child's satiety signals to increase the likelihood that these mechanisms will become sufficiently sensitive to allow them to adjust food intake to needs.

A newer, somewhat speculative theory suggests that obesity may be associated with defective thermogenesis (heat production) and increased storage of food energy as fat. Defective brown adipose tissue, a specialized form of adipose tissue, is thought to be responsible. The function of brown adipose tissue, which is present in highest concentrations in newborns and individuals exposed to cold, is to increase heat production for maintaining body temperature. Brown adipose tissue metabolism is mediated by norepinephrine, and it acts to shift oxidative metabolism to fatty acids for heat production. During adult life, the quantity of brown adipose tissue declines and may be responsible for the age-related decline in basal metabolism and the increased prevalence of obesity in middle-age and older people.[9] Several different types of defects in thermogenesis in brown adipose tissue have been identified in animals, but the extent of the contribution to human obesity of defective energy buffering by brown adipose tissue is uncertain.

Assess for disorders in endocrine function that may be important in the development of obesity. Hyperinsulinism and hypercorticism are notable among these disorders. Insulin is a lipogenic substance that promotes fat synthesis and deposition. High insulin levels thus promote obesity; obesity in turn is associated with insulin resistance, and thus a vicious cycle is initiated that may be important in the perpetuation of obesity. Treatment with glucocorticoids or endogenous overproduction of these steroids (Cushing's syndrome) may be a factor in obesity. In clients with Cushing's syndrome, assess for altered body fat distribution with truncal obesity and relatively thin extremities. Endocrine changes in pregnancy are associated with deposition of body fat, and lack of growth hormone reduces the mobilization of stored fats.

Many attempts have been made to associate the development of obesity with hypothyroidism. Advanced hypothyroidism leads to fluid accumulation and puffiness of the tissues (myxedema) but not obesity. Be aware that thyroid hormone has little longterm value in the treatment of obesity.

Many hormonal changes and changes in intermediary metabolism occur with obesity. Although it is not totally clear whether these abnormalities precede or follow the obesity, observe that the endocrine and metabolic profile becomes more normal following weight reduction, suggesting a secondary rather than a causal relationship. As fat cell size approaches normal with weight reduction, the usual cellular metabolic and hormonal response appears to be restored.

Excessive Kilocaloric Intake during Critical Periods of Adipose Cell Division. As noted in Chapter 13, it is hypothesized that kilocaloric excess during critical phases of adipose cell division may result in adipose cell hyperplasia. The resulting excessive numbers of fat cells may be permanent. This hypothesis has been questioned, however, because of the method used for measuring fat cells, and there is some discussion among investigators about the timing of fat cell proliferation in obese and nonobese subjects.

Although the hypothesis is thus very tentative, it may provide an explanation for some of the difficulties encountered in weight reduction efforts, especially in obesity with onset early in life. Weight reduction in all obese clients, regardless of age of onset or degree or duration of the obesity, is achieved solely by a decrease in adipose cell size. Cell number remains constant, even with massive weight loss. Weight loss in extremely obese persons in whom the obesity had an early onset is extremely difficult. If successful, the weight loss is almost inevitably followed by a recurrence of the previous degree of obesity. At all age levels, obese children have a larger number of larger-size fat cells than do nonobese children—in some instances, the number may be two to four times greater.

Because of the apparent irreversibility of early-onset obesity, be involved with interventions for early detection, early treatment, and prevention to increase the potential for preventing lifelong obesity. Since the prenatal period, the first 2 years of life, and adolescence represent periods of fat cell proliferation, be particularly aggressive in assessing excessive weight gain during these periods.

Drugs. Pharmacologic agents can lead to an increase in body weight. Cyproheptadine and the phenothiazines are probably the major agents associated with an increase in body fat. Advise users of oral contraceptives that they may experience weight gain; much of this gain may be fluid retention, but some women may have an increase in appetite.

Environmental and Social Factors in the Etiology of Obesity. Factors related to food availability and use, along with the sedentary lifestyle of modern society, may promote the development of obesity. Socioeconomic factors and cultural and ethnic views of overweight appear to influence the incidence of the disorder.

In an affluent society, food is readily available, and individuals are constantly being induced to buy a wide array of food products. Social customs that promote the use of food for various events (such as weddings, funerals, holidays) and occupational uses of food (such as coffee breaks, office parties, study breaks for students, and the business lunch with cocktails) all may contribute to excess kilocaloric intake. Along with the affluence of American society has come a sedentary pattern of living. Automobiles, public transportation systems, escalators, and elevators are the modes of transportation and movement. Labor-saving devices are abundant at home and in the workplace. A great proportion of the population engages in spectator sports rather than participatory sports.

To be sure, the effect of physical activity on energy balance is uncertain. Whether reduced physical activity is a cause or a result of obesity is not clear; nonetheless, it serves to perpetuate it. Physical activity is important for maintaining energy balance in two ways: (1) it facilitates the use of excessive kilocalories and (2) it facilitates the regulation of appetite and food intake. It appears that energy intake and expenditure can be balanced only in the presence of moderate physical activity. When sedentary, obese people increase their level of physical activity, observe that they may actually eat less rather than more. The ability to regulate energy balance precisely may be compromised at both extremely low and extremely high levels of energy expenditure. The extremely inactive person, for instance, tends not to decrease food intake sufficient to prevent weight gain. The converse situation is true in that extremely active persons find it difficult to eat enough to prevent weight loss.

Cultural and ethnic views of body size or particular food patterns may affect the incidence of obesity. Some cultures view overweight as a sign of prosperity, and, in others, a round, plump woman is preferred to a thin one. For some, the strength symbolized by a large body may be a source of security. Many cultures consider a fat baby a healthy one, and the food patterns of some cultures promote obesity (see Chap. 19.)

Psychologic and Emotional Factors. Psychologic factors have been thought to be important in the etiology of obesity. However, it has not been possible to identify specific personality factors common to the obese or to establish a firm psychologic cause for most obesity. Assess the contribution of psychologic factors to the etiology of obesity on an individual basis—in some clients it may play little or no role and in others a dominant role. In the latter situation, however, it is difficult to determine whether the psychologic manifestations are a cause or an effect of the obesity. For example, one may question whether the obese adolescent becomes obese because he or she feels worthless or feels worthless because he or she is fat.

For some, overeating may be a balancing factor in adjusting to life. Provide other forms of emotional support before attempting to control the overeating. For others, overeating or compulsive eating may be a response to nonspecific emotional tensions, a symptom of underlying emotional tension, or a form of addiction.

Assess for the contribution of psychologic aspects of parent–child interactions to obesity in childhood. Since food is strongly associated with the emotions, parents often use it for numerous nonnutritive purposes—for reward or punishment, as a comfort measure, or as a means of showing love or relieving guilt and ambivalence. For example, children of unwanted pregnancies may be overfed to relieve parental guilt; food may be used to reward good behavior, to comfort a frustrated child, or to compensate for a handicapping problem. When food is used in this manner, children may learn to view food as a way to manipulate, or be manipulated, by other people or they may use food to compensate for emotional or social difficulties. This pattern may persist throughout life.

Psychologic trauma may precipitate obesity. Probe for a precipitating event, such as surgery, a prolonged period of enforced bedrest, a move to a new neighborhood, mother starting to work, or the death of a family member, that can often be identified with the onset of obesity in the school-age period.

Compulsive food intake patterns have been identified in two small subgroups of obese persons: the night eaters and the binge eaters. Both patterns represent reactions to stressful situations. Once initiated, the night eating syndrome tends to recur daily until the stress is alleviated; with binge eating, the bouts are not usually periodic. Night eaters are commonly females who experience a triad of morning anorexia, evening hyperphagia, and insomnia.

Binge eaters suddenly and compulsively eat large quantities of food to the point of abdominal pain and self-induced vomiting. With night eaters, attempts to lose weight may precipitate severe emotional stress, and it may be wiser to allow the client to remain obese than to precipitate emotional illness. Antidepressants may be useful in treatment. It has been suggested that the small percentage of obese persons who later develop anorexia nervosa appear to be binge eaters; binge eaters may benefit from psychotherapy.

Pathologic Manifestations. Obesity is associated with an increase in health risks, mechanical problems associated with excessive fat accumulation, and various psychosocioeconomic pressures that lower the quality of life and lead to a more restrictive lifestyle. In general, the greater the obesity, the greater the risks. In adults, obesity increases the risks of morbidity and mortality. An inappropriate weight status in children and adolescents appears to be associated not only with physical problems but also with problems of psychosocial development.

Notice that obesity is often associated with various metabolic disorders, including cardiovascular disease, diabetes mellitus, respiratory disorders, gastrointestinal disorders, skeletal and joint disorders, skin disorders, surgical complications, and reproductive disorders. Be aware, however, that association with a disease does not necessarily prove cause and effect. In some cases, the obesity appears to contribute directly, whereas in others, obesity is a commonly associated factor (Table 23–2). An important example is the association of obesity with coronary heart disease, although evidence to directly implicate obesity as a causal agent in coronary heart disease is not clear-cut. Obesity may lead to elevated blood pressure, hyperlipidemia, and glucose intolerance, all factors thought to promote heart disease. The influence of weight loss on coronary risk is thought to be mediated by influences on blood pressure, blood lipids, and glucose tolerance.

In most epidemiologic surveys, the risk of premature death and serious health problems begins to increase when body weight is about 20 to 30 percent above the average for age, sex, and height. A body weight less than 20 percent over the average weight for age, sex, and height does not appear to be associated with increased mortality and the health risks associated with moderate overweight appear to be modest.

Most life insurance statistics show that lean persons live longer and that a reduced life expectancy is associated with obesity. The increased mortality may result from the association of obesity with coronary heart disease, hypertension, and diabetes mellitus. Studies with experimental animals show that kilocaloric restriction leads to an increase in longevity.

Obesity with an onset prior to adulthood has potentially long-term consequences. The potential

TABLE 23–2
HEALTH PROBLEMS DIRECTLY AND
INDIRECTLY ASSOCIATED WITH OBESITY

Disorders in which obesity appears to contribute directly to the expression of the disease
  Respiratory disorders: hypoventilation, dyspnea, and in extreme form the pickwickian syndrome
  Complications of anesthesia and surgery: mechanical problems in the surgical procedure posed by excess fat; thrombophlebitis, wound dehiscence, and atelectasis
  Diabetes mellitus: insulin resistance and glucose intolerance
  Hypertension

Disorders in which obesity is an associated factor
  Coronary heart disease (probably mediated by effects on blood pressure, blood lipids, and glucose tolerance)
  Cerebrovascular accident (probably mediated by effects on blood pressure)
  Skeletal and joint disorders: backache, foot problems, and osteoarthritis of the lower spine and weight-bearing joints; hyperuricemia and gout
  Reproductive disorders: menstrual irregularities and possibly infertility in females; increased risk of toxemia, complications at delivery, and stillbirths in pregnancy; cancer of the breast and endometrium in females; hypogonadal syndromes in males
  Gastrointestinal disorders (gallstones, fatty liver)
  Skin disorders (thickening of the skin and proneness for skin disorders, such as intertrigo—rashes in the creases or overlapping areas of the skin—and yeast and fungal infections that may be aggravated by excessive friction and moisture)

exists for the obesity to persist into adulthood, with the associated changes in organ function, predisposing this particular group of the obese population to considerable health risks. Some overweight children become overweight adolescents and adults, although this is not an invariable consequence. Observe that many obese children have disturbed personality characteristics and altered self-concept and body image, although it is not known whether these characteristics precede or follow the obesity. The alteration in body image may persist into adulthood. An overdependency syndrome is seen occasionally. Assess for this particularly when obesity involves the youngest child of the family. The child may continue to be emotionally dependent on the mother and vice versa.

Intervention

Treatment of obesity is based on one or a combination of six basic approaches: dietary modification, physical exercise, behavior modification, pharmacologic agents, surgery, and psychotherapy. Less commonly used approaches include acupuncture and hypnosis. Each type of treatment may be successful in given individuals, but no one approach is successful in all obese clients. Although there are approaches that have some potential for success, a considerable amount of quackery and faddism surround the notion of weight reduction, and one finds devices or techniques, such as sweat suits, massage parlors, hormone creams, miracle drugs, and an endless ar-

ray of fad diets and other schemes promoted in the pursuit of thinness. In many cases, the obese client will pursue one approach after another and continue adding to the list of failures.

Behavior modification is one of the newer approaches, and currently a three-faceted program that combines an appropriate dietary regimen, regular physical activity, and behavior modification directed at both eating and exercise habits is gaining recognition as potentially the most successful approach to weight reduction and maintenance. Fasting, surgical intervention, and psychotherapy are reserved for the relatively small number of individuals who cannot be managed by other mechanisms.

Self-help groups that provide peer support, such as Weight Watchers, TOPS (Take Off Pounds Sensibly), Overeaters Anonymous, Diet Kitchen, and Diet Workshop, are now widespread in the United States. These groups were the first to appreciate the behavioral correlates to eating and weight reduction, and some are as successful as most medically managed programs (or more so). Overall success, however, appears to be only slightly better than that of the diet programs alone, and few diet approaches to weight reduction seem to have much long-term success in achieving weight loss of more than 20 pounds. The various groups tend to use reasonably sound dietary principles. Assess the attributes of local self-help groups before referring clients to particular ones.

Just as there are numerous complications associated with obesity, so are there complications associated with its treatment. The complications, which may be major or minor, include various metabolic and emotional or behavioral changes that accompany weight reduction. The specific metabolic complications depend on the specific regimen followed and may include such problems as negative nitrogen balance, ketosis, hypertension, cardiac irregularities, and even death. Dieting may also be accompanied by depression, and even psychotic reactions have been observed in those who lose a considerable amount of weight. Assess for adverse behavioral reactions in high-risk groups, including those whose obesity began in childhood (as opposed to adult-onset obesity) and those who follow kilocaloric-restricted regimens (rather than total fasting). Because of the overall low success rate and the frustrations and disappointment that accompany failure, nurses should be cautious and propose weight reduction only when there is a clear indication of need. Provide continuing support during the process.

Teach clients that control of obesity mandates not only weight loss but also permanent maintenance of the reduced state. Many treatment programs require drastic changes in lifestyle that are often difficult to continue on a permanent basis. Weight reduction entails a change in energy intake and expenditure to reverse the state of kilocaloric excess to one of negative kilocaloric balance. One pound of stored fat is the equivalent of 3500 kcal of stored energy—to lose 1 lb of fat in 1 week, the client must theoretically incur a daily deficit of 500 kcal. The prognosis for successful weight control appears to vary inversely with the degree and duration of obesity and with the number of previous failures at dieting. Use these guidelines to aid in achieving success:

1. Promote a high level of primary motivation: the obese are often more successfully motivated by potential socioeconomic gains, such as cosmetic changes, improved employability, or better relations with the opposite sex, than by physical risks. Scare tactics or promises to reduce risk factors may not be effective.

2. Establish a realistic short-term weight loss goal, that is, a small rate of loss, to be continued over a prolonged period. A weekly loss of 1 lb will lead to an annual loss of over 50 lb. A loss of 2 lb per week is usually considered the upper safe limit of loss unless the individual is under close medical supervision.

3. Make needed changes in eating habits and exercise patterns on a gradual incremental basis to assist the individual in shifting from current patterns to more suitable ones.

4. Provide a system of social support on a long-term basis: establish a family-based weight control program rather than one that is individually based, allow for regular medical visits to monitor weight, and encourage the recording of food intake to serve as a constant reminder of the amount of food consumed. People often eat less when recording food consumption.

5. Incorporate nutrition education as part of the weight control program to better enable the individual to make suitable food selections (e.g., provide information on appropriate food selection, menu planning, portion sizes and techniques for judging portion sizes, shopping techniques, interpretation of food labels, and cooking procedures, such as trimming visible fat from meat). With regard to portion sizes, people often tend to underestimate the kilocaloric value of meat and to overestimate the kilocaloric value of starchy foods. This underlying bias may make it difficult to estimate portion sizes and thus hinder efforts to lose weight. Food models may be a useful educational tool in helping clients learn to visually estimate portion size and kilocalorie content.

6. Consider the broader sociocultural environment in which the client lives and to which he or she returns after termination of formal treatment. Determine if a particular client has the ability to become actively involved in a weight control program that promotes efforts to alter his or her personal environment and to adopt a new lifestyle. Obese persons may have developed a lifestyle that enables them to cope with their over-weight—interacting with other obese persons, for example—and may find it difficult to give up this lifestyle.

Dietary Management. Dietary approaches to weight reduction include the traditional method of restricting kilocaloric intake while maintaining a relatively balanced nutrient intake, formula diets, fasting, and a wide array of fad diets—ever increasing in number—based on manipulation of the ratio of carbohydrate, protein, and fat, those based on so-called virtues of particular foods in bringing about weight loss, or those based on other faddist notions. Though obese persons are often attracted to fad diets that promise quick, painless weight loss, restriction of kilocaloric intake remains the mainstay in the treatment of obesity. Fasting regimens are sometimes used as the first phase in a program of long-term weight reduction for the grossly obese.

Kilocaloric Restriction. The rationale for kilocaloric restriction to reduce weight is that achievement of a state of negative energy balance requires the body to draw on its fat stores. The rate at which the body loses fat, however, depends almost entirely on the size of the energy deficit, whereas the rate at which the body loses weight depends on the type of nutrients lost, particularly the water content of the substances lost. With kilocaloric restriction, short-term fluctuations in body weight occur, and these can usually be attributed to changes in water balance. The change in water balance accounts for the plateau observed with weight reduction, i.e., a period of about a week of rapid weight loss may be followed by a period of about a week or 10 days of no weight loss—or even a weight gain. To avoid discouragement, teach clients to expect this plateau and to expect the diet to bring results the following week. Water balance can be affected by the nutrient compositon of the diet (a low-carbohydrate intake induces a water diuresis, whereas consumption of carbohydrate results in retention of sodium and water) as well as by the water composition of the nutrients lost (approximately 70 percent of the fat-free body mass is water). In the initial stages of kilocaloric restriction, both fat and protein are lost. Protein catabolism leads to loss of lean body mass and a water diuresis. The initial weight loss reflects primarily body water loss, and fat loss makes a smaller contribution. During prolonged kilocaloric restriction, the body adapts by increasing the relative contribution of its fat stores to the energy deficit and by conserving protein and water. Water weighs more than fat, and weight gain may occur as the body reconstitutes the early large fluid losses. Subsequent weight loss, which occurs at a much lower rate, reflects an increase in fat catabolism. Restriction of sodium and water is not usually indicated to offset the fluid retention that accompanies weight reduction unless complications occur. However, reducing the sodium intake may decrease the tendency to excessive fluid retention sometimes seen in sedentary clients or in middle-age and older women.

Explain to the dieter that weight loss is accompanied by a decrease in the metabolic rate, which may explain the decreased rate of weight loss with time that may be experienced, in spite of careful adherence to the diet. When this occurs, it will be necessary to further reduce kilocalorie intake or increase physical exercise for weight loss to continue.

Use these basic principles of kilocaloric restriction to establish the dietary regimen:

1. Establish a kilocaloric level that brings about a slow, steady loss of approximately 1 to 2 lb (0.5 to 1.0) per week
2. Provide a nutritionally balanced low-kilocalorie diet that contains conventional amounts of the energy-producing nutrients (carbohydrate, protein, and fat)
3. Plan a diet that is palatable and conforms to individual cultural patterns and usual patterns of eating
4. Readjust the kilocalorie intake to maintain the lost weight after the desired weight level is achieved

The amount of energy that should be consumed to achieve weight loss will depend on age, sex, body size, and activity. It is based on recommended body weight. To arrive at an appropriate energy level, first, determine the client's recommended body weight from tables provided by the Metropolitan Life Insurance Company given in Appendix 7 or use the rule of thumb method given in Chapter 2; second, assess the client's level of physical activity; and third, use the following guidelines to arrive at the specific number of kilocalories for a daily adult plan:

1. Determine basal kilocalories: allow 10 kcal/lb recommended body weight
2. Determine activity level and add kilocalories for activity to basal kilocalories:
   a. Sedentary: 3 kcal/lb recommended body weight
   b. Moderate activity: 5 kcal/lb recommended body weight
   c. Strenuous activity: 10 kcal/lb recommended body weight

Since the kilocalorie requirement of clients of similar body size and activity can vary, use these figures as a guideline only and adjust for individual differences. Taking into account different body builds and levels of activity, most adult males with a sedentary-to-moderate activity level will achieve weight loss on a kilocalorie intake ranging from 1500 to 1800 kcal/day, and adult females with the same activity level will usually be able to lose on 1000 to 1500 kcal/day. It has been suggested, however, that one of the reasons obese persons do not lose weight is that they become more efficient users of energy on a weight reduction diet. A daily kilocaloric intake that is less than 1000 in ambulatory females and less than 1500 in ambulatory males is not likely to be well tolerated over a long period of time. Supplement diets containing fewer than 1200 kcal daily with vitamins and minerals.

Different authorities recommend different percentages of carbohydrate, protein, and fat to comprise the total kilocaloric intake. At present, many recommend the prudent diet approach that not only restricts kilocalories but also reduces other dietary components that are thought to pose a risk of coronary heart disease (see Chap. 29). The prudent diet approach emphasizes a decrease in use of saturated fat and cholesterol, substituting some polyunsaturated fat for some saturated fat, using fish and poultry more often than red meat, and substituting vegetables and fruits for sweets. Suggested approximate percentage compositions of carbohydrate, protein, and fat for weight reduction diets that reflect this approach are:

Carbohydrate   45–50 percent
Fat   30–35 percent
Protein   20 percent

In general, the protein level should not be below 12 to 15 percent of total kilocalories, or the fat level above 35 percent. Carbohydrate should compose the remainder of the diet. Recommend to clients that sucrose should be restricted and a variety of complex carbohydrates (starches and fibrous foods) be used.

TABLE 23–3
DAILY FOOD PLANS BASED ON THE EXCHANGE SYSTEM FOR VARIOUS KILOCALORIE LEVELS

	1000 kcal	1200 kcal	1500 kcal	1800 kcal
Milk (nonfat) exchanges	1	2	2	2
Vegetable exchanges	2	2	2	2
Fruit exchanges	3	3	3	3
Bread exchanges	4	5	7	9
Meat (lean) exchanges	5	5	6	7
Fat exchanges	4	6	8	10
Free foods	◄——————————— As desired ———————————►

(Source: From North Carolina Dietetic Assoc: Diet Manual, ed. 2. Charlotte, NC, 1978, pp 131–161.)

The exchange lists for meal planning (Appendix 2) can be used as a basis for establishing a daily meal plan for weight reduction diets. Once the daily meal plan is established, assist the client to establish a meal pattern and to plan menus based on substitutions from the exchange lists to meet individual needs.

Table 23–3 provides sample meal plans for various kilocaloric levels. These plans are calculated to provide 45 percent of kilocalories from carbohydrate, 20 percent from protein, and 35 percent from fat. A sample meal plan and a sample menu for the 1200 kcal meal plan given in Table 23–3 are found in Table 23–4. Let the client know that the Basic Four Food Groups (see Chap. 2) can also serve as a basis for planning a weight reduction diet. Use of the recommended servings from each food group provides approximately 1200 to 1500 kcal and supplies most of the needed nutrients.

No consensus exists as to the desired frequency of food intake. Some may like small meals with one or two snacks, whereas others respond better to a rigid meal schedule.

Consider alcohol consumption in the weight reduction regimen because of its high kilocaloric content (1 g alcohol provides 7.1 kcal or about 200 kcal/oz). Kilocalories provided by alcohol comprise about 7 to 10 percent of the total kilocaloric intake of the average American. Beer, ale, and wine contain carbohydrate as well as alcohol, whereas distilled spirits contain only alcohol. In addition, sugar- or carbohydrate-containing beverages are often added to distilled spirits as a mixer. For clients who consume alcohol, substitute the beverages for fat or bread exchanges—consider the carbohydrate as bread exchanges and the alcohol as fat exchanges. Some examples of substitutions are given below:[10]

Distilled spirits (e.g., gin, rum, vodka, scotch, whiskey)	1½ oz	3 fat exchanges
Martini	3½ oz	3 fat exchanges
Ale	8 oz	½ bread and 1½ fat exchanges
Beer	12 oz	1 bread and 2 fat exchanges
Cordials (e.g., anisette, benedictine, creme de menthe, curaco)	⅔ oz	½ bread and 1 fat exchange
Wine		
Dry table (12% alcohol)	3 oz	1½ fat exchange
Dry sherry	3 oz	½ bread and 2 fat exchanges
Port or muscatel	3½ oz	1 bread and 2 fat exchanges
Mixed drinks		
Old fashioned	4 oz	½ bread and 3½ fat exchanges
Daiquiri	3½ oz	½ bread and 2 fat exchanges

**TABLE 23–4
SAMPLE MEAL PLAN AND MENU FOR A 1200 KCAL DIET**

Exchange List	No. of Exchanges	Menu Item
Breakfast		
Fruit	1	½ grapefruit
Meat (Lean)	1	Soft-cooked egg, 1 (omit 1 fat exchange)
Bread	1	Toast, 1 slice
Fat	2	Margarine, 1 tsp
Milk (nonfat)	1	Nonfat milk, 1 c
Coffee or tea (with sugar substitute)		As desired
Lunch		
Meat (lean)	2	Tuna, ½ c
Vegetable	1	Tomato, 3 slices
Bread	2	Bread, 2 slices
Fat	2	Mayonnaise, 2 tsp
Fruit	1	Unsweetened canned pineapple, ½ c
Coffee or tea (with sugar substitute)		As desired
Dinner		
Meat (lean)	2	Chicken (no skin), 2 oz
Vegetable	1	Green beans, ½ c
Bread	2	Mashed potato, ½ c Roll, 1
Fat	2	Margarine, 2 tsp
Fruit	1	Dates, 2
Coffee or tea (with sugar substitute)		As desired
Bedtime		
Milk (nonfat)	1	Nonfat milk, 1 c

What does the dieter do when dining out? Even when trying to lose weight, dining out can be pleasurable if a few simple guidelines are followed. For most people, dining out means cafeteria and coffee shop lunches. Vending machines and fast-food establishments tend to provide high-kilocalorie meal items, snacks, and beverages. Cafeterias may display the kilocaloric content of various menu items, and a salad bar or diet plate is often available. For restaurant dining, advise the client to order a la carte to avoid tempting side dishes and, in anticipation of the event, to eat a small but adequate breakfast and lunch. Specific guidelines in food selection when eating out are given in Table 23–5.

Formula Diets. Formula products, available from pharmaceutical, dairy, and food companies in liquid, powder, or solid form periodically became popular as an adjunct to weight reduction. Recommended daily intake provides approximately 900 kcal, with a percentage composition of carbohydrate, protein, and fat of 50, 20, and 30, respectively. Formula diets provide the advantages of convenience and standardized nutrient composition. The disadvantages, however (which include monotony and failure to learn new eating habits), lead to a high rate of dropout after 3 to 4 weeks. Suggest their usefulness to clients in certain situations, such as in the beginning stages of a weight reduction program, for those who wish to lose only a few pounds, and for those requiring immediate weight reduction before surgery or because of a serious medical disorder. On a long-

term basis, they may be used to replace one meal a day during a weight control program.

The efficacy of defined formula diets (see Chap. 21) has been tested in treating obesity. Although the use of these products for obesity control requires further evaluation, some feel that their use may be a safe and acceptable treatment for those with severe or refractory obesity.

Fasting. Fasting regimens, which include total fasting for short or prolonged periods, intermittent fasting, and supplemented fasting, are used in the management of obesity. The safety of total fasting is now much in doubt, and it has lost much of its earlier popularity. The overall results are disappointing in that most clients tend to regain the lost weight after 1 to 2 years. Intermittent fasts—that is, short-term fasts for periods up to 14 days followed by 1 or 2 fast days per week until recommended body weight is achieved—have not proven superior to continuous reduction of kilocalorie intake. Long-term data are not yet available on the efficacy of supplemented fasting, but the technique is still deemed experimental and should be considered only for the morbidly obese.

Total fasting should be conducted only in hospitalized clients, and close medical supervision is mandatory for those following the supplemented fasting regimen. Assess for conditions in which fasting is contraindicated, including clients with a history of gout, cardiac, hepatic, or renal disease, during periods of growth, or in the elderly. When fasting is

---

TABLE 23–5
A GUIDE TO FOOD SELECTION WHEN EATING OUT ON A KILOCALORIE-CONTROLLED DIET

Category	Recommended Selections
Appetizers	Clear broth, consommé, plain seafood cocktail, fresh fruit, pickles, or vegetable relishes
Main dishes	Poultry (with the skin removed), seafood, or red meat (with visible fat removed) that is broiled or roasted and served plain, i.e., with no gravies, glazes, or breadings; low-fat cheese (such as uncreamed cottage cheese or farmer cheese); eggs should be used in moderation and prepared by boiling or poaching
Vegetables, fruits, and salads	Fresh, steamed, or boiled and served without sauces or toppings; substitute starchy vegetables for bread; if legumes are substituted for meat they should be combined with a grain product to assure protein of high quality; bean curd and sprouts provide a source of protein that is practically free of fat; avoid rich salad dressings and limit the quantity of mixed salads (such as tuna, chicken, or potato salad and cole slaw) that may contain a large amount of mayonnaise
Beverages	Skim milk; plain, low-fat yoghurt (fruit-flavored yoghurt may provide twice as many kcal as plain yoghurt); beverages (including alcoholic beverages) should be selected in accordance with the exchange lists

contemplated, review concomitant drug therapy to establish contraindications or determine the need to alter drug dosage. The extent to which drug action is altered by starvation is uncertain.

After the termination of the fast, institute refeeding slowly to allow for adjustment in insulin secretion and fluid and electrolyte balance—potassium and water balance tend to change rapidly. Refeeding is usually accompanied by a marked weight gain due to expansion of the fluid spaces. However, expect a spontaneous diuresis usually after 10 days to 3 weeks. Fasting is accompanied by a lowering of the BMR, which returns to normal after a period of time, therefore monitor food intake closely to prevent weight gain.

With total fasting there is a rapid weight loss and anorexia. Let the client know that little hunger will be experienced after 36 to 48 hours. Anorexia is thought to occur secondary to the ketosis that develops. With total fasting, a weight loss of 4 to 8 lb in 24 hours is not uncommon. After the first days of the fast, however, weight loss tapers off to 1 to 2 lb per day until a plateau is reached after 2 to 3 weeks, presumably due to water retention. Allow water ad libitum. Some regimens also allow nonkilocaloric liquids and limited quantities of low-calorie foods, such as lettuce. Administer multivitamin and mineral supplements to minimize deficiencies.

Total fasts for periods of a few weeks do not appear to be accompanied by serious metabolic disturbances, although there is some weakness associated with a negative nitrogen balance. Although prolonged fasting produces greater weight loss, serious metabolic disorders and psychologic reactions have been reported. Metabolic disorders include dehydration, ketosis, loss of lean body mass, hyperuricemia and gout, vitamin and mineral deficiencies, hypokalemia, atrial arrhythmias, orthostatic hypotension, anemia, increased serum bilirubin concentration, fatigue, and apathy. Sudden death has occurred during and after fasting, presumably as a result of cardiac complications.

The loss of lean body mass in fasting is of primary significance. During the first month, one half of the tissue loss is loss of lean tissue, and thereafter, the loss lessens to one fourth to one third. The loss of lean tissue occurs secondary to the use of muscle protein to provide glucose for the brain via gluconeogenesis. After the first month of fasting, however, adaptation occurs, and the brain uses ketones to supply approximately two thirds of its energy need. Thus the need to use the lean body mass for energy lessens.

Supplemented fasting arose out of concern for the metabolic complications of total fasting and in order to provide a mechanism for replacing muscle and visceral protein being catabolized, thus promoting loss of only adipose tissue. Supplemented fasting uses the concept of nitrogen sparing. However, it is postulated that exogenous protein is preferred to glucose to spare body protein. Whereas glucose in-

gestion leads to a rise in blood glucose and stimulation of insulin secretion—insulin in turn promotes fat synthesis and inhibits fat breakdown—protein ingestion is associated with a decrease in insulin secretion, which in turn is associated with a rise in plasma free fatty acids and ketones. Thus, muscle tissue and perhaps other components of the lean body mass are spared while fat is burned for energy.

Supplemented fasting has been used in controlled clinical situations to bring about weight reduction. Some regimens use a supplement mixture of casein and glucose that provides about 300 kcal/day as the first phase of a program of long-term weight reduction in the grossly obese. A regimen called the **protein-sparing modified fast** (PSMF) combines diet, behavior modification, nutrition education, and exercise training for lifestyle modification as the approach to weight reduction. The diet consists of lean meat protein (1.0 to 1.5 g/kg recommended body weight per day), nonkilocaloric liquids, and mineral and vitamin supplements (including potassium supplements). Monitor blood pressure closely, make frequent biochemical assessments of blood and urine electrolytes, and observe for side effects, including halitosis, hyperuricemia, postural hypotension, gastrointestinal side effects (constipation, nausea, or vomiting), dehydration, amenorrhea, transient hair loss, dry skin, and muscle cramping in clients following this regimen.

Fad Diets. A wide array of nutritionally unbalanced diets are promoted for weight reduction, and periodically a new diet scheme surfaces or resurfaces. For example, 1975 saw the high-fat diet revolution; 1976, the high-fiber, save-your-life diet; 1977, the predigested liquid protein, last-chance diet; 1978 the Scarsdale diet (a modification of the principles underlying the high-fat diet). Some fad diets are relatively safe and can be followed effectively for a short period of time, but others are potentially dangerous (especially when followed for prolonged periods) and require medical supervision. Teach obese clients that a feature common to all fad diets is that no reeducation about eating habits occurs, and after the diet is abandoned—"going on a diet" implies "going off" at some future time—the previous pattern of eating may lead to regaining of weight lost. Such numerous fluctuations of body weight may be more deleterious than maintenance of a stable, though excessive, body weight. Some of the common fad diets are discussed here.

Low-carbohydrate Ketogenic Regimens. The low-carbohydrate ketogenic regimen has been in vogue since the mid-1800s (then known as the Banting diet), and it resurfaces periodically under a new name. In the 1950s and early 1960s, it was called the "Calories Don't Count Diet," the "Dupont Diet," the "Air Force Diet," and the "Drinking Man's Diet." More recently it has resurfaced as the "Doctor's Quick-Weight-Loss Diet" and as "Dr. Atkins' Diet Revolution."

A common feature of the ketogenic diet is its low-carbohydrate content, although the particular diets differ in the amount of protein and fat allowed. Frequently, the diets allow for unlimited kilocaloric consumption and unlimited consumption of protein and fat. The Scarsdale diet, however, uses the low-calorie approach—the daily menu is calculated to provide 1200 to 1500 kcal—and restricts fat to low to moderate levels, markedly restricts carbohydrate, and is high in protein.

The rationale given for the weight loss resulting from ketogenic diets varies, but such notions as "excessive calories are excreted as ketones," "obese clients alter their metabolism in response to the diet by secreting a fat-mobilizing hormone," or "it's the carbohydrate, not fat, that adds fat" are often cited. It has been noted, however, that urinary ketone losses rarely exceed 100 kcal/day, and there is no evidence of the existence of a fat-mobilizing hormone in humans. Furthermore, fat has a much greater kilocaloric density than has carbohydrate—9 kcal/g as opposed to 4 kcal/g. Individuals do lose weight when following the regimen—one reason for the weight loss is the spontaneous consumption of fewer kilocalories because of the monotony of the diet. However, the amount of weight loss is no greater than when following a conventional low-kilocalorie diet of equal kilocaloric content, although the initial rate of weight loss is higher because of a transient diuresis associated with the consumption of a low-carbohydrate diet. A high protein intake also promotes diuresis.

Assess for side effects in clients following a ketogenic diet regimen, including hyperlipidemia, elevated blood uric acid (which may lead to gout and renal stones in some individuals), postural hypotension, and fatigue. The increase in protein metabolism may be hazardous or stressful to those with existing or potential liver or kidney disease.

Low Protein Diets. On the other end of the spectrum are the low-protein diets that do not restrict carbohydrate. These are sometimes recommended as a quick way to reduce unsightly fatty spots on the hips, thighs, or legs. Examples of low-protein diets are the "Doctor's-Quick-Inches-Off-Diet" and the rice diet. A low-protein diet may lead to excessive loss of lean body mass.

Diets that Emphasize the Repetitious Use of One Food. Diets that emphasize the virtues of a particular food (such as grapefruit) are numerous. While the grapefruit diet, also called the Mayo diet, consists of other foods as well as grapefruit, it is promoted on the premise that grapefruit has an enzyme that burns up fat. No food is known to have a property of this nature.

The Liquid Protein Modified Fast. This diet, a modification of the principles underlying the PSMT, has been promoted as a popular diet and advertised as the last-chance diet. It received considerable notoriety after extended use of the diet (with and without medical supervision) became associated with serious complications and even death. The products used as the basis for the diet are generally based on partially hydrolyzed protein in liquid, powdered, or tablet form. Most of the protein used in the early stages of popularity of the diet was of low nutritional value, based on collagen and gelatin, and more than 50 deaths were associated with its use. The people whose deaths were associated with the diet all died suddenly of heart irregularities while on the diet or soon after discontinuation. Close monitoring of serum electrolytes or use of intensive cardiac care techniques did not anticipate or correct the abnormalities. Several possible mechanisms have been suggested for the relation of the dietary regimen to the deaths, however autopsy findings were compatible with protein–calorie malnutrition. Although more recent modifications of the very low kilocalorie regimen have not been associated with excessive mortality to date, their use should still be considered experimental.

The Cambridge Diet Plan. This is another extremely low kilocalorie diet regimen that provides a total of 420 kcal daily as a powdered milkshake-type formula. This milk-based protein powder contains about 75 percent of the legal standards for protein established by the Food and Drug Administration and 100 percent of the standards for minerals and vitamins. It also contains a small amount of carbohydrate and fat. After a maximum of 4 weeks on the program, the client is allowed 1 or 2 weeks of maintenance meals providing 800 kcal/day before resuming the 420 kcal/day plan, which is continued until desired body weight is achieved. At this point, the maintenance regimen is established, whereby the client keeps a record of his or her weight and adds or subtracts foods until the daily energy intake necessary to maintain weight is determined.

Predictably the intake of only 420 kcal/day initially induces rapid weight loss primarily because of water loss. Although the diet plan may not be dangerous if used as a replacement for one or two meals a day, the Food and Drug Administration has received reports of illness associated with its use and has issued a warning that users of these products should be under the care of a physician who has experience with modified fast diets.

Lecithin–Kelp–Vitamin B_6–Cider Vinegar Diet. A diet composed of a mixture of lecithin, kelp, vitamin B_6, and cider vinegar in combination with a 1000 kcal diet has been suggested for weight reduction and for redistributing fat deposits in obese persons. A controlled study of the diet found the regimen useless in promoting weight loss beyond that due to restriction of energy intake.[11] Advise clients following this regimen that overuse of kelp (dried seaweed) may result in iodine toxicity.

Simeon's Regimen. This regimen consists of daily injections of human chorionic gonadotropin (HCG), a placental hormone obtained from the urine of pregnant women, in conjunction with a 500 kcal diet. It has been postulated that weight loss with the diet–hormone combination is more efficient than with diet alone, as HCG suppresses the appetite, improves the mood, and redistributes fat. While HCG may influence lipolysis indirectly through thyroid stimulation, it has no advantage to a very low kilocalorie diet beyond that of a placebo. The 500 kcal diet is actually a semistarvation regimen regarded as unphysiologic and unsafe, especially under conditions where medical supervision may be minimal. The regimen has the added shortcoming of expense.

Physical Exercise. An increase in energy expenditure is a useful, though often neglected, adjunct to decreasing energy intake in creating a negative energy balance. Exercise in combination with dietary restriction results in a greater weight loss than that achieved by diet restriction alone. Often, however, as food intake is reduced, so is physical activity. Exercise alone is not an effective means of weight reduction; a concurrent low kilocalorie intake is essential. Obesity in childhood and adolescence, however, is best controlled by increasing the level of physical activity, with little change in the diet. Teach obese clients about these other benefits of physical exercise: it improves muscle tone, shifts body composition in the direction of increasing lean body mass at the expense of adipose tissue, improves cardiopulmonary efficiency, aids in controlling hyperlipidemia and hypertension, increases HDL cholesterol, regulates satiety and appetite, improves glucose tolerance, and promotes a sense of well-being.

Although it is true that most exercises, such as walking, bicycle riding, and swimming, result in only modest increases in energy expenditure, advise clients that the additive effects of mild-to-moderate exercise performed on a consistent daily basis can make a significant contribution. For example, one must walk approximately 35 miles in order to lose a pound of fat. If, however, one walks about a mile a day (approximately 8 to 10 blocks), this will result in an annual weight loss of 10 lb, provided kilocaloric intake remains constant. Physical activity aids in regulating appetite and food intake and, in sedentary persons, appetite is not regulated by kilocaloric requirements. Unfortunately, moderate physical activity may increase the appetite although demanding and sustained physical effort often results in reduced appetite. Moreover, strenuous activity is accompanied by an increase in the metabolic rate for up to 24 hours and, thus, kilocaloric expenditure continues after cessation of the exercise.

For exercise to be effective, teach clients that it must be a consistent daily discipline and should involve continuous use of large muscle groups and be rhythmic and aerobic in nature, for example, running or walking. A program of exercise performed in the home is more likely to be performed daily than are group exercise classes. Advise medical clearance by a physician before increasing activity, since the practice may be contraindicated for certain people. Activity should be increased slowly and gradually to build up endurance. For some, activity stress tests should be performed to determine the appropriate starting and target intensities of the exercise program. Since fat is an insulator and restricts the rate of heat loss, stress to the client the importance of giving particular attention to rest periods and hydration during the summer months.

The energy costs of activity in relation to the energy values of representative foods are available in a variety of publications.[12] For example, to use the kilocalories provided by a glass of carbonated beverage (106 kcal) requires 20 minutes of walking, 13 minutes of bicycle riding, 9 minutes of swimming, 5 minutes of running, and 82 minutes of reclining. Figures for a malted milk shake (502 kcal) are 97, 61, 45, 26, and 386 minutes, respectively.

Just as dietary management of obesity is subject to faddism, so is the role of exercise. For example, the notion exists in some that vibrating machines can spot-reduce by mobilizing body fat. This notion has not been supported by scientific evidence.

Behavior Modification. In recent years, behavior modification techniques have been increasingly applied in the treatment of obesity. A multifaceted treatment program is aimed at altering eating and exercise habits and may be an effective approach for some obese persons. The long-term effectiveness of the technique has not been demonstrated, however, and results are less enthusiastic than on a short-term basis. Behavior modification should be used as part of a combined approach to treat obesity.

In the behavior modification approach, obesity is viewed as a learned behavior disorder. The basic assumption is made that the connection between environmental stimuli and the eating response is learned—and thus it can be unlearned. The obese person is triggered to eat more by environmental stimuli than by internal mechanisms that regulate appetite and satiety. Behavior modification involves helping the obese client learn self-management techniques for controlling the environmental stimuli related to food buying, food preparation, food intake, and exercise behavior. Control of overeating and exercise behavior—not weight reduction per se—is the primary goal.

Attempts are made to modify eating through manipulating both the stimuli that precede eating (antecedents) and those that follow it (consequences) and thus serve to potentiate the eating pattern. By the use of recordkeeping, techniques to control the stimuli (both antecedent and consequence), and contingency management, the frequency of desired behaviors is increased and that of undesired behaviors decreased. The ultimate goal is to establish a permanent set of eating habits that result in weight loss and maintenance of the loss.

In applying the technique, first assist the client to identify those environmental conditions that trigger inappropriate eating. Then focus on techniques for modifying these patterns, establish a contract, and agree on a set of rules. If the rules are followed, provide rewards; if not, withhold the rewards. Design all activities within the framework of daily routines and lifestyle.

Steps in Behavior Modification. Follow these four progressive steps in a behavior modification program:

1. Describe the behavior to be controlled
2. Modify the stimuli that govern eating
3. Develop techniques to control the act of eating
4. Provide prompt reinforcement for behaviors that delay or control eating

The overall program must be evaluated continuously as well as terminally when specific objectives are reached.

Description of Behavior to Be Controlled. To initiate the program, ask the client to record baseline data giving specifics related to time of eating, foods eaten and amounts, place of eating and associated activity, with whom client eats, and feelings while eating, such as mood and degree of hunger. A sample form for recording this information is given in Figure 23–1. Second, analyze these data with the client to pinpoint specific habit patterns that may trigger or cue eating, e.g., does eating take place in all rooms or a specific room in the house? While watching TV? When bored? Finally, identify behavior patterns that should be eliminated, decreased in incidence, or strengthened.

Modify or Control the Discriminatory Stimuli that Govern Eating. With the client, design techniques for eliminating or decreasing the incidence of cues that trigger inappropriate eating behavior and strengthening those cues that signal appropriate behavior. These techniques should be implemented in a series of small steps rather than all at once.

Many obese clients report that eating occurs in a wide variety of rooms at home and at many different times during the day. Through repeated association with food, these rooms and times become stimuli that trigger eating. For those who eat while watching TV, talking on the phone, or playing cards, the TV, phone, and cardtable are signals for food. To modify or control the stimuli to eat, narrow the span of stimuli—have the client move the TV or favorite reading chair to another room, designate only one room in the house for eating, and use special table settings to make the eating area as distinctive as possible. Encourage the client to make eating a pure experience unaccompanied by other activities, such as watching TV, reading, or arguing with the family. If an emotional response, such as boredom, anxiety, or depression, is the cue to eating, assist the client to plan alternate activities, such as singing, taking a shower, or working on art projects, for times when these emotional reactions are experienced. Some cues cannot be totally eliminated and can only be suppressed. For example, social stimuli to problem eating may be controlled by standing or sitting away from the food table, holding a drink with both hands while at a party, and similar behavior.

Strengthen cues to appropriate eating behavior. For example, share with the client food records that indicate desirable behavior. Provide tips on how to make appropriate foods attractive in appearance and distribute them in an appropriate meal and snack pattern.

Develop Techniques to Control the Act of Eating. Specific techniques can be developed to decrease the speed of eating, to become aware of all components of the eating process, and to gain control over each of these components. For example, advise the client to delay the start of the meal after being seated,

Food: Amount and preparation method	Time	Location	Alone or with whom	Activity and physical position	Mood and degree of hunger	kcal

Figure 23–1
Food record for behavior modification treatment of obesity.

to eat only one bite at a time, and to chew slowly to allow the sensory feelings of taste and texture awareness to develop, to put utensils on the plate after each bite, and to introduce 2-minute interruptions periodically during the meal.

Provide Prompt Reinforcement for Behavior that Delays or Controls Eating. The taste of food is a potent and immediate positive reinforcer of eating. Since an object of behavior modification is to displace food as the reinforcer, provide alternatives. The reinforcers may be positive or negative in nature—in either instance they should be immediate and meaningful. For example, positive reinforcement for exercising the designated techniques for controlling the act of eating may consist of rewards, such as verbal praise and points or tokens to be later exchanged for something desired by the client, e.g., a dress or a weekend trip. Negative reinforcement for failure to follow the agreed-upon procedures might consist of subtraction of points or a neutral response.

The suggested changes should be livable, so that they can become a permanent part of the lifestyle. When making a change, encourage the client to ask: "Can I live with this the rest of my life?" If the answer is "No," it is a waste of time to make the change. Encourage family members to participate in cue identification and techniques for rewarding the client.

Hypnosis is another behavioral approach to weight reduction, although its use is not widespread and there are few data to determine its effectiveness. Sometimes it is used inappropriately, with the hypnotic suggestion that one will no longer feel hungry, even though it has been noted that persons do not necessarily overeat because they are hungry. When used, hypnosis should be part of an overall treatment program designed to change eating behavior.

Pharmacologic Therapy. Numerous drugs have been used in weight reduction programs. In general they fall under the categories of appetite suppressants, hormones, bulking agents, diuretics, and laxatives. The use of drugs for the treatment of obesity in adults is at best only a temporary adjunct to dietary restriction, and drug therapy is usually contraindicated in treating childhood obesity. Only a few of the drugs have been reported to be more effective than placebos in a weight reduction program. Considering the minimal short-term efficacy of drug therapy and the potential for side effects, including dependence and abuse, drugs, if used at all, should be used only on a short-term basis and in conjunction with an energy-restricted diet. In a few cases, drug therapy may stimulate motivation, but the effect is usually short-lived, and there is a strong tendency for people to regain weight after cessation of drug therapy. The principal drugs used in the management of obesity are summarized in Table 23–6.

Surgical Management. Surgical procedures used for the treatment of obesity include surgical excision of localized fat deposits, wiring the jaws, and procedures that bypass large portions of the gastrointestinal tract.

Excision of localized areas of fat is not effective for overall reduction in body weight but is useful under certain circumstances.

Solid food intake can be prevented by applying bands to connect the upper and lower teeth so that the client must consume liquids through a straw. Assist clients with wired jaws to maintain the nutrient quality of the diet by the judicious use of soups, fruit and vegetable juices, milk, liquid formula diets, and supplements of vitamins and minerals. This procedure is not only hazardous—wire cutters must be carried to prevent the possibility of aspiration should vomiting occur—but it is also generally ineffective, since weight loss can be precluded by consuming high-kilocalorie liquids, such as blenderized foods.

Gastrointestinal bypass procedures include jejunoileal shunting and gastric bypass. More recently, gastroplasty, a modification of the gastric bypass, has been developed. The objective of jejunoileal shunting is to create a state of chronic malabsorption by decreasing the intestinal absorptive surface and transit time. About 90 percent of the intestine is converted into a blind loop, leaving approximately 1.5 ft of absorbing surface. In contrast, the gastric surgical procedures limit the amount of food consumed by occluding a large part of the stomach. The remaining pouch, which has a small outlet, limits gastric volume to approximately 2 percent of the original stomach volume and will hold approximately 50 ml of food. Both procedures allow for reversal of the operation. Figure 23–2 illustrates the gastric procedures.

The surgical procedures lead to large amounts of weight loss. For example, with the jejunoileal bypass, initial weight losses have been 60 to 100 lb or more during the first year. The weight loss tapers off during the second year, however, and a plateau is reached within 12 to 18 months, after which weight stabilizes at a point somewhat above recommended body weight. Intestinal adaptation, with hypertrophy and increased absorptive capacity of the functional bowel segment, is cited as the reason for the weight stabilization. Many clients eventually return to their presurgical weights. Clients with a gastric bypass also tend to stabilize at a weight somewhat above the recommended weight. Malabsorption contributes to the weight loss with the jejunoileal shunt. However, in all the procedures the client is conditioned to eat less, and decreased consumption accounts for much of the loss. The postprandial discomfort—the diarrhea and abdominal distention with a jejunoileal shunt, and the nausea, vomiting, and distention that accompany excessive food intake with the gastric surgical procedures—leads to a decrease in the amount of food consumed.

TABLE 23–6
DRUGS USED IN THE TREATMENT OF OBESITY

Drug	Comment
Appetite suppressants Amphetamine and its derivatives (no longer available by prescription for treating obesity)	Anorexic effect is short-term and requires increasing dosage for sustained weight loss; side effects include insomnia, cardiac arrhythmias, excitability, hypertension, dry mouth, impotence, constipation, allergy, blood disorders, paranoid reactions
Nonamphetamine drugs, such as fenfluramine	Produce fewer side effects than amphetamine and may prove useful as an adjunct for weight reduction for certain clients
Hormones Thyroid hormone	Prolonged treatment with high doses brings about weight loss, although the effect is transient; produces negative calcium balance and negative nitrogen balance (loss occurs at the expense of lean body mass); large doses lead to cardiac arrhythmias and other cardiovascular effects
Human chorionic gonadotropin (HCG)	Doubtful effect
Human growth hormone	Mobilizes body fat without concomitant nitrogen loss; efficacy and safety of treatment have not been established; small supplies limit its use to research studies at present
Progesterone	Reduces pulmonary complications of obesity; effectiveness not clearly established
Indigestible bulking agents, such as methylcellulose and alginic acid	Adsorb water and expand stomach to produce satiety; may be useful adjunct to diet therapy
Diuretics	Promote fluid loss and thus weight loss; may be useful if there is excessive fluid retention
Laxatives	Promote fluid and nutrient malabsorption and thus weight loss; can lead to fluid and electrolyte malabsorption

Most gastric bypass clients report a change in food preferences and show an intolerance for sweet foods, with a preference for vegetables, fruits, and salads.

Both gastric and jejunoileal bypass operations can create life-threatening operative and postoperative complications, since surgical risks are always greater in obese clients. The complications of the jejunoileal bypass are particularly significant. There is a 3 to 5 percent mortality associated with the surgery itself or from postoperative complications. Liver disease, a late complication, leads to the majority of deaths. Protein malnutrition is thought to contribute to the liver disease, but other etiologic factors, such as accumulation of bile acids, have been considered. Malnutrition and liver disease are the major reasons for reanastomosis. The complications of gastric bypass are lesser. Lean tissue loss is minimal (15 percent), and organ dysfunction, particularly liver disease, is avoided. Surgical risks are fewer with gastroplasty, since the operation can be done in less time. For this reason, the gastric bypass

procedures are assuming greater importance in the management of the morbidly obese and the intestinal bypass operation is no longer considered acceptable. With the original gastric bypass procedure, the dumping syndrome (see Chap. 27) developed in some clients whose stoma had stretched and allowed rapid passage of food from the stomach to the jejunum. With newer surgical procedures, this complication does not appear to be a problem. Because of the associated complications, all types of gastrointestinal surgery for obesity remain investigational and should be reserved for highly motivated, morbidly obese clients who are refractory to the traditional methods of weight reduction. Usually criteria specify that the client be at least double recommended body weight. The procedure should be performed only in a medical center with specialized facilities and specialized surgical teams.

There are benefits of the surgery. The weight loss leads to improved psychosocial functioning, such as improvement in mood, self-esteem, body image,

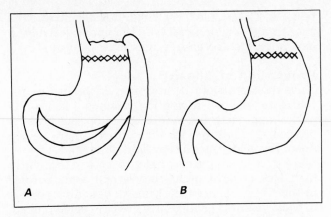

Figure 23–2
*Gastric surgical procedures for obesity. **A**. Gastric by-pass. **B**. Gastroplasty. In both procedures the stomach is divided into a small upper segment and a large lower segment. With gastric bypass, the upper segment of the stomach is anastomosed to the upper jejunum, and a small stoma forms a passageway for food to empty into the jejunum. Gastroplasty involves stapling the stomach almost closed, and a small stoma allows food to empty into the lower stomach. With the latter procedure, there is normal passage of food through the entire stomach and small bowel.*

interpersonal relations, and vocational effectiveness, as well as an increase in activity level, and a decrease in risk factors for heart disease, including a lowering of blood pressure, a decrease in blood lipids, and improved glucose tolerance.

Following gastric bypass procedures, emphasize the following dietary principles:

1. Eat small meals and stop eating when full
2. Eat slowly and chew foods to a mushy consistency (a bolus of food or large food particles may obstruct the stoma)
3. Drink low-calorie beverages and water between meals to meet fluid needs (high-calorie beverages and frequent snacking should be avoided)
4. Select a nutritionally balanced diet that emphasizes protein-containing foods
5. Avoid foods that are not well tolerated (food intolerance will vary with individuals; foods that are difficult to chew to the proper consistency, such as apple peels or membranes of citrus fruit, should be avoided)
6. Provide multivitamin supplements in liquid or chewable form (during the first few months it may not be possible to consume sufficient food to meet nutrient needs)

Following surgery, the diet is progressed according to tolerance. When eating is resumed following surgery, initially provide clear liquids. When solid foods are tolerated, some authors[13] suggest the use of blenderized foods for several weeks, which decreases the possibility of stomal obstruction, helps educate the client about appropriate food consistency, and is more likely to encourage clients to mod-

ify eating habits. After 2 to 3 weeks, cautiously add soft, solid foods to the diet, and well-chewed foods of any texture are usually tolerated after 6 weeks. Since the stomach pouch may stretch with time, educate clients about necessary changes in eating habits to avoid regaining weight.

Psychotherapy. Psychotherapy involves individual counseling with a therapist. The aim is to assist the client to gain insight into the basis of the problem. Rarely has psychotherapy been effective, and it is time-consuming and expensive. Two groups of clients may benefit from psychotherapy: binge eaters and those with severe disturbances of body image. Emotional support is an important adjuvant to therapy in all types of obesity, however.

Client Education. For successful treatment of obesity, include the client as an active participant rather than a passive recipient. Establish an ongoing communication network that ideally will allow for weekly contact at least for the first 6 months and preferably for the first year. If it is not possible to see the client in the health care facility on a weekly basis, establish a system of home visits or telephone or mail contact for monitoring the effectiveness of treatment.

During the counseling sessions provide information not only on how to eat and exercise properly for a thin lifestyle but also on how to cope with stress and how to deal with family and friends. Assist the client to gain insight into the reasons for overeating and to develop a plan for gradual changes in lifestyle, with self-management being the final goal. At each visit provide only a small amount of information, give the client homework assignments between visits, and assess these assignments at each visit. Each brief lesson should be supplemented with visual materials, such as charts. Proceed from simple to complex tasks and repeat content as necessary. Approach the topic of weight maintenance in initial counseling sessions, and at all times deemphasize scale weights on a weekly basis but focus on the long-term goal of self-management.

First, have the client define present eating habits by keeping a record of foods eaten and the amounts consumed. Stress accuracy by having the client measure all foods initially and record food intake directly after eating rather than at the end of the day. Then, assist the client to develop an awareness of the kilocaloric value of foods by providing simple tables for calculating the energy values. Some therapists have had success assigning points to energy values, for example, 1 point for each 25 kcal. A pocket table is available for this purpose.[14] Later, a similar approach can be used to teach nutritive values.

As the client completes these tasks, add more complex ones, such as identifying the circumstances and cues associated with eating. It may be helpful to have the client inventory foods at home and identify those that are best left out of the house or suggest that they be stored in places that are not readily accessible. From these records, identify with the client the problem areas associated with eating and develop a weekly plan for dealing with them. Develop strategies for dealing with the simplest ones first to allow for a feeling of success on the client's part, and suggest that the strategies be tested initially only three to four times per week rather than daily.

Stress the importance of increasing physical activity in the early counseling sessions. Suggest walking initially at a time of the client's own choosing and at a pace that can be managed. When this is accomplished, encourage the client to lengthen the time and increase the briskness of the walks and to increase the overall level of physical activity, such as using the stairs rather than elevators and standing rather than sitting to do certain tasks.

Provide information as necessary on meal planning and food preparation techniques to reduce the intake of concentrated carbohydrates and fats. Some suggestions are as follows:

1. Eliminate sugar, honey, and soft drinks and substitute an artificial sweetener and sugar-free sodas and beverages
2. Substitute fresh fruit or water-packed canned fruit for regular canned fruit
3. Select lean meat with little fat marbling
4. Substitute broiling, stewing, and roasting for frying as a method of cooking meat
5. Remove the skin from chicken before eating (preferably before baking)
6. Refrigerate meat broth and drippings to allow the fat to come to the surface; remove the fat before use in making soup or gravy
7. Substitute diet margarine for regular margarine (diet margarine provides about one half the kilocalories of regular margarine)
8. Prepare a substitute for whipped cream from evaporated skim milk or nonfat dry milk
9. Use skim milk to prepare cream soups and sauces and to prepare creamed cottage cheese from dry cottage cheese
10. Prepare a low-calorie salad dressing from lemon juice, vinegar or tomato juice, and seasonings

Encourage the client to read food labels in order to determine low-calorie items. Stress the importance of control of portion sizes; use food models or actual foods to teach this concept. Provide the client with a list of foods that are kilocalorie free or low in kilocalories, such as bouillon, plain coffee and tea, tomato juice, and raw vegetables, such as celery.

Once the desired amount of weight has been lost, give the client guidance in the transition from a reducing diet to a maintenance diet by adding foods gradually until weight is kept constant. Maintenance of desirable body weight is difficult, and the client must understand that the changes made in food habits to decrease weight must continue.

Prevention of Obesity

Since the results of the treatment of obesity are discouraging at best, prevention remains a logical potential approach. Because of the numerous obesity-promoting measures in our culture, many people are at risk of developing a weight problem. However, there are some groups that are at a particularly high risk of developing obesity and some periods in the life cycle in which the risk of adding pounds to body weight is particularly great. Provide preventive counseling for high-risk groups, which include children of obese parents, infants with a high birth weight or those whose weight increase is proportionately greater than that appropriate for height, and children with a heavy body build. The importance of childhood and adolescent weight gains in establishing lifelong patterns is well recognized. Direct health and nutrition education particularly to young adults during the childbearing years, with primary emphasis on establishing nutritionally sound infant feeding practices and development of good eating habits during childhood and adolescence. Assist parents to dispel such notions as "a fat baby is a healthy baby" or a fat baby will "outgrow his baby fat." In the adult, periods of increased risk occur in circumstances associated with marriage (i.e., changes in eating habits and activity patterns), pregnancy (associated with physiologic fat deposition), stressful situations (such as unemployment or other life stresses), and periods of recurrent minor disability that impairs regular physical activity.

UNDERWEIGHT

Assessment

Obesity implies a positive energy balance, whereas underweight implies a negative balance. An adult client whose body weight falls below 10 percent of recommended body weight is said to be "underweight." Standards for evaluating underweight in children are given in Table 23–7.

Underweight can be serious, since it may be a symptom of an illness, or it may predispose the individual to illness. In underweight clients, observe for a decrease in resistance to infection, growth retardation in children, and an increase in complications for the pregnant woman (see Chap. 14). There are likely to be multiple endocrine disorders (such as a decrease in glandular function—the adrenal, thyroid, pituitary, and gonads). Further, underweight persons are plagued with other physical problems, such as lack of endurance, weakness, and sensitivity to cold.

Underweight may result from a variety of physical and psychologic disorders as well as from irregular eating habits and poor food choices. Assess for

TABLE 23-7
STANDARDS AND EVALUATION OF WEIGHT FOR AGE AND WEIGHT FOR STATURE, FROM BIRTH TO AGE 18

Age	Standards	Evaluation
Birth–36 months	National Center for Health Statistics Growth Charts (see Appendices 8A and C); plot weight for age and weight for length	Probable weight deficit: 5th–15th percentile on either graph
3 years–18 years	National Center for Health Statistics Growth Charts (see Appendices 8B and D); ages 3–18, plot weight for age; ages 3–10 in girls and 3–11½ in boys, plot weight for stature[a]	Significant weight deficit: <5th percentile on either graph

[a] Body compositional changes with the pubertal growth spurt render plotting weight for stature invalid.

underweight in clients with acute or chronic disease conditions that may predispose to the condition: those that decrease the appetite (e.g., cancer), those that decrease digestion and absorption (e.g., malabsorption syndromes), those that increase nutritional requirements (e.g., fevers, hypermetabolic states, and hyperthyroidism), and those that lead to decreased intake secondary to psychologic disorders (e.g., anorexia nervosa). In addition, various psychologic and emotional stresses may lead to a decrease in food intake. Those of a certain personality type—tense, nervous, and active—may regard eating as a bother. Determine the basic cause of the underweight in order to institute effective treatment.

Intervention

Dietary management for underweight includes a high-kilocalorie, high-protein diet with an adequate supply of vitamins and minerals. Use the principles described for obesity in determining the exact kilocalorie levels, that is, the levels based on recommended body weight. Just as a daily 500 kcal deficit is needed to achieve a weekly loss of 1 lb of weight, so is a daily 500 kcal excess needed to gain 1 lb per week. However, higher levels are needed in those whose underweight results from hypermetabolism or poor nutrient use. For most moderately active individuals, 3000 to 3500 kcal daily will bring about the desired weight gain. Keep the protein content of the diet high (100 g or more daily) to replace body protein, and in order to achieve the desired kilocalorie level, increase the carbohydrate and fat content. Avoid excessive fat intake, however, as it may dull the appetite or be unpalatable. Generally, clients can tolerate uncooked fats, such as salad dressings, butter or margarine, and cream, better than fried foods. Give supplements of vitamins, especially the B-complex, to metabolize the increased kilocalories. They may also stimulate the appetite.

Use the principles outlined below for implementing a high-kilocalorie, high-protein diet for the underweight client:

1. Use the Basic Four Food Groups discussed in Chapter 2 as the basic pattern for the diet.
2. Add additional foods from each of the Basic Four Food Groups to provide a balanced addition of nutrients.
3. Increase nutrient intake gradually and in a stepwise fashion to avoid gastric discomfort and periods of discouragement (in the severely malnourished, parenteral feeding may be necessary initially, since the gastrointestinal tract may not tolerate the usual foods).
4. Adjust the type of feeding (i.e., larger portions of traditional foods or concentrated supplements) and the frequency of feeding to individual preferences. Determine the amount of traditional foods that can be ingested at meals or snacks and provide the remainder as a concentrated supplement, such as a beverage prepared by adding cream to whole milk. Children may prefer between-meal feedings, men may prefer larger portions of foods served at meals, and women may prefer a concentrated beverage served with a meal or as a snack. For some, a bedtime feeding that provides the desired kilocalories may be desirable to avoid dulling the appetite for meals during the day.
5. Increase the use of foods of high-kilocaloric density and limit the excessive use of foods of low-kilocaloric density. Foods of high-kilocaloric density include butter, margarine, salad dressings, heavy cream, gravy, sauces, cereal, bread, starchy vegetables (such as corn, potatoes, and legumes), dried fruits, jelly, jam, sugars, high-kilocalorie desserts (such as ice cream, custard, pudding, and cake), nuts, meat, fruit-flavored yoghurt,

milk (fortified with skim milk powder, cream, or undiluted evaporated milk), malted milk, milkshake, and eggnog. Low-kilocalorie foods (such as clear soups) and foods high in fiber (such as salads) should not be eaten at the beginning of a meal as they tend to give temporary satiety and diminish the appetite for the more substantial part of the meal.

6. Plan a definite eating schedule and conform to it.
7. Use behavior modification techniques to increase food consumption.

Some examples of foods or food combinations that supply approximately 500 kcal are:

	Kcal
Milk (3 c)	480
Malted milk (2 c)	488
Commercially prepared, nutritionally complete liquid formulas—1 kcal/ml (2 c)	480
Combination of:	
Milk beverage: ½ milk and ½ light cream, 20% fat—(1 c)	330
Bread (1 slice)	70
Margarine (2 tsp)	90
	490
Combination of:	
Ice cream (1 c)	250
Potato (1 small)	70
Margarine (2 tsp)	90
Banana (1 large)	80
	490

It will be easier for the client to consume extra food if at least three regular meals are eaten and if the client has regular exercise, relaxation, and sleeping patterns.

REVIEW QUESTIONS AND ACTIVITIES

1. Distinguish among the terms "overweight," "obesity," and "underweight."
2. Describe techniques used in the assessment of obesity.
3. Differentiate between developmental and reactive obesity.
4. Explain the rationale for a postulated genetic–environmental interaction in the etiology of obesity.
5. Discuss the possible role of three major metabolic abnormalities in the development of obesity.
6. Discuss the importance of preventing obesity during infancy, childhood, and adolescence.
7. Distinguish between social and psychologic factors in the development of obesity.
8. Identify four disorders to which obesity is

directly related and six disorders to which obesity is indirectly related.
9. List six guidelines that are important to consider in achieving successful weight reduction.
10. Calculate the number of kilocalories needed to achieve a slow, steady rate of weight loss in an adult male whose ideal body weight is 70 kg and who follows a sedentary lifestyle.
11. Explain the use of the six food exchange lists in planning a weight reduction diet.
12. Describe the appropriate use of alcohol in a weight-reduction diet.
13. List potential hazards associated with each of the following weight reduction regimens: (a) prolonged total fast, (b) low-carbohydrate, ketogenic diets, (c) liquid protein modified fast, (d) thyroid hormone, and (e) use of laxatives and diuretics.
14. Discuss the use of behavior modification in the treatment of obesity.
15. Discuss the dietary management following gastric bypass surgery.
16. List three categories of health problems that may lead to underweight.
17. Describe the principles of diet therapy for clients who are underweight.

REFERENCES

1. Thomas AE, McKay DA, Cutlpe MB: A nomograph for assessing body weight. Am J Clin Nutr 29:302, 1976.
2. Bray GA, Jordan HA, Sims EA: Evaluation of the obese patient. I. An algorithm. JAMA 235:1487, 1976.
3. Frisancho AR: New norms of upper limb fat and muscle area for assessment of nutritional status. Am J Clin Nutr 34:2540, 1981.
4. Cronk CE, Roche AF: Race- and sex-specific reference data for triceps and subscapular skinfolds and weight/stature. Am J Clin Nutr 35:347, 1982.
5. Abraham S, Johnson CL: Overweight adults 20–74 years of age: United States, 1971–74. Vital and Health Statistics, Advance Data No. 51, Hyattsville, Md, 1976.
6. DHEW: Obesity in America. NIH Publication No. 79–359, 1979, pp 3, 34.
7. National Academy of Sciences: Summary of a Workshop: Fetal and Infant Nutrition and Susceptibility to Obesity. Washington, DC, National Academy Press, 1978, p 3.
8. Schacter S: Obesity and eating. Science 161:751, 1968.
9. Bray GA: Brown tissue and metabolic obesity. Nutr Today 17:23, 1982.
10. Cinnamon PH, Swanson MA: Everything You Always Wanted to Know About Exchange Values for Food. Moscow, Idaho, University Press of Idaho, 1976, pp 34–35.
11. Dobbs JC, Kime Z, Wilmore J: Evaluation of a lecithin–kelp–vitamin B₆–cider vinegar weight reduction diet in human females (Abstr). Fed Proc 35:760, 1976.
12. U.S. Department of Agriculture: Food. Home and Gar-

den Bulletin No. 228, Pueblo, Colo, Consumer Information Center, 1979.

13. Bukoff M, Carlson S: Diet modifications and behavioral changes for bariatric gastric surgery. J Am Diet Assoc 78:158, 1981.

14. Linder PG, Linder DC: The Point Food Program, ed 10. Hollywood, Calif, Wilshire Book, 1977.

BIBLIOGRAPHY

Franklin BA, Rubentire M: Losing weight through exercise. JAMA 244:377, 1980.

Holm RP, Qaussig MT, Carlton E: Behavioral modification in a weight reduction program. J Am Diet Assoc 83:171, 1983.

Knapp TR: A methodological critique of the ideal weight concept. JAMA 249:506, 1983.

Langford RW: Teenagers and obesity. Am J Nurs 81:556, 1981.

Lansky D, Brownell KD: Estimates of food quantity and calories: Errors in self-reporting among obese clients. Am J Clin Nutr 35:727, 1982.

Newmark SR, Williamson B: Survey of very low-calorie weight reduction diets. Arch Intern Med 143:1195, 1983.

Newmark SR, Williamson B: Survey of very low-calorie weight reduction diets: II. Total fasting, protein-sparing modified fasts, chemically defined diets. Arch Intern Med 143:1423, 1983.

Sansone RA: Complications of hazardous weight loss methods. Am Family Phys 30:141, 1984.

Stewart AL, Brooks RH: Effects of being overweight. Am J Public Health 72:171, 1982.

Timmons KH: Metabolic effects of liquid protein. J Am Diet Assoc 82:53, 1983.

Van Itallie TB: Obesity: Adverse effects on health and longevity. Am J Clin Nutr 32 [Suppl]:2723, 1979.

Woo R, Garrow JS, Pi-Sunyer FX: Effect of exercise on spontaneous calorie intake in obesity. Am J Clin Nutr 36:470, 1982.

CHAPTER 24

Nutrition and Endocrine Disorders:
Diabetes Mellitus and Hypoglycemia

Objectives

After completion of this chapter, the student will be able to:

1. Develop a nursing care plan for all stages of the treatment of a patient with reactive hypoglycemia.

2. Adapt the nursing care plan for a patient with reactive hypoglycemia to make it appropriate for a client with fasting hypoglycemia.

3. Differentiate between the etiologic factors in insulin-dependent and non-insulin-dependent diabetes mellitus.

4. Differentiate between the acute complications of diabetes mellitus in relation to precipitating factors, symptoms, and treatment.

5. For a diabetic client, construct a diet plan that contains a relatively high percentage of kilocalories from complex carbohydrate, moderate amounts of protein, and a relatively low percentage of kilocalories from fat.

6. Adjust the diet of the insulin-dependent diabetic client in each of the following situations and compare the adjustments with those needed by a noninsulin-dependent diabetic: (a) unusual exercise, (b) delayed meals, (c) periods of acute illness that decrease food tolerance, (d) use of alcohol, and (e) use of special dietetic food.

7. Manage the diet of a diabetic client who is using the six Food Exchange Lists.

8. Develop a teaching plan for the dietary management of an insulin-dependent diabetic client and adjust the teaching plan to make it appropriate for a noninsulin-dependent diabetic client.

Disorders of blood glucose metabolism, both hyperglycemia and hypoglycemia, require the attention of the health team in management. Appropriate nutritional care calls for basic knowledge of the causes, manifestations, and treatment of the disorders.

Hyperglycemia, an elevation of the blood glucose level, is one manifestation of diabetes mellitus, a disease now recognized as a group of chronic metabolic disorders that is among the 10 leading causes of death in the United States. Diabetes has both acute and chronic manifestations. A major goal of treatment is to attempt to control the late complications that appear with increasing frequency as the person becomes older. Although it is not possible to correct totally the metabolic alteration with current treatment strategies, proper dietary management can diminish the day-to-day fluctuations that occur in blood glucose and other nutrients and may be important in delaying or preventing the long-term complications. Diet therapy, an integral part of the plan of treatment for any type of diabetes, is the major type of treatment for the noninsulin-dependent obese diabetic in whom weight reduction can alleviate many of the symptoms. A much smaller percentage of the diabetic population requires insulin or other hypoglycemic agents to control the disease.

Changing concepts in dietary treatment of diabetes mellitus have appeared in recent years. In the past, carbohydrate restriction was recommended, although the diet for the diabetic client now tends to be more liberalized in carbohydrate, with emphasis given to the complex carbohydrates, starch, and fiber. Because of the propensity for the diabetic client to develop atherosclerosis at an earlier age and more extensively than occurs in the general population, control of fat intake is also recommended.

Diet therapy is an important component of the control or treatment of some types of hypoglycemia, which is characterized by a low blood glucose level. Although hypoglycemia that occurs in the fasting state cannot be treated satisfactorily by diet alone, diet therapy is important in controlling reactive hypoglycemia and hypoglycemia that occurs as an acute complication of diabetes mellitus.

HYPOGLYCEMIA

In recent years, hypoglycemia has been popularly thought of as a common disorder accounting for various abnormalities. Hypoglycemia, however, is not a disease process but rather a symptom of other disorders. Under normal conditions the blood glucose level is regulated within a narrow range by hormonal control. The rise in blood glucose that follows food intake is brought back within normal limits by the secretion of insulin. Conversely, the blood glucose level is maintained at physiologic levels during food deprivation by a drop in insulin secretion and release of hormones that stimulate glycogenolysis and gluconeogenesis. It is important to maintain the blood glucose within a normal range because glucose is the major fuel source for the central nervous system. Prolonged or repeated episodes of hypoglycemia can lead to irreversible brain damage. When the blood glucose falls below a critical level, insulin secretion is turned off, and catecholamines, glucagon, glucocorticoids, and growth hormone are secreted. These hormones raise the blood glucose level by controlling the hepatic release of glucose. Hypoglycemic disorders may arise from any one of the mechanisms involved in maintenance of a normal blood glucose level.

Assessment

Classification. Two types of hypoglycemia are (1) food stimulated (or **reactive hypoglycemia**) and (2) food deprived (**fasting hypoglycemia**). Reactive hypoglycemia results from an exaggerated insulin response to ingestion of carbohydrate-containing foods. Individuals with this type of hypoglycemia

will experience symptoms that include tachycardia, sweating, pallor, anxiety, weakness, hunger, nausea, and vomiting 2 to 4 hours after the ingestion of a high-carbohydrate meal. The carbohydrate is quickly digested and absorbed, and an excessive amount of insulin is secreted in response to the resulting high blood glucose level. Suspect this type of hypoglycemia if the client's history includes a gastrectomy or gastroenterostomy, or it may be an early sign of diabetes mellitus in a client. In the early stages of diabetes mellitus, hypoglycemia occurs as a result of a delayed and excessive secretion of insulin in response to postprandial hyperglycemia. In general, reactive hypoglycemia is less serious than those disorders associated with hypoglycemia occurring in the fasting state.

Fasting hypoglycemia often occurs after a period of fasting (e.g., 8 or more hours), and it may be associated with conditions that either increase the secretion of insulin or otherwise alter the mechanisms involved with maintaining glucose homeostasis. Anticipate hypoglycemia secondary to hyperinsulinism in clients with pancreatic beta-cell hyperplasia or neoplasms and in those who are sensitive to leucine (an amino acid). Hypoglycemia that occurs in the fasting state secondary to altered glucose homeostasis (e.g., diminished glycogen storage, gluconeogenesis, or glucose absorption) is sometimes seen in clients with hepatic damage or hepatic enzyme deficits, endocrine disorders (such as pituitary and adrenocortical insufficiency), some malabsorption syndromes, and alcoholism. Salicylates (such as aspirin) may also interfere with enzyme systems involved with glucose homeostasis and produce hypoglycemia.

A nurse who sees a diabetic client with hypoglycemia may suspect management errors, for example, the improper spacing of food intake, the skipping of meals, participation in unplanned exercise, or excessive administration of insulin or oral hypoglycemia agents. By far the most common cause of hypoglycemia is the improper use of hypoglycemic drugs (e.g., insulin or sulfonylurea) used for treating diabetes. Other causes of hypoglycemia are relatively rare.

In addition to the above types, there are some hypoglycemic disorders that are observed only in infants and children. Transient neonatal hypoglycemia may occur as early as the first 6 hours of life in infants of diabetic mothers and infants with erythroblastosis fetalis or by the second or third day of life in infant giants and infants who are premature or small for gestational age. Idiopathic hypoglycemia may occur in children under the age of 2 years, and ketotic hypoglycemia is a self-limited disorder affecting children between 18 months and 5 years. The disorder remits spontaneously.

Symptoms and Diagnosis. The precise blood glucose level at which symptoms are likely to occur is difficult to pinpoint, since the relationship between the blood glucose level and the development and severity of symptoms varies in different individuals and even in the same individual at different times. The rate of fall, rapid or gradual, appears to affect the onset and severity of symptoms. Symptoms may or may not be evident when the blood glucose level falls below 40 mg percent. The symptoms and their severity increase as the blood sugar level falls to very low levels.

The symptoms of hypoglycemia (regardless of the cause) result from the combined effect of the hypoglycemia on the adrenal glands and the central nervous system. When the blood sugar falls to approximately 40 mg percent, there is an increase in secretion of catecholamines by the adrenals. Observe for the symptoms of the hyperepinephrinemic syndrome. These symptoms are not specific to hypoglycemia, however, and can be observed secondary to catecholamine release from any cause, including anxiety.

Should the blood glucose level fall further, a decrease in cerebral cortical function becomes manifest. Because of insufficient glucose for the brain's energy, the client may complain of headache, drowsiness, and blurred vision. Amnesia and alteration in behavior, such as confusion, negativism, and psychotic behavior, may be seen. If the hypoglycemia is severe, hypothermia, seizures, and coma often occur. (Again, these symptoms are not specific to hypoglycemia and may be observed during cerebral anoxia.) With diabetic clients, it may be difficult to distinguish the coma of hypoglycemia from that of hyperglycemia. However, observation for rapid, deep breathing and an acetone odor to the breath that is characteristic of hyperglycemic coma will aid in the differentiation.

The adrenal symptoms predominate in reactive hypoglycemia in association with an acute fall in blood glucose, whereas the neurologic symptoms are most noticeable in fasting hypoglycemia, in which the fall in blood glucose is more gradual. In fasting hypoglycemia, the hyperepinephrinemic syndrome often goes unrecognized, and impairment of brain function occurs mainly during the hypoglycemic episodes. In diabetes, the taking of an excessive dose of a short-acting insulin brings about the rapid appearance of adrenal gland-related symptoms, whereas neurologic symptoms are more evident when there is overdosage with the intermediate- or long-acting insulins, and the onset of symptoms is more gradual. A summary of signs and symptoms to assess for is found in Table 24–1.

The client is assessed for hypoglycemia by laboratory evidence of low blood glucose levels in association with the occurrence of symptoms and demonstrated relief of symptoms by food or sugar intake. Further testing is necessary to identify the specific type of hypoglycemia. Plasma cortisol levels are measured, and a glucose tolerance test is performed in which the blood glucose level is determined for a period of 5 hours following the administration of

TABLE 24–1 **SYMPTOMS OF HYPOGLYCEMIA**	
Hyperepinephrinemic Symptoms	*Neurologic Symptoms*
Tachycardia	Headache
Sweating	Drowsiness
Pallor	Blurred vision
Anxiety	Depressed intellectual function
Weakness	Amnesia
Trembling	Alteration of behavior
Hunger	Confusion
Nausea	Negativism
Vomiting	Psychotic behavior
	Hypothermia
	Seizures
	Coma

oral glucose. Hypoglycemia is usually accompanied by a significant rise in plasma cortisol levels.

In preparation for the glucose tolerance test, instruct the client to follow, for a period of 3 days, a regimen of unrestricted physical activity and diet (consuming a minimum of 150 g of carbohydrate daily) and to fast for a period of at least 10 hours (but not more than 16 hours) prior to the test. Water is permitted during this period. At the time of the test, the client should be free of illness and consuming no drugs that affect the blood glucose. During the test, tell the client to remain seated and refrain from smoking. Perform the test in the morning, since afternoon testing may bring aberrant results. Emotional disturbances may account for a symptomatic response without documented hypoglycemia during the test. Normal and abnormal glucose tolerance curves are shown in Figure 24–1.

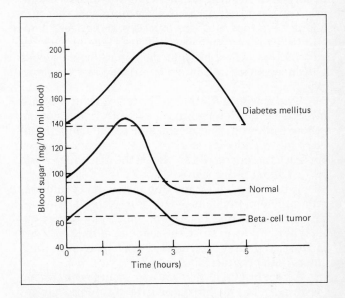

Figure 24–1
Normal and abnormal glucose tolerance curves.

Intervention

The treatment for hypoglycemia depends on the blood glucose pattern observed and the cause of the disorder. Diet therapy is an important part of this treatment.

Dietary management for reactive hypoglycemia is directed toward preventing a marked rise in blood sugar, which stimulates the pancreas to secrete an excessive amount of insulin, by restricting the intake of foods high in simple carbohydrates that are quickly digested and absorbed, such as candy, jelly, and sweetened soft drinks. Some physicians restrict total carbohydrate content to less than 40 percent of the total kilocalorie level, but others note that certain clients may benefit from a diet that provides 50 to 55 percent of the total kilocalorie intake as carbohydrate, primarily in the complex form and including liberal amounts of fiber.[1] With either regimen, assist the client to differentiate between simple and complex forms of carbohydrates and to emphasize the use of the complex forms, such as starches and vegetables. Fruit and milk are high in simple carbohydrates and must be restricted, and all forms of sugar and concentrated sweets must be avoided. Emphasize the necessity for reading labels to determine whether sugar has been added to such processed foods as peanut butter. The client can freely use protein- and fat-containing foods, which are more slowly digested and absorbed and are thus less rapidly available as sources of blood glucose. The protein allowance should be approximately 2 g/kg daily, with the remaining kilocalories supplied as fat.

Instruct the client to consume small, frequent meals that include a similar division of carbohydrate and protein to avoid extremes in the blood sugar level. High-protein foods, such as boiled eggs, cheese, meat, or nuts, in conjunction with a small amount of carbohydrate food, such as tomato juice or crackers, can be used as snacks. Recommend that the client have food, such as crackers and cheese, constantly available to control attacks should they occur and omit alcohol from the diet. Alcohol blocks gluconeogenesis and may potentiate the hypoglycemia.

The six Food Exchange Lists (Appendix 2) are often used for determining the kinds and amounts of foods allowed. The method for calculating an energy-controlled diet is given later in this chapter. Instruct the client in the use of the Exchange Lists for planning daily meals.

Assess the diet for nutritional adequacy and provide supplements if necessary. For example, calcium and riboflavin intake may be inadequate, particularly for children, since the amount of milk allowed is restricted, and the restriction of fruit may limit the intake of vitamins A and C.

Hypoglycemia that typically occurs with fasting (as in adrenal, pituitary, or liver disorders) cannot be treated satisfactorily with diet alone, and treatment should be directed at the causes. Carbohydrate restriction is not appropriate, and carbohydrate supplements may be necessary in some cases. Recommend that the client consume small, frequent meals.

Intervention guidelines for diabetic clients who have an insulin reaction are given later in the chapter.

DIABETES MELLITUS

Diabetes mellitus is one of the major health problems of modern society. Currently, the disease is thought to affect as many as 10 million Americans, with perhaps as many as 4 million cases going undetected. The number of cases appears to be increasing at a rate of 6 percent annually. The incidence is greatest in middle-age and older adults. It most commonly appears after the age of 40 (and especially in those 50 years of age and more). In the older age group, the disorder affects more women than men and more married women than single women. In contrast, there are more young male diabetics than young female diabetics.

Diabetes mellitus is a chronic, systemic disorder involving the endocrine system, particularly the islets of Langerhans of the pancreas. The heterogeneous nature of the disorder has led some authorities to conclude that the disorder represents a number of different diseases characterized by an abnormally high circulating blood glucose level. Two types of cells within the islets secrete hormones that control the blood glucose level by their opposing effects: the beta-cells secrete insulin, which has a hypoglycemic action, and the alpha-cells secrete glucagon, which has the opposite (hyperglycemic) effect on blood glucose. Insulin exerts its hypoglycemic effect by promoting the cellular transport of glucose (except perhaps in neural tissue and the liver) and stimulating hepatic glycogenesis. Both actions draw glucose from the blood. Moreover, insulin promotes lipogenesis and enhances amino acid deposition in muscle tissue, has an antilipolytic effect, and decreases the rate of glycogenolysis and gluconeogenesis. Thus, insulin is classified as an anabolic hormone. In contrast, **glucagon** increases the blood glucose level, stimulating the hepatic production of glucose by promoting glycogenolysis and gluconeogenesis. In normal situations, the blood glucose level is kept within the physiologic range of 60 to 120 mg percent by the opposing action of these two hormones working in a balanced fashion dictated by the particular needs of the individual. The secretion of both glucagon and insulin is controlled by the blood glucose level. For example, the rise in blood glucose that follows the ingestion of carbohydrate-containing foods stimulates the secretion of insulin and decreases the secretion of glucagon. When the blood glucose falls (as with fasting), insulin secretion is diminished, and glucagon secretion is enhanced in order to provide the needed glucose.

Other hormones also affect the blood glucose

concentration. Growth hormone, catecholamines, glucocorticoids, and thyroid hormone—like glucagon—are antagonists to the action of insulin and have an opposing, hyperglycemic effect. Growth hormone may, with insulin, have an anabolic effect. Another hormone, somatostatin, inhibits the release of both insulin and glucagon as well as growth hormone.

Diabetes mellitus is characterized by an alteration in the system of regulating the blood sugar and an imbalance of insulin and glucagon that leads to hyperglycemia. There is an absolute or relative deficiency of the metabolic effectiveness of insulin and, in nearly all types of diabetes, an excess of glucagon. These findings have led some investigators to hypothesize that diabetes mellitus is a bihormonal disease. Although this concept is controversial, it has received support by findings that injection of a synthetic glucagon antagonist into diabetic rats produced a significant and sustained reduction in blood glucose concentration.[2] Increased levels of growth hormone have also been observed in uncontrolled diabetes. Precise regulation of the blood sugar level in diabetic patients is difficult because of the problems encountered in delivering insulin in a truly physiologic fashion. Even with insulin replacement, there may be wide swings in serum levels of glucose and insulin.

Assessment

Pathologic Manifestations. The metabolic consequences of uncontrolled diabetes mellitus result from both the insulin deficiency and the glucagon excess, and when a client's symptoms include hyperglycemia, glucosuria, muscle wasting, negative nitrogen balance, rapid weight loss, fat catabolism, and accumulation of ketone bodies, the disorder should be suspected. Hyperglycemia occurs secondary to insulin deficiency (with failure of cellular transport of glucose into muscle, heart, and adipose cells and failure of suppression of gluconeogenesis) and glucagon excess (with an increase in hepatic synthesis of glucose from amino acids from muscle via gluconeogenesis). Observe for glucosuria when the renal threshold for glucose is reached. The normal renal threshold for glucose is approximately 160 to 180 mg percent. However, a nurse may see glucosuria at a higher level (e.g., 250 mg percent) in older people with poorly functioning kidneys in whom the renal threshold is higher. Thus, significant hyperglycemia in the absence of glucosuria can be observed in some individuals. Moreover, if the renal threshold is normally low, glucosuria may not be indicative of diabetes. Large amounts of water are excreted with the glucose (osmotic diuresis), and there is also urinary loss of sodium and potassium. The urine volume may be large (polyuria), and the associated electrolyte losses contribute to dehydration. Anticipate excessive thirst (polydipsia), which occurs secondary to the polyuria.

Because of the inability to use glucose and the loss of glucose in urine, observe for an increase in appetite and food intake (polyphagia). Also observe for muscle wasting, negative nitrogen balance, and weight loss, as muscle tissue is being used as a source of glucose. Since insulin also affects the entry of amino acids into cells, protein metabolism is further adversely affected.

Adipose tissue anabolism is diminished and catabolism accelerated. Release of fatty acids provides a source of energy in the absence of glucose, and many body tissues, including muscle cells, can use fatty acids for energy. However, excess fat catabolism leads to the overproduction of ketone bodies (β-hydroxybutyric acid, acetoacetic acid, and acetone) by the liver. Test for the accumulation of the ketone bodies, which may result in diabetic ketoacidosis, a type of metabolic acidosis (see Chap. 10). The acidosis resulting from the accumulation of ketones is compounded by the depletion of such basic ions as sodium, since these ions are excreted with the ketones in the urine. Suspect ketoacidosis in (1) the presence of ketones in the urine (detected by a positive Acetest reaction), (2) Kussmaul respirations (deep, rapid breathing and increased expiration of carbon dioxide), (3) a fruity odor to the breath (due to the excretion of acetone by the lungs—this finding is useful in differentiating diabetic ketoacidosis from a hypoglycemic reaction), (4) excretion of large quantities of chloride by the kidneys (as an additional compensatory mechanism for correction of the acidosis), and (5) a marked decrease in the bicarbonate content of the extracellular fluid. Shifts in the fluid compartments may lead to hypovolemia, coma, and death—this occurs only in severe degrees of uncontrolled diabetes, however.

Classification. Three types of diabetes mellitus are generally recognized: insulin-dependent, noninsulin-dependent, and diabetes associated with certain other conditions and syndromes. There are major clinical and physiologic differences among the types. The first two types are sometimes referred to as juvenile-onset (insulin-dependent or IDDM) and maturity-onset (noninsulin-dependent or NIDDM). However, the dependence on insulin is a better criterion for classification since overlaps exist within age categories. There are insulin-dependent diabetics who become symptomatic after middle age, and there are noninsulin-dependent diabetics who develop the disease before the age of 20 years. Some authorities consider the two types as two separate entities, but most agree that the two forms are different aspects of pancreatic disturbance.

In **insulin-dependent diabetes,** endogenous insulin production is absent or very minimal, and these individuals require daily injections of insulin to prevent ketosis. Clients who require insulin therapy constitute approximately 20 percent of all known diabetes cases. Suspect this type of diabetes in affected individuals who are thin or of normal body weight and in whom the disease appears abruptly in childhood, adolescence, or young adulthood. The peak age of onset is between ages 6 and 11, with a declining incidence at puberty and beyond, and usually progresses to a total absence of beta-cell function after several years. However, insulin-dependent diabetes can develop in adults of any age who are of normal or below normal body weight. Onset of the disease is sudden in most cases. Therefore, observe for acute symptoms, such as polyuria, polydipsia, polyphagia, and often, acute ketoacidosis. Severe weight loss and growth retardation may be noticeable. The disease is very labile, with the blood glucose fluctuating widely, especially during periods of stress, and affected individuals are prone to develop both hypoglycemia and ketoacidosis. The disease can progress rapidly, chronic complications tend to develop frequently, and life expectancy tends to be decreased. As many as 80 to 90 percent of juvenile-onset diabetic clients manifest some chronic complication after 20 to 25 years of illness.

▶ The **noninsulin-dependent** type is the more common form of the disease. This type becomes manifest most commonly after the age of 40, with the highest incidence in the 50s and 60s. The insidious development, milder symptoms, and control by diet modifications are characteristics that a nurse can anticipate in clients with this form of the disease. Because these clients continue to produce insulin, they are not prone to develop ketosis. However, many become transiently insulin-dependent during the stress of trauma, infection, or other conditions that may precipitate ketoacidosis. Within the noninsulin-dependent type, two subclasses have been distinguished: nonobese and obese. In most Western societies, obese noninsulin-dependent diabetics constitute 70 to 90 percent of noninsulin-dependent diabetics. Caution clients whose body weight is above 20 percent of recommended weight that they have twice the risk of developing diabetes. Obese noninsulin-dependent diabetics are usually asymptomatic with appropriate diet therapy and seldom require insulin administration. Persons in the noninsulin-dependent subclass may use insulin for correction of symptomatic or persistent hyperglycemia, however. In these clients a relative, rather than absolute, deficiency of insulin exists. In obesity, peripheral tissues become resistant to the action of insulin, and it is theorized that in obese diabetics the insulin does not bind properly to receptor sites on the cell membrane or that there is a reduction in the number of insulin receptors. Tissue insulin resistance results in compensatory hypertrophy and hyperinsulinism, placing a strain on the beta-cells. Continued hyperinsulinism often results in eventual decompensation of beta-cell function, and if decompensation progresses, insulin levels may eventually become subnormal (i.e., the insulin deficiency becomes absolute). However, complete beta-cell failure is not common. Determine the serum insulin levels in obese diabetics; they may be normal, depressed, or

high depending on the degree of beta-cell dysfunction. The serum insulin level is seldom as high as in obese nondiabetics but is usually higher than in nondiabetics of normal weight. Weight reduction in obese diabetics reduces their insulin level, increases insulin metabolic efficiency, and leads to a drop in the blood glucose level. Nearly all produce enough insulin to keep the plasma glucose normal when they have lost their excess weight. A nurse will see mild to moderate hyperglycemia and mild symptoms, such as nocturnal polyuria and fatigue, in clients with noninsulin-dependent diabetes mellitus. Complications tend to develop, and life expectancy may be decreased if the hyperglycemia persists. Complications may be present at the time of diagnosis.

Observe for the third type of diabetes mellitus, that associated with other diseases, in clients with such conditions as pancreatic disease, hormonal imbalances, and certain genetic syndromes. This type of diabetes often has many clinical features not generally associated with the diabetic state.

▶ The term **brittle diabetes** is sometimes applied to diabetes that does not respond well to the usual methods of treatment (i.e., diet, insulin, exercise). This type may occur in children or adults. In brittle diabetes, there may be frequent swings from hypoglycemia to ketosis and even coma. The disease is often labile during childhood because of emotional stresses, variations in physical growth, and the demands of growth and maturation. Those with the labile form of the disease must be keenly alert to the symptoms of these acute complications and be very astute in management principles.

In some instances, the clinical manifestations of diabetes mellitus may remain latent, although the disorder can be demonstrated by laboratory methods. In other cases, the diabetes may disappear temporarily. For example, in the insulin-dependent–juvenile-onset type, a period of remission called the "honeymoon phase" often occurs. Following the initial period of acute symptoms (often manifest as acute ketoacidosis) necessitating large doses of insulin in management, the exogenous insulin requirement gradually declines as some of the insulin requirement is met by an increase in endogenous insulin secretion. This period of remission is variable in (1) time of onset (within several weeks to a year), (2) intensity (barely noticeable in some to total remission of overt disease in others), and (3) duration (in some, it may last a year or longer). Following the period of remission, the insulin requirement gradually increases and the disease becomes somewhat more difficult to control. Forewarn the child and the parents about this phenomenon, or they may suspect a cure or misdiagnosis.

Etiology. In some cases, diabetes mellitus occurs secondary to disorders that lead to destruction or resection of the pancreas or to overproduction of hormones that are antagonistic to the action of insulin. In other cases, physiologic stress, such as pregnancy, aging, trauma, or infectious diseases, may precipitate symptoms of diabetes. Glucose intolerance with onset during pregnancy is termed gestational diabetes. Observe for an increased incidence of perinatal complications in gestational diabetes, and counsel affected women of an increased risk for their developing diabetes mellitus within 5 to 10 years after parturition. Many elderly persons appear to have diabetes mellitus, since there is some evidence of a lessened peripheral action of insulin with aging and that beta-cells, like other body cells with limited replicative capacity, gradually decrease functioning. Be aware of the uncertainty surrounding diagnostic standards used to assess for diabetes in individuals above 40 years of age.

In the majority of cases, however, an interplay between genetic and environmental factors is involved in the etiology, and it is now hypothesized that insulin-dependent and noninsulin-dependent diabetes have causes that are distinct from each other. A genetic predisposition to diabetes mellitus is generally considered to contribute to the risk of developing the disease. However, the hereditary pattern is different in the two disorders. The genetic component may be stronger in the noninsulin-dependent type than in the insulin-dependent type. Studies with identical twins have shown that if one twin develops diabetes after the age of 40, the other twin has a greater chance of developing the disease than if the diabetes appeared before age 25. In practically 100 percent of the cases in which one identical twin develops noninsulin-dependent diabetes, the other twin will develop the disease. The situation is different with insulin-dependent diabetes, however, in which the genetic input allows for expression of the disease in only about one fourth of the cases. Observe the unaffected sibling of a twin who develops diabetes mellitus and note that unless the unaffected twin develops the disorder within 2 years after the affected twin, the former does not get the disease at all.

It is now hypothesized that noninsulin-dependent diabetes is inherited as a dominant trait with almost complete penetrance. This type may be unmasked by overweight or physical inactivity. Present evidence suggests that the most important nutritional factor that increases the risk of developing diabetes mellitus is an excessive kilocaloric intake[3] leading to obesity, although chromium deficiency may be associated with glucose intolerance. Obesity appears to place an additional burden on insulin reserves. Observe that obese people will require two to three times more insulin than their thin counterparts to maintain normal basal metabolism. Furthermore, obesity brings a decrease in insulin effectiveness, and physical inactivity decreases the effectiveness of insulin.

Conversely, it is now hypothesized that insulin-dependent diabetes is an autoimmune disease associated with a hereditary immune disturbance that may be unmasked by a viral infection, such as intrauterine rubella, mumps, and Coxsackie virus. Immune system defects causing the system to attack not only the virus but the beta-cell membranes as well are being investigated as possible factors in the development of the disorder. Note that the abrupt onset is highly suggestive of an infectious process, and there have been a few reports in which the onset was associated with a prior viral infection. The disease is associated with certain HLA (human leukocyte group A) histocompatibility antigens. Observe for the presence of islet cell antibodies during assessment.

Diagnosis. In general, the diagnosis of diabetes mellitus should be based on:

1. Unequivocal elevation of blood glucose concentration in conjunction with the classic symptoms of diabetes, or
2. Elevated fasting blood glucose on more than one occasion, or
3. Elevated blood glucose concentration after an oral glucose challenge on more than one occasion

In view of the many factors that can elevate the blood glucose and impair glucose tolerance, it is necessary to observe an elevation in blood glucose on more than one occasion before a clinical diagnosis can be made. The diagnosis of diabetes mellitus in children is generally relatively clear-cut. Observe for the usually rapid onset of the acute manifestations of polyuria, polydipsia, polyphagia, rapid weight loss, and acute ketoacidosis. These findings in conjunction with an unequivocal elevation of the plasma glucose are usually sufficient to make the diagnosis of diabetes. The diagnosis of the noninsulin-dependent form, however, is sometimes more difficult. Use several blood and urine tests in screening and diagnosis. Test the urine for volume, specific gravity, presence of glucose, and presence of ketones, and test the blood for sugar in the fasting state (fasting blood sugar). The finding of an elevated fasting blood sugar on more than one occasion (i.e., 140 mg/dl or more using venous plasma) is diagnostic of diabetes. The fasting blood sugar is usually elevated in all except the mildest cases.

An abnormal response to a glucose tolerance test (with glucose administered orally or intravenously) is also used to diagnose diabetes mellitus. The glucose tolerance test is indicative of the body's ability to use a specific amount of glucose (75 g carbohydrate in nonpregnant adults and 1.75 g/kg body weight in children, not to exceed 75 g). A commercial preparation, Glucola, glucose flavored with lemon, is commonly used. In diabetes, the blood sugar rises higher and returns to normal more slowly than in nondiabetics (see Fig. 24–1). To perform the test, determine the plasma glucose in the fasting state and then at 30-minute intervals for a period of 2 hours (or 3 hours in the case of pregnant subjects) after administering the glucose. A plasma glucose concentration that exceeds, on more than one occasion, 200 mg/dl (using venous plasma) both at 2 hours after administration of the glucose dose and at some other time point between 0 and 2 hours during an oral glucose tolerance test is diagnostic of diabetes.[4] For valid evaluation, proper preparation is necessary (see text discussion on hypoglycemia). Explain all procedures to the client, including the diet, glucose administration, and collection of blood samples. It is not recommended that the glucose tolerance test be administered when the client is hospitalized, since the sedentary routines associated with hospitalization may lead to higher-than-normal blood sugar. The test is usually unnecessary for a diagnosis of diabetes when the fasting blood sugar is elevated on more than one occasion.

An important screening method, as well as a method for monitoring the adequacy of control of the disease, is measurement of the level of hemoglobin A_{1c}, a part of the hemoglobin molecule that becomes bound to glucose in the red cells in venous blood. Hemoglobin A_{1c} levels vary directly with the plasma glucose level, and values at any time reflect the plasma glucose for the previous 4 to 8 weeks or longer.

Complications. The complications of diabetes include not only the short-term complications (ketoacidosis, hypoglycemia, hyperglycemia) but also chronic complications (growth retardation in children, cardiovascular disease, neuropathy, and susceptibility to infection). These are discussed below along with their implications for management of diabetes.

Ketoacidosis. Diabetic ketoacidosis is the most important cause of mortality and serious morbidity in the child with diabetes mellitus. However, this syndrome does not usually appear in noninsulin-dependent diabetics, in whom there is usually sufficient insulin present to prevent excessive fat mobilization and the development of ketonemia and ketonuria. Ketoacidosis is usually provoked by physical stress (trauma or infection) or emotional stress or by management errors, i.e., inadequate insulin therapy. Ketoacidosis is not induced by excessive food intake—the excessive consumption of carbohydrates may lead to hyperglycemia and glucosuria but not ketoacidosis. Ketoacidosis is often the first manifestation of diabetes.

The symptoms of ketoacidosis and coma are glucosuria and dehydration, abdominal pain, nausea, and vomiting. Assess for signs of dehydration, including dry mouth, thirst, flushed face, low blood pressure, and cold, dry skin. Kussmaul respirations may be present, and there may be an acetone odor to the breath. Other signs may include progressive drowsiness, pain in the back and legs, diminished reflexes, headache, extreme weakness, and dizziness. Since some of the signs of ketoacidosis are similar to those of hypoglycemia, check for an acetone odor to the breath and use results of blood and urine tests and information about the client before the onset of symptoms to aid in making the distinction.

Rapid treatment is essential, since the resulting coma may be fatal. Initial treatment is emergency treatment, requiring constant nursing care. The treatment involves insulin therapy and correction of the dehydration and acidosis with fluid and electrolyte replacement. When the client can tolerate oral foods, first give clear liquids, adding fruit juices, skim milk, and finally solid foods as food tolerance increases. Intravenous infusion should be maintained until an adequate oral intake is assured.

In maturity-onset diabetics, observe for another type of syndrome, nonketotic hyperosmolar coma, which occurs infrequently in children. Nonketotic hyperosmolar coma has an insidious onset and may be seen in adults with mild or undiagnosed disease in whom an acute stress, such as an acute infectious process, precipitates symptoms. The syndrome is characterized by marked hyperglycemia (e.g., blood glucose of 600 to 3000 mg percent), hyperosmolality, osmotic diuresis, marked dehydration, and hypovolemia. The hypovolemia may lead to diminished renal blood flow, thromboemboli, cerebral dysfunction, and coma. Acidosis is absent; this phenomenon is not understood. Therapy is similar to that for ketoacidosis, but the rate of correction of the dehydration should be slower in order to prevent rapid osmotic changes that may further disturb central nervous system function.

Hypoglycemia. A hypoglycemic reaction may be precipitated by a temporary excess of insulin as a result of (1) administration of an excessive amount of insulin, (2) a decrease in blood glucose due to skipping a meal, vomiting, or diarrhea, or (3) an increase in exercise without the necessary adjustment in food intake. Exercise decreases the need for insulin and increases the need for food. The timing of the appearance of symptoms is related to the characteristics of the particular insulin being used, i.e., its duration and peak action (see the discussion of insulin below). Instruct clients to drink an oral glucose solution, such as fruit juice or sweetened carbonated beverage, or take some form of sugar when these symptoms are experienced. To avoid a recurrence of the reaction after a few hours in those taking one or more of the slowly acting insulins, the initial carbohydrate therapy should be followed in 1 or 2 hours and at later intervals with slowly absorbed carbohydrate foods, such as milk or bread. If the client is unconscious and swallowing ability is impaired, inject glucagon subcutaneously to stimulate gluconeogenesis and glycogenolysis, followed by intravenous glucose infusion. When the client is conscious, offer an oral glucose solution. Insist that clients who use insulin keep sugar or hard candy available at all times to control attacks.

Hyperglycemia. In addition to causing glucosuria, hyperglycemia and concomitant hyperosmolality may lead to blurring of vision in diabetic children. Rapid shifts in osmolality lead to changes in visual acuity. Hyperglycemia may contribute to infection; for example, the associated glucosuria may lead to vaginal yeast infection in females, since the glucose provides a good culture medium for the growth of *Candida.* There is some evidence of impaired leukocyte function and a diminished ability to handle infection in the presence of hyperglycemia. However, an increased incidence of infection (with the exception of yeast infection) is usually not evident until the disease has been present for 10 or more years.

The chronic complications of diabetes mellitus include an increased incidence of infection, possible growth retardation in children, and degenerative changes in the cardiovascular system and peripheral nerves.

Infections. Diabetic clients are more prone to infection, which tends to be severe and difficult to control. There is some evidence that resistance to infection may be impaired by hyperglycemia, but it is not clear at what level of hyperglycemia this defect is evident. Impaired leukocyte function and vascular disease may contribute to the proneness to develop infections. Infection makes diabetes more difficult to control.

Growth Retardation. Overall growth in diabetic children appears to be related to the degree of control of the disorder. However, the physiologic release of endogenous insulin, which is a dynamic phenomenon integrated with dietary intake, other hormonal secretions, and the demands of physical and emotional stress, cannot be mimicked by the release of exogenous insulin given by subcutaneous injection. Therefore, optimal diabetic control is difficult to achieve, and the extent to which control should approximate normoglycemia is not known. Observe for episodes of hypoglycemia when the regimen calls for tight control. The question then becomes whether the benefits of tight control are sufficiently proven to warrant the risks of hypoglycemia. The demands of physical and emotional growth, particularly at adolescence, make control particularly difficult. Provide continuing support to adolescent clients to assist them in meeting not only their physical needs but their emotional needs as well. Uncontrolled diabetes leads to weight loss, and underweight is more common in diabetic children than in adults. Moreover some delays of growth in stature have been noted in juvenile diabetics, though they tend to attain an adult height that is well within the range of normal (but below the mean for the United States). Full growth potential may not be achieved, however, when the onset of diabetes is just before the adolescent physical growth spurt. Assess the growth of diabetic children by monitoring height and weight on growth charts, skinfold thickness, and radiologic films of the hand showing bone age.

Degenerative Changes in the Cardiovascular and Nervous System. With the advent of insulin therapy and increased life span of diabetics, there has been a steady increase in chronic complications caused by vascular and neural changes. The tendency to develop chronic degenerative changes of the cardiovascular and nervous systems appears to be related to the duration of the illness. For example, complications are rare in juvenile diabetics until the disease has been present for 10 years. The onset of complications gradually increases after this period of time, and after 20 years, 80 to 90 percent of affected clients may show signs of complications, such as vascular changes. Since it is not possible to pinpoint the time of onset of the disease in maturity-onset diabetics, it is not possible to relate the duration of the illness to the appearance of complications. In fact, complications may be present at the time of diagnosis.

The cardiovascular complications include angiopathy (disease of the blood vessels) of two types: (1) macroangiopathy (atherosclerosis of the large arteries, particularly those supplying the heart, head, and legs) and (2) microangiopathy (disease of the capillaries that brings a thickening of the basement membrane and reduction in the number of supporting cells, leading to weakening, plugging, and leakiness of the capillary walls; capillaries particularly affected include those in the eyes and kidneys, although a form of microangiopathy may affect the small vessels of the heart muscle and the walls of large arteries, leading to disease in these structures). Complications of the nervous system include interference with nerve conduction in the peripheral nervous system, leading to peripheral neuropathy particularly affecting the nerves of the feet and legs and, less frequently, the viscera.

The degenerative complications can be further grouped into two major classes: (1) those that affect diabetics and nondiabetics alike, and (2) those that affect predominantly diabetics. The first group includes macroangiopathy (notably atherosclerosis and peripheral vascular disease), whereas microangiopathy and peripheral neuropathy are relatively specific to diabetics. It is not known whether the complications differ in the two types of diabetes, but there are severe consequences of both types.

Vascular disease, particularly coronary arterial disease, is the leading cause of death in diabetic clients. Approximately 75 percent of all deaths among diabetics are due to cardiovascular disease (as opposed to 50 percent in the general population). Coronary heart disease alone accounts for well over half of the mortality in diabetes, with nephropathy accounting for the bulk of the remainder.

The underlying causes of the complications and the efficacy of treatment modalities in preventing or delaying their appearance are the subject of considerable research interest. It has been hypothesized that microvascular lesions may result from glucose toxicity, and some investigations have shown in animal experiments that control of blood sugar can prevent or minimize the development of diabetic lesions.[5] Unfortunately, many of the lesions in animals are pathologically distinct from those in humans, although epidemiologic evidence correlating control of blood sugar with a diminution of complications in the human is now appearing. Conversely, most diabetologists believe that hyperglycemia bears a very weak or no relationship to development of the macrovascular complications. These lesions may result from other factors, such as obesity and abnormal lipid metabolism. Since there is some evidence that good control of the blood sugar may prevent, delay, or slow the progression of some of the complications, it appears prudent to provide good blood sugar control in all diabetic clients.

The relationship between diabetes mellitus and atherosclerosis is not simple. There are many risk factors connected with atherosclerosis that are known to occur with greater frequency in the diabetic population, e.g., a greater tendency toward obesity, hypertension, and hyperlipidemia. The hyperglycemia associated with diabetes may increase the risk. Hyperglycemia tends to induce hypertriglyceridemia and, in some cases, hypercholesterolemia as well. Thus, control of the hyperglycemia may lead to lower blood lipid levels.[3] The hyperlipidemic tendency may contribute to the development of premature atherosclerosis, and it has been suggested that diabetics with hyperlipidemia are most susceptible to atherosclerosis. Although there is no conclusive evidence that control of the disease reverses the propensity to atherosclerosis, many investigators feel that proper attention to diabetic control—including the hyperglycemia and hyperlipidemia—has great potential for reducing the extent of atherosclerotic lesions.

Colwell and colleagues suggest a comprehensive approach directed at the major known risk factors in the macrovascular system, i.e., efforts to reduce obesity, hypertension, cigarette smoking, and hyperlipidemia.[6] These risk factors and their management are discussed in Chapter 29.

Long-standing diabetes produces a characteristic lesion of the kidneys, called the Kimmelstiel–Wilson syndrome, that eventually leads to renal failure. In the early stages, the disorder is usually asymptomatic and is detectable only by the occurrence of albuminuria. The disorder may progress to the nephrotic syndrome, however, with extensive proteinuria and edema. Hypertension becomes evident as the disease further progresses to chronic renal insufficiency. Once end-stage renal disease is reached, the Kimmelstiel–Wilson syndrome is not clinically distinguishable from other types of renal disease. Dietary management for the diabetic with renal disease follows the principles outlined in Chapter 30. Renal transplantation has become the preferred method to chronic hemodialysis for treating diabetics with end-stage renal disease.

Vascular changes in the eye (retinopathy) are common, and diabetes is now the leading cause of new blindness in the United States. Light coagulation, using a xenon or argon laser photocoagulator, is used as a method for preventing hemorrhage and development of more extensive scar tissue in those with retinopathy, although pituitary ablation, scleral buckling, vitrectomy, or sometimes a combination of these techniques is necessary. The early development of cataracts (as well as the propensity to develop peripheral neuropathy, discussed below) is considered by some to result from an increased conversion of glucose first to sorbitol, a sugar alcohol, and then to fructose in the eye, nerve cells, and certain other cells. In certain tissues (such as the lens of the eye, liver cells, the aorta, and Schwann cells of the peripheral nerves), glucose can enter the cells without insulin. Sorbitol and fructose exert an osmotic effect in the cell, drawing water into the tissue and producing disruption and damage. Careful control of the blood sugar is most important in reducing the formation of increased amounts of sorbitol and fructose in the tissues. Experimental efforts are being directed toward blocking the enzyme that leads to the formation of sorbitol.

In a significant number of individuals with long-standing diabetes, peripheral neuropathy of the lower extremities and, to a lesser extent the viscera, develops. Diabetic neuropathy is treated symptomatically, and in some cases, the symptoms may disappear. Diets high in myoinositol, a polyhydric alcohol found in high concentration in the myelin sheath of nerves and excreted in large amounts in the urine of diabetic clients, may have promise for improving motor nerve conduction in neuropathic diabetic clients.[7]

Intervention

The goals of management of diabetes are:

1. To achieve as normal a state of metabolism as possible
2. To prevent the acute complications (hyperglycemia, hypoglycemic reactions, and ketoacidosis) and the chronic complications (macrovascular disease, microvascular disease, and peripheral neuropathy) of the disease
3. To control preexisting diseases or complications of diabetes that may develop
4. To provide a diet that is nutritionally adequate, that allows for normalization of body weight, and that allows for a normal growth rate in children and pregnant women and adequate nutrients for lactating women
5. To provide for each patient an individualized program of education and follow-up

Although keeping the plasma glucose as near the physiologic range as possible is a goal, current techniques of management do not permit the maintenance of plasma glucose within normal physiologic limits at all times and in all clients. Achievable goals include prevention of some of the symptoms, e.g., polyuria, vaginitis, ketoacidosis and coma, and hyperosmolar coma. At the same time, hypoglycemia can be avoided and hypertriglyceridemia can be reduced. The question of whether the chronic complications can be controlled has not been unequivocally answered.

At all times in management, the client plays a central role, since adherence to the management regimen requires a sense of purpose and self-discipline. Assist clients in understanding the objectives of treatment and provide them with the information needed to assume day-to-day responsibility for self-care. The cornerstone of control is a regimen of dietary regulation, alone or in combination with insulin or oral hypoglycemic agents. A regimen of regulated, regular exercise is also important.

Insulin-dependent diabetics require both dietary regulation and insulin therapy. These individuals are usually of normal weight or lean. Regulated exercise is particularly important in the management of these clients. The oral hypoglycemic agents have no role in the management of insulin-dependent diabetes. Diet, and not insulin, is the treatment of choice for noninsulin-dependent diabetics who are asymptomatic and obese. Approximately 50 percent of those who develop the disease after maturity can be treated with diet alone. Dietary management consists of control of kilocaloric intake to control the obesity. With kilocaloric restriction, other parameters affected by diet will normalize, i.e., the plasma glucose, glucosuria, and plasma lipids (cholesterol and triglycerides). Because of the correlation of obesity and diabetes, there is a tendency to associate diabetes control with kilocaloric restriction. This can be detrimental for growing children, however, as growth retardation may result from kilocaloric restriction. If diet alone is not sufficient, insulin or one of the oral hypoglycemic agents is added to provide symptomatic relief of the hyperglycemia. Current controversy regarding the long-term effects and safety in the use of the oral hypoglycemic agents (see below) leads some authorities to suggest that their use should be reserved for symptomatic clients who cannot be controlled by diet alone and who are unable or unwilling to take insulin.

Insulin Therapy. In the insulin-dependent diabetic, daily administration of commercial insulin preparations is necessary to control the illness. The insulin must be given by subcutaneous injection because oral ingestion will result in its digestion, since insulin is a protein. Improved methods of insulin therapy in recent years, including the use of highly purified insulin preparations, providing multiple insulin injections (split dose) rather than a single daily dose, and providing mixtures of insulin rather than a single type, have made control of blood sugar a more achievable goal for insulin-dependent diabetics than in the past.

Commercial insulin preparations are extracted from the pancreases of pigs and cattle, and pork, beef, and mixed pork–beef insulins are now available in purified forms. Two of these more nearly pure preparations currently available are single-peak insulin (SPI) and single component-insulin (SCI). Conventional insulins contain several other pancreatic hormones, including proinsulin, which can cause allergic reactions. Some clients develop antibodies to the contaminants and may become insulin resistant. Purification removes the contaminants, thus reducing the potential for insulin allergy and resistance as well as for the development of lipoatrophy (localized lipid atrophy or induration) at the injection site. Instruct clients to rotate insulin injection sites among the upper arm, thigh, buttocks, back, and abdomen as a further precaution against lipoatrophy. Purified insulin appears to have greater biologic effectiveness than conventional insulin. Caution clients who switch from conventional to purified insulin to observe for hypoglycemia unless the dose is reduced.

Three general types of insulin are available, and they differ primarily in their rate of onset (related to the rate of absorption and release), time of peak action, and duration of the hypoglycemic effect. The three general types and characteristics are listed in Table 24–2. It should be noted that there may be individual variations in the pattern of release and use of insulin, for example, NPH action usually

---

TABLE 24–2
TYPES AND CHARACTERISTICS OF INSULIN PREPARATIONS

Types (Rate of onset and Duration)	Peak Action (hr)	Duration (hr)
Rapid onset and short duration		
Regular (crystalline)	2–4	6–8
Semilente	4–6	12–16
Intermediate		
Globin	6–10	12–18
NPH[a]	8–12	18–24
Lente[a]	8–12	18–28
Slow onset and long duration		
Protamine zinc[b]	14–20	24–36+
Ultralente	16–18	24–36+
Combinations		
Regular and NPH	2–10	18–24
Regular and lente	2–10	18–24
Semilente and lente	4–10	18–24
Semilente and ultralente	2–24	30–36

[a] Most popular.
[b] Rarely used today.

peaks 8 to 12 hours after injection. Observe, however, the peak action for each individual client by reviewing the pattern of urine glucose or blood glucose test results and adjust the diet to match the observed peak.

In order to approximate glycemic equilibrium throughout the 24-hour period a combination of two types of insulin is frequently used and often given in split doses. For example, NPH or lente insulin may be combined with regular insulin; two thirds of the total dosage may be given in the morning and one third in the evening, with two thirds of each dose as the intermediate-acting insulin and one third as the regular insulin. The regular insulin enhances the effort of the intermediate-acting insulin in preventing hyperglycemia throughout the day, and splitting the dose prevents hyperglycemia during the night.

When insulin is used, consideration should be given to its balance with food intake and physical activity. Since the daily insulin injection is constant, there is not the freedom of food intake that exists for the nondiabetic. Food intake must be planned to correlate with the time of onset, peak action, and duration of the particular types of insulin used. Unless food intake is properly spaced (assuming the individual receives an insulin injection before the morning meal), a period of hypoglycemia might be expected before the noon meal if regular insulin is used, in the afternoon before the evening meal with an intermediate insulin, and later if protamine zinc insulin is used. Caution the client to eat within a 2 to 3 hour period after taking insulin. The roles of diet and exercise are discussed below.

Observe for the Somogyi phenomenon, progressive deterioration in diabetic control, in clients who receive increasing doses of insulin. The phenomenon is characterized by symptomatic or inapparent hypoglycemia followed by reactive hyperglycemia, glucosuria, and ketonuria, despite high levels of circulating insulin. The problem is not uncommon in diabetic children and frequently results from efforts to completely eliminate glucosuria. The child becomes overinsulinized. The Somogyi phenomenon should be suspected in a child who is receiving more than 1.5 units of insulin/kg and in whom there is persistent or recurrent marked hyperglycemia and ketonuria. A possible explanation is that subclinical hypoglycemia stimulates the secretion of insulin antagonists, such as glucagon, cortisol, growth hormone, and catecholamines—that make insulin ineffective, and rebound hyperglycemia occurs. Gradual reduction in the total insulin dosage and splitting the dose are usually effective in management.

Severe food restriction in an attempt to lose weight may lead to the biochemical pattern of hypoglycemia, with concomitant ketonuria.

Oral Hypoglycemic Agents. Sulfonyluria compounds (Table 24–3) are effective in lowering the blood sugar in a significant number of diabetic

TABLE 24–3
DURATION OF HYPOGLYCEMIC EFFECT OF SULFONYLUREA COMPOUNDS

Oral Agent	Duration of Action (hr)
Tolbutamide (Orinase)	6–24
Acetohexamide (Dymelor)	12–24
Tolazamide (Tolinase)	12–24
Chlorpropamide (Diabinese)	Up to 60

clients with mild-to-moderate disease. These drugs sensitize the beta-cells to glucose and stimulate the cells to secrete endogenous insulin. They are effective only in those who have beta-cells that can respond to the stimulus. Analogs of several of the sulfonylurea compounds are also available.

At present, continuing use of the oral hypoglycemic agents is controversial since one study (the University Group Diabetes Program) concluded that there was a small but significant increase in mortality in groups using certain of these compounds. Although the study has been widely criticized, some investigators support the conclusion that the use of oral hypoglycemic agents may endanger a small number of diabetics.

Other Therapies. Because somatostatin leads to hypoglycemia by decreasing the secretion of glucagon, somatostatin therapy may be a useful adjunct to insulin therapy in the treatment of insulin-dependent diabetics in whom control of the blood sugar is often difficult. Somatostatin also inhibits growth hormone, which may be present in excess in diabetic clients. The suspicion that excess growth hormone secretion may be related to the development of microangiopathy increases the potential for the use of somatostatin. However, the growth hormone-inhibition property of the hormone may make its use inappropriate for children.

Two additional approaches to better control of blood sugar are under extensive study: (1) the use of an artificial pancreas and (2) transplantation of whole pancreases, pancreatic segments, or cultured islet cell tissue. Many authorities believe that if the minute-by-minute regulation of blood sugar that is achieved by the normal pancreas could be achieved by other means, the long-term complications could be minimized or avoided. An artificial pancreas in the form of an insulin pump is currently being used to provide insulin to some diabetic clients. The device can be clipped to a belt or carried in underclothing and provides a continuous low-dose infusion of insulin, with stepped-up delivery during meals, through a tube into the injection site of choice, subcutaneous or intravenous. A subcutaneously implanted intravenous insulin pump has been developed.[8] Use of these devices has allowed for the achievement of improved control of hyperglycemia in a small number of highly supervised clients, and some researchers conclude that this type of insulin delivery system is acceptable to clients and can be applied successfully to clinical practice.[9]

Although islet cell transplantation has been achieved in experimental animals and produces interesting results, there are predictable problems of tissue rejection necessitating large doses of steroids and immunosuppressive drugs, and the results of long-term transplants in humans have been disappointing to date. At present, the risks are not justified for diabetics who can be controlled by regulated insulin or infusion.

Long-term oral supplements with chromium have been found to improve glucose tolerance in some noninsulin-dependent diabetics, presumably in those with a marginal chromium deficiency. Chromium deficiency renders insulin less effective, and its efficiency is improved when the deficiency is alleviated.

Exercise. A regimen of regular exercise has long been considered an important adjunct to other therapy in the treatment of diabetes, not only because exercise aids in the management of adiposity but also because exercise stimulates total body glucose use. In normal individuals, muscular work is accompanied by an increase in glucose uptake by exercising muscles and several hormonal changes, including a decline in plasma insulin levels and a rise in the levels of insulin antagonists, including glucagon, cortisol, growth hormone, and the catecholamines that stimulate hepatic glucose production to meet the demands for glucose. If the exercise is prolonged, lipids are mobilized from adipose tissue and used for energy. Thus, the situation is one of an increase in glucose use in association with a fall in insulin concentration. Exercise may increase tissue sensitivity to insulin.

The interactions between exercise and diabetes are multiple and complicated, however, and the effect of exercise on the blood glucose level will depend on the degree of control of the diabetes (i.e., the presence of a critical amount of insulin during the exercise) and the effect of mechanical factors on blood glucose alterations during the exercise (i.e., the effect of exercise on mobilizing the insulin from the injection site). A small amount of insulin appears to be necessary for exercise to have a stimulating effect on glucose turnover and glucose uptake by the muscle. The alteration in blood sugar that is induced by exercise appears to be different in poorly controlled and well-controlled diabetics, and exercise cannot be viewed as a substitute for proper insulin management. Alert diabetics who are poorly controlled (i.e., blood sugar in excess of 300 mg percent) due to relative insulin deficiency at the time of exercise to the fact that the exercise may aggravate the hyperglycemia and lead to ketosis. This is presumably due to an exaggerated rise in plasma catecholamines and growth hormone. In contrast, in individuals with adequate circulating insulin, exercise brings a reduction in the blood glucose concentration. A critical amount of insulin is needed to stimulate glucose uptake and prevent the overstimulation of the hormones that are antagonistic to insulin. Sustained activity may lead to hypoglycemia, since hepatic glucose production and lipolysis are inhibited while glucose use continues.

Diabetics receiving insulin injections should be aware of the possible effects of exercising the insulin injection site on mobilization of insulin and alterations in blood glucose during exercise. The rate of mobilization of insulin is increased when the injection site (e.g., the leg) is exercised. This brings an exaggerated fall in blood sugar and exercise-induced hypoglycemia. This phenomenon does not occur when insulin is injected into a nonexercised site, such as the abdomen. At present, it is not possible to make precise recommendations regarding exercise relative to insulin injection site, but two general recommendations may be appropriate: (1) teach diabetics who are prone to develop exercise-induced hypoglycemia to inject insulin into a nonexercised site, and (2) teach those who are prone to hyperglycemia (but do not experience exercise-induced hypoglycemia) to inject insulin into an exercised site to provide better control.

For those who are prone to develop hyperglycemia, a program of regulated exercise performed at times during the day when blood glucose levels tend to be high can optimize therapy. For example, exercise performed after meals can be useful in preventing postprandial hyperglycemia. The American Diabetes Association and the American Dietetic Association suggest that in the absence of contraindications, a good plan is to walk a total of about 5 miles a day by walking at a fairly brisk pace for 30 minutes (covering a distance of approximately 1.5 miles) after each meal.[10]

Since exercise increases the potential for hypoglycemia, give all insulin-dependent clients specific instructions regarding regulation of insulin dosage and food intake during periods of unusual or sporadic exercise. In many situations, it is usually easier to provide extra kilocalories without adjusting the insulin dosage. The number of extra kilocalories required before and during the exercise depends on the intensity and duration of the activity, degree of physical conditioning, and size, age, and sex of the individual. Moreover, increased kilocalorie requirements may be offset by increased insulin sensitivity. Estimates can be made by referring to tables that list average kilocalorie expenditure for various types of activity.[11,12] This should be individualized according to previous experience. Periods of moderate activity may increase kilocalorie requirements by 2 to 3 kcal/kg body weight per hour. A general rule is to provide about 15 g carbohydrate for 1 hour of moderate exercise or a half hour of strenuous exercise. A more substantial snack, such as half a sandwich, may be necessary if the exercise is to be prolonged, and additional food may be required for up to 12 hours after strenuous exercise to replete glycogen stores.

Diet. The optimal diet in the management of diabetes mellitus is not known, and controversy about the efficacy of various types of diets has existed for some time. Various strategies, including low-carbohydrate, normal carbohydrate, high-carbohydrate, and numerous other diet combinations have been promoted. It is clear that no one diet is of unique therapeutic value for all diabetic clients. No long-term studies on the effect of various types of diets on morbidity and mortality have been conducted. Diabetics have usually been excluded from dietary studies related to atherosclerosis, since their inclusion would complicate the study.

Weight reduction of obese diabetics is strongly advocated in treatment, but there are few data available to assess the influence of persistent obesity on the outcome of diabetes or the effect of secondary weight reduction on morbidity and mortality. It has long been thought that the principal aim of diet therapy is to reduce the consumption of total carbohydrate and refined sugar. However, changes in energy sources have recently been recommended in the diet for diabetics, and there is now a trend toward increasing the carbohydrate content and decreasing the fat content of the diet. These recommendations are based on observations that high carbohydrate intake can improve carbohydrate tolerance, and fat restriction may alter the macrovascular complications. However, the long-range effects of these changes are not known. Restriction of refined sugar is based on the rationale that sugar is absorbed rapidly, causing higher blood sugar peaks. Evidence to support restriction of glucose in the diabetic diet is good, since blood glucose levels are higher after an oral glucose load than an equicaloric starch load in both normal individuals and persons with diabetes. In contrast, in normal and diabetic subjects, fructose causes less of a rise in blood glucose than do some types of starch, sucrose, or glucose. Little difference has been found in the blood glucose response to equicaloric amounts of sucrose and starch in normal and diabetic subjects. At present, it is difficult to draw firm conclusions from studies about the effect on blood glucose of specific carbohydrates when consumed as part of a mixed diet or by individuals in different metabolic states.

Dietary fiber may improve glucose tolerance as well as decrease serum lipid levels.[13] It has been shown that when carbohydrate is ingested in conjunction with soluble plant fibers in fruits and vegetables (guar gum and pectin), postprandial levels of glucose, insulin, and other hormones decrease, glucosuria may be diminished, and insulin requirements may be lowered. Various mechanisms have been proposed to explain the improved glucose tolerance with the ingestion of soluble plant fibers, including slower carbohydrate absorption secondary to delayed gastric emptying and gel formation properties or interaction with gut hormones. The long-term effectiveness and safety of purified fibers, such as guar and pectin, are not known, however, and the role of fiber in the diabetic diet is under study. There is some initial evidence to indicate that chronic high fiber intake may induce histologic changes in the intestinal mucosa that may alter the absorption of carbohydrate as well as other nutrients. Further study is needed to determine the extent of the effects and whether the changes are beneficial or detrimental.

For the present, it appears prudent to substitute natural foods containing unrefined fiber-containing carbohydrate foods, such as whole grains, legumes, and vegetables, for highly refined carbohydrates that are low in fiber if the foods are acceptable to the client. Since changes in fiber content of the diet may alter the insulin requirement, call the physician's attention to any change in the fiber content of the client's diet.

Dietary Strategies. Dietary strategies are different for nonobese insulin-dependent and noninsulin-dependent obese diabetics. With both types, however, attention is given to nutritional requirements, kilocaloric level, timing and constancy of food intake, and distribution of the kilocalories (i.e., percentage composition of carbohydrate, protein, and fat at meals). The timing and constancy of food intake and distribution of the kilocalories are less important in those not taking insulin.

In general, the nutritional requirements for diabetics are the same as for nondiabetics of the same age, sex, height, and activity. The diet should be planned so that it is nutritionally adequate and allows for attainment or maintenance of recommended body weight and for growth in children and pregnant women. When diabetes is poorly controlled or there is infection, malabsorption, or other complications, provide a diet that is higher in protein to counteract negative nitrogen balance, and supplement with vitamins and minerals. Also provide vitamin and mineral supplements for clients who follow a weight reduction diet containing less than 1200 kcal daily. Evaluate carefully diets that contain less than 1500 kcal for nutritional adequacy.

The particular kilocaloric level depends on age and current weight of the client. For the young insulin-dependent diabetic who is underweight, sufficient kilocalories should be provided to attain desirable weight and to allow for normal growth and development. For the insulin-dependent diabetic of any age who is of normal weight, give attention to weight maintenance and avoidance of weight gain with age. Weight reduction to achieve and to maintain recommended body weight is indicated for obese diabetics and is the single most important objective in dietary management of obese, noninsulin-dependent diabetics. Weight reduction not only reduces hyperglycemia, hyperlipidemia, and hypertension (all risk factors for atherosclerosis) but also returns glucose tolerance to or toward normal. Thus insulin or oral glucose-lowering agents may not be needed. In order to bring about long-term changes in eating habits associated with obesity, a professionally supervised weight and exercise control program with strong reinforcement by qualified health professionals is of primary importance. Fad diets for weight reduction should be avoided.

The RDA (see Chap. 2) can be used as a guide for determining the kilocaloric level during the growth cycle. A more precise method is to determine current intake based on a 3 to 7 day diet history and food recall. Educate the parents and child in measurement of portion sizes and record keeping to assure accuracy of the diet history. Children's diets need frequent revision to allow for growth. Repeat the diet history with each revision and adjust the prescription as necessary for weight gain or loss. The protein requirement ranges from 1 to 2 g/kg of body weight depending on the child's age. Table 24–4 provides a method for calculating the kilocalorie level for obese, adult diabetics. Some authorities consider it advisable to keep the weight of diabetics 5 to 10 percent below average.

Meal regularity and diet composition (especially kilocalories from carbohydrate) of meals and snacks are an important consideration, particularly for those taking hypoglycemic agents (insulin or oral agents). The time of day when meals are eaten, the number of meals eaten, and the composition of the meals should be not only consistent from day to day but also balanced with the kind and amount of insulin or oral agent taken and the usual pattern of physical activity. In order to prevent hypoglycemia, instruct individuals taking insulin to avoid spans of time between meals that exceed 3 to 4 hours. There should be at least five daily feedings, if not more. Most children under 10 years are best managed with three meals and three snacks (midmorning, midafternoon, and before retiring), whereas older children and adults may wish to omit the midmorning snack. Foods containing protein and complex carbohydrates, such as starch and fiber, are preferred to rapidly absorbed simple carbohydrates, such as sugars; for example, bread is a better choice

than fruit juice for a bedtime snack. To assure constancy in the blood sugar level, each meal should usually contain about 0.2 to 0.4 of the kilocalorie and carbohydrate content and each snack should usually contain about 0.1 of the kilocalories and carbohydrate. Since the conversion of protein to carbohydrate is slow, to prevent early morning hypoglycemia it is advisable to include protein-containing foods as well as complex carbohydrate (such as a sandwich and milk) at the bedtime snack when using intermediate-acting insulins. When protamine zinc insulin with its prolonged action is used, it is advisable to include about one half of the protein in the evening and bedtime meal to allow for continuous input of glucose during the night. The remaining 50 percent of the protein is then divided to include one sixth at breakfast and one third at noon. If the patient taking insulin tends to be hyperglycemic or hypoglycemic at a given time of day, alleviate the problem by instructing the client to shift portions of food from one meal to another. If the patient is taking two to three injections of short-acting insulin daily or using short-acting insulin as a supplement to the longer-acting insulins, adjustment of the insulin dosage may allow greater meal flexibility.

The regularity of meals and the diet composition are less important for the noninsulin-dependent diabetic. A meal pattern should be established that is congruent with the lifestyle, and the number of meals should usually be three, but not less than two, per day. A large carbohydrate load at one time should be avoided, however, to avoid swings in blood sugar. There is no need for special snacks between meals.

The composition of the kilocalories, particularly the carbohydrate and fat content, and their effect on glucose homeostasis and long-term complications have been the subject of much debate. If the carbohydrate content is kept low, the fat content will necessarily be high to provide sufficient kilocalories. Conversely, if the carbohydrate content is high, the fat content must be low to remain in kilocalorie equilibrium. Although carbohydrate has traditionally been restricted in the diet of diabetics, new approaches are now being advised that liberalize the intake of carbohydrate and limit the intake of fat (Table 24–5). This approach is based on the association between dietary saturated fat and cholesterol consumption and the development of atherosclerosis. Atherosclerotic lesions are the major cause of morbidity and mortality in diabetic clients. Moreover, the insulin requirement is more closely correlated with total kilocalorie intake than with the level of dietary carbohydrate. Provided total kilocalories are controlled at an appropriate level, increasing the total carbohydrate allowance does not seem to affect the insulin requirements of insulin-dependent diabetics. Nor does it appear to lead to fluctuations in the blood sugar level in the postprandial period or to induce hypertriglyceridemia. In some adult clients with endogenous hypertriglyceridemia,

---

TABLE 24–4
KILOCALORIC REQUIREMENT OF ADULTS

Activity Level (Add to Basal)[a]	Kcal/kg Recommended Body Weight[b]
Sedentary activity	3 kcal/lb recommended body weight
Moderate activity	5 kcal/lb recommended body weight
Strenuous activity	10 kcal/lb recommended body weight

[a] Basal kcal: 10 kcal/lb ideal body weight.
[b] Subtract 500 kcal from estimate for each pound of weekly weight loss desired.

TABLE 24–5
PERCENTAGE NUTRIENT COMPOSITION OF NORMAL AND DIABETIC DIETS

Nutrient	Nutrient Percentage Composition		Current Recommendations for Diabetic Diets[a]
	Typical U.S. Diet	Traditional Diabetic Diet	
Carbohydrate	46	35–40 (⅔ polysaccharides and ⅓ mono- and disaccharides)	50–60
Protein	12	15–20	12–20
Fat	42	40–50	Fat to supply the remainder (saturated fat decreased to <10% of total kcal, polyunsaturated fat should supply up to 10% of total kcal and the remainder of food fat derived from monounsaturated fat sources)

[a] (Source: Principles of Nutrition and Dietary Recommendations for Individuals with Diabetes Mellitus, 1979. J Am Diet Assoc 75:527, 1979.) These are general recommendations and should not be construed as rigid requirements, since it is more appropriate to adapt the dietary plan to the individual's usual diet provided it meets the nutritional needs of the individual.

however, basal triglyceride levels may rise sharply in response to an increase in carbohydrate—the hypertriglyceridemia responds to kilocalorie and carbohydrate restriction as in nondiabetic clients. Finally, it has been demonstrated that diets providing a high percentage of kilocalories from carbohydrate lead to an improved glucose tolerance in diabetics who maintain control of total kilocalorie intake. This maneuver leads to a deterioration in glucose tolerance in untreated diabetics, however. The increased sensitivity of the tissues to insulin with a high carbohydrate intake appears to be an adaptive response to the increased proportion of carbohydrate. As much as 60 percent of the kilocalories may be derived from carbohydrate, mainly as complex carbohydrates from starch and vegetables. Since the effect of specific carbohydrates on blood glucose remains unsettled, the recommendation to limit simple sugars and emphasize complex carbohydrates can be more rationally based on the fact that complex carbohydrates make more significant nutritional contributions than do simple sugars. Moreover, there are differences of opinion as to whether any sucrose at all should be allowed on a diabetic diet, although its exclusion poses problems of compliance, since sucrose is present in many prepared foods. The American Diabetes Association has recommended that a moderate amount of sucrose is acceptable contingent upon maintenance of metabolic control.[14] Although a plan for exchanging various carbohydrates in the diet based on their effect on blood glucose has been suggested, more data are needed before this suggestion can be implemented. More emphasis should be placed on those foods that produce the smallest rise in blood glucose, however, and less emphasis on those that are associated with higher glycemic responses.[15]

Both insulin-dependent and noninsulin-dependent diabetics may benefit from a diet liberalized in carbohydrate content and limited in content of saturated fat and cholesterol. Diabetics, like nondiabetics, respond to fat restriction with a reduction in serum levels of cholesterol and triglyceride. The kilocalories supplied by saturated fat can be replaced by complex carbohydrates, protein, and unsaturated fat. There appears to be no additional advantage to adding polyunsaturated fat, since the kilocalorie level may be excessive, and there are uncertainties regarding the long-term effects of large quantities of polyunsaturated fat. With the liberalization of the carbohydrate intake, however, kilocaloric control must not be relaxed.

In practice, one sees a variety of dietary approaches used in treatment, and there is no standard diet therapy. Since controversy still exists as to whether strict control of blood sugar and blood lipids does indeed delay or reduce the incidence of complications, currently prescribed diets vary on a continuum from extremely strict to moderate to liberal diet control. Thus one may find a weighed or carefully measured diet (strict approach), a middle of the road approach using the six Food Exchange Lists described in Chapter 2 (moderate approach), or a free diet—free in the most liberal sense or a free diet that restricts concentrated sweets (liberal approach).

A diet based on the exchange system provides a moderate degree of consistency in intake of kilocalories, carbohydrate, protein, and fat, while allowing for flexibility of food choices. The professional organizations that prepared the 1976 revision of the traditional six Food Exchange Lists recognized the need for both kilocaloric control and fat control by diabetics, and the new Exchange Lists are helpful in planning low-kilocalorie, low-fat diets.[16]

Physicians and dietitians, with input from

nurses, are usually responsible for setting up the diet plan for the diabetic. However, it is the diabetic client himself or herself who must plan daily meals. Therefore, if the exchange system is used, give adequate education in its use, including the method of making substitutions. Five steps are involved in processing a diabetic diet, from the setting up of the diet plan to the planning of the daily menus. These steps are:

1. Determining the appropriate kilocalorie level
2. Determining the percentage distribution of carbohydrate, protein, and fat and the amounts of each in grams
3. Determining the number of exchanges from each of the six Food Exchange Lists needed to achieve the desired amounts of carbohydrate, protein, and fat
4. Distributing the exchanges into a daily meal plan
5. Planning daily menus on the basis of the meal plan

Use the techniques described above for determining the appropriate kilocalorie level. A sample calculation using the distribution percentage of carbohydrate, protein, and fat given in Table 24–5 to determine the specific number of grams of carbohydrate, protein, and fat to use in the diet prescription for an adult, overweight, sedentary diabetic is given in Table 24–6.

In order to calculate the number of exchanges needed from each list, it is necessary to review the carbohydrate, protein, and fat content of the six Food Exchanges given in Chapter 2 and listed in Table 24–7. As noted in Table 24–7, carbohydrate is contained in foods from milk, vegetables, fruit, and bread exchanges, protein in foods from milk, vegetables, bread, and meat exchanges, and fat in meat and fat exchanges. If milk other than the non-

---

TABLE 24–7
CARBOHYDRATE, PROTEIN, AND FAT CONTENT OF THE EXCHANGE LISTS

Exchange	Carbohydrate (g)	Protein (g)	Fat (g)
Milk (nonfat)	12	8	
Vegetable	5	2	
Fruit	10		
Bread	15	2	
Meat			
Low-fat		7	3
Medium-fat		7	5
High-fat		7	8
Fat			5

---

fat form is used, fat is also present. In calculating the number of exchanges needed to fulfil a given diet prescription, follow these three steps:

1. Calculate the number of exchanges of milk, vegetable, fruit, and bread needed to fulfil the carbohydrate prescription
2. Calculate the number of exchanges of meat needed to complete the protein prescription
3. Calculate the number of fat exchanges needed to complete the fat prescription

A sample calculation for a 1500 kcal diet (185 g carbohydrate, 75 g protein, and 50 g fat) is given in Table 24–8, the total exchanges derived from the calculation are given in Table 24–9, and Table 24–10 provides a sample meal plan. With the meal plan, the client uses the substitutions possible in the six Food Exchange Lists to plan daily menus. Various alternatives are possible when calculating the number of exchanges to include from the various lists, and the end result should be tailored to individual food preferences. For example, if an individual is not a milk drinker, milk need not be calculated into the exchange pattern. Rather, the carbohydrate and protein content of the milk can be used to include foods that the individual will eat on a regular basis; for example, additional fruit or bread exchanges can replace the carbohydrate of milk, and meat exchanges can replace the protein content. When distributing the exchanges into the meal pattern, give consideration once again to food habits and lifestyle, as well as insulin therapy and exercise patterns. Teach the client regarding substitutions possible in the exchange system and free foods (see Appendix 2), so that he or she can plan menus that are economical and appealing.

Some clinicians use food grouping systems other than the exchange system in planning the diabetic diet. One alternate food grouping system is (1) protein foods, (2) low-carbohydrate foods, (3) high-carbohydrate foods, (4) fats and oils, and (5) free foods. Appendix 1 provides a listing of the nutrient composition of the most frequently served foods.

TABLE 24–6
DIET CALCULATION BASED ON ENERGY NEEDS OF ADULT, OVERWEIGHT, SEDENTARY DIABETIC WHOSE RECOMMENDED WEIGHT IS 70 KG

Client: Recommended body weight = 70 kg (154 lb)[a]
      Activity = sedentary
Total kcal need = 1500 [(10 × 154) + (3 × 154) − 500] kcal for estimated weight loss of 1 lb per week (see Table 24–4)
Grams of carbohydrate = 185 (1500 × 0.50 ÷ 4)
Grams of protein = 75 (1500 × 0.20 ÷ 4)
Grams of fat = 50 (1500 × 0.30 ÷ 9)
Diet prescription: Kcal, 1500
              Carbohydrate, 185 g
              Protein, 75 g
              Fat, 50 g

[a] Percentage distribution of carbohydrate, protein, and fat is 50, 20, and 30, respectively; grams calculated to the nearest 5.

TABLE 24–8
SAMPLE CALCULATION OF NUMBER OF FOOD EXCHANGES TO USE IN A DIABETIC DIET PRESCRIPTION[a]

Calculation of Carbohydrate, Protein, and Fat	Sample Calculations	Exchange List and Number of Exchanges	Final Diet Plan		
			Carbohydrate (g)	Protein (g)	Fat (g)
Carbohydrate 1. Determine the amount of milk, vegetables, and fruit to be included in diet plan based on individual's food habits and preferences		1. Milk, lowfat (2) Vegetables (2) Fruit (2)	24 10 20	16 4	
2. Determine the number of bread exchanges needed to complete the carbohydrate prescription by: a. Totaling the amount of carbohydrate available from milk, vegetables, and fruit	a. Total carbohydrate from sources other than bread exchanges = 54 g				
		Subtotal—carbohydrate	54		
b. Subtracting the total derived from (a) from the total carbohydrate prescription	b. 185 g − 54 g 131 g				
c. Dividing the result of (b) by 15— the number of grams of carbohydrate provided by one bread exchange—to determine the number of bread exchanges needed to complete the carbohydrate prescription	c. 131 ÷ 15 = approx 9 bread exchanges				
		2. Bread (9) Total carbohydrate (g)	135 189	18	
Protein 1. Determine the number of meat exchanges needed to complete the protein prescription by: a. Totaling the protein provided by milk, vegetables, and bread	a. Total protein from sources other than meat exchanges = 38 g				
		Subtotal—protein		38	
b. Subtracting the total derived from (a) from the total protein prescription	b. 75 g −38 g 37 g				
c. Dividing the result of (b) by 7— the number of grams of protein provided by one meat exchange—to determine the number of meat exchanges needed to complete the protein prescription	c. 37 ÷ 7 = approx 5 meat exchanges				
		1. Low-fat meat (5) Total protein (g)		35 73	15
Fat 1. Determine the number of fat exchanges needed to complete the fat prescription by: a. Totaling the amount of fat provided by milk (if other than skim milk is used) and meat	a. Total fat from sources other than fat exchanges = 15 g				
		Subtotal—fat			15
b. Subtracting the total derived from (a) from the total fat prescription	b. 50 g −15 g 35 g				
c. Dividing the result of (b) by 5— the number of grams of fat provided by one fat exchange—to determine the number of fat exchanges needed to complete the fat prescription	c. 35 ÷ 5 = 7 fat exchanges				
		1. Fat (7) Total fat (g) GRAND TOTAL	189	73	35 50 50

[a] 1500 kcal (185 g carbohydrate, 75 g protein, and 50 g fat)—end result within 5 g of prescription for each nutrient.

TABLE 24–9
TRANSLATION INTO FOOD EXCHANGES

Exchange List	Total No. for Day	Carbohydrate (g)	Protein (g)	Fat (g)	Kcal
Milk, skim	2	24	16		160
Vegetable	2	10	4		56
Fruit	2	20			80
Bread	9	135	18		612
Meat, low-fat	5		35	15	275
Fat	7			35	315
TOTAL DISTRIBUTION		189	73	50	1498

Other Special Dietary Concerns. Such situations as traveling, eating out, acute illness, surgery, use of alcohol, use of salt, and use of special foods pose additional considerations in dietary management.

Instruct the client to give consideration, when eating out, to the kilocaloric content and portion size of kilocalorie-containing foods selected and to avoid foods for which a reasonable estimate of kilocalorie content cannot be made. Suggestions given to the obese client when eating out (see Chap. 23) are also appropriate for the obese diabetic. Teach diabetic children and their families to study the school lunch menus a week in advance and prepare packed lunches for those days when the selection at school in inappropriate. Remind insulin-dependent diabetics to carry nonperishable foods (such as peanut butter or cheese crackers or packets of table sugar) when traveling, since traveling may entail delayed or missed meals. The individual should also inquire in advance about meal schedules on planes and in hotels. Air travel time changes may disturb the rhythm of insulin injection and meals, and jet lag in itself may add control problems. Should meals be unavoidably delayed, the ingestion of 15 to 30 g of carbohydrate protects from hypoglycemia for 1 to 2 hours.

Special measures are required should there be a period of acute illness that curbs the appetite or food intake. Acute situations, such as infections, trauma, and severe emotional stress, will usually aggravate the metabolic disturbance and put the diabetic out of control. It may be necessary to consult a physician immediately, and if the illness is pro-longed, particularly if there is vomiting and persistent ketonuria, hospitalization may be a safer approach to therapy. The increased insulin requirement occasioned by acute metabolic disturbances is balanced to some degree by the lessened insulin requirements that accompany the associated diminished kilocalorie intake.

With illness there is usually a temporary revision in dietary priorities and strategies. However, caution clients taking insulin to continue its administration and encourage them to eat if possible to avoid ketosis. Priority should be given to the avoidance of vomiting and starvation. Adjust plans temporarily to include a more easily tolerated and more easily digested regimen that contains a higher proportion of simple carbohydrates and lesser amounts of complex carbohydrates, proteins, and fats. Foods of a liquid or soft consistency (such as soups, fruit juices, carbonated beverages, milk beverages, cooked cereal and cereal gruel, eggs, and cottage cheese) are usually tolerated best. Substitute these for the standard exchanges. For example, cereal diluted with milk as a gruel or milk toast may substitute for part of the milk and bread allowance; eggnog for milk and meat; pureed vegetable diluted with milk and served as a vegetable–milk soup for vegetable and milk, and fruit juices, carbonated beverages, or sweetened gelatin for fruit exchanges. The insulin-dependent diabetic in particular may need to consume sweetened carbonated beverages and sweetened gelatin. It is most important that some portion of the carbohydrate and kilocalorie allowance be consumed even on a limited kilocalorie in-

TABLE 24–10
EXAMPLE OF A MEAL PLAN

Exchange List	Morning Meal	Noon Meal	Evening Meal	Snack
Milk, skim	1		1	1
Vegetable		1	1	
Fruit	1	1		
Bread	2	3	3	1
Meat, low-fat	1	2	2	
Fat	2	2	2	1

take, and a protocol of eating small frequent feedings of carbohydrates that provide 50 to 75 g for each 6 to 8 hour period will help prevent hypoglycemia or ketosis. Usually a missed meal may be satisfactorily replaced by 50 g of carbohydrate taken by mouth over a 4 to 6 hour period. If oral intake in not possible, it may be necessary to give glucose intravenously. The carbohydrate content of selected foods is given in Table 24–11.

During acute illness, instruct all diabetics to test the urine for sugar and acetone more frequently than usual. The noninsulin-dependent diabetic may require transient insulin therapy during the illness. For the diabetic, planned surgery is usually managed with intravenous glucose infusions with concomitant administration of short-acting insulin injections to control the blood glucose. The postoperative period is managed in a similar manner (or even with continuous insulin infusion) until food can be taken orally.

Alcohol accounts for 7 to 10 percent of the kilocalories consumed by the general U.S. population, but its consumption presents a special problem to the diabetic not only because of its rapid absorption and possible contribution to weight gain (alcohol provides 7.1 kcal/g) but also because of its effects on blood glucose. It may have either a hyperglycemic or hypoglycemic effect, depending on the metabolic state when ingested. In the nonfasting state, large doses of alcohol may cause a small, transient rise in the blood sugar, occurring late in the course of alcohol intake and frequently when the plasma alcohol concentration is declining. In contrast, alcohol consumption may induce hypoglycemia in the fasting state. Although alcohol alone does not stimulate insulin secretion or require insulin for metabolism, consumption of alcohol by those taking insulin or oral hypoglycemic agents tends to promote hypoglycemia, especially if meals are missed or delayed, presumably by reducing gluconeogenesis. Additionally, alcohol in moderate amounts appears to enhance the glucose-lowering action of insulin or other hypoglycemic agents and prolong the effect of a single insulin injection. Alcohol may promote hypertriglyceridemia in predisposed subjects, ketoacidosis, and, in some persons taking sulfonylureas, annoying symptoms of flushing, palpitations, tingling, and chest tightness have been noted due to alcohol–sulfonylurea interactions. The mechanism underlying the latter syndrome is not understood, but it is similar in some respects to the alcohol–Antabuse (disulfiram) interaction. Further, alcohol consumption may be associated with irregularities in eating, and the symptoms of intoxication are not dissimilar to those of hypoglycemia. For these reasons, instruct clients to use alcohol only when the diabetes is under control, to use it in moderation only, and to take it with meals or snacks to avoid hypoglycemia. Many alcoholic beverages contain appreciable amounts of sugar or carbohydrate. Whereas hard liquor (i.e., gin, vodka, rum, whisky) contains no carbohydrate, it does contain a considerable amount of alcohol that can be substituted occasionally for an appropriate number of fat exchanges by the noninsulin-dependent diabetic, since alcohol is metabolized like fat. Insulin-dependent diabetics of normal weight whose diabetes is well controlled may regard as an extra the occasional use of alcoholic beverages that do not contain carbohydrate. If alcohol is used daily, however, its energy value must be included in the meal plan. Advise clients to avoid drinks that contain a lot of sugar, such as sweet wines, liqueurs, and sugar-containing mixes. Beer, ale, and wine, which contain carbohydrate, can be substituted for fruit or bread exchanges. The following formula can be used to calculate the kilocalories provided by alcohol:

$$0.8 \times \text{proof} \times \text{no. oz} = \text{kcal}$$

See Chapter 23 for examples of substitutions.

The average American eats more salt than is necessary, and in some, this excessive salt consumption may promote hypertension. Hypertension is not uncommon in obese diabetics, and in these individuals, consider sodium restriction. Moreover, modest reduction in the intake of salt should be considered for well-controlled diabetics who do not have other medical problems.

A great many special dietetic foods are available for use with numerous diet modifications, but many of these foods are not designed for kilocalorie-controlled diets. Some products are prepared without sugar, salt, or other ingredients. In general these special foods are more expensive than standard products, and even though the food may be prepared without added sucrose, it may contain appreciable amounts of carbohydrate and kilocalories. Various dietetic cakes, cookies, candies, ice cream, and pud-

TABLE 24–11
CARBOHYDRATE CONTENT OF SELECTED FOODS

Food	Amount	Carbohydrate Content (g)
Orange juice	½ c	10
Banana	½	10
Regular soft drink	½ c	10
Popsicle	½ twin pop	10
Regular Jello	¼ c	10
Lifesaver candy	6	10
Sugar cubes	5 small	10
Sugar	2½ tsp	10
Honey	2 tsp	10
Milk	1 c	12
Unsweetened eggnog	1 c	12
Cream soup	1 c	12
Yoghurt	1 c	12
Sugar	3 tsp	12

ding mixes are available, but these frequently contain a larger number of kilocalories and may contain more fat than the products they were designed to replace.

Many diabetics have the mistaken notion that special dietetic foods are a necessary component of the diabetic diet. Moreover, labeling information may be confusing and misleading, giving the erroneous impression that the foods do not contain a significant number of kilocalories and can be used freely. When used, these foods should be substituted for regular foods in the diet. Alternate sweetening agents, such as fructose, sorbitol, mannitol, and xylitol, are sometimes mistakenly assumed to be noncaloric, but the kilocalories they provide must be calculated in the diet.

Give diabetics information about the correct interpretation of nutrition information available on food labels. The ingredient listed first on the label is present in the largest quantity and other ingredients are listed in descending order of proportionate quantity. Those ingredients ending in "ose" are sugars, i.e., lactose, sucrose, fructose, and the use of foods with these ingredients must be limited appropriately. Food labels that state the amount of kilocalories, carbohydrate, protein, and fat can be used to estimate food exchanges.[17] When composition and portion size are known, various convenience foods can be incorporated into the exchange system. Some food processors and fast-food chains provide detailed lists of Food Exchange equivalents of their products. In other instances, the client may request specific information about nutrient composition from the manufacturer.

In most instances, it should be unnecessary to purchase special foods. The diet can be selected from the same food prepared for the rest of the family. Some may wish to use an artificial sweetener to sweeten beverages, such as coffee and tea, and to buy artificially sweetened or water-packed fruit, fruit packed in its own juice, and artificially sweetened gelatin, puddings, and soft drinks. When using fruits packed in their own juice, allowance should be made for the carbohydrate contained in the juice. An alternate approach to the use of artificial sweeteners is to encourage the client to become accustomed to a low-sugar regimen. After a period of time, the craving for sweets may diminish.

At present, saccharin is the only nonnutritive sweetener available in the United States, and its fate is uncertain. Aspartame, the low-calorie nutritive sweetener available in tablets or single-serving packages, can be used as a sweetener for cold or warm beverages, gelatin, puddings, fillings, and toppings but is not suitable for baked products, since it loses its sweetening power at high cooking temperatures. Although aspartame contains 4 kcal/g, it is 180 to 200 times sweeter than sucrose. Therefore, it need be used in only small amounts, and its kilocalorie contribution is insignificant. Fructose, sorbitol, and xylitol are also used as sugar substitutes. These sugars are absorbed from the gastrointestinal tract more slowly than glucose and do not significantly raise blood glucose when consumed as pure substances in modest amounts by clients with well-controlled diabetes. In poorly controlled diabetics, however, the use of these substances may lead to a significant rise in blood glucose concentration. Long-term studies are needed to evaluate the effects of adding a substantial quantity of these sugars to meals. Large intakes of the substances are known to produce an osmotic diarrhea, and xylitol has been reported to be a possible tumor-causing substance. Unlike saccharin, these are kilocalorie-containing substances, providing equivalent kilocalories as an equal amount of sucrose. Since fructose is sweeter than sucrose, slightly less may be required to give the same sweetness as table sugar. However, its sweetness decreases as temperature, concentration, and acidity increase. The sweet taste is also altered by incorporation into food, cooking, and the taste threshold of the individual. Further studies are needed in order to draw firm conclusions about the metabolic effects of these sweeteners before significant use in diabetic diets can be recommended. As an alternate to the use of sweetening agents, suggest to the client that fruits and spices may satisfy the taste for sweets. Fruit consumption, however, must be limited to the allowed amount.

Table 24–12 provides a summary of dietary strategies for control of insulin-dependent and non-insulin-dependent diabetes.

Monitoring the Control of Diabetes. Daily urine testing for glucose and acetone, along with periodic blood glucose and hemoglobin A_{1c} determinations, form the basis for determining the adequacy of diabetic control. Urine testing is done before meals and before breakfast, and a double-voided specimen (emptying the bladder and testing the next voided specimen) is used. Periodically, fractional (or block) urine specimens are collected over a 24-hour period. This represents the amount of glucose excreted in the urine at different periods during the day. Concomitant use of certain drugs can cause false-positive or false-negative tests for glucose, and large doses of vitamin C can cause a false-positive result. Some diabetics monitor their own blood glucose several times daily by smearing a drop of blood from a pricked finger on a chemically treated reagent strip, Chemstrip bG, or by use of a reflectance meter. When blood glucose is checked daily, the urine does not have to be tested for glucose, although acetone levels should still be checked. Insulin dosage, exercise, or food intake can be adjusted depending on the blood and urine results.

Client Education. Instruct the client regarding the basic nature of diabetes mellitus and the rationale for the treatment, including the role of diet in controlling the disorder. Surveys tend to show that a significant percentage of diabetic clients do not fol-

TABLE 24–12
SUMMARY OF DIETARY STRATEGIES FOR CONTROL OF DIABETES

Strategy	Obese Diabetics Who Do not Require Insulin	Nonobese, Insulin-dependent Diabetics and Those Taking Oral Agents
Nutritional requirements	Same as nondiabetics of same age, sex, height, activity; decrease kcal	Same as nondiabetics of same age, sex, height, activity
Regularity of meal time	Not essential but may aid weight loss	Yes (planned to correlate with pattern of insulin and exercise)
Increased frequency and number of meals	Usually no (four to five daily feedings may be desirable if this can be done without exceeding kilocalorie allowance)	Yes (planned to correlate with pattern of insulin and exercise)
Consistency of meal composition relative to carbohydrate, protein, and fat content and consistency of meal size	Not crucial; distribution of carbohydrate among meals may minimize swings in blood sugar, however	Yes
Allow extra food for unusual exercise	No diet adjustments necessary	Usually appropriate (increase carbohydrate intake before and during unusual exercise)
Use food to treat hypoglycemia	Not necessary	Yes
During complicating illnesses, provide small frequent carbohydrate feedings or give carbohydrate IV to prevent starvation ketosis	Often not necessary because of resistance to ketosis	Yes
Alcohol	Use discouraged because of its high kcal value and its appetite-stimulating effect; if used, substitute for fat exchange	If allowed, take with food; occasional use may be considered as extra; avoid if taking sulfonylurea, which may cause intolerance

(*Source: Adapted from West KM: Diet and diabetes. Postgrad Med 60:210, 1976.*)

low their prescribed diet on a long-term basis. One factor contributing to this is misunderstanding by the client of the aims of diet therapy and the mechanics of the diet, including the Food Exchange Lists. Another is diet prescriptions that do not fit the clients' needs relative to age, sex, occupation, cultural, social, and economic status, level of intelligence and education, and degree of incentive and self-discipline. Success rates for weight reduction are also low. Even with an ongoing supervised weight reduction program, the results of weight reduction in diabetics are not necessarily better than in the nondiabetic obese population. These findings point to a need for more effective nutritional care, including individualized diet prescriptions and effective counseling. Assist the health team in tailoring the diet prescription to the client's eating habits and lifestyle; for example, supply a vegetarian diet pattern for a vegetarian, plan sufficient quantities of a particular food that is staple to a given cultural

or ethnic group, and plan for the use of low-cost foods when income is low. Integrate the insulin and diet therapy; for example, adjust the administration of insulin in relation to the usual eating schedules. If an individual is accustomed to eating the main meal at noon, that pattern should be continued, and insulin administrations should be adjusted to that timing. Insulin-dependent diabetics often find it easier to adjust the insulin regimen than to change basic eating habits.

Vegetarianism can be an acceptable way to eat, and lacto-vegetarian and lacto-ovo-vegetarian diets (see Chap. 20) can be nutritionally adequate. Nutritional adequacy is jeopardized, however, if dairy products or eggs are omitted, and some supplementation with vitamins and minerals may be necessary. Additional supplements are necessary for vegan diets.

Focus nutrition education on the level of individual needs. Begin the initial counseling session by taking a diet history, thus providing information about eating patterns and the extent of changes in these patterns that will be necessary. Emphasize these points about the diet in instruction:

1. The purpose of the diet
2. The relation of the diet to the overall management of the disease
3. The potential for reducing the acute and long-term complications
4. The specific characteristics of the diet, including:
   a. A list of foods to avoid
   b. A list of foods that can be used in any amount
   c. The number of daily meals
   d. The number and size of servings of foods to use at each meal
   e. Substitutions that are possible, i.e., the Food Exchange Lists (see Appendix 2), if this system is used
   f. The interpretation of food labels
   g. The methods of food preparation that are appropriate
   h. The degree of flexibility possible in interpreting the diet

Make dietary recommendations as flexible as possible—a flexible meal plan may be more acceptable to less compulsive persons, whereas, compulsive persons may find a rigid dietary regimen more suitable. Interpretation of the diet should be liberalized, particularly for children, to allow for occasional party dishes. However, emphasize the difference between occasional overconsumption and persistent dietary indiscretion. The weighing of food portions is seldom necessary on a long-term basis, although the practice of weighing and measuring foods may be useful initially to gain precision in estimating weights and amounts. For some it may be desirable to teach the carbohydrate, protein, and fat content of common foods to allow a greater degree of options in food choices than provided by the Exchange Lists alone. Moreover, the Food Exchange Lists can be modified to meet the needs of individual clients, for example, allowing unlimited use of vegetables except those exceptionally high in kilocalories or allowing substitutions between the bread and fruit list (a bread exchange is roughly equal to one and one-half fruit exchanges).

Give the client specific instructions regarding special situations that may arise. Regular exercise should be stressed, but give guidance on how to regulate insulin dosages or food intake during periods of increased or erratic exercise or when regularly scheduled exercise is decreased. Guidelines should be given for other special situations, such as dietary adjustments needed when eating out, when alcohol is used, and when variations in appetite occur from day to day or with acute illness. To avoid hypoglycemia by those taking hypoglycemic agents when meals are unavoidably delayed, instruct the client to eat a readily available source of carbohydrate. Also advise diabetic clients to increase exercise during times of emotional upset to avoid hyperglycemia.

Many clients ask about the use of special dietetic foods, fast foods, convenience foods, and mixed dishes, and appropriate information should be provided.

Be sensitive to the timing of the instruction. For example, after diagnosis, the client must learn to cope with a long-term chronic illness and may not be able to initially integrate the information needed to make the necessary behavioral changes. Use meal trays as a teaching aid for the hospitalized client. With guidance the client can learn the size of portions allowed and become familiar with items in each exchange group. Those foods that do not appear on the tray, such as sugar, jelly, pies, cakes, and fruits canned in sugar syrup, can also be emphasized. Selective menus, food models, and other visual devices, such as measuring cups and spoons and various sizes of glasses and cups, are useful teaching aids. It is imperative that an appropriate family member understand and be able to implement the daily meal plan if this becomes necessary. Since adequate instruction takes a considerable amount of time, follow-up counseling is particularly important.

Coping with a chronic disease, superimposed upon the emotional conflicts of childhood and adolescence, poses additional problems for the child and family. Give children with diabetes the responsibility of planning their own diets from family meals. By so doing, they learn to plan their diets for meals eaten away from home.

A variety of educational resources are available, and many printed materials have been prepared by health agencies, pharmaceutical firms, such professional organizations as the American Diabetes Association, the American Dietetic Association, and others. Problems encountered when using printed materials include insufficient education on the part of the client, inability to read English, and failing vision. Some diet plans have been specially prepared for people of different ethnic backgrounds, such as Mexican-Americans, Chinese, Italians, and others.

REVIEW QUESTIONS AND ACTIVITIES

1. Describe the hormonal control of the blood glucose concentration.
2. Describe the symptoms of hypoglycemia.
3. Differentiate between reactive hypoglycemia and fasting hypoglycemia in relation to time of onset of symptoms and examples of conditions that precipitate them.
4. Identify the protocol for a glucose tolerance test.
5. Compare dietary strategies for control of reactive hypoglycemia and fasting hypoglycemia.

6. Classify the principal types of diabetes mellitus.
7. Explain the rationale for the pathologic manifestations of diabetes mellitus.
8. Identify the postulated etiologic factors in diabetes mellitus.
9. Differentiate between hypoglycemia, hyperglycemia, ketoacidosis, and nonketotic hyperosmolar coma in relation to precipitating factors, symptoms, and treatment.
10. Explain the honeymoon phase of diabetes in children and the Somogyi phenomenon.
11. Identify the relationships among exercise, diet, and hypoglycemic agents in the management of diabetes mellitus.
12. Compare and contrast the dietary strategies used in treating insulin-dependent diabetes mellitus and noninsulin-dependent diabetes mellitus.
13. Identify the appropriate proportions of carbohydrate, protein, and fat in a diabetic diet.
14. Use the six Food Exchange Lists in assisting diabetic clients with dietary management.
15. Describe dietary adjustments for each of the following situations in diabetic clients: (a) unusual exercise, (b) delayed meals, (c) periods of acute illness, (d) use of alcohol, and (e) use of special dietetic foods.

REFERENCES

1. Leichter SB: Alimentary hypoglycemia: A new appraisal. Am J Clin Nutr 32:2104, 1979.
2. Bihormonal theory of diabetes gets solid backing. JAMA 26:1685, 1982.
3. West KM: Diet and diabetes. Postgrad Med 60:209, 1976.
4. National Diabetes Data Group: Classification and diagnosis of diabetes mellitus and other categories of glucose intolerance. Diabetes 28:1039, 1979.
5. Levin ME, Boniak I, Anderson CB, Avioli LV: Prevention and treatment of diabetic complications. Arch Intern Med 140:692, 1980.
6. Colwell JA, Halushkay PV, Sanji KE, et al.: Vascular disease in diabetes: Pathophysiological mechanisms and therapy. Arch Intern Med 139:225, 1979.
7. Clement SR, Vourganti B, Darnell B, et al.: Effect of low and high dietary myoinositol content upon nerve conduction velocities in neuropathy diabetes. Diabetes 27 [Suppl 2]:436, 1978.
8. Rupp WM, Barbosa JJ, Blackshear PJ, et al.: The use of an implantable insulin pump in the treatment of type II diabetes. N Engl J Med 307:265, 1982.
9. Mecklenburg RS, Benson JW, Becker NM, et al.: Clinical use of the insulin infusion pump in 100 patients with type I diabetes. N Engl J Med 307:513, 1982.
10. American Diabetes Association, American Dietetic Association: A Guide to Professionals: The Effective Application of Exchange Lists for Meal Planning. New York and Chicago, 1977, p 4.
11. Franklin BA, Rubenfine M: Losing weight through exercise. JAMA 244:377, 1980.
12. Konishi F: Food energy equivalents of various activities. J Am Diet Assoc 46:187, 1965.
13. Vahoney GV: Dietary fibers, lipid metabolism, and atherosclerosis. Fed Proc 41:2801, 1982.
14. Glycemic effects of carbohydrates. J Am Diet Assoc 84:1487, 1984.
15. Diabetes Care and Education Practice Group of the American Dietetic Association: Diabetes mellitus and glycemic responses to different foods: Summary and annotated bibliography. Chicago, American Dietetic Association, 1983.
16. American Diabetes Association, American Dietetic Association: Exchange Lists for Meal Planning. New York and Chicago, 1976.
17. U.S. DHEW, Food and Drug Administration: Using Nutrition Labels with Food Exchange Lists. HEW Publication No. FDA 77–2072, Rockville, Md, 1977.

BIBLIOGRAPHY

Hypoglycemia

Crapo PA, Scarlett JA, Kolterman OG, et al.: The effects of oral fructose, sucrose, and glucose in subjects with reactive hypoglycemia. Diabetes Care 5:512, 1982.

Foä PP, Dunbar JC, Klein SP, et al.: Reactive hypoglycemia and A-cell ("pancreatic") glucagon deficiency in the adult. JAMA 244:2281, 1980.

Hale F: Hypoglycemia. Biol Psychiatry 17:125, 1982.

Johnson DD, Dorr KE, Swenson WM, Service FJ: Reactive hypoglycemia. JAMA 243:1151, 1980.

Diabetes Mellitus

Anderson JW, Chandler C: High fiber diet benefits for diabetics. Diabetes Educ 7:34, 1981.

Craig JW: Clinical implications of the new diabetes classifications. Postgrad Med 68:122, 1980.

El-Beheri Burges BRB: Rationale for changes in the dietary management of diabetes. J Am Diet Assoc 81:258, 1982.

Franz MJ: Diabetes mellitus: Considerations in the development of guidelines for the occasional use of alcohol. J Am Diet Assoc 83:147, 1983.

Grinvalsky M, Nathan DM: Diets for insulin pump and multiple daily injection therapy. Diabetes Care 6:241, 1983.

Khachadurin AK, Noronha JL, Amorosa LF: Management of noninsulin-dependent diabetes mellitus. Am Fam Phys 21:154, 1980.

Koivisto V, Soman V, Nadel E, et al.: Exercise and insulin: Insulin binding, insulin mobilization, and counterregulatory hormone secretion. Fed Proc 39:1481, 1980.

Kulkarni K: Advice from the dietitians. Vegetarian diets. Diabetes Educ 9:35, 1983.

Olefsky JM, Crapo P: Fructose, xylitol, and sorbitol: A review. Diabetes Care 3:390, 1980.

Prater B: Educational guidelines for self-care living with diabetes. J Am Diet Assoc 82:283, 1983.

Rosenbloom AL, Kohrman A, Sperling M: Classification and diagnosis of diabetes mellitus in children and adolescents. J Pediatr 99:320, 1981.

Wylie-Rosett J: Development of new educational strategies for the person with diabetes. J Am Diet Assoc 81:268, 1982.

Client Resources

American Diabetes Association: Diabetes Forecast (Bimonthly magazine).

American Diabetes Association, American Dietetic Association: Exchange Lists for Meal Planning. New York and Chicago, 1976.

American Diabetes Association, American Dietetic Association: Family Cookbook. Englewood Cliffs, NJ, Prentice-Hall, 1981.

American Diabetes Association, Washington, DC, Area Affiliate, Inc: Supplement to Exchange Lists for Meal Planning, Jewish Cookery. Washington, DC, 1978.

Brown A: The Diabetic Gourmet. New York, Barnes & Noble, 1980.

Cinnamon PA, Swanson MA: Everything You Always Wanted to Know About Exchange Values for Food. Moscow, Idaho, University Press of Idaho, 1976.

Exchange Lists for the Blind, 1978. Volunteer Braille Services, 3017 Harvard Ave., Suite 203, Metairie, La, 70002.

Finsand MJ: The Complete Diabetic Cookbook. New York, Sterling, 1980.

Middleton K, Hess MA: The Art of Cooking for the Diabetic (paperback). Chicago, Contemporary Books, 1979.

U.S. DHHS: Cookbooks for People with Diabetes, Selected Annotations. NIH Publication No. 81–2177, Bethesda, Md, 1981.

Wason CD, Coyle VC, Moss FT: Select-A-Meal (A Personal Meal Plan). Rocky Mount, NC, American Diabetes Association, NC Affiliate, Inc, 1978.

CHAPTER 25

Nutrition and Endocrine Disorders:
Thyroid, Parathyroid, Adrenal, and Pituitary Disorders

Objectives

After completion of this chapter, the student will be able to:

1. Compare and contrast the nutritional effects of hyperthyroidism and hypothyroidism.

2. Develop a nursing care plan for the nutritional management of a client with hyperthyroidism and adjust it to be appropriate for a client with hypothyroidism.

3. Distinguish between the dietary strategies for controlling the abnormal blood calcium concentration in clients with hyperparathyroidism and hypoparathyroidism.

4. Compare and contrast the nutritional effects and dietary management of Addison's disease and Cushing's syndrome.

5. Distinguish among the nutritional management of primary aldosteronism, pituitary diabetes insipidus, and the syndrome associated with inappropriate secretion of the antidiuretic hormone.

6. Plan an appropriate diet for an infant during the first year who has nephrogenic diabetes insipidus.

The thyroid, parathyroid, adrenal, and pituitary are endocrine glands that perform vital body functions, including control of metabolic processes and integration of the body's response to stress. Metabolic abnormalities associated with their dysfunction are extensive and encompass various nutritional imbalances, including imbalances of body weight. Fortunately, surgery and hormonal replacement can restore functional capacity in many instances. Dietary modifications, however, are a component of the treatment of the acute phase of some of the disorders and of the supportive therapy that is necessary for the ongoing management of others.

In order for nurses to give responsible nutritional care and diet counseling for clients with endocrine disorders and to interact with other members of the health care team from a theoretical base that supports effective nutritional care, it is necessary to have an understanding of the hormonal–nutrient metabolism interrelationships and of the specific diet modifications necessitated by the hormonal imbalance and its treatment.

ABNORMALITIES IN FUNCTIONING OF THE THYROID GLAND

Abnormal functioning of the thyroid gland may result from either an oversecretion or an undersecretion of the thyroid hormones (thyroxine, or T_4, and triiodothyronine, or T_3) needed to regulate a variety of body processes. Because of the role of these hormones in regulating the metabolic rate, the metabolism of carbohydrate, protein, and fat, and their effects on growth and bone maturation, an imbalance

361

will have far-reaching effects. The effects of T$_3$ and T$_4$ on the biochemical processes of the body as they relate to nutrient metabolism are:

1. Regulation of the metabolic rate. Increase oxygen consumption and metabolic activity of most body tissues.
2. Regulation of the metabolism of protein, carbohydrate, and lipid.
   a. *Carbohydrate.* Increase glucose absorption from the gastrointestinal tract and oxidation of glucose by the cells. They also stimulate gluconeogenesis and glycogenolysis to increase the supply of glucose for oxidation.
   b. *Lipid.* Enhance mobilization of lipids from adipose tissue with an increase in plasma free fatty acid concentration and accelerated oxidation of free fatty acids by the cells. Fatty acid synthesis is enhanced to a lesser degree. In contrast, thyroid hormones lead to a lowering of the serum cholesterol by increasing the conversion of cholesterol to bile acids and increasing the excretion of cholesterol and bile acids in the feces. Cholesterol synthesis is enhanced to a lesser degree. With diminished thyroid secretion, the concentrations of cholesterol, phospholipids, and triglycerides are increased, and there is excessive fat deposition in the liver.
   c. *Protein.* Increase the rate of both protein anabolism and catabolism. Because they stimulate protein synthesis, thyroid hormones are necessary for growth. Excessive secretion of thyroid hormones can, however, stimulate protein catabolism and negative nitrogen balance by depleting energy resources from carbohydrate and fat, necessitating the use of protein for energy by enhanced gluconeogenesis.
3. Alternation of vitamin metabolism. Increase the production of various enzymes, and since some vitamins such as those needed for energy oxidation are an essential part of coenzymes, the hormones bring an increase in the need for certain vitamins.
4. Effects on growth and bone metabolism. Promote protein anabolism; they are therefore essential for normal growth, including bone growth. Thyroid hormones lead to rapid closure of the epiphyses (ossification centers at extremities of long bone) and to an increase in osteoclastic (bone destruction) activity. Thus excessive secretion can lead to premature closure of the epiphyses in young people, and final height achieved may be below normal, and the enhanced activity of osteoclasts may result in porous bones.
5. Effect on gastrointestinal function. Increase the rate of nutrient absorption, the rate of secretion of digestive juices, gastrointestinal motility, and the appetite.

With excessive secretion of the thyroid gland, all body processes are speeded up, whereas the opposite is true when the gland fails to secrete a normal amount of hormones. Diseases of the thyroid gland include (1) hyperthyroidism, (2) hypothyroidism, and (3) thyroid enlargement—goiter—without evidence of abnormal thyroid hormone production.

Hyperthyroidism

Assessment. Also called toxic goiter, thyrotoxicosis, Graves' disease, and Basedow's disease, **hyperthyroidism** may lead to an increase in the basal metabolic rate (BMR) by as much as 60 to 100 percent above normal, but more often the increase in BMR ranges between 40 and 60 percent. The condition, which is characterized by an accelerated rate of all metabolic processes, is more common in women than in men. Hyperthyroidism is thought to be a manifestation of an autoimmune disorder, although the condition occasionally results from a localized tumor in thyroid tissue that secretes large quantities of thyroid hormone.

Observe for marked hyperplasia of the thyroid gland and evaluate for excessive secretion of T$_3$ and T$_4$ and for these signs and symptoms in clients with hyperthyroidism: (1) weight loss, muscle wasting, weakness, and fatigue (even in the presence of an excessive appetite and increase in food intake) due to catabolism of endogenous protein and fat, (2) varying degrees of diarrhea associated with an increase in bowel motility, (3) demineralization of bone secondary to an increase in bone resorption, (4) glucose intolerance associated with an increase in intestinal glucose absorption, glycogenolysis and gluconeogenesis, and increased insulin degradation, and (5) depressed serum cholesterol due to increased conversion of cholesterol to bile acids and increased excretion of cholesterol and bile acids in the feces. Many clients develop a protrusion of the eyeballs (exophthalmos), which is thought to result from an increased accumulation of extracellular fluid. Assess the growth records of hyperthyroid children. Early manifestations of hyperthyroidism may be an acceleration of linear growth and bone maturation; should the hypermetabolic state continue to the point of weight loss, growth retardation may be the end result. Moreover, the epiphyses close at an early age so that eventual height achieved may be reduced.

Intervention. Until the disorder is controlled by medical management, diet considerations are important. These include management in the use of energy, protein, carbohydrate, fluids, and stimulants. Energy requirements may increase 15 to 25 percent above the normal recommended levels in mild cases and as much as 50 to 75 percent above normal in severe cases. Provide a diet that contains up to 4500 to 5000 kcal daily for clients with severe hyperthyroidism and increase the protein content in the diet of all hyperthyroid clients to 1 to 2 g/kg recommended body weight to offset the negative nitrogen balance. To compensate for the disordered carbohydrate metabolism, to supply energy, and to spare protein, liberalize the carbohydrate intake. Be aware, however, that thyroid hormones increase intestinal glucose absorption, and the blood glucose level will rise after carbohydrate-rich meals. Spacing the food into six feedings may be necessary in order to attain the desired kilocalorie and protein level. Be aware that the judicious use of cream, butter, jelly, jam, and sugars will quickly increase the kilocaloric level, but excessive use may provoke nausea and loss of appetite. Further guidelines for implementing a high-kilocalorie, high-protein diet are given in Chapter 23 (about underweight clients). The B-complex vitamins required for energy oxidation are needed in larger amounts concomitant with the larger kilocalorie intake, and for reasons not well understood, the use of vitamins A and C is also increased. Consider the option of recommending a vitamin supplement should the client not receive adequate amounts of these vitamins in the diet. Compensate for the increased fluid losses that occur with the increases in perspiration, BMR, and respiration by providing an average of 3000 to 4000 ml/ day. In the presence of exophthalmos, however, restrict the intake of both sodium and fluid. Extra calcium and phosphorus are needed to counteract the osteoporosis, and vitamin D is needed for intestinal absorption of calcium. Encourage the liberal use of vitamin D-fortified milk; calcium salts may also be necessary. Discourage the use of stimulants, such as coffee, tea, and cola beverages, and monitor the use of alcohol and tobacco, since these may aggravate nervousness. Replace regular coffee with decaffeinated coffee. Instruct the client to avoid highly seasoned and fibrous foods, since these will increase peristalsis and aggravate the diarrhea.

Involve the client in all aspects of the diet plan to ensure an understanding of its rationale. Provide a mealtime environment that is quiet to encourage an adequate intake of food. Once the condition has been treated, take measures to prevent excessive kilocalorie consumption so as to avoid obesity. The appetite does not necessarily decrease as the disease is controlled.

Hypothyroidism

Assessment. Deficient production or activity of thyroid hormones brings **hypothyroidism** (myxedema or Gull's disease), a disorder more common in women than in men. Depending on the age of onset, hypothyroidism may be classified as (1) adult hypothyroidism or myxedema, (2) juvenile hypothyroidism (if occurring in childhood), or (3) congenital hypothyroidism or cretinism (if it develops in fetal life or shortly after birth). The disorder may result from chronic thyroiditis (Hashimoto's disease), surgical removal of the thyroid gland or its destruction by radiation therapy or disease, a congenital defect, iodine deficiency, or excessive intake of goitrogenic substances (see Chap. 9).

In general, the effects of hypothyroidism are the opposite of those of hyperthyroidism. A decrease in thyroid activity is reflected in depressed thyroid function tests. Observe for these manifestations, which have implications for nutritional therapy, in adult hypothyroid clients: (1) a decline in the BMR (as much as 30 percent below normal), (2) fluid retention secondary to mucoprotein deposition in subcutaneous and extracellular spaces that pulls fluids into these spaces, (3) constipation, (4) elevated blood triglycerides and cholesterol, and (5) moderate anemia resulting from depressed bone marrow metabolism and depressed intestinal absorption of vitamin B_{12}. Weight gain is not an essential feature of the disease. Although catabolism is reduced, so is the appetite. Weight gain may be evident in some clients, however, who fail to reduce food intake proportionate to the reduced metabolism, and part of the excess weight may be due to fluid retention.

In children, hypothyroidism results in delayed growth and bone maturation and delayed epiphyseal closure. Both physical and mental growth are greatly retarded in cretinism, the congenital or infantile form of advanced hypothyroidism. Observe that cretins are often significantly heavier at birth than normal newborns, prenatal osseous development is retarded, and neonatal jaundice is prolonged. Cretinous children may have large tongues that obstruct swallowing and breathing. The abdomen is large, and an umbilical hernia is usually present.

Intervention. Hypothyroidism is treated by the administration of thyroid extracts. In treating children, exert caution to assure a balance of hormones that allows for a positive nitrogen balance without precipitating protein catabolism and growth deficits. Treat cretins soon after birth to diminish the degree of retardation. Since feeding difficulties are prominent during the first month of life, provide ongoing support for the child's parents.

Reduce the kilocalorie level in the diet of hypothyroid clients in accordance with the low metabolic rate and the degree of overweight (if present). Principles of kilocalorie reduction are discussed in Chapter 23. Counteract the constipation by assuring that the diet contains an adequate amount of fluid, fiber, and natural laxative foods, such as bran and prunes. Encourage the client to drink six to eight glasses of water daily. Monitor fluid intake carefully, however, since excessive fluids could lead to fluid retention. Since the client's appetite may be poor, provide suggestions for serving food attractively.

For those at risk of developing hypothyroidism because of low iodine intake, encourage the use of iodized salt. Assess the adequacy of iodine intake in pregnant women, particularly when a sodium-restricted diet is imposed. Under normal conditions of use, intake of goitrogens in such foods as cabbage and turnips presents no problems, but the potential exists for the development of goiter and hypothyroidism when large quantities are consumed with a concomitant low iodine intake. Encourage thorough cooking of these vegetables to inactivate the antithyroid agents.

PARATHYROID GLAND DISORDERS

Because of the role of the parathyroid (PTH) in maintaining a constant level of ionized calcium and phosphorus in the blood and a correct ratio of calcium to phosphorus, parathyroid gland abnormalities are associated with problems related to imbalance of these two minerals.

Assessment

Excessive or deficient secretion of PTH (hyperparathyroidism and hypoparathyroidism) lead to abnormal blood levels of calcium and phosphorus. Hyperparathyroidism leads to hypercalcemia and hypophosphatemia and may result from primary hyperparathyroidism (secondary to a tumor or hyperphasia of the gland) or from the secretion of parathyroid-like hormones by nonparathyroid malignancies. Secondary hyperparathyroidism is a usual accompaniment of vitamin D deficiency or renal failure, but hypercalcemia is not seen in these situations. In contrast, damage to the parathyroid gland during thyroid surgery, accidental removal of the glands with thyroidectomy, or other disorders, such as congenital defects and autoimmune destruction, lead to hypoparathyroidism with hypocalcemia and hyperphosphatemia. Observe in affected clients for manifestations of hypercalcemia and hypocalcemia that are summarized in Table 9–8. In addition, prolonged hypocalcemia can cause ectodermal lesions, such as changes in the skin (coarse, dry, scaly), hair (alopecia), and nails (thin, brittle, transverse grooves), as well as cataracts and changes in the teeth (delayed eruption with a hypoplastic appearance).

Intervention

Treatment of hyperparathyroidism and hypoparathyroidism involves medical management of the underlying disorders and pharmacologic measures to normalize the blood calcium level. Assist clients with hypercalcemia to drink 3000 to 4000 ml fluid daily to maintain a dilute urine and thus guard against a propensity to develop renal stones. Consider the intravenous administration of sodium to promote the renal clearance and excretion of calcium. A calcium-restricted diet should be considered only in the event that the imbalance is complicated by excessive absorption of calcium (see idiopathic hypercalciuria, Chap. 30).

To treat hypocalcemia provide a high-calcium, low-phosphorus diet. Since dairy products that are high in calcium are also high in phosphorus, this may be difficult to do, and it may be necessary to administer calcium salts and medications to decrease the intestinal absorption of phosphorus. Provide a supplement of vitamin D or its synthetic analogs to promote the intestinal absorption of calcium. Monitor the client closely, however, for signs of hypercalcemia. The physician may prescribe a magnesium supplement, since a deficiency of magnesium can impair the release of parathyroid hormone.

ABNORMALITIES OF THE ADRENAL GLANDS

Abnormalities of adrenal function are due to an excess or deficit in the secretion of glucocorticoids (primarily cortisol) and mineralocorticoids (primarily aldosterone), resulting from a variety of congenital or acquired diseases of the hypothalamus, pituitary gland, or adrenal cortex. Excessive and prolonged steroid therapy may also lead to adrenal hyperfunction or hypofunction. Symptoms associated with adrenal malfunction may be mild or severe, insidious or abrupt in onset, and temporary or permanent, and they may begin in infancy or later in life. The nutritional ramifications of these imbalances are widespread because of the effects of glucocorticoids and mineralocorticoids on nutrient metabolism. The effects of glucocorticoids are:

- *Carbohydrate.* Increase blood glucose level by enhancing hepatic gluconeogenesis (in concert with glucagon) and diminished cellular glucose use; enhance hepatic glycogenesis.
- *Protein.* Provide substrates for hepatic glucose synthesis by (1) increasing protein catabolism (particularly in muscles, skin and connective tissue, and lymphoid tissue) and (2) decrease protein synthesis; stimulate the synthesis of hepatic enzymes that synthesize glucose.
- *Lipid.* Inhibit lipogenesis and permit the lipolytic effect of catecholamines and other hormones.
- *Calcium.* Exert an antagonistic effect on the intestinal absorption of calcium by vitamin D (this property makes glucocorticoids useful in treating certain types of hypercalcemia).
- *Vitamin C.* Considerable amounts of vitamin C are present in adrenal tissue; oversecretion of the hormones may deplete adrenal tissue of the vitamin.

Although glucocorticoids have minimal effects on fluid and electrolyte balance, excessive quantities have mineralocorticoid effects. Gastric secretory activity is increased by the glucocorticoids, and there may be an increase in hydrochloric acid and pepsin secretion in individuals who take large doses of glucocorticoids for therapeutic purposes. It has been suggested that steroids may alter gastric mucosal protective factors, contributing to ulcer formation in those taking steroids. Moreover, glucocorticoids enhance red blood cell formation, and excessive quantities stimulate the appetite and can contribute to obesity.

Because glucocorticoids have the property of suppressing the inflammatory response, these hormones and their synthetic analogs are widely used in treating a host of conditions that have an allergic or inflammatory component. They are therapeutically effective, but various side effects related to metabolic activity and action on various organ systems have been noted. The products used vary somewhat in the degree of their effects on metabolism. Some of the synthetic analogs, such as dexamethasone, have enhanced glucocorticoid activity and minimal mineralocorticoid activity. Thus, it is important to consider the implications of diet–drug relationships when there is long-term use of the hormones. Additionally, the immunosuppressive and antiinflammatory effects of large doses of steroids may lead to an inability to withstand the stress of acute infections. Prolonged pharmacologic doses of glucocorticoids lead to persistent suppression of the release of ACTH by the pituitary and Cushing's syndrome. In response to stress or acute withdrawal of the drug, adrenal insufficiency may result.

Mineralocorticoids maintain sodium balance and extracellular fluid volume. The basic mechanism of action of aldosterone is to increase the renal reabsorption of sodium, although there are many secondary effects, such as an increase in water reabsorption and an increase in urinary potassium loss.

Adrenal Insufficiency

▶ *Assessment.* **Addison's disease,** or **adrenal insufficiency,** is associated with a failure of the secretion of the adrenocortical hormones due to atrophy, disease, or surgical removal of the glands or acute corticosteroid withdrawal after long-term treatment. The manifestations are those of mineralocorticoid and glucocorticoid deficiency. Observe for an increased urinary loss of sodium, chloride, and water, causing a decrease in extracellular fluid volume and hypotension due to the lack of aldosterone secretion. The kidneys retain potassium, causing high serum potassium levels, and there is a concomitant metabolic acidosis. Assess for these signs of cortisol deficiency: (1) altered mobilization of protein and fat, (2) fasting hypoglycemia (due to failure of gluconeogenesis and glycogenesis), (3) increased sensitivity of peripheral tissues to insulin, and (4) increased susceptibility to the deteriorating effects of stress, such as infection, surgery, or trauma. Anorexia, nausea, weight loss, and a low taste threshold

for salt are common in addisonian clients. Unless the disease is treated, or if there is a concomitant trauma, the client is susceptible to addisonian crisis. Suspect this complication if the client's symptoms include hypoglycemia, hyponatremia, hyperkalemia, and shock. Precrisis symptoms include poor heat tolerance, abdominal discomfort, diarrhea, anorexia, vomiting, and weight loss.

Intervention. Treatment involves a combination of hormonal replacement and nutritional management. Hormonal management involves replacement of glucocorticoids, such as cortisol, cortisone, and prednisone, that exert glucocorticoid and mineralocorticoid activity. Should orthostatic hypotension persist, a synthetic sodium-retaining hormone, such as fludrocortisone, may be added. Nutritional management requires attention to the sodium and potassium content of the diet as well as measures to control the fasting hypoglycemia. In acute situations, encourage the client to consume a liberal amount of sodium (174 mEq or more or 4 g or more) to replace urinary losses and to restrict the intake of foods high in potassium to prevent hyperkalemia. Also instruct the client to consume adequate fluids to prevent dehydration and provide supplements of the B-complex vitamins and vitamin C to support the increased metabolism associated with the disease management. These same interventions are appropriate when replacement therapy includes only the glucocorticoids with minimal mineralocorticoid activity, such as cortisol or cortisone. With combined therapy, no change is usually required in the sodium or potassium content of the diet. Foods of high salt content (such as condiments, potato chips, and cold cuts) and salt tablets can be used to achieve the desired sodium level, and foods extremely high in potassium should be avoided (see Chap. 9 for foods high in potassium). The use of salt tablets to provide sodium is questioned, however, since they do not dissolve well and may cause intestinal problems. Since fasting leads to hypoglycemic episodes, instruct the client to eat small frequent meals that are high in protein and low to moderate in carbohydrate content, restricting simple sugars. To prevent early morning hypoglycemia, include a bedtime snack and keep available such snacks as crackers and cheese if hypoglycemia occurs frequently. The practice of skipping meals should be avoided. When procedures are contemplated that necessitate fasting, the health care team should carry them out with caution.

Instruct the client to take glucocorticoids with milk or antacids to minimize gastric irritation and to weigh themselves at periodic intervals to ascertain progress. Excess weight may reflect fluid retention secondary to the medication or weight gain associated with a stimulation in appetite. Prolonged therapy may necessitate the opposite modifications: a potassium supplement and a diet restricted in sodium to prevent potassium depletion and sodium retention. Stress to the client the importance of keeping appointments for blood chemistry tests.

Adrenal Hypersecretion

Hypersecretion of the adrenal cortex can lead to Cushing's syndrome and primary hyperaldosteronism.

Cushing's Syndrome

Assessment. Cushing's syndrome may be associated with intrinsic defects in the adrenal cortex itself, or the disorder may be iatrogenic, i.e., occurring as a result of prolonged exogenous administration of pharmacologic doses of corticosteroids. The effects of administration of glucocorticoids resemble the effects of excess endogenous secretion of cortisol. Most of the abnormalities of the disorder are associated with glucocorticoid excess, but there may also be significant effects due to excesses of mineralocorticoids.

The effects of the glucocorticoid excess are:

1. Abnormal glucose tolerance, insulin resistance, and hyperglycemia (adrenal diabetes) resulting primarily from the enhanced gluconeogenesis and inhibition of glucose use. Latent diabetes may become unmasked, and diabetic clients may require additional insulin (if the glucose intolerance is a result of steroid therapy, it may be permanent in some clients but may diminish in others after withdrawal of drug therapy).
2. Negative nitrogen balance, severe muscle wasting, weakness, poor wound healing, growth retardation in children, and depressed immune function and increased susceptibility to infection (cortisol also has an immunosuppressive effect). Therapy has, on occasion, induced zinc deficiency and a resultant delay in wound healing (this is correctable by zinc supplements).
3. Osteoporosis and a tendency toward vertebral fractures due to lack of deposition of protein in bone, enhanced protein catabolism, and negative calcium balance due to the antagonistic effect of glucocorticoids on vitamin D metabolism and glucocorticoid-induced increase in the renal excretion of calcium in association with an increased glomerular filtration rate.
4. Truncal obesity secondary to redistribution of body fat; i.e., fat accumulates in the face, supraclavicular areas, and over the cervical vertebrae of the trunk (moonface and buffalo hump).
5. Sodium and water retention, hypertension, hypokalemia, and hypokalemia-associated metabolic alkalosis accompany the mineralocorticoid effect of high cortisol levels, even though aldosterone levels are not elevated.
6. Appetite stimulation and weight gain resulting from the high cortisol levels; weight gain may also occur secondary to fluid retention.

Intervention. To promote a positive nitrogen balance in clients with Cushing's syndrome, provide a diet high in protein content (1 g/kg body weight) that includes sufficient kilocalories from carbohydrate and fat for protein sparing. Evaluate for glucose intolerance. Control carbohydrate intake in the presence of mild intolerance and provide an individualized, structured diet (Chap. 24) if diabetes is diagnosed. Sodium restriction (40 to 85 mEq or 1 to 2 g daily) may be useful for decreasing sodium and water retention. To prevent potassium depletion and hypochloremic alkalosis, instruct the client to ingest high-potassium foods, such as fruit and fruit juices, vegetables, and whole grain cereals, or to use potassium supplements. The same measures to prevent peptic ulceration as described for hormonal replacement therapy for adrenal insufficiency also apply. Refer to Chapter 23 for measures to control excessive weight gain.

Primary Hyperaldosteronism

Assessment and Intervention. Hyperaldosteronism may result from primary lesions of the adrenal glands (i.e., tumor or hyperplasia)—primary hyperaldosteronism—or from factors that activate the renin–angiotensin system—secondary aldosteronism. The latter occurs in many common disorders in which edema is prominent, such as the nephrotic syndrome, congestive heart failure, and cirrhosis of the liver. The clinical consequences of aldosterone excess in primary aldosteronism are sodium and fluid retention with hypertension, and hypokalemia with metabolic alkalosis and tetany. Severe hypernatremia and edema are not common. Before definitive treatment by surgery, provide foods of high potassium content or potassium supplements.

PITUITARY DISORDERS

Abnormalities of both the anterior and posterior portions of the pituitary gland may bring clinical syndromes that sometimes necessitate nutritional intervention. Since several of the anterior pituitary hormones stimulate the secretion of other endocrine glands, such as the adrenal cortex and the thyroid gland, their imbalance can lead to manifestations that are analogous to those previously described.

Anterior Pituitary Abnormalities

Assessment and Intervention. Clinical syndromes associated with abnormal function of the pituitary gland include diseases of hormone deficit and hormone excess. For example, deficiencies in release of the adrenocorticotropic hormone (ACTH, which controls the secretion of the adrenocortical hormones by the adrenal cortex) and thyroid-stimulating hormone (TSH, which controls the release of thyroid hormones from the thyroid gland) lead to adrenal insufficiency and hypothyroidism, respectively. Follow the nutritional care guidelines previously presented in treating clients with these pituitary disorders. Excess secretion of the pituitary hormones brings characteristics of hormonal excess. For example, hypersecretion of ACTH results in adrenocortical hyperfunctioning—Cushing's syndrome. Nutritional intervention is similar to that for treating Cushing's syndrome resulting from other causes.

Several of the anterior pituitary hormones—growth hormone, ACTH, and TSH—have the property of increasing the blood glucose concentration. A generalized increase in secretion of the anterior

▶ pituitary hormones, then, leads to **pituitary diabetes.** This condition differs from diabetes mellitus in several ways: (1) the rate of glucose use is only moderately depressed in pituitary diabetes, whereas there is little or no use in diabetes mellitus, (2) there is a relative refractoriness to insulin in pituitary diabetes as opposed to lack of insulin in some types of diabetes mellitus, and (3) many of the side effects associated with glucose intolerance in diabetes mellitus are absent in pituitary diabetes. Treat the condition by controlling carbohydrate intake or by providing a diabetic diet as necessary.

Posterior Pituitary Abnormalities

Abnormalities of secretion or use of the antidiuretic hormone (ADH or vasopressin) from the posterior pituitary gland may necessitate nutritional management.

Diabetes Insipidus

Assessment and Intervention. Failure of the secre-
▶ tory mechanism for ADH leads to the disorder **pituitary diabetes insipidus.** Although diabetes insipidus arises from a number of disorders, most frequently it occurs in clients with a tumor of the hypothalamus or hypophysis that destroys the mechanism for control of ADH. The hormone deficit may be partial or total.

Assess for polyuria and polydipsia in affected clients. Large volumes of dilute urine are excreted. The tendency toward dehydration is usually offset by an increase in thirst resulting from the rapid loss of fluid in the urine. Under conditions of circulatory stress, lack of an available supply of water, or absence of an intact thirst mechanism, water loss can be serious.

▶ **Nephrogenic diabetes insipidus** closely mimics vasopressin deficiency, but in this disorder there is a congenital failure of the renal tubular reabsorption of water. The polyuria and polydipsia may go unnoticed in affected infants, and the client's pre-

senting symptoms may be severe dehydration, fever, and failure to thrive.

Pituitary diabetes insipidus is treated with hormonal replacement, whereas nephrogenic diabetes insipidus does not respond to hormonal replacement therapy. Caution clients with pituitary diabetes insipidus against restricting fluids to decrease urine volume. Their fluid intake must be increased to prevent dehydration. Suggest low-calorie beverages for use in fluid replacement to guard against obesity. Remind clients to weigh themselves periodically to ascertain the effectiveness of therapy.

Treatment of nephrogenic diabetes insipidus consists of administration of fluids at frequent intervals and in amounts sufficient to prevent dehydration and fever and provision of a low-solute diet (restricting protein, sodium, and chloride) to decrease obligatory fluid loss in order to maintain normal serum electrolyte levels. During the acute phase of treatment, use 2.5 to 3 percent dextrose solutions to correct dehydration; since the existing hyperosmolality may be aggravated by solutions containing 5 percent dextrose.

Provide strict diet control for affected infants during the first year. Restrict dietary protein to 1 to 2 g/kg body weight per day and limit the intake of meat, fish, milk and milk products (except salt-free butter), eggs, and salt. Initially, provide all of the allowed protein as formula—a high-calorie low-protein formula, such as PM 60/40 (Ross Labs), can be used. When solid foods are added, suggest the use of fortified cereals, fruits, and vegetables, avoiding canned vegetables, canned meats, and canned soups. Remind the parents to provide generous amounts of water to prevent dehydration. As the infant becomes older, assess the ability to satisfy fluid requirements without assistance. When this is accomplished, liberalize the dietary regimen.

Inappropriate Secretion of ADH

Assessment and Intervention. On occasion, the secretion of ADH is inappropriately high for concurrent osmolality of the blood, and secretion is not suppressed by further dilution of body fluids. The
▶ condition is termed **inappropriate ADH syndrome**—SIADH. This disorder is associated with conditions involving the central nervous system, such as meningitis, encephalitis, brain tumors or abscesses, and trauma. The condition is particularly prevalent in oat cell carcinoma of the lung and has been observed in clients using chlorpropamide in treatment for diabetes mellitus. This drug potentiates vasopressin.

The major defect is a marked decrease in the sodium concentration of the extracellular fluid, and the symptoms are those of water intoxication (see Chap. 10). There is usually only a slight increase in the extracellular fluid volume. Treat the hyponatremia by restricting fluid, and assist clients with the appropriate distribution of allowed fluids throughout the day.

REVIEW QUESTIONS AND ACTIVITIES

1. Compare the clinical manifestations and principles of dietary management of hyperthyroidism and hypothyroidism.
2. Plan a day's menu that would be suitable for a client with hyperthyroidism; list five ways in which the kilocalories can be increased in the diet for this client.
3. What adjustments would you make in the menu in Question 2 to make it appropriate for a client with hypothyroidism?
4. Discuss the role of diet therapy in the treatment of hypercalcemia and hypocalcemia associated with hyperparathyroidism and hypoparathyroidism.
5. Differentiate between the etiology of hypocalcemic tetany and alkalotic tetany.
6. Identify the principal glucocorticoid and the principal mineralocorticoid secreted by the adrenal cortex and distinguish between their metabolic effects.
7. Relate the clinical manifestations and dietary treatment of Addison's disease to the hormonal deficiency associated with the disorder.
8. List five foods that could be used to increase sodium intake in a client with Addison's disease.
9. Identify the clinical manifestations of glucocorticoid excess.
10. Describe diet modifications that are appropriate for clients with glucocorticoid excess.
11. Describe the clinical manifestations of primary hyperaldosteronism and its dietary management.
12. Why is a diabetic diet sometimes necessary for clients with hyperfunction of the pituitary gland?
13. Differentiate between the etiology and treatment of pituitary diabetes insipidus and nephrogenic diabetes insipidus.
14. Plan a diet for a newborn with nephrogenic diabetes insipidus and adjust the diet during the first year of life.

BIBLIOGRAPHY

Austin LA, Heath H III: Calcitonin: Physiology and pathophysiology. N Eng J Med 304:269, 1981.

Hallal JC: Hyperthyroidism. Am J Nurs 77:419, 1977.

Hallal JC: Hypothyroidism. Am J Nurs 77:427, 1977.

Jung RT, Shetty PS, James WP: Nutritional effects on thyroid and catecholamine metabolism. Clin Sci 58:183, 1980.

Kozak GP: Primary adrenocortical insufficiency (Addison's disease). Am Fam Phys 15:124, 1977.

O'Brian JT, Bybee DE, Burman KD, et al.: Thyroid hormone homeostasis in states of relative caloric deprivation. Metabolism 29:721, 1980.

Pittman CS: The effects of diabetes mellitus on thyroid physiology. Thyroid Today 4:647, 1981.

Richmand DA, Molitch ME, O'Donnell TF: Altered thyroid hormone levels in bacterial sepsis: The role of nutritional adequacy. Metabolism 29:936,1980.

CHAPTER 26

Nutrition and Upper Gastrointestinal Tract Disorders

Objectives

After completion of this chapter, the student will be able to:

1. Develop a nursing care plan for the nutritional care of clients with oral lesions that are secondary to nutritional deficiencies and for clients with inadequate ability to chew.

2. Distinguish between the nutritional management of esophagitis and esophageal stricture.

3. Develop a nursing care plan for the nutritional management of a client with achalasia and adjust the plan so that it is appropriate for a client with hiatus hernia complicated by an incompetent lower esophageal sphincter.

4. Manage the diet for a client with peptic ulcer disease.

5. Manage the diet for a client during all stages of the dumping syndrome.

6. Compare and contrast the dietary strategies for acute and chronic gastritis and dyspepsia.

The clinical manifestations of diseases of the upper gastrointestinal tract, which includes the mouth, esophagus, and stomach, present a potential threat to the client's nutritional status. The nurse's objectives in nutritional care should therefore be to maintain or restore good nutritional status while alleviating annoying or painful symptoms that accompany the underlying disease process. Historically, diet therapy has played an important role in supporting the medical–surgical management of gastrointestinal disorders, although in many instances the specific protocols used were based on tradition and folklore rather than on a sound, scientific rationale. Research findings now provide a basis for a more scientific approach to dietary treatment, and many long-held notions are being refuted. This is particularly true in the case of peptic ulcer disease, and current trends are toward a liberalized dietary approach in the ongoing management of this chronic disorder.

ORAL CAVITY

Assessment and Intervention

The functional capacity to chew and swallow and the condition of the mouth affect food consumption and thus nutritional status. Management of oral diseases necessitates treating the underlying disorders while providing supportive nutritional therapy in some cases.

Lesions of the mouth may affect the soft tissues or the teeth. Soft tissue lesions are not uncommon with nutritional deficiency, particularly a deficiency of the B-complex vitamins or secondary to anemias of nutritional origin. Ascorbic acid deficiency produces abnormal dentine formation, and vitamin A deficiency produces hypoplasia of the dental enamel and dentine. Defective calcification occurs with vitamin D deficiency, and dental caries (also characterized by hypoplasia) is associated with a low intake

TABLE 26–1
ORAL MANIFESTATIONS OF NUTRIENT DEFICIENCY

Manifestation	Nutrient Deficiency
Cheilosis (flaking, crusting and cracking of the epithelium of the lips) and bilateral angular stomatitis (inflammation and fissuring at the angles of the mouth)	Riboflavin, niacin, and iron
Glossitis (inflammation of the tongue)	B-complex vitamins, iron, and zinc
Changes in papillae on the tongue (atrophy of the filiform papillae and hypertrophy of fungiform papillae)	B-complex vitamins, iron, and zinc
Gingivitis (inflammation of the gums)	Vitamin C
Loss of taste	Zinc, copper, niacin, vitamin A

of fluoride and excessive consumption of refined carbohydrate, particularly sucrose. Lesions of the mouth occur with cancer of the mouth and pharynx, as well as with the chemotherapy and radiotherapy applied in treatment.

Alterations in taste (dysgeusia) and smell (hyposmia) are a manifestation of nutrient deficiency. These alterations may also occur secondary to aging, therapy with certain drugs, and a variety of chronic diseases, including cancer and renal failure. Altered taste and smell may lead to anorexia; therefore, provide more highly flavored foods to increase food intake when these conditions are present. Assess for the oral manifestations of nutrient deficiency summarized in Table 26–1. If it is reasonably clear that the manifestations are due to nutritional deficiency, administer the appropriate supplements.

Unless treated, dental caries may lead to tooth loss, and tooth loss can occur secondary to periodontal disease, a common disorder among the elderly. Clients who lose teeth without adequate replacement often consume a nutritionally inadequate diet. With poorly fitting dentures, the consumption of adequate amounts of a variety of foods is either difficult or impossible. For clients who are edentulous, provide a variety of soft foods; some clients without teeth may be able to handle foods of normal consistency, as well. Except for a lack of fiber, a nutritionally adequate diet can be prepared from blenderized foods for clients whose jaws are wired shut in order to facilitate healing of broken bones.

Radical surgery of the head and neck region often interferes with chewing or swallowing. With training, oral feeding is possible in some clients, but in others, tube feeding may be required.

DISEASES OF THE ESOPHAGUS

Diseases of the esophagus, which include obstruction, inflammation, and alteration in the swallowing mechanism, are less common than diseases of the stomach or intestine. Clinical features common to many esophageal disorders are heartburn (burning, epigastric, substernal pain) and dysphagia (difficulty in swallowing).

Esophagitis

▶ *Assessment and Intervention.* Inflammation of the esophagus, **esophagitis,** may occur in clients secondary to an upper respiratory infection, prolonged gastric intubation, excessive vomiting, radiation of the mediastinal area for cancer, ingestion of such toxic substances as lye, or extensive burns. Chronic esophagitis usually results from the irritating effect of gastric reflux (such as from a hiatus hernia) on the mucosa of the lower esophagus. A rare cause of esophagitis is the Plummer–Vinson syndrome. This disorder occurs principally in middle-age women and is usually a consequence of long-standing iron deficiency. Atropic changes in the esophageal mucosa secondary to the iron deficiency make the tissue vulnerable to the minor trauma of food. In addition to the esophagitis, which occurs in the upper esophagus, there is also dysphagia, glossitis, and achlorhydria.

Assess clients with acute esophagitis for substernal pain during swallowing. With chronic esophagitis, however, clients will often complain of heartburn, and as the condition progresses, they will experience dysphagia. Also observe for mucosal erosion, hemorrhaging, and narrowing of the lumen.

The treatment of esophagitis depends upon the cause: the objective is to avoid further trauma to the esophagus. In acute esophagitis, consider restricting the following types of foods: fibrous foods, spicy and acid foods, and foods that are very hot or very cold. A liquid diet may be desirable. If there is excessive trauma to the esophagus, as with lye ingestion, there is a risk of perforation. Provide tube feeding by gastrostomy or parenteral feeding for a period of time. Should the esophagus become perforated, restrict oral food intake and provide parenteral feeding. Provide iron supplements for clients with the Plummer–Vinson syndrome. Treatment of chronic esophagitis resulting from gastric reflux is discussed later.

Esophageal Stricture

Assessment and Intervention. Esophageal stricture or obstruction occurs secondary to pressure from adjacent organs, hiatus hernia (diaphragmatic hernia), achalasia (also called cardiospasm), scar tissue formation, diverticula (herniations of the mucosa), foreign bodies, or malignant disease. Observe for difficulty in swallowing (first of solids and later of semisolids) and weight loss in clients with the disorder. Treatment by dilatation, surgery, or radiotherapy may be necessary. Depending on the degree of obstruction, the diet may be of liquid consistency served at frequent intervals, a solid diet restricted in fiber, or tube feeding by gastrostomy. If the client can take foods orally, advise drinking liquids with meals to facilitate swallowing. If debilitation is present, provide nutritional rehabilitation before and after surgical treatment or radiotherapy.

GASTROESOPHAGEAL SPHINCTER ABNORMALITIES

Three esophageal disorders are associated with abnormalities of the gastroesophageal sphincter: achalasia, gastroesophageal reflux, and hiatus hernia.

Achalasia

▶ ***Assessment and Intervention.*** **Achalasia** is a disorder of lower esophageal motility in which there is failure of esophageal peristalsis in the upper two thirds of the organ (the body of the esophagus tends to constrict in unison rather than peristaltically) and failure of the lower esophageal sphincter to relax and open during swallowing. Thus, the passage of foods and fluids from the esophagus to the stomach is impeded. The physiologic basis for the disorder is considered to be neural, due to either damage or absence of the myenteric plexus in the lower portion of the esophagus. With progression of the disease, the esophagus becomes dilated above the stricture because of the long-continued intraesophageal pressure, and the sphincter opening narrows in diameter. The client experiences dysphagia and complains of a feeling of fullness in the chest after eating. Food collects in the esophagus, and fermentation may occur. Esophagitis may be present, and weight loss may occur, especially in those with advanced esophageal stasis complicated by aspiration pneumonia.

Treatment necessitates weakening the lower esophageal sphincter so that gravity can aid passage of food to the stomach. This is usually accomplished by dilatation of the sphincter or surgical intervention to split the circular muscle of the cardiac sphincter. Esophageal motility is not restored by the treatment, however. Following treatment, foods enter the stomach by gravity and oropharyngeal pressure. Since the loss of the sphincter allows reflux of gastric contents, take measures to prevent ulceration.

Before treatment, provide a semifluid diet served in small, frequent feedings. Liquids do not require peristalsis, although they may be difficult to swallow. Avoid temperature extremes in foods; neither very hot nor very cold foods are well tolerated. Instruct the client to eat slowly and chew food well. Provide plenty of fluids with meals and instruct the client to sip fluids concurrently with consumption of the more solid components of the diet.

Since the competence of the lower esophageal sphincter is thought to be controlled by gastrointestinal hormones and influenced by diet, emphasize foods that tend to lower esophageal sphincter pressure (Table 26–2). The diet should emphasize fat and moderately restrict protein. Use whole milk rather than skim milk for oral feedings to increase the fat content of the diet. Also provide chocolate and a moderate amount of alcohol for their effect on lowering the sphincter pressure. Avoid spicy foods, citrus fruits, and tomato juice, since these foods may be injurious to the esophageal mucosa.

TABLE 26–2
INFLUENCES ON LOWER ESOPHAGEAL SPHINCTER PRESSURE

Substances that Decrease Lower Esophageal Sphincter Pressure	Substances that Increase Lower Esophageal Sphincter Pressure
Alcohol	Protein foods (stimulate gastrin release)
Chocolate	Antacids
Cigarette smoking	Bethanechol
Fatty foods (the release of cholecystokinin may be the mechanism)	Metoclopramide
Peppermint and spearmint	
Estrogens and progesterone	
Anticholinergic drugs	

Gastroesophageal Reflux

Assessment and Intervention. The primary function of the lower esophageal sphincter is to prevent reflux of gastric contents into the esophagus following food ingestion. Lower than normal pressure of the sphincter results in sphincter incompetence, and the sphincter does not close as it should between swallows. The consequent gastric reflux into the lower esophagus results in esophagitis in affected clients. Chronic esophagitis can lead to bleeding, inflammatory stricture, and dysphagia. The client's most common clinical symptom is heartburn, although there may be regurgitation of gastric contents into the mouth during the night or when bending over. The condition is often complicated by the presence of hiatus hernia, although the two conditions are not synonymous. An incompetent sphincter and symptomatic reflux can exist without a hiatus hernia, and a hiatus hernia can exist without an incompetent sphincter and symptoms. Hiatus hernias may aggravate reflux by interfering with esophageal clearing of acid, especially in the recumbent position.

Various neural and hormonal factors control the pressure of the lower esophageal sphincter, and the gastrointestinal hormones (gastrin, secretin, and cholecystokinin) are thought to be important in altering the pressure. Gastrin increases the lower esophageal sphincter pressure, and secretin and cholecystokinin decrease it. Reflux and heartburn are also associated with ingestion of certain foods in some individuals. The effects of various substances on the lower esophageal sphincter pressure are summarized in Table 26–2. Studies on the effect of caffeine on lower esophageal sphincter pressure have yielded conflicting results.

Dietary management of the disorder is not clear-cut. However, the foods and other factors listed in Table 26–2 that decrease sphincter pressure should be avoided or restricted in the diet. Assist the client to select a high-protein diet while limiting fat to less than 45 g per day. Stress to the client that esophageal irritation can be lessened by avoiding irritating foods, such as citrus fruit juices, tomato juice, and coffee (restricting coffee reduces the effect of gastric acidity). Recommend small, frequent meals to decrease the volume of gastric reflux, and encourage weight reduction for overweight clients. Advise the client against reclining, bending over, or straining immediately after meals and against eating during the 2 to 3 hours before bedtime. To further improve esophageal clearing and decrease the volume and frequency of reflux, suggest sleeping with the head of the bed elevated by 6 to 8 in, using blocks. Clothing that is tight around the abdomen should be avoided. Since citrus fruits and tomato juice are restricted in the diet, assess the diet for other sources of vitamin C and provide supplements if indicated. Antacids are used in treatment, and those that contain calcium or aluminum tend to be constipating. Consider including laxative foods and increasing fluid intake to combat constipation in clients who take these medications. In contrast, magnesium-containing antacids tend to cause diarrhea. Consider the alternate use of the calcium–aluminum and magnesium agents or provide antacids that combine both types of agents to avoid side effects.

Hiatus Hernia

▶ ***Assessment and Intervention.*** **Hiatus hernia** is a common disorder in which there occurs a herniation, or outpouching, of a portion of the stomach through the hiatus of the diaphragm (the opening in the diaphragm through which the esophagus passes from the thoracic cavity to the abdominal cavity) and into the thoracic cavity. The herniation occurs at the juncture of the stomach and esophagus.

Assess for the etiologic significance of these factors in clients with the disorder: (1) congenital weakness or trauma to the diaphragm, (2) weakened musculature associated with aging, and (3) situations that increase the intra-abdominal pressure, such as pregnancy, obesity, chronic cough, ascites, tight-fitting clothes, and such postural changes as stooping, lifting, or straining. Epidemiologic data suggest that consumption of a low-fiber diet may be an important etiologic factor. The hypothesis has been proposed that a low fiber intake predisposes to constipation and straining at stool, and the resulting increase in abdominal pressure forces the abdominal components against the diaphragm and leads to protrusion of the stomach. There is no evidence to show that a high-fiber intake is useful in treating the disorder, however.

The disorder causes illness in only a small portion of affected individuals. Underlying the symptoms is reflux of gastric contents into the esophagus, producing esophagitis. Heartburn is the most common complaint, although dysphagia, secondary to esophagitis or stricture, and ulceration and bleeding may also occur. The symptoms tend to occur when the herniated portion is irritated. The wearing of tight garments or belts appears to provoke symptoms, and symptoms also occur after meals and when lying down.

Treatment is directed toward reducing those factors that provoke gastric reflux and neutralizing the gastric acid. Antacids and anticholinergic drugs are used when esophagitis or ulceration is present. In severe cases, surgical repair becomes necessary.

GASTRIC DISORDERS

Gastric disorders that necessitate attention to the diet include peptic ulcer disease, gastric surgery, gastritis, and dyspepsia.

Peptic Ulcer Disease

▶ *Assessment.* **Peptic ulcers** are defined as sharply circumscribed lesions of the digestive tract resulting from the digestive action of gastric juice. Ulcers can develop in the lower end of the esophagus (esophageal ulcers), in the stomach (gastric ulcer), in the duodenum (duodenal ulcer), or at the site of abnormal gastrointestinal openings, such as a gastrojejunostomy (anastomosis of the stomach to the jejunum). The most common site is the first few centimeters of the duodenum; ulcers also occur along the lesser curvature of the antral end of the stomach and, more rarely, in the lower esophagus secondary to gastric juice reflux. Marginal ulcers develop at the site of abnormal openings.

Although gastric and duodenal ulcers are considered by some investigators as separate diseases, they are grouped together under the general term, peptic ulcer. Peptic ulcer may be acute (with or without bleeding) or chronic, with periodic recurrence of acute pain. Permanent cure of ulcers is rare, and the condition tends to recur in 75 to 80 percent of cases.

Incidence and Predisposing Factors. Peptic ulcer disease affects approximately 10 percent of the U.S. population, with duodenal ulcer being roughly 10 times more prevalent than gastric ulcer. Although the mortality rate for the two types is comparable, duodenal ulcer is associated with greater morbidity. Prior to the 1900s, duodenal ulcer was rare. Its incidence increased in the early 1900s, reached a peak in the 1950s, and has declined significantly since that time. The decline is more marked for men than for women. The reasons for the changes in incidence are unknown.

Ulcers are more common in men than in women. The incidence of both gastric and duodenal ulcers increases with age, although gastric ulcers occur more frequently in older age groups.

Assess for these factors that may predispose to ulcers: (1) smoking, (2) use of certain drugs, (3) heredity, and (4) physiologic stress. Smokers have a higher incidence of ulcer disease (particularly gastric ulcer) than do nonsmokers. The underlying mechanism is not clear, as nicotine does not have a definite effect on acid or pepsin secretion. Caution clients that individuals who ingest large amounts of aspirin on a regular basis have an incidence of gastric ulcer that is approximately three times that of individuals who are not large users of aspirin. Suggested causes for this are inhibition of prostaglandin synthesis and disruption of the mucosal barrier by aspirin. Prolonged use of large doses of corticosteroids (with the exception of ACTH) is associated with an increase in the incidence of ulcer.

Examine the family history of clients with ulcer. Heredity has been implicated, since ulcers are about three times more common in relatives of affected individuals than in the general population. Moreover, persons with type O blood (and who are nonsecretors into the intestinal tract of blood group substances—mucopolysaccharides with antigenic properties, present in the red cell) have a 2.5 times greater likelihood of developing ulcer than those with blood types A, B, and AB (who are secretors of blood group substances). Physiologic stress (such as shock, sepsis, burns, surgery) causes an ulcer lesion that is histologically different from chronic peptic ulcer.

Psychosomatic factors are often cited as important in the etiology of ulcers. Although emotions can alter gastrointestinal function, and acute psychologic stress precedes the development of ulcer in some clients, it has not been shown that personality traits or situations that create tension are a cause of ulcers. Further studies are needed to clarify the role of psychologic factors in the pathogenesis of peptic ulcer disease.

Although dietary factors are thought to be involved in ulcer pathogenesis, there are no studies to document this, and the influence of diet has not been studied satisfactorily.

Pathogenesis. Peptic ulcer disease reflects an imbalance between the amount of gastric juice secreted and the degree of mucosal resistance—acid-pepsin secretion is excessive relative to the degree of protection provided by mucus and the neutralization of gastric acid by the duodenal secretions. All areas of the gastrointestinal tract normally exposed to gastric juice are well supplied with mucus-secreting glands, including the mucus-secreting glands of the lower esophagus and the Brunner glands of the upper duodenum, which secrete a highly alkaline mucus. The duodenum is further protected from the effects of acid by the alkalinity of the small intestinal secretions. In the alkaline environment pepsin is inactivated and cannot digest the mucosa. Any factor that increases the rate of production of gastric juice or blocks these normal protective mechanisms can predispose to peptic ulcer.

Test for hypersecretion of gastric acid in clients with duodenal ulcer. With duodenal ulcer, there is a greater than normal secretion of both gastric acid and pepsin during the interdigestive phase and in response to gastric stimulation. For example, whereas normal individuals secrete approximately 18 mEq hydrochloric acid (HCl) in the 12-hour interdigestive period during the night, those with duodenal ulcer occasionally secrete as much as 300 mEq HCl during this same period. In contrast, clients with gastric ulcers often exhibit normal or low secretion of hydrochloric acid. The tissue insult in gastric ulcer may result from damage to the gastric mucosal barrier, and thus reduced resistance of the stomach mucosa to digestion, rather than from an excess secretion of gastric juice. The mucosal barrier consists of mucous cells and very tight junctions between the adjacent epithelial cells, which serve to protect the gastric mucosa.

Hypersecretion of gastric acid is seen in the Zollinger–Ellison syndrome, which is characterized by the presence of gastrin-secreting tumors of the non-beta-islet cells of the pancreas and leads to intractable peptic ulceration of the duodenum, jejunum, or esophagus. The high serum gastrin level causes hypersecretion of gastric acid and the development of multiple recurrent peptic ulcers with symptoms similar to the usual duodenal ulcer. There is also maldigestion and malabsorption, which may be due to deactivation of pancreatic enzymes and bile acids by the increased acidity or structural and functional changes of the intestinal mucosa. Intestinal hypermotility is present and leads to diarrhea and hypokalemia.

Symptoms and Complications. Although chronic ulcer tends to produce characteristic symptoms, occasionally the symptoms may be absent or indefinite, and hemorrhage or perforation may be the first sign of illness.

The most common symptom is chronic and periodic pain in the epigastrium (to the left of the midline) that is gnawing, aching, burning, or boring in nature and sometimes described as heartburn. In clients with duodenal ulcer, assess for the occurrence of pain more or less regularly from 1 to 4 hours after a meal and during the night. The pain is relieved by food or nonabsorbable antacids. The pattern of pain–food–relief is more variable with gastric ulcers, and clients may complain of epigastric pain while eating. The basis for the pain may be the action of unneutralized HCl on nerve fibers at the site of the ulcer, hypermotility of the stomach, or gastric distention following ingestion of large amounts of foods or liquids.

Clients with ulcer may experience other symptoms. Observe for anorexia, nausea, vomiting, and weight loss particularly in clients with gastric ulcer. Also assess dietary intake, since the client may reduce food intake because of self-imposed dietary restrictions. In contrast, nurses may see weight gain in clients with duodenal ulcer. These clients often have a good appetite and may eat excessively to avoid discomfort. They often experience other gastrointestinal symptoms, such as heartburn, regurgitation, constipation, or diarrhea.

In some clients with ulcer, the first symptoms that nurses observe may be those that occur secondary to a complication, such as hemorrhage, perforation, or obstruction. If an ulcer bleeds slowly, observe for melena (black stools) and anemia. If the ulcer erodes a blood vessel, the hemorrhage may be massive, with hematemesis (vomiting of blood) and sudden weakness. Should the ulcer perforate the gastric or duodenal wall, the client will experience severe pain and peritonitis. Both hemorrhage and perforation require emergency treatment. Scar tissue formed by the healing of repeated ulceration may obstruct the pyloric valve of the stomach. In the presence of vomiting in otherwise asymptomatic clients, suspect this complication.

Intervention. Considerable controversy has surrounded the therapeutic modalities affecting the symptoms, healing, recurrence, and complications of ulcer. Antacids and anticholinergic drugs are the primary agents used in management. Healing may also be expedited by hospitalization and rest, discontinuance of smoking, and avoidance of aspirin. Traditional diet modifications have not been demonstrated to be of definite value in ulcer management,[1] although in the past relatively strict restrictions were applied. At present there is no evidence that the traditional bland diet, i.e., a diet designed to rest the stomach by avoiding foods thought to be chemically, mechanically, and thermally irritating, alters the symptoms, healing rates, recurrence, or complications of ulcer. Actually, very few foods are thought to be harmful to the ulcer client, and diets used in treatment are now more liberal. Effective drug therapy is now preferred over less rational forms of diet therapy. Definitive treatment for the Zollinger–Ellison syndrome is total gastrectomy or, on occasion, resection of the pancreatic tumor.

Antacids are given to buffer or neutralize gastric acid, and anticholinergics are used to decrease the secretion of HCl and pepsin by decreasing the vagal stimulation of gastrin. Anticholinergics are more effective in inhibiting basal or nocturnal gastric secretion than food-induced secretion, and they are, therefore, more useful for relieving nocturnal pain. Other drugs in current use that are potent inhibitors of acid secretion are prostaglandin E_2 and the H_2-receptor or histamine antagonists, e.g., cimetidine (Tagamet), which blocks the specific histamine receptor site for gastric secretion. Be aware of the nutritional side effects of these medications (see Table 21–9) and of the sodium content of the antacids should the client also be following a sodium-restricted diet. The sodium content varies from 0.7 mg/5 ml for Riopan to 8.0 mg/5 ml for Amphojel and Mylanta II. Stress to the client the importance of consuming laxative foods if antacids that are constipating are prescribed.

In general, clients with an ulcer expect to be placed on some type of diet restriction. However, it is not possible to generalize the dietary treatment for all clients. Individualize the regimen according to stage of the illness (i.e., acute or chronic), presence of other medical complications, nutritional status, and individual food tolerances. Provide a diet that:

1. Is nutritionally adequate
2. Decreases and neutralizes acid
3. Maintains resistance of the gastrointestinal mucosa to acid
4. Is nonirritating to the gastrointestinal mucosa

In designing the diet, give attention to both the buffering and acid-stimulating properties of particular categories of food and the size of the meals served. When trying to reduce acidity, consider both the immediate and delayed effects of food. Foods have characteristic secretory and neutralizing properties, and most foods, even water, stimulate gastric secretion to some extent. Foods also tend to provide a degree of buffering. Protein foods are the most potent stimulant to secretion, but they also have the greatest buffering capacity because of their amphoteric nature. The buffering effect is only temporary, however, and the digestive products of protein (amino acids and polypeptides) stimulate the secretion of gastrin, which in turn stimulates the secretion of gastric acid. In the individual with active disease, the initial relief of pain on eating is provided by the buffering effect of protein. The recurrence of pain 1 to 4 hours later results from the drop in gastric pH due to the acid-stimulating effects of the products of protein digestion. Both the acid-stimulating and acid-neutralizing properties of carbohydrate and fat are less. However, fat reduces both gastric motility and gastric secretion. Carbohydrate neither stimulates nor inhibits gastric secretion. The diet should contain a moderate amount of protein for its buffering effect and a moderate amount of fat to decrease gastric motility and secretion.

Milk is sometimes used for its buffering effect, but this effect is slight, and the acid-neutralizing effect may be outweighed by its acid-stimulating property (acid rebound). Milk is a potent stimulus to gastric acid secretion because of its content of both calcium and protein. It stimulates acid secretion to approximately 30 percent of maximal output, and the effect may last for approximately 3 hours and often coincides with the onset of postprandial pain in ulcer clients. For this reason, avoid using milk as a substitute for antacid therapy. Use of large amounts of milk may also predispose the client to obesity, atherosclerosis, and myocardial infarction because of the high kilocalorie content and content of saturated fat. Moreover, it may lead to hypercalcemia and a type of alkalosis referred to as the milk–alkali syndrome.

Advise the client to restrict foods or beverages that increase the secretion of gastric acid or that are irritating to the gastric mucosa. Alcohol, caffeine, and theobromine all stimulate gastric acid secretion. Caffeine is a natural constituent of a number of plants, including coffee beans, tea leaves, kola nuts, cocoa beans, and maté, and is found in products made from these plants, such as coffee, cocoa, chocolate, cola, and pepper-type drinks. The average amount of caffeine in these products is listed in Table 26–3. Aspirin and some stay-awake preparations also contain caffeine. Decaffeinated coffee has been found to stimulate an amount of gastric acid equivalent to regular coffee, and in one study it was found to elicit a higher acid secretion response than protein.[2] Both regular and decaffeinated coffee ap-

TABLE 26–3 AVERAGE CAFFEINE CONTENT OF SELECTED PRODUCTS	
Beverage or Food[a]	Average Caffeine Content (mg)
Regular coffee (5 oz)	128
Instant coffee (5 oz)	66
Decaffeinated coffee (5 oz)	3
Cola drinks (12 oz)	
Coca-Cola	65
Pepsi-Cola	43
Tab	50
Sweet chocolate bar (1 oz)	20
Cocoa (5 oz)	13
Tea	
Black	46
Green	32

[a] The strength of the brew and length of brewing time for hot beverages influence the content; domestic teas contain less caffeine than imported black teas.

pear to be more potent stimuli to gastric secretion than caffeine per se. Theobromine is present in cocoa and chocolate.

Teach clients that in addition to being a mild stimulant of acid secretion, alcohol damages the mucosal barrier and leads to mucosal irritation. Although one study showed that ingestion of red chili powder by clients with duodenal ulcer had no effect on the rate of ulcer healing,[3] it is advisable to restrict chili powder and black and red peppers, which are gastric irritants.

The size of meals served is an important consideration, since distention of the antrum stimulates the secretion of gastrin. When symptoms are acute, advise the client to consume small or moderate-size feedings to avoid excessive distention and enhancement of gastric secretion. In such cases, use frequent feedings (e.g., every 2 hours) to provide constant buffering and to achieve a reasonable nutrient intake. Some investigators feel, however, that small feedings are contraindicated when the ulcer is healed, especially in individuals with duodenal ulcer and hypersecretion, to avoid the repeated stimulus to gastric secretion provided by food ingestion.[4] Some authorities recommend against a bedtime feeding because of its stimulatory effect on acid secretion during the night.[5] Assess for the effect of bedtime snacks on the client's degree of pain and recommend that they be omitted if they cause pain during the night. Regardless of the buffering capacity of foods, no diet will maintain 24-hour neutralization of gastric contents. The amount of acid returns to a high level within ½ to 2 hours following a meal.

There is no evidence that fibrous foods, if well chewed and mixed with saliva, will traumatize an ulcer. Recommend grinding or straining food only in the event that teeth are in poor condition or miss-

---

TABLE 26-4
LIBERAL DIETARY REGIMEN FOR PEPTIC ULCER DISEASE

Avoid foods capable of stimulating gastric acid secretion when symptomatic; use in moderation when asymptomatic:
   Caffeine-containing beverages (tea may be better tolerated than coffee)
   Decaffeinated coffee
   Alcohol

Avoid foods or drugs that are mucosal irritants when symptomatic; use in moderation when asymptomatic:
   Alcohol
   Pepper and chili, including chili powder and chili pepper
   Aspirin

Reduce or eliminate smoking

Avoid foods that contribute to symptoms on an individual basis

Adjust meal size to the stage of the disease (i.e., eat small meals at frequent intervals when symptomatic)

Provide vitamin supplements if dietary adequacy is questionable; thiamine supplements may be needed if antacids are used extensively, since antacids destroy or prevent absorption of the vitamin

Chew foods well

Eat meals on a regular basis and in as relaxed an environment as possible

---

ing. Homogenization, mincing, or pureeing of food may actually increase rather than decrease gastric acid secretion.[6]

Guidelines for a liberalized dietary regimen for clients with peptic ulcer disease are summarized in Table 26–4. Since clients who are accustomed to traditional diets may have difficulty accepting a liberalized regimen, explain the rationale for the change. After the individualized changes have been incorporated into the dietary pattern, evaluate the diet for nutritional adequacy. Table 26–5 provides a listing of foods allowed and foods restricted when symptoms are acute. The latter regimen may be used with other acute gastrointestinal problems, such as severe esophagitis, gastritis, upper gastrointestinal bleeding, and symptomatic hiatus hernia.

Nutritional Management of Hemorrhaging Ulcer.
The nutritional management of hemorrhaging ulcer is controversial. Some use a conservative approach and withhold oral food until the bleeding has stopped, whereas others favor oral feeding as soon as symptoms, such as nausea, hematemesis, or shock, have passed. With the conservative approach, milk or milk supplemented with such foods as egg, toast, crackers, tender cooked fruits and vegetables, and simple puddings are offered at 1 to 2 hour intervals after the bleeding has stopped. Subsequently, other foods are added according to tolerance. However, if the hemorrhage is not severe and nausea and vomiting are not a problem, the clients may tolerate oral foods sooner. Those who favor early feeding note that hemorrhaging clients progress more satisfactorily when fed than when starved. A soft or regular diet with small, frequent feedings may be appropriate for most clients being treated for bleeding ulcers.

Gastric Surgery

Assessment. Surgery for peptic ulcer may be necessary in the event of hemorrhage, perforation, obstruction due to scar tissue formation, or intractability. Surgical techniques include gastrectomy (total or partial) and vagotomy, the latter frequently combined with a drainage procedure. When the gastrectomy is total, the esophagus is anastomosed to the jejunum. Subtotal gastrectomy procedures include Billroth I or antrectomy (the gastric remnant is anastomosed to the duodenum) and Billroth II (the gastric remnant is anastomosed to the jejunum, and an afferent, or blind, loop is created). Vagotomy entails partial or total severance of the vagus nerve innervating the gastrointestinal tract. Depending upon the extent of the vagotomy, the secretion of HCl and pepsin is reduced and gastric emptying is slowed. Gastric atony with stasis, distention, and a feeling of fullness usually result from vagotomy. To facilitate drainage, the pyloric sphincter is enlarged (pyloroplasty) or another suitable procedure is performed.

Gastric surgery is followed, to a greater or lesser degree, by disturbances in gastric function, including:

1. Rapid emptying of the gastric remnant and increased intestinal motility
2. Reduced secretion of HCl, pepsin, intrinsic factor, and pancreatic enzymes
3. Inadequate mixing of food with digestive secretions
4. Changes in pH in the alimentary tract
5. Alteration in the intestinal flora
6. Reduced nutrient absorption, e.g., calcium, iron, folic acid, vitamin B_{12}, and fat
7. Rapid absorption of glucose

TABLE 26-5
STRICT BLAND DIET FOR ACUTE PHASE OF GASTROINTESTINAL DISORDERS

Category	Foods Allowed	Foods Avoided
Beverages	Milk (whole, low-fat, skim, buttermilk), eggnog, milkshakes, cereal beverages	Coffee, decaffeinated coffee, tea, carbonated beverages, alcoholic beverages, cocoa
Bread	White bread, saltines, soda crackers, rusk, melba toast, zwieback	All others not tolerated
Cereal	Refined cooked cereal (strained oatmeal, grits, cream of wheat, farina), refined dry cereals (Corn Flakes, Rice Krispies, Puffed Wheat, Puffed Rice), cornmeal	All others not tolerated
Dessert	Plain cake (angel, sponge), plain cookies (vanilla wafers), custard, gelatin, and rennet desserts, cornstarch, rice, and tapioca pudding, vanilla ice cream	Pastries, chocolate desserts, desserts containing raisins or nuts
Fat	Butter, margarine, cream (sweet and sour), cream cheese, vegetable fat and oils	All others not tolerated
Fruit[a]	Canned peaches, pears, cherries, applesauce, ripe banana, grapefruit and orange sections, cooked plums, fruit juices	All others not tolerated
Meat, fish, poultry, eggs, cheese[b]	Eggs, cottage cheese, mild American and cheddar cheese, creamy peanut butter	Fried eggs, strong or sharp cheeses, nuts, and all others
Potato or potato substitute	Baked or boiled potato (without skin), macaroni, noodles, spaghetti, refined rice	Fried potato, potato chips, all others
Soup	Strained cream soup made with vegetable puree: asparagus, green and wax beans, beets, carrots, peas (not dried), potato, spinach, squash	Meat stock, broth, bouillon, soups prepared from meat, fish, poultry, dry peas or beans, all others
Sweets	Sugar, hard candy, and clear jelly in moderation	Chocolate candy, all others
Vegetables[a]	Cooked asparagus tips, beets, carrots, green peas, spinach, squash, green and wax beans, tomatoes and tomato juice, pumpkin	All others not tolerated
Miscellaneous	Moderate amounts of salt, extracts, allspice, cinnamon, caraway seeds, mace, sage, paprika, thyme	Pepper, chili powder, cloves, mustard seeds, nutmeg, all other spices, pickles, olives, relishes, gravy, popcorn, chocolate

[a] With acute symptoms, fruits and vegetables may be limited to the use of purees and juices.
[b] The use of meat, fish, and fowl is restricted according to the severity of symptoms; i.e., their use is restricted when symptoms are acute, and they are allowed as tolerated with less acute symptoms.

The altered gastric function is accompanied by nutritional complications, and the more extensive the resection, the greater the incidence of complications. For instance, such sequelae as steatorrhea, weight loss, dumping syndrome, and bacterial overgrowth occur more frequently with Billroth II than with Billroth I operations. Some of the complications occur in the early period following surgery and are associated with discomfort upon eating; others develop later due to the long-term effects of the disturbed function. Weight loss is a common complication and is due to inadequate food intake secondary to discomfort related to eating, and to malabsorption.

Four factors may contribute to discomfort of clients when eating and their subsequent reduction of food intake:

1. Distention of the gastric remnant
2. The dumping syndrome
3. Late postprandial hypoglycemia
4. Afferent loop obstruction

Usually, at least 50 percent of the stomach is removed when gastrectomy is performed. Assess clients with a gastrectomy for an early sensation of fullness while eating due to distention of the gastric remnant. Discomfort may also be associated with gastric irritation due to a reflux of bile.

► The **dumping syndrome** is a combination of vasomotor symptoms and diarrhea that may occur shortly after surgery. The intensity of the symptoms varies from mild to severe, and the condition tends to improve with time. In some clients, however, severe symptoms persist. The disorder occurs because of the reduction in the reservoir capacity of the stomach and the diluting effect of its secretions—ingested material enters the intestine more rapidly and in a more concentrated form than normally (usually the stomach intermittently empties small quantities of liquid chyme into the proximal intestine and thus guards against massive and acute changes in osmotic load). Although proof is lacking, the symptoms of the dumping syndrome may be mediated by gastrointestinal hormones or by a decrease in the hydrogen ion concentration of gastric contents.[7]

Within approximately 15 to 30 minutes after the client has ingested food, observe for one or more of the following symptoms of dumping: flushing, faintness, sweating, sensation of epigastric fullness, nausea, and abdominal cramping followed by diarrhea. The rapid dumping of osmotically active substances, primarily sugars, into the proximal intestine leads to a transient, sharp reduction in blood volume as extracellular fluids are drawn into the intestine to dilute the hypertonic material. The vasomotor symptoms (flushing, faintness, and sweating) are attributed to adrenosympathetic stimulation due to the drop in blood volume. Abdominal cramping, hypermotility, and diarrhea may occur because of the resulting intestinal distention or the release of serotonin in response to the distention.

Two to three hours after a meal, observe for weakness, perspiration, hunger, nausea, anxiety, and tremors. The rapid movement of carbohydrate into the intestine and the high concentration of sugars lead to rapid absorption of glucose, hyperglycemia, glucosuria, overproduction of insulin, and eventually, late postprandial hypoglycemia, a type of reactive hypoglycemia. In a few clients, late postprandial hypoglycemia occurs 1½ to 3 hours after meals without previous symptoms of dumping.

In clients with Billroth II operations who complain of pain after meals or who vomit bilious material, suspect obstruction of the afferent loop. Transient obstruction of the afferent loop allows food and secretions to become trapped and distend the loop.

Assess for signs of nutritional deficiency associated with malabsorption of nutrients, particularly fat, fat-soluble vitamins, iron, calcium, folate, and vitamin B_{12}, that occur postgastrectomy. The degree of malabsorption varies greatly, but the majority of clients experience some steatorrhea. Fat malabsorption and concurrent malabsorption of fat-soluble vitamins may occur secondary to (1) bacterial overgrowth from afferent loop stasis or obstruction (bacteria deconjugate the bile salts needed for fat absorption), (2) relative pancreatic enzyme insufficiency (passage of food into the intestine may not evoke an adequate stimulus to pancreatic secretion, there may be inadequate mixing with enzymes, or there may be pancreatic atrophy if marked weight loss has occurred), and (3) unmasking of the celiac–sprue syndrome (see Chap. 27) due to failure of gastric dilution of stomach contents. Impaired absorption because of the dumping syndrome, bile regurgitation, or other reasons, further impedes a good nutritional status.

With the bypass of the proximal portion of the intestine, as in the Billroth II procedure, absorption of calcium and iron is impaired, since the duodenum and proximal intestine are the site of maximal transport of these two nutrients. Iron absorption is also reduced because rapid stomach emptying prevents thorough mixing of food with gastric HCl, and thus iron is not changed to its absorbable ferrous form. Iron deficiency anemia is common after gastric resection and is the most common cause of anemia postgastrectomy. Chronic malabsorption of calcium and vitamin D leads to osteomalacia in a considerable number of clients.

The absorption of vitamin B_{12} may be reduced as a result of (1) intrinsic factor deficiency in near-total or total gastrectomy and (2) competition for and binding of the vitamin by bacteria should bacterial overgrowth occur with afferent loop obstruction or stasis. These bacteria also bind with folate and decrease its absorption. There may be a time lag in noting a lowering of the serum vitamin B_{12} level because of liver stores of the vitamin. Deficiencies of folate and vitamin B_{12} also contribute to anemia.

Gastrectomy may unmask lactase deficiency. The high concentration of lactose in the intestine that results from failure of gastric dilution may precipitate symptoms of lactose intolerance (see Chap. 27).

Intervention. Direct dietary management after gastric resection toward preventing and treating the early complications and preventing the deterioration of nutritional status associated with the late complications. Institute nutritional measures early to ensure an adequate nutrient intake, since the development of nutritional deficiency may be slow and insidious and thus escape attention.

Authorities disagree on the optimum feeding regimen during the acute postoperative period. It has been suggested, however, that the feeding of choice is small amounts of dry, low-fiber foods rather than liquids. The rationale for this is that the stomach empties itself more readily with this type of feeding, and liquids may cause distention and dumping. When oral feeding is established, progress the diet according to individual tolerance and give attention to foods that are less likely to prevent symptoms of dumping and malabsorption. This is particularly important in clients in whom the pyloric sphincter was not preserved during the surgery. There is virtually no need for diet restrictions to prevent dumping if the pyloric sphincter is intact.

The symptoms of dumping and postprandial hypoglycemia are related to the type and amount of food ingested, and the aim of treatment is to reduce the osmolality and volume of the solution entering the intestine. Restrict total carbohydrate intake by eliminating simple carbohydrates, which are osmotically active, and restricting the total amount of

---

TABLE 26–6
DIETARY PRINCIPLES IN THE TREATMENT OF THE
DUMPING SYNDROME

Eat a high-calorie (35–45 kcal/kg recommended body weight), high-protein (1.5–2 g/kg recommended body weight), high-fat diet; restrict carbohydrate to less than 140 g and use protein and fat to meet kcal needs

Avoid simple carbohydrate: sweetened fruits, juices and soft drinks, baked products with added sugar, desserts made with regular gelatin, ice cream, candy, chewing gum, sugar-coated cereals, table sugar, jam, syrup, molasses, and honey

Eat meals of small size (e.g., 4–5 oz) at frequent intervals (e.g., six times daily)

Avoid liquids at meal time: liquids can be taken ½–1 hour before or after meals

Lie down for a short period after meals

Check tolerance for milk: it may be better tolerated in small amounts than in large amounts or it may not be tolerated at all

Keep concentrated sweets available in the event of postprandial hypoglycemia

---

fruits, most vegetables, bread, and cereal. Unless contraindicated because of concomitant overweight, cardiovascular disease, or renal disease, increase the intake of protein and fat to provide an adequate kilocalorie intake. To decrease the volume of foods entering the proximal intestine, use small, frequent feedings and provide fluids ½ to 1 hour after meals rather than with meals. Add milk to the diet cautiously because of potential lactose intolerance. Fermented forms of milk, such as buttermilk, may be better tolerated.

Supplement the diet routinely with vitamins and minerals and provide these parenterally if malabsorption is present. With steatorrhea, medium-chain triglycerides may be better tolerated than traditional fats, and pancreatic enzyme supplements may be useful. If diarrhea results from bacterial overgrowth in an afferent loop with stasis, administer antibiotics. Table 26–6 provides a summary of the dietary principles to control the dumping syndrome and postprandial hypoglycemia. The six Food Exchange Lists (see Appendix 2) can be used as a basis for calculating the diet and to teach the client carbohydrate control. Advise the client to monitor body weight closely to detect changes early.

Gastritis

▶ *Assessment and Intervention.* **Gastritis** is an inflammation of the gastric mucosa that may be acute or chronic. Assess for symptoms of gastritis, including anorexia, nausea, vomiting, fever, epigastric pain, or feeling of fullness, and possibly gastric hemorrhage in clients who have ingested chemical irritants, who are exposed to gastric irradiation, or who have bacterial or viral infections or a history of food allergy. Drugs, such as aspirin, antibiotics, steroids, and alcohol, or agents, such as strong acids and alkali, can lead to acute gastritis. Moreover, acute gastritis may result from the ingestion of food contaminated with *Staphylococcus* or *Salmonella* as well as conditions associated with the accumulation of metabolic toxins, such as uremia.

The etiology of chronic gastritis is not known, but it may follow repeated attacks of acute gastritis and is more common in clients who smoke and drink heavily. Suspect chronic gastritis in clients with gastric lesions, such as ulcer and cancer, and in clients with pernicious anemia and chronic iron deficiency, since the condition frequently occurs in association with these disorders. Damage to the gastric mucosal barrier may be important in the etiology of chronic gastritis. Reflux of duodenal contents brings the irritating effects of bile salts on the mucosa. Immunologic factors may be an additional cause.

Recurrent inflammation of the gastric mucosa can lead to atrophy of gastric glands with reduced secretion of acid, pepsin, and intrinsic factor. Assess the client's vitamin B_{12} status. Although vitamin B_{12} deficiency may not progress to pernicious anemia, the associated clinical manifestations (including weakness, loss of memory, and mental depression) frequently respond to vitamin B_{12} therapy. Iron deficiency anemia is also common and is due to inadequate iron intake, poor absorption, and recurrent bleeding from minor gastric erosions.

Acute gastritis usually heals in several days. Direct treatment toward resting the stomach and replacing fluid and electrolytes lost in vomiting. Initially, withhold oral foods, and provide nourishment by the parenteral route. If the physician approves, give the client ice chips to hold in the mouth. When the client can tolerate oral feeding, give a liquid diet with gradual progression to a normal diet, using foods listed in Table 26–5 during the transition.

Manage chronic gastritis by individualizing treatment to the underlying cause. In some cases a soft diet that excludes hot spices, served in small, frequent feedings, may be tolerated. Determine if there is a possibility of damage to the mucosal barrier. If so, use the same dietary principles as for peptic ulcer; that is, administer antacids and advise the client to restrict gastric irritants, such as alcohol, coffee, and hot spices. Assess for constipation or diarrhea, depending on the type of antacid being taken.

Dyspepsia

▶ *Assessment and Intervention.* **Dyspepsia,** an-
▶ other word for **indigestion,** is a nonspecific term
used to describe various gastrointestinal symptoms,
such as nausea, heartburn, epigastric pain, and distention, associated with taking food. Assess for the
concurrent presence of disease conditions, such as
peptic ulcer, renal disease, or heart disease. In their
absence, analyze the client's food habits and lifestyle
for other possible causes, including (1) psychologic
pressures (e.g., tension and anxiety), (2) individual
food intolerances, or (3) poor lifestyle and habits
(e.g., overeating, bolting food without proper chewing, overindulgence in smoking or alcohol). Relate
the treatment to the cause; a therapeutic diet for
simple indigestion is seldom necessary. Assist the
client to correct faulty food habits if they are found
to be a contributing factor.

REVIEW QUESTIONS AND ACTIVITIES

1. Describe the five major manifestations of
   nutritional deficiency on soft tissues of the
   oral cavity.
2. Discuss nursing interventions for increasing food intake in clients with poor chewing
   ability.
3. Identify foods that may be tolerated by
   clients with esophagitis.
4. Describe the nutritional management of
   esophageal stricture.
5. Identify the clinical manifestations and dietary management of achalasia.
6. Distinguish between substances that increase and decrease pressure in the lower
   esophageal sphincter.
7. Discuss dietary, medical, and mechanical
   measures directed toward controlling gastric reflux and neutralizing gastric acid in
   clients with hiatus hernia.
8. Identify four predisposing factors in the
   etiology of peptic ulcer disease.
9. Differentiate between the postulated mechanisms that lead to gastric ulcer and duodenal ulcer.
10. Compare the symptoms of gastric and
    duodenal ulcer as they occur relative to food
    intake.
11. Explain the rationale for the dietary restric-
    tions in treating peptic ulcer disease.
12. Explain the rationale for each of the follow-

ing problems that may become manifest in
clients following a gastrectomy: (a) dumping
syndrome, (b) postprandial hypoglycemia,
(c) lactose intolerance, (d) fat malabsorption,
(e) anemia, and (f) osteomalacia.
13. Describe the principles of dietary manage-
    ment of the dumping syndrome.
14. Discuss the dietary management of acute
    and chronic gastritis and dyspepsia.

REFERENCES

1. American Dietetic Association: Handbook of Clinical
   Dietetics. New Haven, Conn, Yale University Press,
   1981, p B24.
2. Fieldman EJ, Isenberg JI, Grossman MI: Gastric acid
   and gastrin response to decaffeinated coffee and a pep-
   tone meal. JAMA 246:248, 1981.
3. Kumar N, Vij JC, Sarin SK, Anand BS: Do chilies influence healing of duodenal ulcer? Br Med J 288:1803,
   1984.
4. Peterson WL, Fordtran JS: In Sleisenger MH, Fordtran
   JS, eds: Gastrointestinal Disease, ed 2. Philadelphia,
   WB Saunders, 1978, Vol 1, pp 891–913.
5. Richardson CT: Pharmacotherapy: A perspective.
   South Med J 72:260, 1979.
6. American Dietetic Association, op cit, p B27.
7. American Dietetic Association, op cit, p D3.

BIBLIOGRAPHY

Arvanitakis C: Diet changes in gastrointestinal disease.
A commentary. J Am Diet Assoc 75:449, 1979.
Cohen S: Pathogenesis of coffee-induced gastrointestinal
symptoms. N Engl J Med 303:122, 1980.
Elashoff JD, Grossman MI: Trends in hospital admissions
and death rates for peptic ulcer in the United States
from 1970 to 1978. Gastroenterology 78:280, 1980.
Feinberg LE: Recurrent duodenal ulcer—A new nonsurgi-
cal alternative. Drug Therapy 10:45, 1980.
Grossman MI: New medical and surgical treatments for
peptic ulcer disease. Am J Med 69:647, 1980.
McArthur K, Hogan D, Isenberg J: Relative side effects
of commonly used beverages on gastric acid secretion
in humans. Gastroenterology 83:199, 1982.
Rune SJ, Greibe J, Møllman KM, et al.: Recurrence of
duodenal ulcer pain after treatment with cimetidene
for four and eight weeks. Gut 21:151, 1980.
Stolinsky DC: Sugar and saccharin content of antacids.
N Engl J Med 305:166, 1981.
Symposium on duodenal peptic ulceration. Mayo Clin Proc
15:1, 1980.
Thomas J, Greig M, Piper DW: Chronic gastric ulcer and
life events. Gastroenterology 78:905, 1980.

CHAPTER 27

Nutrition and Lower Gastrointestinal Tract Disorders

Objectives

After completion of this chapter, the student will be able to:

1. Distinguish among diarrhea, steatorrhea, maldigestion, and malabsorption in terms of etiology, clinical manifestations, and dietary management.

2. Develop a nursing care plan for the nutritional management of an 18-year-old female client with Crohn's disease and adapt the plan to be appropriate for a 30-year-old female client with ulcerative colitis.

3. Plan a day's menu for an elderly male client with asymptomatic diverticulosis and adjust the menu for this client, who is receiving oral food intake, during an acute attack of diverticulitis.

4. Compare and contrast the dietary management of asymptomatic diverticular disease, irritable bowel syndrome, and atonic constipation.

5. Compare and contrast the following disorders in relation to etiology, clinical manifestations, and dietary management: (a) gluten-induced enteropathy, (b) tropical sprue, (c) glucose–galactose intolerance, (d) sucrose–isomaltose intolerance, and (e) lactose intolerance.

6. Plan a diet for an adult female homemaker with gluten-induced enteropathy and adjust the diet to be appropriate for an adult male nurse with the same disorder who eats lunch at the hospital cafeteria.

7. Manage the diet for a client during the first year following massive bowel resection.

8. Develop a nursing care plan for an 18-year-old female with an ileostomy (that involves resections of a large portion of the terminal ileum) and adjust the plan to be appropriate for a 70-year-old male client with a colostomy (that involves resection of the sigmoid colon).

The small intestine is the site of digestion of food and absorption of nutrients. Therefore, disease of this organ or loss of functioning intestine secondary to surgical restriction or bypass has effects on nutritional status that may vary from minor to profound. Since the duodenum, jejunum, and ileum have specialized functions, the type of problem depends on the particular area of intestine involved. Although the colon has no digestive function and only a minor absorptive function, colonic disease can alter nutritional status by influencing food intake and nutrient use. Even a disorder as simple as constipation can lead to nutrient depletion if it causes anorexia or leads a client to develop "the laxative habit." Nurses must have an understanding of the manifestations and treatment of intestinal disorders in order to anticipate possible nutritional problems and detect them early in clients. Corrective action based on sound nutritional principles thus can be provided before nutritional deficits become severe. As research findings are better delineating the underlying pathophysiology, dietary approaches to treating intestinal disorders are being improved.

OVERVIEW OF DIARRHEA, STEATORRHEA, AND MALABSORPTION

Diarrhea, which is a symptom of a disease rather than a disease per se, refers to the frequent passage of loose, watery, and unformed stools. Diarrheal stools consist of water, electrolytes, and frequently undigested or unabsorbed food. The more acute the diarrhea, the greater the loss of water and electrolytes, such as sodium, potassium, chloride, and bicarbonate. Steatorrhea is a type of diarrhea characterized by excess fat in the stools. The stools are frothy, bulky, and shiny in appearance, are foul-smelling, and float in water.

▶ The term **steatorrhea** is often used synony-
▶ mously with the term **malabsorption syndrome.** Steatorrhea, however, applies strictly to the passage of excess fat in the stool, whereas in the malabsorption syndrome multiple nutrient malabsorption occurs. Malabsorption may also refer to failure of absorption of a specific nutrient, such as vitamin B_{12}, or failure of reabsorption of biologically useful substances, such as bile salts that undergo enterohepatic circulation or absorption and circulation to the liver for reuse. The term malabsorption also encompasses maldigestion of food nutrients. The specific substances affected in malabsorption depend upon the area of the intestinal tract involved. Involvement of the proximal intestine may lead to malabsorption of multiple nutrients, whereas involvement of the distal ileum may induce malabsorption only of bile salts and vitamin B_{12}. Malabsorption may be accompanied by diarrhea or steatorrhea. Malabsorption of multiple nutrients contributes to a vicious cycle since the consequent nutrient deficiency leads to degeneration of intestinal mucosal cells.

Diarrhea

Assessment. Diarrhea may be acute or chronic in nature. In clients with acute diarrhea, assess for its cause, which may be (1) bacterial toxins, such as *Salmonella* or *Staphylococcus* food poisoning, (2) bacterial infections, such as *Streptococcus, Escherichia coli,* or *Shigella,* (3) drugs, such as neomycin and quinidine, (4) food sensitivity, (5) chemical toxins, such as arsenic or lead, or (6) psychologic factors, such as nervous irritability. Salmonellosis and shigellosis are probably the most common causes of gastroenteritis in the United States. Mucosal changes in the terminal ileum secondary to *Salmonella* invasion can alter the absorption of fats, fatsoluble vitamins, and other nutrients, whereas shigellosis primarily affects the colon.

Causes of chronic diarrhea include chronic le-

sions of the gastrointestinal tract associated with anatomic or mucosal defects, metabolic disorders, such as diabetic neuropathy, alcoholism, cancer of the gastrointestinal tract and its associated treatment, cirrhosis of the liver, laxative abuse, and enzyme deficiency states, such as deficiency of disaccharidases. Lesions that range from congestion and erythema to ulceration and chronic diarrhea are associated with the inflammatory bowel disorders discussed later in this chapter.

Mechanisms that underlie the net increase in intestinal fluid production and lead to diarrhea are (1) increased secretion of water and electrolytes, (2) increased concentration of osmotically active substances in the intestine, and (3) hypermotility.

Secretory diarrhea refers to an increased delivery of water and electrolytes to the rectum, resulting from increased secretion from the mucosa due to hormonal or toxic stimulation or due to inflammatory states. Moreover, a high concentration of fatty acids or bile acids in the colon may stimulate the colonic secretion of water and sodium or inhibit sodium and water reabsorption by the colon. Bacterial degradation of fatty acids produces hydroxy acids, which stimulate colonic secretion of water and sodium. This mechanism is responsible for the cathartic action of castor oil. The presence of bile acids in the colon inhibits colonic absorption of water and electrolytes and, to some extent, increases in the secretion of potassium.

Osmotic diarrhea results from an increased solute load in the intestinal lumen that draws fluid into the lumen from the extracellular fluid, as in the dumping syndrome following gastric surgery. The passage of osmotically active dietary components (such as disaccharides) into the colon may further increase osmotic activity of the substrate as a result of bacterial action.

Enhanced motility of the intestinal tract leads to rapid movement of nutrients through the tract and consequent malabsorption. Hypermotility may occur secondary to the action of certain laxatives and bowel disorders, such as the irritable bowel syndrome and diverticular disease.

Nutritional and metabolic consequences of intractable diarrhea are due to loss of water, electrolytes, and specific nutrients as well as the superimposed systemic effects of a precipitating illness. Fulminant (acute onset with great intensity) diarrhea or severe exacerbations of a chronic diarrhea may produce profound dehydration (either hypertonic or hypotonic) and equally profound electrolyte and acid–base disturbances. The fluid loss in acute inflammatory states tends to resemble the composition of plasma, and, thus, loss of protein as well as fluid and electrolytes occurs. Be aware that severe diarrhea can be more serious in infants, small children, and the elderly, who may become dehydrated rapidly. Monitor electrolyte levels closely, since losses, especially of potassium, account for the profound weakness associated with severe diarrhea.

Moreover, potassium depletion may alter bowel motility and induce anorexia. Potassium loss may reflect tissue depletion rather than specific changes in the blood potassium level, however. In clients with chronic illnesses associated with diarrhea, test for depletion of other nutrients, such as calcium, fat-soluble vitamins, iron, folic acid, and vitamin B_{12}, in addition to a generalized protein–calorie malnutrition. The nutrient depletion may occur secondary to diminished food intake (often associated with fear of precipitating symptoms with eating) and secondary to increased nutrient requirements associated with the excess stool losses. Should antibiotic therapy become necessary to control the precipitating illness, expect a temporary reduction in the intestinal synthesis of vitamin K and the B-complex vitamins. Iron deficiency is not uncommon in conditions associated with chronic diarrhea, not only because of diminished intake and increased intestinal loss but also in conjunction with chronic gastrointestinal bleeding in some diseases.

Intervention. Manage diarrhea by replacing fluid, electrolytes, vitamins, and minerals and by restoring and maintaining adequate kilocalorie and protein intake. The nutritional management of diarrheal disease depends on its acuteness and on individual food tolerance in each situation. For mild, acute diarrheal attacks, which are usually self-limited, minimal or no treatment may be necessary. Clear fluids and soft, nonirritating foods, such as refined bread, cereals, and soups, are often tolerated until the condition resolves. In severe conditions, restrict oral food intake for a period of 24 to 48 hours to allow for total bowel rest and maintain fluid and electrolyte balance by the parenteral route. Keep meticulous records of intake and output to aid in prescribing fluid replacement. It may be desirable to weigh the client daily as an indicator of fluid status. Should the period of oral food intolerance persist for more than 2 or 3 days, the addition of amino acids to the parenteral solution may be desirable. With persistent diarrhea, total parenteral nutrition may be necessary, especially if the precipitating condition warrants, or may warrant, surgery.

When the diarrhea subsides, progress the diet according to individual tolerance. Initially give small amounts of clear liquids. When tolerance for oral fluids is established, increase gradually the amounts and types of foods, first using full liquids, then a soft or low-residue diet, and finally a normal diet as tolerated. With oral food intake, adequate fluid and electrolytes should be provided, especially sodium and potassium. Fruit juices (high in potassium) and broth and bouillon (high in sodium) may be tolerated (see Chap. 9 for other foods high in potassium and Chap. 29 for foods high in sodium). Warm foods may be better tolerated than very hot or very cold foods. Determine if carbonated beverages result in gas or cramps. If this is the case, substitute flat beverages. As the diet progresses, assess for tolerance for individual food items, such as milk, fat, and foods high in fiber.

Impaired absorption secondary to anatomic changes or mucosal alterations in the small bowel is a common feature of many chronic diarrheal states. In these situations, provide a high-kilocalorie, high-protein intake to prevent losses of body weight and protein depletion. In some situations a daily intake that includes as much as 4000 kcal and 150 g protein may be necessary. With this diet regimen, include concentrated sources of kilocalories and protein (such as milk fortified with skim milk powder or nutritionally complete commercial liquid supplements, see Chap. 21).

Diets low in residue and fiber may be advocated as part of the diet progression in acute diarrheal states in order to reduce intestinal irritation. **Pectin,** a component of dietary fiber, may be of value in treating diarrhea. Pectin (as well as guar gum) has been reported to delay gastric emptying significantly, and this effect may contribute to its therapeutic value.[1] Moreover, pectin, like other components of dietary fiber, absorbs water in the gut and may prove beneficial in returning the stool to a soft consistency without the loss of free water. Give foods high in pectin content, such as peeled raw apple and applesauce, every 2 to 4 hours to improve the uptake of free water and to improve the consistency of stools. Pectin can also be added to water (1 tsp of pectin to 1 quart of water).

The nutritional management of diarrhea associated with specific intestinal disorders is included in the discussion of the specific disorders.

Steatorrhea

Assessment. Steatorrhea is a major clinical and biochemical manifestation of maldigestion and malabsorption. This is attributable to the fact that the steps involved in digestion and absorption of fats are more complex than for other nutrients. Healthy individuals excrete about 2 to 6 g of fat in the stool that is derived from unabsorbed dietary lipids, desquamated cells, and bacteria. In the severest form of steatorrhea, which occurs in clients with pancreatic disease, the client may excrete as much as 100 g.[2]

Observe for steatorrhea in clients with these intestinal disorders:

1. Mucosal lesions or damage, such as gluten-induced enteropathy, Crohn's disease, radiation damage to the intestine, and excessive alcohol consumption
2. Enteral infections, such as acute enteritis and blind loop stasis
3. Maldigestion secondary to a deficiency of bile salts or pancreatic enzymes
4. Surgery, such as ileal resection, massive small bowel resection (i.e., resection of over 50 percent of the intestine), and gastric resection

5. Biochemical abnormalities, such as the Zollinger–Ellison syndrome and lipoprotein deficiency (i.e., abeta-lipoproteinemia)
6. Impaired intestinal lymphatic drainage

With severe steatorrhea, maintenance of energy intake may present a problem. Observe for weight loss as a common manifestation. Moreover, with fecal fat loss there is a concomitant loss of nitrogen, water, fat-soluble vitamins, magnesium, and calcium (calcium and magnesium ions may form insoluble soaps with fatty acids in the intestine). The consequent vitamin D and calcium loss makes calcium depletion a significant problem.

Intervention. Since steatorrhea is a symptom of many organic diseases, treatment of the primary disease will bring secondary relief. Dietary management includes restricting fat (discussed in Chap. 28) or substituting medium-chain triglycerides (MCT), such as MCT oil (Mead Johnson) for traditional fats, and providing supplements of fat-soluble vitamins (in a water-miscible form), calcium, and magnesium. Formulas that contain MCT oil are available for infants (Pregestimil and Portagen—Mead Johnson). If steatorrhea is caused by a bile salt deficiency, redistribution of the fat in the day's meals may be helpful. Since the intestinal concentration of bile is greater after the morning meal—the gallbladder retains all circulating and newly synthesized bile salts overnight—an increase in the fat content of the morning meal is indicated. Fat digestion may be adequate in the morning but inefficient at meals later in the day.

By virtue of their smaller molecular size and greater solubility in water, MCT are hydrolyzed more rapidly than normal fat despite pancreatic lipase deficiency (hydrolysis can occur intracellularly), and they do not require bile acids for micelle formation, a prerequisite to fat digestion and absorption. Moreover, MCT are transported directly to the liver through the portal circulation. Thus, these lipids bypass the triglyceride resynthesis, chylomicron formation, and lymphatic transport necessary for conventional fats.

These special properties make MCT useful in treating malabsorptive disorders in which long-chain fats are poorly digested and absorbed. They provide a rapidly available source of energy (8.3 kcal/g), resulting in weight gain in adults, growth in children, and enhanced absorption of calcium and magnesium.[3] Another interesting feature associated with MCT are a lower tendency to be deposited as body fat.

Observe for side effects of nausea, abdominal distention or cramps, and diarrhea in clients who take MCT supplements. The symptoms are attributed to the hyperosmolar load associated with the rapid hydrolysis of MCT and the irritating effects of high levels of free fatty acids in the intestinal tract. To minimize these adverse reactions, advise clients to consume MCT slowly and in small amounts at a time. No more than 60 percent of the total fat kilocalories (or 20 percent of total kilocalories) should be given as MCT. Since large amounts may cause ketosis, be cautious in administering MCT to pregnant women or to diabetic clients, particularly if they are ketosis-prone. Be aware that MCT contain no essential fatty acids nor do they promote absorption of fat-soluble vitamins. They, therefore, should not be given as the sole source of fat in the diet.

Allot a considerable amount of time to the hospitalized client for teaching the principles of the diet and MCT cooking. MCT can be used for seasoning vegetables and in preparing baked goods, casseroles, salad dressings, puddings, sauces and seasonings, and fried foods. Provide recipes for preparing these foods.[4-6] Blended with skim milk or fruit juice, MCT can be used as a beverage.

Malabsorption

Assessment. The causes and clinical manifestations of the malabsorption syndrome vary widely. Clinical manifestations depend on the site and severity of the pathology, the specific nutrients affected, and the nutrient stores present at the onset of the illness. Causes of maldigestion and malabsorption are listed in Table 27–1. Observe clients with these disorders for the clinical manifestations that may arise (Table 27–2).

Intervention. The general management of maldigestion and malabsorption varies according to diagnosis and may involve surgery, medications, and diet modifications. Nutritional management of severe malabsorption entails replacement of electrolytes, minerals, and vitamins (give a water-miscible form of fat-soluble vitamins). In clients with disease or resection of the terminal ileum, give vitamin B_{12} by injection. Assess the adequacy of kilocalorie and protein intake and supplement with commercial liquid formulas (see Chap. 21) if necessary. In some situations, total parenteral nutrition is indicated. Since gastric emptying is affected by the volume of intragastric contents, provide small meals of low volume to slow gastric emptying and intestinal motility.

Other dietary manipulations depend on the underlying illness, as discussed here.

INFLAMMATORY BOWEL DISEASES

Inflammatory bowel disease refers to several conditions of nonspecific etiology and with variable manifestations, whose course is characterized by intermittent remissions and recurrences, ranging from mild intermittent exacerbations to unremitting, devastating illness. Included in this group are

---

TABLE 27–1
CAUSES OF MALDIGESTION AND MALABSORPTION

Maldigestion

Gastric resection leading to
    Decreased volume of gastric secretions
    Relative pancreatic and hepatic insufficiency
    Inadequate mixing of secretions
    Bacterial overgrowth in an afferent loop of intestine
Pancreatic insufficiency
    Decreased enzymes: chronic pancreatitis, cystic fibrosis, carcinoma of the pancreas with duct obstruction, pancreatic resection
    Decreased pH (a pH above 6 favors digestive action of pancreatic enzymes); decreased bicarbonate output by pancreas; Zollinger–Ellison syndrome (gastric hypersecretion alters the gut pH)
Hepatobiliary insufficiency leading to bile salt deficiency and a decrease in lipolysis and micelle formation
    Extrahepatic biliary obstruction, e.g., stones or carcinoma
    Congenital defects (biliary atresia)
    Hepatitis, cirrhosis, and chronic intrahepatic cholestasis
    Intestinal bacterial overgrowth syndromes
    Cholestyramine treatment

Malabsorption

Inadequate absorbing surface
    Extensive intestinal resection (i.e., resection of 50% or more of the intestine)
    Partial or total resection of the terminal ileum leading to malabsorption of vitamin B_{12} and bile acids
    Intestinal bypass (e.g., jejunoileal bypass for morbid obesity)
Microbial effects
    Stasis and bacterial overgrowth (blind loop syndrome) leading to malabsorption of fat, folate, and vitamin B_{12} (bacteria bind folate and vitamin B_{12} and deconjugate bile salts) due to
        Abnormal gut motility (diffuse as in amyloidosis and scleroderma or localized as in the blind duodenal pouch created in Billroth II reconstruction)
        Jejunal diverticulosis
        Strictures and fistulas (as in radiation enteropathy or Crohn's disease)
    Parasitic infestation (such as tapeworm or hookworm)
Inflammatory small bowel disorders (such as regional enteritis, radiation enteritis, and infections)
Vascular insufficiency and small bowel ischemia
Lymphatic obstruction leading to malabsorption of fat (due to congenital defects or tumors)
Severe malnutrition
Drug-induced effects on the intestine (such as alcohol, neomycin, and colchicine)
Metabolic diseases or diseases of uncertain origin (such as endocrine disorders, diabetes mellitus, Paget's disease, collagen diseases, amyloidosis, and skin disorders)
Specific cellular disorders, such as gluten-induced enteropathy, tropical sprue, congenital and acquired lactase deficiency, glucose–galactose malabsorption, sucrase–isomaltase deficiency, cystinuria, Hartnup disease, abeta-lipoproteinemia, and gastrointestinal allergy

---

Crohn's disease (also referred to as regional enteritis, granulomatous enteritis, and granulomatous colitis), ulcerative colitis, and diverticulitis. Crohn's disease and ulcerative colitis usually develop in young adults, often beginning in the second or third decade, and the incidence in males and females is about equal. The incidence of these disorders has increased worldwide during the past several decades, and in the United States it is more common among Jewish people.[7] The incidence of diverticular disease, which is the most common colonic disease of Western nations, increases with age. Epidemiologic data suggest that its incidence has increased during the last century and relate the increased incidence to consumption of a low-fiber diet.

Both Crohn's disease and ulcerative colitis are chronic, progressive, inflammatory processes involving the intestines. Unlike Crohn's disease, which can affect any part of the gastrointestinal tract and which affects the entire thickness of the bowel wall, ulcerative colitis is essentially a disease of the colon and rectum and involves the mucosal and submucosal segments. In contrast, diverticulitis occurs when a diverticulum (a herniation of the intestinal mucosa through the muscle fibers of the bowel wall) becomes inflamed in clients with the chronic disorder, diverticulosis. Like ulcerative colitis, the colon is most often affected, however, and like Crohn's disease, diverticula can occur in any part of the gastrointestinal tract.

TABLE 27-2
CLINICAL MANIFESTATIONS OF MALDIGESTION AND MALABSORPTION

Manifestation	Cause
Weight loss	Malabsorption; voluntary restriction of food intake to decrease symptoms; anorexia
Diarrhea and abdominal pain	Increased secretion or decreased reabsorption of water and electrolytes; increased concentration of osmotically active substances in the intestine; hypermotility
Nocturia	Delayed water absorption
Muscle weakness	Electrolyte depletion (particularly potassium depletion)
Peripheral edema	Hypoalbuminemia secondary to reduced hepatic synthesis of albumin due to protein malabsorption, leakage of serum proteins through the damaged intestinal mucosa, or passage of lymph from the intestinal lymphatics
Anemia	Malabsorption of protein, iron, folate or vitamin B_{12}; chronic blood and iron loss; secondary to chronic inflammatory or neoplastic disease
Capillary fragility, hemorrhagic tendencies, purpura, and petechiae	Vitamin K or vitamin C malabsorption
Bone pain, osteoporosis, osteomalacia	Malabsorption of calcium and vitamin D; impaired activation of vitamin D (if liver disease is present)
Tetany and paresthesia	Calcium and magnesium malabsorption
Impaired dark adaptation	Vitamin A malabsorption
Glossitis, cheilosis, skin changes, peripheral neuritis	B-complex vitamin malabsorption
Gallstones	Impaired enterohepatic circulation of bile salts, reduction in the bile salt pool, and saturation of bile with cholesterol
Renal stone formation (oxalate and uric acid)	*Oxalate stones:* enhanced oxalate absorption in the colon secondary to fat malabsorption and binding of fat with calcium—less calcium is thus available in the gut to form insoluble calcium oxalate *Uric acid stones:* secretion of a persistently acid urine in those with inflammatory bowel disease

(*Source: Adapted from Holt PR: Nutrition in Disease: Malabsorption. Columbus, Ohio, Ross Laboratories, 1977, p 10.*)

Assessment

Etiology. The etiology of inflammatory bowel diseases is unknown, although a number of etiologic factors have been implicated. It has been speculated, for example, that genetic and immunologic factors and infectious processes may be important in the etiology of Crohn's disease and ulcerative colitis. Allergic conditions and psychologic stress have been implicated in the etiology of ulcerative colitis.

An altered motility pattern in the colon and the amount of dietary fiber ingested have been implicated in the etiology of diverticular disease. Development of diverticula has been attributed to chronic ingestion of a low-fiber diet leading to small, compact stools. According to this theory, the small stools cause the colon to contract more tightly around it, thus causing the colonic lumen to narrow and the intraluminal pressure to rise. This high pressure may lead to herniation of the colonic muscles and the diverticular characteristic of the disorder. In contrast, the soft, bulky stools that accompany a high fiber intake are propelled more easily, require very little pressure for ejection, and are not conducive to diverticular formation. At this time, however, there is no direct proof of any cause and effect relationship between a low fiber intake and diverticular disease.

Crohn's Disease (Regional Enteritis): Pathologic Manifestations. Inflammation of the intestine with granuloma formation (growths usually of lymphoid and epithelial cells) is characteristic of Crohn's disease. Progression of the disease and diffuse granuloma formation lead to edema, thickening, fibrosis, narrowing, and stenosis of the intestine, creating the possibility of obstruction. Diseased areas of the bowel may alternate with healthy ones— hence, the term **regional enteritis**. It commonly affects the terminal ileum, but the colon and anorectal area may also be involved. Assess for the signs and symptoms summarized in Table 27–3, which will

TABLE 27–3
MANIFESTATIONS OF INFLAMMATORY BOWEL DISEASE

Crohn's Disease

Insidious onset with intermittent diarrhea, tenderness, pain, and cramping in the right lower quadrant of the abdomen

Blood in the stool (less prominent than in ulcerative colitis); increased secretion of mucus by the bowel

Low-grade fever

Complications include external fistulization, scarring with obstruction, perforation with abscess formation and hemorrhage, arthritis, and intestinal carcinoma

Selective or diffuse malabsorption and malnutrition associated with mucosal defects or induced by fecal bile salt losses or bacterial overgrowth
  Widespread involvement of the small bowel results in variable degrees of malabsorption of fat, protein, carbohydrate, vitamins, and minerals and weight loss
  Impaired absorption of vitamin B_{12} and impaired reabsorption of bile salts with terminal ileal involvement
  Vitamin B_{12} deficiency may lead to macrocytic anemia and neurologic damage
  Bile salt losses lead to diarrhea, steatorrhea, oxaluria, and gallstone formation

Small intestinal stasis and bacterial proliferation
  Vitamin B_{12} and folate deficiency
  Secretory diarrhea and steatorrhea

Anemia secondary to bleeding

Retarded growth in children

Ulcerative Colitis

Onset usually insidious

Lesions begin in the rectum and progress backward

Anorexia

Abdominal pain, diarrhea, blood in the stool, and altered colonic mucus

Complications include abscesses, arthritis, toxic megacolon (paralysis of the motor function and dilatation of the transverse colon), massive hemorrhage, and carcinoma of the colon

Malabsorption and weight loss

Anemia secondary to bleeding

Diverticulitis

Flatulence, intermittent diarrhea or constipation, and discomfort in the lower left quadrant of the abdomen

Complications include bleeding, perforation, and peritonitis, abscess and fistula formation, and intestinal obstruction from stenosis resulting from acute or chronic diverticulitis

Stasis and bacterial overgrowth
  Diarrhea, steatorrhea, and vitamin B_{12} deficiency (when the small bowel is involved)

---

vary considerably depending on the stage of progression of the disease and the area of the gastrointestinal tract involved.

The malabsorption may be selective or diffuse. When the terminal ileum is involved, absorption of vitamin B_{12} and bile salts may be impaired. Both of these substances undergo enterohepatic circulation. Macrocytic anemia and neurologic damage may result from vitamin B_{12} malabsorption, and diarrhea, steatorrhea, oxaluria (increased excretion of oxalate in the urine with an increased tendency to form oxalate renal stones) and gallstone formation may be side effects of the increased bile salt loss in the colon. The presence of bile salts in the colon produces a laxative effect, leading to a secretory diarrhea. With extensive disease, the liver cannot keep pace with bile salt losses, and the bile salt pool is lowered, leading to inadequate micelle formation and steatorrhea. Oxaluria is thought to occur because of (1) an increase in the concentration of

free oxalate reaching the colon, and (2) an increase in colonic permeability to oxalate in the presence of fatty acids and bile salts. The binding of calcium in the small intestine by intraluminal fat leads to a diminished production of insoluble calcium oxalate. The colon must be present for oxaluria to occur; free oxalate is readily absorbed by the colon. The increased tendency to form gallstones occurs secondary to the bile salt loss. The bile then has a tendency to become lithogenic; i.e., the cholesterol tends to come out of solution.

More widespread involvement of the small bowel results in variable degrees of malabsorption of multiple nutrients, leading to malnutrition.

Ulcerative Colitis: Pathologic Manifestations.
Nonspecific ulcerative colitis is a diffuse, inflammatory, and ulcerative disease of the colon and rectum, which generally follows a prolonged course with alternating periods of remissions and exacerbations

and, occasionally, spontaneous recovery. Initial pathologic lesions are confined to the mucosa and consist of abscess formation in the crypts. Edema and congestion may lead to extreme friability and bleeding even with minor trauma. With progression of the disease, the abscesses spread to the submucosa, which becomes ulcerated. Assess for the signs and symptoms summarized in Table 27–3 in affected clients.

Diverticulitis: Pathologic Manifestations. Diverticular disease or diverticulosis is a condition characterized by the presence of single or multiple herniations (diverticula, or blind outpouchings) of the gastrointestinal mucosa through the muscular wall. Diverticula, which may be congenital or acquired, usually develop at points in the intestinal wall where it is weakened by the penetration of blood vessels. Infection and inflammation of the diverticula can occur as a result of bacterial action on food residues or fecal matter that may accumulate
▶ in the sacs. This condition is called **diverticulitis.**

The symptoms (see Table 27–3) are similar to the spastic or irritable colon syndrome. Assess for a previous history of the latter disorder, which may precede the development of diverticulosis in some clients. The pressure changes in diverticular disease are similar to those found in the irritable colon syndrome. Whereas diverticulosis occurs most often in the elderly and is generally attributed to general muscle tone weakness, the so-called spastic colon diverticulosis occurs with increasing frequency beginning with the third decade of life as a result of unusually high intraluminal pressure.

Effects on Nutrition. Chronic malnutrition is common in inflammatory bowel disease, particularly Crohn's disease and ulcerative colitis, in association with inadequate intake, excess fecal losses, malabsorption, and increased requirements. Expect these mechanisms, particularly the malabsorption, to be more accentuated in Crohn's disease than in ulcerative colitis, since the small intestine is often involved in Crohn's disease. In contrast, diverticular disease usually does not present nutritional complications unless it is accompanied by inflammation, formation of abscesses or fistulae, perforation, or obstruction.

Assess the energy and nutrient intake and evaluate the effect of each of the following as potential causes of inadequate intake in affected clients: (1) anorexia (secondary to long-standing inflammatory disease), (2) altered taste (due either to drug therapy or to abnormalities in heavy metal metabolism, particularly zinc), (3) increased abdominal pain (in association with the disease itself or in response to food intake), and (4) diarrhea (triggered or exacerbated by food intake or even independent of food intake).

Gastrointestinal bleeding, steatorrhea (particularly in Crohn's disease), diarrhea, and protein-losing enteropathy bring an increase in fecal loss

of nutrients. In the last condition, there is excessive loss of plasma protein into the gastrointestinal tract by exudation through the inflamed and ulcerated mucosa. The protein loss may lead to edema and hypoproteinemia. The net absorption of sodium and water may be diminished in inflammatory bowel disorders, and low serum folic acid levels, vitamin B_{12} malabsorption, and calcium depletion are common. Calcium deficiency occurs as a result of steatorrhea as well as mucosal malabsorption of vitamin D and calcium. In general, the malabsorption in Crohn's disease is a reflection of the degree of small bowel involvement, and electrolyte losses, dehydration, folic acid deficiency, and mineral and fat-soluble vitamin deficiency parallel the severity of the steatorrhea. The folate depletion occurs because of mucosal malabsorption, dietary inadequacy, and competition for absorption between the vitamin and sulfasaline (Azulfidine), a medication used in treatment of inflammatory bowel disease.[8] Severe diarrhea in ulcerative colitis leads to varying degrees of dehydration and losses of sodium, potassium, and chloride. Test for iron deficiency anemia, which is common in both Crohn's disease and ulcerative colitis. The degree of anemia reflects the extent of bleeding as well as the extent of the inflammatory bowel disorder.

Assess for the presence of fever in clients with inflammatory bowel disease. Energy and nutrient requirements increase when fever is present.

Intervention

Treatment of inflammatory bowel disorders is largely symptomatic and empirical. There is no specific or curative treatment. Take measures to prevent infection, control inflammation, attain remission, and maintain nutritional status. Surgical intervention is usually reserved for unremitting disease and for complications, such as obstruction, perforation, hemorrhage, and fistulation.

In Crohn's disease and ulcerative colitis, corticosteroids may be used to control inflammation and promote remission, and antibiotics and antibacterials are used in the presence of fever, sepsis, and so on. The laxative effect of bile salts in the colon can be diminished by binding the salts with a sequestrant, such as cholestyramine. Acute diverticulitis necessitates bedrest, antibiotics, and stool softeners.

In providing nursing care for clients with Crohn's disease and ulcerative colitis, provide emotional support on a continuing basis, since the disorders are chronic, the prognosis is variable, and the etiology is unknown. Moreover, the client is often a young person who frequently feels resentful about having a chronic illness in this particular period of life. There may be apprehension about triggering symptoms with the intake of particular foods. Therefore, provide constant reassurance about the content of the diet.

Follow these five objectives in planning nutritional care for clients with inflammatory bowel disorders:

1. Restore metabolic homeostasis to as nearly normal as possible
2. Replace obvious losses, e.g., blood, protein, electrolytes
3. Correct deficits
4. Promote energy and nitrogen balance
5. Stimulate growth (should the disorder occur in children)

Types of nutritional support include traditional table foods, oral supplements (such as nutritionally complete liquid formulas), nasogastric feedings administered by continuous drip, and total parenteral nutrition (TPN). Table 27–4 provides a summary of the principles of nutritional management for clients with Crohn's disease and ulcerative colitis. Observe the client's response to the various feeding strategies and establish an individualized regimen.

Assess for tolerance of fibrous foods, milk, fat, and iced fluids and provide dietary advice based on this assessment. For example, restrict milk and provide lactose-free commercial formulas if there is an intolerance to lactose. No more than 50 g of conventional fat may be tolerated, particularly in clients with Crohn's disease. Use MCT as a source of additional energy in clients with steatorrhea. Also advise

---

TABLE 27–4
NUTRITIONAL MANAGEMENT OF CROHN'S DISEASE AND ULCERATIVE COLITIS

Crohn's Disease (Regional Enteritis)	
Dietary Factor	**Comments**
1. Kcal 2. Protein	1 and 2. 3500–4000 kcal and at least 125 g protein to overcome losses due to malabsorption and protein-losing enteropathy; kcal derived largely from carbohydrate and protein; amino acid supplements may be necessary
3. Fat	3. Restricted to 10–25% of kcal in presence of steatorrhea; MCT may be substituted for long-chain fats
4. Vitamins and minerals	4. Supplemented according to client need; particularly need supplements of vitamin C, B-complex (including B_{12} and folate), vitamin K, calcium, magnesium, iron, and potassium; vitamin K, vitamin B_{12}, and iron are not well absorbed and should be administered parenterally at intermittent intervals when indicated by low blood levels
5. Oxalate	5. Restricted to prevent oxaluria (see Chap. 30 for oxalate content of foods); oxalate restriction should be accompanied by fat restriction and calcium (or magnesium or possibly aluminum) supplements to decrease colonic absorption of oxalate; since ascorbic acid may be metabolized to oxalate in some individuals, intakes of large doses of the vitamin should be avoided; oxalate-binding agents may also be used
6. Meal size and frequency	6. Six or more small meals
7. Feeding method	7. *With severe symptoms:* Provide bowel rest; TPN or DFD may be useful in those who have undergone considerable weight loss; if oral feedings are used, a clear liquid or low-residue diet may be indicated *With mild or moderate symptoms:* After initial period of bowel rest, provide low-residue oral feedings with eventual return to normal diet, restricting only those foods known to aggravate symptoms (for some a degree of fiber restriction may be desirable)[a]
Ulcerative Colitis	
Dietary Factor	**Comments**
1 and 2. Kcal and Protein	1 and 2. 2500–3500 or more kcal and 125–150 g protein to replace losses from diarrhea and protein-losing enteropathy; high-kcal, high-protein liquid supplements may be necessary
3. Fat	3. Restricted if steatorrhea is present; substitute MCT
4. Vitamins and minerals	4. Supplement as necessary; blood transfusions or intramuscular iron injections may be necessary to correct the anemia, since oral iron supplements may cause gastrointestinal disturbances even when taken with meals; potassium supplements are necessary with exacerbations of diarrhea
5. Meal size and frequency	5. Six or more small feedings
6. Feeding method	6. The diet is individualized according to the severity of the disease; TPN or DFD may be necessary in acute stages to induce weight gain, positive nitrogen balance, and healing of ulcerated lesions (if oral feedings are used, clear liquid or low-residue diet may be indicated); following the period of bowel rest, the diet may progress to one of low-residue content and later to a regular diet that excludes foods for which intolerance is established (e.g., some may not tolerate raw fruits and vegetables or fruit juices, others may not tolerate milk—in some there seems to be an allergy to cow's milk protein) (see Chap. 32 for a milk-free diet)

[a] A low-residue diet is advocated by some as the maintenance diet to reduce peristalsis and diminish the possibility of obstruction. Others note that in some individuals an increase in the fiber content may decrease the diarrhea.

**TABLE 27-5
A LOW-RESIDUE DIET**

Category	Foods Allowed	Foods Avoided[a]
Beverages	Carbonated; coffee, cereal beverages, tea, decaffeinated coffee; milk, if tolerated (limit to 2 c daily, including that used in cooking)	Milk or milk beverages in excess of 2 c daily; yoghurt with seeds or fruit
Bread and cereal	Refined, enriched white or light rye bread or rolls without seeds; saltine crackers; rusk or melba toast; English muffins; zwieback; matzo; bagels; Italian or French bread; cornbread made with refined cornmeal; refined cooked or ready-to-eat cereals made from rice, corn, oats, or wheat, such as farina, Cream of Wheat, strained oatmeal, grits, Corn Flakes, Puffed Rice, Rice Flakes; macaroni, noodles, spaghetti, white rice	Bran or bran products; whole grain products; graham flour products; products containing seeds, nuts, coconut, or dried fruits such as granola-type cereals; quick breads and pastries; brown rice
Dessert	Plain cakes with plain frosting, such as angel food, sponge, chiffon, and plain pound cake; plain cookies; pies made from allowed fruit or pureed fruit; gelatin; fruit ice; fruit whips and sherbet; ice cream, junket, milk-flavored sherbet and pudding within milk allowance	Desserts made with nuts, coconut, seeds, dried fruit, fruit with skins or raw fruit other than those allowed
Eggs	Eggs prepared any way except fried	Fried eggs
Fat	Butter, margarine, mayonnaise, vegetable oil, cream (limit to ½ c per day); crisp bacon; mild salad dressings; plain gravy; cream cheese	Rich or spiced gravies
Fruit	Tender canned or cooked fruits without seeds or tough skin such as applesauce, peaches, pears, and peeled apricots; peeled raw apple, banana, and demembraned citrus fruit sections; ripe avocado; fruit juices; jellied cranberry sauce	Raw fruits other than those allowed; any fruit with seed or tough skin; dried fruit; prune juice
Meat or substitute	Tender meat, fish, or fowl prepared by roasting, baking, boiling, broiling, creaming, or stewing; less tender meat should be chopped or ground; canned tuna and salmon; sweetbreads; canned ham without gristle; creamy peanut butter; mild American or cheddar cheese and cottage cheese (when cheese is used, reduce milk ½ c for each oz of cheese used)	Fried meats; tough meats with gristle; highly spiced and seasoned meats; smoked meat or fish; corned beef; frankfurters; luncheon meat; sharp or strongly flavored cheese; cheese with seeds or fibrous ingredients
Soup	Broth, bouillon, strained cream soups made with allowed foods and within daily milk allowance	Soups containing tough meats or fibrous vegetables; highly seasoned soups; cream soups in excess of milk allowance
Sweets	Granulated and brown sugar; clear jelly; honey; hard candy; gumdrops; marshmallows; corn and maple syrup and light, refined molasses	Chocolate candy or candy made with coconut, seeds, dried fruit, nuts; jam; preserves; marmalade
Vegetables	Canned or well-cooked asparagus tips, beets, carrots, pumpkin, squash, green and wax beans, spinach, other tender leafy greens, strained tomatoes; white and sweet potatoes without skins; vegetable and tomato juice	All other vegetables; dried peas, beans and other legumes; fried potatoes; potato chips; potato skins; raw salads
Miscellaneous	Salt; mild herbs and spices in moderation; simple sauces such as white sauce; vinegar; lemon juice; catsup; mild mustard; flavoring extracts	Pepper and other hot spices; garlic; olives; pickles; popcorn; relishes; excessive seasonings; chili sauce, Worcestershire sauce

[a] The residue content of the diet can be reduced to minimum levels by eliminating milk and milk products and substituting strained fruit and vegetable juices in the fruit and vegetable categories.

clients with Crohn's disease to restrict the intake of foods high in oxalate (see Chap. 30). This measure in combination with fat restriction and calcium supplementation tends to diminish the colonic absorption of oxalate and the propensity for oxalate stone formation.

When anorexia is present, use nursing strategies for making meals attractive and mealtime pleasant. Clients recognize the relationship between food intake and discomfort and need continuing support. Consider the use of defined formula diets (DFD) as a supplement, and improve their palatability by adding fruit juice.

Avoid giving folic acid supplements concomitantly with sulfasaline, since the vitamin will not be well absorbed when given with the drug. Increase fluid intake to 2500 ml daily as an adjunct to sulfasaline therapy. Assess for fluid retention as a side effect of corticosteroid therapy and restrict sodium in its presence.

During periods when the disorder is asymptomatic, encourage a further increase in food intake to replace losses in conjunction with exacerbations. Deficits must be corrected before catch-up growth can occur in children. Observe the growth records of children with inflammatory bowel disorders to evaluate the effectiveness of treatment. When symptoms are acute and oral intake is impossible, provide total parenteral nutrition.

Diets identified as low-residue, low-roughage, and low-fiber are used at times in the management of inflammatory bowel diseases. Much confusion and misunderstanding surround the definitions of these terms. The terms **fiber** and **roughage** are used synonymously, but these are not synonymous with **residue.** Dietary fiber refers to the indigestible content of food, whereas residue denotes all material that remains in the lower intestinal tract after digestion and absorption have occurred proximally. Residue includes not only the undigested and unabsorbed food but also metabolic and bacterial products (e.g., desquamated cells from the mucosa and bacterial residues). All foods provide some residue. Whole grain cereal and bran are considered to be high-residue foods because of their high fiber content. It does not necessarily follow, however, that a low-fiber food is also low in residue. For example, there is some evidence that milk, a fiber-free food, indirectly contributes some residue to the fecal contents, and controversy surrounds its use in residue-restricted diet plans. Despite the fact that prune juice leaves no residue upon chemical digestion, it is classified as a high-residue food, since it contains a laxative that indirectly increases stool volume. The elastin fibers of meat are also restricted in low-residue diets to decrease the volume of fecal material.

A low-residue diet is indicated in conditions in which the presence of bulky fecal materials in the bowel is undesirable, e.g., in acute phases of inflammatory bowel disorders or if stenosis of the bowel has occurred. The diet is not ordered on a routine basis for Crohn's disease, ulcerative colitis, or chronic diverticular disease. Residue-restricted diets are ordered at various levels of restriction—minimal residue, moderate residue, and low residue. Foods that produce the least residue are gelatin, sucrose, dextrose, Karo syrup, concentrated broth, hard-cooked eggs, meat, rice, farina, and cottage cheese. In contrast, nuts, seeds, fruits, vegetables, and whole grains are among those that produce the largest amount of residue. A diet low in residue is given in Table 27–5.

In clients experiencing symptoms of acute diverticulitis, limit feedings to clear liquids, with a gradual progression in texture to a low-residue diet until the inflammatory crisis has subsided. It may be necessary to restrict oral intake for a period of time if there are signs of obstruction. For asymptomatic diverticular disease, however, emphasize the use of a high-fiber diet. A low-fiber regimen is thought to perpetuate a vicious cycle and is therefore contraindicated for routine, long-term use unless the colon is narrowed or stenosed. With an increase in the fiber content of the diet, there is an increase in the velocity and volume of residue passing through the gut (transit time is shortened, and stool volume and weight are increased). The distention of the bowel wall from within should therefore correct to some extent the abnormal intraluminal colonic pressure that is thought to contribute to the disorders. When a high-fiber diet is prescribed, the diet should contain approximately 13 g or more of crude fiber daily. Table 27–6 provides a list of the crude fiber content of selected foods. A list of the dietary fiber content of selected foods has been published.[9]

When increasing the fiber content of the diet, assure the client of its potential efficacy. The client

TABLE 27–6
CRUDE FIBER CONTENT OF SELECTED FOODS

Food	Crude Fiber/100 g
Bran flakes (100% bran)	7.8
Bran flakes (40% bran)	3.6
Raisin bran	3.0
Bran muffin	1.8
Puffed Wheat	2.0
Shredded Wheat	2.3
Whole wheat bread	1.6
Peanuts (with skins)	2.7
Filberts	3.0
Pecans	2.3
Brazil nuts	3.1
Pistachio nuts	1.9
Peanut butter	1.9
Almonds	2.6
Raisins (uncooked)	0.9
Prunes (dried, uncooked)	1.6
Currants (black European)	2.4
Raspberries (raw, black)	5.1
Apple (raw, unpared)	1.0
Strawberries (raw)	1.3
Pear (raw including skin)	1.4
Orange (peeled)	0.5
Artichoke (raw or cooked)	2.4
Beans (red)	1.5
Brussels sprouts (cooked)	1.6
Carrots (raw or cooked)	1.0
Cabbage (raw or cooked)	0.8
Celery (raw or cooked)	0.6
Cucumber (not pared)	0.6
Turnip greens (cooked)	0.7
Tomato (raw)	0.5
Spinach (raw or cooked)	0.6

(*Source:* USDA: *Handbook of the Nutritional Content of Foods.* New York, Dover Publishing, 1975.)

may be apprehensive about this dietary approach, since diverticular disease was formerly treated with a low-residue diet. Assist the client to plan menus using the high-fiber foods listed in Table 27–7. Low-fiber foods, such as meat and eggs, should be selected to complete the nutritional adequacy of the diet. Encourage the client to increase fiber content gradually, since starting with a large amount may give rise to considerable abdominal discomfort and flatus. When increasing the fiber content, stress the importance of consuming adequate water (at least 2000 ml daily) because of fiber's water-absorbing capacity.

The laxative effect of unprocessed wheat bran is superior to that of vegetable and fruit fibers because of its higher fiber content and greater indigestibility. Coarsely ground bran is preferable to finely ground bran. Daily consumption of bran supplements is the most widely recommended way of achieving a high-fiber diet. However, the laxative effect of fruits and vegetables is quantitatively important and should not be discounted, and unrefined breakfast cereals and whole wheat and rye flour contain significant amounts of fiber. If bran supplements are used, advise the client to start with small doses (e.g., 1 tsp twice a day) and gradually increase the amount to about 6 tsp a day (the precise amount will depend on client tolerance and the amount of other fiber sources in the diet). Bran can be mixed with foods, such as cereals and soups, or added to baked goods. Be aware, however, that the large amount of phytates in bran and unprocessed flour may chelate minerals, such as calcium, iron, and zinc and possibly folate as well. To achieve a high-fiber diet without the use of bran, encourage the client to use whole grain bread and cereal in lieu of their refined counterparts and to include generous amounts of fruits and vegetables, such as raw carrots, apples, oranges, and cooked, unpeeled potatoes.

TABLE 27–7
FIBER CONTENT OF FOODS

Category	Foods High in Fiber	Foods Low in Fiber
Beverages		All are low in fiber[a]
Bread and cereal	Bread, rolls, muffins, and pancakes made from 100% whole wheat or whole rye flour; graham, wheat, or rye crackers; Rye Krisp; whole grain bread with seeds; buckwheat bread; cracked wheat bread; cornbread made with course-ground meal; oatmeal; Shredded Wheat; whole wheat and bran cereal, unprocessed bran (in moderation); Puffed Wheat; brown rice; granola cereal with dried fruit added; Grapenuts; wheat flakes; wheat germ; millet	White bread, sourdough bread; French bread; English muffins; saltines and soda crackers; refined flours; refined wheat, corn, rice, and oat cereal; white rice; macaroni; noodles; spaghetti
Dessert	Fresh fruit and fruit pies; fruitcake; desserts made with dried fruit, nuts, or coconut, e.g., fig bars and macaroons; bran muffins and cookies; oatmeal cookies	Ice cream, pudding and custard[a]; cream pies, plain cakes and cookies
Eggs and cheese		All are low in fiber
Fat		All are low in fiber
Fruits	Fresh fruits with skin and seeds, e.g., apples, figs, apricots, peaches, pears, plums, berries, grapes, avocados, oranges, quinces, bananas; dried fruit, e.g., raisins, prunes, figs, apricots, pears, apples, dates, currants	Canned fruit
Meat and meat alternates	Legumes, seeds, crunchy peanut butter, nuts	Meats are low in fiber
Soups	Vegetable, green pea, and bean soups; chili; minestrone soup	Broth and soup made from low-fiber foods
Sweets	Candy with coconut, nuts, dried fruit; candied and glazed fruit; jam; marmalade; preserves	Clear jelly, honey, sugar, plain candy
Vegetables	Fresh or frozen vegetables, such as artichoke, peas, parsnips, winter squash, brussels sprouts, pumpkin, leafy greens, carrots, cauliflower, beans (green and wax), potatoes (sweet and white) in skin, beets, radishes, broccoli, corn, celery, okra, asparagus, green pepper, cucumber, mushrooms, cabbage, summer squash (eat raw when possible or steam in small amounts of water)	All overcooked vegetables
Miscellaneous	Coconut, pickles, olives, popcorn	

[a] Milk and milk-rich products tend to increase residue in the diet.

Provide recipes for preparing foods of high fiber content, such as pies, cookies, and muffins containing bran, seeds, and nuts. Stress to the client that if acute abdominal pain occurs while consuming a high-fiber diet, the diet should be temporarily discontinued and the physician notified.

BACTERIAL OVERGROWTH (BLIND LOOP SYNDROME)

Assessment and Intervention

Stasis of the small intestine and retarded drainage from a part of the small intestine may result from (1) anatomic changes (associated with degenerative or inflammatory disease or surgical intervention), (2) loss of neuromuscular activity, or (3) impairment of secretory activity. Stasis provides an environment conducive to bacterial overgrowth. In contrast to the colon, the proximal segments of the small bowel have only a small population of bacteria, which do not interfere with nutrient absorption. With stasis and stagnation, however, the substrates upon which bacteria feed are increased, and the bacteria flourish and form large colonies. Anticipate problems related to malabsorption secondary to bacterial overgrowth in clients with the following conditions that lead to stasis in the intestine:

1. Dilatations, proximal to strictures
2. Jejunal diverticula
3. Afferent loop of the duodenum that is created with a Billroth II gastrectomy that drains improperly
4. Fistulas
5. Disease states that alter motility, such as scleroderma and amyloidosis

In clients with these disorders, observe for signs and symptoms attributable to bacterial overgrowth, including nausea, postprandial colicky pain, flatulence, diarrhea, and steatorrhea, and test for malabsorption of vitamin B_{12} and folate. If the jejunum is involved, defective carbohydrate absorption may also be noted. The steatorrhea may be accompanied by a failure to absorb fat-soluble vitamins and some minerals, such as calcium and magnesium. The mechanisms underlying vitamin B_{12}, folate, and fat malabsorption with bacterial overgrowth involve binding of bile salts, vitamin B_{12}, and folate by bacteria. The bacteria deconjugate bile salts, making them less efficient in fat digestion and absorption, and use the vitamins for their own growth.

Treatment varies with the cause. Surgical correction of anatomic derangements, such as obstruction or stenosis, may be necessary. Broad-spectrum antibiotics are administered intermittently; administer vitamin B_{12} parenterally. Restrict conventional fats, supplement with MCT, and administer supplements of calcium, magnesium, folate, and fat-soluble vitamins. If the duodenum is involved, iron supplements may be necessary.

GLUTEN-INDUCED ENTEROPATHY

Gluten-induced enteropathy, a disorder affecting both children and adults, gives rise to the characteristic clinical manifestations of intestinal malabsorption in response to the ingestion of a specific protein component of certain cereal grains. The disease, which is genetic in origin, is known by several terms—celiac disease, nontropical sprue, and idiopathic steatorrhea. The onset of symptoms may occur in early childhood (primarily between the ages of 1 and 5) or may be delayed until adulthood (usually in the third to fourth decade). In children, the disease may be called childhood celiac disease. It is the second most common cause of chronic malabsorption in childhood (cystic fibrosis is first). In adulthood, the disorder is sometimes referred to as adult celiac disease or nontropical sprue. The term **gluten-induced enteropathy** was introduced when it was discovered that a protein fraction in gluten (protein-bound glutamine—glutenin and gliadin) occurring in some cereal grains was the specific toxic agent responsible for the symptoms. The term gluten-induced enteropathy more aptly describes the etiologic and functional abnormalities found in affected clients.

Assessment

Gluten-induced enteropathy is a disease of the small intestinal mucosa characterized by villus cell damage and consequent malabsorption. In sensitive individuals, the ingestion of gluten (contained in such grains as wheat, rye, oats, barley) induces morphologic changes in the villi of the intestinal mucosa. Instead of maintaining their normal appearance (i.e., fingerlike projections) they assume a blunted or flat appearance and appear minimal in number or absent.

Although the mechanism whereby gluten induces damage to the intestinal mucosa is not known precisely, both a biochemical and an immunologic basis have been hypothesized. Neither of the two theories is without criticism, however, and one or both mechanisms may be involved. The biochemical school of thought suggests that the disorder may represent an inborn error of metabolism characterized by a peptidase deficiency, accumulation of undigested peptides of gluten, and consequent mucosal damage. The other suggestion is that the mucosal damage represents an immunologic reaction to gluten, and it has been demonstrated by some researchers that there is an increased synthesis of immunoglobulins in the intestine and an increase in serum and tissue levels of IgA and IgM. Whether these changes are primary or secondary is not known.

Pathologic Manifestations. The clinical manifestations of the disorder are the end result of malabsorption. Keep in mind, however, that the manifestations are not specific to gluten-induced enteropathy but can occur with any disorder characterized by malabsorption. The specific symptoms are related to the severity of the malabsorption; not all clients have all of the symptoms.

The onset of the disorder is gradual. In the early stages malabsorption of fat, with diarrhea and steatorrhea, is usually more significant than malabsorption of other nutrients. Observe the character of the stools, which are loose, pale, frothy, and malodorous—the latter due in part to their content of fatty acids. The client may complain of abdominal distention due to excessive gas production. Malnutrition may be progressive, and the signs and symptoms reflect the degree of the malabsorption. Test for anemia, which can result from malabsorption of either iron, folic acid, or vitamin B$_{12}$. In severe cases, assess for weight loss and wasting of tissues, retarded

growth in children, hypoalbuminemia, tetany, osteomalacia, decreased prothrombin level, and ecchymoses (bruises). Exacerbations and remissions are common; anticipate exacerbations in association with emotional stress, infection, surgery, pregnancy, or the ingestion of gluten.

Diagnosis. There are no diagnostic tests that are specific to gluten-induced enteropathy. Criteria for diagnosis are (1) demonstration of malabsorption based on the client's history and certain diagnostic tests (e.g., measurement of stool fat), (2) finding of characteristic morphologic changes in the duodenal–jejunal mucosa with a peroral biopsy, and (3) a positive response to a gluten-free diet. In the last case, expect dramatic clinical improvement to occur in a matter of days or weeks. Failure to improve on

---

TABLE 27–8
GLUTEN-RESTRICTED DIET

Category	Foods Allowed	Foods Avoided
Milk	Milk (skim may be better tolerated initially); homemade ice cream; custard; puddings of rice, cornstarch, or tapioca; sherbet; cocoa made of chocolate or pure cocoa	Check labels on chocolate drink and cocoa to be sure they are free of gluten products; commercial ice cream; pudding
Meat and meat substitutes	Beef, lamb, pork, veal, fish, poultry prepared without wheat, rye, oat, or barley products; eggs; nuts; legumes; cheese	Prepared meats, such as bologna, frankfurters, luncheon meat, and commercial hamburger that may contain cereal fillers; creamed or breaded meats; meat loaf, sausage, scrapple, or croquettes that contain cereals; canned meat mixtures; thickened stews; pizza; cheese spreads or cheese food; egg omelet made with flour
Vegetables–fruit	Fresh, frozen, dried, or canned fruit and vegetables and juices; potatoes (white, sweet, yams, potato chips); vegetable soups	Breaded or creamed vegetables; canned fruit pie fillings
Bread–cereal and bakery products	Any made from rice, corn, and allowed flours (potato, soybean, buckwheat, lima bean, gluten-free wheat starch); pasta made from gluten-free wheat starch; cornmeal; hominy; rice; Puffed Rice; Rice Krispies; rice flakes; rice wafers; cakes or cookies made from allowed flours (such as rice cake)	Wheat germ; flour (whole wheat, graham, gluten, white); bread, biscuits, rolls, muffins, crackers, pretzels, doughnuts, pancakes, and waffles made from wheat or rye or prepared mixes; Rye Krisp; rusks; zwieback; breaded foods; bread crumbs; oatmeal; bran or bran cereals; Cream of Wheat; farina; Grapenuts; oatmeal; Shredded Wheat; Puffed Wheat; Pablum or other cereal from wheat, rye, or barley; dumplings; macaroni; noodles; spaghetti; cakes; cookies; pastry; prepared mixes with permitted flours; some packaged rice mixes
Miscellaneous	Bacon; butter; cream; cream cheese; oil (corn, cottonseed, olive, sesame, soybean); meat or poultry fat; pure mayonnaise or salad dressing made with allowed flours or fillers; honey; jam, jelly; preserves; marmalade; candy (homemade with allowed ingredients); molasses; sorghum; sugar (brown, white, maple); syrup; carbonated drinks; pure coffee; tea (containing no gluten products); gelatin; fruit ice or sherbet; rennet dessert; clear soups; other soups thickened with allowed ingredients; coconut; flavoring extract; marshmallows; pickles; herbs; condiments and spices; salt; pepper; homemade catsup and chili sauce; olives; arrowroot starch; cornstarch; meringues	Mayonnaise-type salad dressings containing flour or gluten stabilizer; commercial candies containing cereal products; ale; beer; root beer; malted beverages; Ovaltine; Postum; check labels on decaffeinated coffee to be sure they are free of gluten products; chewing gum; gravy and cream sauces thickened with prohibited flour; commercial meat sauces; commercially prepared soups and soups thickened with wheat, rye, oats, or barley; brewer's yeast

(*Source:* Adapted from North Carolina Dietetic Association: Diet Manual, ed 2. Charlotte, NC, 1978, pp 1–3J.)

the diet may be due to an incorrect diagnosis, failure to eliminate all sources of gluten from the diet, or a secondary deficiency of intestinal lactase. The mucosal damage may create a secondary lactase deficiency. Retest while restricting lactose in the diet (see the discussion of Lactose Intolerance for food sources of lactose).

Intervention

Manage the disorder by restricting all sources of gluten from the diet, and, during the first few months of treatment, restrict fat and lactose as well. These nutrients may be tolerated when the mucosa recovers, however. Correct deficiency states and compensate for the potential deficits of the diet (which may be low in B vitamins and iron) by administering vitamin and mineral supplements.

A gluten-free diet (Table 27–8) excludes the use of all forms of wheat (except gluten-free wheat starch), rye, oats, and barley. Corn and rice are the only grains permitted. Although the diet does not cure the disease, the symptoms can be relieved completely when gluten is entirely excluded from the diet. Although it may take several weeks for normal mucosal integrity to be restored and for the symptoms to disappear completely, tell the client to expect subjective improvement within the first few days after the removal of gluten. A longer period may be required in those who have been ill for years and who may have badly damaged mucous membranes. Following treatment, there is generally good catch-up growth in children.

Give the client and family a detailed list of foods to be omitted and explain carefully why certain foods must be avoided. Since the diet is very restrictive, use the same type of guidelines described for allergy in Chapter 32 with regard to label reading, menu planning, and use of recipes. Foods without listed ingredients and recipes of unknown composition must be checked before being incorporated into the diet. Instruct the client in the use of substitute bread and flour products made from wheat starch, potato, buckwheat, soybean, lima bean, arrowroot, cornmeal, and rice. Flours used as a substitute for wheat flour produce a product of lower volume and a more crumbly texture. Tips on baking with gluten-free flour have been published.[10] Moreover, gluten-free flours are comparatively expensive. Suggest that the client contact milling companies to obtain products, such as rice flour, directly. For variety, suggest other sources of acceptable products, such as gluten-free forms of bread or pasta at gourmet or Oriental shops. When eating away from home, advise the client to eat plain foods that do not contain breading, gravy, cream sauces, and other foods to be avoided.

Stress to the client that the diet must be followed for life. While remissions do occur, there is no cure for the disorder. For unexpected relapses, assess food intake for the previous several days to detect intake of possible sources of gluten. Many clients find it difficult to follow the diet indefinitely without continuing dietary advice and counseling, and ongoing follow-up is necessary. The American Celiac Society serves as a valuable resource for clients with this disorder; other resources for clients are listed at the end of the chapter.

TROPICAL SPRUE

Assessment and Intervention

Another of the malabsorption syndromes, tropical sprue, is indigenous to certain tropical and subtropical areas of the world, notably Puerto Rico and countries of the Far East. While there are important differences between gluten-induced enteropathy and tropical sprue, the two disorders closely resemble each other in clinical manifestations (i.e., malabsorption) and morphologic changes in the bowel (i.e., villous atrophy of the intestinal mucosa). Gluten-induced enteropathy and tropical sprue respond to different therapy, however. The former responds to a gluten-free diet, whereas the latter responds to folic acid supplementation. Moreover, the manifestations of tropical sprue are milder than those of gluten-induced enteropathy.

The etiology of tropical sprue is unknown, although it has been postulated that a folic acid-deficient diet or infectious processes may be important. The disorder reflects an alteration in bacterial flora, but the nature of the flora and the mechanisms whereby morphologic changes in the bowel are produced are the subject of debate.

Manifestations may include diarrhea, steatorrhea, and malnutrition. In the majority of clients with tropical sprue, the absorptive defects are of ileal origin. Observe for these signs of malnutrition on physical examination: pallor, weight loss, submucosal and subepidermal hemorrhage, edema, cheilosis, glossitis, hyperpigmentation of the skin at pressure points, and generalized loss of muscle tone. Study the results of the laboratory tests that show a megaloblastic anemia due to malabsorption of folic acid or vitamin B_{12}, hypoalbuminemia, and low blood levels of calcium, magnesium, phosphorus, and vitamin D.

Treat the disorder by administering broad-spectrum antibiotics and folic acid supplements. Vitamin B_{12} injections may also be necessary to correct the anemia. Counteract the malnutrition and weight loss by providing a diet that contains 2400 to 3000 kcal and 100 to 150 g protein. With steatorrhea, reduce the fat intake to 50 to 60 g initially and supplement with MCT to provide sufficient energy. Encourage good food sources of folic acid, including organ meats, beef, eggs, whole grains, and green leafy vegetables. Animal protein foods also provide vitamin B_{12}. Lactase deficiency may be present, and, therefore, delete lactose-containing foods from the diet initially. Give supplements of potassium, calcium, magnesium, phosphorus, and vitamin D. Multivitamin supplements may also be given. With treatment, the client becomes asymptomatic and the intestinal mucosa returns to normal. To prevent relapses, the treatment should be continued for a minimum of 6 months.

CARBOHYDRATE INTOLERANCE

Assessment

Defective digestion and absorption of dietary carbohydrate is common in infants and children and may occur in adults. Carbohydrate intolerance may be primary (i.e., an inherited defect that may be permanent) or secondary (i.e., a response to mucosal damage or bacterial colonization of the intestine, which is transient).

Intolerance may occur with monosaccharides or disaccharides, both as primary and secondary phenomena. Monosaccharide intolerance is a rare condition that is usually manifest at birth and requires prompt attention for survival of the infant. Congenital glucose–galactose malabsorption has been described and appears to result from an alteration in the intestinal and renal transport mechanisms for glucose and galactose. Affected clients are unable to tolerate carbohydrates, such as table sugar, starch, or milk, that yield glucose or galactose upon hydrolysis. Transient monosaccharide malabsorption may occur following neonatal surgery and in protein–calorie malnutrition.

More often, carbohydrate intolerance is precipitated by a deficiency or a low level of brush border enzymes that hydrolyze the disaccharides (sucrose, maltose, isomaltose, or lactose) and allow the absorption of monosaccharides. Disaccharidase enzyme activity, which occurs in the microvilli of the brush border of the intestinal mucosa, normally takes place over the entire length of the small intestine. Peak enzyme activity occurs in the jejunum or proximal ileum, and disaccharidase activity is low in the first part of the duodenum and in the distal ileum. Maltase and sucrase enzyme activity reaches maximal activity at 8 months of intrauterine life, whereas lactase activity does not reach its full potential until the end of the ninth month. Premature infants thus have a lessened ability to digest the lactose in milk for a period of time. In the adult, hydrolysis of lactose occurs at a slower rate than hydrolysis of maltose and sucrose.

Disaccharidase deficiency may occur as a single enzyme deficiency or as a deficiency of more than one enzyme. The intolerance may be congenital or acquired secondary to small intestinal diseases. Secondary deficiencies usually involve lactase and occur in such diseases as cystic fibrosis and gluten-induced enteropathy that damage the small bowel mucosa.

Isolated sucrose and combined sucrose–isomaltose intolerance have been reported in infants and children as a primary defect. Sucrase–isomalase deficiency is a rare form of disaccharidase deficiency occurring in infancy in which both sucrase (needed to hydrolyze sucrose) and isomaltase (needed to hydrolyze the 1–6 linkage of the amylopectin of starches) enzyme activity is lacking. Starch appears to play a less important role in the pathogenesis than sucrose, since the 1–6 linkage accounts for only a small percentage of the total linkages in the starch molecule.

Lactose intolerance is the most frequently reported carbohydrate intolerance, occurring in both primary and secondary forms, and appears to be the most common congenital form of disaccharidase intolerance in infants. Nonetheless, it is seen more often in adults as a delayed manifestation of an inherited enzyme defect or as an acquired deficiency. Lactose intolerance is discussed in detail in the next section.

Observe for abdominal discomfort, bloating, flatulence, nausea, vomiting, watery-acid diarrhea, dehydration, and weight loss following the ingestion of the offending monosaccharide or disaccharide in clients with carbohydrate intolerance. The diarrhea, which is more severe in infants and children than in adults, is osmotic in nature and caused by an increased solute load in the intestine.

Intervention

Treat the intolerance by eliminating the offending carbohydrate from the diet. For infants with glucose–galactose intolerance, provide a formula that is free of glucose and galactose and in which fructose is used as the carbohydrate replacement. An appropriate formula is RCF (Ross Labs). Older children may be able to tolerate limited amounts of milk and starch in the diet, although an unrestricted diet leads to recurrence of symptoms. If a galactose-free diet is ordered, refer to the food lists for a galactose-free diet given in Table 22–2.

Manage sucrase–isomaltose deficiency in an infant by recommending breastfeeding or a formula free of sucrose or starch, such as Enfamil (Mead Johnson) or Similac (Ross Labs). When solid foods are added, restrict those high in starch and sucrose. Fruits and vegetables containing less than 2 percent sucrose may be tolerated, and a list of these foods has been published.[11] Tolerance for starch improves with age, and small quantities can be added to the diet. Supplement the diet with vitamin C, since fruits and fruit juices that are good sources of the vitamin are restricted.

LACTOSE INTOLERANCE

▶ **Lactose intolerance,** a term often used interchangeably with lactase deficiency or milk intolerance, denotes a syndrome characterized by various gastrointestinal symptoms following ingestion of lactose-containing foods by individuals who do not digest this compound in a normal manner. The underlying pathology usually involves a total lack or a deficiency of lactase, the disaccharidase that is needed for the chemical hydrolysis of lactose to its component monosaccharides, glucose and galactose, during digestion.

Assessment

Classification. Three major classifications of lactose intolerance are generally recognized: congenital, primary, and secondary (or acquired). The congenital form, which is inherited and sometimes referred to as an inborn error of metabolism, is a rare, severe form of the disorder in which there is a total lack of the enzyme. Other disaccharidases may be missing as well. The enzyme lack, which is evident at birth, persists throughout life. A transient form of lactose intolerance may be evident at birth in premature infants (and in some normal full-term infants). In full-term infants, the lactase levels generally rise at birth. However, this rise may be inadequate in premature infants, and low lactase levels may be evident for the first few weeks of life. Assess for the symptoms of carbohydrate intolerance described previously when initiating feeding, particularly in premature infants.

Primary lactose intolerance is characteristic of most of the world's population and has been described as the norm for adults. In most mammals (including man), lactase activity is maximal during infancy, and in all but a few ethnic groups, the activity of the enzyme declines at weaning. The phenomenon may be genetic or adaptive in origin or a combination of the two. The disorder is genetically determined (as an autosomal recessive trait) with a delayed expression. When present, the incidence is low in children and high in adults. Assess for signs of diminishing lactase levels between the ages of 3 and 7 years in high-risk groups. Lactase levels typically diminish to the point of deficiency during late childhood and adolescence. As an adaptive response, lactose intolerance may be related to the long-term habits of milk consumption of a population, i.e., the continued ingestion of milk after weaning and into adulthood. The incidence is particularly low in cultural groups that are traditionally herdsmen or who keep milk-producing animals.

Observe for distinct racial and geographic differences in the incidence of the disorder, and be aware of the various ethnic groups in the United States in which it may pose a problem. In Caucasians of Scandinavian, northern European, or western European descent and in some African tribes with a long history of dairying, the incidence is relatively low (5 to 15 percent). In contrast, the incidence is 60 to 90 percent in non-Caucasians, such as adult American blacks, native American Indians, Jewish people, Arabs, Asians, and some Eskimo tribes. The incidence is particularly high in people originating from the Mediterranean basin.

Assess for secondary lactose intolerance in clients whose history includes conditions that dam-

age the gastrointestinal epithelial tissue, such as acute gastroenteritis, chronic intestinal diseases, such as gluten-induced enteropathy, cystic fibrosis of the pancreas, tropical sprue, protein–calorie malnutrition, and the use of such drugs as colchicine and antibiotics (including neomycin and kanamycin). The rapid transit of nutrients through the intestinal tract that occurs in postgastrectomy patients or with intestinal resection may also induce lactose malabsorption, even with normal lactase levels. In severe cases of lactose intolerance, a general deficiency of disaccharidases may occur. Expect lactose tolerance to return to normal levels with control of the disease process, although the return is not always immediate.

Symptoms. In infants, lactose intolerance may induce severe diarrhea, acid stools, dehydration, and failure to thrive. In children and adults, note that the symptoms are less dramatic and include flatulence, bloating, abdominal pain, and diarrhea, although the intensity of symptoms will vary among clients. The degree of severity and the number of symptoms depend on differences in the amount of lactase present and the amount of lactose ingested. Assess for the timing of the appearance of symptoms relative to the ingestion of lactose-containing foods. Symptoms usually appear within 1 to 2 hours after lactose intake and disappear by about the third hour. The onset of symptoms may be delayed when the lactose is consumed as part of a meal, however.

The symptoms occur as a result of a net secretion of fluid into the intestinal tract, a diminished absorption of fluid from the intestinal tract, and gas production, all induced by the presence of undigested lactose in intestinal contents. The osmotic effect of the hypertonicity produced by the lactose results in an increased fluid load in the small intestine, with resulting distention, cramps, and increased peristalsis. The increased motility may result in diminished nutrient absorption and diarrhea, although the published data about this are conflicting and inconclusive. Once in the colon, the lactose is fermented by bacteria, with the production of acids and gases that lower pH, further enhance the osmotic effect of the lactose, and interfere with the absorption of water and electrolytes from the colon. Gas production contributes to bloating, flatulence, and frothy diarrhea. It has been suggested that milk avoidance in affected clients, and thus low calcium intake, may be related to the development of osteoporosis. These people usually spontaneously limit milk consumption to levels that can be tolerated.

Diagnosis. Individuals with lactose intolerance can sometimes be identified by a clinical trial. Observe for the presence of symptoms following the ingestion of lactose-containing foods or for the absence of symptoms with withdrawal of the foods. Alternately, there are several laboratory tests that may be used. In infants, test for a high level of reducing sugars in the stool and an acid pH, which may denote the presence of undigested carbohydrate and products of their fermentation. In adults, determine the rise in blood glucose following an oral lactose tolerance test or measure breath hydrogen after lactose ingestion. Clients with lactose malabsorption will have a low rise in blood glucose following the lactose tolerance test and have an increased level of hydrogen production in the intestinal tract and thus an increased level in the expired air. Measurement of lactose activity from a biopsy of a segment of the small intestine can also identify the lactase-deficient client.

Intervention

Treat the disorder by either eliminating or restricting the intake of lactose, depending upon whether the deficiency is partial or complete. Since milk and other dairy products are the major dietary source of lactose, lactose-intolerant clients can use these products in varying degrees.

For infants with the congenital form of lactase deficiency, provide a lactose-free formula, such as RCF or Isomil (Ross Labs), MFB (Gerber Products Company), or Nutramigen or ProSobee (Mead Johnson). Breastfeeding is contraindicated for feeding infants with congenital lactose intolerance because of the high lactose content of breast milk. For clients with primary or secondary forms of the disorder, individualize the lactose content of the diet according to tolerance. Many can ingest nutritionally valuable amounts of milk or dairy products when given under these conditions:

1. In small amounts throughout the day (rather than a large amount at one time)
2. With meals
3. At body temperature
4. In a sweetened form, such as chocolate milk (the added sugar may delay gastric emptying)
5. In a fermented form, such as yoghurt, buttermilk, or cheese. Hard, ripened cheese, such as cheddar, Swiss, and mozzarella, contains only a small amount of lactose. Although fermented milks, such as buttermilk and yoghurt, contain an amount of lactose similar to regular milk (Table 27–9), these products appear to be better tolerated by some individuals. It may be that the bacteria added during the culturing process exert lactase activity in the gastrointestinal tract (Acidophilus milk has been recommended for use, but a recent study failed to demonstrate its value[12])
6. As lactose-hydrolyzed milk in which at least 90 percent of the lactose has been hydrolyzed (Lact-Aid—SugarLo Company, Atlantic City, NJ—is a powdered lactase enzyme that can be added to milk)
7. By gradual introduction over a period of time

TABLE 27–9
APPROXIMATE LACTOSE CONTENT OF SELECTED DAIRY PRODUCTS

Product	Unit	Lactose (g)
Milk		
Whole	1 c	11
Skim	1 c	12–14
Low-fat (2%)	1 c	9–13
Chocolate	1 c	10–12
Buttermilk	1 c	9–11
Yoghurt (low-fat)	1 c	10–15
Ice cream	1 c	9
Sherbet	1 c	4
Liquid breakfast mix	1 envelope	12
Cheese		
Cottage (creamed)	1 c	5–6
Cottage (low-fat, 2%)	1 c	7–8
Cheddar	1 oz	0.4–0.6
Process	1 oz	0.5

(Although lactase is not an adaptive enzyme, i.e., it does not increase its activity with a continued lactose challenge, clients may adapt in some way to moderate levels of lactose and not have symptoms even when lactase levels remain low)

The lactose content of various dairy products is given in Table 27–9, and a lactose-controlled diet is presented in Table 27–10.

Take a comprehensive dietary history to ascertain the level of lactose that the client can usually tolerate and use Tables 27–9 and 27–10 as guides for establishing the dietary plan. Advise the client that he or she may remain symptom free while limiting the amount of milk consumed to perhaps 1 c per day. Tell the client that more discomfort may be experienced when ingesting skim milk than whole milk. If nutritionally complete formulas are used for oral supplements or for tube feeding, select formulas that are free of lactose, such as Ensure or Osmolite (Ross Labs).

Remind the client to expect milk that has been treated with enzymes to be somewhat sweeter than untreated milk. Kosher foods that are labeled *pareve* do not contain milk and can serve as a source of commercial foods, since Jewish laws prohibit the consumption of milk and meat at the same meal. In addition to stressing the importance of reading labels to detect hidden sources of lactose, suggest that the client consult a pharmacist to identify the presence of lactose in pharmaceutical products.

When milk and dairy products are restricted, assess the diet for adequacy of other nutrients, such as calcium and riboflavin, and provide supplements if necessary. Encourage the client to challenge himself or herself with lactose-containing foods at intervals, since adaptation may occur, permitting a moderate consumption without provoking annoying symptoms.

TABLE 27–10
LACTOSE-CONTROLLED DIET

Category	Foods Allowed	Foods Avoided
Milk	1 c milk (whole, low-fat, skim, chocolate) if tolerated; fermented milk (yoghurt, cultured buttermilk) if tolerated; lactose-free commercial products (e.g., Ensure, Lact-Aid, soya milk)	Skim milk if lactose added; milk (whole, low-fat, skim, or chocolate) in excess of 1 c; malted milk; cocoa; custard, ice cream, ice milk, milk puddings, sherbet (unless counted as part of milk allowance)
Meat and meat substitutes	Beef, veal, lamb, pork, poultry, fish, organ meats, and eggs prepared without milk; all-meat cold cuts, sausage, and frankfurters; ripened cheese (American and Swiss) if tolerated; legumes; nuts; peanut butter; seeds	Creamed or breaded meats, fish, poultry; eggs cooked with milk; cold cuts, sausage, and frankfurters with milk products added
Vegetable–fruit	Fresh, frozen, canned and dried vegetables, fruits, and juices prepared without milk or lactose; vegetable soups prepared without milk; potatoes (white, sweet, yams, potato chips)	Commercially prepared creamed or breaded vegetables; check labels on canned or frozen vegetables; fruits, juice, or soup processed with lactose, milk, or sauces; instant potato; commercially prepared French fries
Bread–cereal and baker products	Bread prepared without milk (includes Kosher bread, Roman Meal bread, sourdough, French rolls, Vienna bread); bakery products marked *pareve;* limit bread and rolls made with milk to 4 slices per day; crackers; cooked and dry cereals; rice; pasta; cakes, pies, desserts, and cookies made without milk; angel food cake; pecan pie; lemon meringue pie	Commercial baking mixes; pancakes, waffles, or French toast unless used as part of milk allowance
Miscellaneous	Vegetable oils; meat fat; mayonnaise; margarine or butter for table use (use a milk-free margarine such as Nucoa or Mazola and unsalted sweet margarine for cooking); olives, avocado; lactose-free salad dressing mixes; sour cream (if tolerated); sugar; syrup (including corn syrup); pure jam and jelly; honey; molasses; cane sugar candy; German baking chocolate; semisweet chocolate; coffee; tea; carbonated beverages; fruit-flavored drinks; gelatin; water ices and popsicles; broth soups; pure spices and seasonings; pickles; vinegar; catsup; popcorn; nondairy creamers	Cream (unless counted as part of milk allowance); lactose-containing salad dressings; blackstrap molasses; milk chocolate; candy (caramel, butterscotch, toffee, and peppermint); Ovaltine; check labels for addition of lactose to soft drinks, instant tea and coffee, freeze-dried and powdered coffee; dried soups; cream soups and chowder; cream sauces and gravies unless made with allowed foods; check labels on dietetic foods

(Source: Adapted from North Carolina Dietetic Association: Diet Manual, ed 2. Charlotte, NC, 1978, pp 21–23J.)

NONINFLAMMATORY DISORDERS OF THE COLON

Irritable Colon Syndrome

Assessment and Intervention. The irritable colon syndrome (also called spastic colitis and mucous colitis) is a common disorder of unknown cause associated with irregular and uncoordinated bowel motility that can lead to constipation or diarrhea. Clients who complain of diarrhea may have a decrease in sigmoid segmental contractions, whereas the converse may be true for those with constipation. Affected clients often experience predominantly left lower quadrant abdominal pain varying from mild to severe. There may be concurrent anorexia, nausea, vomiting, distention, flatulence, or heartburn. Mucus may be present in the stool.

Since the disorder is common in population groups consuming a low-fiber diet, it has been attributed by some to fiber deficiency. Some authorities consider the irritable colon syndrome to be a forerunner of diverticular disease of the colon and have termed the disorder **spastic colon diverticulitis.** Colonic pressure abnormalities have been described that are similar to diverticular disease. The irritable colon syndrome occurs with increasing frequency after the third decade of life.

Assess for the possible role of other factors that have been implicated in the etiology of the disorder, which include abuse of laxatives, alcohol, tobacco, and coffee, antibiotic therapy, food sensitivity, emotional stress, and poor habits of personal hygiene related to rest, bowel evacuation patterns, and food and fluid intake.

Counsel the client about measures for controlling stress and assist with correction of any faulty health habits identified during the assessment. Recommend an increase in physical activity for sedentary clients with constipation and postprandial rest periods for clients with diarrhea. Rest periods after meals may decrease the exaggerated hypermotility state.[13] Recommend a diet high in fiber content (Table 27–7). Some clients may benefit from the addition of unprocessed bran, and this measure may lead to a decrease in intraluminal pressure and thus restore segmental activity to a more normal pattern. Teach the client to add additional fiber and bran to the diet gradually and to increase fluid intake concomitantly. Stress the importance of planning a regular time for eating and for bowel evacuation. With recurrent diarrhea, the low-residue diet described in Table 27–5 may be appropriate. A low-fiber diet may actually aggravate the symptoms of the irritable bowel syndrome and is contraindicated in long-term management unless the colon is narrowed or stenosed.

Constipation

Assessment. Constipation is a disorder of the colon characterized by infrequent or difficult evacuation of feces. Residues are retained in the colon beyond the normal colonic emptying time, and the feces are small in volume and of a hard, dry consistency. Defecation normally occurs 24 to 72 hours after food intake, but with constipation, transit time in the colon is delayed, bringing removal of excessive amounts of water and hardening of the stool. Constipation may be accompanied by generalized abdominal discomfort and even pain on defecation.

Include an assessment of the normal bowel patterns of clients—for some a daily bowel movement is normal, whereas for others bowel evacuation every second or third day may be the normal pattern. Be aware that normal bowel habits may be temporarily disrupted by changes in diet or a change in the routine elimination schedule. Suppression of the stimulus to defecate, for instance, may affect the conditioned bowel reflexes. The stimulus to defecate occurs as the feces enter the rectum from the colon. This is initiated by mass peristalsis of the colon, which is stimulated by the entry of food into the stomach (gastrocolic reflex) or by the morning activities following arising. When a client complains of chronic constipation, assess for its causes, which may include the following mechanisms:

1. Weakness of the intestinal musculature, causing weak peristaltic waves, loss of rectal sensibility, and stasis in the colon (Atonic constipation, or the so-called lazy bowel, occurs in the elderly, in the obese, and in pregnant women and secondary to fevers, surgery, or debilitating diseases)
2. Spasm of the colon and retardation of the forward movement of intestinal contents. This may be due to the presence of irritating substances or psychologic stress or other factors
3. Abnormal consistency of the feces. For easy expulsion, colonic contents must be semisolid; assess the fluid and fiber content of the diet, the two factors that must be present in adequate amounts for normal stool consistency
4. Colonic obstruction by tumor, diverticula, stenosis, and so on (obstructive constipation)
5. Presence of organic diseases (such as hypothyroidism), malnutrition (such as thiamine deficiency), or secondary drug therapy (such as nonabsorbable antacids)
6. Lifestyle factors, such as failure to establish regular patterns of eating, rest, and elimination, i.e., a hurried lifestyle; lack of exercise, which decreases intestinal muscle tone; abuse of cathartics, which leads to structural changes in the terminal ileum and colon; and emotional stress

In young children, voluntary withholding of stools leads to chronic constipation with rectal leakage of watery fecal matter. This condition is called ▶ **encopresis** and often arises in association with issues involved with bowel training.

Probe for the excessive use of cathartics or enemas in clients with recurrent constipation or those who express anxiety over missed bowel movements. Excessive use of cathartics or enemas may bring fluid and electrolyte (especially potassium) depletion, weakness, and bowel damage. A vicious cycle may ensue, making it difficult for the client to establish a normal elimination routine. A common side effect of constipation, straining at defecation, or abuse of cathartics or enemas is hemorrhoids (ruptured blood vessels around the anal sphincter that may be internal or external and may or may not cause pain and discomfort). The passage of dry, hard stools in clients with hemorrhoids who are constipated often causes bleeding and severe pain.

Intervention. Treat constipation by dealing with its cause. Dietary modifications may be beneficial in atonic and spastic constipation. In atonic constipation, dietary treatment is preferable to the use of laxatives. Advise the client to use laxatives only if absolutely necessary. If the problem is related to irregular eating habits, lack of exercise, or suppression of the stimulus to defecation, advise the client to make the necessary changes. Encourage an increase in physical activity and a regular morning routine, with perhaps consumption of hot liquids, such as hot water and lemon juice, upon arising to stimulate the gastrocolic reflex. Reassure the client that a daily bowel movement is not necessary for everyone. Stress the use of high-fiber foods (Table 27–7) for their laxative effect in forming soft, passable stools. Bacterial formation of volatile acids as fiber moves through the colon is thought to contribute to the laxative effect of dietary fiber.

Follow the intervention guidelines described for increasing fiber intake for clients with diverticular disease in educating the client about dietary management. If the client is an elderly person, advise the use of cooked vegetables and canned or stewed fruits initially, with the addition of fresh fruits and vegetables and bran as colonic function improves. Although bran is the most concentrated source of food fiber, it should be used in moderation. Large quantities may produce gas and diarrhea and may cause impaction, especially in the elderly. Stress the need for an adequate fluid intake (approximately 8 to 10 glasses daily) and use of foods that stimulate intestinal motility by pharmacologic means— prunes and prune juice contain the chemical laxative, diphenylisatin. Concentrated sugars, such as sugar syrup, produce an osmotic effect by drawing fluid into the intestine, distending the rectum, and promoting defecation. A moderate amount of fat may be desirable in view of the laxative effect of fatty acids. However, excessive fat intake may induce diarrhea.

Assist a client (and the parents) with encopresis to develop a routine toilet regimen and to train the muscles involved with defecation. Advise the use of a high-fiber diet in conjunction with mineral oil until bowel movements are regulated.

NUTRITIONAL CONSIDERATIONS FOLLOWING INTESTINAL SURGERY

Many clients require intestinal surgery, e.g., small or large bowel resection, hemorrhoidectomy, ileostomy (surgical removal of the lower bowel and varying segments of the ileum with attachment of the proximal end of the remaining ileum to an opening on the abdominal wall for excretion of wastes), or colostomy (surgical removal of part of the colon and attachment of the proximal end of the remaining colon to an opening on the abdominal wall for excretion of wastes). For example, extensive inflammatory disease, bowel trauma, vascular insufficiency with infarction, volvulus, widespread neoplasm, and radiation enteritis (intestinal inflammation due to radiation therapy) with fistula formation and obstruction may necessitate resection or bypass of the affected segment. Total colectomy (removal of the colon) requires an ileostomy, whereas partial colectomy or lower bowel bypass procedures are managed, temporarily or permanently, by formation of a colostomy.

Short Bowel Syndrome

Assessments. There is an increasing population of clients who require extensive small bowel resection, with consequent reduction in the intestinal absorbing surface. With extensive resection, the short bowel syndrome follows—a metabolic imbalance characterized by diarrhea, malabsorption, weight loss, and other secondary complications. The short bowel syndrome also occurs secondary to the jejunoileal bypass surgery for morbid obesity (see Chap.

23). The degree of malabsorption is related to (1) the extent and site of resection, (2) the presence or absence of the ileocecal valve, (3) the condition of the remaining bowel, and (4) the degree of adaptation of the bowel remnant.

Most nutrient absorption occurs in the proximal two thirds of the small intestine. The larger the resection, the greater the extent of malabsorption. Moreover, many substances can be absorbed only by active transport in localized areas of the small intestine, and resection of these portions of the small bowel often results in depletion of the specific metabolites. Table 27–11 specifies nutrients most likely to be lost by the specific area of bowel resected.

If a client's resection involves only a short segment of the bowel, expect little or no disturbance in function, and provided the duodenum, distal ileum, and ileocecal valve remain intact, the client will not experience significant impairment even when up to 40 percent of the small intestine is removed. Variable malabsorption becomes apparent, however, with a greater degree of resection, i.e., 50 percent or more, or distal ileal or with ileocecal valve resection. When more than two thirds of the small bowel is removed in an adult, severe metabolic disturbance and malnutrition supervene—with a residual of 3 ft or less, the problems are serious and long-term. If less than 15 to 18 in remain, it is likely that permanent parenteral nutrition will be necessary to supplement oral intake.

In clients with the short bowel syndrome, glucose and most water-soluble vitamins are absorbed relatively efficiently unless hypermotility is induced by the entry of extremely hypertonic solutions into the intestine. Provided no more than 8 ft of proximal jejunum is resected, malabsorption of protein and fat is minimal, since the ileum has large functional

---

TABLE 27–11
SITE OF ABSORPTION OF SELECTED NUTRIENTS

Area of Small Bowel	Nutrients Absorbed
Proximal segment	Iron
	Calcium
	Magnesium
	Sugars
	Amino acids
	Water-soluble vitamins (except vitamin B_{12})
	Electrolytes
	Fats
	Fat-soluble vitamins
Middle segment	Sugars
	Amino acids
	Fats
	Fat-soluble vitamins
Distal segment	Bile salts
	Vitamin B_{12}
	Cholesterol

reserves and can assume some of the function of the upper small bowel. Where there is resection of more than 8 ft, however, test for impaired absorption of fat, protein, fat-soluble vitamins, calcium, and magnesium. Clients with resection of the terminal ileum malabsorb vitamin B_{12} and bile salts, and the bile salt losses eventually lead to malabsorption of fat and fat-soluble vitamins. With the short bowel syndrome, absorption of amino acids may improve with time, but tolerance for fats may be permanently impaired.

Determine if the ileocecal valve is retained following intestinal surgery. This valve is located at the junction of the ileum and cecum. It limits the amount of small bowel contents that enter the colon at one time as well as hinders the retrograde movement of colonic bacteria that may stimulate bacterial overgrowth in the intestine. When it is removed with surgery, the degree of malabsorption is greater, and the malabsorption is complicated by the bacterial overgrowth syndrome.

Assess the condition of the remaining portions of the gastrointestinal tract in affected clients. For instance, expect the malabsorption to be intensified if intestinal resection is complicated by pancreatic or hepatic insufficiency.

With time, the remaining bowel adapts by dilatation, elongation, and hyperplasia, and nutrient absorption is improved. Most clients require a period of 6 months or more to adapt to an extensively shortened bowel. The presence of nutrients in the intestinal lumen appears to stimulate hyperplasia (the hormone gastrin may be involved).

In addition to malabsorption, observe for these additional complications of the short bowel syndrome: gastric hypersecretion, hypermotility, increased incidence of gallstones, hyperoxaluria and the potential for oxalate calculi, bacterial overgrowth, primary pancreatic atrophy, and extensive weight loss. The immediate postoperative course may be complicated by ileus (obstruction due to absent peristalsis) and infection.

Gastric hypersecretion is associated with an increased concentration of gastrin. The hypersecretion induces chemical injury to the remaining mucosa, inactivates pancreatic enzymes, and potentiates excess fluid loss, leading to acidic diarrheal stools. The increase in gastrointestinal motility and peristalsis leads to a decrease in gastrointestinal transit time. Observe that gastric emptying and intestinal peristalsis are most markedly affected in clients whose distal small bowel has been resected. Gallstone formation is favored if the terminal ileum is affected. The resulting bile salt losses create lithogenic bile. Hyperoxaluria depends on the presence of the colon, and if it remains with surgery, the potential for oxalate stones is increased.

Intervention. Nutritional management is usually divided into three stages: first, provide a period of parenteral feeding alone, second, use combined par-

enteral and enteral feeding, and finally, with intestinal adaptation, use enteral feeding alone. Provide adequate nutrition in the early phases to encourage intestinal adaptation. Although it is desirable to initiate oral or tube feeding as early as possible to facilitate the process, refrain from giving oral feedings prematurely, since hypermotility, diarrhea, and fluid and electrolyte loss may be accelerated. With extensive bowel resection, delay oral feeding until the volume of diarrhea diminishes to less than 2 liters/day (or seven to eight bowel movements).

The three phases of nutritional management are as follows:

- Phase 1 (immediate postoperative period). Use total parenteral nutrition as the sole source of nutrients for about 3 to 4 weeks (if 20 to 30 percent of the small bowel is left intact) or for about 2 to 3 months (with resections of greater magnitude). To prevent excoriation from the frequent, acidic, diarrheal stool, provide good personal hygiene during this period.
- Phase 2 (intermediate transition period). As diarrhea and fluid and electrolyte losses subside and appetite returns, introduce oral feeding gradually (Table 27–12), using both the enteral and parenteral routes to maintain sufficient kilocalorie intake. As oral intake increases, decrease the amount of parenteral feeding to a level that allows the client to maintain or gain weight as needed while preventing interference with appetite. Observe for malabsorption when oral feeding begins. Although defined formula diets may be used during the diet progression, clients generally prefer ordinary table foods. Encourage the client to keep a food diary to identify the pattern of food tolerance and use trial and error to establish a progressive increase in food intake. Some authors suggest that low-fiber carbohydrate foods should be added first and no other foods should be given until 50 to 100 g are tolerated. Protein foods such as lean meat are then added. After tolerance for carbohydrate- and protein-containing foods is established, introduce small amounts of fat. Initially, give oral feedings every 2 hours; later increase the amount and lengthen the interval between feedings. Advise the client to expect temporary setbacks, minor complications, and some discomfort during this phase. Be patient in planning and implementing the progressive program.

Phase 3 (late transition period). Within 3 to 6 months, it is usually possible to provide the total nutritional requirements by mouth, and the diet can then be more varied. Weight stabilizes during this phase (usually at a substantially lower level, generally within 20 percent of the recommended value) as balance with

TABLE 27–12
GENERAL PRINCIPLES OF NUTRITIONAL MANAGEMENT FOLLOWING EXTENSIVE SMALL BOWEL RESECTION

Dietary Factor	Comment
Kcal	Provide 3500–4000 daily (derived primarily from carbohydrate and protein)
Protein	Provide at least 100 g/day (provided kcal intake is adequate, this amount is consistent with positive nitrogen balance)
Fat	Restrict oral intake to approximately 40 g initially to decrease steatorrhea and lessen the loss of fat-soluble vitamins, calcium, magnesium, and other electrolytes; as the condition stabilizes, fat intake can usually be increased to 50–60 g daily; substitute medium-chain triglycerides if conventional fats are poorly tolerated
Vitamins and minerals	Supplement as needed (particularly fat-soluble vitamins, vitamin B_{12}, calcium, magnesium, and potassium)
Oxalate	Restrict oral intake (if the colon is present) to decrease oxaluria
Volume and frequency of oral feedings	Small, frequent feedings
Consistency of the diet	Initiate oral feeding with a cautious trial of isotonic fluids, followed by progression to dilute feedings of a defined formula diet; this may be given as a tube feeding, using 24-hour continuous drip, as a beverage, or frozen as popsicles

the disability is achieved. Diarrhea may continue to be a problem, but with time the colon adapts. Advise the client to continue with the food diary during this period. Some clinicians advise the avoidance of alcohol, excessive caffeine, extremely spicy foods, and foods high in fat for at least a year following massive bowel surgery. Six to eight small feedings are usually better tolerated than larger, less frequent meals.

Diarrhea and dehydration of a life-threatening nature may occur secondary to gastroenteritis in those with extensive small bowel resection. Advise the client to seek immediate medical attention if symptoms of enteritis are present.

Enterostomy

Assessment. With improved diagnostic procedures for recognition of bowel disorders, enterostomy, including ileostomy and colostomy, is increasingly used in surgical management. Inflammatory or obstructive processes, congenital or traumatic disruption, and malignant tumors within the intestinal tract may necessitate an enterostomy. Most ileostomies are performed for ulcerative colitis or Crohn's disease that fail to respond to medical management. In contrast, colostomy may be indicated in the treatment of various anomalies localized in the colon.

Assess the nutritional status of enterostomy clients at the time of surgery. A state of negative nutritional balance may coexist with the underlying disorder that necessitated the surgical procedure. Moreover, clients with a long-standing enterostomy may subject themselves to malnutrition by voluntarily limiting food intake to decrease the stomal discharge. Conversely, a significant number of ileostomy clients tend to become obese following surgery. The improved appetite and nutrient use associated with control of the inflammatory bowel disease may lead to obesity.

There are major differences in the problems encountered by clients with left-sided ostomies (those involving the left transverse, descending, or sigmoid colon), right-sided ostomies (ileostomy or those involving the cecum, ascending, or right transverse colon), and ileostomy that includes resection of a significant portion of the terminal ileum. The fluidity, frequency, and enzyme content of the stomal drainage are less in left-sided ostomies than in right-sided ostomies, making the former easier to control. Observe that, in contrast to a client with an ileostomy, reflex control and dietary regulation by a client with a left-sided colostomy may allow for regular, predictable evacuation, and an appliance need be worn only at the time of expected evacuation. Many ileostomy clients do develop a reasonably regular elimination pattern relative to meals. Assess for the presence of constipation, which is not uncommon in a client with a long-standing left-sided colostomy.

Considerable amounts of water and electrolytes, particularly sodium and postassium, are lost initially in the stomal drainage in a client whose stoma is located in close proximity to the duodenum and in whom the discharge is fluid and constant. Adaptation occurs with time, however, and the discharge becomes progressively thicker as fecal losses are minimized, although the client frequently borders on negative fluid and electrolyte balance. The highly fluid nature of the ileostomy drainage may prompt some clients to limit fluid intake because of the misconception that this restriction thickens the drainage or decreases the amount. Expect the client to have difficulty coping with excessive losses associated with vomiting, diarrhea, or excessive sweating. Severe diarrhea is especially serious because of the probability of developing dehydration and electrolyte depletion. Use urinary volume as a guide to hydration status in the presence of diarrhea. A drop in volume to below 1 quart daily is indicative of dehydration. The ileostomy client tends to secrete a persistently acid urine, a condition that favors precipitation of uric acid stones (see Chap. 30).

Clients with an ileostomy occasionally have their stomas obstructed by partially digested food. Common offenders are fibrous foods, especially celery, cabbage, dried fruit and nuts, and foods with kernels, such as corn and popcorn.[14]

The problems experienced by clients with an ileostomy associated with resection of a significant portion of the terminal ileum are similar to the problems of clients with Crohn's disease with terminal ileal involvement—vitamin B_{12} deficiency, bile-salt related disorders, steatorrhea, an increased tendency to form gallstones, and bacterial overgrowth. Oxaluria generally does not occur, since the colon must be intact for excessive oxalate absorption to take place.

Absence of sphincter control and lack of sensations in the stoma are characteristic of all enterostomy clients, and therefore discharge of intestinal gas and fecal odor can be especially troublesome. Many foods are classified as gas-formers, but with few exceptions there is no solid link between the ingestion of specific foods and the production of gas and odor.[15] There is evidence that gas is produced in the colon from bacterial fermentation of nonabsorbable carbohydrate, including lactose and the complex carbohydrates found in beans, such as navy beans and lima beans. Assess for other factors that can lead to gas and odor formation, such as air swallowing associated with eating, anxiety, chewing gum, bolting food, or drinking large amounts of liquids while eating. Clients with poor dentition tend to drink more liquids while eating. Skipping meals in an attempt to reduce bowel movements leads to an empty bowel that still produces gas.[15] An altered intestinal motility pattern and an abnormal pain response are also associated with bloating, pain, and gas. Vitamin preparations and some drugs may produce odor.

Bowel patterns are not changed by the surgical procedures, and, therefore, responses to specific foods do not change. Assist clients to trace their own food histories to determine personal idiosyncracies. If a food caused gas, constipation, or diarrhea prior to surgery, the response will be the same after surgery.[16]

Intervention. During the immediate postoperative period, provide intravenous and clear liquid regimens, progressing to a soft or low-residue diet. Long-term use of a low-residue diet is not indicated, however, and following recovery from surgery, most clients are able to eat a regular diet with modifications made on an individual basis. Assist the client to return to a nutritionally adequate diet with the nutritional and psychologic advantages of few restrictions. With an adequate oral intake, additional vitamins or other food supplements are unnecessary, except in individual cases.[17]

Provide a diet high in kilocalories and protein supplemented with vitamins and minerals for clients who are malnourished at the time of surgery. Consider the use of defined formula diets that are low in residue content.

Encourage colostomy clients to progress as rapidly as possible to a completely normal diet and ileostomy clients to resume a normal diet gradually to allow for intestinal adaptation. Advise all enterostomy clients that if a particular food causes problems shortly after surgery, they should try it again at a later time, since it may be tolerated later. Encourage clients to establish a regular routine of care that includes regular eating habits, to eat meals leisurely, at regular times, and to chew foods well. Regulation of the number and spacing of meals can allow for a predictable pattern of evacuation for the colostomy client and, to some degree, for the ileostomy client.

Stress the importance of adequate fluid intake to prevent dehydration and the propensity to develop uric acid stones in the ileostomy client and to prevent constipation in the colostomy client. The ileostomy client may require as much as 3000 to 4000 ml of fluid daily. Reassure the client that the extra fluid will not make care of the ostomy more difficult. When losses are increased in association with gastroenteritis or excess sweating, stress the importance of replacing both fluids and electrolytes. Suggest that extra salt be added to foods and that the client consume foods rich in sodium, such as bouillon and broth, and foods rich in potassium, such as milk and fruit juices. Beverages designed for athletes that contain water, glucose, and electrolytes are useful in replacing losses. Advise against the use of salt tablets because they are difficult to dissolve and some clients experience additional gastrointestinal problems with their use. Replacing losses is especially critical in ileostomy clients because of their diminished fluid and electrolyte reserves.

Inform clients that the foods that may cause gastrointestinal problems, such as gas, constipation, or diarrhea, are those that caused these problems before the illness that necessitated surgery. Encourage clients to be adventurous in testing food tolerance rather than rely on the experience of others. Tell clients that problems related to gas and odor can be reduced by avoiding excessive air swallowing, meal skipping, and foods that they have found to produce excessive gas or an offensive odor. Allow clients to decide for themselves whether they wish to avoid foods that cause discomfort. Assist clients to establish an appropriate balance of fiber intake, i.e., an amount that will avoid diarrhea (which may be a problem for the ileostomy client) or constipation (which may be a problem for the colostomy client). Advise clients that it is necessary to use more discretion in the intake of fibrous foods during the first 1 or 2 months after surgery than will be necessary later.

To avoid the possibility of stomal blockage by undigested food, advise the ileostomy client that such foods as corn, popcorn, dried fruit, coconut, mushrooms, membranes of citrus fruit and other fibrous fruits and nuts must be thoroughly chewed. Some ileostomy clients have fewer problems by eliminating these food items.

Rectal Surgery

Intervention. Nutritional care following rectal surgery, such as hemorrhoidectomy, aims at delaying bowel evacuation until healing has begun and preventing wound infection by fecal contamination. Depending on the severity of the surgery, provide a clear liquid diet, a defined formula diet, or a low-residue diet (Table 27–5) that eliminates milk and milk products and uses strained fruits and vegetables and juices until a normal diet is tolerated. The use of constipating drugs may be indicated. Following recovery from surgery for hemorrhoids, instruct the client to follow a high-fiber diet (Table 27–7) to aid in preventing recurrence.

REVIEW QUESTIONS AND ACTIVITIES

1. Identify the following in relation to diarrhea, steatorrhea, maldigestion, and malabsorption: (a) mechanisms underlying their occurrence, (b) gastrointestinal disorders associated with each, and (c) rationale for the occurrence of disorders in each instance.
2. Discuss the causes of the following manifestations of gastrointestinal disorders: (a) edema, (b) anemia, (c) tetany, (d) hemorrhagic tendencies, (e) gallstones, (f) kidney stones, (g) muscle weakness, (h) bone disorders, (i) oral and skin lesions, (j) altered vision, and (k) vitamin B_{12} deficiency.

3. Explain the rationale for the use of the following treatment regimens: (a) a low-residue diet and pectin to control diarrhea, (b) a low-fat diet and substitution of medium-chain triglycerides to control steatorrhea, and (c) vitamin and mineral supplements in malabsorptive disorders.
4. Compare and contrast the clinical manifestations and dietary management of Crohn's disease, ulcerative colitis, and symptomatic and asymptomatic diverticular disease.
5. Distinguish between a low-fiber and a low-residue diet.
6. *Case study:* Your client is a 50-year-old female (Mrs. J.) with long-standing diverticulosis who has been following a low-residue diet for many years. She is being discharged with an order to follow a high-fiber diet with bran supplements. She is confused about the change in diet, concerned about its cost, and asks for assistance in making the change.
   a. Explain the rationale for the current diet order, including the use of bran.
   b. List three examples of high-fiber foods in each of the following categories: bread and cereal, fruits and vegetables, and desserts.
   c. How would you advise Mrs. J. to implement the diet?
   d. Considering the expense of bran and fruits and vegetables, what suggestions could you make for increasing the residue content of the diet without their use?
   e. What would you tell Mrs. J. about fluid intake?
7. Explain the rationale for the development of folate and vitamin B_{12} deficiency and steatorrhea in clients with intestinal disorders associated with bacterial overgrowth.
8. Identify the etiologic agent and clinical manifestations in gluten-induced enteropathy and tropical sprue.
9. Describe the significance of secondary lactose deficiency in clients with gluten-induced enteropathy.
10. List foods that are high in gluten content.
11. Compare the dietary management of gluten-induced enteropathy with that of tropical sprue.
12. Distinguish between the etiology, clinical manifestations, and dietary treatment of primary and secondary forms of carbohydrate intolerance.
13. Identify the incidence of primary lactose intolerance in various ethnic groups.
14. Identify the circumstances under which dairy products may be tolerated by clients with primary or secondary lactose intolerance.
15. *Case study:* Your client is a 70-year old male (Mr. B.) who is complaining of constipation.

He has no diseases that could lead to this disorder.

   a. Identify three possible causes of Mr. B.'s constipation.

   b. What is the appropriate dietary regimen for constipation that is not associated with disease?

   c. How does this diet regimen compare to the regimen used for the irritable bowel syndrome and asymptomatic diverticular disease?

16. Describe the three phases of nutritional management following extensive resection of the small intestine and the nutritional management following hemorrhoidectomy.

17. Distinguish between a left-sided colostomy, an ileostomy, and a right-sided colostomy relative to (a) ease of regulation and (b) problems related to maintenance of fluid and electrolyte balance.

18. Describe the appropriate dietary adjustments needed to control each of the following problems in clients with an enterostomy: (a) diarrhea, (b) constipation, (c) gas and odor, and (d) stomal obstruction.

19. Describe additional problems and measures to control problems unique to clients with an ileostomy that involves resection of a significant portion of the terminal ileum.

REFERENCES

1. Vahouny GV: Conclusions and recommendations of the symposium on Dietary Fibers in Health and Disease, Washington, DC, 1981. Am J Clin Nutr 35:152, 1982.
2. Bliss CM: Fat absorption and malabsorption. Arch Intern Med 141:1213, 1981.
3. Bach AC, Babayan VK: Medium-chain triglycerides: An update. Am J Clin Nutr 36:950, 1982.
4. Howard BD, Morse EH: Muffins and pastry made with medium-chain triglycerides. J Am Diet Assoc 62:51, 1973.
5. Bowman F: MCT cookies, cakes, and quick breads; quality and acceptability. J Am Diet Assoc 62:180, 1973.
6. Recipes using MCT oil and portagen. Evansville, Ind, Mead Johnson.
7. Kirsner JB, Shorter RG: Recent developments in nonspecific inflammatory disease. Part 2. N Engl J Med 306:837, 1982.
8. Halsted CH, Gandhi G, Tamura T: Sulfasaline inhibits the absorption of folates in ulcerative colitis. N Engl J Med 305:1513, 1981.
9. American Dietetic Association: Handbook of Clinical Dietetics. New Haven, Conn, Yale University Press, 1981, p B-11.
10. Hartwig MS: Sticking to a gluten-free diet. Am J Nurs 83:1308, 1983.
11. Ament ME, Perera DR, Esther LJ: Sucrase–isomaltase deficiency—A frequently misdiagnosed disease. J Pediatr 83:721, 1973.
12. Payne DL, Welch JD, Manion CV, et al.: Effectiveness of milk products in dietary management of lactose malabsorption. Am J Clin Nutr 34:2711, 1981.
13. Burns TW: Colonic motility in the irritable bowel syndrome. Arch Intern Med 140:247, 1980.
14. Lewis CM: Diet planning for ostomates. Patient Care 11:163, 1977.
15. Ibid, p 162.
16. Ibid, p 159.
17. Ibid, p 152.

BIBLIOGRAPHY

Almy TP, Howell DA: Diverticular disease of the colon. N Engl J Med 302:324, 1980.

An evaluation of children with gluten-sensitive enteropathy. Clinical and laboratory data compared with jejunal biopsy findings. Nutr Rev 39:365, 1981.

Brauer PM, Grace M, Thomson ABR: Diet of women with Crohn's and other gastrointestinal disease. J Am Diet Assoc 82:659, 1983.

Chernoff R, Dean JA: Medical and nutritional aspects of intractable diarrhea. J Am Diet Assoc 76:161, 1980.

Coale MS, Robson JRK: Dietary management of intractable diarrhea in malnourished patients. J Am Diet Assoc 76:444, 1980.

Drude RB Jr, Hines JC: The pathophysiology of intestinal bacterial overgrowth syndrome. Arch Intern Med 140:1349, 1980.

Fagundes-Neto U, Stump MV: Catch-up after the introduction of a gluten-free diet in children with celiac disease. Arch Gastroenterol 18:30, 1981.

Hillman LC, Stace NH, Fisher A, et al.: Dietary intake and stool characteristics of patients with the irritable bowel syndrome. Am J Clin Nutr 36:626, 1982.

Hodges P, Gee M, Grace M, Thomson ABR: Vitamin and iron intake in patients with Crohn's disease. J Am Diet Assoc 84:52, 1984.

Jones VA: Food intolerance. A major factor in the pathogenesis of irritable bowel syndrome. Lancet 2:1115, 1982.

Kirshner JB, Shorter RG: Recent developments in "Nonspecific" inflammatory bowel disease. (Part I). N Engl J Med 306:13, 1982.

Lennard-Jones JE: Current concepts: Functional gastrointestinal disorders. N Engl J Med 308:431, 1983.

Malnutrition in regional ileitis. Nutr Rev 41:57, 1983.

Metabolic bone disease and vitamin D deficiency in Crohn's disease. Nutr Rev 41:213, 1983.

Reasoner J, Maculan TP, Rand AG, Thayer WR Jr: Clinical studies with low-lactose milk. Am J Clin Nutr 34:54, 1981.

CLIENT RESOURCES FOR GLUTEN-INDUCED ENTEROPATHY

Organizations

American Celiac Society, 45 Gifford Avenue, Jersey City, NJ, 07304.

Gluten Intolerance Group, 26604 Dover Court, Kent, WA 98031.

Midwestern Celiac–Sprue Association, P.O. Box 3554, Des Moines, IA 50322.

Distributors of Gluten-free Food Products

Chicago Dietetic Supply, Inc., P.O. Box 529, La Grange, IL 60525.

Ener-G Foods, Inc., P.O. Box 24723, Seattle, WA 98134.

Henkel Corporation, Dietary Specialties, 4620 W. 77th Street, Minneapolis, MN 55435.

Others

Hills HC: Good Food, Gluten Free. New Canaan, Conn, Keats Publishing, 1976.

Pointers for Parents Coping with Celiac Sprue. Chicago, Clinical Dietetics Department, Children's Memorial Hospital, 1982.

Wood MN: Gourmet Food on a Wheat-free Diet. Springfield, Ill, Charles C Thomas, 1972.

CHAPTER 28

Nutrition and Disorders of the Liver, Biliary Tract, and Exocrine Pancreas

Objectives

After completion of this chapter, the student will be able to:

1. Distinguish among fatty degeneration of the liver, type A hepatitis, type B hepatitis, and toxic hepatitis with regard to etiology, clinical course, and dietary management.

2. Compare and contrast the clinical manifestations and dietary management of hepatobiliary insufficiency and pancreatic insufficiency.

3. Develop a nursing care plan for the nutritional management of uncomplicated cirrhosis and adapt the plan for each of the following complications: (a) ascites, (b) esophageal varices, and (c) hepatic encephalopathy.

4. Distinguish between the nutritional management of acute and chronic pancreatitis.

5. Develop a nursing care plan for the nutritional management of an infant with cystic fibrosis and adjust the plan to be suitable for a school-age child and an adolescent with the disorder.

6. Distinguish between the dietary strategies for treating obese clients with gallstones during asymptomatic and symptomatic phases and postcholecystectomy.

Acute and chronic diseases of the liver, pancreas, and gallbladder produce nutritional problems and necessitate diet modification in management. Diet therapy is generally accepted as one of the most important aspects of the management of clients with liver disease, although a conclusive scientific basis for such therapy is lacking. Since liver cells can regenerate, successful treatment of early liver disease may result in recovery of adequate function. Nutritional care in liver disease, particularly in chronic progressive disease leading to end-stage hepatic failure, shares many of the characteristics of nutritional care in renal disease and involves modification of energy, protein, fluid, and electrolytes.

LIVER DISEASE

Assessment

The liver, the largest glandular organ in the body, performs highly complex activities that include metabolic, synthetic, storage, and detoxification functions. The metabolic activities of the liver account for approximately one fourth of the basal metabolism and use 35 to 40 percent of the cardiac output. The liver is served by two vascular systems, the hepatic arterial circulation and the portal venous circulation. Functions of the liver are summarized below.

1. Nutrient metabolism
   a. Carbohydrate. Maintains blood glucose homeostasis by glycogenesis, glycogenolysis, gluconeogenesis, and lipogenesis
   b. Protein. Regulates the distribution of amino acids to body cells; synthesizes plasma proteins, such as albumin, globulins, fibrinogen, heparin, prothrombin; synthesizes urea; deaminates and transaminates amino acids; maintains protein reserves to replace serum proteins as needed
   c. Fat. Synthesizes triglycerides, phospholipids, lipoproteins, cholesterol; converts some cholesterol to bile salts; oxidizes fatty acids, with production of ketones
   d. Alcohol. Metabolizes over 90 percent of ingested alcohol
   e. Vitamins. Activates certain vitamins, e.g., converts carotene to vitamin A, hydroxylates vitamin D, and converts thiamine to thiamine pyrophosphate
2. Synthetic function. Synthesizes bile in addition to the compounds described above
3. Storage function. Stores considerable amounts of fat-soluble vitamins, vitamin B_{12}, iron, copper, and other minerals, and stores lesser amounts of vitamin C and other B-complex vitamins
4. Detoxification function. Detoxifies metabolic by-products (e.g., inactivates hormones), exogenous drugs and toxins, toxins produced by bacteria in the body, and ammonia produced as a by-product of amino acid metabolism

Because the liver is the central organ of metabolism of most nutrients, liver disease can have a profound effect on nutritional status, leading to deficiency states, intolerance of dietary constituents, and change in nutrient requirements.

Liver disease may be acute or chronic, progressing to end-stage hepatic failure. However, acute stages may or may not progress to a chronic phase. The liver has a great reserve and compensatory capacity and responds to treatment even under adverse conditions. The capacity of liver cells to regenerate permits survival even after severe damage.

Assess for factors that may precipitate liver disease in clients, including infectious and parasitic agents, toxins, metabolic or nutritional factors, biliary obstruction, and carcinoma. Regardless of the cause, the pathologic processes are similar and may include (1) fatty infiltration, (2) inflammatory necrosis, and (3) fibrosis (cirrhosis). The earliest and generally reversible stage of liver damage is fatty infiltration, whereas cirrhosis is the most advanced and least reversible stage of liver disease.

▶ **Fatty infiltration** is characterized by deposition of fat droplets in liver cells. The process is completely reversible, but if damage is severe or long-

standing, it may be followed by necrosis or fibrosis.
▶ Inflammatory processes (e.g., hepatitis) lead to **necrosis** of hepatic cells. The necrosis may be mild or massive, causing widespread destruction of the organ. Regenerative activity in liver cells is maintained, however.

The end result of liver damage leading to ne-
▶ crosis is fibrosis, giving rise to the term **cirrhosis.** (Cirrhosis can also occur in the absence of obvious necrosis.) Although regenerative activity occurs in cirrhosis, the progressive loss of cells exceeds their replacement. There is fibrosis of supporting tissues and the vascular bed, and inactive fibrous connective tissue replaces the liver cells. In contrast to the enlarged fatty liver, the fibrotic liver contracts in size with time. Progressive distortion of the vascular system may obstruct the flow of blood in the portal venous system and lead to portal hypertension. The outflow of bile may be obstructed, leading to jaundice—a yellow pigmentation of the skin and body tissues due to the accumulation of bile pigments in the blood. With the formation of dense vascular and fibrous bands, the scarring is reported to be permanent, although further damage can be prevented.

Cirrhosis is a generic term that describes all forms of liver disease characterized by significant cell loss. Thus it includes Laennec's, postnecrotic, biliary, and cardiac or congestive cirrhosis. Cirrhosis may occur as a result of congenital defects of the liver or metabolic abnormalities, such as hemochromatosis (associated with an increase in tissue iron) or Wilson's disease (associated with an increase in tissue copper). Alcohol abuse is often associated with Laennec's cirrhosis, and viral hepatitis is a factor in some cases of postnecrotic cirrhosis.

Controversy surrounds the role of nutritional factors in the pathogenesis of hepatic disease, although some are well known. Without appropriate treatment for clients with Wilson's disease or hemochromatosis, for example, cirrhosis will occur. Ingestion of foods containing toxic substances, such as peanuts contaminated with *Aspergillus flavus* or contaminated shellfish, can also lead to liver damage. Dietary deficiency has been implicated, and although it is agreed that malnutrition may be a factor in the etiology of fatty liver, there is no convincing evidence that cirrhosis is caused by malnutrition.

Alcohol abusers develop fatty livers, and malnutrition (particularly protein deficiency) has been proposed as a predominant factor in alcoholic liver disease. Although there is indirect evidence to support this contention, current evidence supports the view that alcohol's direct toxic effect on the liver is the major factor and that alcohol can produce cirrhosis even when dietary intake is adequate. Liver damage occurs in about 20 percent of alcoholics, and it appears to be dose related even in those who are susceptible. Genetic and immunologic factors may be involved. The interactions between alcohol and nutritional factors (e.g., the malnutrition that may result from the substitution of alcohol for food and the maldigestion and malabsorption that result from alcohol's effect on the gastrointestinal tract) in the pathology of alcoholic liver disease remain largely unexplored. It appears prudent to assume, particularly from a therapeutic point of view, that malnutrition may be a contributing factor.

Nutritional problems in liver disease arise from the failure of liver function and obstruction of the portal circulation, leading to edema and ascites, esophageal varices, and chronic congestion of the gastrointestinal tract. Assess for such symptoms as anorexia, nausea, vomiting, diarrhea (or constipation), weight loss, lassitude, weakness, fever, abdominal distention, gas, and heartburn. Jaundice is a symptom common to many diseases of the liver and biliary tract. Determine the origin of the jaundice, which may be (1) obstructive (due to blockage of the flow of bile by stones, tumors, inflammation, or congenital defects), (2) toxic (due to effects of poisons, drugs, or viral infections), or (3) hemolytic (due to excessive destruction of red blood cells).

The effects of liver disease on nutritional status vary widely. Some clients may demonstrate little obvious clinical evidence of malnutrition, whereas others have signs of severe nutritional deficiency, such as beriberi, scurvy, and peripheral neuropathy. Expect nutritional alterations to be more severe in those with alcoholic liver disease than in those with liver disease due to other causes, although weight loss may occur in any client who is acutely ill. Although clinical evidence of malnutrition may be sparse, numerous alterations in biochemical indices of nutritional status may be evident, and it is appropriate to correct reversible deficiencies when this is possible.

Assess for the causes in alterations in nutritional status, which may be deficient dietary intake (due to anorexia, alcoholism, or other factors), associated drug therapy (cholestyramine), or alterations in nutrient absorption, storage, or metabolism in association with the liver disease. Use the summary of complications of liver disease given in Table 28–1 to aid in the assessment and to guide nutritional therapy.

Fatty Degeneration of the Liver

Assessment and Intervention. Suspect fatty degeneration of the liver if the client's history reveals severe malnutrition (particularly protein malnutrition), alcohol abuse, exposure to toxic agents, such as DDT and carbon tetrachloride, or if the client is obese. The condition may also be a complication of total parenteral nutrition, jejunoileal bypass for obesity, poorly controlled diabetes mellitus, or long-standing heart failure. Although many believe that fatty liver is the forerunner of cirrhosis, its progression to cirrhosis is still questionable. In contrast to other types of liver disease, fatty liver represents a relatively benign condition, and prompt treatment may dramatically reverse the situation, and

the liver returns to a normal architecture and function. For example, the fatty degeneration and ▶ **hepatomegaly** (liver enlargement) that accompany obesity are rarely associated with significant impairment of liver function, and the condition improves rapidly with weight reduction. Toxic agents, such as alcohol or hepatotoxins, however, may cause hepatic cell necrosis or autoimmune responses that produce further damage. Moreover, the level of some enzymes, such as alkaline phosphatase, may be elevated with hepatomegaly associated with total parenteral nutrition. When this occurs, reduce the proportion of carbohydrate to protein in the infusate.

Treatment of fatty liver necessitates removal of alcohol or toxic agents and treatment of the precipitating disorder. Provide an appropriate diet to control or correct the underlying disorder, i.e., diabetes, obesity, or malnutrition. Instruct the client to eat a diet high in protein and adequate in other nutrients and energy to promote liver cell regeneration. The amount of fat accumulation in alcohol-induced fatty liver may decrease when long-chain triglycerides are replaced with medium-chain triglycerides. A possible mechanism is that medium-chain triglycerides are not stored but oxidized to carbon dioxide.[1]

Hepatobiliary Insufficiency

Assessment and Intervention. Hepatobiliary insufficiency results from conditions that decrease bile acid synthesis or diminish its release into the intestine. The ensuing steatorrhea and malnutrition are the result of fecal losses of fat, fat-soluble vitamins, and such minerals as calcium and magnesium. Observe for steatorrhea as a complication in clients with acute viral hepatitis, cirrhosis, and biliary obstruction. Chronic biliary obstruction may be due to primary biliary cirrhosis, postoperative traumatic biliary stricture, biliary atresia (congenital lack of a normal opening in the bile ducts), or blockage of the bile ducts by stones, cysts, or tumors. Since the stores of vitamin K are small, observe for hypoprothrombinemia (low blood prothrombin) and bleeding disturbances as an early phenomenon. Long-standing malabsorption may lead to calcium and vitamin D depletion with osteomalacia in some clients. In clients with severe depletion of vitamin A, observe for night blindness, hyperkeratosis, and impairment of taste and smell. Vitamin E deficiency appears to have no obvious consequences.

If the condition is correctable by surgery (i.e., removal of the cause of obstruction), there is little indication for specific dietary measures, since the metabolic disturbances are reversed following surgery. Restrict dietary fat, however, during the period before surgery. In clients with chronic hepatobiliary insufficiency, nutrient modifications are often necessary to decrease the steatorrhea and associated nutrient losses. Restrict long-chain fats to approximately 40 g daily. If additional kilocalories are

---

TABLE 28–1
COMPLICATIONS OF LIVER DISEASE WITH IMPLICATIONS
FOR NUTRITIONAL STATUS AND THERAPY

Complication	Explanatory Comments
Impaired protein and amino acid metabolism and alteration of amino acid profile	Decrease in albumin synthesis; alteration in the ratio of the aromatic and branched-chain amino acids (aromatic amino acids—tyrosine, phenylalanine, and tryptophan—are increased in the blood, and branched-chain amino acids—valine, leucine, and isoleucine—are decreased)
Disordered metabolism of water and minerals	Sodium and water retention lead to accumulation of fluid in the abdominal cavity (ascites), pleural effusion, and edema; increase in urinary excretion of zinc and decrease in serum zinc levels; potential for hepatic injury due to iron excess secondary to an increase in iron absorption (alcohol increases iron absorption, and some alcoholic beverages contain significant amounts of iron); portal-systemic shunting increases iron absorption
Impaired glucose tolerance (symptomatic diabetes mellitus less common)	Altered carbohydrate metabolism associated with hyperinsulinemia and insulin resistance
Fat malabsorption and steatorrhea with secondary malabsorption of fat-soluble vitamins, calcium, and magnesium	Occurs secondary to diminished bile synthesis or biliary obstruction; in clients with Laennec's cirrhosis, pancreatic insufficiency may be a contributing factor
Impaired storage and activation of vitamins	Decreased storage of vitamins and diminished conversion of vitamins to their metabolically active forms, leading to a diminished response to vitamin therapy
Varices (varicose veins) in the esophagus or abdominal region	Occurs as a consequence of distortion and obstruction of the vascular bed, leading to portal hypertension and shunting of portal blood into the portal-systemic venous collateral circulation; varices pose danger of rupture and hemorrhage; hemorrhage may precipitate hepatic encephalopathy
Renal failure	May be vascular in origin; may be precipitated by severe infection, massive gastrointestinal hemorrhage, or dehydration
Hepatic encephalopathy (cerebral dysfunction with disorders of consciousness and motor function of hepatic origin occurs particularly with severe liver disease or secondary to natural or surgically induced vascular shunting of blood from the portal to the systemic circulation)	Cause uncertain but may be due to altered metabolism of amino acids and nitrogenous compounds or altered ratio of amino acids, leading to an intolerance to protein (particularly protein of high aromatic amino acid content)

---

needed to maintain or gain weight, consider adding medium-chain triglycerides (MCT). However, use of MCT may be contraindicated in clients with cirrhosis of the liver,[1] particularly if the disorder is associated with hypoproteinemia and shunting, although there is no general agreement on this point. If the steatorrhea is complicated by pancreatic insufficiency, administer pancreatic supplements as well.

Provide fat-soluble vitamins and calcium supplements on a long-term basis. If there is hepatocellular damage, be aware that the response to vitamin K therapy may be poor, since the liver may not be able to synthesize prothrombin and other clotting factors.

Hepatitis

Assessment. Hepatitis is an inflammation of the liver leading to necrosis and degenerative changes in the liver and, in some individuals, bile stasis with jaundice. In mild cases the tissue injury is reversible, but occasionally what appears to be an acute, uncomplicated hepatitis suddenly takes a fulminant form, leading to massive liver necrosis, liver failure, and death. Hepatitis, which may be viral or toxic in origin and acute or chronic in nature, is caused by infectious agents, such as viruses and bacteria, or toxic agents, such as alcohol and certain drugs.

▶ The term **viral hepatitis** encompasses three

conditions caused by three different types of viruses, type A, type B, and type non A–non B.

1. Type A hepatitis (previously called "infectious hepatitis") caused by type A virus: This condition is the most common cause of liver disease in Western societies, is readily transmitted (by the intestinal–oral route) through contaminated drinking water, food, or sewage, although it can be transmitted parenterally, and is mildly contagious

2. Type B hepatitis (previously called "serum hepatitis") caused by type B virus: This condition is transmitted primarily by blood transfusions using blood from a person who is a carrier (either symptomatic or nonsymptomatic) of the virus or by use of contaminated skin-puncturing equipment, such as needles, syringes, dental drills, or tattooing needles; the virus can also enter the body by the oral route or by intimate contact

3. Type non A–non B hepatitis: This type cannot be traced to either the A or B virus and is believed to be caused by at least one and probably several viruses and is often spread by blood transfusions

If the client's history reveals abuse of alcohol or hard drugs, hypersensitivity to such drugs as penicillin, or exposure to other hepatotoxic agents, such as carbon tetrachloride and chloroform, suspect toxic hepatitis. The term **alcoholic hepatitis** is used to describe the liver cell necrosis and necrotic inflammation that develop in some alcohol abusers. Some authors hypothesize that alcoholic hepatitis is a forerunner of alcoholic cirrhosis (Laennec's cirrhosis), although in many instances, cirrhosis gradually develops in the absence of this intermediate stage. In its more overt form, alcoholic hepatitis is frequently fatal in spite of hospitalization, abstinence from alcohol, and consumption of an adequate diet.

Chronic hepatitis may result from acute viral or toxic hepatitis or from autoimmune phenomena. While acute type A hepatitis is almost always a self-limited disorder, clients with type B and type non A–non B hepatitis are more likely to develop the chronic form of the disease.

Regardless of the cause of acute hepatitis, observe for its typical symptoms, including anorexia, nausea, vomiting, fever, headache, weight loss, fatigue, and abdominal discomfort. Observe for hepatomegaly and splenomegaly, which is present in a significant number of clients, and for jaundice, which usually becomes apparent after 2 to 5 days. In the presence of jaundice, observe for dark-colored urine and light-colored stools.

Intervention. Treat acute hepatitis by instituting nursing measures to promote comfort and rest to counteract fatigue and by providing an adequate diet to aid in the regeneration of liver tissue and to pre-

vent further liver damage. During the period of acute nausea, vomiting, and anorexia, infuse 5 to 10 percent glucose. Consider the addition of amino acids or protein hydrolysates to the intravenous feeding or the use of tube feeding if the client cannot consume oral feedings for a prolonged period. When oral feeding is possible, provide a diet that contains (1) 35 to 40 kcal/kg of body weight in an adult, (2) 1 g or more of protein/kg of body weight (with selections from animal and vegetable sources) to allow for liver cell regeneration, (3) 300 to 400 g carbohydrate to spare the dietary protein for synthetic purposes and to promote glycogenesis, and (4) moderate to high fat content (30 to 40 percent of kilocalories) to increase palatability and kilocaloric density. Restrict fat intake, however, if there is steatorrhea in association with intrahepatic biliary obstruction. Serve small, frequent meals to diminish the nausea and anorexia that may appear with larger, fewer meals. Consider the client's food preferences and serve foods attractively to enhance the appetite. Milkshakes and eggnogs can be used as interval feedings, and these appear to be well tolerated. If food intake is adequate, vitamin and mineral supplements are not routinely needed, but with steatorrhea, administer a vitamin K supplement. Some authorities advocate the avoidance of alcohol for a period of 6 months to 1 year after illness to avoid further liver cell injury. Others, however, note that there is no evidence that moderate use of alcohol has a deleterious effect. To avoid contracting the disease, use disposable tray services during the infectious period and follow routine anti-infective precautions.

The dietary management of chronic hepatitis (viral or toxic in origin) and acute fulminant hepatitis follows the principles described below for cirrhosis. Recognize, however, that nutritional requirements in persons suffering from fulminant disease are different from those with chronic liver disease. In the former, nutritional status was most likely previously normal in contrast to the nutrient depletion that may be present in those with cirrhosis. In acute fulminant hepatitis, a high or even normal protein intake may induce hepatic encephalopathy. Observe for signs of hepatic encephalopathy in these clients, including euphoria, apathy, confusion, disturbed sleep patterns (i.e., awake and confused at night and asleep during the day), severe depression and mania, drowsiness and stupor, leading to coma. There may be a flapping tremor of the hands (asterixis) and an offensive odor to the breath (fetor hepaticus). If any of these signs are present, restrict dietary protein.

Cirrhosis

Assessment. Cirrhosis is the end-stage of liver disease, characterized by chronic hepatic insufficiency. Cirrhosis may develop secondary to such factors as chronic alcoholism, biliary obstruction, exposure to toxic agents, metabolic abnormalities, and infection, but Laennec's cirrhosis (generally associated with alcohol abuse) is the most common form. Not all alcoholics develop Laennec's cirrhosis, however, and the disorder also occurs in nonalcoholics.

Regular evaluation of liver function and nutritional status and cautious nutritional support are required in cirrhosis, since during this stage of liver disease, such complications as sodium and fluid retention, esophageal varices, hepatic encephalopathy, and nutritional deficiency may occur in association with a variety of secondary metabolic changes.

Intervention. Provide a dietary regimen to counteract malnutrition and promote liver regeneration. At the same time avoid provoking symptoms of hepatic encephalopathy—this problem often prevents attainment of the nutritional goal. In the absence of complications, an ad libitum diet can be given, but be sure to assess tolerance for protein, which can vary in individual clients. Give attention to the kilocalorie, protein, carbohydrate, fat, mineral, and vitamin content of the diet (Table 28–2). Moreover, if sodium and water retention and upper gastrointestinal bleeding are complications, further modifications are necessary.

If the client has anorexia, nausea, vomiting, or abdominal pain associated with eating, consumption of an adequate amount of food may be difficult. Make a concerted effort to serve attractive food, and allow the client to select those foods that are most appealing. Obtain a record of food likes and dislikes from the client or a relative. Serve small, frequent meals, with the largest meal given at the time when the appetite is best, which for many is the morning meal. The client with severe ascites needs small meals to avoid further distress and a further increase in portal pressure that may occur with large meals. Monitor food intake closely and record estimates of foods and supplements consumed for the previous 24 hours in the medical record. If an inadequate amount of food is being consumed, consider alternative feeding methods, such as tube feedings or parenteral supplements of formulas designed for clients with liver disease. However, tube feeding (by a nasogastric tube) is contraindicated in the presence of esophageal varices. If supplements of MCT are being used, provide them in small, well-chilled servings to increase acceptability. Adjust the dietary regimen as dictated by the client's changing clinical status, and advise the client to abstain from alcohol. If alcoholism is the underlying cause, the client may be helped by a self-help group, such as Alcoholics Anonymous.

Sodium and water retention leading to edema and ascites necessitates the use of diuretics and dietary sodium (and possibly fluid) restriction. Use daily body weight and frequent measurement of serum electrolytes as a guide to therapy—a reasonably safe guideline is a weight loss that does not exceed

TABLE 28–2
NUTRIENT RECOMMENDATIONS FOR CIRRHOSIS

Nutrient Factor	Comment
Kilocalories	Increase to 35–45 kcal/kg (for adults) to minimize endogenous tissue catabolism and achieve maximal nitrogen sparing
Protein	Balance the intake between increased need for liver regeneration and limitation to avoid precipitation of hepatic encephalopathy; the ultimate goal is 1 g/kg of body weight, giving emphasis to protein of high biologic value; attain optimal intake gradually in response to client tolerance as measured by neurologic status; increased protein intake is contraindicated in the presence of symptoms of hepatic encephalopathy
Carbohydrate	Increase to 300–400 g daily to achieve the desired energy level and maximal nitrogen sparing
Fat	Regulate intake according to the presence or absence of steatorrhea; in absence of steatorrhea, fat content should be moderately high to provide palatable meals and to achieve desired energy level; in presence of steatorrhea (which accompanies cirrhosis in about one half of cases), restrict fat intake; use MCT to supply additional energy except in advanced cases (this point is controversial)
Vitamins and minerals	Evaluate nutritional intake and malabsorption and determine the need for supplements; in particular evaluate B-complex vitamins (especially thiamine and folic acid), fat-soluble vitamins (especially vitamin K), potassium, zinc, magnesium, and calcium; routine iron supplements are contraindicated because of the potential of further liver injury

5 kg/week. The degree of sodium restriction that is necessary is judged by the severity of the retention. In severe, refractory retention, severe sodium restriction (i.e., 230 mg or 10 mEq daily) may be necessary, and a diet containing 500 to 2000 mg (approximately 20 to 85 mEq) of sodium daily may be sufficient in less severe cases. Low-sodium diets are discussed in Chapter 29. When obvious clinical improvement is demonstrated, liberalize the sodium intake. Hyponatremia is not an infrequent finding in cirrhosis (presumably due to an increase in the secretion of the antidiuretic hormone), and with mild hyponatremia and severe, refractory edema or ascites, the severe sodium restriction is still advocated. The sodium restriction promotes water loss, with an increase in serum sodium. If the hyponatremia is symptomatic, administer hypertonic saline and restrict fluid. Also observe for hyponatremia as well as hypokalemia secondary to diuretic therapy and provide supplements as indicated. Hypokalemia and associated alkalosis may precipitate hepatic encephalopathy. With severe sodium restriction, low-sodium milk must often be used. Increase its palatability by the addition of honey, vanilla, or other flavoring. Fluid restriction may sometimes be necessary to control the sodium and water retention. The amount of fluid allowed may be restricted to daily fluid losses.

Upper gastrointestinal bleeding may occur in cirrhotic clients secondary to rupture of esophageal varices or associated gastritis or peptic ulcer. The hemorrhage may be fatal, or the large protein load from the digested blood in the gut may precipitate hepatic encephalopathy. To prevent or minimize the potential for hemorrhage, use these nursing interventions:

1. Provide small, frequent feedings
2. Use antacid therapy
3. Avoid gastrointestinal irritants, such as nicotine and hot spices
4. Provide a diet of smooth texture and avoid fibrous and sharp-edged foods (such as raw fruits and vegetables and foods with bone fragments)

Should bleeding occur, substitute a liquid diet. Surgical intervention may be necessary if the bleeding is recurrent. A portacaval shunt may be performed to relieve pressure on the esophageal and stomach veins. Construction of a portacaval shunt involves connecting the portal vein to the vena cava. In this way, nutrients are not carried to the liver but instead enter the general circulation directly. Following this surgical procedure, assess tolerance for protein carefully. Transient encephalopathy may be evident in the immediate postoperative period due to depressed liver cell function secondary to surgery. Restrict protein immediately after surgery and gradually increase the amount to normal levels (e.g., in 20 g increments) during the following week. These clients exhibit a high prevalence of chronic hepatic encephalopathy within 3 years following surgery.

Hepatic Encephalopathy (Hepatic Coma)

Assessment. Observe clients with severe parenchymal liver disease and those with portacaval shunts carefully for signs of encephalopathy and impending hepatic coma. A number of factors are implicated in the etiology of this disorder, although the topic remains controversial. Failure of the liver to detoxify products of protein catabolism and the altered amino acid profile (increase in aromatic amino acids and decrease in branched-chain amino acids) have both been offered as explanations for the cerebral dysfunction associated with severe liver disease. Failure of the damaged liver to synthesize urea from ammonia during protein catabolism or shunting of portal blood (containing ammonia and other nitrogenous compounds formed by bacterial action on exogenous or endogenous protein sources, such as blood) into the systemic circulation allows nitrogenous compounds to flood the central nervous system. The disrupted balance between the aromatic and branched-chain amino acids may allow a decreased transport of branched-chain amino acids and increased movement of aromatic amino acids into the brain, altering neurotransmitter metabolism.[2] Although the etiologic mechanism is not definitive, the blood ammonia concentration is usually elevated in the disorder. If the laboratory findings show an increased ammonia level, suspect impending hepatic coma. Since the condition is characterized by protein intolerance, hepatic coma is generally the limiting factor in providing an adequate protein intake in clients with liver disease.

Intervention. The aims of treatment in clients who show clinical signs of hepatic failure are to decrease the exogenous and endogenous protein load and prevent the absorption of noxious substances from the gastrointestinal tract. A combination of diet and drug therapy is used to achieve the desired goals. Restrict dietary protein to tolerance levels, control gastrointestinal bleeding (if present), administer nonabsorbable drugs to decrease the degradation of protein by the gut bacteria and to prevent the absorption of the products of their metabolism, and administer enemas to remove blood and protein from the bowel. Tolerance for dietary protein can be enhanced by the concurrent administration of neomycin, a nonabsorbable antibiotic, to suppress the population of intestinal bacteria (and thus reduce the bacterial conversion of protein to ammonia and other toxic products), and lactulose, a nonabsorbable synthetic disaccharide, to promote the retention of ammonia in the colon through lowering of the luminal pH and inducing diarrhea. With progression of the liver disease, however, protein tolerance diminishes gradually, despite treatment with these agents. Observe for side effects of neomycin therapy, including malabsorption of fat, fat-soluble vitamins, and carbohydrate.

To minimize the exogenous protein load with hyperammonemia, restrict the protein intake to 0.5 g/kg of body weight or less. With coma, eliminate protein entirely for a short period of time. Protein intake should be resumed as soon as possible, however, to minimize body protein loss. Supply at least 1600 kcal daily from carbohydrate and fat during the period of protein restriction to minimize endogenous protein catabolism and enhance the anabolic use of dietary protein. If oral intake is not possible because of coma during the period, administer tube feeding or parenteral nutrition. Intake of protein can be appropriately controlled with these forms of nutritional therapy.

During recovery, gradually reintroduce dietary protein with small progressive increments (e.g., with absence of symptoms for 1 week, increase protein intake by 10 g every 3 to 5 days if tolerated until the desired goal of 1 g/kg is reached—higher protein levels increase the risk of precipitating coma without necessarily leading to improved protein status). Monitor clinical status and laboratory findings regularly during this period, and reduce protein again if symptoms recur. Hepatic coma may be delayed by up to a week after increasing the protein. In those with chronic hepatic failure, the desired level of protein intake may not be achieved, although many clients tend to stabilize at a level of 50 g or more daily. Distribute the protein fairly evenly in meals during the day to prevent a sudden overload of protein. Provide protein of high biologic value, and assist the client to maintain an adequate kilocalorie intake. With this regimen, it is possible to attain nitrogen balance with a daily protein intake of 35 to 40 g daily. Foods of high biologic value not only supply the essential amino acids but also theoretically have a lower ammonigenic potential than have foods rich in nonessential amino acid content. Milk and eggs are said to produce less ammonia than does meat. The concept of varying ammonigenic potential of different foods is not widely accepted, since no relationship between the nitrogen and ammonia content of food has been proven. The protein content of foods listed in the six Food Exchange Lists (see Appendix 2) can be used to construct a low-protein diet. Table 28–3 provides the composition of sample 30 and 40 g protein diets. Low-protein diets are discussed further in Chapter 30.

Protein supplements in the form of branched-chain amino acids, administered by oral or tube feeding or parenterally, are being used to restore amino acid balance in the plasma, to prevent or ameliorate encephalopathy, to support overall nutrition, and to prevent catabolism of lean body mass. Hepatic-Aid (McGaw) and Travasorb Hepatic (Travenol) are oral supplements that are rich in branched-chain amino acids, and a high-nitrogen product (Traum-Aid HN, McGaw) is available for use in clients who are experiencing catabolic stress. Because of their

TABLE 28–3
CONTENT OF 30 G AND 40 G PROTEIN DIETS

Exchange List	No. of Exchanges and g Protein Provided	
	30 g Protein Diet	40 g Protein Diet
Milk	1 (8 g)	1 (8 g)
Meat	2 (14 g)	3 (21 g)
Bread	3 (6 g)	3 (6 g)
Vegetables	2 (4 g)	3 (6 g)
Nonprotein foods (such as sugar, jelly, fruit, oil, salt-free butter or margarine, low-protein wheat starch products, low-electrolyte supplements—see Chap. 30—sufficient to provide the desired number of kcal)		
Total	32 g	41 g

hypertonicity, if these are used as a tube feeding, administer by continuous drip to avoid the complications of a hyperosmolar solution. Oral or parenteral alpha-keto-analogs (see Chap. 30) of the branched-chain amino acids are being tested for their effectiveness. These derivatives of amino acids can be transaminated to form the corresponding amino acids. Although the clinical usefulness of these protein supplements is not now clear, prospective studies are underway to evaluate their effectiveness.[3] These supplements do not provide vitamins and minerals in quantities sufficient to maintain normal nutrition. Provide supplements if the client's diet is restricted in protein.

There is some limited clinical evidence that vegetarian diets may be useful in treating clients with encephalopathy, although a recent study failed to document this.[4] Theoretical considerations for the effectiveness of such diets include their reduced content of aromatic amino acids and their high content of complex carbohydrate, which may alter insulin response and bacterial metabolism.

PANCREATIC DISEASE

Pancreatic Insufficiency

Assessment. The pancreas, which is located in the upper abdomen behind the stomach, has both an exocrine and an endocrine function. Its exocrine function is related to secretion of digestive enzymes by the acini tissue to aid in the digestion of carbohydrate, protein, and fat. The endocrine function is provided by the islets of Langerhans, which secrete hormones directly into the blood. The islets of Langerhans consist of at least four types of cells: the alpha-cells, which secrete glucagon; the beta-cells, which secrete insulin; the delta cells, which secrete

---

TABLE 28–4
SIGNS AND SYMPTOMS OF PANCREATIC INSUFFICIENCY

Defects in the digestion and absorption of carbohydrate, protein, and fat (starch digestion is less affected than protein and fat)

    Diarrhea, steatorrhea, azotorrhea, and malabsorption of fat-soluble vitamins and vitamin B_{12} (deficiency symptoms of fat-soluble vitamins are rarely seen, however, in contrast to other forms of malabsorption)

Lowered serum levels of calcium, potassium, and sodium

Weight loss

Disturbances of carbohydrate metabolism (transient)

Glucose intolerance occurs in acute pancreatis; diabetes mellitus may occur in the late stages of chronic pancreatitis, following massive pancreatic resection, and pancreatic carcinoma

---

somatostatin; and the pancreatic polypeptide cells (or F cells), which secrete pancreatic polypeptide. Digestive enzymes are secreted into a system of ducts. The major pancreatic duct joins the common bile duct, forming the hepatopancreatic ampulla of Vater as it opens into the duodenum, and the sphincter of Oddi controls the opening.

The pancreas has a large functional reserve, and considerable diminution of function must occur before clinical manifestations are apparent. For example, pancreatic secretory function may be reduced to 10 percent of normal without the appearance of azotorrhea (excretion of excessive amounts of nitrogenous substances in the stool) or steatorrhea. However, progressive malabsorption occurs with a greater loss of function. As much as 80 percent of the pancreas may be removed without interfering with fat digestion or absorption.

Pancreatic insufficiency refers to diminution or absence of the enzymes secreted by the exocrine acinar cells. Observe for signs and symptoms (Table 28–4) of enzyme deficiency in clients with the following conditions:

1. Chronic pancreatitis (inflammation of the pancreas) secondary to alcoholism, gallbladder disease, trauma, or other disorder
2. Pancreatic carcinoma with obstruction of the ductal system or localized areas of pancreatitis
3. Cystic fibrosis
4. Pancreatic resection (pancreatectomy necessitates a partial gastrectomy, which complicates the clinical course)

Intervention. Treatment of pancreatic insufficiency depends on the severity of the defect, and diet modifications may be unnecessary in uncomplicated cases. Use the degree of glucose intolerance and fat malabsorption to guide management following resection and treat symptomatic pancreatic insufficiency by:

1. Oral replacement of the missing enzymes in the form of pancreatic extracts; the action of the enzymes may be enhanced by the concomitant administration of antacids (to prevent enzyme inactivation by gastric acid) or gastric antisecretory agents, such as cimetidine (to decrease gastric acid secretion)[5]
2. Supplementation with fat-soluble vitamins (in a water-miscible form), calcium, and possibly vitamin B_{12} (the defect in vitamin B_{12} absorption is partially corrected by administration of oral bicarbonate and fully corrected with oral pancreatic extracts)
3. Restriction of dietary fat (e.g., 50 to 60 g or less daily) or use of medium-chain triglycerides to control steatorrhea
4. Control of carbohydrate intake if glucose intolerance and diabetes mellitus are present (see Chap. 24); the diabetes is usually of the brittle type, requiring relatively small quantities of insulin; the disorder is difficult to control with precision

Tolerance for fat varies from client to client. If fat intake must be restricted, maintain kilocalorie intake at a high level (3000 to 6000 kcal/day) by increasing the carbohydrate (400 g or more daily) and protein (100 to 150 g daily) intake. The amount of protein and fat absorbed can be increased by increasing the amount consumed, although excessive fat intake is not desirable. With concomitant enzyme replacement, provide 50 g of fat in the daily diet and gradually increase the intake to 200 g or until steatorrhea becomes clinically apparent. Small, frequent feedings are preferred to large meals. Defined formula diets (see Chap. 21) may be useful in severe cases, since these products provide only a minimal stimulus to pancreatic secretion. With prolonged severe pancreatitis, nutritional support by total parenteral nutrition may become necessary. Discourage the use of alcohol in clients with pancreatitis, since it serves as a gastrointestinal irritant and encourages recurrence of the disorder.

Adequate dosage and proper timing of the pancreatic enzyme replacement are essential, although there are varying opinions about the ideal enzyme replacement, dosage, and administration schedule. The supplements most commonly used are pancreatin (Viokase), pancrelipase (Cotazym), and most recently pancrease, although several others are available. The available preparations vary widely in enzyme activity. The administered enzymes help to moderate problems related to malabsorption but do not entirely alleviate the malabsorption. Instruct the client to take the prescribed medication dosage with meals and snacks. For infants and children, the outer capsule of enteric-coated preparations can be broken open and the microspheres mixed with food without changing taste and consistency. With nonenteric-coated preparations, however, this procedure adds an unpleasant flavor and causes a consistency change as the food begins to be digested in the dish.[6] Modify the supplement regimen according to individual client response. For some, it may be desirable to give part of the dose before the meal and part during the meal or the medication may be given hourly.

Pancreatitis

Assessment and Intervention. Pancreatitis may be acute or chronic, and the acute form may or may not progress to the chronic state. In chronic pancreatitis, inflammation and fibrosis of the enzyme-secreting acinar glands produce the syndrome of pancreatic insufficiency.

The etiology of pancreatitis is poorly understood, although the condition is associated with a number of disorders, including chronic alcoholism, biliary tract disease, infection, ingestion of certain drugs, trauma, hypercalcemia, and hyperlipoproteinemia (types 1, 4, and 5; see Chap. 29). Pancreatitis is related to many etiologic factors that lead to obstruction of pancreatic secretions (such as gallstones), accumulation of these secretions in the pancreas, and subsequent autodigestion by its activated enzymes. Fat tissue surrounding the pancreas may be digested, leading to sequestering of calcium by fatty acids. Chronic alcoholism is a common cause of pancreatitis. Alcohol may have a direct toxic effect on the pancreas, or it may lead to obstruction secondary to an associated duodenitis (inflammation of the duodenum), with edema of the ampulla of Vater, reflux of bile and pancreatic secretions, and subsequent destruction of pancreatic tissue.

The symptoms of pancreatitis range from mild to severe. Assess for the presence of pain in the upper abdomen that may be moderate to severe (lasting for hours or days), fever, nausea, vomiting, and jaundice. In the presence of severe pain, shock, and paralytic ileus, suspect that caustic juices have escaped into the abdominal cavity. Evaluate the biochemical findings, which include an elevation in serum amylase and lipase (these pancreatic enzymes pass from the inflamed pancreas into the circulatory system), hyperlipidemia, and hypocalcemia. Assess for signs of tetany.

Treat acute pancreatitis by avoiding the stimulation of pancreatic secretions and bile—no oral feeding is allowed initially, and nutrients are provided parenterally. As oral feeding is tolerated, begin feeding with a clear liquid diet composed of simple carbohydrates, with gradual progression to a normal diet. The average client with acute, uncomplicated pancreatitis is free of pain, nausea, and vomiting within 2 to 3 days, and by the end of the first week, most clients tolerate a six-meal light diet.

To treat chronic pancreatitis associated with symptoms of pancreatic insufficiency follow the principles outlined above. In addition, instruct the client to avoid caffeine-containing beverages and decaf-

feinated coffee. Evaluate the client for signs of diabetes mellitus, since some islet involvement may occur.

Cystic Fibrosis (Mucoviscidosis)

Assessment. Cystic fibrosis is a generalized, progressive, hereditary disorder in which there is widespread dysfunction of the exocrine glands. Either the glands are obstructed by thick, sticky mucus, or they excrete abnormal amounts of sodium and chloride. Normally, mucous secretions are thin and flow easily, but in cystic fibrosis they are thick and sticky and lead to most of the clinical manifestations of the disease: the bronchi, bronchioles, nasal sinuses, salivary ducts and glands, pancreatic ducts, bile ducts, intestinal glands, and seminiferous tubules become obstructed with viscous or solid material, and the enzyme-secreting glands of the pancreas become fibrosed and nonfunctional. The involvement of the mucus-secreting glands has the most serious consequences, but the excretion of large amounts of sodium and chloride by the sweat and salivary glands also presents problems.

Cystic fibrosis is believed to be an inborn error of metabolism, although the defect underlying the dysfunction is not understood. The disease is one of the most common chronic diseases of children and adolescents and represents the most serious lung disease among American children. Cystic fibrosis is transmitted as an autosomal recessive trait, and the gene responsible for the disorder is carried by approximately 3 to 6 percent of the population. Although primarily a disorder occurring among Caucasians, it is also well documented in other ethnic groups, including black Americans, Native Americans, Chinese, and Japanese.

Pulmonary insufficiency, which is present in almost all clients at some time in the course of the illness and which is frequently severe and progressive, presents the most significant clinical problems and ultimately determines the client's fate. Pancreatic insufficiency occurs in 85 to 90 percent of cases, although the resulting maldigestion and malabsorption can usually be managed successfully. Although pancreatic insufficiency is often evident soon after birth, it may not be expressed until later in infancy or in childhood.

In recent years, newer methods of diagnosis and treatment have brought about a dramatic change in the prognosis for affected individuals, and the life span has lengthened considerably. For example, the average age of death from cystic fibrosis was age 4 in the 1940s; this is in contrast to age 17 in the 1970s. Moreover, over 50 percent of children with cystic fibrosis now reach age 21. The prognosis is determined by the degree of lung involvement and the speed with which treatment is instituted.

The complications of cystic fibrosis include chronic pulmonary disease, pancreatic insufficiency, increased concentration of electrolytes in sweat, and occasionally, cirrhosis of the liver. Many of the gastrointestinal manifestations result from pancreatic insufficiency leading to steatorrhea and generalized malabsorption. Observe for the physiologic manifestations of the disease summarized below:

- *Respiratory manifestations.* Thick mucous plugs in the bronchi and bronchioles lead to recurrent infection, chronic progressive lung disease, pulmonary insufficiency, and ultimately right-sided heart failure; obstruction of the upper airway leads to nasal congestion, chronic sinusitis, and nasal polyps
- *Gastrointestinal manifestations.* Obstruction of the pancreatic duct leads to pancreatic atrophy and fibrosis with pancreatic insufficiency, steatorrhea, and generalized malabsorption, abdominal pain (sometimes severe, associated with the presence of undigested food, gas, and fecal obstruction), malnutrition, growth retardation, and rectal prolapse (due to large bowel movements); destruction of the insulin-secreting cells results in diabetes mellitus in older clients; obstruction of the intestinal glands may lead to meconium ileus in the newborn and fecal masses, constipation, and intestinal obstruction in the older child, adolescent, and young adult; hepatic duct obstruction produces focal fibrosis of the liver that occasionally leads to cirrhosis with portal hypertension and esophageal varices
- *Sweat gland manifestations.* The sodium and chloride concentration in sweat is increased (two to five times normal) and may lead to salt depletion and heat prostration (the nature of the defect in the sweat gland is not known but is thought to be due to a decrease in the absorption of sodium and chloride from the ducts); the sodium and chloride concentration of saliva is also increased, although not to the same degree as in the sweat
- *Reproductive complications.* Fertility is generally reduced in females due to the presence of cervical mucous plugs; loss of potency or obliteration of the vas deferens in males usually results in sterility
- *Other metabolic manifestations.* The majority of clients experience glucose intolerance; only a small percentage require insulin therapy, but the stress of an acute infection may increase the severity of glucose intolerance and lead to significant glucosuria.[6]

Be sensitive to the psychosocial effects of the disease on the child and family. Although modern treatment has prolonged the life span of affected clients, it is still decreased, and the anxiety and frustration of coping with the illness are great. Financial aspects of the disease add to the strains. Parents may overprotect the child. Assess for retarded socialization and other developmental skills. Moreover, the developmental tasks of adolescence and young adulthood are complicated by the illness.

The most useful and reliable diagnostic test for the disease is a quantitative analysis of sweat for sodium and chloride. More than 95 percent of affected clients have a positive sweat test regardless of other clinical manifestations. Consider the finding of a sweat chloride concentration above 60 mEq/liter or a sweat sodium concentration above 70 mEq/liter as diagnostic of cystic fibrosis. The concentration of either may range as high as 150 mEq/liter. Also consider the presence of meconium ileus at birth (an obstruction of the small intestine by sticky meconium) as diagnostic of the disease. Meconium ileus occurs in about 15 percent of affected infants.

Assess the nutritional status of all clients with cystic fibrosis using the techniques for anthropometric, biochemical, clinical, and dietary evaluation outlined in Chapter 11 as a basis for the nutritional care plan.

In contrast to the usual textbook description of the voracious appetite of the child with cystic fibrosis, the kilocalorie intake of the majority of clients is inadequate for their needs.[6] There may be marked signs of malnutrition, with wasted buttocks and protuberant abdomen, and many clients are remarkably underweight for height and age and fail to grow normally. Observe the condition of the teeth; affected children often have poor teeth because of nutritional deficiencies.

Children with cystic fibrosis usually have lower blood levels of vitamin A, carotene, vitamin E, cholesterol, and essential fatty acids than have unaffected children. These children often have symptoms of vitamin A and vitamin E deficiency, yet clinical evidence of vitamin D deficiency with associated rickets is lacking. This finding has puzzled investigators, since rickets is seen in most other forms of steatorrhea. However, in one study of vitamin D and mineral metabolism in 21 adolescents and young adults with cystic fibrosis, a reduction in serum 25-hydroxyvitamin D and calcium concentration, evidence of calcium malabsorption with secondary hyperparathyroidism, and a reduction in bone mass were reported.[7] These findings suggest that currently accepted modes of pancreatic enzyme replacement and vitamin D supplementation may be inadequate to maintain normal mineral homeostasis. Screen cystic fibrosis clients for vitamin D deficiency and provide additional vitamin D supplements if needed. An adequate calcium intake is essential. The frequent finding of essential fatty acid deficiency has led some investigators to study the effects of essential fatty acid supplements on the clinical manifestations. These attempts have yielded variable results.

Intervention. Direct the treatment of cystic fibrosis toward controlling the pulmonary and pancreatic insufficiency and improving psychosocial functioning. Frequent evaluation of pulmonary function is vital. To control infection, clear secretions, and keep secretions thin, wet, and mobile, antibiotics, bronchodilators, inhalation therapy, postural drainage, and chest physiotherapy are used. When iodides are used as liquefiers, evaluate for iodide sensitivity and goiter. Schedule chest postural drainage before meals to minimize vomiting, and provide mouth care after the procedure. Encourage an increase in fluid intake as a means of liquefying secretions.

Control of pancreatic insufficiency by dietary manipulations and pancreatic enzyme replacement is an essential part of management. With appropriate nutritional support and control of the respiratory complications, marked catch-up growth is possible. Even if there has been a period of malnutrition during infancy, children can be expected to grow at about the 50th percentile.

Dietary management for those with pancreatic involvement follows the principles outlined previously for pancreatic insufficiency. However, the diet should be regulated according to individual needs. In particular, encourage the client to increase energy intake. The need for kilocalories and nutrients exceeds the RDA. The energy requirement is about 150 percent of the RDA for a person of the same age and sex. In addition to the increased nutritional losses associated with pancreatic insufficiency, clients have an increased energy expenditure because of the hypermetabolic state associated with fever and infection, labored respirations, and extra expenditure during chest physiotherapy.[6] In general, there is lesser tolerance of dietary fat than of protein and carbohydrate, although tolerance of fat varies in individual cases. The diet should be kept as normal as possible, within limits, to provide

some degree of stability for the child who requires many restrictions in other areas. Lactase deficiency necessitating lactose restriction (see Chap. 27) is a frequent complication of cystic fibrosis. The principles of dietary management are given in Table 28–5.

Teach the client to use the character of the stools to determine tolerance for fat. Some can manage by eliminating the more obvious fats from the diet (e.g., 30 to 40 g daily may be tolerated), whereas others may need a greater degree of restriction (e.g., 20 to 30 g). Counsel the client about foods that are more likely to cause distress, but encourage experimentation for tolerance to different foods. Many clients voluntarily limit fatty foods because of the associated discomfort, whereas others would rather experience some discomfort in order occasionally to enjoy foods that they may not normally eat. They usually learn the amount of fat and specific food combinations that precipitate gastrointestinal distress. Stress to the client that mild to moderate steatorrhea is not necessarily harmful. Achievement of an increase in kilocalories retained by the body is the goal.[6] With rectal prolapse, fat restriction is essential, and rectal prolapse tends to abate with improved nutritional status. If the desired rate of growth is not occurring, consider the use of medium-chain triglycerides and protein supplements. Polycose (Ross Labs) can be used as a carbohydrate supplement.

Although pancreatic supplements improve nutrient absorption, they do not completely resolve the malabsorption. The optimal dosage is not currently

---

TABLE 28–5
PRINCIPLES OF DIETARY MANAGEMENT OF CYSTIC FIBROSIS

Nutrient Factor	Age		
	Infants	*1–9 Years*	*9–18 Years*
Kcal/kg/day	150–200	130–180	Males: 100–130 Females: 80–110
Protein (g/kg/day)	4	3	3 (2½–3 for young adults)
Fat	Restrict according to tolerance		
Carbohydrate	Increase quantities (simple carbohydrates are usually easily assimilated, although there are some who cannot use concentrated sweets)		
Vitamin supplements	Give multivitamins: vitamin K must be given separately (vitamin K given to all infants on prophylactic basis and given to older children when prothrombin is low); fat-soluble vitamins given in a water-miscible form		
Sodium chloride	Give liberal amounts with food particularly in hot weather, with fever, or with heavy exercise; may sprinkle extra salt on food or give salt tablets (⅛ tsp table salt is the sodium equivalent of a 1 g salt tablet); salt tablets on a regular basis not usually necessary nor recommended		
Lactose	Restrict if intolerance is manifest; use of Lact-Aid in milk before ingestion is suggested		
Pancreatic enzyme replacement	Give supplements with meals and snacks (e.g., pancreatin, pancrelipase, pancrease)		

known, and response to enzyme therapy varies. If the client complains of persistent, frequent, foul-smelling stools, flatulence, and abdominal distention, consider a change or increase in the replacement therapy. Increase enzyme dosage only to the point of diminishing benefits, since excessive dosage can lead to anorexia, constipation, and increased uric acid levels. The latter can be nephrotoxic.[6]

Assist parents of infants to select an appropriate formula such as Portagen, Pregestimil, or Nutramigen (Mead Johnson). Portagen and Pregestimil contain medium-chain triglycerides and, in Pregestimil, the nutrients are in an easily absorbable form. Nutramigen contains hydrolyzed casein. All three formulas are lactose-free.

Breastfeeding is usually not advocated, since breast milk does not provide adequate protein for growth. Breast milk also contains lactose.

Give parents guidelines for adding solid foods to the infant's diet. Solids are usually added earlier (between 4 and 8 weeks) than for an unaffected child, and small, frequent feedings throughout the day should be encouraged. Cereals should be delayed until after 1 year to encourage the use of foods higher in protein content. Ripe bananas and applesauce can be given initially, followed by lean meat. Strained and pureed meats are better sources of protein than are vegetable–meat mixtures. Prunes and plums have a laxative effect and should not be given. Carrots, green beans, and squash are usually well tolerated. Increase the variety of fruits, vegetables, and meats as the child gets older.

After the use of formula, at about 1 year of age, instruct parents to use skim milk (made double strength by the addition of ¼ to ⅓ c skim milk powder to 1 c of fluid skim milk) until later childhood, when plain homogenized milk can be given if tolerated. Digestion and absorption frequently become more efficient with increasing age, and less dietary regulation may be required.

Encourage the client's family to treat the child as normally as possible during meals and to prepare meals for the entire family at once rather than focusing on the need for special foods.

Begin preventive teaching early, reassess nutritional status at regular intervals, and revise the care plan accordingly. Stress to the client the importance of monitoring intake, especially when appetite is poor, and provide motivation to keep intake as adequate as possible on a consistent basis. Provide snack ideas to supplement protein and kilocalorie intake, including the necessary recipes, and encourage the client to be responsible for his or her own dietary needs.

BILIARY TRACT DISEASE

Assessment

The gallbladder is a pear-shaped organ attached to the underside of the liver. Its main function is to concentrate and store bile secreted by the liver. Be-

tween meals, the gallbladder is full and relaxed, but at mealtimes, the bile is released into the duodenum. The intake of fat and protein stimulates release of the hormone cholecystokinin, which in turn stimulates contraction of the gallbladder and reciprocal relaxation of the sphincter of Oddi.

The most common disease of the biliary tract is **cholelithiasis** (gallstones) complicated by acute and chronic **cholecystitis** (inflammation of the gallbladder). Cholecystolithiasis refers to stones in the gallbladder; choledocholithiasis develops when a stone slips into the common bile duct, causing obstruction and cramps. Although many view cholecystitis as an infectious disease, this is now being challenged. The disorder is the result of chemical inflammation of the wall of the gallbladder, which usually occurs in association with obstruction of the cystic duct of the neck of the gallbladder, usually by a gallstone. Secondary bacterial infection and ischemia may develop.

Gallstones are composed of cholesterol crystals, bile salts, or bile pigments, or a combination of these. Most stones (approximately 80 percent) have a high percentage of cholesterol. Pigment stones result from hemolytic phenomena (much of the bile pigment is derived from the breakdown of the red blood cells). A prerequisite to the formation of cholesterol gallstones is bile saturated with cholesterol. The lithogenicity of hepatic bile may be related to its cholesterol, bile salt, and phospholipid concentration. The lithogenicity may be increased if the cholesterol concentration is increased or the content of bile salt or phospholipid is reduced. The tendency for stones to form in the gallbladder presumably is enhanced by a lithogenic bile or prolonged stasis of bile in the gallbladder due to inefficient or infrequent emptying. For example, fasting tends to increase the lithogenicity of bile. Moreover, the lack of hormonal stimulation in the fasting state will lead to stagnation of bile in the gallbladder.

Diet, heredity, and female sex hormones have all been implicated in the incidence of cholelithiasis and cholecystitis. Cholelithiasis is common in Western countries and is strongly associated with obesity, diabetes mellitus, and hyperlipidemia. The incidence of gallstone disease varies from country to country and appears to be high in areas where high-kilocalorie, high-fat diets are consumed. Populations with a low fat intake may be less vulnerable to gallstone formation. The incidence of gallstones may increase if the polyunsaturated fat intake is greatly increased. Observe that gallstone disease occurs more commonly in women than in men, and women with a history of the disease tend to have had more live births than women without the disease. The incidence of the disorder is generally considered to increase with age, although it is being found in younger segments of the population than previously. A very high incidence of gallstones has been observed in Native Americans, and a genetic predisposition has been postulated.[8] Assess for an increased inci-

TABLE 28-6
FAT-RESTRICTED DIET: 30–40 G FAT

Category	Foods Allowed	Foods Avoided
Beverages	Skim milk (fluid, evaporated, and dry); buttermilk and yoghurt made from skim milk; low-fat chocolate drink; carbonated beverages; lemonade; punch and fruit drinks; coffee; tea; cereal beverages	Whole milk; condensed or evaporated milk; eggnog; malted milk; milkshakes; chocolate milk; buttermilk made from whole milk; low-fat milk (1% and 2%); yoghurt made from whole milk or 2% milk
Bread and cereal	White, rye, whole grain, or pumpernickel bread; plain yeast rolls; bagels; oatmeal, raisin, Italian, or French bread; English muffins; matzo; saltines; graham crackers; pretzels; bread sticks; melba toast; tortillas; all breakfast cereals (cooked and dry); grain products, such as rice, noodles, spaghetti, macaroni, and flour	Quick breads; sweet rolls; pastries; doughnuts; egg or cheese bread; pancakes; waffles; French toast; corn chips; potato chips; cheese crackers and other flavored crackers; other products containing whole milk, egg yolk, or fat
Dessert	Gelatin dessert; desserts made with skim milk and egg white; popsicles, fruit ices; sherbet; angel food or sponge cake; fruit whip made without cream; fruits; meringue; thin vanilla wafers	Ice cream; ice milk; desserts that contain whole milk, fat, cream, egg yolks, nuts, or chocolate; cookies; cake; pastries; pies
Fat[a]	1 tbsp daily of butter, mayonnaise, margarine, oil, lard, or shortening	More than 1 tbsp fat; bacon; bacon fat; fatback; cream sauces; gravy (unless all fat is removed); cream; cream cheese; sour cream
Fruit	Any fresh, canned, frozen, or dried fruit (except those not allowed); fruit juice	Avocado; coconut; olives
Meat and meat substitute	4 oz daily: lean, well-trimmed meat (beef, lamb, pork, ham, organ meats, veal), fish and shellfish (fresh or water-packed), poultry (note poultry not allowed), dried or chipped beef—prepare by baking, boiling, broiling, roasting, stewing, or simmering; 1 egg[a] daily (egg whites as desired): prepare by boiling, poaching, or scrambling without fat; any cheese made with skim milk; cottage cheese without cream (regular cheese may be substituted for meat or egg)	More than 4 oz of meat and 1 egg; cheese except as listed; fried meat or egg; fatty meat, such as duck, squab, poultry skin, goose, bacon, spareribs, sausage, cold cuts and luncheon meats, corned beef, pastrami, frankfurters; fatty fish, such as sardines, eel, mackerel, herring, anchovies, swordfish, or fish canned in oil; peanut butter; canned pork and beans; scrapple; nuts
Soup	Clear soup and broth with fat removed; soup made from skim milk; bouillon cubes; consommé; broth-based packaged dehydrated soup	Soup or broth with fat, cream, or whole milk
Sweets	Sugar, jelly, honey, marmalade, syrup, hard candy, sugar candy made without nuts, chocolate, or coconut; gumdrops; marshmallows	Candy made with nuts, chocolate, or coconut
Vegetables	All fresh, frozen, canned, or dried vegetables; vegetable juices; unbuttered popcorn (daily fat allowance may be used in preparation)	Vegetables cooked with meat or additional fat; fried potatoes; potato chips; buttered popcorn; any that cause digestive distress
Miscellaneous	Herbs; lemon juice; horseradish; vinegar; pepper; salt; spices; extracts; condiments, such as catsup, mustard, chili sauce, pickles, relish; limited amounts of powdered cocoa	Chocolate; any spices or condiments not tolerated; fried foods; highly seasoned food if not tolerated

[a] The fat content of the diet can be reduced to 20 g by omitting the fat and egg. The diet can also be adjusted for use in type I hyperlipoproteinemia by omitting the fat and limiting egg yolk to 3 per week.

dence of the disorder in other clients, such as those taking certain drugs, including clofibrate, cholestyramine, and birth control pills, those with ileal resection or ileal disease, postvagotomy patients, and siblings of persons with gallstones.

With regard to specific dietary factors in the etiology of the disorder, the evidence is insufficient at present to justify widespread dietary modifications to reduce gallstone disease.

Gallstones may be symptomless unless there is obstruction of the cystic duct, causing inflammation of the gallbladder. In this instance, assess for upper right quadrant abdominal pain, nausea, vomiting, flatulence, belching, and fever. Jaundice and steatorrhea may appear with duct obstruction. In this case, observe for light-colored stools because of the absence of bile pigment. If the obstruction is not corrected, chronic cholecystitis may result. The reflux of bile can also lead to biliary cirrhosis or pancreatitis.

Diagnosis of gallstone disease is by cholecystography (x-ray examination of the gallbladder) and cholangiography (x-ray examination of the bile ducts). Serve a fat-free test meal (avoiding meat, fat, and greasy and fried foods) the evening before the test and allow no food by mouth after midnight of the day preceding the test and until after the test is performed.

Intervention

Treatment of gallstones and cholecystitis may involve a combination of dietary management, drugs to dissolve the gallstones, and surgical removal of the stones or the gallbladder. Asymptomatic gallstones do not require treatment.

Individualize dietary management according to the symptoms and individual food tolerance. There is no evidence that dietary manipulations (e.g., cholesterol restriction) can dissolve gallstones or that individuals with gallstones have a greater intolerance for fat than those with other digestive complaints. However, assess for intolerance of specific foods (manifest by epigastric pain or distention after eating), such as onions, sauerkraut, cabbage, cucumbers, turnips, relishes, spicy foods, chocolate, rich pastry, and fatty foods, and use the client's input to plan the diet to ensure that these foods are avoided. A fat-restricted diet may provide symptomatic relief in clients with gallbladder disease. The purpose of the diet is to prevent biliary colic by decreasing the fat-induced gallbladder contractions. The ingestion of fat stimulates cholecystokinin secretion and gallbladder contraction, and high-fat diets theoretically increase discomfort. However, amino acids have the same effect, and discomfort may result from taking almost any type of food.

With acute illness, use intravenous nutritional support, or if oral intake is possible, provide a low-fat, clear liquid regimen for a short period of time. In chronic conditions, suggest moderate fat restriction (to 25 percent of total kilocalories or 45 to 75 g/day) (see Table 28–6). The rationale for drastic fat restriction in gallbladder disease has been questioned. With fat restriction, evaluate the diet for adequacy of fat-soluble vitamins and provide tips on methods of food preparation. Frying of foods should be avoided. If obesity is a complication, restrict kilocalories and use the regimen described for hepatobiliary insufficiency if there is associated biliary obstruction.

Drugs are used to dissolve the gallstones. Dissolution depends on the proper relationship of cholesterol, bile acids, and phospholipids in bile. The administration of chenodeoxycholic acid, (CDCA),[9] a primary bile salt and a normal component of human bile, is effective in dissolving gallstones, but complete dissolution may require 6 to 50 months of treatment. It is hypothesized that CDCA expands the bile salt pool, returning the bile to normal so that it is no longer supersaturated with cholesterol. It is not presently known whether clients have to continue taking CDCA to prevent the recurrence of gallstones. Side effects of the drug include diarrhea, altered liver enzymes, and elevation of the serum cholesterol;[9,10] therefore, careful client selection is necessary. Other compounds, including ursodeoxycholic acid, are also being tested for effectiveness

in dissolving gallstones. Dietary modifications are unnecessary for clients receiving this therapy.

When the stones are large in number or size, surgical excision may be necessary. With removal of the gallbladder, bile is temporarily stored in the common bile duct, which stretches to accommodate the volume of bile. Fat digestion appears to be unimpaired following cholecystectomy, and there is little reason to restrict fat in any way. Advise clients that following a cholecystectomy, they should be able to tolerate a diet of normal composition. Some clients have limited fat intake for a number of weeks or months after surgery, and they seem to do better by gradually increasing fat intake to a normal amount.

REVIEW QUESTIONS AND ACTIVITIES

1. Explain the functions of the liver relative to each of the following processes: (a) nutrient metabolism, (b) synthesis of body compounds, (c) nutrient storage, and (d) detoxification of endogenous and exogenous substances.
2. Differentiate between the etiologic agents in viral and toxic hepatitis.
3. Describe the possible interaction between alcohol consumption and malnutrition in the etiology of liver disease.
4. Compare the dietary management of fatty degeneration of the liver and acute and chronic hepatitis.
5. Discuss the clinical manifestations of chronic hepatobiliary insufficiency and chronic pancreatic insufficiency.
6. Explain the rationale for use of a fat-restricted diet and nutrient supplements in clients with chronic hepatobiliary insufficiency.
7. Explain the basis for the development of each of the following clinical manifestations of liver disease: (a) edema, (b) steatorrhea, (c) esophageal varices, and (d) hepatic encephalopathy (coma).
8. Explain the significance of the ratio of aromatic amino acids to branched-chain amino acids in clients with liver disease.
9. Distinguish among the types of diet used in treating each of the following stages or manifestations of cirrhosis: (a) uncomplicated cirrhosis, (b) cirrhosis complicated by edema and ascites, (c) cirrhosis complicated by esophageal varices, and (d) cirrhosis complicated by hepatic coma.
10. Compare the dietary modifications used during the acute and recovery phases of hepatic coma.
11. Identify the rationale for the administration of neomycin and lactulose to clients with hepatic coma.

12. Discuss four principles of treatment (including dietary management) of symptomatic pancreatic insufficiency.
13. Identify the pathologic basis for the clinical manifestations of cystic fibrosis.
14. Describe the gastrointestinal and sweat gland manifestations of cystic fibrosis.
15. Compare the kilocalorie and protein requirements of infants, young children, and adolescents with cystic fibrosis.
16. Assess the need for adjusting the intake of each of the following nutrients by individuals with cystic fibrosis: (a) fat, (b) carbohydrate, (c) vitamins, (d) sodium chloride, and (e) lactose.
17. *Case study:* Your client is a 60-year-old obese female of Hispanic origin who has been following a 1200 kcal, fat-restricted (25 g) diet to control cholelithiasis. Currently, she is in the hospital with complaints of abdominal pain, nausea, and vomiting. Her physician has indicated that a cholecystectomy may be needed.
    a. Identify factors from the client's history that you would want to assess for their possible role in the etiology of cholelithiasis.
    b. Identify the rationale for the diet order prior to admission to the hospital.
    c. Discuss common food practices of Hispanic clients who follow the traditional dietary pattern.
    d. List problems that might be encountered by clients who follow a 25 g fat diet.
    e. Adjust the diet order in accordance with the client's current symptoms.
    f. Identify an appropriate dietary regimen following a cholecystectomy.

REFERENCES

1. Bach AC, Babayan VK: Medium-chain triglycerides: An update. Am J Clin Nutr 36:950, 1982.
2. James JH, Jeppsson B, Ziparo V, Fischer JE: Hyperammonaemia, plasma amino acid imbalance, and blood–brain amino acid transport: A unified theory of portal-systemic encephalopathy. Lancet 2:772, 1979.
3. Fischer JE: Panel report on nutritional support of patients with liver, renal, and cardiopulmonary diseases. Am J Clin Nutr 34:1235, 1981.
4. Shaw S, Worner TM, Lieber CS: Comparison of animal and vegetable protein sources in the management of hepatic encephalopathy. Am J Clin Nutr 38:59, 1983.
5. Cameron DJS, Pitcher-Wilmott R, Milla PJ, et al.: The effect of cimetidine on meal-stimulated gastric function and exogenous pancreatic enzymes in cystic fibrosis. Human Nutr Clin Nutr 36C:475, 1982.
6. Hubbard VS, Mangrum PJ: Energy intake and nutrition counseling in cystic fibrosis. J Am Diet Assoc 80:127, 1982.
7. Hahn TJ, Squires AE, Halstead LR, Strominger DB: Reduced serum 25-hydroxyvitamin D concentration and disordered mineral metabolism in patients with cystic fibrosis. J Pediatr 94:38, 1979.
8. Morris DL, Buechley RW, Key CR, Morgan MV: Gallbladder disease and gallbladder cancer among American Indians in tricultural New Mexico. Cancer 42:2472, 1979.
9. Update: Chenodeoxycholic acid and gallstones. JAMA 245:2378, 1981.
10. Schonfield LJ, Lachin JM: The National Cooperative Gallstone Study Group: Chenodiol (chenodeoxycholic acid) for dissolution of gallstones. Ann Intern Med 95:257, 1981.

BIBLIOGRAPHY

Balart LA, Ferrante WA: Pathophysiology of acute and chronic pancreatitis: Arch Intern Med 142:113, 1982.

Barthel JS, Butt JH II: Ascites. Am Fam Phys 27:248, 1983.

Borowsky SA, Strome S, Lott E: Continued heavy drinking and survival in alcoholic cirrhotics. Gastroenterology 80:1405, 1981.

Bunout D, Gattás V, Iturriaga H, et al.: Nutritional state of alcoholic patients: Its possible relationship to alcoholic liver damage. Am J Clin Nutr 38:469, 1983.

Chase HP, Long MA, Lavin MH: Cystic fibrosis and malnutrition J Pediatr 95:337, 1979.

Fischer JE, Bower RH: Nutritional support in liver disease. Surg Clin North Am 61:3, 1981.

Gannon RB, Pickett K: Jaundice. Am J Nurs 83:404, 1983.

Heaton KW: The role of diet in the aetiology of cholelithiasis. Nutr Abstr Rev 54:549, 1984.

Landon C, Kerner JA, Castillo R, et al.: Oral correction of essential fatty acid deficiency in cystic fibrosis. J Parent Enter Nutr 5:501, 1981.

Larter N: Cystic fibrosis. Am J Nurs 81:527, 1981.

Malnutrition and anergy in liver disease. Nutr Rev 40:105, 1982.

Muscle protein catabolism in cirrhotic patients reduced by branched-chain amino acids. Nutr Rev 41:146, 1983.

Rossi-Fanelli R: Effect of glucagon and/or branched-chain amino acid infusion on plasma amino acid imbalance in chronic liver failure. J Parent Enter Nutr 5:414, 1981.

CHAPTER 29

Nutrition and Cardiovascular Disease

Objectives

After completion of this chapter, the student will be able to:

1. Differentiate between the dietary factors that are implicated in the etiology of coronary heart disease and hypertension.

2. Distinguish between elevated blood levels of low-density lipoprotein (LDL), very low-density lipoprotein (VLDL) and high-density lipoprotein (HDL) as predictors of risk for developing coronary heart disease.

3. Develop a teaching plan for the dietary management of type IIa hyperlipoproteinemia and adjust the plan to make it appropriate for clients with type IIb and type IV hyperlipoproteinemia.

4. Develop a teaching plan for a hypertensive client of normal weight who has recently been placed on an 85 mEq sodium dietary regimen.

5. Formulate a plan for nutritional care for an obese client of Jewish background with angina and adapt it to be appropriate for this client during the acute phase of myocardial infarction and, later, when the client develops congestive heart failure and is placed on a 40 mEq sodium dietary regimen.

6. Compare and contrast the dietary management of clients with rheumatic fever and clients with edema.

7. Plan the diet of an infant with a congenital heart defect.

Cardiovascular disease is a health problem of considerable magnitude in all affluent societies, including the United States. Diseases of the cardiovascular system account for approximately 50 percent of all deaths in the United States. Myocardial infarction and cerebrovascular accident are the major causes of cardiovascular system-related deaths. Atherosclerosis is the underlying disease or pathologic process causing most of these deaths. The percentage of deaths from cardiovascular disease rises steadily with age, reflecting, in part, the continued progression of atherosclerotic changes with age.

Although cardiovascular disease appears to be a growing problem in some areas of the world, data from the National Center for Health Statistics show a slow, consistent decline in the death rate from these disorders in the United States since the early 1960s. The decline is evident in all age, sex, and race groups except the group older than 85 years. The reasons for the decline are not known, but many attribute it to changes in lifestyle emphasizing prevention, i.e., reduction in smoking, control of hypertension, increase in physical activity, and consumption of diets lower in kilocalories, cholesterol, and saturated fat. In particular, there is a trend toward consuming less fat from animal sources (saturated fat) and more from vegetable sources (polyunsaturated fat). The average American's level of blood cholesterol has also dropped 5 to 10 percent since the early 1960s. An elevated blood cholesterol level is a major risk factor.

Cardiovascular diseases that contribute to human mortality and morbidity in the United States are coronary heart disease, hypertension, acute myocardial infarction, congestive heart failure, rheumatic heart disease, and congenital heart disease. These are discussed in this chapter. Major emphasis is given to coronary heart disease because of its especially high incidence and the direct implications for dietary intervention in prevention and treatment.

CORONARY HEART DISEASE

▶ **Coronary heart disease,** also called **ischemic heart disease,** is the leading cause of death in the United States and Western Europe. The underlying
▶ disease process is **atherosclerosis,** or fatty degeneration, with plaque formation in arterial walls. Atherosclerotic arteries become thickened, with consequent narrowing of the lumen and diminished blood circulation to the organs supplied. As the disease progresses, the fatty plaques may undergo additional changes, including calcification, internal hemorrhage, ulceration, and thrombosis. Atherosclerosis with superimposed thrombosis is a common cause of myocardial infarction, cerebrovascular accident, and gangrene of the lower extremities.

The etiology of coronary heart disease is multifaceted—genetic, metabolic, anatomic, and environmental factors all contribute. The important role of environmental factors is suggested by the decline in the incidence of the disease in the United States in recent years in association with lifestyle changes. Noteworthy is the fact that there was no similar worldwide decline. Although the evidence is strong that nutrition has an important influence, the complexity of etiologic factors makes it impossible to delineate a definite and unquestionable relationship.

Atherosclerosis may have its origin in childhood, since fatty streaks appear in the intimal lining of major arteries even in the first years of life. As children age, the number and size of the streaks increase. Controversy surrounds the prognosis of the fatty streaks—the opinion has been expressed that the streaks vary in their potential, i.e., some regress, some are static, and some progress to form plaques.

Research studies have identified a number of modifiable risk factors associated with susceptibility to coronary heart disease. Although current evidence is insufficient to predict the benefits of modifying these risk factors, the magnitude of the problem is sufficient to justify taking all reasonable measures to reduce the risk factors associated with coronary heart disease.

Assessment

Relationship of Diet to Risk Factors. Risk (or predisposing) factors commonly cited in association with the development of atherosclerosis and coronary heart disease (Fig. 29–1) include (1) an inher-

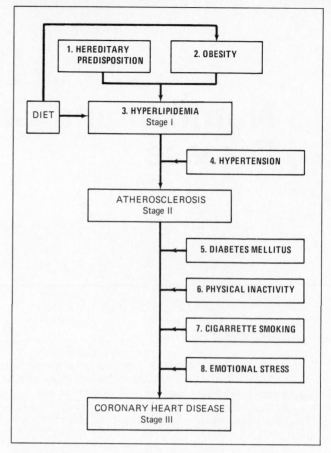

Figure 29–1
Risk factors related to coronary heart disease.

ited predisposition, (2) obesity, (3) hyperlipidemia (a general term denoting elevation of any blood lipid, such as cholesterol and triglycerides), (4) hypertension, (5) presence of diabetes mellitus, (6) physical inactivity, (7) excessive cigarette smoking, and (8) emotional stress, including type A behavior pattern, characterized by a sense of time urgency, excessive competitiveness, and feelings of hostility or aggression. These risk factors have been identified on the basis of epidemiologic, experimental, and clinical studies.

Although diet is associated directly or indirectly with several risk factors in the development of atherosclerosis and coronary heart disease, it is especially significant in relation to obesity and hyperlipidemia. For example, a diet high in saturated fat and cholesterol may lead to an elevated blood cholesterol level. Assess a client's history for an inherited tendency. Familial forms of hyperlipidemia exist and family screening is an important diagnostic tool. Other clients may consume excessive kilocalories and become obese or may inherit a tendency toward obesity; this, in turn, is a risk factor for hyperlipidemia.

Dietary excesses of five specific food factors are possibly implicated in hyperlipidemia. These food factors are (1) cholesterol, (2) saturated fat, (3) car-

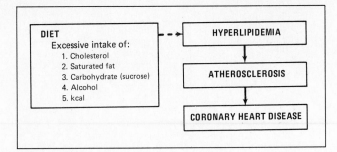

Figure 29–2
Possible relationship of dietary factors to coronary heart disease.

bohydrate, especially sucrose, (4) alcohol,* and (5) kilocalories. Figure 29–2 shows the possible relationship of these factors to hyperlipidemia (the coronary risk factor), atherosclerosis (the underlying disease process), and the subsequent development of coronary heart disease.

With few exceptions, it has been noted that population groups consuming diets high in saturated fat and cholesterol have a high mean blood level of cholesterol and a high incidence of death from atherosclerotic disease. However, it has not been possible to establish relationships between dietary consumption of fat and cholesterol and the serum cholesterol in individuals within populations.[1,2] Heredity may be important in determining the variability of the serum cholesterol response to diet, and dietary and genetic factors may interact with numerous other variables in determining the plasma lipid levels.

Nurses can assist clients to alter plasma lipid levels by modifying the level and kind of dietary fat and the amount of dietary cholesterol, although the effect is less in subjects from free-living populations than in those living in metabolic wards under rigid dietary control. A high intake of saturated fat and a high intake of polyunsaturated fat as a percentage of total kilocalories are important factors, respectively, in elevating and lowering the serum cholesterol. Dietary cholesterol is least important, particularly in the range of 300 to 600 mg/day. In order of importance, without regard to the direction of the effect, the dietary factors affecting serum cholesterol concentration are saturated fat, polyunsaturated fat, and cholesterol. The effect of saturated fat in raising serum cholesterol is about two times greater than the cholesterol-lowering effect of polyunsaturated fat. The average serum cholesterol concentration in adults increases with increasing dietary cholesterol intake when the total intake is in the range of 0 to 600 mg/day. Dietary cholesterol above about 600 mg/day produces no additional effect in most persons. The response tends to be

greater if dietary cholesterol is combined with saturated fat.[3] To date, no significant correlation between cholesterol intake and serum cholesterol concentration has been demonstrated in free-living persons in the United States.[4]

Carbohydrates may also influence the serum lipid levels; the effect is less on serum cholesterol than on triglycerides.[5] Some epidemiologic data have related the increasing death rates from coronary heart disease in industrialized nations to an increased dietary intake of carbohydrate, especially sucrose. However, the epidemiologic data, in contrast to the data for dietary fat and cholesterol, are not supplemented by a large amount of additional evidence relating dietary carbohydrate components to atherosclerosis and heart disease. Assess clients for their tolerance of sucrose, since some people appear to be sensitive to a large amount of sucrose, and a high-sucrose diet may bring an elevation of serum triglycerides.

Alcohol ingestion has generally been shown to be associated with an elevation of serum triglycerides. This effect of alcohol ingestion in normal individuals appears to be small, but observe for a striking rise in triglycerides with alcohol ingestion in those clients with preexisting hypertriglyceridemia. Studies indicate that within the general population there are those who are markedly susceptible to this effect, which may be seen with only moderate amounts of alcohol. The effects disappear when alcohol is discontinued.[6]

Kilocalorie excess leading to obesity has long been suspected as an important risk factor for coronary heart disease. It has not been possible to pinpoint the obese state as an independent risk factor, however, since overweight is related to several other coronary risk factors, including hyperlipidemia (particularly elevated triglycerides), diabetes mellitus, and hypertension.

The influences of other dietary characteristics in the etiology of coronary heart disease are now being investigated. Research related to dietary fiber and vitamins C and E is presented in Chapters 5 and 8, respectively. The role of other factors, such as protein, trace minerals, caffeine, hardness of the drinking water, *trans* fatty acids, dairy products, garlic, fatty acids from fish and other marine life, and meal frequency, are not well understood. Some of these possible relationships are discussed here, and others are addressed in sources listed in the bibliography at the end of the chapter.

Some studies have shown that the ingestion of animal protein produces hypercholesterolemia in experimental animals.[7] In general, protein of vegetable origin is less hypercholesterolemic than protein of animal origin, and vegetarians tend to have lower blood cholesterol levels than do omnivores. The mechanisms underlying these differences are not clear. They may result as much from differences in the intake of saturated fat as from differences in the source of protein. Some authorities suggest

---

Although alcohol is not a specific food factor, it is often consumed with foods and, therefore, will be treated as a food factor in this discussion.

that adopting a vegetarian diet may be a prudent measure in the treatment of hypercholesterolemia.

Although there is no evidence for a direct cause–effect relationship between mineral and trace element status and atherosclerosis in humans, many elements exert a strong influence on individual risk factors for cardiovascular disease, such as blood pressure and glucose tolerance. Optimal intake of elements, such as sodium, magnesium, calcium, chromium, copper, zinc, and iodine, can reduce these individual risk factors.

Consumption of caffeine-containing beverages leads to an increase in serum free fatty acids, and some data show a positive correlation between the amount of coffee consumed and the level of total blood cholesterol and triglycerides and, in women, an inverse relationship with high-density lipoprotein (HDL) cholesterol.[8] Moreover, cardiac arrhythmias may occur in some clients following coffee consumption.

Control of risk factors is essential in any program designed to prevent or treat atherosclerosis and coronary heart disease. However, do not interpret the concept of risk to indicate a direct cause-and-effect relationship. Although individuals with hyperlipidemia are at a statistically greater risk of developing heart disease than those with normal blood lipids, many individuals with heart disease have normal lipid levels, and others with elevated blood lipids may escape heart disease. Diet and drug therapy can lower blood lipids, but a corresponding lowered susceptibility to coronary heart disease has not been unequivocally established. It is not known whether the atherosclerotic process is retarded or reversed by lowering elevated blood lipids. However, there is increasing evidence that atherosclerosis may be potentially both preventable and reversible.[9]

The efficacy of lowering blood cholesterol by drugs and diet to reduce the risk of coronary heart disease was tested in the Lipid Research Clinic's coronary primary prevention trial over a period of approximately 7½ years. The results showed that reducing blood cholesterol diminished the incidence of coronary heart disease morbidity and mortality in men at high risk of coronary heart disease because of elevated low-density lipoprotein (LDL) cholesterol levels. Coronary risk decreased 2 percentage points for each 1 percent drop in cholesterol level, regardless of how the decrease in blood cholesterol was achieved (drugs or diet).[10,11] Nonetheless, the role of specific dietary components in the prevention and treatment of atherosclerosis remains controversial, and clinicians do not agree totally on the relative importance of the various dietary relationships in the disease process. Consequently, nurses will see various types of modifications used in both prevention and treatment programs.

Hyperlipidemia. The major blood lipids and their sources are summarized in Figure 29–3. Cholesterol and triglyceride are the two lipids whose elevation

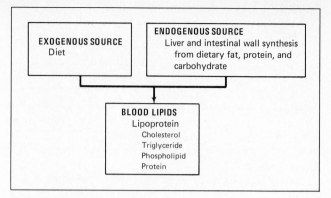

Figure 29–3
Major blood lipids and their sources.

is most commonly associated with atherosclerosis. The serum cholesterol level is a potent indicator of risk of coronary heart disease; the risk of developing a premature coronary attack rises continuously as serum cholesterol is elevated. Above the age of 50 to 60, however, the predictive power of serum cholesterol weakens, suggesting that vigorous lipid-lowering efforts should be carried out in the younger age groups. Triglyceride levels are thought by some to be an independent risk factor for coronary heart disease, whereas other investigators note that triglyceride is not an independent risk factor.[12] It has been observed that in many parts of the world with a low incidence of coronary heart disease mortality, there are substantially higher triglyceride values than in high incidence areas.[13] However, triglyceride and cholesterol are associated through mutual lipoprotein carriers, and elevated triglyceride blood levels are frequently associated with obesity, impaired glucose tolerance, and high levels of LDL and low levels of HDL, which do affect risk.

Mean blood cholesterol and triglyceride levels vary with age and sex, and both tend to increase with age. Although there are no absolute blood values for cholesterol and triglyceride that are considered abnormal, some authorities believe that the average blood cholesterol level, in particular, among Americans is too high and contributes to the risk of heart disease. A consensus panel convened by the National Institutes of Health noted that a blood cholesterol level less than 180 mg/100 ml for adults in their twenties and less than 200 mg/100 ml for those 30 years of age is a desirable goal.[14] This group urged cholesterol-lowering measures for adults in their twenties with levels above 200 mg/100 ml, for adults in their thirties with levels above 220 mg/100 ml, and for those 40 years old and over with levels above 240 mg/100 ml. Other groups suggest that the upper limit of normal for adults under age 55 is 220 mg/100 ml and values in excess of this may require treatment. The corresponding value for triglyceride is 150 mg/100 ml.[15]

Hyperlipidemia may be of primary or secondary origin. Hyperlipidemia of primary origin may be inherited or acquired. An inherited defect leads to excessive endogenous lipid synthesis or to defective lipid clearance. Acquired hyperlipidemia may result from environmental factors, such as a high-fat diet with a low ratio of polyunsaturated fat to saturated fat (P:S ratio) and a sedentary lifestyle. Hyperlipidemia sometimes occurs secondary to diseases that alter lipid metabolism, such as hypothyroidism, nephrotic syndrome, diabetes mellitus, and obstructive liver disease, or the use of certain drugs, such as oral contraceptive agents.

Classification. Lipids circulate in the blood bound to plasma proteins as lipoproteins. Four major groups of lipoproteins have been identified in the plasma in normal individuals. These four classes all contain cholesterol, triglyceride, phospholipid, and protein, but in varying amounts. They may be separated by ultracentrifugation, and with this technique they are classified by density according to their content of lipid and protein. Those containing most lipid and least protein are the least dense (chylomicrons) and those containing least lipid and most protein are the most dense (HDL). Lipoproteins may be separated by electrophoresis, and separation in this manner is dependent upon the differences in electrical charges of the components of the molecule. When separated in this manner, lipoproteins are classified as chylomicrons and pre-beta, beta, and alpha lipoproteins. The four major lipoprotein groups and the major lipid class transported by each group are listed from least to highest density below. The percentage composition of the major lipoprotein groups is given in Table 29–1.

1. Chylomicrons: Transport exogenous triglyceride absorbed from the intestine to adipose tissue and the liver
2. Very-low density lipoprotein (VLDL) or pre-beta-lipoprotein: Transports endogenous triglyceride synthesized by the liver to adipose tissue; is converted first to an intermediate-density lipoprotein (IDL), and then to low-density lipoprotein (LDL) through loss of triglyceride
3. LDL or beta-lipoprotein: Metabolic end product of VLDL catabolism; transports cholesterol to peripheral tissues and possibly promotes entry of cholesterol into cells

4. HDL or alpha-lipoprotein: Function not totally clear; may enhance the exit of cholesterol from cells and may transport excess cholesterol from peripheral tissues to the liver for catabolism and excretion

A fifth type of lipoprotein, intermediate-density lipoprotein (IDL), is an intermediate type formed in the conversion of VLDL to LDL. IDL has physical characteristics that are intermediate between VLDL and LDL. In certain familial disorders of lipid metabolism, this remnant form of lipoprotein accumulates as a result of a block in the normal conversion of VLDL to LDL.

Although abnormally high levels of chylomicrons, VLDL, and LDL are associated with various pathologic manifestations (including a high risk of coronary heart disease when LDL and possibly VLDL are elevated), various studies now suggest that HDL levels are inversely related to coronary heart disease prevalence: the higher the level of HDL, the lower the risk of coronary heart disease. Thus, the concentration of cholesterol carried in LDL and HDL may be more specific risk factors (positive for LDL and negative for HDL) than the total plasma cholesterol concentration. Expect relatively small changes in HDL cholesterol (e.g., 5 to 10 mg) to be associated with significant changes in coronary risk. Although the exact function of HDL and its possible protective effect against heart disease remain speculative, the concentration of HDL is receiving increasing attention as a predictor of risk, particularly because it appears to continue to be discriminative with advancing age, whereas serum cholesterol becomes less predictive after age 50.

Assess for these factors that appear to influence the HDL level:

1. Race: Blacks have higher HDL levels than whites
2. Sex: Females have higher HDL levels than males (until adolescence, there is little difference in HDL levels between the sexes; following puberty and thereafter, even after menopause, the HDL level is higher in females than males)
3. Body weight: Obesity is associated with lower HDL levels; weight reduction leads to a decrease in VLDL and a reciprocal rise in HDL

TABLE 29–1
CHARACTERISTICS OF PLASMA LIPOPROTEINS

	Chylomicrons	*VLDL*	*LDL*	*HDL*
Protein (%)	1	10	25	50
Triglyceride (%)	90	65	10	2
Cholesterol, as free cholesterol and cholesterol esters (%)	5	13	43	18
Phospholipid (%)	4	12	22	30

TABLE 29–2
ABNORMALLY ELEVATED LIPIDS AND LIPOPROTEINS IN HYPERLIPIDEMIA AND HYPERLIPOPROTEINEMIA

Lipoproteinemia Type[a]	Elevated Serum Lipid (Hyperlipidemia)	Elevated Lipoprotein (Hyperlipoproteinemia)
Type I	Triglyceride[b]	Chylomicrons
Type IIa	Cholesterol	LDL (or beta)
Type IIb	Cholesterol and triglyceride	LDL (or beta) and VLDL (or pre-beta)
Type III (broad-beta disease)	Cholesterol and triglyceride	IDL
Type IV	Triglyceride[b]	VLDL (or pre-beta)
Type V	Triglyceride[b]	Chylomicrons and VLDL (or pre-beta)

[a] See reference 15 for other clinical features of the disorders.
[b] Cholesterol may be normal or elevated.

4. Cigarette smoking: Lowers HDL levels
5. Alcohol use: Moderate use of alcohol (e.g., no more than a couple of ounces of whiskey, or its equivalent, per day) increases HDL
6. Physical activity: Exercise increases HDL levels
7. Hormones: Estrogens increase HDL levels, and androgens lower them
8. Drugs: Clofibrate, nicotinic acid, and heparin increase HDL levels; zinc supplements lower HDL levels.

Speculations regarding HDL have led some investigators to theorize that HDL levels should be measured when other lipids are measured in screening programs. However, the ratio of HDL to LDL, denoting the balance between the cholesterol delivery and removal systems, may be more important than serum levels. A high HDL:LDL ratio, signifying a higher percentage of the HDL fraction, is desirable. When there is an increase in blood cholesterol or triglyceride or both (hyperlipidemia) due to either primary or secondary causes, the corresponding lipoproteins are also increased (hyperlipoproteinemia). For example, clients with hypercholesterolemia will also have LDL elevations, and VLDL is elevated in clients with hypertriglyceridemia.

Six types of hyperlipoproteinemia have been identified[15] based on abnormal blood levels of cholesterol, triglyceride, and the associated abnormal lipoprotein patterns. These are type I, type IIa, type IIb, type III, type IV, and type V. Types IIa, IIb, and IV are relatively common patterns, and all three are associated with premature atherosclerosis. Types I, III, and V are rare.

Many health care professionals are now using these classifications of hyperlipoproteinemia, since they provide a more rational and often more successful basis for diet and drug therapy. By identifying the specific type of hyperlipoproteinemia, the fat transport mechanism that is overloaded can be pin-pointed. Diet and drug therapy can then be tailored to treat the disorder. Measurement of blood levels of cholesterol and triglycerides is nonspecific, and it is necessary to identify the specific lipoprotein abnormality by interpreting hyperlipidemia in terms of hyperlipoproteinemia to increase the chance for successful therapy. Visual observation of a plasma sample obtained in the fasting state and stored at 4°C overnight, in combination with determination of total plasma cholesterol and triglyceride levels, allows diagnosis of a lipid abnormality in 95 percent of subjects. Quantitation of lipoprotein classes by electrophoresis or ultracentrifugation facilitates the diagnosis of type II and type III hyperlipoproteinemias.

Hypercholesterolemia and hypertriglyceridemia may occur alone or in combination in the various types of hyperlipoproteinemia. Table 29–2 provides a summary of the lipids and corresponding lipoproteins that are elevated in the six types of hyperlipoproteinemia.

Intervention

Use a combination of diet and drug therapy to treat both inherited and acquired primary hyperlipidemia. Treat secondary hyperlipidemia by managing the underlying disease process rather than the hyperlipidemia per se. A summary of the dietary management for hyperlipoproteinemia is given in Table 29–3. Nurses can find detailed descriptions of the diets, which incorporate suggestions that they can give to clients for buying and cooking foods, in publications available upon request from the National Institutes of Health.[15] The rest of this section focuses on specific diet therapy for types II and IV, since these disorders are common and are associated with premature atherosclerosis.

For hypercholesterolemia (apparent in type IIa, type IIb, and to a lesser degree in type IV—cholesterol may be slightly elevated in type IV, and in some individuals with type IV who are undergoing weight reduction, there may be a reciprocal change

TABLE 29–3
SUMMARY OF DIETS FOR HYPERLIPOPROTEINEMIA

	Type I	Type IIa	Type 11b and Type III	Type IV	Type V
Diet prescription	Low fat 25–35 g	Low cholesterol; polyunsaturated fat increased	Low cholesterol; approximately 20% kcal protein, 40% kcal fat, 40% kcal carbohydrate	Controlled carbohydrate (approximately 45% of kcal); moderately restricted cholesterol	Restricted fat 30% of kcal; controlled carbohydrate, 50% of kcal; moderately restricted cholesterol
Kilocalories	Not restricted	Not restricted	Achieve and maintain recommended weight, i.e., reduction diet if necessary	Achieve and maintain recommended weight, i.e. reduction diet if necessary	Achieve and maintain recommended weight, i.e., reduction diet if necessary
Protein	Total protein intake is not limited	Total protein intake is not limited	High protein	Not limited other than control of client's weight	High protein
Fat	Restricted to 25–35 g; kind of fat not important; medium-chain triglycerides may improve palatability	Saturated fat intake limited; polyunsaturated fat intake increased	Controlled to 40% kcal (polyunsaturated fats recommended in preference to saturated fats)	Not limited other than control of client's weight (polyunsaturated fats recommended in preference to saturated fats)	Restricted to 30% of kcal (polyunsaturated fats recommended in preference to saturated fats)
Cholesterol	Not restricted	As low as possible; the only source of cholesterol is meat in diet	Less than 300 mg; the only source of cholesterol is meat in diet	Moderately restricted to 300–500 mg	Moderately restricted to 300–500 mg
Carbohydrate	Not limited	Not limited	Controlled; concentrated sweets are restricted	Controlled; concentrated sweets are restricted	Controlled, concentrated sweets are restricted
Alcohol	Not recommended	May be used with discretion	Limited to 2 servings (substituted for carbohydrate)	Limited to 2 servings (substituted for carbohydrate)	Not recommended

(*Source: U.S.DHEW: The Dietary Management of Hyperlipoproteinemia: A Handbook for Physicians and Dietitians. DHEW Publication No. (NIH) 80–100, Bethesda, Md., National Heart, Lung, and Blood Institute, 1980.*)

in LDL) provide a low-cholesterol, low-saturated fat diet with substitution of polyunsaturated fat. For hypertriglyceridemia (apparent in type IIb and type IV), provide a controlled carbohydrate diet that restricts alcohol and allows for weight reduction. If the client is obese, stress weight reduction for control of both types of lipid elevations. However, weight reduction is much more important in the control of hypertriglyceridemia than of hypercholesterolemia. In obese clients with hypertriglyceridemia, weight loss alone normalizes blood triglycerides in some cases.

The type of dietary fat has a much greater effect on serum cholesterol levels than on triglyceride levels. Saturated fatty acids, particularly lauric, myristic, and palmitic acids (which contain 12 to 16 carbon atoms), and cholesterol increase the level of serum cholesterol, and polyunsaturated fatty acids, particularly linoleic acid, decrease the level. Stearic acid, a saturated fatty acid that contains 18 carbon atoms, appears to have little effect on the blood cholesterol level. Monounsaturated fatty acids, such as oleic acid, also lower blood cholesterol but to a lesser degree than polyunsaturated fat.

Since saturated fatty acids are twice as powerful in raising serum cholesterol as polyunsaturated fatty acids are in lowering them, 2 g of polyunsaturates are needed to counteract the effect of 1 g of saturates. An overall P:S ratio of 2.0 is considered desirable in diets designed to lower blood cholesterol. Many investigators are in disagreement with this P:S ratio, however, considering it unnecessary to increase the polyunsaturated fat content of the diet when the total saturated fat content can be kept very low. Some studies have associated an increased incidence of malignant disease and of gallstones with the ingestion of diets high in polyunsaturated fat, although the evidence is not conclusive. Moreover, if weight reduction is indicated, the use of large amounts of polyunsaturated fat is impossible. Current blood cholesterol-lowering regimens emphasize restricting saturated fat and, within the fat limitation, to use polyunsaturates in the diet.

A number of studies have been conducted to show the effect of egg consumption on the blood cholesterol level—egg yolks are high in cholesterol—but the results have not been consistent. Some subjects show a rapid rise in plasma cholesterol in response to a high cholesterol intake, whereas others can ingest up to 700 to 800 mg per day without any effect on plasma lipid levels, at least for short periods of time. The great differences in response to egg consumption reported by various investigators emphasize the desirability of evaluating dietary changes on an individual basis rather than assuming that a certain dietary component will automatically elevate the blood cholesterol level.

Excessive kilocalorie consumption leading to overweight also raises serum lipids. At recommended body weight, the client with type IV hyperlipoproteinemia always has lower triglyceride concentrations, and sometimes the loss of excessive weight returns the triglycerides to normal. Carbohydrate and alcohol may increase endogenous triglyceride synthesis. Sucrose and fructose are more effective than starch as inducers of endogenous hypertriglyceridemia. Sugar intolerance has been thought to be genetic in origin, but the condition may be due to associated overweight or impaired glucose tolerance and diabetes mellitus. Although alcohol is not metabolized in the same manner as carbohydrate, it also leads to excessively high levels of VLDL in hypertriglyceridemic individuals.

Dietary management of type IIa hyperlipoproteinemia, with elevation of blood cholesterol, involves cholesterol-lowering measures only. Since both cholesterol and triglyceride are usually elevated in both types IIb and IV, a combination of measures to lower both cholesterol and triglyceride is necessary. Table 29–4 gives general descriptions of diet modifications for the three types. Although diets for types IIb and IV appear similar, there are differences in the proportion of kilocalories derived from carbohydrate and fat, the ratio of saturated

to polyunsaturated fat, and the total amount of cholesterol allowed in the diets. A listing of foods allowed and foods to avoid for a fat-controlled diet (restricted in cholesterol and saturated fat, with substitution of polyunsaturated fat) designed to lower the blood cholesterol (for type IIa and type IIb hyperlipoproteinemia) is given in Table 29–5. Table 29–6 provides further guidelines for type IIb, which are also appropriate for type III, in which triglyceride-lowering measures (restriction of kilocalories, sucrose and other concentrated sweets, and alcohol) and cholesterol-lowering measures are necessary. Food listings for type IV hyperlipoproteinemia, which requires the same triglyceride-lowering measures as type IIb and type III but less stringent cholesterol-lowering measures than type IIa, are shown in Table 29–7. Assist clients with lipid disorders to develop daily food plans, such as the examples given below for clients on a type IIa, type IIb (and type III), and type IV diet.

Type IIa

Breakfast	Lunch and Dinner	Between Meal Snack
Citrus fruit juice	Cooked poultry, fish, or lean, trimmed meat	Fruit
Cereal		Skim milk (if desired)
Toast	Potato or substitute	
Allowed fat	Vegetables	
Jelly and sugar	Bread	
Skim milk	Allowed fat	
Coffee or tea	Fruit or allowed dessert	
	Skim milk	
	Coffee or tea	

TABLE 29–4
HYPERLIPOPROTEINEMIA AND DIET

Type and Lipid Pattern[a]	Diet
Type IIa (C high; TG normal)	To lower cholesterol: 1. Restrict cholesterol intake to less than 300 mg daily (maximal is 100 mg/day) 2. Decrease saturated fat intake (to less than 10% of kcal) 3. Substitute polyunsaturated fat for saturated fat
Type IIb (C high; TG slightly elevated)	To lower cholesterol: Same as above To lower triglyceride: 1. Restrict kcal if obese 2. Restrict carbohydrate intake by eliminating sucrose and concentrated sweets 3. Restrict alcohol intake
Type IV (C normal or slightly elevated; TG high)	To lower triglyceride: Same as in type IIb To lower cholesterol: 1. Moderately restrict cholesterol intake to 300–500 mg daily 2. Decrease saturated fat intake 3. Substitute polyunsaturated fat for saturated fat

[a] C, cholesterol; TG, triglyceride.

TABLE 29–5
FAT-CONTROLLED DIET: LOW CHOLESTEROL, LOW SATURATED FAT, INCREASED POLYUNSATURATED FAT

Category	Foods Allowed[a]	Foods Avoided or Used Sparingly
Meat	Lean, well-trimmed cuts of fresh or frozen meat. Emphasize use of chicken, turkey, fish (except shrimp), and veal in meat meals with less frequent use of beef, pork, ham, lamb	Heavily marbled meat; fatty meat including regular ground beef, bacon, spareribs, frankfurters, sausages, luncheon meats, fatty corned beef, goose, duck, mutton; commercially prepared foods containing fat (unless polyunsaturated fat specified), including fried meat, frozen or canned meat in sauce or gravy; frozen or packaged dinners; shrimp; fish roe; organ meats
Egg	Egg white only (some regimens allow two or three egg yolks per week); egg substitutes containing no cholesterol	Egg yolk
Other meat alternates	Legumes, soy protein meat alternates, peanut butter, nuts such as walnuts, pecans, almonds (note nuts to avoid)	Canned pork and beans; cashew and macadamia nuts
Milk and cheese	Skim milk and products made from skim milk (liquid, powdered, and evaporated skim milk); buttermilk; low-fat chocolate drink; cocoa made with non-fat milk; cheese, cottage cheese, and yoghurt containing up to 1% fat; sapsago cheese; specially prepared cheese high in polyunsaturated fat; sherbet (1–2% fat)	Whole milk and whole milk products, including chocolate, evaporated, condensed milk; whole milk yoghurt; malted milk and milkshake; cream (sweet and sour); ice cream and ice milk; nondairy substitutes for cream, sour cream, and whipped toppings that contain coconut or palm oil; cheese made from cream or whole milk
Vegetables and fruits	Any fresh, canned, frozen, dried vegetables and fruits; juices; vegetables prepared without animal fat or solid vegetable shortening; vegetarian baked beans	Buttered, creamed, or fried vegetables unless prepared with allowed fat; pork and beans; use avocado sparingly
Bread and cereal	All cooked and dry cereal; rice, flour, pasta (except egg noodles); breads made with a minimum of saturated fat, including white, whole wheat, rye, pumpernickel, raisin, oatmeal, Italian, and French bread; English muffins; hard rolls; matzo; melba toast; pretzels; rye wafers; saltines; graham crackers; homemade products made without whole milk, egg yolk, or saturated shortening	Egg noodles, egg bread; commercial biscuits, muffins, sweet rolls, donuts, coffee cake, cornbread, pancakes, waffles, butter rolls, and commercial mixes containing dried eggs, whole milk, or fat; corn chips, potato chips, and other deep fried snacks; cheese crackers and other flavored crackers
Fat	Vegetable oils, including safflower, corn, soybean, sunflower, sesame, cottonseed; soft margarine that lists an allowed liquid oil as the first ingredient on the label; commercial mayonnaise and other salad dressings not containing sour cream or cheese	Other margarine, including low-calorie margarine; butter; hydrogenated vegetable shortening, lard, bacon, meat drippings; salt pork; suet; cream; coconut and palm oil; olive and peanut oil; gravies and cream sauce unless made with allowed fat and skim milk
Desserts and sweets	Angel food cake; fruit ices, sherbet (1–2% fat); fruit whip made with egg white or gelatin; gelatin dessert; meringues; junket made with skim milk; cake, pie, cookies, pudding and frosting made with allowed fat, skim milk and egg white; pure sugar candy (gumdrops, jellybeans, hard candy, marshmallows, mints—not chocolate, Lifesavers, sour balls, plain fondant); jam; jelly; honey; syrup (containing no fat); molasses; sugar	Commercial cakes, pies, cookies, mixes; desserts and candy containing nonallowed fat, egg yolk, and whole milk; chocolate; coconut
Soup	Bouillon; clear broth; fat-free vegetable soup and pot liquor; cream soup made with skim milk and allowed fat; packaged dehydrated soup	All other soups
Miscellaneous	Coffee; tea; caffeine-free coffee; carbonated beverages; olives, pickles, relishes; fat-free barbecue sauce, catsup; chili sauce; salt; pepper; spices; herbs; extracts and flavorings; lemon juice; vinegar	

[a] No specific kcal limitation. If kcal and carbohydrate are restricted, additional modifications are necessary.

TABLE 29-6
CONTROLLED CARBOHYDRATE, CONTROLLED MODIFIED FAT, LOW-CHOLESTEROL DIET FOR TYPE IIB AND TYPE III HYPERLIPOPROTEINEMIA[a]

	Quantity Allowed						
Kilocalories	1500	1800	2000	2200	2400	2600	2800
Protein (g)[b]	75	80	90	115	120	120	125
Fat (g)	70	80	95	100	110	120	130
Carbohydrate (g)	135	180	195	210	225	255	285
Food groups (servings)							
Lean, cooked meat (3 oz)	2	2	2	3	3	3	3
Skim milk or buttermilk (1 c)	2	2	3	3	3	3	3
Bread–cereal (1 slice or ½ c cooked cereal)[c]	5	8	8	9	10	12	14
Fat (1 tsp)	10	12	15	15	17	19	21
Fruit (½ c)[d]	3	3	3	3	3	3	3
Vegetables (½ c)[e]	As desired						

[a] See Table 29–3 for general diet prescriptions for type IIb and type III hyperlipoproteinemia; see Table 29–5 for low-cholesterol, low-saturated fat, high-polyunsaturated fat food selections.
[b] 1 oz of meat, fish, poultry = 8 g protein and 3 g fat.
[c] Any one of the following may be substituted for 1 serving from the bread–cereal group (limit to 2 servings/day): 1½ in cube angel food cake; ⅓ c gelatin dessert; ¼ c sherbet or fruit ice; ½ c plain pudding prepared with skim milk; 1 tbsp sugar, honey, molasses, syrup, jam, or ½ oz jellybeans, gumdrops, hard candy, marshmallows, and mints (not chocolate) or 6 oz of carbonated sweetened beverage (such as carbonated water, cola type, ginger ale, or root beer) or 3 oz fruit flavored sodas and Tom Collins mixes may be substituted for 1 serving of the desserts listed above. No more than once daily if approved by the physician); up to 2 servings of alcoholic beverages may be substituted for bread–cereal if approved by the physician: 1 serving = 1 oz distilled spirits, 1½ oz dessert or sweet wine, 2½ oz dry table wine, 5 oz beer.
[d] ½ c unsweetened fruit or juice = 10 g carbohydrate.
[e] Starchy vegetables, such as potatoes, corn, lima beans, dried peas and beans, should be substituted for bread–cereal.
(*Source: Adapted from U.S.DHEW: Dietary Management of Hyperlipoproteinemia. A Handbook for Physicians and Dietitians. DHEW Publication No. (NIH) 80–110, Bethesda, Md., National Heart, Lung, and Blood Institute, 1980, p 28.*)

Type IIb, Type III, and Type IV

Breakfast	Lunch and Dinner
Citrus fruit or juice	Cooked poultry, fish, or lean, trimmed meat
Cereal or toast	Potato or substitute
Allowed fat	Vegetables
Skim milk	Bread
Coffee or tea	Allowed fat
	Fruit
	Skim milk (at lunch or dinner)
	Coffee or tea

If diet therapy fails to normalize blood lipids, drug therapy is added. The diet is continued with drug therapy, since the effect of diet and drugs is additive.

Client Education. Stress to the client that a permanent change in eating habits is necessary if diet therapy is to be effective in lowering blood lipids and maintaining normal levels. Avoid the term "special diet" because of its connotations. Rather, approach change as food choices for a more healthful lifestyle. Assess the client's present eating habits and food practices as a first step from which necessary modifications evolve. Detailed instructions are necessary about food selection and preparation techniques consistent with the diet. Nurses should present a positive approach to the diet by emphasizing the foods that are allowed as well as those to avoid.

Coordinate the plan for nutritional care with all other aspects of treatment in the nursing care plan. Since the combined changes in lifestyle needed to control atherosclerosis may overwhelm even the most highly motivated client, introduce the diet modifications gradually if the client is free of symptoms. Refrain from simply giving the client a printed list of foods to avoid. Rather, be involved in an ongoing process of education and encouragement that includes help with food preparation, selecting foods when eating away from home, and flavoring the diet to make it palatable. During periodic check-ups, provide increasingly comprehensive instruction. When the diet modifications bring about a fall in blood lipids, bring this to the client's attention for positive reinforcement. Use these guidelines to assist clients in selecting foods for the fat-controlled diet:

1. Use low-fat foods as desired. Low-fat foods include vegetables, fruits, legumes, cereals, and flour. Use baked products prepared with a minimum amount of fat, such as loaf bread and hard rolls.

TABLE 29–7
CONTROLLED CARBOHYDRATE, CONTROLLED MODIFIED FAT, MODERATELY RESTRICTED CHOLESTEROL DIET FOR TYPE IV HYPERLIPOPROTEINEMIA

Category	Foods Allowed	Foods Avoided or Used Sparingly
Meat	Lean beef, veal, pork, ham, chicken, turkey, fish, shellfish, canned drained fish, lean game meats; 2 oz of liver or organ meats may be substituted for 1 egg yolk	All fatty meats, mutton, duck, goose, canned meat products, luncheon meats, cold cuts, frankfurters, bacon, sausage, fish roe, spare ribs, poultry skin, commercially fried meats and fish, frozen and packaged dinners, meats canned or frozen in gravy or sauces; organ meats as specified
Egg	Limit to 3 whole eggs per week (including those in cooking), egg whites as desired; cholesterol-free egg substitutes	All others
Other meat alternates	Legumes, soy protein meat alternates, peanut butter, nuts (note nuts to avoid)	Canned pork and beans; cashew and macadamia nuts
Milk and cheese	Skim milk, buttermilk (made from skim milk), powdered skim milk, evaporated skim milk; low-fat yoghurt; creamed cottage cheese, low-fat cheese, 2 oz cheddar cheese per week	Whole milk, condensed milk, evaporated whole milk, dried whole milk, chocolate milk; milkshakes; all other cheeses
Vegetables and fruit	Unsweetened fruits or juices of any type (in reasonable amounts); any fresh, frozen, or canned vegetables (without added animal fat, solid shortening, or sauces); starchy vegetables should be used in limited amounts	Sweetened fruits and juices; buttered, creamed, or fried vegetables unless prepared with allowed fat
Bread and cereal	Biscuits, cornbread, hot-bread, loaf bread, pancakes, waffles, yeast rolls (all made with allowed oils and allowed milk), crackers (graham, soda, saltine, oyster); hamburger or frankfurter rolls; rye wafers; matzo; English muffins; bread sticks, pretzels, hard roll, melba toast; pasta (except egg noodles); any hot cereal prepared without whole milk, cream or butter; any dry cereal that is not presweetened; flour, cornmeal	Hot breads (unless made with allowed oils); cheese or egg breads; egg noodles; corn chips, potato chips, flavored crackers; commercial biscuits, muffins, doughnuts, sweet rolls, pancakes, waffles (unless prepared as specified); granolas that are presweetened or that contain chocolate; presweetened dry cereal
Fat	Any vegetable oil (except palm and coconut oil); special margarines that specify a liquid allowed oil as the first ingredient on the label; mayonnaise and commercial salad dressing not containing sour cream or cheese	Butter; solid vegetable shortenings; palm and coconut oil; bacon; cream; nondairy substitutes; lard; bacon grease, suet, salt pork; gravies and cream sauces (unless made with allowed margarine or oil)
Desserts and sweets	*Small* portion of angel food cake; gelatin, sherbet, fruit ice; pudding made with skim milk[a]	All sugar, candy, jelly, honey, syrup; cake, sweet rolls, pie, cookies; ice cream or ice milk; molasses; chocolate
Soup	Fat-free broth or bouillon, fat-free pot liquor; milk soups made with skim milk and special margarine	Soups made with meat fat, whole milk, cream, or butter
Miscellaneous	Sugar-free drinks (carbonated or other); coffee, tea, postum; extracts; flavorings, herbs, spices, lemon juice; salt, pepper, vinegar, catsup, chili sauce; sour pickles, relishes, barbeque sauce (made with allowed oil); cocoa powder; olives; avocado; unflavored gelatin; mustard; rennet tablets; soy sauce, Worcestershire sauce	Sweetened sodas or other beverages; coconut; alcohol[a]

[a] Sugar-containing desserts and alcohol, when used, should be substituted for bread and cereal and limited to no more than 2 servings per day. Alcohol should be used only with the approval of the physician.

2. Select poultry (chicken and turkey), fish, and veal more often than beef, lamb, pork, and ham for the latter contain more saturated fat. Restrict other fatty meats, such as sausage, frankfurters, and luncheon meats.

3. Select lean cuts of meat with only a small amount of visible fat within the flesh (low marbling). Lower grades of meat contain less fat marbling than prime grades. Most regular ground beef is too high in fat to be used.

A light pink color indicates an excessive fat content. For ground beef, use ground round ground-to-order from well-trimmed stew beef or round steak.

4. Restrict the use of egg yolks. Some regimens eliminate egg yolks altogether, whereas others allow two or three per week. Use egg whites as desired.

5. Select fat-free or low-fat milk, yoghurt, and cheese. Fluid skim milk, skimmed milk pow-

der, evaporated skim milk, and buttermilk may be used. Cheese made from skim or partially skim milk, such as uncreamed cottage cheese, is acceptable. Cheese made from polyunsaturated fat is also available.

6. Use polyunsaturated vegetable oils, such as safflower, corn, and soybean oils, in lieu of saturated fats. Sunflower, sesame, and cottonseed oils are also acceptable. Commercial mayonnaise and other salad dressings contain the above oils and can be used unless they also contain cheese or sour cream. Coconut oil and palm oil, both saturated vegetable oils, should not be used; peanut and olive oils, monosaturated vegetable oils, should not be used when a high P:S ratio is desired. Contrary to common belief, there is no justification for the recommendation that such oils as corn oil used in lipid-lowering diets should not be heated more than once or twice. Studies with corn oil have shown that heating several proprietary brands seven times to temperatures as high as 250°C (much higher than usually recommended for frying in oil) produced no loss of linoleic acid, the main polyunsaturated fatty acid in corn oil.

7. Use only soft margarine with a desirable P:S ratio that lists a recommended liquid vegetable oil as the first ingredient on the label, followed by one or more partially hydrogenated vegetable oils. The following label indicates an acceptable margarine:

> Liquid corn oil, partially hydrogenated corn oil, nonfat dry milk, water, salt.

The degree of hardness of the margarine frequently reflects the degree of unsaturation. Margarine packed in a plastic tub tends to be softer and more unsaturated than stick margarine.

8. Use convenience foods (packaged or prepared foods) only if they:
   a. Are fat-free or allow for fat addition during preparation. Examples include canned or frozen vegetables, some dehydrated foods, such as potatoes, and some packaged mixes, such as pancake mix. Polyunsaturated fat can be added during preparation.
   b. Contain polyunsaturated fat. An example is sardines packed in soybean oil. Many convenience foods must be eliminated because they are prepared with whole milk, egg yolk, or other sources of saturated vegetable or animal fat. Examples include frozen dinners and other canned or frozen food mixtures, nondairy substitutes for cream, sour cream, and whipped topping that use a coconut oil base, baked prod-

ucts, such as butter rolls, biscuits, sweet rolls, cakes, pies, and many mixes, and snack foods, such as potato and corn chips.

9. Interpret food labels carefully. Should the label include statements such as "margarine made from 100 percent corn oil," "contains no animal fat," or "nondairy product," the list of ingredients should be checked thoroughly. Even if the term "partially hydrogenated corn oil" is the first ingredient listed on the margarine label, the margarine may not have a suitable P:S ratio. If coconut oil, palm oil, or partially hydrogenated vegetable oil is listed on the label, the product is unsuitable. Coconut oil is frequently substituted for butterfat in nondairy creamers, whipped topping, and imitation cheeses. A few nondairy creamers that contain primarily polyunsaturated fat are available; an example is Poly Perx.

Food selection for the fat-controlled diet requires a great deal of food preparation from scratch. Many excellent cookbooks are available that include methods for adopting favorite recipes for use with vegetable oil. Some cooking tips that can be suggested to clients on a fat-controlled diet are given below.

1. Trim all visible fat from meat and remove the skin from poultry. If poultry is cooked in the skin to retain moisture, the skin should not be eaten because it contains more fat than the flesh.

2. Remove excess fat from meats during food preparation in the following ways:
   a. Use cooking methods that require little additional fat and remove excess fat contained in the meat. Methods include baking, roasting, broiling, sauteeing, braising, and stewing. Although frying with polyunsaturated oil is acceptable, less excess fat will be removed from the meat with this method.
   b. Brown meat under a broiler rather than in a pan when the recipe requires initial browning.
   c. Roast and bake meat on a rack so that fat can drain. Wine, tomato juice, or bouillon can be used for basting while cooking. The meat drippings can be refrigerated and the hardened fat subsequently skimmed and discarded. The resulting broth is fat-free and can be further used in cooking.
   d. Cook stews and soup stock the day before use and refrigerate them. The hardened fat can then be skimmed and discarded. Canned soup and broth can be reduced in fat by refrigeration and removal of visible fat before use.

3. Prepare gravy from fat-free meat stock, fat-

free meat drippings, or bouillon with flour and vegetable oil.

4. Season cooked vegetables with oil and any favorite herbs or spices.

5. Use special recipes to prepare baked items with vegetable oils or soft margarine, egg whites, and skim milk.

6. Use evaporated skim milk or triple-strength skim milk (made from nonfat dry milk) as a substitute for cream.

7. Incorporate vegetable oil in cooking in the following ways:

   a. Substitute oil for an equivalent amount of solid fat in recipes for pancakes, waffles, muffins, and yeast bread. Special recipes are available for use of oil in pie crust, cakes, and cookies.

   b. Use oil in meat preparation by brushing meat with oil before baking, roasting, or broiling. Use oil for frying meat, and use it as an ingredient for meat marinade, barbecue sauce, and cream sauce.

   c. Use oil in vegetable preparation as a cooked vegetable seasoning with herbs or spices, in frying or sauteeing, or as an ingredient for cream sauce, soup, and salad dressing.

   d. Use oil in preparation of snack foods, such as popcorn.

Should the client on a fat-controlled diet eat out daily, suggest that he or she choose a restaurant that can best meet the dietary requirements and become a regular customer of that restaurant. Some restaurants may be able to give regular customers special consideration.

Teach the client that a good general rule to follow in restaurant meals is to order simply prepared foods rather than mixed dishes. A general meal pattern with some examples of specific food choices is given in Table 29–8 for those who enjoy an occasional or frequent meal out.

Several booklets have been prepared by the National Institutes of Health for the dietary management of hyperlipoproteinemia, and the American Heart Association has published booklets that outline fat-controlled meal patterns. These booklets, listed in the bibliography, are available to clients through the physician or dietitian/nutritionist and are useful aids for nutrition counseling sessions. The American Heart Association has developed manuals designed for the dietitian or nutrition counselor and a client treatment manual featuring a stepwise approach to lowering serum lipid levels.*

The American Heart Association has published a cookbook with recipes for fat-controlled, low-

---

* Manuals for the professional: Heart to Heart, and Counseling the Patient with Hyperlipidemia (1984); Manual for the Client: Eating for a Healthy Heart (1984). Available from the American Heart Association National Center, Dallas, Tex.

TABLE 29–8 A MEAL PATTERN FOR EATING OUT ON A FAT-CONTROLLED DIET	
Meal Pattern	**Food Choices**
Appetizer	Fruit, fruit or vegetable juice, clear soup
Entree	Chicken, fish, chop, steak (remove visible fat, no sauce or gravy, no added fat)
Vegetables	Any vegetables, no sauce
Salad	Any fruit or vegetable salad; avoid cheese, sour cream, whipped cream
Fat	Soft margarine, mayonnaise, and salad dressings, such as Italian, French, and vinegar, with or without allowed oil
Bread	Saltines, plain sliced bread, hard rolls; avoid hot bread
Dessert	Fruit, fruit gelatin, sherbet, fruit ices, angel food cake; avoid desserts containing fat, egg yolks, whole milk, or cream

cholesterol meals (see bibliography); this book and other reliable recipe books and leaflets designed for fat-controlled meals allow for preparation of foods from basic ingredients that are suitable for the diet. Nurses should caution clients who are also following a low-calorie diet for obesity or a low-sodium diet for hypertension that some of the recipes may contain too many kilocalories or too much sodium. A number of food products that are especially designed for fat-controlled diets are available commercially. These include egg substitutes, fabricated meat analogs, margarine that is high in polyunsaturated fat, and imitation cheese and ice cream. Stress to the client the importance of label reading to determine if these items are appropriate. Some are high in sodium content (particularly the meat analogs and cheese) and should not be used if there is concomitant sodium restriction. Others may contain ingredients not allowed on the diet, such as plant sources of saturated fat, or they may provide an unfavorable P:S ratio. Whereas these special foods may add variety to the diet, in most cases their use is not essential to the diet's success. Emphasize to the client that drug therapy is not a substitute for diet modifications for hyperlipidemia; rather, drugs may be needed in addition to diet modifications.

For clients who must restrict sugar and concentrated sweets, use client education guidelines related to this given in Chapter 24. Since regular weight measurements are important, encourage the client to establish regular weighing times and to seek assistance if weight loss is not achieved or maintained.

The Role of Diet in Decreasing Susceptibility to Atherosclerosis. As noted earlier, there is a lack of agreement on the role of specific dietary factors in the incidence of atherosclerosis and coronary heart disease, on the benefits to be gained by lowering elevated blood lipids, and on the benefits and risks associated with specific diet modifications for prevention of atherosclerosis and coronary heart disease. Although specific food components, including fat, carbohydrate, alcohol, and kilocalories, are implicated in the etiology of the disorders, their roles remain controversial.

Regarding the benefits to be gained by lowering blood cholesterol levels, some authorities contend that the weight of evidence supports energetic efforts to lower cholesterol in persons with high levels as well as supporting the case for reducing cholesterol levels in the population as a whole.[16] Others continue to debate the issue, including the cholesterol level above which a major risk exists for coronary heart disease. With diet alterations, consideration must be given to potential risks resulting from possible nutrient imbalance, and diets designed to lower blood lipids should be carefully evaluated for both nutrient deficiency and excess. The recommendations of various groups for preventing heart disease are summarized in Table 2–7 and recommendations of the National Research Council are given in Chapter 7.

Must the general public eat no fat? Although scientific opinion varies, there is general agreement on five preventive measures that should provide health benefits. These five measures, applicable throughout the life cycle, are the following:

1. Eat a balanced diet consistent with nutritional needs for one's age.
2. Maintain recommended body weight by an appropriate balance of kilocalories and physical activity.
3. Use moderation in the consumption of sugar and alcohol. These substances may contribute to overweight, in addition to their possible effect on blood lipids in susceptible persons and other health factors.
4. Use moderation in the total amount of fat consumed. Although the correlation with heart disease is greater with the type of fat than with the amount of fat, high-fat diets tend to contain a large amount of saturated fat, cholesterol, and kilocalories. There is no agreed-upon definition of moderation, but many individuals may need to reduce the amount of fat used in food preparation and at the table to reduce total fat consumption.
5. Use a variety of types of fat. This can be achieved by moderation in the amounts of foods containing saturated fat and cholesterol and by use of some fat from polyunsaturated sources, such as vegetable oils.

For individuals at risk of coronary heart disease because of hyperlipidemia, diet modifications to lower cholesterol and triglycerides are indicated. However, dietary changes must be made on an individual basis, with other risk factors considered.

It has been hypothesized that interventions designed to reduce multiple risk factors, such as hypertension, cholesterol levels, and smoking habits—when applied in combination—may retard the atherosclerotic obstructive process. The Multiple Risk Factor Intervention Trial (MRFIT) was initiated in 1972 and completed in 1982 to determine whether a comprehensive preventive program directed at the combination of these three factors in high-risk men in the United States would significantly reduce mortality from coronary heart disease. Because of many intervening factors, the fundamental research questions from the study were not answered. Both the experimental and control groups experienced substantially lower mortality than expected, and mortality did not differ significantly in the two groups. In the experimental group, surprisingly, a subset of clients with initial hypertension and electrocardiographic abnormalities sustained a higher death rate from coronary heart disease than did comparable clients in the control group. It was found that men who stopped smoking had fewer deaths from heart disease.[17]

HYPERTENSION

Assessment

▶ **Hypertension** is defined as a sustained elevation in arterial blood pressure (systolic or diastolic). The disorder results from an increased arteriolar resistance to circulating blood and leads to thickening and narrowing of the blood vessels, with altered blood flow and consequent damage to body organs, such as the kidneys and heart. The condition may ▶ be primary or secondary in origin. **Primary hyper-** ▶ **tension,** also called **essential hypertension**—accounts for approximately 90 percent of hypertensive incidence. The cause of the disorder is not known, although it is theorized that renal humoral factors, autonomic nervous system or adrenocortical dysfunction, or mineral imbalance may be involved. The ▶ causes of **secondary hypertension** include renal parenchymal disease, peripheral vascular disease, endocrine disorders, coarctation of the aorta, and toxemia of pregnancy, among others.

Hypertension may be asymptomatic or, in other cases, symptoms such as morning headache may be evident. In its mild form, hypertension may remain undiagnosed for years. Severe, untreated hypertension may result in severe damage to the eye, kidney, heart, and brain. In the Framingham study, hypertension was found to be the most important of the major risk factors influencing morbidity and mortality in cardiovascular disease.[18] Control of blood pressure reduces the incidence of stroke and congestive heart failure.

Blood pressure increases with age and fluctuates widely even in one individual. Difficulties in diagnosing hypertension are compounded by lack of a natural cutoff point between normal and elevated blood pressure, and there may be difficulty in deciding what value denotes hypertension and necessitates treatment.

Hypertension affects approximately 15 to 20 percent of the adult population, and approximately 20 percent of American children are at risk of developing hypertension as adults. Assess for the relationships among age, sex, race, and family background in the incidence of the disorder. Although hypertension may occur at any age, it is progressively more common as age increases, with essential hypertension being most common between the ages of 35 and 50. Proportionately more women (18.5 percent) than men (12.5 percent) have hypertension. However, men are thought to tolerate hypertension less well than women. This may be related in part to the propensity of men to develop arteriosclerosis. The prevalence of the disorder is not only higher among American blacks than among whites (about double) but also is more severe in blacks. A strong familial incidence is also apparent. The likelihood that a child with hypertensive parents will develop hypertension is high. The familial occurrence of hypertension suggests a genetic basis, but genetic tendencies are thought to be modified by environmental factors, including diet and other elements of lifestyle, such as cigarette smoking, degree of stress, and degree of physical activity. Thus a diet high in sodium, kilocalorie excess, cigarette smoking, stress, and a sedentary lifestyle are associated with the incidence of hypertension, although none of these factors alone has been shown to cause the disorder.

A number of dietary factors have been implicated in the etiology of hypertension, although the strongest relationships exist with salt (sodium) intake and kilocalorie excess (leading to obesity). Other factors that have been suggested as affecting blood pressure include caffeine, alcohol, animal protein, essential fatty acids, and certain other minerals, including potassium, calcium, and magnesium.

Many studies, both in human populations and in animals, strongly implicate a high sodium intake as a causative agent in hypertension. However, observe that there appears to be a strong genetic factor in this association and that persons with a high salt consumption do not necessarily develop hypertension. Hypertension occurs rarely in populations with a low sodium intake. The age at which excess sodium consumption begins appears to be a factor in the development and severity of hypertension. Animal studies have shown that the consequences of feeding salt to young, salt-sensitive subjects are more severe than if the excess salt was consumed later in life. There is, however, no direct evidence to support the hypothesis that hypertension in humans results from excess sodium intake in the absence of genetic susceptibility.

In normal physiology, sodium is closely related to potassium, calcium, and magnesium, and attention is now focused on the role of deficiencies of these minerals in the development of hypertension. A reciprocal relationship between sodium and potassium in the development of hypertension has been noted,[19] and cultural studies show that populations consuming diets high in sodium and who have a high incidence of hypertension also consume diets low in potassium, and vice versa. Potassium supplements have been tested for their effect on blood pressure, with both positive[20] and negative results.[21]

Similar associations have been made with dietary calcium intake and development of hypertension, and calcium supplements have been used experimentally to lower blood pressure in healthy subjects.[22] Magnesium balance is closely related to calcium, and some experimental evidence exists for development of hypertension in association with magnesium deficiency. An explanation that has been offered for the protective effect of calcium and magnesium is that they contribute to the hardness of drinking water, and some findings have shown that individuals living in communities with hard water have lower blood pressure and cardiovascular mortality.[23]

A direct relationship between body weight and blood pressure has been shown by many investigators. For example, longitudinal studies of large populations have shown that an increase in relative weight over a period of years is associated with a rise in blood pressure. In contrast, populations that do not gain weight with age have a low prevalence of hypertension. Other studies have shown that weight gain during early adult life is an important risk factor for subsequent development of hypertension. The mechanism for the association between obesity and hypertension is not well understood. In relation to obesity, it is noteworthy that the tendency to develop hyperlipidemia and diabetes mellitus (both of which influence morbidity and mortality in hypertensive clients) is greater in obese clients.

There are speculations that the essential fatty acids may exert a protective effect on blood pressure; the effect of linoleic acid is not direct but mediated through prostaglandins.[24] Thus, equalizing the P:S ratio in the diet may reduce moderately elevated blood pressure to normal ranges.

Excess protein consumption may be implicated in the etiology of hypertension. Excess protein may lead to renal excretion of calcium. Interestingly, vegetarian diets have been found to have a blood pressure-lowering effect.[25]

Although the effect of caffeine on blood pressure is unpredictable, consider the recent consumption of caffeine-containing beverages when evaluating clients for hypertension. Coffee consumption, for instance, has been shown to elevate blood pressure in some individuals. People who consume large amounts of alcohol consistently exhibit higher blood pressure than nondrinkers.[26] Therefore, evaluate alcoholics for hypertension.

Other elements of lifestyle, such as cigarette smoking, sedentary living, and stressful living conditions, may also be factors in the etiology of hypertension. In some people, cigarette smoking may lead to an acute elevation in blood pressure, although most heavy smokers do not exhibit blood pressure increments. Sedentary individuals tend to have higher blood pressure than those who are physically active. However, this may be related to obesity, since body weight is usually greater in sedentary individuals. Additionally, physical fitness programs may lead to physiologic responses that lower blood pressure. The role of stress in hypertension is not well understood. Although population studies suggest that prolonged stressful situations may be associated with an elevation in blood pressure, and psychologic factors often cause an immediate and temporary rise in blood pressure, it is uncertain whether the stresses and strains of life lead to permanent rises.

Intervention

Early diagnosis and treatment are the key to prevention of end-organ damage. Stress to clients that treatment must continue indefinitely, even after normalization of the blood pressure. Treatment of hypertension includes a combination of drug and diet therapy.

The potential side effects and hazards of the long-term use of antihypertensive medications make dietary and other nonpharmacologic approaches to treatment attractive alternatives. Sodium restriction and weight reduction if the client is obese are important in dietary management. Blood pressure can be reduced with weight reduction alone, with sodium restriction alone, or with the two approaches combined. Exercise and biofeedback (relaxation therapy) are helpful in some circumstances.

Weight Reduction. For obese clients with hypertension, suggest weight reduction as the initial step in treatment. A kilocalorie level of 1000 to 1200 may be appropriate. Inform the client that the weight reduction not only reduces blood pressure (it is not necessary to achieve recommended body weight for results to be evident, and the results will be approximately the same in the very obese as in the moderately overweight) but also reduces the dosage level of drugs required or may eliminate the need for them altogether. Although weight reduction diets are likely to contain less sodium than usual diets, sodium restriction is not necessary for the blood pressure reduction that accompanies weight loss.

Sodium Restriction. Rigid sodium restriction (~10 mEq or 230 mg daily) significantly reduces blood pressure in many hypertensive clients, and even mild sodium restriction (~70 mEq or 1610 mg daily) produces a modest reduction in blood pressure in mildly to moderately hypertensive clients. Sodium restriction is most often used in combination with antihypertensive drug therapy. Not all hypertensive clients respond to sodium restriction: clients whose hypertension responds to diuretic drugs also respond well to sodium restriction. Moreover, sodium restriction enhances the effectiveness of antihypertensive drugs and lessens the potential for hypokalemia, a

common side effect of taking thiazide and loop diuretics. Advise all clients taking these diuretics to reduce their sodium intake to moderate levels (60 to 90 mEq or 1380 to 2070 mg daily) to aid in blood pressure reduction and enhancement of the antihypertensive effect of the diuretic as well as possibly to spare them from taking potassium supplements or the relatively expensive potassium-sparing diuretic combinations. When potassium supplements are required, remind clients that they may be irritating to the gastric mucosa. When possible, suggest dietary sources of potassium, such as additional fruits and vegetables, in lieu of a potassium chloride supplement. Salt substitutes are an economical source of potassium for those with normal renal function who become hypokalemic. Sodium-restricted diets are discussed in detail in the next section. In addition to observing for signs of hypokalemia in clients taking diuretics, observe for signs of other imbalances, such as hypochloremia (reduced blood chloride), hyponatremia, hyperglycemia, and hyperuricemia. Salt substitutes and potassium chloride are good sources of chloride to counteract the hypochloremia that is a common side effect of diuretic therapy.

Fluid restriction is not necessary if cardiac and renal function is adequate, and coffee and tea are permitted unless cardiac arrhythmias or such symptoms as nervousness and irritability are complicating factors.

The Sodium-restricted Diet. Restriction of dietary sodium may be indicated to control both hypertension and edema. These syndromes may occur alone or together in various medical problems, such as cardiovascular, renal, or endocrine disorders, or secondary to therapy with steroid hormones.

Levels of Sodium Restriction. To provide a degree of standardization for low-sodium diets, the American Heart Association has outlined four levels of sodium-restricted diets. These levels, shown in Table 29–9, are applicable for any client requiring a restricted diet. Sodium-restricted diets should be prescribed in a specified amount of sodium rather than in such general terms as salt-poor, low-salt, salt-free diet, or no added salt.

Sources of Sodium. The two major sources of sodium intake are (1) food and water and (2) medications and dentifrices.

Food and Water. With few exceptions, all food and water contains some sodium, either as (1) a naturally occurring mineral or (2) as sodium chloride (salt) or other sodium compound added in food processing, preparation, or service. In some areas, water supplies have sodium added. Sodium is present, either naturally or by addition, in many of the foods providing other nutrients essential for an adequate diet. The amount added in food preparation and service is an individual matter and depends on the seasoning habits of the cook and on how heavy a hand

TABLE 29–9
LEVELS OF SODIUM RESTRICTION

Sodium Level[a]	Descriptive Term	Disease
87 to 174 mEq (2000 to 4000 mg)	Mild	Hypertension, steroid hormone therapy, maintenance diet to *prevent* edema in cardiac and renal disease
43 mEq (1000 mg)	Moderate	Eclampsia (if sodium restriction is indicated), hypertension, clients with edema resistant to higher sodium levels
22 mEq (500 mg)	Strict	To *eliminate* edema of congestive heart failure, cirrhosis with ascites, occasionally in renal disease
11 mEq (250 mg)	Severe	Cirrhosis with ascites, congestive heart failure when edema is resistant to higher levels of sodium

[a] Amounts usually rounded (i.e., 87 to 85, 43 to 40, 22 to 20, and 11 to 10).

an individual has with the salt shaker when eating. This amount is controllable by influencing the seasoning habits of the cook or consumer. The amount that occurs naturally in foods or is added in food processing is controllable only by having a knowledge of the amounts of sodium in specific foods.

SODIUM ADDED TO FOOD. The sodium-containing compounds that add the largest amount of sodium to foods are (1) table salt, (2) baking soda (sodium bicarbonate), (3) monosodium glutamate, (4) baking powder, and (5) brine. The actual amounts of sodium contained in four of these compounds are:

Salt (1 tsp or 5 g)	87.0 mEq Na
Baking soda (1 tsp or 4.9 g)	58.0 mEq Na
Monosodium glutamate (1 tsp)	32.6 mEq Na
Baking powder (1 tsp or 3.7 g)	17.4 mEq Na

Tables 29–10 and 29–11 contain lists of processed foods containing these five sodium compounds in either (1) relatively large amounts or (2) smaller yet significant amounts. The lists refer to commonly available foods and not to dietetic foods. **Dietetic foods** are those in which the content of some nutrient, such as sodium or fat, or of kilocalories has been altered or reduced. For example, Tab and other low-calorie soft drinks are dietetic foods. Dietetic foods prepared for the sodium-restricted diet contain lesser amounts of sodium than regularly processed products.

In addition to containing the five major sodium compounds already named, the foods in these lists may contain lesser amounts of other sodium compounds, such as sodium benzoate, sodium citrate, sodium propionate, sodium alginate, sodium sulfite,

TABLE 29–10
PREPARED FOODS AND FLAVORING AGENTS CONTAINING RELATIVELY LARGE AMOUNTS OF SODIUM

Flavoring Agents	Prepared Foods
Vegetable salts and flakes, such as onion, garlic, celery; seasoned salts; chili sauce; catsup; prepared mustard; horseradish prepared with salt; meat extracts and tenderizers; meat sauces, such as soy and Worcestershire; commercial mayonnaise and salad dressings; bacon grease	Relishes: Salted pickles, olives, pickle relishes Snacks: Potato chips, pretzels, salted nuts, salted popcorn. Vegetables: Sauerkraut, vegetables cooked with salt pork Bread–cereal: Bread, rolls, crackers with salt toppings; bran, bran flakes Cheese: Processed cheese and cheese spreads Soup: Canned, frozen, and dehydrated soup; bouillon cubes Meat: Canned meat and fish, such as Vienna sausage, tuna; salt-cured meat, such as ham, bacon, tongue, herring; corned beef; chipped beef; luncheon meats, such as frankfurters, bologna; sausage; salt pork; salt-koshered meat; frozen fish fillets; low cholesterol breakfast meat substitutes

TABLE 29–11
FOODS CONTAINING SMALLER BUT SIGNIFICANT AMOUNTS OF SODIUM

Milk–Meat–Substitutes	Bread–Cereal	Vegetable–Fruit	Miscellaneous (Fats, Beverages, Desserts)
Commercial buttermilk with salt added, frozen dinners, peanut butter	Loaf bread and other prepared bakery products; self-rising flour, self-rising cornmeal, biscuits and cornbread made with these products; packaged mixes; most packaged breakfast cereals; quick-cooking cereals, such as quick Cream of Wheat	Canned vegetables; frozen peas, frozen lima beans; boil-in-bag frozen vegetables with butter added; whole hominy; commercially prepared citrus sections; maraschino cherries; glazed and crystallized fruit; dried fruit, such as prunes, raisins, figs	Butter and margarine; gelatin desserts; commercial candy; Dutch-process cocoa; beverage mixes, such as Tang, Start, some Kool-Aid; carbonated beverages; beverages with sodium saccharin

sodium hydroxide, disodium phosphate, and sodium saccharin. These latter compounds are added to foods for a variety of reasons. They can act as a preservative, flavor enhancer, bleach, softener, or sweetener, retard mold growth, produce a smooth texture, or reduce cooking time. In most instances, these compounds are added in relatively small amounts.

The foods that are naturally high in sodium (Table 29–12) also contain other essential nutrients, especially protein, calcium, iron, and vitamin A. All meats contain significant amounts of sodium, and shellfish (except oysters) are especially high in sodium content. Organ meats contain more sodium than muscle meat, and the dark meat of poultry contains more than white meat. Although all fish contain natural sodium, salt-water fish contain no more sodium than fresh-water fish.

SODIUM IN WATER. In some areas of the United States, drinking water may contain significant amounts of sodium due to two factors: (1) a high natural sodium content of the water supply and (2) an addition of softeners to the water in hard water areas. In water systems, sodium is substituted for the minerals responsible for the hardness of water.

Since the total amount of water used for drinking in beverages, such as coffee and tea, and in food preparation is approximately 2½ quarts per person per day, water supplies high in sodium content have a definite effect on the sodium content of the diet. In areas where water contains more than 20 mg of sodium per quart, persons on restricted sodium diets should make allowance for this in their diet or drink only distilled water. Information concerning the sodium content of community water supplies can be obtained from the local chapter of the American Heart Association or the Public Health Department.

Bottled soft drinks may be high in sodium if manufactured in areas where sodium in the water supply is high. Low-calorie beverages may contain sodium due to the addition of sodium saccharin, a noncaloric sweetener. These drinks should, therefore, be restricted in the diet, especially where strict or severe sodium restriction is indicated.

Medications, Dentifrices, and Other Substances. Variable amounts of sodium may be ingested through the use of the following substances:

1. Medications, including proprietary medications
2. Dentifrices and mouthwashes
3. Chewing tobacco and snuff

Medications that may contain sodium include (1) barbiturates, (2) sulfonamides, (3) antibiotics, (4) cough medicines, (5) laxatives, and (6) antacids.

To prevent absorption of the sodium contained in toothpastes and mouthwashes, instruct clients on a low-sodium diet to thoroughly rinse the mouth after using these substances.

The food exchange system (described in Chaps. 2 and 24) that is used for calculating kilocalorie-controlled diets has been adopted for use in calculating sodium-restricted diets as well. The average sodium content of each exchange group has been calculated. However, the sodium values apply only to foods produced, processed, and prepared without the addition of salt or any other sodium compound. The values reflect the quantity of sodium that the foods naturally contain. Table 29–13 gives the sodium composition of the Food Exchange Lists.

TABLE 29–12
FOODS NATURALLY HIGH IN SODIUM

Animal Protein Foods	Vegetables	
Milk	Beets and their greens	Celery
Eggs	Carrots	Chard
Meat, including fish and poultry	White turnip roots	Spinach
	Artichokes	Kale
Cheese		

TABLE 29–13
SODIUM CONTENT OF FOOD EXCHANGE LISTS

Food Group	Quantity for 1 Exchange	Sodium[a] (mg)
Milk exchange	8 oz (1 c)	120
Vegetable exchange	½ c	9
Fruit exchange	Varies	2
Bread exchange	Varies	5
Meat exchange Low-fat, medium-fat and high-fat	1 oz	25
Fat exchange	1 tsp	Negligible

[a] Food produced, processed, or prepared without the addition of sodium.

Dietary Adjustments for Sodium Restriction. Clients with any degree (mild to severe) of sodium restriction must consider the sodium intake from all sources. A client on mild sodium restriction, for example, may have no restrictions on intake of foods naturally high in sodium. The client should be aware of their sodium content, however, so that these foods can be used in moderation. The sodium content of most incidental sources of sodium and that present in water supplies become a critical factor only in strict and severe levels of sodium restriction. Clients on these two levels of restriction are usually hospitalized and have an unusually low sodium tolerance.

The important factor for nurses to keep in mind when trying to help a client adjust food intake to a specific level of sodium is that it is the total sodium intake for the day (and not the restriction of intake of specific foods) that is significant. For example, if a dietitian–nutritionist can work a slice of bacon into the diet plan without increasing the intake above the prescribed level, this is acceptable. Likewise, some clients prefer a small amount of salt added to their food. By working with the dietitian to reduce the intake of sodium-containing foods that might otherwise be allowed in their diets, nurses can help clients make this adjustment.

There are five major adjustments that can be made in a normal diet to reduce the sodium intake. Depending on the level of restriction desired, clients may need to make as few as two or as many as all five of these adjustments. These adjustments are:

1. Add no salt to foods at mealtime
2. Add no salt to foods in cooking
3. Omit processed foods containing large amounts of added sodium
4. Omit or restrict processed foods containing smaller but significant amounts of added sodium
5. Omit or restrict some foods naturally high in sodium

The adjustments that must be made in a normal diet to achieve the four levels of sodium restriction are illustrated in Figure 29–4. Use these adjustments as guidelines for helping clients to achieve the desired level of sodium intake. Since the mild low-sodium diet represents a wide range (from 85 to 174 mEq), this is broken down into two separate levels.

Maintaining Normal Food Intake. An increasing number of foods or methods of food preparation must be deleted in the four levels of sodium restriction. The restrictions range from simple to complex, that is, from (1) restricting only the addition of salt to foods at mealtime and the intake of processed foods that contain large amounts of added sodium for the mildest degree of sodium restriction to (2) omitting intake of all processed foods containing added sodium and restricting foods naturally high in sodium at the severe level of restriction. In between, a variety of adjustments can be made aimed at keeping the intake of one's usual foods as nearly normal as possible. Examples are given below.

Mild Sodium Restriction
- *130 to 174 mEq (3000 to 4000 mg).* Even though no salt is added at meals and processed foods with large amounts of added sodium are eliminated, moderate amounts of salt may be used in cooking.
- *85 mEq (2000 mg).* For this diet, while no salt is added at meals or in cooking and foods especially high in sodium are eliminated, some processed foods with smaller but significant amounts of added sodium are allowed. The usual foods and amounts allowed from this group are listed in Table 29–14.

Moderate Sodium Restriction
- *40 mEq (1000 mg).* Although this diet is restricted in terms of adding salt to meals, in cooking, and in intake of foods containing large amounts of added sodium, a small amount of food containing smaller, yet significant amounts of sodium may be allowed. The daily allowance of usual foods includes two slices of regular bread plus 5 tsp of regular margarine or butter, or one serving of a prepared dessert.

Control of Intake of Foods Naturally High in Sodium. Control of the intake of foods naturally high in sodium becomes increasingly important with the stricter levels of sodium restriction. Amounts usually allowed daily are listed in Table 29–15.

Client Education. A client adapting to a sodium-restricted diet must have discipline, willingness to change, and willingness to experience some degree of unpleasantness. Sodium restriction entails a long-term modification, often represents a drastic change in eating habits, and for many people is unpleasant. The flat taste of food prepared without salt is an ever-present reminder of the person's illness. Food

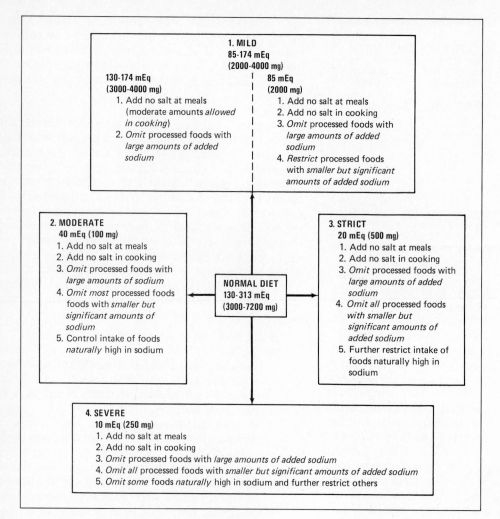

Figure 29–4
Dietary adjustments to achieve various levels of sodium intake.

does not taste the same, even though it may be camouflaged and otherwise well seasoned. Acknowledge to the client that food may taste different rather than overemphasizing the positive.

A client may follow a diet in the hospital and when not feeling well but, when discharged and feeling better at home, may think that it is no longer necessary. When intrinsic motivation is lacking, ap-

ply the four principles of diet modification given in Table 29–16 to encourage a client to follow the diet rather than simply telling him or her to change lifelong eating habits. If, after thorough application of these principles, a client is unable to follow the diet because of cost or inability to change eating habits, inform the physician, who may choose to increase the medication dosage. Practical aspects related to changes in meal planning, shopping, and food preparation are discussed below.

Meal Planning. Foods that can be included in a sodium-restricted diet include fresh foods, foods processed without added salt, and low-sodium dietetic foods. Fresh foods and foods processed without sodium are listed in Table 29–17.

A number of low-sodium dietetic foods are available in the special diet foods section of many groceries, but stress to clients that they are more expensive than regular processed foods. In addition, they are not a necessary component of the low-sodium diet. Although they contribute to variety in meals, an adequate diet can be achieved without their use. If vegetables naturally high in sodium, such as beets and carrots, are not allowed in the diet, instruct

TABLE 29–14
REGULAR FOODS ALLOWED ON MILD SODIUM-RESTRICTED DIETS

Food	Amount Daily
Regular loaf bread	6 slices (1 *small* biscuit or cornbread = 2 slices bread)
Regular margarine or butter	6 tsp (1 tsp margarine or butter = 1½ tsp mayonnaise)
Dry cereal, such as Corn Flakes	1 serving (no bran or bran flakes)
Prepared dessert	1 small serving (such as pie or cake)
Vegetable	1 serving canned (if frozen or fresh, may add small amount of salt in cooking)

TABLE 29–15
AMOUNTS OF FOODS NATURALLY HIGH IN SODIUM ALLOWED DAILY

Food	Moderate Restriction (40 mEq or 1000 mg)	Strict Restriction (20 mEq or 500 mg)	Severe Restriction (10 mEq or 250 mg)
Meat	5 to 6 oz	5 to 6 oz	2 to 4 oz
Eggs	1	1	3/week
Milk	2 to 3 c	2 c	None (substitute low-sodium milk)
High-sodium vegetables	2–3 servings/week	None	None

Note that greater control is necessary at the strict and severe levels than at the moderate level.

clients that the low-sodium dietetic canned vegetables should not be used either. Dietetic foods are equivalent in sodium content to the ingredients used.

Shopping. Instruct the client to read labels more carefully to look for salt or other sodium compounds among the list of ingredients. Because of this, shopping time is usually increased.

Food Preparation. The degree of change in methods of food preparation and service depends not only on the degree of sodium restriction but also on the individual's usual food habits. Clients requiring mild levels of restriction or those accustomed to using small amounts of salt in cooking or at meals require less change than those with a greater degree of restriction or those accustomed to using large amounts of salt. The food habits of some groups in the South, for example, are characterized by the consumption of large amounts of smoked pork, green leafy vegetables high in sodium, salt pork seasonings for vegetables, cornbread, and biscuits and necessitate a great deal of change. Clients using large amounts of packaged convenience foods and snack foods must make considerable changes in food preparation methods.

The two major changes in food preparation usually necessitated by a low-sodium diet are:

1. Use of more food prepared from basic ingredients
2. Development of alternate means to improve the palatability of the diet

FOOD PREPARED FROM BASIC INGREDIENTS. Since most packaged foods have salt added, sodium-free ingredients must be used in preparing homemade foods, such as salt-free bread, cakes, and cookies. The usual methods for cooking meats, eggs, and vegetables can still be used, including boiling, broiling, roasting, stewing, and even frying, if there is no kilocaloric restriction. However, bacon fat or salt pork should not be used for seasoning. Instruct the client to use vegetable oil, shortening, and fresh pork as substitutes for bacon fat or salt pork and to rinse fresh fish purchased commercially thoroughly before cooking. Homemade baked beans can be prepared from dry lima beans.

To avoid preparing separate meals for the individual on a diet, all family foods may be prepared without added salt, and other family members can salt their food individually. An alternate to this is

TABLE 29–16
PRINCIPLES OF DIET MODIFICATION

Principle	Application
Client understands significance of the restriction	Explain how diet helps to control disease process
A realistic goal is set and accepted	The prescription should be at a level that is realistic for client
	Explain exact level to client, rather than tell him/her just to "cut down on salt"
The goal is realistically adapted to client's life situation	On the basis of diet history, adjust diet to economic, cultural, and social situation
Client has sufficient knowledge about diet to follow it	Explain sources of sodium, changes in meal planning, shopping, and preparation, and habits of eating out necessitated by the restriction

TABLE 29–17
FOODS TO USE ON LOW-SODIUM DIETS

Meat	Vegetable–Fruit	Bread–Cereal	Miscellaneous
Unsalted fresh, frozen, or low-sodium dietetic canned meats, including beef, veal, lamb, pork (ham, chops, variety products such as feet), liver, chicken, turkey, fresh wild game, fish, oysters, legumes, dietetic cheese and peanut butter, nuts prepared without salt	Most fresh, frozen or dried fruits and vegetables, canned fruits, low-sodium dietetic canned vegetables	Cereals processed without salt, including rice, grits, oatmeal, macaroni, spaghetti, noodles; prepared cereals without salt, including puffed wheat and rice, Sugar Smacks, Shredded Wheat, Muffets; homemade baked goods made from sodium-free ingredients including (1) plain cornmeal and flour (not self-rising), (2) sodium-free baking powder, (3) oil or unsalted shortening, such as Spry and Crisco, (4) yeast, (5) cream of tartar, low-sodium dietetic bakery products	Coffee, tea, most cola beverages, lard, vegetable oils, such as corn oil, hydrogenated vegetable shortenings, such as Spry and Crisco, low-sodium dietetic flavorings, such as mustard, catsup, mayonnaise

to suggest to the client that low-sodium portions be removed before salt seasonings are added. Individual homemade TV dinners and casseroles may be prepared in advance and frozen for later use.

ALTERNATE MEANS TO IMPROVE PALATABILITY OF DIET. If one has never tried tasting foods prepared without salt, to do so would greatly increase the understanding of the client's problems. Eating foods, such as broiled chicken and mashed potatoes, without salt will demonstrate more vividly than can be described in writing the eating enjoyment that is lost. All available ideas should be used to improve the palatability of the diet. Since eating involves a composite of the five senses (sight, sound, smell, touch, and taste), appealing meals can be served by giving attention to color, flavor, and texture in meal planning. Additionally, experimentation with alternate flavorings that stimulate the sweet, sour, and bitter taste sensations will help compensate for the lost salt taste.

Suggest the use of sodium-free seasoning agents to use as alternatives to salt: (1) sodium-free fats, (2) herbs and spices, (3) fruits, including lemon juice, (4) fresh vegetables, (5) sugar, (6) alcoholic beverages, (7) vinegar, and (8) salt substitutes. In addition, some special diet products, such as low-sodium bouillon cubes, catsup, and mustard, are available. Examples of the use of some of these seasonings are:

1. Use dry mustard, cornstarch, and vinegar to prepare a mustard sandwich spread
2. Serve a fruit sauce with meat
3. Add sugar, honey, or fresh fruit to cooked cereal
4. Add a small amount of sugar to cooked vegetables, such as green beans or tomatoes, to bring out the natural flavor
5. Use an acidic food, such as vinegar, lemon juice, or low-sodium tomato juice, to replace commercial meat tenderizer

6. Serve low-sodium milk icy cold or with nutmeg, cinnamon, or chocolate

Salt substitutes consist chemically of potassium or ammonium chloride. Since potassium may be contraindicated in renal disease and ammonium in hepatic disease, salt substitutes should be used only by prescription from a physician. In this case, they may be used in cooking or for seasoning at the table; however, they do not taste like salt. Some clients enjoy them, and others find the taste unsatisfactory. They should be used sparingly, seasoning small amounts of food at one time, since too much makes the food taste bitter. Seasoned salt substitutes are available and preferred by some clients. Another product sometimes confused with salt substitutes is Lite Salt. This substance contains approximately one-half the sodium of table salt but should not be used unless it has been planned in the diet.

The American Heart Association has published booklets (and leaflets in a more simplified form) describing sodium-restricted diets at three levels of restriction—500 mg, 1000 mg, and mild sodium restriction. These teaching materials can be obtained from local chapters of the American Heart Association. Many low-sodium cookbooks are available; also consult with a dietitian–nutritionist for suggestions for altering recipes from basic cookbooks so that they can be used in the diet.

ANGINA PECTORIS, MYOCARDIAL INFARCTION, AND CONGESTIVE HEART FAILURE

Assessment

Acute manifestations of cardiovascular disease are angina pectoris, acute myocardial infarction, and congestive heart failure. Each of these entities necessitates dietary modifications.

▶   **Angina pectoris** is a symptom complex that is a common warning signal of coronary heart disease. The symptoms, which include acute substernal chest pain, usually with a characteristic radiation to the left arm, result from a transient ischemic deprivation of the blood flow to the myocardium. Atheromatous lesions in the coronary arteries impede coronary blood flow and diminish the blood supply to the heart. Symptoms may be precipitated by physical exercise or other exertion that increases the oxygen requirements of the heart.

   Heart failure may result from a defect in the heart itself (myocardial infarction) or from circulatory congestion because of abnormal retention of sodium and water (congestive heart failure). Myocardial infarction is a syndrome characterized by permanent damage to a portion of the myocardium due to sudden, overwhelming ischemia secondary to a complete obstruction of one of the branches of an atherosclerotic coronary artery. This total permanent deprivation of the blood supply is in contrast to the transient diminished blood flow that is characteristic of angina pectoris. The severity of the heart attack is related to the site and extent of the obstruction, the degree of collateral circulation established, and the condition of the myocardium itself. The syndrome is accompanied by severe chest pain, dyspnea, sweating, and weakness. Arrhythmias, shock, cardiac failure, and death may ensue.

▶   **Congestive heart failure** (CHF), which may be acute or chronic, compensated or decompensated, left-sided or right-sided, results from congestion of the pulmonary or systemic circulation with an abnormal amount of blood. In CHF, the weakened myocardium fails to maintain a cardiac output sufficient to propel blood through the circulatory system. In order to maintain an adequate cardiac output, the heart compensates by increasing both its size (cardiomegaly) and its rate (tachycardia). Acute CHF results from a sudden, severe insult, such as myocardial infarction, whereas chronic CHF develops over a long period of time. Chronic CHF can occur in all forms of heart disease, including ischemic, hypertensive, rheumatic, or congenital heart disease. If compensatory mechanisms are adequate (compensated heart disease), the organ is able to maintain an almost normal circulation. However, in decompensated heart disease, compensatory mechanisms are insufficient to maintain normal circulation. Cardiac output falls, renal blood flow is decreased, and sodium and water are retained in abnormal amounts (edema).

   CHF may be left-sided (left ventricular failure) or right-sided (right ventricular failure). Both may coexist in the same individual. The diminished cardiac output results in a diminished venous return, leading to venous stasis and an increase in venous pressure in the weakened side of the heart, either right or left. It also results in a decrease in the renal blood flow, leading to a decrease in glomerular filtration and excretion of sodium, an increase in hormonal stimulation and secretion of renin, and consequent retention of sodium and water in the body. Left ventricular failure produces acute pulmonary edema, cyanosis, and dyspnea. In contrast, right ventricular failure produces systemic edema, hepatomegaly, ascites, and hydrothorax (fluid in the pleural cavity).

Intervention

Assist clients with angina pectoris to plan fat-controlled diets at a kilocaloric level that will achieve recommended body weight and to consume small, frequent meals. In the case of surgical intervention to bypass the occluded vessels, these same dietary considerations are necessary after the surgery to forestall recurrence and progression of coronary arterial disease.

   Base the nursing care plan for clients with acute cardiac conditions, such as myocardial infarction, cardiac surgery, and acute congestive heart failure, on these objectives: (1) provide maximum rest for the heart, (2) prevent or eliminate edema, and (3) provide the minimum nutritional requirements. Since weight reduction in obese clients decreases metabolic demands and thus the cardiac work load, stress to obese clients the importance of reducing body weight. Some physicians advocate a mild degree of weight loss even with normal weight. For obese clients at bedrest, a diet that provides 1000 to 1200 kcal is usually sufficient to bring about weight loss. During periods of stress, such as that imposed by congestive heart failure, providing nutritionally adequate amounts of kilocalories, protein, vitamins, and minerals is desirable but often impossible because of anorexia and use of restricted diets. Provide vitamin and mineral supplements and use foods of high kilocalorie content, such as concentrated carbohydrates. Avoid foods high in fat, however, because of their possible role in atherogenesis. Clients with well-compensated heart disease should be told that diet modifications are not usually necessary other than attention to avoiding obesity. Mild sodium restriction may be necessary in order to avoid edema, however.

   Clients who have suffered a myocardial infarction are at a high risk for developing arrhythmias, heart failure, and cardiogenic shock. Anticipate the following metabolic response in these clients, although it varies from individual to individual and may be influenced by such factors as nutritional status, related clinical problems, and associated drug therapy:

- Reduced cardiac output
- Hypotension
- Lactic acidosis (the severity of which appears related to mortality associated with hypotension and arrhythmias)
- Increased secretion of epinephrine, norepinephrine, and cortisol
- Suppression of insulin secretion

- Elevated plasma glucose
- Elevated free fatty acids in the plasma, which may lead to arrhythmias

Consider the following aspects of nutritional therapy during the period following an infarction (which is at present based on limited research data): (1) timing of initiation of oral feeding, (2) consistency of food served, (3) size, frequency, and temperature of meals served, (4) use of stimulants (e.g., caffeine), and (5) restriction of sodium and fat. These are summarized in Table 29–18.

Some authorities advocate a period of undernutrition during the first few days after a heart attack.[27] The goal is to provide kilocalories sufficient to meet basic metabolic requirements and to provide as optimal a level of essential nutrients as is possible without causing an increase in oxygen uptake. The kilocalorie level recommended during the period is 800 to 1200, with the kilocalories increased gradually according to client progress. Higher kilocaloric intake is usually limited to those who have passed the acute stage and who do not require a lower kilocalorie regimen because of obesity, hyperlipoproteinemia, or diabetes mellitus. Monitor the daily intake of kilocalories carefully, however. An adequate supply of glucose is essential, since there is a preferential oxidation of glucose instead of free fatty acids as the energy source immediately postmyocardial infarction.

A liquid diet is thought to be better tolerated by the client who may be nauseated and whose condition may be complicated by heart failure, shock, severe pain, or arrhythmias. In addition, liquids may reduce gagging (gagging could induce a vasovagal response and lead to arrhythmia and cardiac arrest) or the likelihood of vomiting and aspiration pneumonia. Since typical clear liquid diets provide only about 500 to 600 kcal/day and a source of glucose is critical, some feel that kilocaloric intake should be maintained without regard to consistency.

Small feedings given at frequent intervals are advocated (e.g., six small feedings). This is important to reduce the need for the splanchnic circulation (which serves the stomach, intestines, liver, and spleen) to allow for digestion and absorption. Assess the client's intolerances for specific foods, such as those that cause gas, in order to avoid unnecessary diet restrictions, and take measures to prevent constipation if at all possible. Although research data on the effect of food temperature on the cardiac client are sparse and conflicting, avoidance of temperature extremes in food is often advocated as a measure to prevent arrhythmias.

Xanthine-containing foods and beverages—caffeine, theophylline, and theobromine are examples of methylated xanthines—act as stimulants to the central nervous system and cardiac muscle. Although opinions vary about the use of coffee and other xanthine-containing beverages, these beverages exhibit certain metabolic properties that make it prudent to limit their use in the acute stages when metabolism is altered. Xanthines stimulate the release of catecholamines from the adrenal medulla,

---

TABLE 29–18
SUMMARY OF DIET MODIFICATIONS POSTMYOCARDIAL INFARCTION

Timing of initiation of oral feeding	NPO until evaluated by the physician
Consistency of food served	Liquids, such as clear broth, clear soups, skim milk, tea, ginger ale, and water during the first 24 hours, followed by a soft diet
Size, frequency, and temperature of foods	Small, frequent feedings: initially, provide a daily volume of 1000–1500 ml that contains 500–800 kcal and give only a small amount of liquid at one time; when soft feedings are initiated, provide no more than 1½ c of fluids with meals and avoid foods that are bulky, irritating, or gasforming to prevent gastric distention and stimulation of reflexes that could produce arrhythmias; avoid icy foods and allow hot foods to cool before eating
Use of stimulants	Eliminate xanthine-containing foods or beverages (xanthine in coffee, tea, and cola drinks; theophylline in tea; and theobromine in chocolate and cocoa) initially and add in moderate amounts during the convalescent period; substitute decaffeinated beverages, cereal-based beverages, ginger ale, and other noncola drinks
Sodium content	Restrict only in the presence of CHF or pulmonary edema
Fat content	Maintain fat-controlled diet

and catecholamines in turn cause a rise in the plasma free fatty acid levels. It is hypothesized that the elevation of free fatty acids in the plasma may account for arrhythmias. Most arrhythmias occur within 48 hours after a myocardial infarction. It is postulated that caffeine may decrease the binding of calcium by the cell membrane and thus induce ventricular fibrillation by affecting the action potential.

Individualize the sodium content of the diet to the client's specific condition and avoid routine sodium restriction. The client with a myocardial infarction may become sodium deficient because of sodium losses in conjunction with diaphoresis (profuse sweating) and vomiting and disturbed renal tubular function leading to sodium loss. Moreover, shock can be precipitated or aggravated by sodium restriction. Since many clients who experience a myocardial infarction may be following a fat-controlled diet, it is well to maintain a consistent dietary approach.

Advise the client not to eat when upset or under stress because at these times there may be insufficient blood in the digestive organs for efficient digestion. As soon as possible after admission, ascertain food likes, dislikes, and specific intolerances from a relative or close friend. Promptly explain all dietary modifications. Written as well as verbal explanations may be necessary because the client may be preoccupied at the time of verbal explanation. Allow clients to feed themselves unless they are physically handicapped.

Anticoagulants, such as heparin, warfarin, and dicumarol, are often used to prevent clot formation in the client with an infarction. With anticoagulant therapy (especially with dicumarol), monitor the intake of vitamin K in the diet or in supplements. Vitamin K promotes blood clotting by prompting hepatic synthesis of prothrombin. Food sources of vitamin K are listed in Chapter 9.

For clients with acute CHF, restrict sodium intake to aid in preventing or eliminating edema, and provide foods that are easy to chew and digest. The dietary sodium intake may range from 250 mg (10 mEq) to 1000 mg (40 mEq). As the edema is eliminated, an intake of 1000 mg or more may be satisfactory. Assess for an associated renal disease with inability to reabsorb sodium normally (salt wasting), and in its presence avoid severe sodium restriction to prevent sodium depletion.

If renal function is normal and sodium intake is restricted, fluid restriction is unnecessary. Provision of 2000 to 3000 ml of fluid daily may lessen the renal workload in excreting wastes and may even enhance diuresis. With dilutional hyponatremia (a low serum sodium level with an associated increase in total body water content), restrict fluid intake rather than increase the sodium intake. Dilutional hyponatremia may result from hormonal imbalance, severe sodium restriction, or excessive use of diuretics and leads to refractoriness to diuretic therapy. With fluid restriction, consider those foods that are liquid at room temperature (e.g., gruel, ice cream, and Jello) or high in water content (e.g., fresh fruits) as part of the total fluid allowance.

Dyspnea and chewing are incompatible in the client with severe CHF, since mouth breathing may be necessary. Therefore, provide liquid or soft foods that require little chewing in the initial diet. To prevent exertion, to decrease the cardiac workload, and to decrease abdominal distention, provide small, frequent feedings of nongasforming foods. To avoid constipation, the judicious use of foods with laxative properties (e.g., prune juice, raisins, apricots, and foods with fiber, such as fruits, vegetables, and whole grain bread and cereal) is recommended. Proper positioning for eating is important, and the client should eat or be fed slowly to prevent aspiration.

Malnutrition is not uncommon in clients with advanced cardiac disease because of poor circulation of nutrients to the tissues. Weight loss may be masked by edema; the face may be puffy and the extremities edematous. Record weight daily before and during treatment to serve as an index of fluid loss and to establish the client's dry weight to serve as a baseline for nutritional care.

RHEUMATIC HEART DISEASE AND CONGENITAL HEART DISEASE

Rheumatic heart disease and congenital heart disease are both relatively common entities. **Rheumatic heart disease** results from inflammation of the heart valves and heart muscle secondary to rheumatic fever. Rheumatic fever is one of the leading causes of chronic illness in children and is the commonest cause of heart disease in persons under age 50. Rheumatic heart disease ranks third (behind hypertension and coronary heart disease) in overall incidence of heart disease. Congenital heart disease accounts for approximately 12 percent of the major congenital anomalies found in newborns and for about 2 percent of all heart disease in adults.

Rheumatic Heart Disease

Assessment. Rheumatic fever is an inflammatory disease initiated by infection with group A β-hemolytic *Streptococcus*. The disease may be self-limiting or lead to slowly progressing cardiac valvular deformity. Rheumatic fever is the major cause of valvular heart disease. Acute rheumatic fever may be complicated by myocarditis, pericarditis, or pulmonary embolism. Chronic rheumatic heart disease results from single or repeated episodes of rheumatic fever.

The complications of rheumatic heart disease may be congestive heart failure, arrhythmias, hypertension, obesity, subacute bacterial endocarditis, and atherosclerosis. Treatment is governed by the symptoms and complications and is medical, nutritional, or surgical.

Intervention. Nutritional therapy for rheumatic fever is directed toward (1) providing a nutritionally adequate diet, (2) replenishing nutrient stores, and (3) compensating for losses imposed by the stress of illness and elevated body temperature. Bedrest is required until all signs of active infection have disappeared. With corticosteroid therapy, mild sodium restriction may be necessary to prevent edema. Assist the client to develop patterns of eating that serve to maintain recommended body weight and limit sodium intake. By doing so, it will be easier to deal with complications that may arise in later years when habit changes are more difficult.

Congenital Heart Disease

Assessment. Congenital anomalies of the heart and great vessels, which include such conditions as atrial or ventricular septal defect, coarctation of the aorta, transposition of the great vessels, tetralogy of Fallot, and aortic stenosis, result from arrested or defective prenatal development. The conditions may or may not be detected at birth. The lesions may occur in isolation or as part of multiple structural or physiologic abnormalities. In many cases the causative factors are unknown and are probably multiple, involving both genetic and environmental factors that to date have not been well identified. One known causative factor is maternal rubella, which results in a specific syndrome. Prevention of rubella with vaccine prior to the first trimester of pregnancy is an important preventive measure. Based on animal experiments, maternal dietary deficiency has been suggested as a cause, although no significant evidence of such a causal relationship has been shown in humans.

Clients are subject to various complications, such as congestive heart failure, cyanosis, arrhythmias, pulmonary hypertension, bacterial endocarditis, recurrent infections, and growth retardation. Treatment is primarily surgical. Medical management is directed toward prevention and treatment of complications. Newer surgical techniques have dramatically improved the extended outlook for some individuals with cardiac abnormalities, and thus the incentive is great to provide meticulous management. Surgical intervention is technically easier in a larger child, and the current trend is to apply corrective surgery at the age of 12 to 15 months.

The majority of infants who require hospitalization in the first month of life are full term, and, thus, they do not have the complicating factors associated with prematurity. Further, most of the infants are of appropriate size at birth. Growth failure is a recurrent problem, and the severity of the growth impairment is related to the hemodynamic effect of the cardiac lesion. In those with mild symptoms of heart disease, normal growth may occur. Though a number of hypotheses have been proposed

to explain the growth retardation, in many instances it is clearly related to inadequate kilocalorie intake. Rapid fatigue while feeding and labored respiration leading to difficulty in swallowing often result in a decreased volume of food consumed. Assess for inadequate nutrition, particularly in clients with chronic hypoxia, acidosis, pulmonary hypertension, and repeated infection. Increased metabolic requirements and deficient gastrointestinal absorption are further complications of congestive heart failure. With congestive failure, evaporative losses and oxygen consumption are increased. Sodium restriction and use of diuretics to treat congestive failure may create additional dietary inadequacy in the child already consuming an inadequate intake.

Intervention. Nutritional management[28] involves providing sufficient kilocalories and other nutrients and maintaining fluid and electrolyte balance in a manner that does not stress the precarious fluid balance. Select formulas and foods other than formula on the basis of kilocaloric density, sodium content, renal solute load, and digestibility. Explain to parents the difference between their infant's condition and adult atherosclerotic disease to avoid their inappropriately limiting the child's intake of fat and cholesterol by using skim or low-fat milk and avoiding eggs and visible fats.

The kilocaloric requirement per kilogram of body weight is greater in those who fail to thrive than in normal infants of the same age. The increased kilocaloric requirement and small volume of formula that the infant is able to take (many under 1 year of age can take only 450 ml per day) necessitate a formula of high kilocaloric density. The kilocaloric content of commercial formulas can be manipulated by adding carbohydrate (such as Karo syrup or Polycose, Ross Labs) and fat (such as MCT oil, Mead Johnson). See Table 29–19 for a summary of feeding techniques.

When carbohydrate or fat is added to formula or other foods, however, assess carefully to determine the child's ability to tolerate increasing levels of carbohydrate without developing diarrhea or increasing levels of fat without developing ketoacidosis or steatorrhea. When semisolids are added, assure that 8 to 10 percent of total kilocalories is provided by high-quality protein.

The digestibility of the foods served also merits consideration. Medium-chain triglycerides are easily digested and absorbed and should be used in the early months. Fruits are readily digested and should be the first type of semisolid food offered. Cereal should be reserved for older infants who can better digest starchy foods.

The renal solute load and sodium and potassium balance are important considerations in maintaining fluid and electrolyte balance when giving concentrated foods. Assess urine osmolality to monitor the renal solute load. If an increase in kilocaloric density of commercial formula is achieved by adding less

---

TABLE 29–19
FEEDING TECHNIQUES FOR INFANTS WITH CONGENITAL HEART DEFECTS

Kilocaloric requirement	120–135 kcal/kg daily; some infants may require up to 150–175 kcal/kg to maintain sustained growth
Techniques to increase kilocaloric density of the infant's diet before solid food additions	Add sufficient carbohydrate and fat to commercial premature formulas to increase kilocaloric density from the usual 24 kcal/oz to 30 kcal/oz; addition of these ingredients to standard formulas that contain 20 kcal/oz may excessively dilute the protein content
Techniques to increase kilocaloric density of the infant's diet after solid food additions	When solid foods containing carbohydrate and fat are being consumed, eliminate these additives from the formula and increase kilocaloric density of the diet in either of two ways: (1) add sugar and oil to solid foods such as cereal and fruit or (2) increase the kilocaloric density of standard commercial formula from 20 kcal/oz to 30 kcal/oz by diluting the concentrated liquid formula with half the usual amount of water
Digestibility of foods	Use easily digested foods, such as MCT oil and fruits
Renal solute load	Provide sufficient water to counteract a high renal solute load as evidenced by a high urine osmolality; limit meat in the diet to no more than 1 oz, or eliminate it when fluid balance is precarious, otherwise allow meat in the diet of older infants to provide protein and essential electrolytes
Sodium and potassium balance	Avoid both deficits and excesses of sodium; provide potassium supplements when diuretics are used
Other nutrients	Supplement the diet with multivitamins, calcium, iron, and folic acid to compensate for the infant's limited intake

---

water to commercial concentrates, this may precipitously increase the renal solute load and be hazardous for the infant who has excessive water losses from diarrhea or vomiting. Provide sufficient fluid to allow for the excretion of those nutrients not used for growth.

Sodium balance presents several problems: on the one hand, sodium is an essential nutrient for growth; on the other hand, sodium excess may precipitate congestive heart failure or lead to an excessively high renal solute load. Low-sodium formulas are available (SMA, Wyeth Labs, and PM 60/40, Ross Labs). However, these formulas may provide an insufficient amount of sodium for growth and obligatory losses because of the small volume of formula that may be taken. Moreover, the addition of pure fat or carbohydrate to the formula or solid foods supplies energy with only a trace amount of electrolytes. Low-sodium formulas are reserved for periods of severe cardiac failure or for the infant who is particularly sensitive to sodium. Standard formulas may be used and solid foods of high sodium content avoided.

Hypokalemia may occur secondary to the use of diuretics to control congestive heart failure and may lead to diminished renal tubular concentrating capacity as well as a predisposition to digitalis toxicity. Potassium supplementation should be considered with regular use of diuretics.

Be sensitive to parental anxiety about feeding. Anxious parents may equate food intake with the child's survival. Assure them that limited amounts of solid foods can be introduced at the appropriate ages, although the volume of solids may need to be limited to avoid diluting the dietary protein intake to below acceptable levels. The psychologic ramifications of congenital heart disease are numerous. For example, it may be difficult for parents of a child who becomes cyanotic with prolonged crying to set limits on behavior. Provide anticipatory guidance regarding mealtime management to all parents of children with congenital defects. Assist them with selecting and preparing a formula or diet that is adequate in kilocalories and protein, that is easily digested, and that does not bring an excessive solute load. Also stress the importance of taking the prescribed supplements. Explain to the parents what constitutes normal feeding behavior and encourage them to use a consistent approach.

REVIEW QUESTIONS AND ACTIVITIES

1. Identify the two lipids whose elevation is most commonly associated with atherosclerosis.
2. Identify the major lipid transported by each of the four major classes of lipoproteins.
3. Identify the upper limits of normal for blood cholesterol and blood triglyceride.
4. Compare the use of the serum level of cholesterol and triglyceride as indicators of risk of developing coronary heart disease.
5. Differentiate among elevated blood levels of LDL (low-density lipoprotein), VLDL (very low-density lipoprotein), and HDL (high-density lipoprotein) as predictors of risk of developing coronary heart disease.
6. Discuss the relationship between excessive amounts of saturated fat, cholesterol, sucrose, alcohol, and kilocalories and the blood level of lipids and lipoproteins, and compare these effects with that of polyunsaturated fat.
7. Identify the effect of each of the following on the blood level of HDL: (a) cigarette smoking, (b) alcohol, (c) physical activity, and (d) body weight.
8. Identify the following in relation to hyperlipoproteinemia: (a) the six major types, and (b) the three types that are both common and associated with premature atherosclerosis.
9. Identify specific lipids that are elevated and appropriate diet modifications for each of the following types of hyperlipoproteinemia: type IIa, type IIb, and type IV.
10. Select appropriate foods for use by clients who are following a fat-controlled diet to reduce the blood level of cholesterol.
11. Discuss the relationship between sodium intake and obesity in the etiology of hypertension.
12. Identify three mineral elements that may play a protective role in preventing hypertension.
13. Discuss the role of diet modification in the treatment of hypertension.
14. Differentiate among four levels of sodium restriction as classified by the American Heart Association.
15. List five examples of foods that contain significant amounts of sodium in each of the following categories: (a) foods that contain relatively large amounts of added sodium, (b) foods that contain smaller but significant amounts of added sodium, and (c) foods that are naturally high in sodium.
16. List dietary adjustments that are necessary in order to plan a mild (85 mEq) and a moderate (40 mEq) sodium-restricted diet.
17. Plan a day's menu that contains approximately 85 mEq sodium and adjust the menu to contain only 40 mEq sodium.
18. Describe suitable adjustments in food preparation methods for sodium-restricted diets.
19. List foods that may present problems in planning sodium-restricted diets for Jewish clients (see Chap. 19 for Jewish dietary patterns).
20. Compare and contrast the nutritional care for clients with angina, myocardial infarction, and congestive heart failure.
21. Describe the dietary management of rheumatic fever.
22. Identify techniques for supplying an adequate intake of calories and nutrients for an infant with a congenital heart defect.

REFERENCES

1. McGill HC: Appraisal of cholesterol as a causative factor in atherosclerosis. Am J Clin Nutr 32 [Suppl]:2632, 1979.
2. Glueck CJ: Appraisal of saturated fat as a causative factor in atherosclerosis. Am J Clin Nutr 32 [Suppl]:2637, 1979.
3. McGill HC: The relationship of dietary cholesterol to serum cholesterol concentration and to atherosclerosis in man. Am J Clin Nutr 32 [Suppl]:2664, 1979.
4. National Research Council: Toward Healthful Diets, Washington, DC, National Academy of Sciences, 1980, p 11.
5. Story JA: Dietary carbohydrate and atherosclerosis. Fed Proc 41:2797, 1982.
6. Spritz N: Appraisal of alcohol consumption as a causative factor in liver disease and atherosclerosis. Am J Clin Nutr 32 [Suppl]:2655, 1979.
7. Carroll KK: Hypercholesterolemia and atherosclerosis: Effects of dietary protein. Fed Proc 41:2792, 1982.
8. Thelle DS, Arnesen E, Forde OH: The Tromso heart study. Does coffee raise serum cholesterol? N Engl J Med 308:1454, 1983.
9. Gotto AM: Is atherosclerosis reversible? J Am Diet Assoc 74:551, 1979.
10. The Lipid Research Clinic Program: The Lipid Research Clinic's coronary primary prevention program results: I. Reduction in incidence of coronary heart disease. JAMA 251:351, 1984.
11. The Lipid Research Clinic Program: The Lipid Research Clinic's coronary primary prevention program results: II. The relationship of reduction in incidence of coronary heart disease to cholesterol lowering. JAMA 251:365, 1984.
12. Hulley SB, Rosenman RH, Bawol RD, Brand RJ: Epidemiology as a guide to clinical decisions—The association between triglyceride and heart disease. New Eng J Med 302:1383, 1980.

13. Kannel WB: Status of coronary heart disease risk factors. J Nutr Educ 10:10, 1978.
14. National Institutes of Health Consensus Development Conference Statement: Lowering blood cholesterol. Nutr Today 20:13, 1985.
15. U.S. DHEW: The Dietary Management of Hyperlipoproteinemia: A Handbook for Physicians and Dietitians. DHEW Publication No. (NIH) 80–110, Bethesda, Md, National Heart, Lung, and Blood Institute, 1980, p viii.
16. Is reduction of blood cholesterol effective? Lancet 1:317, 1984.
17. Multiple Risk Factor Intervention Trial Research Group: Multiple risk factor intervention trial. JAMA 248:1465, 1982.
18. Kannel WB: Role of blood pressure in cardiovascular disease: The Framingham Study. Angiology 26:1, 1975.
19. Parfrey PS, Vandenburg MJ, Wright P, et al.: Blood pressure and hormonal changes following alteration in dietary sodium and potassium in mild essential hypertension. Lancet 1:59, 1981.
20. MacGregor GA, Smith SJ, Markandu ND, et al.: Moderate potassium supplementation in essential hypertension. Lancet 2:567, 1982.
21. Burstyn P, Hornall D, Watchorn C: Sodium and potassium intake and blood pressure. Br Med J 281:537, 1980.
22. Belizan JM, Villar J, Pineda O, et al.: Reduction of blood pressure with calcium supplements in young adults. JAMA 249:1161, 1983.
23. Neri LC, Johansen HL: Water hardness and cardiovascular mortality. Ann NY Acad Sci 304:203, 1978.
24. Iacono JM, Judd JT, Marshall MW, et al.: The role of dietary essential fatty acids and prostaglandins in reducing blood pressure. Prog Lipid Res 20:349, 1981.
25. Rouse IL, Beilin LJ, Armstrong BK, Vandongen R: Blood-pressure-lowering effect of a vegetarian diet: Controlled trial in normotensive subjects. Lancet 1:5, 1983.
26. Arkwright PD, Beilin LJ, Rouse J, et al.: Effects of alcohol use and other aspects of lifestyle on blood pressure levels and prevalence of hypertension in a working population. Circulation 66:60, 1982.
27. Hemzacek KI: Dietary protocol for the patient who has suffered a myocardial infarction. J Am Diet Assoc 72:112, 1978.
28. Rickard K, Brady S, Gresham EL: Nutritional management of the chronically ill child. Pediatr Clin North Am 24:158, 1977.

Ellison RC, Newburger JW, Gross DM: Pediatric aspects of essential hypertension. J Am Diet Assoc 80:21, 1982.
Freeland-Graves JH, Friedman BH, Han WH, et al.: Effect of zinc supplementation on plasma high-density lipoprotein cholesterol and zinc. Am J Clin Nutr 35:988, 1982.
Frohlich ED: Physiological observations in essential hypertension. J Am Diet Assoc 80:18, 1982.
Harper AE: Coronary heart disease—An epidemic related to diet? Am J Clin Nutr 37:669, 1983.
Holden RA, Ostfeld AM, Freeman DH Jr, et al.: Dietary salt intake and blood pressure. JAMA 250:365, 1983.
Hofman A, Hazebroek A, Valkenbrug HA: A randomized trial of sodium intake and blood pressure in newborn infants. JAMA 250:370, 1983.
The Joint National Committee on Detection, Evaluation, and Treatment of High Blood Pressure: The 1984 report of the Joint National Committee on Detection, Evaluation, and Treatment of High Blood Pressure. Arch Int Med 144:1045, 1984.
Kritchevsky D: Trans fatty acid effects in experimental atherosclerosis. Fed Proc 41:2813, 1982.
Kumar MR: Nutritional management of the cardiac transplant patient. J Am Diet Assoc 83:463, 1983.
Lewis C: Proteins and Carbohydrates, Lipids. Philadelphia, FA Davis, 1976.
Lewis C: Vitamins and Minerals, Sodium and Potassium. Philadelphia, FA Davis, 1976.
March AC, Koons PC: The sodium and potassium content of selected vegetables. J Am Diet Assoc 88:24, 1983.
McCarron DA, Kotchen TA: Nutrition and blood pressure control: Current status of dietary factors and hypertension. Ann Intern Med 98:697, 1983.
Puska P, Iacono JM, Nissinsen A, et al.: Controlled randomized trial of the effect of dietary fat on blood pressure, Lancet 1:8314, 1983.
Thompson LU, Jenkins DJA, Amer MAV, et al.: The effect of fermented and unfermented milk on serum cholesterol. Am J Clin Nutr 36 [Suppl]:1106, 1982.
Thuesen L, Nielson TT, Thomassen A, et al.: Beneficial effect of a low-fat, low-calorie diet on myocardial energy metabolism in patients with angina pectoris. Lancet 2:59, 1984.
Treatment of hypertriglyceridemia. JAMA 251:1196, 1984.
USDHHS: Report of the Working Group on Critical Patient Behaviors in the Dietary Management of High Blood Pressure. NIH Publication No. 81–2269, Bethesda, Md, 1981.
Vermeulen RT, Sedor FA, Kimm SYS: Effect of water rinsing on sodium content of selected foods. J Am Diet Assoc 82:394, 1983.
Voors AW: Relation between ingested potassium and sodium balance in young blacks and whites. Am J Clin Nutr 37:583, 1983.

BIBLIOGRAPHY

Ackley S, Barrett-Connen E, Suarez L: Dairy products, calcium, and blood pressure. Am J Clin Nutr 38:457, 1983.
Bordia A: Effect of garlic on blood lipids in patients with coronary heart disease. Am J Clin Nutr 34:2100, 1981.
Circulating cholesterol level and risk of death from cancer in men aged 40 to 69 years. JAMA 248:2853, 1982.
Clifford AJ, Ho CY, Swenerton H: Homogenized bovine milk zanthine oxidase: A critique of the hypothesis relating to plasmologen depletion and cardiovascular disease. Am J Clin Nutr 38:327, 1983.

CLIENT RESOURCES

American Heart Association: Cooking Without Your Salt Shaker. Dallas, American Heart Association National Center, 1978.
From the American Heart Association, New York, NY:
  1. Planning Fat-controlled Meals for 1200 and 1800 Calories
  2. Planning Fat-controlled Meals for Approximately 2000–2600 Calories

3. Programmed Instruction for Fat-controlled Diet, 1800 Calories

Bagg E: Cooking Without a Grain of Salt. Garden City, NJ, Doubleday and Co., 1964.

Eshleman R, and Winston M: The American Heart Association Cookbook. New York, David McKay Co., 1979.

From the National Institutes of Health, Bethesda, Md:
1. Diet 1 for Dietary Management of Hyperchylomicronemia (Type 1 Hyperlipoproteinemia), 1978
2. Diet 2 for Dietary Management of Hypercholesterolemia (Type IIa Hyperlipoproteinemia), 1978
3. Diet 3 for Dietary Management of Hypercholesterolemia with Endogenous Hypertriglyceridemia (Type IIb or Type III Hyperlipoproteinemia), 1978
4. Diet 4 for Dietary Management of Endogenous Hypertriglyceridemia (Type IV Hyperlipoproteinemia), 1983
5. Diet 5 for Dietary Management of Mixed Hypertriglyceridemia (Type V Hyperlipoproteinemia), 1981

U.S. Department of Agriculture: The Sodium Content of Your Food. Home and Garden Bulletin No. 233, August 1980.

CHAPTER 30

Nutrition and Renal Disorders

Objectives

After completion of this chapter, the student will be able to:

1. Distinguish between the clinical manifestations of acute and chronic renal failure.

2. Develop a nursing care plan for the nutritional management of a client with chronic renal failure (without dialysis) and adjust the plan to make it appropriate for a client with acute renal failure and for a client on maintenance dialysis.

3. Compare and contrast the dietary modifications necessitated by maintenance dialysis and posttransplant.

4. Plan the diet for a client with the nephrotic syndrome.

5. Develop a nursing care plan for the nutritional management of a client during all stages of acute glomerulonephritis.

6. Compare and contrast the dietary modifications for the four major types of renal calculi that may respond to dietary management.

A wide variety of acute and chronic renal disorders exist, and their causes are both varied and complex. The chronic disorders are most common. Treatment of renal disorders includes conservative medical management (drugs and diet modification) alone or drugs and diet therapy combined with dialysis and transplantation. Most clients with chronic renal disease begin with conservative medical management, but most progress to a program of maintenance dialysis, the cost of which is now borne by the Social Security Medicare program. Advances in surgery and immunosuppression have made transplantation an acceptable form of treatment for those in the terminal phases of the disease, and the number of individuals with a kidney transplant is thus increasing.

Even with the development of newer methods of treatment, however, dietary modifications and nutritional support continue to be an important part of a long-range control program. Diet modifications may serve as a moderate-term substitute for maintenance dialysis in selected individuals in whom the remaining renal function does not deteriorate rapidly. Diet therapy is an important adjunct to treatment for those undergoing dialysis or receiving a transplant. Indeed, much of the clinical success of dialysis depends upon following the prescribed dietary regimen. Finally, diet therapy serves as a major treatment modality in those for whom dialysis or transplant is not feasible. Like other forms of treatment, diet does not cure renal disease. Rather it serves only to control the disorder by ameliorating the systemic abnormalities that result from accumulation of toxic products.

This chapter focuses on the nutritional management of acute and chronic renal diseases. A brief review of normal kidney function and the changes that occur when the kidneys are diseased is included.

455

NORMAL AND ABNORMAL RENAL FUNCTION

Assessment

The kidneys are composed of roughly 2 million functioning units (nephrons) whose chief functions are classified as excretory, regulatory, and endocrine. These functions are summarized below (a diagram of the kidney and a discussion of the processes of excretion, secretion, and reabsorption are found in Figure 10–1).

- *Excretory.* Excretes the waste products of metabolism (i.e., nitrogenous products—urea, uric acid, and creatinine—sulfate, phosphate, and organic acids), drugs, and potentially toxic substances
- *Regulatory.* Maintains the volume and composition of body fluids by selectively excreting, secreting, and reabsorbing substances as the filtrate passes from the glomerulus to the collecting ducts and by conserving essential substances, such as glucose and amino acids
- *Endocrine.* Secretes renin, which aids in controlling blood pressure (renin stimulates the production of angiotensin, which is a potent vasoconstrictor; angiotensin also stimulates the release of aldosterone from the adrenal cortex, which increases blood volume by stimulating the retention of sodium and water); secretes erythropoietin, which stimulates the production of red blood cells by the bone marrow, stimulates the production of the active form of vitamin D (calcitriol or 1,25-dihydroxyvitamin D_3) and thus maintains calcium–phosphorus–bone homeostasis

The healthy kidney filters approximately 120 ml fluid per minute (or approximately 180 to 200 liters in 24 hours). Most of this filtrate is reabsorbed, and the normal urine output is 1 to 2 liters per day in adults. The urine has the following approximate composition:

Water	95 percent
Solutes	5 percent (nitrogenous substances, 60 percent; inorganic salts, 40 percent)

The composition of the final urine is dependent on the secretion of several hormones that regulate the secretion and reabsorption of substances: aldosterone, which stimulates the reabsorption of sodium (in exchange for potassium or hydrogen), antidiuretic hormone (ADH), which stimulates water reabsorption in the collecting duct, and parathyroid hormone, which stimulates calcium reabsorption and phosphate excretion.

The major nitrogenous component of urine is urea, and uric acid, creatinine, and ammonia are present in small amounts. The concentration of urea depends on the client's level of dietary protein and ▶

energy intake. A diet high in protein, one that contains large quantities of protein of low biologic value, or that is low in energy increases the urea level. Conversely, clients with a low protein intake excrete lesser amounts of urea. Clients who experience endogenous tissue catabolism have a higher urinary urea concentration as well as a higher concentration of creatinine—the breakdown product of creatine–phosphate found in muscle tissue. The amount of creatinine excreted is proportional to the muscle mass and is not altered by the diet under normal circumstances. Sodium chloride is the predominant inorganic salt excreted. Phosphate and sulfate salts of calcium, sodium, potassium, and magnesium are excreted in smaller amounts.

The kidneys have a remarkable reserve capacity. The nephrons function independently, and healthy nephrons can compensate for those that fail by hypertrophy and a consequent increase in their efficiency. Moreover, during the slow development of chronic renal failure, the body tissues are continuously bathed in an abnormal fluid and in many cases appear to have adapted to the altered environment. The reserve capacity of the kidney enables it to maintain homeostasis until approximately 75 to 80 percent of the nephrons are destroyed (minimal excretory capacity is even maintained until only about 10 percent of functioning kidney tissue remains). At this point, however, both excretory and regulatory functions are severely compromised, and waste products accumulate in the tissues and blood—a condition called **uremia.** Uremia is the final common pathway of chronic, progressive renal disease.

Once the residual function approaches about 3 percent of normal (a creatinine clearance below 5 ml/minute), the client must begin dialysis or have a renal transplant to maintain life. In clients with **chronic renal failure,** there is a gradual, progressive deterioration of the nephrons that is not reversible. The regulatory, excretory, and endocrine dysfunctions can lead to the uremic syndrome if permitted to progress without appropriate treatment. In contrast, clients with **acute renal failure** will experience an abrupt failure of previously healthy kidneys, which can occur secondary to surgery, trauma, or other causes. Toxic products accumulate, and the condition must be treated aggressively with diet and medications (with or without dialysis). If it takes the form of acute necrosis of the tubules, acute renal failure is reversible, but if the kidney cortex is involved, it is irreversible.

In the course of the development and progression of chronic renal failure—in contrast to acute renal failure—assess for these stages:

1. Decreased renal reserve. Reflects the loss of up to 50 percent of nephron function without significant loss of homeostatic function (usually no dietary restrictions are required)
2. Renal insufficiency. Reflects a decrease in homeostatic function (i.e., mild **azotemia**—

accumulation of nitrogenous products); make dietary adjustments in accordance with signs or symptoms (e.g., sodium restriction if there is hypertension); protein restriction is not usually required

3. Renal failure. Reflects a significant decrease in homeostatic function with a decrease in renal concentrating ability, moderate to severe azotemia, and marked anemia; modify the protein, electrolytes, and fluid content of the diet

4. Uremia (end-stage renal disease). Reflects a severe decrease in homeostatic function and is characterized by severe azotemia, progressive acidosis, fluid retention, electrolyte disturbances, anemia, and manifestations of dysfunction in many body organs; institute strict diet modifications and dialysis

Also assess for the effects of uremia on other body organ systems (Table 30–1). Expect the syndrome to develop in the late stage of chronic, progressive kidney disease after 90 percent or more of renal function is lost. It may develop earlier, however, if there is superimposed stress, infection, or hemorrhage. Acute renal failure can abruptly lead to the uremic state.

The breakdown products of protein metabolism are thought to be responsible for the toxicity of the disease; use the blood urea nitrogen level (BUN) as a rough guide to the level of toxins. Although urea itself is generally thought to be nontoxic (at least in the levels usually present), it serves as a marker for the level of toxic products. In general, the severity of the uremia depends on the rapidity of rise of the BUN and on individual tolerance to the chemical imbalance, not on the precise BUN level per se. Some clients may have symptoms with a BUN of 50 mg percent, whereas others may fail to show symptoms with levels above 100 mg percent. If the disorder advances to the comatose stage, it is usually fatal.

Of all the diseases of the kidney, chronic renal disease is the most frequent, and end-stage renal failure exists in greater numbers of clients than any other type of renal disease. Acute renal failure occurs more frequently in adults than in children. Chronic renal failure may be precipitated by systemic disease processes that involve the kidney or by diseases that are intrinsic to the kidney itself. Disease processes that can eventually lead to chronic renal failure differ in their clinical course, and they may progress rapidly or slowly. The disorders can cause progressive destruction of renal functional tissue, and because of the irreversibility of chronic renal failure, death may result unless dialysis or renal transplant is initiated.

Suspect acute renal failure in clients whose history includes (1) the ingestion of substances that are toxic to the kidney and (2) circulatory failure.

TABLE 30–1
MULTISYSTEM DISEASE ASPECTS OF UREMIA

System	Abnormal Manifestation
Gastrointestinal	Anorexia, nausea, vomiting, ammonia taste in the mouth, gastrointestinal bleeding, diarrhea, constipation, gastroenteritis, peptic ulcer, mouth ulcers
Dermatologic	Uremic frost, calcium deposition, pigmentation (yellowish coloration), pruritis, excoriation, ecchymosis
Hematologic	Anemia (from blood loss, toxic suppression of the bone marrow, toxic decrease in the life span of erythrocytes, and decrease in the production of erythropoietin); defective blood clotting
Cardiovascular	Hypertension, pericarditis, cardiomyopathy, congestive heart failure
Respiratory	Pulmonary edema, dyspnea, uremic pneumonitis and pleuritis, urine smell to the breath
Skeletal	Renal osteodystrophy, including osteomalacia, osteitis fibrosa cystica, bone pain, soft tissue calcification, gout
Endocrine	Hyperlipoproteinemia, impaired glucose tolerance, hyperparathyroidism, thyroid abnormalities, menstrual irregularities and amenorrhea, infertility, loss of libido, gynecomastia and impotence in males
Neural	Cerebral edema, headache, drowsiness, coma, lethargy, insomnia, muscular weakness, twitching, convulsions, disorientation, irritability, psychoses, peripheral neuropathy (burning feet, paresthesias, motor weakness, paralysis), depression, anxiety, denial
Immunologic	Increase in susceptibility to infection
Ocular	Hypertensive retinopathy, blindness, nystagmus

The latter condition reduces the renal blood flow and leads to ischemia. Both mechanisms produce acute destruction or degeneration of the renal tubules (acute tubular necrosis, or ATN). With appropriate treatment, acute renal failure resulting from factors other than diseases within the renal parenchema itself may be reversible. The period of time required for regeneration of the renal tubular cells is variable and unpredictable, and the failure may last for 2 to 3 weeks or longer. In spite of extensive advances in the use of intensive care facilities and the ready availability of dialysis, the mortality rate in acute renal failure remains high.

Observe for these signs and symptoms in acute renal failure: an extremely rapid rate of tissue catabolism, hyperkalemia, fluid overload, and oliguria (diminished urine volume) or anuria (absence of urine). While oliguria or anuria is usually present, on occasion urine volume may not decrease, but there is failure to excrete the waste products of catabolism (nonoliguric or polyuric renal failure). Hyperkalemia occurs secondary to the decreased urinary flow and release of potassium from cellular breakdown. The duration of the oliguria appears to be related to reversibility. Should it persist for more than 3 weeks, suspect that total cortical necrosis has occurred and that the condition is possibly irreversible. When the oliguria persists for more than 24 to 48 hours without treatment, the rapid accumulation of metabolic waste products leads to the clinical symptoms of uremia.

Observe for malnutrition in clients with acute and chronic renal failure as well as in those undergoing maintenance dialysis. The metabolism of many nutrients is altered in renal disease, and many clients ingest quantities of nutrients that are not sufficient to maintain good nutritional status. The rigid dietary restrictions that are sometimes necessary and the gastrointestinal and neural complications of the disease may limit food intake. Assess for these signs of malnutrition in uremia: a decrease in body weight (a decrease in body fat and fat-free solids), diminished levels of serum proteins (e.g., albumin, transferrin, and complement), a reduced ratio of essential to nonessential amino acids and of valine to glycine in plasma, a decrease in certain water-soluble vitamins, especially vitamins C, B$_6$, and folic acid, and retarded growth in children with the disease.[1]

Growth retardation is characteristic of children with chronic renal disease. Even with control of uremia by hemodialysis or transplantation, variable improvements in growth have resulted. Impaired growth has been attributed to many causes, including undernutrition, osteodystrophy, acidosis, weakness, electrolyte depletion, chronic infection, hypertension, use of corticosteroids, and somatomedins.[2]

Intervention

Dietary modifications are important in treating both acute and chronic renal failure. Many of the principles described below, which apply directly to chronic renal failure, are also applicable to acute renal failure. Significant differences are discussed in the section on acute renal failure. In both conditions, nurses must assist clients to balance dietary intake with excretory capacity.

CHRONIC RENAL FAILURE

Assessment

In chronic renal disease, when kidney function decreases to approximately 20 to 25 percent of normal, observe for these changes in body chemistry:

1. Nitrogenous waste products (e.g., urea and creatinine) accumulate in the blood
2. Sodium and water are often retained, leading to edema, hypertension, and weight gain (in some cases, sodium may be lost in abnormally large quantities, however)
3. Acids from protein catabolism accumulate in the blood, leading to progressive acidosis
4. Metabolism of various nutrients becomes altered (e.g., the calcium:phosphorus ratio and the metabolism of carbohydrate, protein, fat, minerals, and vitamins become abnormal

There is evidence that in renal disease, the altered nutrient metabolism may change the requirements for some nutrients. Notably, requirements for calcium, iron, zinc, some water-soluble vitamins, and vitamin D are increased in chronic uremia (as well as in clients being dialyzed), and the tolerance for potassium, phosphorus, magnesium, and possibly vitamin A is decreased in renal failure. The requirement for sodium may be either increased or reduced. Uremia leads to altered carbohydrate and lipid metabolism with type IV hyperlipoproteinemia and accelerated vascular disease. In renal failure, many nutrients may be toxic at lower levels of intake, possibly due to kidney retention.

The metabolism of specific amino acids is altered in chronic renal failure and necessitates consideration in management. In addition to the eight amino acids that are essential for adults (see Chap. 6), histidine behaves as an essential amino acid as well. Imbalances of others have been described, and recommendations have been made for providing an appropriate balance of amino acids without giving an excess of tyrosine, histidine, phenylalanine, and the sulfur-containing amino acids that can retard the repletion process.[3]

Intervention

Use these principles of dietary management to minimize the symptoms of uremia:

1. Decrease the nitrogenous load by restricting the dietary protein intake, yet assure a positive nitrogen balance by providing the ideal requirement of the essential amino acids

2. Provide sufficient kilocalories from carbohydrate and fat to assure optimal use of the ingested protein for maintenance of nitrogen balance
3. Control edema and electrolyte imbalance by balancing the intake of fluids and electrolytes with urinary, insensible, and fecal losses
4. Prevent or delay the development of renal osteodystrophy by regulating the intake of calcium, phosphorus, and vitamin D
5. Provide nutrient supplements as needed to assure an adequate nutrient intake
6. Provide a diet that is palatable, attractive, and consistent with lifestyle as nearly as possible

In order to meet these goals, the diet must often be restricted in protein, sodium, and fluid and sometimes in phosphorus and magnesium. When protein is restricted, provide adequate kilocalories with carbohydrate and fat, and supplement the diet with vitamins, calcium, iron, and zinc. Although potassium excretion is usually adequate until the final stages of chronic renal failure, observe for hyperkalemia in the earlier stages in clients who experience a sudden increase in the potassium load (e.g., due to catabolic response to stress or tissue injury, gastrointestinal hemorrhage, severe acidosis, or use of potassium-sparing diuretics, such as spironolactone or triamterene). Use Table 30–2 as a guide for modifications that are often necessary. Specific modifications may vary widely depending on the individual's current nutritional status, degree of progression of the disease, degree of stress, concomitant drug therapy, and other factors. However, do not assume that all clients with renal disease need all of the modifications enumerated above. In addition, the need for diet restriction may change frequently in the same individual. Sometimes day-to-day changes are necessary as a result of changes that take place in renal function, presence of infection, or the influence of medications.

The relevance of the various dietary components in the treatment of renal disease is discussed below.

Protein. When kidney function decreases to approximately 25 percent of normal, initiate a mild protein restriction to reduce the level of toxins (which are thought to be products of protein catabolism), potassium, and acid-producing substances. Sulfur and phosphorus are contained in all protein foods. Not only does the accumulation of these substances in the blood lead to acidosis, but phosphate accumulation is thought to be a factor in the etiology of renal osteodystrophy (metabolic bone disease) and metastatic calcification. Although the precise level of renal function at which protein restriction is indicated has not been clearly established, the decision to adjust protein intake is usually based on the clinical symptoms and the results of certain laboratory tests. Progressive deterioration of renal function is accompanied by gastrointestinal symptoms. The appearance of anorexia, nausea, and vomiting means that protein restriction is highly desirable. Other clues that nurses can use to initiate adjustment of the protein intake are a fall in the creatinine clearance to below 25 ml/minute and a rise of the BUN above 100 mg/dl. Protein restriction is useful when the creatinine clearance is between 4 and 25 ml/minute. Protein restriction is not usually considered necessary when the creatinine clearance is above 25 ml/minute although there is some evidence that restricting protein in the early stages may delay the progression of kidney disease.[4] A rough guide for adjusting daily protein intake in accordance with progressive changes in renal function as gauged by changes in the creatinine clearance is given in Table 30–2. To these amounts should be added gram-for-gram increments to compensate for proteinuria, which may complicate the renal disease: for each gram of protein lost in the urine, add 1 gram to the diet.

When restricting the dietary protein, be sure to provide protein of sufficient quality and quantity to assure the maintenance of nitrogen balance without adding to the nitrogenous load to be excreted. In essence, this means providing the necessary amount of the essential amino acids. Ideally, all of the nitrogen supplied will be used in protein synthesis for synthesis of enzymes, hormones, muscle and visceral protein, and so on, and none will be available for excretion.

Protein foods of high biologic value (HBV) found in egg, meat, fish, and poultry contain a relatively greater amount of essential amino acids and are used more efficiently than foods with lower quality protein, such as vegetables and grains. The biologic value of egg protein is essentially 100 percent. Therefore, with rigid restriction of dietary protein, provide at least 75 percent of the allowance as HBV protein.

Current dietary management of renal failure is based on modifications of principles described by Giordano, Giovannetti, and Maggiore in the early 1960s.[5] These Italian physicians were able to bring about a lowering of the BUN, an improvement of clinical symptoms, and a positive nitrogen balance in uremic clients by providing a diet high in kilocalories (2000 to 3000, supplied primarily as carbohydrate and fat) and containing the required amount of essential amino acids and minimizing the intake of nonessential amino acids. The diet contained 24 g protein, with approximately 70 percent supplied as HBV protein (1 egg and ¾ c of milk—an additional egg or an occasional 1 oz of meat could be substituted for the milk). Although meat has a good balance of essential amino acids, it has large quantities of nonessential amino acids as well, and the diet sharply restricted intake of meat and vegetable protein. Multivitamin and iron supplements were provided, and sodium and potassium were restricted. The rationale for the diet was that the large endogenous urea pool could be recycled for synthesis of

TABLE 30-2
NUTRIENT MODIFICATIONS IN RENAL DISEASE

Nutrient	Normal Daily Intake	Chronic Renal Failure (No Dialysis)	Acute Renal Failure	Dialysis
Protein	Adults: 80–100 g (see RDA, Chap. 2, for recommended amount) Children: See RDA	Adults: Depends on creatinine clearance: creatinine clearance — g/kg body wt/day (ml/min/1.73 m²) 30–20 — 0.7–0.5 19–5 — 0.38 — ~¾ provided as HBV protein <5 — 0.26 Children: Level should not fall ↓1.0–2.0 g/kg [at least 60–70% of protein of ↑ biologic value—animal origin—and essential amino acid supplements may be required]	Adults: approximately 0.2–0.5 g/kg (largely HBV) unless dialyzed	Adults: 1.0–1.25 g/kg for hemodialysis and 1.2–1.5 g/kg for peritoneal dialysis (~50% from HBV protein) Children: 3–4 g/kg
Kilocalories	Adults: 29–41 kcal/kg (see RDA) Children: See RDA	Adults: 35–40 kcal/kg/day (~2000–3000) Children: At least 80% of RDA; some suggest 1500 kcal/m² of body surface area	Adults: 45–50 kcal/kg	Adults: 35–45 kcal/kg [substantial amounts of glucose (78–316 g/day) can be absorbed from the diasylate in CAPD] Children: At least 80% of RDA
Sodium	Adults: 3–4 g or 120–170 mEq	40–130 mEq (920–3000 mg). [20–40 mEq (460–920 mg) if severe edema or hypertension]	20–40 mEq in oliguric phase; replace losses in diuretic phase	60–120 mEq (1380–2760 mg)
Potassium	Adults: 2–6 g or 50–150 mEq	40–70 mEq (1560–2730 mg)	30–50 mEq in oliguric phase; replace losses in diuretic phase	40–70 mEq (1560–2730 mg)
Fluid	Ad lib	Adults: 400–600 ml + output Children: 200–500 ml + output	400–500 ml + output in oliguric phase; replace losses in diuretic phase	400–500 ml + output; 1500–2000 ml daily for CAPD
Other minerals Magnesium	See RDA	Restrict or control intake	During oliguric phase, closely monitor levels of magnesium, phosphorus, and calcium and adjust intake as necessary; phosphate binders may alleviate hypocalcemia; replace losses in diuretic phase	
Phosphorus	See RDA	Restrict to 1 g or less and/or use phosphate binders		Restrict dietary phosphate and use binders
Calcium	See RDA	Supplement with calcium carbonate		Supplement with calcium and ↑ concentration in dialysate
Iron	See RDA	Supplement with ferrous sulfate		Supplement with iron
Vitamins	See RDA	Supplement with water-soluble vitamins with additional folic acid, vitamin B_6, and vitamin C; cautious supplementation with the metabolically active form of vitamin D (calcitriol) if hypocalcemia or osteomalacia present	Supplement with water-soluble vitamins	Supplement with water-soluble vitamins with additional folic acid, vitamin B_6, and vitamin C; cautious supplementation with the metabolically active form of vitamin D (calcitriol) if hypocalcemia or osteomalacia present

the nonessential amino acids. When the urea was thus used, the BUN dropped and the distressing gastrointestinal and other manifestations disappeared or diminished. Provision of adequate kilocalories was essential to allow the ingested protein to be used for purposes of synthesis rather than for energy. At present, however, the nutritional adequacy of such diets and the concept of urea recycling in general are being questioned. The potential for using endogenous urea for amino acid synthesis in uremia may be quite limited, and the mechanism whereby the low-protein diets are effective is not currently known.

Clinical experience has shown that clients may be maintained in nitrogen balance for prolonged periods with a daily protein intake of 37 to 40 g if the kilocalorie requirement is adequately met.[6] When the BUN is very high, the total protein intake can be decreased further to 20 g, provided only egg and milk proteins are used. Although they supply the essential amino acids for internal protein synthesis, milk and egg proteins do not burden the client with excessive nonessential amino acids that add to the nitrogenous pool to be excreted. To prevent protein depletion as the renal failure advances, give uremic clients supplements of the essential amino acids to supply the building blocks needed for daily tissue rebuilding without imposing a burden of nonessential nitrogen for excretion. These may be administered as:

1. Synthetic, crystalline amino acids
2. Analogs (hydroxy or alpha-keto) of the essential amino acids. The analogs consist of the nonnitrogenous carbon skeleton (keto acid) of the amino acids. With dietary essential amino acids restricted, it is hypothesized that the body will synthesize the corresponding amino acid from its analog, using the large urea pool as a source of amino groups (urea + keto acid → amino acid)
3. Defined formula diets as the principal dietary source of amino acids or as a supplement to a low-protein diet. Examples of products available as supplements are Amin-Aid (McGaw Labs) and Travasorb Renal (Travenol)

In general, supplementation with essential amino acids is unnecessary in clients on dialysis in whom protein intake is liberalized.

In view of (1) the evidence that diets that reduce uremic toxicity to a minimum do not always provide optimal nutrition, (2) the ready availability of dialysis, and (3) the liberalization of the diet that is possible with dialysis, some feel that the typical uremic client may fare better with a more liberalized diet and more frequent dialysis.

Low-protein diets, particularly those that stress HBV proteins, tend to be unpalatable. To improve compliance, teach the client to combine allowed HBV and low biologic value (LBV) proteins in a var-

ied diet. Specify exact portion sizes and stress the importance of consuming the amount of protein prescribed. When the amount allowed is small, give assistance with food preparation techniques to vary the form in which the protein is eaten, for example, in casseroles or sandwich spreads.

Kilocalories. Provide sufficient kilocalories when the protein is severely restricted. Without an adequate kilocaloric intake, the dietary protein will be used for energy and body tissue will be catabolized, leading to an increase in the metabolic load of nitrogenous wastes, potassium, and phosphate. Failure of diet therapy is not uncommonly related to insufficient kilocaloric intake due to unpalatable diets and the gastrointestinal complications of uremia. Nurses may find tissue depletion difficult to assess because of concomitant edema.

Select additional kilocalories beyond those supplied by the basic diet from foods low in protein, sodium, and potassium. Emphasize carbohydrate-containing and fat-containing foods that are low in protein content and concentrated in kilocalorie content. The end products of their metabolism (primarily carbon dioxide and water) do not compromise the excretory capacity of the kidney. It is essential that sufficient kilocalories be consumed along with the dietary protein to assure maximum protein-sparing.

Traditional carbohydrate- and fat-containing foods as well as special products can be used to supplement the kilocalorie intake. A listing is found in Table 30–3. Since consumption of large amounts of these foods, such as hard candy, sugar, honey, and fats, may be objectionable to some clients, it may be necessary to suggest special products, such as low-protein pasta and wheat starch and carbohydrate supplements such as Polycose, Hy-Cal, Cal-Power, and Controlyte, to maintain kilocalorie intake. Provide recipes or directions for use of special products and information as to where they can be obtained and their cost. Many medical and renal centers have devised special recipes to make a number of the products more palatable. Since low-protein baked foods differ in taste and texture from regular baked products, assist the client with ways to make them more palatable, such as toasting bread and serving it with margarine and jelly. If sodium and potassium are both restricted, it is necessary to use yeast as a leavening agent, since regular baking powder contains excessive sodium and low-sodium baking powder contains excessive potassium.

Be particularly aggressive in insisting that children consume adequate kilocalories. In a large proportion of children, growth failure often results from malnutrition. Catch-up growth may be possible with adequate kilocalorie consumption.

Sodium. The ability of the kidney to conserve sodium in the presence of sodium depletion and to dispose of sodium when there is an excess is im-

TABLE 30–3
SUPPLEMENTAL SOURCES OF KILOCALORIES
FROM CARBOHYDRATE AND FAT

Carbohydrates	Fats
Candy: Stick candy, lollipops, jellybeans, Lifesavers, gum drops, sour balls, chewing gum, homemade fondant and taffy (made without salt), marshmallows	Coffee-Rich, salt-free butter and margarine, cooking oil, shortening, heavy whipping cream, sour cream, salt-free salad dressing and mayonnaise, fat part of fresh pork siding
Sugar: Pure white sugar, honey, jelly, jam, corn syrup	Special products:
Beverages (used within the fluid allowance; use sugar-containing beverages, not dietetic beverages): Colas, Dr. Pepper, Sprite, 7-Up, ginger ale, root beer, lemonade, limeade, Kool-Aid, fruit-flavored sodas, cranberry juice, fruit-iced popsicles, tea with sugar, beer and liquor (if allowed by physician)	Lipomul oral—corn oil emulsion, 3 kcal/ml (Upjohn)
Starches: Cornstarch, tapioca, arrowroot	
Special products:	
Liquid, deionized glucose supplements (2+ kcal/ml): Hy-Cal (Beecham), Cal-Power (Henkel Corporation)	
Protein-free, low-electrolyte carbohydrate polymers (30 kcal/tbsp and can be stirred into beverages, puddings, cereals): Controlyte (Doyle), Polycose (Ross)	
Paygel wheat starch and baking mix (Henkel Corporation) and Cellu Low Protein baking mix and wheat starch (Chicago Dietetic Supply, Inc., La Grange, Ill)—high in kcal and low in protein and electrolytes; for use as a flour substitute in baked products	
Other prepared products: Aproten pasta (macaroni, noodles), rusks, semolina (a cereal), low-protein cookies, low-protein bread, and Prono (a low-protein gelled dessert mix) (Henkel Corporation)	

Recipes are provided by the manufacturers of the special products.

paired in chronic renal failure. Thus both sodium excess and deficiency are poorly tolerated. Excess sodium intake leads to overhydration, hypertension, edema, congestive heart failure, and aggravation or precipitation of nausea and vomiting. Conversely, a sodium deficit brings dehydration, hypovolemia, hypotension, a decrease in glomerular filtration, and deterioration of the clinical state. Further, muscle cramping and convulsions may occur.

The exact sodium prescription depends on the ability to both excrete and conserve sodium, on the presence or absence of hypertension and edema, and on the sodium content of medications that are used. In the absence of hypertension or edema, dietary sodium restriction may not be necessary. In general, the amount of sodium required is that amount necessary to prevent or control edema and hypertension while maintaining adequate hydration. Some control of sodium intake may be desirable if there is a concomitant fluid restriction. Sodium intake and

thirst are closely related; thirst accompanies a high sodium intake.

Some clients with renal failure are salt retainers (i.e., they do not excrete sodium adequately), and others are salt wasters (i.e., they do not conserve sodium adequately). Assess for salt-wasting tendencies in clients whose renal failure stems from such conditions as polycystic kidney disease, disease affecting the renal tubules, chronic pyelonephritis, and analgesic nephropathy. Hypertension is more likely to occur in clients with glomerulonephritis.

Assess frequently serum and urinary sodium, body weight, blood pressure, and degree of edema (if present) to establish the correct diet prescription. Sodium intake must balance sodium output. The daily amount allowed in the diet must be equal to the amount excreted in the urine for a 24-hour period plus any additional losses that occur in visible perspiration, vomiting, or diarrhea. Provide additional sodium for clients who lose large quantities in the urine to prevent the complications of hyponatremia. Use fluctuations in body weight as a general guide to the adequacy of intake. Teach clients to weigh themselves daily as well as to examine the eyelids and ankles for edema.

Table 30–2 provides a general guide to the degree of sodium restriction necessary to control edema and hypertension. Even those with salt-losing nephropathy may develop edema and require some control of sodium intake. When sodium is severely restricted, monitor renal function closely.

Make necessary adjustments in the dietary prescription to compensate for the sodium contained in certain medications. Those that contain sodium include some antacids, alkalizing agents used to treat acidosis, such as sodium bicarbonate (2 g sodium bicarbonate contains 24 mEq sodium), Scholl's solution (1 ml contains 1 mEq sodium), and Kayexalate (a cation exchange resin used to lower blood potassium—1 g Kayexalate removes 1 mEq potassium and adds 1 mEq sodium). Conversely, overuse of diuretics, especially in combination with a sodium-restricted diet, may lead to sodium depletion.

Chapter 29 details the dietary modifications and client education guidelines necessary for the various levels of sodium restriction. The use of potassium-containing salt substitutes is contraindicated in renal disease.

Potassium. Chronic renal failure may be complicated by either hyperkalemia or hypokalemia. Test the level of serum and urinary potassium at frequent intervals to determine the proper treatment. Hyperkalemia is not a common problem until the renal failure becomes severe and urine volume falls to oliguric levels. However, individuals with deteriorating renal function may be unable to tolerate a sudden increase in the potassium load. Suspect hyperkalemia in these situations:

1. Excessive intake of dietary potassium
2. Use of potassium-containing medications (such as the potassium-sparing diuretics spironolactone and triamterene)
3. Rapid administration of potassium salts (oral or intravenous) to correct hypokalemia
4. Tissue injury or stress (leading to tissue catabolism and potassium leakage from cells)
5. Gastrointestinal hemorrhage
6. Blood transfusion
7. Metabolic acidosis
8. Dehydration with a decline in glomerular filtration (e.g., from nausea and vomiting or severe sodium restriction)

Clients with advanced renal failure can tolerate moderate hyperkalemia (5.0 to 6.5 mEq/liter), but if the potassium level rises rapidly or exceeds 7.0 mEq/liter, the potential for cardiac arrhythmias, abnormal electrocardiogram, and cardiac or respiratory arrest is great. The precise level at which these side effects occur varies greatly from individual to individual.

Treat hyperkalemia by restricting the dietary intake to approximately 40 to 70 mEq daily. If diet restriction alone is ineffective, a cation exchange resin (Kayexalate—sodium polystyrene sulfonate) that exchanges sodium for potassium in the large bowel may be given orally or by retention enema. To increase the palatability of this substance, some centers have incorporated it into candy.

When potassium is restricted, teach the client that potassium is widely distributed in foods and that even small amounts from single foods can quickly lead to consumption of excessive amounts. Foods that are highest in potassium are those of HBV (milk, meat) and fruits and vegetables (see Appendix 1). Concomitant protein restriction limits the potassium intake to a considerable degree. With hyperkalemia, eliminate or restrict the amount of fruits and vegetables containing more than approximately 6 mEq/serving (230 mg). Foods that are high in potassium should be distributed at meals throughout the day to avoid a large potassium load at any one time that might lead to a transient but marked rise in the serum potassium level.

Fruits and vegetables contain potassium in amounts ranging from relatively small to as much as 25 to 40 mEq per serving. For example, canned green beans contain approximately 1.6 mEq per serving, whereas a baked potato contains 20 mEq per serving. Teach clients on diets restricted to 50 mEq or less daily the following food preparation techniques to reduce the amount of potassium foods so that they can occasionally be used.

1. Use cooked or canned fruits and vegetables instead of raw produce, which is higher in potassium content
2. Drain the liquid from canned fruits and vegetables before eating or cooking
3. Extract the potassium from hard fruits and vegetables by:
   a. Peeling and slicing thinly
   b. Soaking in a large volume of water and discarding water
   c. Cooking in a large volume of water and discarding water

The third procedure may reduce the potassium content of fruits and vegetables by approximately 50 percent. Meat can be reduced in potassium content by simmering in a large volume of water. Since this method removes considerable amounts of other nutrients in addition to potassium, it is recommended only for those who need to reduce the potassium in certain foods in order to be able to eat them.

Assess for hypokalemia in association with these factors:

1. Potassium-losing nephropathy, e.g., in those with renal disease stemming from chronic pyelonephritis

2. Excessive use of diuretics that induce secondary potassium loss
3. Excessive use of cation exchange resins
4. Vomiting and diarrhea

Potential adverse effects of hypokalemia include vascular degeneration of the renal tubules with loss of concentrating ability and myocardial damage. Treat hypokalemia with potassium salts or high-potassium foods.

Fluid. In the early stages of renal failure, fluid is not ordinarily restricted, since loss of renal concentration capacity may lead to large fluid losses that must be replaced. Nonetheless, restrict fluid as the failure progresses and oliguria becomes apparent.

When fluid is restricted, balance intake and output to avoid dehydration on the one hand and overhydration on the other. The goal is to allow the maximum amount of fluid in 24 hours that the client can excrete without developing signs of edema and congestive heart failure. In clients with some urine output, a high fluid intake may pose less of a danger than fluid deprivation.

In oliguric clients, the daily fluid allowance of 400 to 600 ml plus an amount equivalent to the volume of urine excreted during the previous 24 hours (Table 30–2) is calculated to compensate for the difference between insensible fluid losses (approximately 800 to 1000 ml) and the endogenous water gained by the metabolism of foods (approximately 350 to 400 ml). If there are other fluid losses (such as vomiting, diarrhea, or visible perspiration), an equivalent amount is added to the fluid allowance.

With fluid restriction, consider the water content of foods in the daily plan. Food sources of water include:

1. Liquid beverages, soups, and juices (visible fluid)
2. Foods that are liquid at room temperature (such as ice cream, sherbet, Jello, ice, and popsicles) (visible fluid)
3. Water contained in solid foods—some fruits and vegetables may be in excess of 90 percent water by weight (invisible or hidden fluid). If vegetable and fruit servings are limited, it is usually not necessary to calculate the hidden fluid. With this limitation, hidden fluid accounts for approximately 500 to 750 ml. With no more than this amount of hidden fluid, fluid intake can be 500 to 800 ml in addition to the amount of urinary output, rather than 400 to 600 ml as stated in Table 30–2

Instruct clients to drain all foods well before eating. Develop the plan for regulating fluid intake with the client, giving reasonable consideration to his or her preferences for use of fluids at meals and throughout the day and to the need for fluids to drink when taking medications. Clarify with the health team whether the fluid allowance includes liquid medications, since these medications, especially if consumed at frequent intervals throughout the day, can add substantially to the daily fluid intake.

Daily recording of intake and output and body weight is essential for determining the fluid allowance and for assessing hydration status. Teach clients to assess these parameters on a daily basis. Some clients may prefer to follow a pattern in which a fixed amount of fluid is consumed at specified times throughout the day, whereas others may prefer more flexibility by measuring their allowed amount of fluid for 24 hours and keeping it refrigerated in a graduated container. Clients on severe fluid restriction often complain of thirst. Thirst is usually decreased and control of fluid intake is easier when dietary sodium intake is also restricted. The following interventions may be helpful in controlling thirst:

1. Stretch the fluid allowance by freezing water and other beverages since frozen beverages tend to be more thirst-quenching
2. Add lemon juice to water or ice cubes to make the beverages more refreshing
3. Suck on hard, sour candies that are sugar-free
4. Relieve oral dryness with mouthwash that has been refrigerated or saliva-stimulating gums such as Quench or Gatorgum
5. Reduce the thirst-producing effect of dry air by controlling the room humidity and temperature
6. Avoid dry, thirst-producing foods, such as crackers or popcorn
7. Space fluids properly throughout the day
8. Schedule the medication dosage so as to use as little fluid as possible in this manner; a small amount of strained applesauce may assist in swallowing medications

Modification of Other Nutrients. Other nutrients that require consideration in chronic renal failure are calcium, phosphorus, magnesium, fluoride, iron, zinc, vitamins (especially vitamin D, vitamin B_6, vitamin C, and folic acid), carbohydrate, and lipids.

Abnormalities of calcium, phosphorus, and vitamin D metabolism occur in progressive renal failure and lead to secondary hyperparathyroidism and renal osteodystrophy. Bone disease may also be related to magnesium and fluoride excess. The bone disease may take several forms: osteitis fibrosa cystica, osteomalacia, and metastatic calcification. Symptoms include bone pain, bone deformities, fractures, loss of height, and extraosseous calcification. Although significant advances have been made in the pathogenesis of the bone disorders, the mechanisms are still not clearly understood and the topic remains controversial.

When creatinine clearance falls below 25 ml/minute, changes occur in the calcium:phosphorus ratio. Phosphate excretion decreases and phosphate is retained. The blood calcium level drops; this is thought to occur secondary to (1) a reciprocal decline as the blood phosphorus level increases, (2) failure to form sufficient quantities of the metabolically active form of vitamin D needed for increasing the intestinal absorption of calcium and for bone resorption, and (3) a dietary lack of calcium (if the diet is restricted). In normal situations, hypocalcemia induces a series of compensatory changes that lead to an elevation in the blood calcium level. However, these mechanisms become less efficient in renal disease.

Persistent hypocalcemia leads to secondary hyperparathyroidism and, in advanced cases, osteitis fibrosa cystica characterized by dull, aching bone pain. Since metabolically active vitamin D contributes directly or indirectly to bone mineralization, osteomalacia and rickets may also result. Should the calcium × phosphorus product (see Chap. 9) exceed 70, metastatic calcification occurs in such diverse areas as the conjunctivae of the eye, conduction system of the heart, lung, and extremities.

Hypermagnesemia (elevated blood magnesium) can exacerbate existing bone disease, and although the role of fluoride remains uncertain, high serum levels of fluoride seem to aggravate existing bone disease by enhancing demineralization. Excessive fluoride in the dialysis bath for dialysis clients has been implicated in producing osteosclerotic bone lesions.

Treat renal osteodystrophy using a combination of diet and drug therapy to "turn off" the secondary hyperparathyroidism that is implicated in the development of bone disorders. Take measures to increase the blood calcium level by (1) providing calcium supplements and (2) restricting dietary phosphorus and using substances that bind phosphorus in the intestinal tract and thus prevent its absorption. Initiate treatment early to prevent or delay hyperparathyroidism. Give supplements of vitamin D to treat severe hypocalcemia and osteomalacia. Therapy designed to increase blood calcium is contraindicated if hypercalcemia exists or if the calcium × phosphorus product is above 70.

The goal of phosphate restriction is to keep the serum phosphorus level in the range of 3 to 4 mg/100 ml to prevent serum calcium suppression. Hypophosphatemia should be avoided as this condition can result in osteomalacia. Dietary phosphorus restriction may follow a stepwise reduction proportional to the decline in creatinine clearance. Actually, the low-protein diet reduces phosphorus ingestion, since the mineral is present in large concentration in protein, foods particularly dairy products (see Chap. 9 for other sources of phosphorus). Phosphate binders, which include nonabsorbable aluminum hydroxide and aluminum carbonate, may lead to constipation, which is usually controlled by stool softeners or laxatives because of the concomitant restricted diet. Improve palatability by crushing the medication and mixing it with food or a small quantity of beverage. Recipes for cookies and other products that incorporate the substances have been developed (e.g., Amphogel cookies by Vita-wheat, available through Erika). The safety of prolonged usage of aluminum phosphate-binding gels is uncertain. It has been associated with accumulation of aluminum in the tissues and brain and may contribute to encephalopathy and osteodystrophy. Aluminum hydroxide may also bind iron in the gastrointestinal tract.

Use of small amounts of a synthetic form of the metabolically active form of vitamin D, Rocaltrol, corrects the abnormal calcium and phosphorus metabolism and ameliorates the secondary hyperparathyroidism due to failure of the diseased kidney to produce the metabolically active form of vitamin D. Therapy with Rocaltrol has led to bone remineralization, decreased bone pain, and increased muscle strength in selected clients with renal osteodystrophy.[7] Therapy with this drug should not be initiated until serum phosphorus has been reduced to normal levels. Monitor serum levels of both calcium and phosphorus during drug therapy.

The excretion of magnesium is impaired in chronic renal disease, and the damaged kidney is unable to adjust to a large magnesium load. Hypermagnesemia may be precipitated by excessive ingestion of magnesium (in the diet or as magnesium-containing medications, such as magnesium-containing antacids, by an increase in tissue catabolism, or by acidosis). The disorder is best treated by dialysis, although control of dietary intake is a necessary preventive measure.

The anemia of chronic renal failure is relatively asymptomatic, although fatigue is usually present. The defect in erythropoiesis may be complicated by the low iron content of the protein-restricted diet. Iron supplements are frequently given (the parenteral route is preferred) and erythropoietic-stimulating substances, such as androgens, are sometimes used. Zinc supplements may improve the altered taste acuity and abnormal sexual function observed in clients with uremia.[8]

Supplementation with water-soluble vitamins is recommended for the following reasons: (1) diets severely restricted in protein, sodium, potassium, and phosphorus restrict the vitamin intake (water-soluble vitamins are particularly abundant in fruits, vegetables, and high-protein foods), (2) cooking methods designed to extract the potassium from foods reduce their water-soluble vitamin content, (3) altered metabolism and concomitant drug administration may alter vitamin requirements, and (4) gastrointestinal absorption may be decreased in uremia. Although the current trend is to liberalize protein intake, the other dietary restrictions still prevent an adequate dietary intake.

Little is known about the particular vitamin

TABLE 30–4
NUTRIENT COMPOSITION OF MEAL PLAN FOR DIETS IN RENAL FAILURE

Nutrient	Amount		
Protein	40 g	60 g	80 g
Sodium	74 mEq (1700 mg)	80–85 mEq (1850–1950 mg)	87–91 mEq (2000–2100 mg)
Potassium	41–44 mEq (1600–1700 mg)	49–51 mEq (1900–2000 mg)	56–59 mEq (2200–2300 mg)
Calcium	360–375 mg	415–440 mg	490–500 mg
Phosphorus	575–600 mg	775–800 mg	1000–1050 mg
Kilocalories[a]	1300	1450	1700

[a] Kilocaloric intake can be increased to desired levels by increasing the use of sugars (from the allowed sweets group), fats, and allowed beverages (within the fluid allowance). Between-meal eating is encouraged.
(*Source:* North Carolina Dietetic Association: Diet Manual, ed 2. Charlotte, NC, 1978, p 13G.)

requirements of uremic clients, although there is evidence that the metabolism of some is altered and the requirements thus change. Blood levels of the water-soluble vitamins, particularly vitamin B_6, vitamin C, and folic acid are often decreased. The blood levels are frequently lower in both dialyzed and nondialyzed clients. Several authors have suggested that some of the clinical symptoms and biochemical alterations of uremia, such as altered amino acid levels and altered lipid metabolism,[9] may

TABLE 30–5
SUGGESTED MEAL PLAN AT THREE LEVELS OF PROTEIN CONTENT

	40 g Protein (No. of Servings)	60 g Protein (No. of Servings)	80 g Protein (No. of Servings)
Breakfast			
Fruit or juice	1	1	1
Egg	1	1	1
Cereal	1	1	1
Bread	1	1	1
Regular margarine	2 tsp	2 tsp	2 tsp
Salt-free margarine	As desired	As desired	As desired
Milk	½ c	½ c	½ c
Sugar/jelly	As desired	As desired	As desired
Coffee	1 c	1 c	1 c
Lunch			
Meat or substitute	1 oz	2 oz	3 oz
Bread	2	2	2
Potato or substitute	1	1	1
Vegetables	1	1	2
Fruit or juice	1	1	1
Regular margarine	2 tsp	2 tsp	2 tsp
Salt-free margarine	As desired	As desired	As desired
Sugar/jelly	As desired	As desired	As desired
Beverage	See food list	See food list	See food list
Dinner			
Meat or substitute	1 oz	2 oz	3 oz
Bread	1	2	2
Potato or substitute	1	1	1
Vegetables	1	2	2
Fruit or juice	1	1	1
Regular margarine	2 tsp	2 tsp	2 tsp
Salt-free margarine	As desired	As desired	As desired
Sugar/jelly	As desired	As desired	As desired
Beverage	See food list	See food list	See food list

(*Source:* North Carolina Dietetic Association: Diet Manual, ed 2. Charlotte, NC, 1978, p 14G.)

be due to vitamin deficiency. The fat-soluble vitamins are least affected by renal failure, and currently there is no evidence to indicate a need to supplement with vitamins A, E, or K; vitamin A supplements should not be given, since serum levels may be elevated in uremia. Clients with chronic anemia who are not dialyzed should receive a daily supplement of vitamin B_6 (5 mg), ascorbic acid (70 to 100 mg), folic acid (1 mg), and the normal RDA for the other water-soluble vitamins. Stress to the client the importance of taking prescribed medications and supplements.

Carbohydrate and Lipid Abnormalities. Glucose intolerance and accelerated atherosclerosis associated with type IV hyperlipoproteinemia occur in chronic renal failure as well as in clients undergoing dialysis. A moderate degree of glucose intolerance is observed in over 50 percent of renal clients. Various explanations have been given for this finding, including peripheral insulin antagonism by the uremic toxins and a defect in insulin secretion. The abnormal state is corrected by dialysis and in most instances is not a contraindication to a high intake of carbohydrate kilocalories.

Approximately 40 to 60 percent of clients with chronic renal failure develop type IV hyperlipoproteinemia associated with elevated triglycerides and a moderate increase in cholesterol. Low levels of high-density lipoprotein (HDL) cholesterol have been reported in uremic clients. Lipid handling is abnormal in acute renal failure but is only significant in the chronic state because of its longer duration. The hyperlipidemia is due primarily to impaired catabolism of triglycerides, although the cause has not been clearly established. The condition is not generally improved with dialysis, and controversy surrounds the effectiveness of dietary management. Since premature atherosclerosis and cardiovascular disease occur frequently in these clients, attempts have been made to correct the hyperlipidemia. A diet containing 35 percent of kilocalories as complex carbohydrate and 55 percent as fat, with a 2:1 P/S ratio, has been shown to reduce triglyceride levels, but its efficacy in reducing or delaying cardiovascular disease is uncertain.[10] Administration of carnitine, an amino acid needed for fatty acid oxidation, may also lower serum triglycerides. If the client is obese, weight reduction should be encouraged when the medical condition permits.

Diet Plan for Chronic Renal Failure. The specific diet modifications for the client with chronic uremia are based on the principles outlined in Table 30–2 and discussed above. Individualize each diet prescription in accordance with clinical findings, such as the level of the BUN, creatinine clearance, serum and urinary electrolyte levels, urinary volume, presence of uremic symptoms, and body weight.

When protein restriction becomes necessary, provide at least 50 to 75 percent of the protein allowance with protein of HBV to assure that requirements for essential amino acids are met. Essential amino acid supplements may be necessary when the diet is restricted to 40 g of protein or less, and extra protein may be needed to compensate for proteinuria. When the client is dialyzed, the protein content is liberalized to compensate for losses of blood proteins or amino acids incurred with the procedure (see the section on dialysis).

Various regimens have been described for control of protein, sodium, potassium, fluid, and phosphorus, and large hospitals and renal centers have set up their own particular regimens for their control. Generally, the regimens are based on a system of food grouping, with all foods in a given group having the same approximate composition of protein, sodium, and potassium. A daily meal plan is devised and menus planned by selecting the specified number of servings and amounts from each group. The broad food groupings for the various regimens are similar (milk and milk products; meat, poultry, fish, egg; starches; vegetables; fruits and fruit juices; fats; and miscellaneous foods). However, the regimens often differ in the specific foods included and in the portion sizes allowed.

Table 30–4 provides the approximate composition of protein, sodium, potassium, calcium, phophorus, and kilocalories for meal plans at three levels of protein content that might be used for renal failure. Table 30–5 gives meal plans on the three levels, and Table 30–6 gives a list of foods allowed and foods avoided. In general, the food lists emphasize the use of regular foods; fluid restriction must be applied as appropriate.

ACUTE RENAL FAILURE

Assessment

Acute renal failure is characterized by many of the same biochemical aberrations as chronic renal failure; however, assess for these differences:

1. An extremely rapid rate of tissue catabolism (the hypercatabolism associated with renal failure itself may be compounded by the accelerated protein catabolism and increased energy demand induced by predisposing conditions, such as surgery or severe trauma)—as much as 100 to 120 g of protein per day may be catabolized
2. Rapid development of hyperkalemia, associated with the tissue catabolism and oliguria, and compounded by complications, such as gastrointestinal hemorrhage or infection
3. Intolerance of oral food intake for several days because of gastrointestinal failure following severe trauma or abdominal surgery (as in chronic renal failure, uremic symptoms may obviate oral intake for a period of time)
4. An oliguric phase that may last up to 2 to

TABLE 30–6
FOOD LISTS FOR RENAL DIET

Category	Foods Allowed	Foods Avoided
Milk	Whole milk, chocolate milk, half and half, cocoa (½ c only)	Dutch process cocoa, commercial buttermilk
Meat, egg, cheese	Meat: beef, lamb, fresh pork, poultry, veal, liver, codfish, haddock, perch, low-sodium salmon, low-sodium tuna, oysters (no more than specified in meal plan—allowance based on cooked weight without bone, fat, skin) Egg: Prepared as desired (1 daily; additional egg if substituted for meat—1 egg substitutes for 1 oz meat) Cheese: Unsalted cheese (1 oz can substitute for 1 oz meat)	Luncheon meat, hot dogs, corned and dried beef, salted fat, salted meat, bacon, ham, sausage, sardines, commercially frozen fish, canned and potted meat, TV dinners, pot pies, meat extenders More than 1 egg unless substituted for meat All other cheeses

Fruit and juices	Canned and fresh fruit, juices (three ½ c servings daily)
	  Canned fruit: apple sauce, sweet cherries, fruit cocktail, grapefruit sections, peaches, pears, pineapple, apple
	  Fresh fruit: apple (1 small), blueberries (½ c), grapefruit (½ small), tangerine (1), strawberries (10), grapes (22)
	  Fruit juice: apple, grape, cranapple, pear nectar, peach nectar
		Apricots, avocados, bananas, dates, dried fruit, elderberries, mulberries, nectarines, melons, oranges, prunes, raisins, rhubarb, plums
		
		All other fresh fruits
		
		All other juices

Vegetables	Fresh, frozen, regular canned (if canned, must be drained of liquid and seasoned with salt-free margarine (½ c = 1 serving and no more should be used than specified in the meal plan) Asparagus, beets, cabbage, cucumbers, cooked carrots, green or wax beans, green pepper, okra, lettuce, onions, rutabaga, turnips, summer squash, cooked tomato, turnip greens, mustard greens	Broccoli, brussels sprouts, dried beans, dried peas, dandelion greens, mushrooms, pumpkin, parsnips, spinach, winter squash, soybeans, lima beans, cauliflower, collards, cresses, pokeweed, green peas, V-8 juice, tomato paste, puree, sauce, and juice, sauerkraut
Potato or substitute	Noodles, spaghetti, rice, macaroni, ½ c; potato—white or sweet—if leached of potassium by methods described, ½ c	Dried peas or beans, white and sweet potato unless prepared as directed, baked potato, more than ½ potato/day
Bread, cereal	Regular white or whole grain bread (5 servings) plus ¾ c dry cereal (unless on foods avoided list) or ½ c grits, oatmeal, or cream of wheat (cooked without salt)	Product 19, Grapenuts, Total, Special K, Raisin Bran, granola-type cereal, protein-enriched cereal
Soup	Made with allowed vegetables and milk	Soup prepared with meat extracts; canned soup, bouillon cubes or granules, soup mixes
Beverages	Cola drinks, Dr. Pepper, gingerale, Sprite, 7-Up, Kool-Aid, lemonade, root beer, cranberry juice, tea, 1 c per day of regular or decaffeinated coffee	Gatorade, alcoholic beverages (unless approved by physician)
Sweets	Gum drops, hard candy, honey, sugar, jelly, jam, jellybeans, marshmallows, peanut-shaped marshmallows, orange candy slices, fondant, Lifesavers	Brown sugar, molasses, butterscotch, all others

TABLE 30–6 (Continued)

Category	Foods Allowed	Foods Avoided
Fats	Regular margarine (6 tsp/day), unlimited amounts of unsalted margarine, butter, oils, hydrogenated shortenings, salt-free salad dressings or salt-free mayonnaise	Bacon, sausage, fatback, and salt pork, drippings from cured meat
Miscellaneous	Herbs and spices, cornstarch, Coffee-Rich, lemon and vanilla extracts, lemon juice, vinegar, pepper, tabasco sauce, plain cocoa, cranberry sauce	Salt, salt substitute, Lite salt, baking powder substitutes, sodium-free baking powder, barbeque sauces, chili sauce, catsup, steak sauce, meat tenderizer, meat sauce, soy sauce, Worcestershire sauce, meat extracts, nuts, olives, chocolate syrup, peanut butter, coconut, prepared mustard and horseradish, pudding mixes, pickles and pickle relish

(*Source: North Carolina Dietetic Association: Diet Manual, ed 2. Charlotte, NC, 1977, pp 15G–17G.*)

3 weeks, followed by a diuretic phase (however, improved medical management has lessened the problems associated with the diuretic phase)

In approximately 50 percent of those who receive adequate care, normal or near-normal renal function can be restored as the renal tubular cells regenerate. The high mortality rate may be associated with the complications of renal failure. There is a predisposition to sepsis, gastrointestinal hemorrhage, aspiration pneumonia, and malnutrition. Antacids are given to prevent gastrointestinal hemorrhage and the concomitant increase in nitrogen and potassium load.

Intervention

Medical therapy during the oliguric phase is directed toward preventing the manifestations of uremia by dietary restriction or dialysis. Dialysis is often employed in the early stages, although some centers prefer to use a regular diet with fluid restriction and to dialyze as necessary. With this approach, the diet can be more liberal in protein content, and negative nitrogen balance may be prevented. If the oliguric phase persists for more than 3 to 4 days, repeated dialysis is necessary to prevent uremic complications.

Apply the same principles of dietary modification outlined for chronic renal failure to acute renal failure (1) to minimize the nitrogenous load by restricting the dietary protein intake, (2) to promote positive nitrogen balance by providing the minimum quantities of the essential amino acids and adequate kilocalories from carbohydrate and fat, (3) to balance fluid and electrolyte intake with losses, and (4) to provide vitamin supplements.

The diet may be given orally or, if oral intake is impossible, intravenously. Guidelines for diet modification are outlined in Table 30–2. Use laboratory determination of urine volume, serum and urinary electrolytes, BUN and creatinine levels, and body weight (daily weighing is recommended) to determine the specific amount of nutrients allowed. Although some recommend 0.2 to 0.3 g protein/kg body weight, others feel that this amount is insufficient and recommend 0.5 g/kg. The protein content is liberalized with intermittent dialysis.

The intravenous route may be employed initially as nausea, vomiting, or ileus may be present. Total parenteral nutrition solutions that combine concentrated glucose and the essential amino acids (or their keto analogs) are preferred to intravenous solutions that provide glucose alone. Although it has been suggested that providing 100 g glucose/24 hours minimizes ketosis and decreases protein catabolism, maximum protein sparing occurs at far higher levels.

With oral feeding, the diet can be based on conventional foods emphasizing HBV proteins or defined formula diets. The basic feedings should be supplemented with concentrated carbohydrates, such as hard candy and protein-free, low-electrolyte supplements (Controlyte, Polycose, Hy-Cal, Cal-Power; see Table 30–3), and fats.

Restoration of kidney function is signaled by a diuretic phase. Observe for a large urinary volume and large urinary losses of sodium, potassium, magnesium, calcium, phosphate, and water-soluble vitamins during this phase. Carry out frequent laboratory assessments and replace losses with medications and food as necessary to prevent hypovolemic shock and electrolyte imbalance. Avoid overreplacement of fluids, however, since this may potentiate the diuretic phase. As urinary volume becomes stabilized and BUN and blood creatinine levels drop (the latter do not necessarily coincide with the diuresis), gradually increase the intake of dietary protein to normal levels.

DIALYSIS

In those with end-stage renal disease for whom transplantation is not suitable, maintenance dialysis becomes necessary. Maintenance dialysis (either continuous or several times weekly) is initiated when conservative medical management supplemented with occasional dialysis is inadequate to prevent complications. The decision to initiate the procedure is based on criteria related to daily urine volume, rate of rise of the BUN, creatinine clearance, and the client's clinical symptoms.

▶ The term **dialysis** refers to the removal of toxic substances from the body fluids by the processes of osmosis and diffusion across a semipermeable membrane. Either of two types of dialysis is used: (1)
▶ **peritoneal dialysis,** which uses the peritoneal
▶ membrane, and (2) **hemodialysis,** which uses an artificial kidney machine with synthetic semipermeable membranes. Solutes and water move across the membrane from the blood to a dialysis solution (which is similar in composition to normal blood plasma) or from the dialysis solution to the blood in accordance with gradients in concentration. The composition of the dialysate is adjusted to allow urea, creatinine, uric acid, potassium, magnesium, and phosphorus to be removed from the blood and calcium and acetate (which is metabolized to bicarbonate) to be added to the blood.

A new form of peritoneal dialysis, continuous ambulatory peritoneal dialysis (CAPD), has been developed and is now being used more extensively for nonhospitalized clients. A permanent catheter is inserted, and in some cases, the client is dialyzed continuously.

Since most clients lose all renal function soon after the initiation of maintenance dialysis, dietary regulation is essential to prevent excessive accumulation of sodium, fluid, potassium, phosphate, and nitrogenous products between dialyses.

Intervention
Guidelines for dietary management are given in Table 30–2. However, the precise management depends on the philosophy of the treatment center, the type and frequency of dialysis, and the physical condition of the client. The diet is more liberal in protein and thus more palatable than the diet used in the conservative management of acute and chronic renal failure. Liberalize the protein content for clients being dialysed to replace those losses that occur in dialysis and to prevent hypoproteinemia and amino acid depletion. Approximate losses incurred by the two dialysis techniques are:

Peritoneal Dialysis	Hemodialysis
Protein (primarily albumin and IgG): 10–30 g or more/dialysis	Protein: Very small amount
Amino acids: 5–10 g or more/dialysis	Amino acids: 6–10 g/dialysis

The losses of amino acids in the dialysate during CAPD are less than with either intermittent peritoneal dialysis or hemodialysis. Yet, since CAPD is performed continuously, overall losses are similar to or slightly greater than those losses from intermittent peritoneal dialysis carried out several times per week or with hemodialysis 3 times per week.[11]

Amino acid profiles tend to change with hemodialysis. There appears to be an overall reduction in essential amino acids with a concomitant rise in the nonessential amino acids and an increase in the phenylalanine:tyrosine ratio. A marked reduction in the branched-chain amino acids (leucine, isoleucine, and valine) has been noted. Although an increase in dietary protein intake is the most practical approach to replacing the losses, amino acid supplements may also be given. Addition of amino acids to the dialysate reduces the amino acid losses. A large percentage of dietary protein should be of HBV, and substantial quantities of carbohydrate and fat (low in protein) should be supplied to meet the kilocalorie need. Milk must be used sparingly because of its high content of fluid, sodium, potassium, and phosphate.

Restrict the intake of sodium, fluid, potassium, and phosphorus to prevent edema, hypertension, hyperkalemia, and hypocalcemia. The fluid and sodium allowances are designed to limit weight gain between dialyses to no more than 1 lb. The use of phosphate binders may be very important in controlling hyperphosphatemia, since the liberal protein intake makes dietary phosphate restriction difficult.

A vitamin supplement that approximates the RDA for the water-soluble vitamins (and provides larger amounts for some) is essential because there are losses of water-soluble vitamins in the dialysis fluid. Folic acid, vitamin B_6, and vitamin C are especially likely to be depleted during dialysis. In contrast, vitamin B_{12}, vitamin A, and vitamin D are bound to protein, and losses are minimal during dialysis. The recommended dosages of folic acid, vitamin B_6, and vitamin C supplements are 1 mg, 10 mg, and 100 mg, respectively. Some authorities recommend larger doses, particularly of pyridoxine. Persistent hypocalcemia or the presence of renal osteodystrophy necessitates treatment with metabolites of vitamin D and calcium. All forms of vitamin D must be used with caution because of the potential for aggravating bone abnormalities. Supplement of vitamin A is not recommended, and supplements of vitamins E and K are probably not necessary.

Iron deficiency is not uncommon because of associated blood loss (the usual external losses that accompany dialysis and frequent venipuncture).

Iron supplements may therefore be required, and androgens (such as nandrolone decanoate) are sometimes given to stimulate erythropoiesis.

Client Education for Clients with Chronic Renal Failure and Dialysis

Diets that involve combined modifications, such as control of protein, sodium, potassium, and fluid intake, are difficult for the client to implement at home, and intensive diet counseling is needed. Young children, in particular, may not be able to understand the need for adherence to the regimen. Initiate diet instruction for both the client and family as soon as possible during hospitalization, reinforce the teaching daily, and continue it on an outpatient basis and when the client returns for dialysis. The basics of the diet can be recorded on tape for the client to replay at a later time.

The food grouping system discussed earlier in the chapter is often used as a basis for developing the individualized diet plan for the client and as a tool for nutrition counseling. It is essential that the client or a family member understand the categories covered by the food lists, the amounts to use from each list, the way to make substitutions within a given food list, and how to plan daily menus based on the lists.

Use the hospital tray as a teaching tool to indicate the types and amounts of foods allowed and those foods to be avoided. Scales may be useful in determining portion sizes. If special food preparation techniques are necessary, give the client an opportunity to practice preparing the foods while hospitalized. Prior to discharge, instruct the client on how to keep a food diary, and use the diary in follow-up visits to determine if food intake is consistent with the diet plans.

Stress to the client and the family that diet modification is a *primary* form of treatment. In contrast to clients with diabetes mellitus and cardiac disease, who may cheat on their diets without immediate serious side effects, clients with renal failure who eat or drink to the point of exceeding the kidney's capacity to excrete the waste products may die as a result of hyperkalemia or pulmonary edema.

Long-term adherence to a stringent treatment regimen is difficult, particularly for clients on maintenance dialysis, and the rate of noncompliance is high. Nurses can help provide motivation to follow the dietary regimen by assisting to make the diet palatable by selecting foods that take into account the client's food choices and economic status. Since taste changes occur in uremia, sharp, distinct flavors may be preferred. When the client does not adhere to the regimen, determine the reason and have the client identify specific areas of nonadherence and changes that he or she can make to follow the diet.

Be sensitive to the sociologic and psychologic problems encountered by the client. Not only must the individual adjust to a diet that sometimes cannot reflect usual eating patterns, but he or she must also cope with the mechanics of dialysis and take medication and still not feel completely well. While the threat of death may be removed with dialysis, changes in lifestyle, economic situation, and levels of independence may lead to depression and mood changes. Some clients may respond by failure to follow the prescribed regimen, i.e., by diet indiscretions, failure to take medications, and similar behavior. The National Kidney Foundation provides information about community support groups that have been established to assist clients on maintenance dialysis.

POSTTRANSPLANT

Successful kidney transplantation can restore normal renal function and end the need for the diet modifications described for renal failure and dialysis. Should the transplant be unsuccessful, however, return to maintenance dialysis is necessary.

Complications can occur at any time following transplantation, and proper nutritional management of the complications becomes important to the success of the transplant. Many transplanted kidneys will suffer episodes of rejection with reduced renal function. This situation necessitates reinstatement of the diet modifications described for uremia. Additionally, adverse side effects of the immunosuppressive medications used to reduce the risk of transplant rejection pose problems in nutritional management. All transplant clients receive immunosuppressive agents, such as azathioprine (Imuran) and corticosteroids (prednisone).

Early transplantation is particularly desirable in children because of the osteodystrophy and growth retardation associated with chronic renal failure. If transplantation is initiated before closure of the epiphyses, growth may improve.

Assessment and Intervention

Common complications during the course of the transplant that necessitate diet modifications are summarized below, along with the specific diet modification indicated. The specific diet therapy is dictated by the particular complaint present.

1. Massive diuresis during the immediate postoperative period: Provide intravenous replacement of urinary fluid and electrolyte losses (observe for circulatory congestion, volume depletion, and electrolyte imbalance)
2. Hypertension (mild hypertension may be observed in the immediate postoperative period, but the hypertension tends to become more severe during a rejection episode): Treat with antihypertensive drugs and a sodium-restricted diet (43 to 87 mEq or 1 to 2 g daily); use of diuretics may induce secondary hypokalemia, necessitating its replace-

ment with high-potassium foods or potassium salts

3. Immunologic rejection of the allograft with diminished renal function (can occur at any time): Restrict protein, sodium, potassium, and fluid—amounts allowed are determined by concentrations of the substances in blood and urine

4. Decreased glucose tolerance: Hyperglycemia, glucosuria, and relative resistance to insulin (secondary to steroid therapy); substitute complex carbohydrates (i.e., bread, cereal, fruit) for sugars

5. Obesity (moderate to massive) and a cushingoid appearance that may lead to psychologic problems associated with an alteration in body image (secondary to steroid therapy—steroids stimulate the appetite and redistribute fat): Restrict kilocalorie intake as necessary to prevent or control obesity

6. Hyperlipidemia (the most common abnormality is hypertriglyceridemia): See Chapter 29 for appropriate diet modifications for hyperlipidemia

7. Oral and pharyngeal infection with difficulty chewing and swallowing (secondary to immunosuppressive agents): Modify food textures (i.e., serve soft foods that require minimal chewing) and serve small, frequent feedings

8. Acceleration of negative nitrogen and calcium balance (secondary to steroids): Provide a high-protein diet (approximately 2 g/kg) with 800 to 1200 mg calcium

9. Gastrointestinal ulceration with possible hemorrhage and perforation (secondary to steroid therapy that may impair the mucosal barrier): Use a liberal bland diet (i.e., restriction of alcohol, caffeine, and decaffeinated coffee) served in small, frequent feedings as a preventive measure as soon as solid foods are taken; should bleeding occur, use a strict bland diet (i.e., exclusion of raw fruits and vegetables, condiments, foods that contain seeds, foods high in residue, and foods that are very hot or very cold)

Other problems may also become apparent in the posttransplant period. Hyperparathyroidism may persist in some, leading to severe bone disease and hypercalcemia (which can damage the transplanted kidney). Adjustments in the intake of calcium, phosphorus, and vitamin D as described for renal failure are necessary to counteract the calcium–phosphorus imbalance, and in some cases parathyroidectomy becomes necessary. Pancreatitis has been attributed to the use of both azathioprine and steroids, and hepatitis has been reported related to azathioprine. Both of these conditions may necessitate adjustment in the fat intake (see Chap. 29). The disease that caused the initial renal failure may also affect the transplanted kidney.

NEPHROTIC SYNDROME

▶ The **nephrotic syndrome** is not a disease entity per se but rather a group of biochemical and clinical symptoms that can be a component of several forms of renal disease as well as other disease conditions. Glomerulonephritis is the most common cause of the nephrotic syndrome, but it may also appear during the progression of chronic renal disease from renal insufficiency to renal failure. The syndrome may be seen in association with metabolic diseases, systemic sensitivity diseases, circulatory disorders, allergies, drug reactions, and infectious processes. The basic defect in the disorder is an increase in the permeability of the glomerular basement membrane to protein. Thus any disease that increases the permeability of this membrane can cause the nephrotic syndrome. Congenital forms of the nephrotic syndrome exist in children.

Assessment
Observe the results of laboratory tests that reveal proteinuria (loss of protein in the urine), hypoalbuminemia (low blood albumin), and hyperlipidemia. The client will exhibit massive edema. Urinary protein losses may vary from 4 to 40 g daily; test for the amount of protein in 24-hour urine collections. Albumin is the major protein lost in the urine, but other proteins, such as immunoglobulins and complement factors and proteins that bind thyroid hormone, iron, copper, zinc, and possibly other minerals, and vitamin D are also lost. The continued loss of albumin leads to hypoalbuminemia and edema, depletion of tissue and cellular protein, and fatty deposits in the liver. The edema is compounded by an increased reabsorption of sodium. The concomitant malnutrition, which may be masked by the edema, leads to an increased susceptibility to infection. There is a severe iron deficiency anemia, and the low level of vitamin D metabolites may lead to defective gastrointestinal calcium absorption, hypocalcemia, secondary hyperparathyroidism, and renal osteodystrophy. Hypercholesterolemia is the primary manifestation of hyperlipidemia, although triglycerides may be elevated. The cause of the lipid abnormality and its influence on the development of atherosclerosis are uncertain, although there is some evidence that clients with the nephrotic syndrome have an increased incidence of coronary heart disease. Hypertension and hematuria (blood in the urine) may occur, depending on the condition of the kidney. The excretion of urea and other metabolic wastes is usually normal, at least initially.

Intervention
Dietary management is directed toward control of edema, malnutrition, and hyperlipidemia. If the glomerular filtration rate (GFR) is normal, the protein intake is calculated to replace the urinary losses of albumin and to provide for positive nitrogen bal-

ance. Since 7 to 9 g of dietary protein may be required to replace 1 g of protein lost in the urine, a long period of time may be required to replace the losses in clients with gross deficiency. Unless the GFR is greatly reduced, provide at least 1.5 g/kg body weight for adults and 2 to 3 g/kg body weight for children with an amount equivalent to urinary losses added to this figure. Depending on the individual's body weight and the amount of protein loss, the diet may contain 100 to 150 g protein daily. A large percentage of the protein should be HBV, and the kilocalorie intake should be 50 to 60 kcal/kg. If the GFR is depressed, modify the protein as for clients with chronic renal failure.

Restrict sodium to 40 to 90 mEq (920 to 2070 mg) daily to control the edema if the edema responds poorly to diuretic therapy. The level of sodium intake should be sufficient to replace the losses incurred in the 24-hour urine output. If sodium is rigidly restricted, it is difficult to maintain the desired protein intake, as protein foods of HBV are also high in sodium. Use commercial products that are low in sodium and high in HBV protein, such as low-sodium milk, to augment the protein intake. Curtail the intake of cholesterol and saturated fat to control hyperlipidemia, and provide supplemental vitamin D. Although anemia is present, iron therapy has been associated with sepsis.

Because the appetite is often poor in clients with massive edema, use all appropriate nursing strategies to promote food intake. Nephrotic children are particularly challenging in this area. Some clients find it difficult to ingest diets containing more than 100 g protein. Position the client for maximum comfort before meals. Parenteral administration of amino acids or protein hydrolysates may be necessary if the anorexia is severe or if nausea and vomiting are pronounced. Use daily weights to evaluate the status of edema and the effectiveness of diuretic therapy or sodium restriction.

GLOMERULONEPHRITIS

▶ **Glomerulonephritis** is a general term used to describe diffuse inflammatory changes in the glomeruli. In the acute form, there is complete recovery in a large percentage of affected individuals. In a few cases, however, the disease becomes chronic. In the chronic form of glomerulonephritis, the glomeruli gradually become fibrotic, and the tubules gradually degenerate, leading to progressive renal insufficiency and renal failure. Another renal disorder, arteriolar nephrosclerosis, is characterized by similar degenerative changes.

Assessment

Acute glomerulonephritis occurs most often in children and young adults. It often follows a beta-hemolytic group A streptococcal infection, although it may be precipitated by syphilis or other infections.

In contrast, chronic glomerulonephritis is insidious in onset. The majority of individuals with the disease have no previous history of acute glomerulonephritis. Observe for these signs and symptoms in clients with the acute form of the disease: hematuria, edema, hypertension, azotemia, albuminuria, oliguria or anuria, anorexia, lethargy, nausea, and vomiting. In contrast, the sole presenting symptoms in clients with chronic glomerulonephritis may be proteinuria and edema, although the progressive destruction of the glomeruli and tubules continues. The clinical course may demonstrate a prolonged latent stage in which the individual is asymptomatic, followed by a nephrotic stage with symptoms characteristic of the nephrotic syndrome. As the disease progresses, renal insufficiency occurs and there are hypertension, proteinuria with hypoalbuminemia, edema, and nocturia. Nocturia occurs because of lack of renal-concentrating capacity. This stage is followed by uremia necessitating long-term diet therapy and dialysis or transplantation.

Intervention

The dietary modification for glomerulonephritis depend on the symptoms that are manifest. In acute glomerulonephritis, control fluid intake to balance the intake with output to prevent overhydration. Allow 500 to 700 ml daily plus an amount equivalent to the previous day's urine output, and add additional fluid to compensate for vomiting or diarrhea. Apportion the limited fluid intake equally over the waking hours, and keep the client's mouth clean and moist.

In the presence of oliguria or anuria, restrict protein to 0.5 g/kg body weight for adults and 0.75 g/kg body weight for children, giving preference to HBV protein, to curtail symptoms of uremia. Add additional protein to compensate for marked proteinuria. With improvement in kidney function, gradually increase the protein to normal levels. Although a high kilocalorie intake is desirable, it may be difficult to achieve when LBV protein, such as grains and breads, is limited. Use concentrated carbohydrates, such as hard candy and jelly, and fats, such as cream and margarine, to increase kilocaloric intake.

Sodium is not restricted unless edema, hypertension, and oliguria are judged to be potential hazards. In these cases, restrict sodium to 20 to 40 mEq (460 to 920 mg). Ascites may make the normal upright position for eating difficult. In this situation, position the client carefully for meals. Potassium restriction may be necessary when urinary output is greatly reduced. When diuresis occurs, replace fluid losses, remove the sodium restriction, and replace electrolytes as indicated by results of laboratory tests.

Diet modifications are not necessary during the latent stage of chronic glomerulonephritis unless signs of edema or proteinuria are apparent. Following the latent period, diet modifications are based on the stage and are the same as those described previously for the nephrotic syndrome and chronic renal failure. The sodium restriction required during the nephrotic stage must be revoked when renal failure becomes evident, since salt wasting occurs. Fluid intake should be in a range of 2500 to 3500 ml daily to assure proper renal clearance. Maintain this level as long as the deteriorating kidneys waste salt and cardiac function is not impaired.

RENAL CALCULI

▶ **Nephrolithiasis** (renal stones or calculi) is one of the oldest recognized maladies of man and is a common disorder in the United States.

Assessment
Most stones originate in the kidney, although they can occur anywhere along the urinary tract. Numerous factors promote stone formation, for example, metabolic disorders (e.g., idiopathic hypercalciuria, cystinuria, oxalosis, and gout), immobilization, dehydration, hormonal imbalance (e.g., primary hyperparathyroidism), osteoporosis, systemic infection, excessive ingestion of vitamin D, and lesions in the urinary tract that obstruct urinary flow and thus lead to stasis.

The constituents of the stones vary with individuals, but the most common are calcium (as calcium oxalate, calcium phosphate, or a mixture of both), magnesium ammonium phosphate (struvite), uric acid, and cystine. Less common constituents are glycine and xanthine. Of the constituents of renal calculi, calcium is the most common, and the largest percentage of these stones are composed of calcium oxalate. A slightly smaller percentage contain a combination of calcium oxalate and calcium phosphate. Pure calcium phosphate stones are less common. Stones composed of magnesium ammonium phosphate occur almost exclusively in clients with recurrent urinary tract infection, whereas stones composed largely of calcium phosphate occur secondary to hyperparathyroidism and immobilization. Uric acid stones are less common than calcium-containing stones, and cystine stones are relatively rare.

Stone formation usually occurs when crystalline materials (such as calcium, uric acid) precipitate on an organic matrix. Four mechanisms that may lead to changes in the quantity or composition of urine and thus enhance crystalloid precipitation are:

1. A decrease in urine volume: A concentrated urine of low volume favors precipitation
2. Persistent extremes in urinary pH, i.e., acid or alkaline: Acid urine may enhance the precipitation of uric acid and cystine stones, whereas alkaline urine favors the precipitation of stones composed of calcium phosphate and magnesium ammonium phosphate
3. An increase in urinary crystalloid output: Although stones may form with normal urinary crystalloid levels, a high level of such substances as uric acid or oxalate favors precipitation
4. A decrease in urinary excretion of agents that inhibit crystalloid precipitation: A number of inhibitors to crystal formation have been identified in normal urine, including urea, citrate, pyrophosphate, magnesium, trace metals, and certain amino acids. For example, pyrophosphate is a potent inhibitor of calcium crystal growth and aggregation

Intervention
Since stones can damage the kidney by predisposing to obstruction, infection, or pressure necrosis, treatment is necessary to prevent permanent damage. Treatment methods include:

1. Encouraging spontaneous passage
2. Surgical removal
3. Methods to decrease the concentration of stone precursors by
   a. Increasing urine volume (by increasing fluid intake)
   b. Using medications to decrease the synthesis or to bind the precursor; e.g., allopurinol prevents uric acid synthesis, and D-penicillamine binds cystine to form a soluble substance
   c. Limiting the dietary intake of precursors, such as calcium or oxalate
4. Altering urinary pH by diet or medications (sodium bicarbonate and sodium citrate are alkalizers, and methionine and ascorbic acid are acidifiers). Acid and alkaline ash diets (see Chap. 9) have been used in the past to alter urinary pH; however, medications offer a much simpler and more effective approach to controlling pH

Various diet modifications have been used in the past for prevention and treatment of kidney stones, but there is no general agreement as to their overall efficacy. The single most important nutritional consideration in the management of kidney stones, regardless of their composition, is maintenance of a high fluid intake (3000 to 4000 ml daily) in order to increase the urine volume and decrease the concentration of precipitating solutes. Advise clients to drink 250 to 300 ml of fluid hourly while awake and to drink fluids before going to bed and if they void during the night. Since urine is both more concentrated and more acid during the night, this practice will maintain a dilute urine on a consistent basis. If a client's history reveals calcium oxalate stones, suggest that a large portion of the fluids should consist of water and restrict fluids that contain excessive calcium (such as milk) or oxalates (such as tea). Caution the client against becoming dehydrated. Excessive perspiration and other fluid losses necessitate an increase in fluid intake. Also advise clients to ingest a nutritionally balanced diet, since deficiencies of certain nutrients, such as pyridoxine, magnesium, and thiamine, have been associated with the development of stones. In specific instances (discussed below) dietary manipulations based on the etiology of the stone formation may be somewhat helpful.

Calcium-containing Stones Associated with Idiopathic Hypercalciuria. Stones composed primarily of calcium oxalate or a mixture of calcium oxalate, calcium phosphate, and uric acid occur in clients who, for unknown causes, excrete excessive amounts of calcium in the urine. Assess for hypercalciuria in clients with renal stones. Urinary calcium excretion > 4 mg/kg body weight (or > 250 mg/24 hours in females and > 300 mg/24 hours in males) indicates excessive excretion. Note, however, that not all clients with calcium-containing stones exhibit hypercalciuria, nor do all persons who exhibit hypercalciuria develop stones. Two mechanisms have been suggested in the etiology of idiopathic (of unknown cause) hypercalciuria: (1) a familial tendency to absorb calcium at an abnormally high rate by

TABLE 30-7
CALCIUM-CONTROLLED DIET (APPROXIMATELY 400 MG OF CALCIUM)

Category	Foods Allowed	Foods Avoided
Beverages	Carbonated beverages, postum, Sanka, coffee, tea, ¾ c milk	Milk (except for the amount allowed) and milk drinks, ice cream, yoghurt, powdered instant breakfast drinks
Bread–cereal	Regular white bread (3 slices), refined cereals, graham crackers, saltines, soda crackers, Italian bread, plain flour	Other breads, crackers, and cereals, commercially prepared baking mixes, self-rising flour, self-rising cornmeal, instant cooking cereals
Desserts	Allowed fruit and fruit pies, fruit whip, gelatin dessert, water ices, angel food cake, popsicles, sherbet made with water	Those prepared with milk and eggs, figs, dried fruits
Fat	Butter, margarine, bacon, oils, vegetable shortening, lard, salad dressings	Almonds, Brazil nuts, olives, cream, cream sauces, gravies
Fruit	Canned, fresh, and cooked fruit except those on foods avoided list	Dried fruit, rhubarb, figs
Meat, egg, and cheese	5–7 oz daily of red meat, poultry, and low-calcium fish (bluefish, cod, flounder, crab, haddock, halibut, shad, tuna), no more than 1 egg daily (including those used in cooking)	Clams, oysters, bass, smoked herring, lobster, mackerel, canned salmon, canned sardines, shrimp, cheese, peanut butter, hot dogs and cold cuts (unless all meat), more than 1 egg daily
Soup	Meat broth and vegetable soups made with allowed vegetables	Cream or milk soups, bean or pea soup
Vegetables	Canned, fresh, or cooked vegetables or juice except those not allowed	Broccoli, dried peas and beans, commercially prepared canned baked beans, lima beans, lentils, endive, kale, mustard greens, turnip greens, dandelion greens, collard greens, spinach, okra, green onions, creamed vegetables; limit use of green beans, cabbage, fresh carrots, parsnips, radishes, sweet potato, sauerkraut, turnips
Miscellaneous	Hard candy, honey, jam, jelly, white sugar, catsup, cornstarch, mustard, pepper, salt, herbs and spices, vinegar, pickles, popcorn, relishes	Brown sugar, chocolate, chocolate candy, caramels, cocoa, molasses, maple or corn syrups, brewer's yeast, foods with calcium preservatives (such as calcium propionate and dicalcium phosphate)

the intestine and (2) a familial tendency for depressed renal tubular reabsorption of calcium.

Drugs used to normalize the urinary calcium level include thiazide diuretics, inorganic phosphate, and cellulose phosphate. Advise clients who take thiazide diuretics to moderate their sodium intake, since the benefit of the drug in reducing calcium excretion can be diminished by a high sodium intake. If the client's hypercalciuria is associated with hyperabsorption of calcium, it may be prudent to control calcium intake by restricting dietary intake to 400 to 600 mg daily (Table 30–7) and to avoid consumption of calcium-containing medications and vitamin D, including vitamin D-fortified foods. Not all investigators agree that calcium restriction is beneficial, however, and some suggest that thiazide therapy is the preferred treatment.[12] Thiazides lower calcium excretion at least partly by increasing calcium reabsorption in the renal tubules. Ascertain the calcium content of the client's water supply when calcium is restricted, and if the concentration is excessive, suggest the use of distilled water for drinking and cooking. Be aware, however, that dietary calcium restriction may be contraindicated in clients who fail to conserve calcium normally, since this may lead to a negative calcium balance and oxalate absorption and excretion with the potential for precipitation of calcium oxalate stones. Since calcium tends to be soluble in an acid urine, medica-

tions to acidify the urine are used. An acid ash diet (see Chap. 9) serves the same purpose, although it is seldom used today. If there is a concomitant increase in the blood and urinary levels of uric acid, drugs are used to bring the uric acid level to normal, since sodium urate and uric acid may promote the growth of calcium oxalate crystals.

Oxalate Stones. Stones composed of calcium oxalate are common in clients with hyperoxaluria. (Excessive oxalate excretion occurs secondary to an inborn error of oxalate metabolism, excessive ingestion of oxalate or its precursors, or chronic inflammatory small bowel disorders, such as Crohn's disease; see Chap. 27.) In the presence of hyperoxaluria and calcium oxalate stones, instruct clients to restrict the dietary intake of oxalate to 40 to 50 mg daily. Foods of animal origin contain negligible amounts of oxalate, although the substance is widely distributed in fruits and vegetables and average daily intake is 80 to 120 mg. Foods that contain more than 10 mg of oxalate per serving should be avoided completely, and those that contain 2 to 10 mg of oxalate should be limited. Foods with an oxalate content greater than 10 mg/serving are listed in Table 30–8. A number of fruits and vegetables, such as bananas, cherries, Thompson seedless grapes, Bing cherries, melons, peaches, pineapple, plums, broccoli, brussels sprouts, cauliflower, cu-

---

TABLE 30–8
FOODS THAT CONTAIN IN EXCESS OF 10 MG OXALATE PER SERVING

Fruits	Vegetables	Miscellaneous
Berries (black, blue, black raspberry, green goose)	Beans (green, wax, dried; or baked beans canned in tomato sauce)	Chocolate
Currants (red)	Beets	Cocoa
Dewberries	Celery	Grits (white)
Fruit cocktail	Collards	Ovaltine
Grapes (Concord)	Dandelion greens	Peanuts/peanut butter
Lemon peel	Eggplant	Pecans
Lime peel	Escarole	Soybean crackers
Orange peel	Kale	Tea
Rhubarb	Leeks	Tofu
Strawberries	Mustard greens	Wheat germ
Tangerines	Okra	
	Parsley	
	Pepper (green)	
	Pokeweed	
	Potatoes (sweet)	
	Rutabaga	
	Spinach	
	Squash (summer)	
	Swiss chard	
	Watercress	

(*Source: Adapted from Nutrition and the M.D., vol 5 (No. 9), Sept 1979; Ney DM, et al.: The Low Oxalate Diet Book. San Diego, University of California Press, 1981.*)

cumber, onions, peas, and white potatoes, contain negligible amounts of oxalate. Advise clients to avoid taking large doses of vitamin C, since oxalate is the end product of vitamin C metabolism. Some authorities suggest supplements of vitamin B$_6$ and magnesium oxide for treating calcium oxalate stones. Urinary pH has little effect. If the hyperoxaluria is associated with excessive intestinal absorption of oxalate and hypercalciuria is not present, limit the dietary fat in the diet and provide calcium supplements (see Chap. 27 for rationale).

► *Uric Acid Stones.* The precipitation of **uric acid**
► (the end product of purine metabolism) is enhanced
► by disorders that cause **hyperuricemia** (elevated **uric acid** in the blood) and **hyperuricosuria** (elevated uric acid in the urine). In conditions such as gout, starvation, or increase in cell turnover secondary to cancer therapy, there is an increase in uric acid production and excretion. Excretion of a persistently acid urine leading to uric acid stones also occurs in gout and in certain malabsorption syndromes. Although used in the past, low-purine diets (see Chap. 37) and alkali ash diets (see Chap. 9) are rarely used today, since medications are effective in reducing uric acid synthesis and in alkalizing the urine. However, both diet and medications may be used in individual cases. A low-purine diet restricts the use of protein. These foods not only increase uric acid excretion but also tend to acidify the urine because of their high acid ash content.

Cystine Stones. Renal stones composed of cystine occur in clients with cystinuria, a rare, hereditary inborn error by metabolism associated with excretion of increased amounts of cystine and other amino acids in the urine. Being less soluble than the other amino acids, cystine precipitates as stones in acid urine. In clients who develop sensitivity to D-penicillamine, the medication used to treat the disorder, a methionine-restricted diet may be ordered. A methionine-restricted diet is impractical for general use, however, because of its severe protein restriction—clients must avoid milk and dairy products, eggs, fish, and certain fruits and vegetables. Since cystine is insoluble in acid urine, an alkali ash diet may sometimes be used.

REVIEW QUESTIONS AND ACTIVITIES

1. Relate the renal symptoms of chronic renal failure to the excretory, regulatory, and endocrine functions of the kidney.
2. Discuss the rationale for restricting protein, sodium, potassium, and fluid in clients with chronic renal failure.
3. Discuss the use of the blood urea nitrogen (BUN) as a clinical marker in renal disorders.
4. Explain the rationale for use of protein of high biologic value (HBV) in the diet of clients with chronic renal failure.
5. Explain the rationale for a liberal intake of kilocalories from carbohydrate and fat in clients following protein-restricted diets.
6. Explain the rationale for phosphate restriction in clients with chronic renal failure and approaches used in treating elevated blood phosphorus levels.
7. Differentiate between salt retention and salt wasting in clients with chronic renal failure and approaches used in treating these clinical problems.
8. Distinguish between conditions that precipitate hypokalemia and hyperkalemia in clients with chronic renal failure and approaches used in treating blood potassium alterations.
9. Discuss the use of vitamin and mineral supplements in clients with chronic renal failure.
10. *Case study:* Mr. B, a 45-year-old carpenter, has the following diet order to control uremic symptoms prior to being placed on dialysis: Protein, 40 g; sodium, 75 mEq (1725 mg); potassium, 40 mEq (1560 mg).
    a. Plan a day's menu that meets this diet prescription (see Tables 30–4, 30–5, and 30–6).
    b. List foods that could be used to increase the kilocalorie intake without increasing the intake of protein, sodium, or potassium.
    c. Describe food preparation techniques that must be followed to assure that the sodium content of the diet is not excessive (see Chap. 29).
    d. Describe food preparation techniques for reducing the potassium content of high-potassium foods.
    Additional information: Two weeks later, Mr. B was placed on intermittent peritoneal dialysis.
    e. Describe adjustments in the diet prescription that are necessary to meet Mr. B's nutritional needs.
    f. Compare Mr. B's nutritional requirements with the requirements of clients with acute renal failure.
11. Describe the techniques of fluid management and ways of dealing with thirst in clients with chronic renal failure.
12. Identify nine posttransplant complications that may occur secondary to associated drug therapy and the diet modifications necessitated by each complication.
13. Relate the dietary management of the nephrotic syndrome and acute glomerulone-

phritis to the clinical problems experienced by clients with these disorders.

14. Identify the constituents of the most common type of renal stones.
15. List four factors that favor renal stone formation.
16. Identify the single most important dietary measure for control of renal stones.
17. Identify situations in which restriction of dietary calcium and dietary oxalate may be indicated for control of renal stones.
18. Describe the dietary management of stones composed of uric acid and cystine.
19. Identify the urinary pH range (acid or alkaline) that favors precipitation of renal stones composed of (a) calcium, (b) uric acid, and (c) cystine.

REFERENCES

1. Burton BT: Nutritional implications of renal disease. J Am Diet Assoc 70:479, 1977.
2. Spinozzi NS, Grupe WE: Nutritional implications of renal disease. IV. Nutritional aspects of chronic renal insufficiency in childhood. J Am Diet Assoc 70:493, 1977.
3. American Dietetic Association: Handbook of Clinical Dietetics. New Haven, Conn, Yale University Press, 1981, p C-11.
4. Brenner BM, Meyer TW, Hostetter TH: Dietary protein intake and the progressive nature of kidney disease: The role of hemodynamically mediated glomerular injury in the pathogenesis of progressive glomerular sclerosis in aging, renal ablation and intrinsic renal disease. N Eng J Med 307:652, 1982.
5. Berlyne GM, Shaw AB: Giordano–Giovanetti diet in terminal renal failure. Lancet 2:7, 1965.
6. Burton BT, Hirschman GH: Current concepts of nutritional therapy in chronic renal failure: An update. J Am Diet Assoc 82:359, 1983.
7. Massry SG: Requirements of vitamin D metabolites in patients with renal disease. Am J Clin Nutr 33:1530, 1980.
8. Mahajan SK, Prasad AS, Rabbani P, et al.: Zinc deficiency: A reversible complication of uremia. Am J Clin Nutr 36:1177, 1982.
9. Kleiner MJ, Tate SS, Sullivan JF, et al.: Vitamin B_6 deficiency in maintenance dialysis patients: Metabolic effects of repletion. Am J Clin Nutr 33:1612, 1980.
10. Sanfelippo ML, Swenson RS, Reaven GM: Reduction of plasma triglycerides by diet in subjects with chronic renal failure. Kidney Int 11:54, 1977.
11. Kopple JD, Blumenkrantz MJ, Jones MR, et al.: Plasma amino acid levels and amino acid losses during continuous ambulatory peritoneal dialysis. Am J Clin Nutr 36:397, 1982.
12. Broadus AE, Insogna KL, Lang R, et al.: Evidence for disordered control of 1,25-dihydroxy vitamin D production in absorptive hypercalciuria. N Eng J Med 311:73, 1984.

BIBLIOGRAPHY

Baldree KS, Murphy SP, Powers MJ: Stress identification and coping patterns in patients on hemodialysis. Nurs Res 31:107, 1981.

Barsotti G, Guiducci A, Ciardella F, Giovannetti S: Effects on renal function of a low-nitrogen diet supplemented with essential amino acids and keto-analogs and of hemodialysis and free protein supply in patients with chronic renal failure. Nephron 27:113, 1981.

Bergstrom J: Proceedings of the Twelfth Annual Contractors Conference. Artificial Kidney—Chronic Uremia Program. NIAMDD, NIH Publication No. 81–1979, Bethesda, MD, National Institutes of Health, 1981.

Chambers JK: Bowel management in dialysis patients. Am J Nurs 83:1051, 1983.

Christiansen C, Christensen MS, Melsen F, et al.: Mineral metabolism in chronic renal failure with special reference to serum concentrations of 1,25$(OH)_2$D and 24,-25$(OH)_2$D. Clin Nephrol 15(1):18, 1981.

Levine SE: Nutritional care of patients with renal failure and diabetes. J Am Diet Assoc 81:261, 1982.

Metheny N: Renal stones and urinary pH. Am J Nurs 82:1372, 1982.

Mitch WE, Walser M, Steinman TI, et al.: The effect of keto acid–amino acid supplement to a restricted diet on the progression of chronic renal failure. N Eng J Med 311:623, 1984.

Moore J Jr, Maher JF: Management of chronic renal failure. Am Fam Phys 30:204, 1984.

Rostand SG: Profound hypokalemia in continuous ambulatory peritoneal dialysis. Arch Intern Med 143:377, 1983.

Schmidt KH, Hagmaiet V, Hornig DT, et al.: Urinary oxalate excretion after large intakes of ascorbic acid in man. Am J Clin Nutr 34:305, 1981.

Shen SY, Lukens CW, Alongi SV, et al.: Patient profile and effect of dietary therapy on post-transplant hyperlipidemia. Kidney Int 24[Suppl 16]:5–147, 1983.

Smythe WR: Trace element abnormalities in chronic uremia. Ann Intern Med 96:302, 1982.

CLIENT RESOURCES

Jones WO: Diet Guide for Patients on Chronic Dialysis. DHEW Publication No. (NIH) 76–685, Bethesda, Md, National Institutes of Health, 1976.

Los Angeles District of the California Dietetic Association: A Guide to Protein-controlled Diets for Patients, Los Angeles, 1977.

Ney DM, Hoffman AF, Fischer C, Stubblefield N: The Low Oxalate Diet Book. San Diego, University of California, 1981.

St. Jeor S, Groves D, Cole R, Rhen R: Meal Planning for People with Kidney Disease. Salt Lake City, University of Utah Press, 1978.

Understanding and Living with Your Renal Diet: A Basic Guide for Patients. Philadelphia, Wyeth Laboratories, 1983.

U.S. Public Health Service: Living with End-Stage Renal Failure. A Book for Patients. Washington, DC, U.S. Government Printing Office, 1976.

CHAPTER 31

Nutrition and Anemia

Objectives

After completion of this chapter, the student will be able to:
1. Distinguish between the three major mechanisms that lead to anemia.
2. Compare and contrast the etiologic factors and clinical manifestations associated with anemia resulting from a deficiency of iron, folic acid, and vitamin B_{12}.
3. Develop a nursing care plan for the nutritional management of a client with iron deficiency anemia and adapt the plan so that it is appropriate for a client with pernicious anemia.
4. Plan a menu that is high in protein and iron and within the kilocalorie restraints for a young adult female with iron deficiency anemia who also has a low income.
5. Differentiate between the clinical manifestations of vitamin B_{12} deficiency anemia due to a lack of intrinsic factor and vitamin B_{12} deficiency anemia due to other causes.
6. Manage the treatment of anemia in clients with a deficiency of folic acid and vitamin B_{12}.
7. Assess the potential for preventing anemia associated with a dietary deficiency of iron, folic acid, and vitamin B_{12}.

Anemia is a common disorder that may arise from various defects in the blood-forming organs and may be nutritional or nonnutritional in origin. Nutritional anemia results from a deficiency of the nutrients needed to form either the red blood cells or hemoglobin. Iron deficiency anemia is an especially prevalent form of nutritional anemia, although anemia due to either folic acid or vitamin B_{12} deficiency is not uncommon. Successful treatment of nutritional anemia is dependent upon diagnosing the disorder correctly and determining its basic cause. In order to assist in establishing the correct diagnosis, nurses should be knowledgeable of the signs and symptoms of anemia as well as be alert to the possible occurrence of anemia in high-risk groups. It is particularly important to distinguish between the anemia resulting from a deficiency of folic acid and

that resulting from vitamin B_{12} deficiency. Although there are similarities in their clinical manifestations, there are also major differences. Moreover, diet therapy is an important intervention in treating most forms of nutritional anemia, and nurses need an understanding of the therapeutic regimen in order to assist the client with successful implementation.

TYPES AND CLASSIFICATION OF ANEMIA

Assessment
Anemia is a reduction in the total quantity of hemoglobin in the circulating blood, with a consequent impairment in the delivery of oxygen to the tissues.

479

Erythrocytes (red blood cells) may be decreased in number, the amount of hemoglobin in the red blood cells may be decreased, or both may occur. Anemia is often a manifestation of one or more underlying conditions rather than a disease entity in itself. For example, iron deficiency anemia is sometimes the first evidence of a malignant disease or other potentially serious illness.

The primary pathology in anemia involves imbalance between red blood cell production and red blood cell loss. If a client's diagnosis includes anemia, assess for the cause of the imbalance, which may be one or more of the following:

1. Increased red blood cell loss due to hemorrhage
2. Increased rate of red blood cell destruction (hemolytic anemia)
3. Decreased red blood cell production due to nutritional deficiency or suppression of the bone marrow (such as that occurring secondary to infection, chronic disease, or irradiation). Nutritional anemia is a major manifestation of deficiency of three nutrients: iron, folic acid, and vitamin B_{12}. A number of other nutrient deficiencies have been implicated in anemia—deficiency of protein, vitamin C, pyridoxine, riboflavin, vitamin E, and copper

Iron deficiency is the most common cause of anemia. As a consequence, anemia due to iron deficiency has been studied more extensively than other types of nutritional anemia. The second most common cause of anemia of nutritional origin is a deficiency of folic acid. Deficiencies of other nutrients, including vitamin B_{12}, play a less important etiologic role. Protein deficiency leads to anemia when gross malnutrition is present. Anemia occurs in scurvy due to severe vitamin C deficiency, although it is not clear whether the anemia is due entirely to ascorbic acid lack or to an associated folic acid deficiency. Although riboflavin deficiency may produce anemia in experimental animals, this finding is rare in humans. Be alert to the possible occurrence of hemolytic anemia in premature infants that may be associated with vitamin E deficiency (see Chaps. 8 and 15). Anemia due to copper deficiency occurs rarely. Suspect it, however, in children with generalized malnutrition, intestinal malabsorption, or episodes of prolonged diarrhea. It has also been observed in premature infants fed a low-copper infant formula, as a complication of total parenteral nutrition, and with administration of excessively high doses of zinc. Pyridoxine is required for heme synthesis, and pyridoxine-response anemia (a sideroblastic anemia characterized by the presence of ringed sideroblasts in the bone marrow) occurs more frequently as a hereditary or acquired defect than as a manifestation of malnutrition. The sideroblastic anemia of pyridoxine deficiency results from defects in heme synthesis that occur in response to toxic agents (such as alcohol, lead, or certain drugs), chronic use of pyridoxine antagonists (including the antitubercular drugs INH, pyrazinamide, and cycloserine), increased dietary requirements for pyridoxine, or deficiencies of enzymes needed for heme synthesis. Individuals with this type of anemia respond only to pyridoxine therapy—in some cases doses far in excess of the normal daily requirement—and are unresponsive to iron, folic acid, or vitamin B_{12}.

Assess for other types of anemia that result from genetically transmitted mutations. Although most individuals inherit the normal form of hemoglobin (HbA, composed of 2 alpha and 2 beta globin chains), clients with sickle cell anemia and thalassemia inherit an abnormal type of hemoglobin. The defect leads to morphologic abnormalities in the red blood cells and clinical manifestations. For example, in sickle cell anemia, which occurs primarily in blacks, there is the substitution of a single amino acid in the beta chains, leading to a structurally abnormal hemoglobin molecule, HbS. The red cells assume a crescent or sickle shape when deoxygenated, and the altered shape prevents their movement through the capillaries, leading to thrombosis and infarction. Observe that the sickle cells also have a shortened life span in the circulation, and affected clients became anemic because blood cell hemolysis exceeds synthesis. Individuals who are homozygous for thalassemia—the thalassemia syndrome results from mutations that affect the rate of synthesis of the globin chains of hemoglobin with a consequent decreased production of either the alpha or beta chain—develop severe hemolytic anemia and may not survive to adulthood. Heterozygotic individuals generally have only mild clinical symptoms. Avoid confusing this disorder with mild iron deficiency anemia.

Classification. Anemias are described and classified according to the size of the red blood cells and their hemoglobin content (Table 31–1). If a client's anemia is due to iron deficiency, observe that the laboratory data show a microcytic hypochromic anemia in which the red cells are small in size and pale in color due to a reduced amount of hemoglobin. In contrast, the red blood cells of clients who are deficient in either vitamin B_{12} or folic acid will be abnormally large (macrocytic). Although red blood cells are sometimes said to be hyperchromic, this generally refers to their appearance on the stained blood film rather than to an increase in hemoglobin per se. However, in one type of anemia, hereditary spherocytosis, the indices that reflect the hemoglobin concentration are increased above the normal range.

Signs and Symptoms. Regardless of the cause, anemias generally give rise to the same clinical features. The symptoms are usually attributed to tissue hypoxia, although there is little evidence to show a relationship between the circulating level of hemoglobin and the severity of symptoms in iron defi-

TABLE 31-1
CLASSIFICATION OF ANEMIA BASED ON SIZE OF THE RED CELLS AND THEIR HEMOGLOBIN CONTENT

Cell Size	Hemoglobin Content
< Normal cell size: microcytic cells	< Normal hemoglobin content: hypochromic cells
Normal cell size: normocytic cells	Normal hemoglobin content: normochromic cells
> Normal cell size: macrocytic cells	> Normal hemoglobin content: hyperchromic cells

ciency anemia. Symptoms differ depending on the acuteness of onset. They tend to be more prominent in conditions leading to rapid onset than in those with an insidious onset. In the latter case, the body has time to physiologically adjust to the diminished oxygen-carrying capacity.

In mild cases of anemia, the client may be relatively asymptomatic. Should symptoms occur, expect them typically to follow strenuous exertion (e.g., the increased cardiac and respiratory effort associated with exercise may produce palpitations, dyspnea, and excess diaphoresis). In more severe cases, assess for symptoms related to the various body systems summarized below. Observe the client's hemoglobin level and note that symptoms develop when the level falls to approximately 7 to 8 g/100 ml.

1. *Cardiac–respiratory.* Increased cardiac and respiratory effort, dyspnea on exertion, palpitations, sensations of pins and needles in fingers and toes (results from pulsating capillaries due to lowered blood viscosity and subsequent rapid blood flow through the peripheral circulation), heart enlargement (in severe cases)
2. *Neuromuscular.* Headache, dizziness or vertigo, tinnitus (ringing in the ears), irritability, lethargy, increased sensitivity to cold, muscular weakness, easy fatigability, decreased physical work capacity, and concomitant reduction in productivity
3. *Gastrointestinal.* Anorexia, loss of muscle tone, pale mucous membranes, dyspepsia, dysphagia, stomatitis, cheilosis, atrophic glossitis (smooth, inflamed tongue), unusual dietary cravings (pica), impaired absorption, loss of plasma protein into the gut (protein-losing enteropathy)
4. *Genitourinary.* In severe cases, amenorrhea in the female and loss of libido in the male
5. *Skin.* Pallor of the skin and conjunctiva, loss of skin elasticity and tone, brittle hair and nails (nails may become concave and spoon-shaped with longitudinal ridges—koilonychia)
6. *Immune system.* Decreased resistance to in-

fection, impaired cellular immunity and phagocytosis

Pallor (of the skin, oral mucosa, nail beds, and conjunctiva) is often a cardinal sign of anemia. Do not assume that a child who is light-skinned and fair-headed is simply pale. Test for anemia in this case. Observe for subtle changes in children, such as easy fatigability and decreased play tolerance, as possibly indicative of a gradually progressive anemia.

Differential Diagnosis. Use the usual nutritional assessment techniques, especially clinical techniques (physical examination, medical history, and social history), biochemical data, and dietary history to aid in diagnosing anemia. A lowered red blood cell count, hematocrit, or hemoglobin level confirms that anemia is present. Hemoglobin levels below which anemia is likely to be present are given in Table 31–2. A number of studies, however, have shown that blacks normally have a lower hemoglobin concentration than whites. Although the cause of the difference is uncertain, it is frequently ascribed to genetic factors. Results of a recent study of this phenomenon suggest that the level of iron intake of the two groups should be considered before drawing firm conclusions.[1] Use findings from other laboratory studies, such as those listed in Table 31–3, to aid in differential diagnosis.

TABLE 31-2
HEMOGLOBIN LEVELS BELOW WHICH ANEMIA IS LIKELY TO BE PRESENT FOR VARIOUS AGE GROUPS AT SEA LEVEL

Age and Sex	Hb/g%
Children	
6 months–6 years	11
6 years–14 years	12
Adults	
Males	13
Females	12
Pregnant women	11

(*Source:* WHO: Nutritional Anemias. Technical Report Series No. 503, Geneva, 1972.)

TABLE 31–3
LABORATORY STUDIES USED IN THE
DIFFERENTIAL DIAGNOSIS OF ANEMIA

Reticulocyte count
Serum iron
Total iron-binding capacity (TIBC)
Bone marrow aspiration and examination
Corpuscular indices (mean corpuscular volume, MCV; mean corpuscular hemoglobin, MCH; and mean corpuscular hemoglobin concentration, MCHC)
Schilling test
Coombs test
Red cell enzyme tests
Electrophoretic examination of hemoglobin
Sickle cell preparation
Serum bilirubin
Fecal–urinary urobilinogen
Serum ferritin
Serum folic acid
Serum vitamin B_{12}

IRON DEFICIENCY ANEMIA

Assessment

Iron deficiency continues to be the most common specific nutritional deficiency seen in both developed and developing countries. Mild and severe cases of iron deficiency anemia have been identified in large segments of the population in surveys such as the Ten-State Nutrition Survey and the NHANES (Fig. 31–1). In general, the prevalence of iron deficiency anemia is greatest in lower socioeconomic groups, although it is by no means limited to this group.

In the Ten-State Nutrition Survey, for example, families with an income of less than half the Poverty Index Ratio (PIR) (less than $1616 per year for a family of four) usually had twice the number of unacceptable hemoglobin values as individuals from families with an income double the PIR (greater than $6000).[2] The disorder is especially prevalent in infants (particularly in premature or low-birth-weight babies), in adolescents, and in girls and women throughout their childbearing years.

Assess the dietary iron intake of women in particular. Even women who consume the RDA for kilocalories find it difficult to ingest an amount of iron sufficient to meet the RDA for this nutrient. Studies have documented the presence of low iron stores in premenopausal females. After menopause, however, iron stores begin to rise, presumably as a result of the cessation of menstrual blood loss.[3] For this reason, equate satisfactory iron status with maintenance of adequate iron reserves, not with the absence of anemia per se. Use the plasma ferritin concentration as a yardstick of the body iron concentration, since this biochemical measure can detect a reduction in the body iron stores.[4] Also assess for anemia in elderly clients, particularly in those persons whose income is low or who have chronic diseases.

The availability of iron in the food supply, food processing techniques, and food usage patterns all contribute to the high incidence of iron deficiency anemia. For example, the usual mixed American diet provides about 6 mg of iron for each 100 kcal or 12 to 18 mg/day depending on the level of kilocalorie intake. Except for heme iron present in meat, poultry, and fish (see Chap. 9), iron from foods is poorly absorbed (5 to 10 percent), although anemic

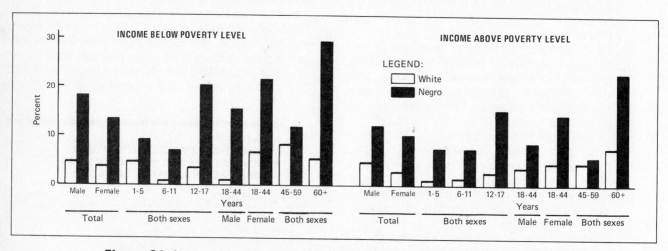

Figure 31–1
Percentage of persons with low hemoglobin values by age, sex, and race for income levels, United States, 1971–1972. (Source: U.S. Department of Health, Education, and Welfare: Preliminary Findings of the First Health and Nutrition Examination Survey, United States, 1971–1972. Dietary Intake and Biochemical Findings. DHEW Publication No. (HRA) 74–1219–1, Washington, DC, Superintendent of Documents, 1974.)

clients increase absorption to a maximum of about 20 percent. Because of high prices, ecologic concern, and health factors related to the use of animal fats, there is a trend toward reduced meat consumption. Assess the client's food preferences. Some foods that are rich sources of iron, such as liver and other organ meats, are often not well liked and are low among individual food preferences. Reduction in kilocalorie consumption is common among weight-conscious Americans. If the client is following a weight-reduction diet, evaluate the iron content of the diet, since reduced iron intake often accompanies a reduction in kilocaloric intake. Changes in food processing techniques that favor refining of foods reduce the amount of available iron and other trace minerals and thus contribute to the problem of meeting requirements. The use of fabricated foods, such as meat analogs, may lower the iron density of the diet unless these foods are fortified with iron at the level contained in meat. A decreased contamination of foods with iron, especially because of decreased use of iron cooking utensils, has been implicated in the lowered availability of iron in the food supply.

Etiology and Diagnosis. If the client's laboratory data indicate iron deficiency anemia, determine its cause, which may be among the following factors:

A. Blood loss (most of the body iron is present in the red cells)
   1. Acute hemorrhage (e.g., from trauma)
   2. Chronic hemorrhage (the continuous loss of a small number of red blood cells will deplete the body iron stores as the bone marrow continuously replaces the cells)
      a. Excess menstrual losses (in excess of 60 ml per cycle). Assist clients to estimate menstrual blood loss properly. Various criteria have been given to suggest excessive losses, e.g., the use of more than 12 pads per period, the damming up of blood behind tampons, the soaking of pads every 1 or 2 hours toward the beginning of a period, the need to use both tampons and pads or double pads, the passage of large clots, and the persistence of blood flow beyond 5 days
      b. Chronic gastrointestinal bleeding (e.g., with ulcers, hemorrhoids, excessive aspirin ingestion, gastrointestinal cancer, alcohol abuse, and hookworm infestation). Chronic blood loss is the most common cause of anemia in the adult male or postmenopausal female; observe for occult blood in the stools in these categories of clients with anemia. Assess the milk intake of young infants with anemia: the ingestion of more than a quart of nonheat-treated homogenized milk may induce chronic blood loss in some infants as well as displace iron-rich foods in the diet
      c. Repeated blood donation (more than three times per year)
      d. Collection of large amounts of blood for diagnostic studies
B. Diminished iron absorption
   1. Malabsorption syndromes and diarrheal states
   2. Diminished gastric hydrochloric acid (e.g., in clients with chronic gastritis, or following gastric resection)
   3. Pica. Although the exact relationship is unclear, there is a strong and persistent link between pica and iron deficiency. Some types of pica are thought to result from iron deficiency, but the pica associated with clay eating is thought to contribute to anemia by inhibiting iron absorption (the ingested clay may chelate or precipitate iron as insoluble compounds in the intestinal lumen). Starch eating may displace iron-containing foods from the diet
C. Dietary deficiency during periods of accelerated demand
   1. Infants and preschool children (a period of rapid growth)
   2. Adolescents (a period of rapid growth)
   3. Women during the reproductive period (a period of chronic iron loss)
   4. Pregnancy (a period of transfer of iron to the fetus)

Because of fetal iron storage (assuming the mother had adequate iron during pregnancy) and the initially high hemoglobin level in infants, iron deficiency is uncommon in infants during the first 6 months. However, an early occurrence of anemia may be evident in those infants with low iron stores (prematures and infants of low birth weight). The occurrence of anemia reaches its peak between 6 and 24 months of age, after which it is relatively infrequent until adolescence. Investigate blood loss as a cause of anemia when it occurs in a child older than 5 years.

In women the iron cost of menstruation and pregnancy combined with a relatively low dietary iron intake frequently produces a negative iron balance. The amount of iron lost in the menstrual blood flow averages about 0.5 mg/day, and pregnancy increases the iron requirement to approximately 3.5 mg/day, with a range from 2 to 4 mg.[5] The use of some intrauterine contraceptive devices increases blood and iron loss, whereas loss is decreased by oral contraceptives. In comparison with adult males, adult females have a higher iron requirement (RDA is 18 mg daily and greater for pregnancy) and a lower kilocalorie requirement. Iron intake of females is not likely to exceed 10 to 12 mg daily. Given

TABLE 31-4
BIOCHEMICAL INDICES OF IRON DEFICIENCY AND ANEMIA

Index	Characteristic
Hemoglobin	Below normal
Hematocrit	Below normal
Red blood cell number	Normal or decreased
Serum iron	Below normal
Serum ferritin	Below normal
Total iron-binding capacity	Above normal
Transferrin saturation	Below normal
Free erythrocyte proto-porphyrin	Above normal
MCV	Below normal with microcytic cells
MCHC	Below normal with hypochromic cells
MCH	Below normal with hypochromic cells
Therapeutic response to iron therapy	Increase in hemoglobin concentration

the inefficiency of dietary iron absorption, the iron intake of females is not likely to provide enough to cover menstrual losses and provide reserves for pregnancy. Treat pregnant adolescents and adults with several successive pregnancies as high-risk candidates for anemia. They are likely to be anemic themselves and to bear infants with low reserves.

Be aware that the need for iron increases considerably during adolescence because adolescents increase their total body iron stores by about 25 percent during their growth spurt. In addition, adolescent girls begin to lose iron in menstrual blood. American teenagers often have poor diets that may not supply enough iron to meet growth requirements. Although iron deficiency anemia is thought to be much less common in men than in women, an unexpected finding of the Ten-State Nutrition Survey was that many adolescent and adult males had low hemoglobin levels.[6]

Expect iron deficiency to develop in these three overlapping stages: (1) depletion of storage iron, (2) decreased transport of iron, and (3) impaired hemoglobin synthesis and a drop in hemoglobin concentration. Stage 3 is the final stage of iron depletion, and at this point iron stores are exhausted. Use the biochemical indices summarized in Table 31-4 to detect the presence of iron deficiency and anemia.

Intervention

Manage iron deficiency anemia by treating its cause, supplementing with iron salts, and manipulating the diet. Iron salts, given in the ferrous form for best absorption, are the most effective and efficient treatment. Replacement therapy for acute hemorrhage (as in surgery) involves emergency measures to restore blood volume. Blood transfusions should be supported by secondary dietary measures to replace iron stores, and medicinal iron supplements may be indicated.

Give clients receiving iron supplements instructions regarding the proper dosage and techniques of administration to reduce gastrointestinal side effects. Although absorption is best when iron is taken on an empty stomach, gastric irritation is a common side effect that can be alleviated by taking the medication with meals. To reduce gastric irritation, instruct the client to increase the dosage gradually until the prescribed dosage is taken. If side effects become a problem, suggest that the dosage be reduced temporarily. Absorption can be enhanced by giving the medication in conjunction with a fruit juice high in vitamin C content. Instruct the client to expect the stools to assume a black, tarry color and, if the medication is taken in a liquid form, that the teeth may become stained. Since oral iron medications interfere with the absorption of tetracycline, instruct clients who are taking both medications to separate their times of administration. Hematinics that contain other vitamins and minerals are not necessary. Although such compounds may bring temporary improvement, they not only increase the expense but may also mask an underlying disease.

If there is no response after a month and the client has taken the medication faithfully, consider another diagnosis, such as occult blood loss or thalassemia, which also cause microcytic anemia. Following normalization of the hemoglobin level, advise the client to continue taking the medication for 2 to 3 months to replenish the depleted iron stores. Repletion occurs as the reverse of depletion with an increase, first, in hemoglobin and, last, in iron stores. Caution the client to keep iron medications out of the reach of small children, since relatively small amounts of iron can be lethal. Clients with malabsorption syndromes or those who are intolerant of oral iron may be given iron parenterally.

Counsel the client to eat a diet high in iron, protein, and vitamins (especially vitamin C) to accompany the iron replacement therapy. Good food sources of iron are lean meat, poultry, fish, organ meats, eggs, legumes, nuts, whole grains and enriched breads and cereals, green leafy vegetables, potatoes, and dried fruits. Many of the iron-rich foods are also good protein sources, although the absorption of iron from whole grains and vegetables may be diminished by the presence of phosphates, phytate, oxalates, and fiber. Since the iron in meat, poultry, and fish not only is well absorbed but also enhances the absorption of iron from plant foods and eggs, suggest the inclusion of some meat at each meal. Since ascorbic acid-containing foods, such as citrus fruits and juices, promote absorption of iron contained in eggs and plant foods, they should also be consumed with meals.

Use the data obtained from assessment of food

preferences as well as the cultural and economic background to assist the client to plan an acceptable iron-rich diet. Although organ meats and legumes are good iron sources, many clients refuse them. Suggest a variety of methods of preparation as a way of possibly increasing their consumption. If these are still unacceptable, suggest suitable alternates, including regional favorites. Baked beans (with added molasses for its iron content) and brown bread (with added raisins), traditional favorites in New England, for example, are rich in iron content. Give the client information or food preparation techniques to preserve the iron content of the foods. Suggest that foods be cut in large pieces and cooked in a small amount of water to decrease the losses of iron and other nutrients. Foods can be steamed to preserve nutrient content, and meat drippings and cooking waters from vegetables can be used to make soups or sauces. Suggest the use of iron cookware, such as a skillet and Dutch oven.

Prevention. The most promising potential for elimination of iron deficiency anemia involves prophylactic supplementation for high-risk groups. Provide an iron supplement for all pregnant women beginning with the second trimester and continuing until 2 to 3 months following delivery. Consider a supplement for women who incur large menstrual blood loss. Full-term infants should receive a supplement by 4 months of age, with the supplement continued throughout the first year. Since the iron in breast milk is better absorbed than the iron in cow's milk, encourage breastfeeding as an important measure in preventing the disorder. Advise nursing mothers that the early introduction of solid foods can impair iron absorption and lead to iron deficiency. For formula-fed infants, consider iron-fortified formula as the standard, to be taken throughout the first year. When solid foods are added to the diet, suggest the use of dry, iron-fortified infant cereal, and encourage use throughout the first year. Discourage the early addition of noniron-containing solid food to the diet of infants and assist parents to balance the amount of milk drunk by infants with iron-containing foods. Should a quart of milk (which contains little iron unless it is fortified with iron as in formula) be consumed daily after 6 months, the infant will have little appetite for other foods. The use of large quantities of fresh cow's milk during the first 6 months of life may be associated with significant occult blood loss. Therefore, infants who are not breastfed should receive a prepared formula rather than fresh cow's milk during this period. If fresh cow's milk is used after 6 months, the amount consumed should be controlled (see Chap. 15).

Other measures that will help in the prevention and control of iron deficiency anemia include appropriate spacing of pregnancies, sanitation measures to control parasites, and astute observation for gastrointestinal bleeding.

ANEMIA DUE TO A DEFICIENCY OF FOLIC ACID AND VITAMIN B_{12}

Assessment

Anemia is a major manifestation of a deficiency of folic acid and vitamin B_{12}. Folic acid deficiency is second only to iron deficiency in frequency of cause of anemia of nutritional origin. In contrast, vitamin B_{12} deficiency is a less frequent cause of nutritional anemia. A deficiency of either nutrient can result from deficient dietary intake or defective absorption. In clinical practice, observe that folic acid deficiency most often arises from deficient intake and that vitamin B_{12} deficiency most often arises from defective absorption. Although malabsorption syndromes lessen the absorption of both vitamins, malabsorption of vitamin B_{12} is often associated with a deficiency of intrinsic factor, a glycoprotein secreted by the parietal cells of the gastric mucosa, needed for absorption of the vitamin. In the stomach, a vitamin B_{12}–intrinsic factor complex is formed. The vitamin B_{12} is subsequently absorbed in the distal ileum (a property unique to this vitamin). In clients with vitamin B_{12} deficiency, distinguish between intrinsic factor deficiency and disease or surgical removal of the distal ileum as the cause of malabsorption.

Expect clients whose anemia results from folic acid or vitamin B_{12} deficiency to experience signs and symptoms similar to those occurring with iron deficiency, e.g., tiredness, lassitude, shortness of breath, and sore mouth and tongue. Note, however, that the biochemical indices are different. Whereas iron deficiency gives rise to hypochromic, microcytic red blood cells, the red cells are greatly increased in size (macrocytic) in folic acid-induced or vitamin B_{12}-induced anemia. Because of their role in nucleic acid synthesis, a deficiency of either results in a defect in nucleic acid metabolism, and this is reflected in the bone marrow as an arrest in the development and maturation of the red cells. Abnormal red cell precursors called megaloblasts—large, nucleated, immature red cells with fragile, easily destroyed cell membranes—are released by the bone marrow. The terms megaloblastic arrest of the bone marrow and megaloblastic anemia refer to the cellular changes observed. The large erythrocytes, which are produced in insufficient numbers, carry a normal complement of hemoglobin. The anemia is thus classified ▶ as **macrocytic** (or megaloblastic), **normochromic anemia.**

A reciprocal relationship exists between vitamin B_{12} and folic acid in the synthesis of nucleic acids, which are formed rapidly in hemopoietic cells. Vitamin B_{12} is needed to maintain normal folic acid function, but the precise biochemical pathways are uncertain. Failure of folic acid function leads to macrocytic anemia; this condition is sometimes called megaloblastic anemia. In some clients anemia may be due to a combined deficiency of folic acid and vitamin B_{12}, and iron deficiency may be present as well. Vitamin C deficiency may be implicated in the anemia, since this vitamin is thought to function in the transformation of folic acid to its biologically active form (tetrahydrofolic acid), and a severe vitamin C deficiency may thus have the same effect as a folic acid deficiency. Actually, nutritional deficiencies of folic acid and vitamin C often go hand-in-hand—both occur in similar foods and both are easily destroyed by overcooking, and so on. Since vitamin C tends to preserve folic acid, it is not surprising that individuals with scurvy (due to severe vitamin C deficiency) are also deficient in folic acid and have megaloblastic anemia.

Vitamin B_{12} deficiency also produces degeneration of nerve tissue. The vitamin is required for the normal function and integrity of nerve tissue. Nervous system disorders may be due to defective myelin synthesis and defective fatty acid metabolism. There is some evidence that folic acid deficiency may also cause neurologic damage, but this is still uncertain.

Correct diagnosis of the cause of macrocytic anemia is essential in order to provide the proper treatment (Table 31–3). If there is a concomitant iron deficiency, however, the morphologic signs of megaloblastic anemia may be masked. Similarly, self-medication with multivitamins containing folic acid may interfere with the correct diagnosis of a vitamin B_{12} deficiency.

Folic Acid Deficiency Anemia. Since folic acid is necessary for nucleic acid synthesis, the requirements are higher during periods of rapid cellular proliferation (e.g., during growth—fetal life, infancy). Requirements are also increased in certain disease states, such as infections and hemolytic anemia. As with iron deficiency, a negative folic acid balance is most often the combined result of a deficient dietary intake and increased demands. Assess for possible folic acid deficiency due to any of the following factors in clients with macrocytic anemia:

1. Deficient dietary intake. Nutritional folic acid deficiency may result from poor food choices or overcooking of food. The water-soluble molecule is labile to heat and is easily destroyed in cooking. Nutritional folic acid deficiency occurs most often in the elderly, pregnant women, premature infants, and alcoholics. The third trimester of pregnancy is a period of particular vulnerability, since fetal growth is especially rapid at this time. Premature infants may be born with reduced folic acid stores. In alcoholism, there may be a reduction in folic acid intake and absorption; in addition, alcohol blocks the response of the bone marrow to folic acid and interferes with the formation of red cells.
2. Malabsorption
   a. Secondary to generalized malabsorption syndromes, such as gluten-induced enter-

opathy, tropical sprue, and Crohn's disease
   b. Secondary to drug therapy, e.g., phenytoin, long-term oral contraceptive therapy, cycloserine, primidone, and phenobarbital
   c. Bacterial competition for folic acid (in anatomic abnormalities, such as the blind loop syndrome, resulting in bacterial overgrowth; the bacteria compete with the host for nutrients)
3. Increased folic acid requirements (e.g., in pregnancy; secondary to hemolytic anemia and tumors)
4. Inactivation or inhibition by folic acid antagonists (such as methotrexate, used to treat cancer)

In addition to the usual signs and symptoms of anemia, also assess for the presence of diarrhea and weight loss in folic acid-deficient clients.

Vitamin B_{12} Deficiency. Suspect vitamin B_{12} deficiency as the cause of macrocytic anemia in clients with the following characteristics:

1. Nutritional deficiency (e.g., when following a diet that restricts animal protein, such as a vegan diet; however, long periods of dietary restriction are necessary to produce any sign of deficiency, since the body has the capacity to store and conserve the vitamin)
2. Malabsorption
   a. Secondary to inadequate or absent secretion of intrinsic factor due to gastric atrophy (pernicious anemia) or gastrectomy
   b. Secondary to malabsorption syndromes, such as gluten-induced enteropathy, tropical sprue, Crohn's disease, and terminal ileal resection
   c. Competition for vitamin B_{12} by intestinal parasites or bacteria (e.g., fish tapeworm, which dissociates the vitamin B_{12}–intrinsic factor complex) and bacterial overgrowth, as in the blind loop syndrome in which bacteria compete with the host for the vitamin

The most important manifestations of vitamin B_{12} deficiency are megaloblastic anemia with its signs and symptoms, glossitis, and neurologic abnormalities. If there is any clue that the client may be deficient in vitamin B_{12}, give particular attention to neurologic assessment, since transient paresthesias (sensations of numbness, prickling, or tingling involving the hands and feet), peripheral neuropathy, and mental disturbances may precede the anemia.

▶ The term **pernicious anemia** is reserved for the megaloblastic anemia resulting from malabsorption of vitamin B_{12} due to gastric deficiency of intrin-

sic factor (not related to surgery). It is associated with gastric atrophy and diminished hydrochloric acid secretion. The finding of specific antibodies to intrinsic factor in the gastric juice, saliva, and blood of clients with pernicious anemia suggests the classi-
▶ fication of the disorder as an **autoimmune disease.** The disorder has a familial incidence that is high in persons of northern European ancestry. It most commonly occurs in people of middle age and the elderly and is rare in children.

In clients with pernicious anemia, observe for typical defects of erythropoiesis characteristic of vitamin B_{12} deficiency and in inadequately treated cases, degenerative changes in the dorsal and lateral tracts of the spinal cord. The onset is insidious, and the degree of anemia may be great before the client consults a physician. In severely anemic clients, observe that the skin may show a lemon-yellow pallor. There is glossitis, anorexia, nausea and vomiting, achlorhydria, abdominal discomfort, and generalized weakness. Pernicious anemia is also associated with infertility.

Intervention

The treatment of megaloblastic anemia must be specific to its cause. Avoid giving folic acid supplements unless it is clear that there is indeed a folic acid deficiency. Folic acid supplements may improve the megaloblastic anemia of vitamin B_{12} deficiency, but it will not alleviate the more serious neurologic symptoms that accompany the disorder. In fact, the insidious development of neurologic damage may be masked. Because of the potential for masking an undiagnosed vitamin B_{12} deficiency anemia, multivitamin preparations may not contain more than 0.1 mg folic acid in a daily dosage.

Correct folic acid deficiency by oral supplementation with the vitamin. If the disorder is due to a dietary deficiency, provide diet counseling that emphasizes the selection of a nutritionally adequate diet containing good food sources of folic acid. Sources include meats and organ meats, legumes, green leafy vegetables, whole grains, brewer's yeast, and orange juice. Since the vitamin is destroyed by heat, advise the client to avoid overcooking food and to eat foods such as fruits and vegetables raw when possible. Since vitamin C converts folic acid to its metabolically active form, foods rich in this vitamin or a vitamin C supplement should be taken. If the underlying problem causing the anemia can be corrected and adequate nutritional status can be maintained on a normal diet, long-term supplementation with folic acid is unnecessary.

In vitamin B_{12} deficiency, oral treatment is not effective except in the management of dietary deficiency. Advise vegans to consume alternate sources of vitamin B_{12}, such as an oral supplement, vitamin B_{12}-fortified foods (soy milk, meat analogs, cereals), or nutritional yeast that has been grown on vitamin B_{12}-enriched media. Although large oral doses of the vitamin may be effective in pernicious anemia, this treatment is seldom used at present. Parenteral administration of the vitamin is indicated in most cases. With severe deficiency, administer the vitamin by injection daily until clinical and biochemical findings have returned to normal. Stress to clients with gastrectomy, ileal resection, and pernicious anemia the importance of a maintenance dose of vitamin B_{12} (usually given at monthly intervals) for the remainder of their lives.

Before treatment, many clients with pernicious anemia are unable to maintain an adequate nutrient intake because of symptoms, such as anorexia, sore mouth, and gastrointestinal discomfort. Counsel the client to consume a soft or liquid diet that restricts tart and spicy foods. Because of the diminished secretion of hydrochloric acid, digestion may be retarded. Thus fats, which further retard gastric emptying, may need to be restricted. Supplement the diet with vitamins and minerals, and suggest the use of high-calorie, high-protein liquid beverages (see Chap. 21) to maintain adequate nutrition. With treatment, the appetite returns and other symptoms lessen. Counsel the client to maintain an adequate food intake and continue the vitamin B_{12} injections.

REVIEW QUESTIONS AND ACTIVITIES

1. Describe the three mechanisms that may lead to the development of anemia.
2. List three nutrients for which anemia is a major manifestation of deficiency.
3. List two types of anemia that are genetically transmitted.
4. Describe signs or symptoms of anemia related to six body systems.
5. Describe clinical manifestations that are relatively specific for vitamin B_{12} deficiency.
6. Describe the characteristics of the red blood cells in the presence of a deficiency of iron, folic acid, and vitamin B_{12}.
7. Distinguish between the causes of iron deficiency anemia and anemia associated with a deficiency of vitamin B_{12} and folic acid.
8. Discuss the differences in the etiology, clinical manifestations, and treatment of pernicious anemia and anemia due to vitamin B_{12} deficiency from other causes.
9. Describe the management of anemia that is due to deficiencies of iron and folic acid, including appropriate pharmacologic and diet therapy.
10. *Case study:* Your client is a 21-year-old Oriental female who has iron deficiency secondary to excessive menstrual blood loss. She is to receive a diet high in protein (75 g) and iron (18 mg). Her kilocalorie requirement is 2000, her income is very limited, and she dislikes organ meats.
    a. Explain the development of anemia in this situation.

b. Describe the rationale for her diet order.

c. Plan a day's menu that meets the diet prescription, using low-cost foods (see Appendix 1 for nutritive values, Chap. 19 for cultural food habits, and Chap. 2 for a description of low-cost foods).

d. Describe techniques for increasing the absorption of the iron from her diet.

11. Describe practices that have a potential for preventing anemia due to dietary deficiencies of iron, folic acid, and vitamin B_{12}.

REFERENCES

1. Jackson RT: Comparison of hemoglobin values in black and white male U.S. military personnel. J Nutr 113:165, 1983.
2. Brown RE, Knittle JL: Prevention of Disease Through Optimal Nutrition. A Symposium. Mt. Sinai Medical Center, New York, and the Institute of Man and Science, Rensselaerville, NY, 1976.
3. Cook JD, Finch CA, Smith N: Evaluation of the iron status of a population. Blood 48:449, 1976.
4. Rothwall TH, Charlton RW: Iron Deficiency in Women (A Report of the International Nutritional Anemia Consultative Group). Washington, DC, The Nutrition Foundation, 1981, p 32.
5. National Research Council: Recommended Dietary Allowances, ed 9. Washington, DC, National Academy Press, 1980, pp 137–138.
6. U.S. Department of Health, Education and Welfare: Highlights, Ten-State Nutrition Survey, 1968–1970. DHEW Publication No. (HSM) 72–8134, Atlanta, Ga, Centers for Disease Control.

BIBLIOGRAPHY

Adler SS: Anemia in the aged: Causes and considerations. Geriatrics 35:49, 1980.

Dallman PR: Iron deficiency: Diagnosis and treatment. West J Med 134:496, 1981.

Dallman PR, Refino C, Yland MJ: Sequence of development of iron deficiency anemia in the rat. Am J Clin Nutr 35:671, 1982.

Dallman PR, Siimes MA, Stekel A: Iron deficiency in infancy and childhood. Am J Clin Nutr 33:86, 1980.

Fischer SL, Fischer SP: Mean corpuscular volume. Arch Intern Med 143:282, 1983.

Haworth C, Evans DIK: Nutritional aspects of blood disorders in the newborn. J Hum Nutr 35:323, 1981.

Herbert V: The nutritional anemias. Hosp Pract 15:65, 1980.

Iron Deficiency in Infancy and Childhood. Report for the International Nutritional Anemia Consultative Group. Washington, DC, Nutrition Foundation, 1979.

Oski FA, Honig AS, Helu B, Howanitz P: Effect of iron therapy on behavior, performance in nonanemic, iron-deficient infants. Pediatrics 71:877, 1983.

Prasad AS, Cossack ZT: Zinc supplementation and growth in sickle cell disease. Ann Int Med 100:367, 1984.

Walter T, Kovalskys J, Stekel A: Effect of mild iron deficiency on infant mental development scores. J Pediatr 102:519, 1983.

CHAPTER 32

Nutrition and Food Sensitivity

Objectives

After completion of this chapter, the student will be able to:
1. Compare and contrast food sensitivity and food intolerance.
2. Compare and contrast immediate-type and delayed-type hypersensitivity relative to (a) time of onset, (b) immunologic basis, and (c) magnitude of symptomology.
3. Develop a nursing care plan for the diagnosis of food sensitivity in a 4-year-old child.
4. Manage the diet during the first year of an infant who is sensitive to milk.
5. Teach a 6-year-old child who is sensitive to wheat and eggs the principles of dietary management.

Adverse reactions are often associated with the ingestion of various foods and are due to a variety of mechanisms. Explanations for these food-induced reactions are several and include intestinal enzyme deficiencies, such as lactase deficiency, presence of noxious constituents, such as pharmacologically active substances, natural toxicants, bacterial toxins, psychologic disorders, and immunologic reactions. The terms food sensitivity, food allergy, and food intolerance are often used interchangeably in referring to food-induced reactions. The term **allergy,** however denotes two components: (1) demonstration of a specific immunologic basis, i.e., an increase in antibody titers resulting from the action of an antigen with a humoral antibody or sensitized lymphoid cell and (2) the concurrent presence of symptoms. In the past, allergy has been the term used to describe immunologically mediated reactions to food, but because the term has often been applied indiscriminately to a wide array of subjective symptoms without proof of an immunologic basis, some health professionals now prefer the term **food sensitivity** to **food allergy.**[1] Food-induced reactions resulting from nonimmunologic mechanisms are referred to as **food intolerance.**

FOOD SENSITIVITY

Assessment

The incidence of allergic disease is high, and allergy is the most common chronic disease affecting children. Allergic reactions result from a number of substances that gain entrance to the body through various routes, namely, ingestion (foods or drugs), inhalation (pollen, dust, molds, animal danders), injection (vaccines, serums, antibiotics, hormones), and direct contact with the skin or mucous membranes (plants, drugs, metals). Even physical agents, such as sunlight or cold, can precipitate allergic reactions.

Although sensitivity to food is considered to constitute a relatively small portion of all allergic reactions, the true prevalence of the disorder is difficult to establish because of the lack of simple and objective means of establishing a clinical diagnosis. As

489

a result, confusion and quackery are widespread in this area.

Although sensitivity to specific foods can appear at any age, observe that its incidence is greatest in infants and young children. The higher incidence at this time is thought to be related to the relative immaturity of immune processes and gastrointestinal function, i.e., the greater permeability of the gastrointestinal mucosa to large molecules, such as intact protein, which can precipitate an allergic reaction. The mucosa becomes less permeable with age. Injury to the intestinal wall as by diarrhea allows intact protein to be absorbed. The predisposition to sensitivity (though not the specific food) is believed to be inherited. Observe for a high incidence in children of parents with a history of the disorder. Sensitivity tends to decrease with age, however, and children often spontaneously recover by the age of 5 or 6, although the prognosis tends to vary with the age of diagnosis and the specific food involved.[2] Take measures to detect food sensitivity in susceptible children at an early age, since the earlier the diagnosis the more likely the child will outgrow the intolerance. Moreover, if the intolerance involves milk, eggs, or soy, expect the symptoms to disappear sooner than if walnuts, peanuts, fish, or shrimp are involved.

Definition and Characteristics of Allergic Responses. Allergy may be defined as an abnormal ▶ or altered tissue reactivity to an **antigen**—a foreign substance that stimulates the immune response— e.g., synthesis of a specific antibody from plasma cells in response to the antigen stimulus. The immune system, which provides protection against foreign substances, such as bacteria and viruses, responds abnormally in allergic individuals.

Most antigens are proteins, antigenic products of protein digestion, or glycoproteins. However, such nonprotein products as polysaccharides and such physical agents as sunlight or cold may initiate an allergic reaction. Some people become sensitized to one or more antigens early in life, whereas others may not become sensitized until adulthood. Still other individuals with the inherited potential may never develop frank allergic symptoms.

▶ Antigens that enter the body are bound by **anti-**
▶ **bodies** (also called immunoglobulins) or **lymphoid cells** that render the antigen innocuous. However, allergic manifestations may result from the interaction of antibody with antigen (humoral response) or from the interaction of antigen with lymphoid cells (cell-mediated or delayed hypersensitivity). The individual with an allergic tendency produces a greater than normal amount of a particular immunoglobulin (IgE). This antibody has the property of binding to the surface membranes of mast cells in tissues or of circulating basophils and of causing the immune mechanism to overreact to an antigen. Allergic individuals may also have defective production of secretory IgA, the component of the immune system that is responsible for surface immunity of mucous membranes. Since cells of the immune system have a memory for foreign antigens to which they have previously been exposed (sensitized), subsequent exposure to the antigen results in an interaction between the antigen (either alone or in combi-
▶ nation with incomplete antigens called **haptens**) and antibody in the general circulation or in specific tissues, causing symptoms such as rhinitis (inflammation of the nasal mucous membranes), asthma, shock, or even death. Much of the symptomology of allergy can be explained by the response of capillaries and surrounding tissues to histamine and other vasoactive mediators released from mast cells or basophils in response to the antigen. IgE is present in high concentrations in so-called allergy shock organs (the gastrointestinal tract, the bronchial tubes, and the nose). Observe that these organs are frequently the site of allergic reactions. Individuals with defective production of secretory IgA are also especially susceptible to allergic responses of the lung and gastrointestinal tract.

Symptoms range from trivial localized effects, such as mild urticaria (also called hives), to generalized effects that may be mild (such as pallor) or severe (life-threatening shock). This latter reaction is
▶ called **anaphylactic shock** and occurs most frequently in clients who receive an injection of a foreign protein substance to which they have been previously sensitized. This type of response accounts for only about 5 percent of food sensitivity, and the causal agent is usually obvious.

Assess for two types of allergic reactions: those that occur immediately after exposure to the antigen (within 4 hours) and those that are delayed (occurring from 4 to 72 hours after exposure). The immediate responses are far more significant because of their rapid onset and possibly life-threatening nature. IgE-mediated reactions are characteristically
▶ rapid in onset and may produce symptoms such as **angioedema** (acute, transitory, localized swelling of subcutaneous tissues or submucosa of the face, hands, feet, genitalia, or viscera), generalized urticaria, asthma, or occasionally shock. Delayed hypersensitivity as opposed to the humoral (B-cell antibody) response occurs in some food allergies, although much less is known about this type than about the immediate responses. This response may involve either immune complexes containing IgG and IgM or cell-mediated immunity. Exposure of sensitized T-lymphocytes to a specific food antigen may transform the cell to a larger cell that releases reaction-causing mediators into the blood. In the case of food allergy, immediate responses are thought to be due to the antigenic properties of intact protein, and delayed responses are thought to be due to the antigenic properties of compounds formed during digestion (evidence for the latter is not convincing, however).

Observe for variability of response to a specific antigen between clients. However, for each client, note that the response to a given antigen is usually specific and characteristic. Reactions can occur at several sites in the same client in response to a single antigen. For example, a sensitivity to egg may produce both asthma and gastrointestinal symptoms. A food antigen may cause immediate symptoms in one individual and delayed reactions in another. Both immediate and delayed reactions can be observed in the same client, though in response to antigens in different foods.

Clinical Manifestations. Since antibodies are distributed throughout the various body cells and tissue fluids, sensitivity reactions can occur in any body tissue. Symptoms, however, are nonspecific for the food sensitivity and can simulate those produced by other conditions. Thus, use caution in diagnosis.

Adverse reactions to foods have been reported to give rise to symptoms in many organs, with different investigators reporting varying frequencies. Table 32–1 provides a partial listing of adverse reactions sometimes attributed to food sensitivity. When food sensitivity is involved, expect respiratory, gastrointestinal, and cutaneous manifestations to predominate. Other organs and tissues are involved only occasionally.

The frequency and severity of symptoms may be influenced by emotional or physical stress, the quantity of food consumed at one time, and the frequency with which a food is ingested. Emotional stress may activate or alter latent sensitivity symptoms, and both physical and emotional stress may increase the severity of the response. Ingestion of excessive amounts of a particular food may initiate a reaction even though consumption of small

amounts may cause no problem. Similarly, a food eaten on a regular basis may cause reactions that do not occur with spasmodic ingestion.

Common Food Antigens. Any food has the potential for producing sensitivity reactions, and investigators disagree on the most important offenders. It is often difficult to demonstrate the presence of food sensitivity and to prove its etiologic significance. The average American diet, characterized by an increasing use of processed foods other than raw foodstuffs, contains many food antigens and other substances, such as food additives, that can produce adverse reactions. Since these reactions can arise from substances added to the food, rather than the food itself, the large use of food additives is of concern. For example, adverse reactions can result from traces of penicillin in cow's milk (an incidental food additive) or from food colors and antioxidants. An example is tartrazine, also known as FD&C Yellow No. 5, which is used in many foods and drugs to impart a distinctive color to the product. Ingestion of tartrazine-containing products can produce such symptoms as urticaria and asthma in susceptible persons, particularly those with a history of both asthma and aspirin sensitivity, although tartrazine sensitivity has been described in nonasthmatic clients without a history of aspirin intolerance. Many foods, such as colored candy, some cake mixes, and some cake icings, contain tartrazine, and a list of the more common foods containing tartrazine has been published.[3] Food and Drug Administration regulations require that the term "FD&C Yellow No. 5" be listed among the ingredients of tartrazine-containing foods and drugs. Another example is sulfite, which is used

---

TABLE 32–1
ADVERSE REACTIONS SOMETIMES ATTRIBUTED TO FOOD SENSITIVITY

Systemic	Neural	Gastrointestinal
Vascular shock	Headache	Cheilitis
Malaise, lethargy	Irritability	Stomatitis
Fever	Hyperactivity	Gingivitis
Retarded growth	Tension fatigue syndrome	Geographic tongue
Pallor	Seizures	Canker sores
	Personality change	Colic
Respiratory	Psychosis	Abdominal pain
Rhinitis	Optic neuritis	Dyspepsia
Cough	Labyrinthitis	Flatulence
Asthma	Neuralgias	Nausea, vomiting
Hay fever		Diarrhea, malabsorption
Sinusitus	Cutaneous	Constipation
Nasal polyps	Urticaria	Colitis
Secretory otitis media	Eczema	Protein-losing enteropathy
Bronchitis	Rashes	Pruritus ani
	Angioedema	Bleeding
Eye	Atopic dermatitis	
Conjunctivitis	Purpura	Genitourinary
Corneal ulcers		Cystitis
	Musculoskeletal	Pruritus vulvae
	Leg pain	Enuresis
	Arthritis	Hematuria
	Hydroarthrosis	Menstrual irregularities

by some restaurants to prevent wilting and discoloration of fruits and vegetables. Persons who are sensitive to this compound may have difficulty determining if it has been used. Interestingly, artificial food colors, artificial flavorings, and salicylates have been implicated as a causative factor in hyperactivity in children. This has been refuted in a recent report, although the effects of food colorings require continuing investigation.[4]

Numerous foods and food components are associated with food sensitivity reactions in susceptible persons, but those most commonly implicated include nuts, peanuts, eggs, cow's milk, soy, wheat, fish, shellfish, mollusks, and chicken.[2,5] Chocolate is reported to be a common cause of clinically significant hypersensitivity, and tomatoes, citrus fruits, and strawberries are commonly believed to be frequent causes of immediate hypersensitivity reactions, although evidence for this is lacking.[5,6]

Foods that belong to the same botanical group may have similar allergenic characteristics. For example, expect that clients who are sensitive to cabbage may also manifest symptoms on eating cauliflower, broccoli, and brussels sprouts. Likewise, lemon and grapefruit may not be tolerated by those who are sensitive to oranges. Interestingly, buckwheat belongs to the same botanical group as rhubarb—it is not a cereal grain. Buckwheat can, therefore, serve as a cereal substitute for those allergic to wheat.

The property of a food to induce sensitivity can be reduced by cooking or processing, since heat denatures the protein. Thus, while raw or pasteurized milk or raw fruit or vegetable may cause symptoms, boiled and evaporated milk and cooked fruit and vegetables may be tolerated.

Frequent offenders in young infants are cow's milk, egg, and wheat. These three foods are often introduced early into the infant's diet. Sensitivity to cow's milk is considered to be the most common cause of sensitivity reactions in infants and children younger than 2 years of age. The onset of milk allergy most commonly occurs before 1 month of age. Each of the four most common proteins in cow's milk—casein, lactalbumin, lactoglobulin, and bovine serum albumin—have been found to produce sensitivity reactions, and two or more proteins are usually responsible for reactions in the majority of affected clients. Sensitivity to cow's milk mimics many other diseases, and any disease associated with gastrointestinal, cutaneous, or respiratory problems may be confused with cow's milk sensitivity. Further, there are several clinical syndromes associated with milk sensitivity, and in many instances an immunologic basis for reactions cannot be identified. For this reason, be cautious in diagnosing milk sensitivity in infants who have such symptoms as colic, diarrhea, irritability, and skin rash.

Egg is capable of being a potent allergen. Although both egg yolk and egg white may precipitate symptoms, the albumin contained in egg white poses greater problems. Severe symptoms may be provoked by even the odor of an egg (as when it is fried) in clients with a high degree of sensitivity. Other clients are less sensitive, and they may be able to eat moderate amounts once or twice a week or eat well-cooked egg, e.g., one that has been boiled for 10 minutes. Vaccines also contain traces of egg, although those grown on chicken embryo now contain much less egg than those previously used.

Wheat is the most common cereal associated with sensitivity reactions, although many children are also sensitive to corn. There are many proteins in wheat that may act as antigens. Gluten-induced enteropathy (see Chap. 27) is manifest as a sensitivity to the alpha-gliadin present in the gluten fraction of wheat. It is not firmly established whether the disorder is a manifestation of sensitivity or of a biochemical defect, however. Wheat is widely used in processed foods, including packaged soup mixes and sauces. Similarly, corn is found in many commercial food products not only as whole corn but also as corn syrup, corn starch, corn flour, corn oil, or corn meal. Sensitivity to soy is common and the increasing use of soy products, such as oil and concentrates, may pose a problem for the sensitive client.

Diagnosis of Food Allergy. Immunologic tests have been developed that will demonstrate hypersensitivity of the immediate, but not the delayed, type. For example, in children more than 3 years of age, immediate-type hypersensitivity can be identified by cutaneous testing involving scratch, puncture, or intradermal tests. Suspect hypersensitivity if a cutaneous wheal and flare reaction is induced by injection of extracts of antigenic material from a suspected food. With this procedure, it is important to have laboratory verification that the extracts do not cause nonspecific or irritant reactions in normal individuals and that they do elicit a specific antibody response in sensitive subjects. Proof that extracts detect specific antibodies ideally requires correlation of positive results from skin tests, food challenges, and other laboratory tests for antibodies. More recently, the radioallergosorbent test (RAST) has been used to estimate the serum IgE levels, and the level of IgE reflects the degree of sensitization. With both the cutaneous and RAST tests, however, only the higher degrees of hypersensitivity correlate with clinical symptoms. At present, the findings of high titers of specific antibodies in serum provide data that is too nonspecific to be useful in the differential diagnosis of food allergy.

Other commonly used methods of diagnosing food allergy include (1) complete clinical studies and (2) restricted diets that involve a period of elimination of suspected allergens followed by a period of oral challenge with the particular foods. The latter technique is not recommended if the client has a history of severe systemic allergic reactions unless the procedure is conducted while the client is hospitalized.

Obtain a complete history that includes family history, history of events that precede attacks, and dietary history. These assessment data, along with a physical examination and laboratory studies, are important for diagnosis. With the diet history, make attempts to correlate symptoms with the repeated ingestion of specific foods to aid in establishing a tentative diagnosis and pinpointing the offending foods. During the dietary interview, question parents as to whether they suspect any food of causing symptoms. Whenever a food is consistently disliked, consider the possibility of sensitivity. Children who avoid specific foods may do so because they are sensitive to them. Parents tend to report immediate reactions to food intake well, but they are less aware of foods that cause delayed responses. In many cases, a detailed food diary is used to aid in diagnosis. In this case tell the client (or the child's parents) to record all foods and liquids consumed, including condiments and ingredients in mixed dishes, and all symptoms manifested for a period of at least a week. Use the results of laboratory studies in conjunction with the diet history and food diary to rule out other disorders that may give rise to symptoms similar to allergy symptoms, such as cystic fibrosis, infections, enzyme defects, or gastrointestinal malformation.

The elimination/oral challenge restricted diets are of two major types. Both types involve elimination of specific foods for a period of time, followed by a period of oral challenge in which gradually increasing amounts of the food are introduced. Observation for the presence or absence of symptoms during the periods of elimination and challenge is essential. The period of observation when a new food is added varies from 4 to 7 days. An antigen may be confirmed by correlating the repeated appearance and disappearance of symptoms with inclusion and exclusion of suspected foods. The precipitation of symptoms by a food on three occasions is accepted by some authorities as evidence of hypersensitivity. Others note, however, that this is misleading, since other mechanisms that may cause adverse food reactions, such as digestive enzyme deficiency, would be expected to behave similarly. Since sensitivity may exist to one or more ingredients of vitamin preparations, treat supplements, if given, in the manner of a new food and observe for possible reactions. Eating out should be discouraged during the trial period to maintain greater control over food intake.

The first type of elimination/oral challenge diet (which is less restrictive) involves the elimination of foods that are suspected of being allergens on the basis of skin tests, diet history, or the food diary. Eliminate suspect foods from the diet for a period of at least a week. Should a remission of symptoms occur, gradually introduce the foods and observe for symptoms. Give the food in a disguised form so that neither the child nor the observer is aware of its identity. If a history of a severe reaction has been reported, hospitalization may be necessary. For infants and young children, mix the challenge food with a familiar, well-liked food. For older children, give capsules containing dried, crushed, or powdered forms of the challenge food. If symptoms occur after the food capsules are given, a placebo (glucose-containing capsule) is not needed. Should equivocal results be obtained, a challenge with a placebo capsule will be needed for verification. When a single dose of 8 g of a food capsule can be tolerated, the food should be given openly in usual portions to evaluate the possible effect of bias, cooking, and digestion. A single unequivocal reaction in a double-blind challenge may be considered as definitive evidence of an adverse reaction to the food but not necessarily to an immunologic process.

A number of elimination diets have been developed that allow only those foods considered unlikely to produce allergic reactions. These highly restricted diets may be used when symptoms occur so frequently that allergy to a commonly eaten food may be justifiably suspected. Modifications of elimination diets developed by Rowe (Table 32–2, for example) are used by some physicians to identify food allergies. The client is placed on one of the test diets for a period of a week to several months. If there is no change in symptoms, another diet is followed for the same period of time. Should symptoms disappear on any of the diets, that diet is followed for an additional week or so. Then new foods are added at intervals of 4 to 7 days, and observation of symptoms is made. If symptoms are noted after the addition of any one food, that food is suspected as the cause of the reaction. If no improvement occurs with the use of elimination diets, assume that nonfood allergens are responsible for the reactions. Defined formula diets have also been used as an elimination diet.

Although the diets are very restrictive, they must be followed carefully if the antigens are to be identified. Provide assistance with meal planning and use of recipes to help alleviate the monotony of the diet. Consider the use of nutrient supplements for infants and children, although optimal nutrition becomes of greater concern after therapeutic interventions are initiated. The nutritional requirements of an infant can be supplied by a defined formula diet (e.g., Pregestimil, Mead Johnson) a meat-based formula (e.g., Meat Base Formula, Gerber Products), or a soy-based formula (e.g., Isomil, Ross Labs). Milk-free margarine made from soy oil and baked products made from soy, potato, lima bean, or tapioca flour are permitted on Rowe's elimination diets. If an allergy to soy products is suspected, they should be eliminated as well.

Intervention

Dietary management entails strict avoidance of the offending foods. Since hypersensitivity tends to decrease with age, the offending foods, unless they are associated with life-threatening symptoms, should be cautiously added to the diet of children and adults from time to time (such as at 6-month or yearly intervals). In some instances, allowing a small amount of the offending food at a social occasion may be psychologically beneficial.

TABLE 32–2
ELIMINATION DIETS

Category	Cereal-free Elimination Diet	Fruit-free, Cereal-free Elimination Diet
Milk	Soy milk: Soy infant formula (free of corn products), soy ice cream, pudding made with soy milk and allowed flours	Same
Meat and meat substitutes	Lamb, chicken (no hens), liver (lamb, chicken), bacon, Canadian bacon	Same
Vegetables	Artichokes, asparagus, carrots, lettuce, lima beans, peas, potatoes (white, sweet, yams), spinach, squash, string beans, tomato, tomato juice	Artichokes, cooked carrots, lima beans, peas, potatoes (white, sweet, yams), squash, string beans
Fruit	Fresh, cooked, or canned (in cane sugar) fruit or juice: Apricots, grapefruit, peaches, pears, pineapple, lemon, prunes; water ices made with allowed fruits	
Bread–cereal and bakery products	Tapioca (pearl), bread, crackers, desserts made with any combination of soy, lima bean, potato, or tapioca flour	Tapioca (pearl), bread, crackers, desserts made with any combination of soy, lima, potato, or tapioca flour
Miscellaneous	Soy oil, sesame oil, milk-free margarine made from soy oil, plain gelatin, sugar (brown, cane, beet), jams, jellies, preserves made from allowed fruits, plain fondant, maple syrup, baking powder (free of cornstarch or tartaric acid), baking soda, cream of tartar, lemon extract, vanilla extract, salt, white vinegar	Soy oil, sesame oil, milk-free margarine made from soy oil, plain gelatin, baking powder (free of cornstarch or tartaric acid), salt, tea, sugar (beet, cane, brown) syrup (made with cane sugar)

(*Source: Adapted from Rowe AH: Food Allergy. Its Manifestations and Control and the Elimination Diets. A Compendium. Springfield, Ill, Charles C Thomas, 1972.*)

Adherence to a restricted diet is much simplified when the allergy involves a single food, especially one that is not usually consumed on a regular basis. Be aggressive in management, however, when the sensitivity involves several foods or if basic foods, such as milk, eggs, or wheat, are not tolerated. Affected clients may be at a high risk of nutritional deficiency. These basic foods are present as ingredients in many other foods and also serve as important sources of nutrients and energy. It is difficult to provide a diet that is adequate in calcium without the use of milk, and the restriction of wheat limits the intake of kilocalories and B-complex vitamins. Nutritional adequacy is less of a problem with egg sensitivity, since other protein sources provide similar nutrients. Monitor the energy and nutrient intake in children on a continuing basis and provide nutrient supplements as necessary to avoid compromising growth and development. Fear of precipitating symptoms by eating, malabsorption induced by certain foods, or the monotony of a restricted diet may also be related to inadequate nutrient intake. Assess for the level of anxiety on the part of the child's parents, since anxious parents may lead the child to use food as a weapon to control the parent's behavior.

Client Education. Diet counseling for the client with an allergy involves (1) providing instruction on reading food labels to detect hidden sources of the offending foods, (2) providing information on the availability of special foods, special recipes, and cookbooks if needed, and (3) giving assistance with menu planning and food preparation.

Some foods or their derivatives, such as milk, eggs, wheat, corn, or soy products, are added to many commercially prepared foods. Therefore, stress the importance of carefully scrutinizing the list of ingredients on food labels for hidden foods. This becomes very significant for those who respond immediately to a food antigen. For example, such terms as lactose, lactalbumin, curds, whey, casein, or caseinate denote the presence of milk, and such terms as albumin, vitellin, ovomucoid, and ovomucin indicate that egg has been added. Encourage the client to study the label each time foods are purchased, since food processors change the formulation of products from time to time. Some processed foods may contain no listing of ingredients, and these foods must be omitted unless information regarding their content is obtained from the manufacturer.

Special foods, recipes, and cookbooks are useful if milk, wheat, or egg must be eliminated (see Client Resources at the end of the chapter). It may be possible to make changes in standard recipes in some instances. For example, ¾ c of rice flour can be substituted for 1 c of wheat flour, and an egg-free cake can be made by replacing the egg with an equal amount of mashed banana and adding an extra ½ tsp of baking powder. Extra flour or cornstarch can be used to replace the thickening action of eggs in other cooked dishes. Stress to the client that improperly washed utensils and use of the same spoon for stirring or serving several foods may be a source of prohibited foods. Give detailed lists of foods to avoid and foods allowed (Tables 32–3, 32–4, and 32–5).

Milk sensitivity in an infant is managed by providing a hypoallergenic feeding. Since the diet is limited to one food, fewer problems are posed than for older children and adults. Breast milk is the best food for infants with a potential for sensitivity, particularly during the first several months, although food antigens can be secreted into breast milk. Discuss this aspect of breastfeeding with nursing mothers and suggest avoidance of offending foods from the diet if symptoms appear in the infant. If breastfeeding is not possible, recommend the use of formulas based on milk substitutes or protein hydrolysates. Soy-based formulas, such as Isomil (Ross Laboratories) and ProSobee (Mead Johnson), are sometimes used as a milk substitute, although the

---

TABLE 32–3
MILK-FREE DIET

Category	Foods Allowed	Foods Avoided
Milk	Milk-free infant formula, pudding and custard made without milk	All forms of milk (buttermilk, evaporated, fresh whole, skim, low-fat, malted, chocolate), yoghurt, cocoa made with milk, ovaltine, all forms of cheese (including dips and spreads), ice milk, ice cream, sherbet, milk-containing custard and pudding
Meat and meat substitutes	Beef, veal, lamb, pork, organ meats, and fish prepared without milk, all-meat cold cuts, sausage, frankfurters, eggs, legumes, nuts, seeds, peanut butter	Frankfurters, luncheon meat, and meat loaf that contain milk solids, meat or eggs prepared with a gravy or sauce that contains milk, cream, butter, or a milk-containing margarine
Vegetable–fruit	All vegetables (including potatoes), fruits, juices, and soups prepared without milk, lemonade, potato chips	Any prepared with milk, cheese, cream, butter, or a milk-containing margarine
Bread–cereal and bakery products	Bread prepared without milk (e.g., kosher, Roman meal, sour dough, French rolls, Vienna bread, rye), crackers, pretzels, corn chips, cereals (dry, cooked) and pasta prepared and served without milk, bread, cookies and crackers marked *pareve*, homemade baked goods prepared without milk (as pies, cakes, cookies), angel food cake	Breads and cereals prepared or served with milk, hot breads (pancakes, waffles, griddle cakes, French toast, muffins, biscuits), commercial baking mixes, pies, cakes, cookies, and doughnuts
Miscellaneous	Vegetable oils, lard, meat fat, milk-free margarine (as Nucoa or Mazola-unsalted, sweet), olives, avocado, milk-free salad dressing mixes, sugar, jam, jelly, lollipops, hard candy, pickles, vinegar, catsup, pure spices and seasonings, meat juice gravy, broth, clear consommé, bouillon, gelatin, fruit and water ices, popsicles, German baking chocolate, semisweet chocolate, coffee, tea, Kool-Aid, carbonated beverages, cocoa made with water	Butter, cream, sour cream, margarine with added milk solids, salad dressing with added milk, candy containing milk (caramels, milk chocolate, fondant, nougat), cream sauces and gravy unless made with allowed foods, hollandaise sauce, cream soups, chowder, and bisque

TABLE 32–4
WHEAT-FREE DIET

Category	Foods Allowed	Foods Avoided
Milk	Milk (most kinds), cocoa (made from wheat-free cocoa or cocoa syrup), custard and pudding made with cornstarch, tapioca, or rice, homemade ice cream and sherbet	Malted milk, cocomalt, commercial ice cream, sherbet
Meat and meat substitutes	Beef, lamb, pork, veal, fish, poultry (prepared without breading and without gravy made with wheat flour), cheese (cheddar, American, Swiss, cottage, farmer), eggs (prepared without wheat or wheat products), legumes, nuts, peanut butter	Processed meats such as bologna, frankfurters, luncheon meat, breaded meats, commercial hamburger with cereal filler, meats prepared with bread fillers such as meat loaf, meat balls, croquettes, sausage, scrapple, pizza, canned meat mixtures such as chili, commercial cheese spread, cheese food or dips, eggs prepared with wheat products such as creamed eggs, cutlets, or omelet
Vegetable–fruit	Fresh, frozen, dried, or canned fruit and vegetables and juices, lemonade, potato (white, sweet, yams, potato chips), vegetable soups	Breaded or creamed vegetable containing wheat products, fruit pies and cobblers prepared with wheat
Bread–cereal and bakery products	Bread made from cornmeal or oatmeal or rye, potato, rice, or soybean flour, pure rye bread and wafers, wheat-free pumpernickel bread, corn, oat, rice, or other nonwheat cereal, cookies made from allowed flour or cereals	Bread, rolls, muffins, biscuits, crackers, dumplings, bread stuffings and breading mixes made from wheat flour (including white, whole wheat, graham, and gluten flour), pretzels, commercial mixes (such as waffle and pancake), matzo, rusk, zwieback, commercially prepared rice, potato or soybean bread with added wheat, all wheat cereals (including Pablum, Allbran, Bran Flakes, Cherrios, Cream of Wheat, Farina, granola type; Grapenuts, Grapenut Flakes, Kix, Krumbles, Maltex, Muffets, New Oats, pettijohns, Puffed Wheat, Special K, ralston, Shredded Wheat, Total, wheatena, Wheat Flakes, wheat germ, Wheaties, Wheat Chex), pastas, cakes, most cookies, dumplings, pastries, ice cream cones
Miscellaneous	Bacon, butter, margarine, cream, cream cheese, animal and vegetable fat and oils, pure mayonnaise and salad dressing made without wheat, honey, jam, jelly, preserves, marmalade, candy (made without wheat), molasses, sorghum, sugar (white, brown, corn, maple) syrup (corn or maple), arrowroot starch, condiments, herbs and spices, salt, pepper, homemade catsup and chili sauce, flavoring extracts, pickles, olives, popcorn, baking soda, baking powder, carbonated beverages, Kool-Aid, coffee, tea, clear soups and others thickened with allowed cereals, Bavarian cream, Indian pudding, fruit ice, mousse, meringues, gelatin and junket desserts	Most commercial salad dressing and some mayonnaise (thickened with wheat flour), commercial candy containing wheat, gravy and cream sauces thickened with wheat, commercial meat sauces, soy sauce, bouillon cubes, most commercial canned soup, soup with noodles, Ovaltine, postum and other coffee substitutes, instant coffee (unless 100% coffee), root beer, beer, ale, gin, vodka, whiskey

(*Source: Adapted from North Carolina Dietetic Association: Diet Manual, ed 2. Charlotte, NC, 1978, pp 14–17J.*)

TABLE 32–5
EGG-FREE DIET

Category	Foods Allowed	Foods Avoided
Milk	Milk (most kinds), cocoa, puddings, ice cream and sherbet prepared without egg	Eggnog, cocomalt, malted beverages, custard, commercial ice cream and sherbet
Meat and meat substitutes	Beef, lamb pork, veal, fish, poultry prepared without the addition of egg, cottage, American, and other plain cheese, legumes, nuts, peanut butter, seeds	Eggs, low-cholesterol egg substitutes, sausage, meat loaf, croquettes, or other meats using egg as a binding or breading agent, cheese dishes made with egg (such as fondue)
Vegetable–fruit	Fresh, frozen, dried, or canned vegetables and fruit and juices, vegetable soups prepared without egg, potato (white, sweet, yams, potato chips)	Vegetables or fruit prepared with egg or egg products, potatoes prepared with egg, as potato cakes and potato salad
Bread–cereal and bakery products	Commercial or homemade bread prepared without egg or egg products, plain crackers, biscuits, cornbread (without eggs), Ry-Krisp, hot and cold breakfast cereals, cornmeal, rice, spaghetti, macaroni, egg-free noodles, homemade cookies and cake, fruit pies and cobblers	Egg-containing bread such as French toast, muffins, waffles, and pancakes, egg-glazed crusts, pretzels, zwieback, crackers, mixes or homemade or commercial products to which egg has been added, egg noodles, commercial cookies, cake, cake frosting, and pie filling containing egg (as cream-filled pies), macaroons, doughnuts, gingerbread, sweet rolls or other homemade or commercially prepared products containing egg, baking mixes, cake flour
Miscellaneous	Butter, margarine, bacon, animal and vegetable fats and oils, French dressing and oil and vinegar dressing to which no egg or egg products have been added, cream cheese, honey, jam, jelly, preserves, marmalade, molasses, sorghum, sugar (white, brown, corn or maple), corn or maple syrup, candy made without egg (such as hard candy), popcorn, olives, pickles, flavoring extracts, herbs, spices, salt, pepper, sauces (such as cream, tomato, white, chili), coffee, tea, some carbonated beverages, cream soups prepared without egg, fruit ices, gelatin, homemade cake frosting	Mayonnaise and most cooked salad dressings, divinity, most commercial candy such as chocolate, fondant, marshmallow, and nougat, hollandaise sauce and other sauces containing egg, baking powder if it contains egg white, root beer, coffee, wine, and soft drinks if cleared with egg white or eggshells, mock turtle, alphabet, and egg noodle soup, consommé, broth, bouillon, or any soup cleared with egg or containing egg as an ingredient, Bavarian cream, meringue, whips

(*Source: Adapted from North Carolina Dietetic Association: Diet Manual, ed 2. Charlotte, NC, 1978, pp 18–20J.*)

usefulness of soy has been questioned because of its antigenicity. Formulas that provide protein in a hydrolyzed form, such as Nutramagen (Mead Johnson), or in an elemental form, such as Pregestimil (Mead Johnson), are sometimes recommended by physicians. The use of soy milk as a calcium-containing beverage can continue as the child grows older. However, protein hydrolysates are often rejected by older infants and children. Goat's milk is not a recommended substitute for cow's milk, since cross-reactions are frequent and use of goat's milk may lead to folic acid deficiency. The milk-sensitive infant may later be able to tolerate heated milk (as in custard, pudding, soup), although heat treatment has no effect on tolerance for some children.

Advise clients who are sensitive to corn of its presence in a great variety of food products. Corn syrup is used in the manufacture of candy, chewing gum, luncheon meats (sausage, frankfurters, bologna, luncheon hams), many types of baked goods (some breads, cakes, cookies, rolls, buns, doughnuts), canned fruits and some brands of fruit juice, ice cream, pancake syrup, sweetened cereals, and some infant formulas. Cornstarch may be found in some salad dressings, sauces, pudding and baking mixes, baking powder, and other prepared food. Corn oil and cornmeal are widely used, and some beer and whiskey contain corn. Monosodium glutamate may be derived from corn.

Soy derivatives are widely used in commercial food preparation. Advise the soy-sensitive client to check food labels for such terms as soy, soybean oil, soy flour, soy milk, soy curd, soy protein isolate, and vegetable protein. These substances are found in such products as soups, cold cuts, baked goods, candy, seasoned sauces such as Worcestershire, and granola-type cereals.

Direct infant feeding practices toward preventing manifestations of sensitivity, particularly in those who are prone to the disorder. In addition to recommending breastfeeding, advise parents to delay the introduction of solid foods until the age of 6 months to permit maturation of the gastrointestinal tract. This is especially true if the child is doing well on breast milk or formula. Moreover, tell parents to exclude foods commonly associated with sensitivity from early additions, to introduce solids one at a time, and to evaluate the response to aid in pinpointing problem foods. Rice cereal is the least allergenic of the commonly used cereals, although rye is the least allergenic cereal. The addition of egg white should be delayed until the end of the first year, although well-cooked egg yolk or commercial strained egg yolk that has been heat sterilized may be added earlier. Noncitrus fruit juices that have been fortified with vitamin C or a synthetic vitamin C supplement may be used in lieu of citrus fruits.

Since food antigens can cross the placenta during pregnancy, advise pregnant women with a history of food sensitivity to avoid the consumption of large amounts of highly sensitizing foods to avoid the risk of sensitizing the fetus in utero.

REVIEW QUESTIONS AND ACTIVITIES

1. Explain the rationale for the preferential use of the term "food sensitivity" to "food allergy."
2. Describe the immunologic basis for the allergic response.
3. Identify the age groups in which food allergy has its highest incidence.
4. List five factors that may precipitate nutritional deficiency in clients who are allergic to several basic foods.
5. Describe the time of onset, immunologic basis, and symptomology associated with immediate-type and delayed-type sensitivity reactions.
6. List the three body systems in which allergic responses to food are most likely to be manifest, and name three characteristic symptoms for each system.
7. Identify the ten foods that are most commonly associated with food sensitivity.
8. Explain the rationale for the reduction in allergic potential associated with cooked or processed food in contrast to raw food.
9. Describe the procedures for diagnosing food sensitivity.

10. Describe the dietary modifications used in the nutritional management of sensitivity to milk, eggs, and wheat.
11. Compare the types of problems that may be encountered by a client who must restrict milk or wheat in the diet to control food sensitivity with the types of problems that may be encountered by a client who must restrict the use of a food, such as strawberries or citrus fruit.
12. Outline a plan of nutritional care for a newborn, a 6-month-old infant, and a 1-year-old infant who is sensitive to milk.

REFERENCES

1. Bock SA: Food sensitivity: A critical review and practical approach. Am J Dis Child 134:973, 1980.
2. Bock SA: The natural history of food sensitivity. J Allergy Clin Immunol 69:173, 1982.
3. Tse CST: Food products containing tartrazine. N Engl J Med 306:681, 1982.
4. National Advisory Committee on Hyperkinesis and Food Additives: Final Report to the Nutrition Foundation. Washington, DC, Nutrition Foundation, 1980.
5. Buckley RH, Metcalf D: Food allergy. JAMA 248:2627, 1982.
6. May, CD, Bock, SA: In E Middleton Jr, EF Reed, EF Ellis, eds: Allergy, Principles & Practice. St. Louis, CV Mosby, 1978, Vol 2, pp 1159–1171.

BIBLIOGRAPHY

Adkinson NF: The radioallergosorbent test: Uses and abuses. J Allergy Clin Immunol 65:1, 1980.

Anderson JA, Sogn DD, eds: Adverse Reactions to Food. Washington, DC, Superintendent of Documents, U.S. Government Printing Office, 1984.

Antibody formation to cow's milk protein or soya protein. Nutr Rev 41:80, 1983.

Atkins FM: The basis of immediate hypersensitivity reactions to foods. Nutr Rev 41:229, 1983.

Belut D, Moneret-Vautrin DA, Nicolas JP, Grilliat JP: IgE levels in intestinal juice. Dig Dis Sci 25:323, 1980.

Check W: Eat, drink and be merry—or argue about food "allergy." JAMA 250:701, 1983.

Grieco MH: Controversial practices in allergy. JAMA 247:3106, 1982.

Iyngkaran N, Abidin Z: One-hour blood xylose in the diagnosis of cows milk protein-sensitive enteropathy. Arch Dis Child 57:40, 1982.

May CD: Food allergy, perspectives, principles, practical management. Nutr Today 15:28, 1981.

Parker C: Food allergies. Am J Nurs 80:262, 1980.

Pearson DJ, Rix KJB, Bentley SJ: Food allergy: How much in the mind? A clinical and psychiatric study of suspected food hypersensitivity. Lancet 1:1259, 1983.

Victoria JC, Camarero C, Sojo A, et al.: Enthopathy related to fish, rice, and chicken. Arch Dis Child 57:44, 1982.

CLIENT RESOURCES

Baking for People with Food Allergies. Home and Garden Bulletin No. 147, Washington, DC, Superintendent of Documents.

Cooking Without Milk. Evansville, Ind, Mead Johnson, 1981.

Crook WG: Tracking Down Food Allergy. Jackson, Tenn, Professional Books, 1978.

Dietary Information for Allergy Diets (available upon request from Chicago Dietetic Supply, Inc., 405 E Shawmut, LaGrange, IL 60525).

125 Great Recipes for Allergy Diets (available from Good Housekeeping, 989 Fifth Ave, New York, NY 10021).

Rudoff C: The Allergy Baker. Menlo Park, Calif, Prologue Pub, 1980.

Thomas LL: Caring and Cooking for the Allergic Child. New York, Sterling Publishing, 1980.

CHAPTER 33

Nutrition and Disorders of the Skin and Other Epithelial Tissues

Objectives

After completion of this chapter, the student will be able to:

1. Compare and contrast the effects on epithelial tissues of a deficiency of each of the following: (a) protein–energy, (b) fatty acids, (c) vitamin A, (d) vitamin C, (e) B-complex vitamins, (f) iron, and (g) zinc.

2. Manage the diet of a client with epithelial manifestations of protein–energy deficiency and distinguish this treatment from that of a client with manifestations of essential fatty acid deficiency.

3. Distinguish between the cutaneous effects of excessive injection of vitamin A and carotene.

4. Plan a day's menu for a zinc-deficient client that is adequate in zinc.

5. Distinguish between the cutaneous manifestations of excessive niacin and cholesterol.

6. Plan the nutritional management of a client who is experiencing nutritional and metabolic effects secondary to a severe skin disorder.

7. Manage the diet for a client with dermatitis herpetiformis.

The quality of the diet influences the integrity of the skin and its appendages, the hair and nails, as well as other epithelial surfaces, including the mucous membranes and mucocutaneous junctions of the anogenital regions. Both nutritional deficits and excesses can induce various disorders of epithelial surfaces. On the other hand, some skin diseases may lead to nutritional and metabolic disorders, and certain skin disorders respond to diet manipulation. These aspects of nutrition and skin disorders are discussed below.

NUTRIENT DEFICIENCY

Assessment and Intervention
Any nutritional deficit that interferes with the rate of growth and maintenance of epithelial tissue will alter the appearance and function of these tissues.

The type, severity, and duration of the abnormality will vary with the specific nutrient that is deficient and with the severity and duration of the malnutrition. Table 33–1 summarizes the clinical manifestations of nutrient deficits. Be aware, however, that clinical manifestations rarely occur as a result of a deficiency of a single nutrient. Rather, multiple nutritional deficiencies are likely to be involved and malnourished clients will exhibit a variety of symptoms. For example, protein deficiency in the absence of other nutrient deficiencies is uncommon. The epithelial abnormalities are often accompanied by other manifestations. For example, a deficiency of either protein, energy, vitamin A, or zinc can lead to growth retardation in children.

Assess for the etiology of the lesions in affected clients. The dietary deficiency may be primary, or it may be conditioned by illness. For instance, the epithelial lesions may arise as a result of failure

TABLE 33–1
SIGNS OF NUTRITIONAL DEFICIENCY IN THE SKIN AND OTHER EPITHELIAL TISSUES

Nutrient Deficit	Pathological Manifestation
Protein–calories	Follicular hyperkeratosis (dry, rough skin with papillae formed by keratotic plugs that project from the hair follicles), changes in pigment (red hair, depigmented skin in blacks, and hyperpigmentation of pressure areas in whites, dermatoses described as ''enamel paint''—(plaques of highly pigmented, shiny skin—or ''flaky paint''—fissuring and scaling of the skin), thinning and loss of hair, decreased nail thickness, edema (these symptoms are characteristic of kwashiorkor)
Essential fatty acid deficiency	Greasy, scaly dermatitis in areas where the sebaceous glands are most abundant (i.e., the face, forehead, and scalp)
Vitamin A	Follicular hyperkeratosis, broken and coiled hairs, seborrheic dermatitis (an inflammatory form of dermatitis in seborrheic zones, Sjogren's syndrome—lack of salivary and lacrimal secretions)
Vitamin C	Follicular hyperkeratosis, broken and coiled hairs, seborrheic dermatitis, Sjogren's syndrome, gingivitis, generalized bleeding into the skin
Folic acid and vitamin B_{12}	Red, smooth tongue
Thiamine	Edema (characteristic of beriberi)
Riboflavin	Increased vascularity of the conjunctivae, angular lesions at the corners of the mouth, seborrheic dermatitis, perioral and perianal inflammation
Niacin	Scaling, hyperpigmented skin in areas exposed to heat or sunlight, perioral and perianal inflammation, erythema of affected areas (characteristic of pellagra)
Pyridoxine	Follicular hyperkeratosis, seborrheic dermatitis, broken hairs
Zinc	Greasy, scaly dermatitis in seborrheic zones, hair loss
Iron	Nail changes (koilonychia, in which the convex surfaces of the nails become concave)

to ingest adequate energy and nutrients because of economic factors, use of fad diets, or alcohol abuse. Metabolic abnormalities, such as a malabsorption syndrome, are also associated with lesions of the skin and other epithelial surfaces, and psychologic disorders, such as anorexia nervosa, lead to malnutrition and associated lesions. A deficiency of zinc may be associated with the inborn error of metabolism, acrodermatitis enteropathica. Recall also that cutaneous lesions, such as urticaria and eczema, may occur as an allergic response in sensitive clients. In some cases, the malnutrition may be iatrogenic; for example, failure to provide essential nutrients, such as essential fatty acids and zinc in solutions used for parenteral feeding.

Once the cause of the lesions has been established, direct treatment toward control of the underlying disorder and correction of any coexisting malnutrition. Assist the client in selecting an adequate diet based on the Basic Four Food Groups, using low-cost foods should low income be contributing to the malnutrition. Also provide information about existing community nutrition resources, such as food stamps, the WIC program, or the Congregate Meals Program.

In the presence of protein–energy deficiency, provide a high-protein, high-calorie diet and use commercial supplements that are high in protein content, such as Citrotein (Doyle Pharmaceutical), Meritene (Doyle Pharmaceutical), or Sustacal (Mead Johnson). The amount of protein required is approximately 1.5 g/kg body weight, or a range of 100 to 120 g protein daily for an adult. The diet is essentially a normal one supplemented with high-protein foods, such as extra milk, meat, and eggs. At least one half of the protein should be of high biologic value (HBV), and some HBV protein should be included at each meal. In some cases, smaller, frequent feedings may be indicated, whereas for others, fewer feedings may result in a better appetite. The optimal kilocalorie:nitrogen ratio is approximately 100 to 200 kcal/g of nitrogen, and 150 kcal/g of nitrogen is commonly used.[1] Very high protein diets lead to an increased urinary loss of calcium and an increased requirement for vitamin A.[2] Therefore, provide adequate amounts of these nutrients. Add powdered skim milk to such foods as mashed potatoes, cream soups, gravies, and cottage cheese to increase the protein and calcium content of the diet.

With deficiencies of B-complex vitamins and vitamin A, supplement with the indicated vitamin and complement this with a high-vitamin diet (see Chap. 8 for vitamin sources). Since the skin lesions are similar in several of the B-vitamin deficiencies, a supplement that includes all of the B vitamins should be given. When there is failure to absorb vitamin B_{12} due to a deficiency of intrinsic factor, administer the vitamin parenterally.

The dermatitis associated with essential fatty acid deficiency occurs most frequently in clients receiving prolonged parenteral feeding devoid of fats. Correct this deficiency with intermittent infusion of a fat emulsion or by a daily cutaneous application of sunflower oil or safflower seed oil in liberal amounts.[3]

Client education guidelines for treating iron deficiency with supplements and diet are given in Chapter 31. In the presence of zinc deficiency, provide a supplement and give the client a list of foods high in this mineral. Good food sources of zinc include animal protein foods (milk, cheese, eggs, meat, shellfish), legumes, nuts, and whole grains. To prevent a deficiency of zinc associated with prolonged parenteral feeding, assure that zinc is included in the infusate.

NUTRIENT EXCESS

Assessment and Intervention

Cutaneous manifestations occur with excesses of kilocalories and some nutrients as well as in disorders, such as hemochromatosis (see Chap. 9). Dermatosis is commonly associated with obesity, and prolonged doses of vitamin A prescribed therapeutically for a variety of dermatologic conditions may lead to hyperkeratosis, dryness of the skin, and possible hair loss. Interruption of therapy for a period of 1 to 2 months after 4 to 6 months of treatment may decrease the likelihood of complications. Occasionally, people consume excessive amounts of foods high in carotene, such as carrots, and their skin takes on an orange-tinged color. This results from the body's inability to convert carotene (provitamin A) to vitamin A rapidly enough to deal with the excessive consumption. Distinguish this type of skin discoloration from jaundice associated with liver abnormalities by noting the absence of the abnormal color from tissues, such as the sclera and buccal membranes, that are spared discoloration when excessive carotene is consumed. The condition is usually asymptomatic. Advise clients that the discoloration gradually disappears when the high carotene intake is reduced.

Tell clients who ingest large amounts (i.e., 500 mg or more daily) of the nicotinic acid form of niacin as part of the treatment regimen for lowering blood cholesterol that flushing, itching, dryness, and thickening of the skin are common side effects. Moreover, this therapy may lead to abnormal liver function tests and an increase in gastric secretion.

Clients with hypercholesterolemia often develop xanthomas—deposits of fatty substances, usually yellow in color—in the skin, often around tendons, and on the eyelids. Use client guidelines given in Chapter 29 for assisting clients with dietary control of hypercholesterolemia.

NUTRITIONAL AND METABOLIC EFFECTS OF SKIN DISORDERS

Assessment and Intervention

Skin disorders may have direct or indirect effects on nutritional status. For example, expect skin disorders associated with excessive scaling (e.g., exfoliative dermatitis) to cause direct losses of nutrients, such as protein, water, and iron. Assess for hypoalbuminemia with concurrent edema in clients who experience chronic protein loss and assess for dehydration, particularly in a hot environment, in clients who experience chronic water loss. Be aware also that normal epidermal desquamation is a source of iron loss, which may be accelerated with excess scaling of skin. Iron metabolism may be altered in certain skin diseases.

The increased use of folic acid that occurs in association with the rapid turnover of the epidermis in certain skin diseases and of vitamin C by the diseased skin may precipitate a deficiency of these nutrients. In addition, the client who is severely ill with a skin disease such as pemphigus (characterized by large water blisters), or lupus erythematosus (a type of collagen disease characterized by lesions of the face, neck, and upper extremities), may be anorexic. When skin disorders are characterized by glossitis or severe oral lesions, eating becomes difficult and secondary nutritional deficiency may arise.

Advise clients with dermatologic diseases associated with excessive scaling of the skin to increase their intake of protein, fluid, iron, folic acid, and vitamin A to prevent deficiencies of these nutrients. When the dermatologic disease is complicated by anorexia, assist the client in planning and preparing palatable foods, and advise small, frequent feedings. If the mouth and tongue are sore, tell the client to avoid acid foods, such as citrus fruits and tomatoes, and highly spiced foods.

DIETARY MANIPULATIONS IN SKIN DISORDERS

Assessment and Intervention

There are a number of skin disorders for which causes are not known, that are chronic, and that respond poorly to medical treatment. Thus, it is not surprising that they are sometimes attributed, by clients and the health team alike, to dietary causes, and diet is used as a mode of treatment or control. For example, various claims have been made for the therapeutic value of diet therapy to treat psoriasis. A number of different types of diets have been tried—low fat, low protein, low taurine, low tryptophan (based on turkey meat, which was later found to be a significant source of tryptophan), low calorie, and supplementation with lecithin, various vitamins, and zinc. To date, however, no diet or diet supplement has shown a consistent beneficial effect on the course of this disease. More recently, restriction of fruits (especially citrus fruits), acid foods (such as coffee, sodas, tomatoes and pineapples), nuts, corn, and milk has been reported to improve the condition,[4] although the effectiveness of this therapy has been debated.[5] Etretinate, an oral analog of vitamin A, has been used successfully in treating psoriasis, although this treatment is associated with a rise in serum lipid levels.[6] Therapy with ultraviolet light and psoralin has proven beneficial for many clients with this disease. Likewise, acne vulgaris, which is common in teenagers, is often attributed to dietary excesses, although there is little evidence that dietary factors are responsible for the disease.

In some situations, dietary management has a rational basis. For example, those disorders induced by nutritional deficiency, such as pellagra and protein–energy malnutrition, respond to therapy with the missing nutrients. The skin disorder dermatitis herpetiformis, which is characterized by an itchy blistery rash and, in some clients, an enteropathy that is indistinguishable from gluten-induced enteropathy (see Chap. 27), responds to a strict gluten-free diet.[7] The rash responds to sulfone drugs, and both the rash and the enteropathy respond to gluten restriction. Use the gluten-free diet and education guidelines described in Chapter 27 to establish a dietary regimen for clients with dermatitis herpetiformis, and advise them that the diet should be continued indefinitely.

Many claims have been made for the beneficial effects of vitamin E for such skin conditions as wrinkling, facilitating wound healing, and preventing scar formation. However, there is no convincing evidence that the vitamin has any beneficial effect.

REVIEW QUESTIONS AND ACTIVITIES

1. Distinguish between the effects of protein–energy deficiency and essential fatty acid deficiency on epithelial tissues.
2. Compare the effects of vitamin A and vitamin C deficiency on epithelial tissues.
3. Describe the effects on epithelial tissues of a deficiency of each of the following B-complex vitamins: (a) folic acid, (b) vitamin B_{12}, (c) thiamine, (d) riboflavin, (e) niacin, and (f) pyridoxine.
4. Identify the effects on epithelial tissues of a deficiency of zinc and iron.
5. Explain the dietary management of protein–energy deficiency.
6. Identify the management of essential fatty acid deficiency.

7. Describe the cutaneous effects of excessive ingestion of vitamin A.
8. Your client (an adult male) is receiving zinc supplements to correct a zinc deficiency. Use Basic Four Food Group guidelines to plan a day's menu that contains good food sources of zinc to complement his therapy.
9. You observe that your client has an orange tint to her skin. On taking a diet history, you find that she is drinking a quart of carrot juice daily. Identify the possible cause of her skin discoloration.
10. Your client has hypercholesterolemia and is taking large doses of nicotinic acid as part of his therapy. List cutaneous manifestations that may occur secondary to the hypercholesterolemia and to the nicotinic acid therapy.
11. Your client has a skin disorder that leads to excessive scaling and shedding of the skin; he also is anorectic and has glossitis.
    a. List three nutrients that may be lost in excessive amounts in association with the excessive scaling of the skin.
    b. List two nutrients that are needed in increased amounts for skin healing and regeneration.
    c. Identify dietary adjustments for dealing with the anorexia and glossitis.
12. Describe the dietary management of dermatitis herpetiformis.

REFERENCES

1. American Dietetic Association: Handbook of Clinical Dietetics. New Haven, Yale University Press, 1981, p C-3.
2. Ibid, p C-4.
3. Ibid, p B-59.
4. Douglas JM: Psoriasis and diet. West J Med 133:450, 1980.
5. Rapaport M: Diet not shown effective in psoriasis. West J Med 134:364, 1981.
6. Cowart VS: Etretinate therapy improves psoriasis but elevates serum lipids. JAMA 247:2647, 1982.
7. Leonard J, Haffenden G, Tucker W, et al.: Gluten challenge in dermatitis herpetiformis. N Engl J Med 308:816, 1983.

BIBLIOGRAPHY

Chandra RK: Acrodermatis enteropathica: Zinc levels and cell-mediated immunity. Pediatrics 66:789, 1980.
Hodges RE: Nutrition and the integument including mucous membranes. In RE Hodges, ed: Nutrition in Medical Practice. Philadelphia, WB Saunders, 1980, p 265.
Hughes S, Williams SE, Turnberg LA: Crohn's disease and psoriasis. N Engl J Med 308:101, 1983.
Rosenberg EW, Spitzer RE, Marley WM, Belew RW: In-

flammatory bowel disease, psoriasis, and complement. N Engl J Med 307:685, 1982.

Sandstead HH: Clinical manifestations of certain classical deficiency diseases. In RS Goodhart, ME Shils, eds: Modern Nutrition in Health and Disease. Philadelphia, Lea & Febiger, 1980, p 685.

Takkunen H: Iron deficiency pruritis. JAMA 239:1394, 1978.

Viteri FE, Torun B: Protein–calorie malnutrition. In RS Goodhart, ME Shils, eds: Modern Nutrition in Health and Disease. Philadelphia, Lea & Febiger, 1980, p 697.

CHAPTER 34

Nutrition and Pulmonary Disorders

Objectives

After completion of this chapter, the student will be able to:

1. Evaluate the relationship between nutrition/nutritional status and pulmonary infection.

2. Develop a nursing care plan for the nutritional management of a client with an acute respiratory infection.

3. Compare and contrast the clinical manifestations and the nutritional management of chronic pulmonary tuberculosis, emphysema, and chylothorax.

4. Evaluate the potential pulmonary hazards of three types of therapeutic regimens.

Nutrition and pulmonary disease may interact in several ways. First, nutrition plays a role in resistance to infection, the most important cause of disease of the respiratory tract. Second, the respiratory tract is often a target organ for the manifestation of other nutrition-related disorders, such as food sensitivity and cystic fibrosis. Third, respiratory disorders may adversely affect nutritional status, and maintenance of adequate nutrition is an important aspect of the management of these disorders. Moreover, some types of therapy, such as tube feeding or parenteral feeding, may lead to pulmonary problems.

The interaction of nutrition and infection, cystic fibrosis, and food sensitivity has been discussed in other sections of the book. The specific relationship between nutrition and pulmonary infection, nutritional considerations in specific lung disorders, and pulmonary hazards of nutritional therapy are discussed here.

RELATIONSHIP BETWEEN NUTRITION AND PULMONARY INFECTION

Assessment

The respiratory system has several defense barriers that provide protection against infection and toxic substances that are inhaled. The tracheobronchial tree is covered by an epithelial surface that provides a mechanical barrier against foreign substances, including microorganisms and, to some extent, toxic gases. The presence of cilia (hairlike projections) and the secretion of mucus and other surface fluids provide mechanisms for clearance of inhaled particles and microorganisms. Phagocytes and immunoglobulins aid in the destruction of microorganisms.

The integrity of the defense mechanisms provided by the respiratory membranes and the immune system is altered by various nutritional and nonnutritional factors. For example, expect them to be depressed in clients who are debilitated and in alcoholics, with resultant impaired clearance of microorganisms and proneness to develop respiratory infections. Assess the client's vitamin A status, since deficiency of vitamin A leads to disintegration of the normal epithelial surface and ciliary loss. Heavy cigarette smoking also leads to loss of cilia. The production of secretions by the epithelial tissue is reduced in clients who are deficient in vitamins A and C.

ACUTE REPSIRATORY INFECTIONS

Assessment and Intervention

Since the organs of the respiratory system are in direct communication with the outside air, they are more susceptible to invading organisms than are other organs, such as the heart or kidney. Infection may be of either viral (e.g., influenza) or bacterial (e.g., bronchitis) origin. Assess for the presence of factors that may decrease nutrient intake in clients with acute respiratory infections, including alterations in the sense of smell and taste, sore throat, nasal obstruction with difficulty breathing, coughing, and dyspnea. Assess the nutritional cost of the infection relative to the presence of these factors and others, such as fever or associated gastrointestinal manifestations of anorexia, nausea, or vomiting. The increased flow of secretion and mouth breathing, with its tendency to dry the secretions, contribute to increased fluid needs. There are increased requirements for kilocalories, protein, vitamins, and minerals, particularly when fever is present. Treat infants and young children, elderly clients, and debilitated clients as high-risk groups, since the infection may tax their homeostatic mechanisms. Since breathing and swallowing cannot occur simultaneously, respiratory obstruction may especially contribute to nutritional problems in infants.

Tailor the diet to the client's ability to tolerate food and base it on his or her age as well as the symptoms, severity, and duration of the infection.

During the acute states when fever is present and the appetite is poor, provide small, frequent feedings of soft or liquid foods. In some cases only liquids may be tolerated. Use the client's appetite and individual desires for particular foods as a guide to what is best tolerated. If the illness persists for more than several days, high-calorie, high-protein foods will need to be emphasized.

Since dehydration promotes the production of thick, tenacious secretions, give close attention to adequate hydration to maintain thin secretions. It does not suffice to tell the client simply that "extra fluids are necessary," particularly if the client is in a high-risk group. Give details about the type and amount of fluids to drink and methods for estimating fluid intake and output. Assist the client to actually work out a schedule of time and needed amount of fluids to consume, then plan for follow-up evaluation of the plan. Fruit juices and milk will provide needed potassium, and salty broth and soups will provide needed sodium chloride. If the throat is sore, however, salty broth, acid-tasting foods, and coarse foods should be avoided. A vitamin supplement may be necessary for a short period.

CHRONIC RESPIRATORY INFECTION

Pulmonary Tuberculosis

Assessment and Intervention. Although tuberculosis most frequently affects the lungs, it may be localized in other organs, such as the lymph nodes or kidney, or it may spread throughout the body (miliary tuberculosis). Invasion of the lungs by the tubercle bacillus brings inflammation with mobilization of white blood cells, which wall off the primary infection. This primary lesion is usually controlled by the body's immune system, but in susceptible clients, it may become reactivated or spread throughout the body. With reactivation, **caseation** (conversion of necrotic tissue into a mass resembling cheese) occurs, with the cheesy formation later dissolving, leaving an open cavity. Healing occurs with calcification of the caseation.

Evaluate for the following manifestations in clients with acute tuberculosis: high fever, cough, expectoration, exhaustion, hypoalbuminemia, and wasting of body tissues. A low-grade fever is characteristic of the chronic phase of the disorder, and the metabolic rate is lower than in the acute phase.

Tuberculosis responds to treatment with drugs, but it is also necessary to include a diet high in kilocalories and protein with supplements of vitamins and minerals as part of the treatment. Provide a diet that contains approximately 2500 to 3000 kcal daily and from 75 to 100 g of protein. The high-protein intake is needed to counteract the negative nitrogen balance and hypoalbuminemia. Since calcium is needed for calcification and healing of the lesions, include the equivalent of a quart of milk in the daily diet or use cheese, yoghurt, or calcium supplements if the client is intolerant of lactose. Calcium and protein intakes can be augmented by adding nonfat milk to beverages, soups, casseroles, and desserts. If the client has a tendency to hemorrhage, administer iron supplements as well. Vitamins that should receive increased attention are (1) vitamin C (to promote wound healing), (2) vitamin D (to promote the intestinal absorption of calcium), and (3) B-complex vitamins (to stimulate the appetite and aid in increasing food intake). Since carotene, the precursor of vitamin A, may be poorly converted to the active form of the vitamin in tubercular clients, assure that adequate amounts of the preformed vitamin, such as milk and egg yolk, are included in the diet.

Isoniazid, one of the chemotherapeutic agents used to treat tuberculosis, is an antagonist of the

B-complex vitamin, pyridoxine. Provide a pyridoxine supplement with prolonged therapy with the drug to prevent the neurologic manifestations of pyridoxine deficiency.

Emphysema

Assessment and Intervention. In emphysema there is an overdistention or rupture of the alveoli of the lung. The disease is characterized by an expiratory type of dyspnea. Air becomes trapped in the alveoli and the lungs become increasingly overdistended. The disorder may result from a number of causes, including air pollution, cigarette smoking, chronic asthma, or chronic lung infection. Nutritional problems may occur because of difficulty in eating an adequate amount of food and because of financial ramifications of the disease. The individual may be unable to function in productive work, and thus income may not be sufficient to purchase adequate food.

Assess for these nutritional problems that are frequently encountered in clients with emphysema: anorexia, a tendency toward dehydration, gastrointestinal distress, and susceptibility to infection. Anorexia, leading to muscle wasting and weight loss, may result from dyspnea, an exhausting cough, and frequent raising of sputum. Because of shortness of breath, the client may lack the strength to purchase, prepare, or otherwise seek food or to chew or swallow a sufficient amount. The dyspnea may be greatest in the morning before arising due to mouth breathing during sleep. This dries the lung secretions and leads to mucous plugs, which obstruct the airways. Many people with emphysema have difficulty eating breakfast. In severe cases, tissue wasting is common, and loss of abdominal fat may cause further breathing problems because this limits the use of the abdominal structures to aid in breathing.

An increased need for fluid results from the mouth breathing, with its drying of secretions, and from an increased volume of respiratory secretions because of the inflamed mucous membranes. The increased fluid need may be coupled with an inadequate fluid intake, leading to dehydration. Dehydration, in turn, increases the tendency to produce thick, tenacious secretions. Thick sputum is an excellent medium for growth of bacteria in the air trapped in the alveoli, and the client may be open to infection due to a decrease in general resistance.

An early compensatory process is the channeling of available energy to vital areas, such as the heart, lungs, and brain, depleting such areas as the muscles and gastrointestinal tract. Peristalsis is slowed, digestion is impaired, and gastric ulceration is a frequent complication. Distention after meals interferes with abdominal breathing. Fear of abdominal distention after meals may further limit food intake.

Advise the client with emphysema to consume small, frequent meals of a diet that is soft (to reduce chewing effort) and free of gas-forming foods (to reduce abdominal distention). Suggest that the client use foods of high-calorie, high-protein density (such as milk-based beverages or high-protein commercial supplements) to supply the greatest nutritional value in the smallest possible volume. Encourage an adequate fluid intake, since liquids help to loosen secretions, and beverages with a distinct flavor (such as acid-tasting fruit juice or well-seasoned broth) may freshen the mouth and improve the appetite. Brushing the teeth before meals may be helpful. Stress to the client that he or she should eat slowly and without talking to reduce air swallowing, which magnifies abdominal discomfort, and that the daily schedule should include a period of rest before and after meals.

A major concern in emphysema is weight loss, but excess weight should also be avoided, since it increases metabolic demands and can impair ventilation and gaseous exchange. Provide support for obese clients in their efforts to lose weight.

Chylothorax

Assessment and Intervention. Chylothorax is a relatively rare condition that may compromise the nutritional status of the affected individual. Impaired lymphatic drainage—due to congenital anomalies of the lymphatic ducts, thoracic trauma and rupture of the thoracic duct, thrombosis of the thoracic duct or the left subclavian vein, or pressure from enlarged lymph nodes or neoplasms—results in the escape of chyle from the thoracic duct into the thoracic cavity. Treatment involves repeated thoracentesis or continuous drainage. These procedures lead to repeated loss of the fat that circulates in the lymphatic system. Manage the diet of affected clients by restricting fat and including adequate amounts of protein (there is also protein loss in the chyle) and kilocalories. Since fat-soluble vitamins are lost, provide supplements, especially vitamins A and D. The use of medium-chain triglycerides that bypass the lymphatic circulation and circulate directly into the portal system may be an alternative to fat restriction. Commercial products containing medium-chain triglycerides include Portagen and MCT oil (Mead Johnson).

Pulmonary Hazards of Various Forms of Therapy

Assessment and Intervention. Hodges describes several practices that have been found to damage or otherwise interfere with the normal functioning of the respiratory system.[1] Mineral oil, which is commonly used as a laxative, can lead to loss of fat-soluble vitamins and essential fatty acids, and its use can also lead to a form of pneumonia. The oil may seep down the trachea, where it immobilizes the cilia and thus reaches the alveoli and leads to inflammation. It may be prudent to discourage the use of mineral oil as a laxative. If it is used, advise clients not to use it in association with meals.

Diminished pulmonary diffusion capacity has been reported in clients who receive intravenous fat emulsions, and ingestion of a fatty meal can impair pulmonary diffusion capacity for a short period. Use fat emulsions in clients with severe pulmonary disease with caution.

The risk of gastric reflux and development of aspiration pneumonia is great in clients whose protective reflexes are diminished and who are being fed by a nasogastric tube. Clients who are at a particular risk include the elderly, those with esophageal or neurologic disorders, debilitated persons, and postanesthetic clients. To reduce the risk of gastric reflux and aspiration pneumonia in clients receiving nasogastric tube feeding, elevate the head of the bed during and after the feeding, and frequently turn clients who are unconscious from side to side. Before feeding, the client's head should be turned to the side to reduce the risk of aspiration should vomiting occur. Provide the feeding by continuous drip, rather than feeding intermittently, to reduce the risk of aspiration. The problem of aspiration is reduced when the feeding site is the duodenum or the jejunum.

REVIEW QUESTIONS AND ACTIVITIES

1. List three mechanisms that protect the respiratory system against infection.
2. Identify the rationale underlying the impairment of respiratory defense mechanisms in clients who are (a) debilitated, (b) heavy cigarette smokers, and (c) alcoholics.
3. Describe the specific effects of a deficiency of vitamins A and C on respiratory defense mechanisms.
4. Identify three categories of clients who may require aggressive nutritional support in the presence of an acute respiratory infection.
5. Describe the principles of dietary management for an acute respiratory infection.
6. Describe the clinical manifestations associ-

ated with chronic pulmonary tuberculosis and discuss the appropriate nutritional therapy.
7. Relate the nutritional management of emphysema to the clinical manifestations of the disorder.
8. Explain the rationale for modifying intake of dietary fat in treating chylothorax.
9. Describe the possible detrimental effect of each of the following practices on respiratory function: (a) use of mineral oil as a laxative, (b) use of fat emulsions given by the intravenous route, and (c) use of tube feedings given by the nasogastric route.

REFERENCE

1. Hodges RE: Nutrition in Medical Practice. Philadelphia, WB Saunders, 1980, p 260.

BIBLIOGRAPHY

Bennett JV: Human infections: Economic implications and prevention. Ann Intern Med 89:761, 1978.
Bernheim HA, Block LH, Atkins E: Fever: Pathogenesis, pathophysiology, and purpose. A review. Ann Intern Med 91:261, 1979.
Dionigi R, Gnes F, Bonera A, Dominioni L: Nutrition and infection. J Parent Enter Nutr 3:62, 1979.
Geppert EF, Leff A: The pathogenesis of pulmonary and miliary tuberculosis. Ann Int Med 139:138, 1979.
Hodges RE: Nutrition and the respiratory system. In RE Hodges, ed: Nutrition in Medical Practice. Philadelphia, WB Saunders, 1980, p 254.
Leff A, Lester W, Addington W: Tuberculosis. A chemotherapeutic triumph but a persistent socioeconomic problem. Arch Intern Med 139:1375, 1979.
Scrimshaw NS: Effect of infection on nutrient requirements. Am J Clin Nutr 30:1536, 1977.
Woodcock AA, Gross ER, Gellert A, et al.: Effects of dihydrocodeine, alcohol, and caffeine on breathlessness and exercise tolerance in patients with chronic obstructive lung disease and normal blood gases. N Engl J Med 305:1611, 1981.

CHAPTER 35

Nutrition and Cancer

Objectives

After completion of this chapter, the student will be able to:

1. Differentiate among the factors that associate substances contained in foods with the (a) etiology, (b) prevention, and (c) treatment of cancer.

2. Compare and contrast the nutrient factors that may be involved in the etiology of cancer of the colon and cancer of the breast.

3. Distinguish among the mechanisms whereby cancer may negatively affect nutritional status.

4. Assess factors associated with weight loss in cancer clients.

5. Distinguish among the side effects associated with the three major treatment modalities for cancer.

6. Develop a nursing care plan for managing cancer clients with each of the following side effects of therapy: anorexia, nausea and vomiting, sore mouth and esophagus, dry mouth, and diarrhea.

Cancer is among the major health problems in the United States today. The death rate from this disease is second only to deaths from cardiovascular disease (including stroke). Although neoplastic disease affects all age groups, the great majority of cases occur in the middle-age and older groups. Approximately one half of all fatal cancers are of three types: lungs, colon, and breast cancer. Although the overall cancer incidence is higher in men than women, the incidence of lung cancer in women has increased in recent years.

Cancer arises from a number of factors—those intrinsic to the individual and those stemming from the environment. In the past, genetic factors related to tumorigenicity received major emphasis. However, sharp differences in the incidence of some varieties of human malignancy in different population groups and in different geographical areas have long been recognized. Further, there have been changes in the incidence of cancer, both internationally and within countries over time. These changes are thought to be related to environmental factors and have led to an intensification of epidemiologic studies in an attempt to delineate the important etiologic environmental agents. Particular attention is being given to those aspects of lifestyle—smoking habits, alcohol consumption, and diet—that may be implicated. Some of the environmental factors implicated in different forms of cancer, such as cigarette smoking in pulmonary cancer, are well recognized.

Data from animal experiments and epidemiologic studies have provided evidence that diet is an important environmental factor in cancer incidence. For example, animal experiments have shown that diet manipulations can influence the development of spontaneous and transplanted tumors. From an epidemiologic perspective, studies with migrant populations, which generally show that the incidence and mortality rates change from those common to the native population to that of the host country, have provided excellent case studies of the relationship between diet and cancer. For instance, these

511

trends have been documented for gastric, colon, and breast cancer in Japanese migrants to Hawaii and the continental United States. After one or two generations, the cancer incidence of the Japanese is similar to that of the population of the host country. The differences in cancer incidence that have been observed in populations living in similar environments but maintaining different dietary habits lend support to the view that diet is a factor in the causation of certain types of cancer. For example, Seventh-Day Adventists and Mormons who consume a diet containing less meat, coffee, and tea than is typical for the American diet have a low risk for colon and breast cancer.[1,2]

These findings tend to support the view that environmental factors, and not genetic factors, predominate in cancer etiology; and since environmental factors can be altered, it is conceivable that cancer incidence can be reduced or even prevented.

The diet is generally associated with cancers of the gastrointestinal tract (i.e., esophagus, stomach, rectum, colon, pancreas, and liver) and cancers of some sex hormone-responsive sites (i.e., breast, prostate, endometrium, and ovary) and to some degree with cancers of the respiratory system and bladder. According to some estimates, diet is responsible for 30 to 40 percent of cancers in men and 60 percent of cancers in women.[3]

In addition to the possible role that nutrition plays in the etiology of cancer, nutrition is vitally important in the treatment of the disorder. The effects of cancer and its treatment (i.e., chemotherapy and radiation therapy) potentiate a cycle of malnutrition. Thus, nutritional support is necessary as an important adjunct to medical or surgical management in order to counteract the complications of cancer and restore the client's nutritional balance.

This chapter focuses on specific dietary factors implicated in the etiology of cancer, the effects of neoplastic disease and its treatment on nutritional status, principles of nutritional management, and use of specific nutrients as a primary form of cancer therapy.

NUTRITION IN CANCER ETIOLOGY

Assessment

Various food factors and substances consumed with food (such as food additives) have been identified as potential etiologic agents in cancer. There are two basic mechanisms by which food or fluid might influence the development of cancer. First, the diet may contain artificial or naturally occurring carcinogens or carcinogenic precursors. Second, a dietary imbalance (deficiency or excess) of specific nutrients or nutrient factors may alter host defense mechanisms, with subsequent susceptibility to carcinogenesis. For example, a positive association exists between excessive dietary fat intake and the prevalence of colon cancer and cancer of the breast. There

is also some evidence that certain substances contained in food may assume a protective role against cancer. It should be kept in mind, however, that none of the potential carcinogens discussed below have been proven to cause cancer in humans. The evidence for classifying a substance as a potential carcinogen is based on its capacity to induce tumors in animals, its induction of mutations in microorganisms, and human epidemiologic studies correlating cancer incidence with prevalence of the substance in the food supply. The evidence provided by these associations is not conclusive, since excessively high doses or unusual routes of administration are used in animal testing. Even though large amounts of a substance causes cancer in animals, one cannot predict how humans will respond to the substances under conditions of ordinary use. Further, there is no proof that microbial mutagens are carcinogens, and many variables other than the food supply separate population groups.

Ingestion of Potentially Carcinogenic Substances. The most obvious mechanism by which food or fluid might influence the development of cancer is by ingestion of potentially carcinogenic substances, such as food additives, environmental contaminants, and toxic substances naturally present in food. Only a small proportion of the substances added to food have been tested for carcinogenicity according to currently accepted standard protocols, and except for the nonnutritive sweeteners, little epidemiologic data on the topic are available. Of the few intentional food additives that have been tested and found to be carcinogenic in animals, all except saccharin have been banned from use in the food supply. For example, some food colors, cyclamate, and diethylstilbestrol (DES), a hormone used as a growth stimulant in the cattle and poultry industries, have been banned because of their potential carcinogenicity or other toxic effects.

Saccharin has been shown to produce bladder cancer in male rats when large amounts were implanted into their bladders or when the rats were fed high-saccharin diets. Moreover, high doses of saccharin have been shown to promote the action of other known carcinogens in rat bladders. In contrast to the experimental studies, most epidemiologic studies have not shown a clear relationship between the use of saccharin and cancer, although one study showed a direct association for men,[4] and other studies have shown possible effects in certain subgroups. The FDA has proposed banning the use of saccharin in food, although it is expected that this decision may be delayed for several years.

Butylated hydroxyanisole (BHA) and butylated hydroxytoluene (BHT) are widely used as food additives primarily because of their preservative and antioxidant properties. Studies with animals have shown BHT to have a tumor-promoting effect, and the FDA has proposed interim regulations on its use pending further studies. There is no indication that BHA has a similar effect, and, in fact, it may be useful in inhibiting the formation of certain types of cancer.

N-nitroso compounds, such as nitrosamines, are strong carcinogens in animals, although there has not been conclusive evidence that they are directly associated with human cancer. The source of N-nitroso compounds is nitrate and nitrite used as preservatives in meats and other cured products and occurring naturally in certain foods. Nitrate can be reduced to nitrite by bacteria during food storage, food preparation, or after ingestion. Nitrite, in turn, reacts with dietary substances, such as amines or amides, to form N-nitroso compounds. Such vegetables as carrots, spinach, and beets contribute most of the ingested nitrate. Other dietary sources include nitrate-rich drinking water and fruit juices. More than one third of ingested nitrite comes from cured meats, and baked goods, cereals, and vegetables also provide nitrite.

While the evidence suggesting that nitrate, nitrite, and N-nitroso compounds play a role in human cancer is largely circumstantial, some epidemiologic studies point to a weak association between consumption of certain smoked or cured meats and an increased incidence of cancers of the esophagus and stomach. The USDA and the FDA have taken steps to reduce the amount of nitrate and nitrite used as food additives.

Very low levels of a number of environmental contaminants, such as pesticide residues and polycyclic aromatic hydrocarbons (PAHs) such as benzo[a]pyrene, may be present in foods, and the FDA monitors the dietary level of some of these. Various PAHs have been shown to cause cancer in laboratory animals, although there are no data to suggest that these compounds individually constitute a risk for human cancer. Polycyclic aromatic hydrocarbons are found in a variety of smoked foods, roasted coffee, and in vegetables and seafood obtained from a contaminated environment. In the absence of contamination, the major sources of these substances are smoked meats and grilled or roasted foods. Smoking of food, as well as charcoal broiling, results in deposition of such compounds as benzo[a]pyrene on the surface of the meat. This compound has carcinogenic and mutagenic properties.

Naturally occurring food contaminants that have been implicated as potential carcinogens are cycasin, a glycoside found in cycad nuts, and aflatoxin, a mycotoxin produced by the mold *Aspergillus flavus*, which grows on peanuts and grains when storage humidity is high. Both cycasin and aflatoxin produce liver cancer in experimental animals. There are epidemiologic data suggesting a correlation between aflatoxin ingestion and liver cancer in humans. Aflatoxins are not a major problem in the United States, where storage conditions are controlled, but it appears prudent to avoid the ingestion of moldy peanuts, seeds, legumes, and cereal grains. Heat processing reduces but does not eliminate the aflatoxin contamination. Aflatoxin levels in foods are monitored by the USDA and the FDA.

Coffee consumption has been associated with an elevated risk of both bladder cancer[5] and pancreatic cancer[6] in humans, although results of studies on the effect of coffee on cancer etiology are not consistent. On the other hand, restriction of caffeine and other methylxanthines (a class of compounds found in coffee, tea, cola beverages, and other carbonated drinks and in some pain medications) is a part of the treatment for fibrocystic breast disease in women. This condition, characterized by benign breast lumps, is associated with a high incidence of breast cancer. A diet free of methylxanthines may significantly reduce breast nodularity in many women with breast lumps.

The observation that cancer mortality is higher in cities with a fluoridated water supply has led to speculation that fluoride is another causal agent in human cancer. Rigorous data analysis has revealed that these cities also had a higher cancer incidence before fluoridation, and there is no evidence implicating fluoride in any change in cancer incidence.[7]

Dietary Imbalance and Cancer Etiology. In some cases, a dietary deficiency of a specific nutrient may contribute to transformation of normal cells to neoplastic cells, although it is also true that in animal studies deficiencies of certain nutrients have been associated with decreased tumor growth. It should be kept in mind, however, that too little scientific evidence exists to draw firm conclusions about any specific cause and effect relationship between nutrient deficiency and cancer. Table 35–1 summarizes the effect of nutrient deficiency on tumor incidence.

Fiber is a dietary component that has received wide attention in recent years for its possible role in the etiology of cancer of the colon and rectum. These cancers have a high incidence in both males and females and are among the leading causes of death from cancer. Some epidemiologic data have linked the consumption of low-fiber diets with cancer of the colon and have shown a protective effect of fiber.[8] It has been hypothesized that differences in colon cancer incidence among different populations are due to differences in fiber intake. This protective role remains a hypothesis that must be studied further. It should be noted that not all data support the hypothesis that fiber intake is inversely related to cancer of the large bowel. The topic is complex, since components of the dietary environment vary together—i.e., diets that are high in kilocalories, animal protein, fat, cholesterol, refined sugar, and food additives are likely to be low in fiber and other complex carbohydrates. Fiber itself is a complex mixture of various compounds with varying properties (e.g., cellulose, lignin, pectin) rather than a single component with a well-defined function.

In other cases, dietary excesses are implicated in the etiology of cancer. The typical American diet, which is considered to contain an excessive amount

TABLE 35-1
EFFECTS OF DEFICIENCY OF SELECTED NUTRIENTS ON CANCER INCIDENCE

Nutrient Factor Deficient in Diet	Effect	Comment
Kilocalories	In animal studies, kcal restriction inhibits the development of transplanted tumors and inhibits the growth of both spontaneous and transplanted tumors	Kcal restriction is not a means of preventing tumor formation in humans, however
Protein	In animal studies, carcinogenesis is suppressed by diets containing protein at or below the minimal level needed for optimal growth and is enhanced by a high protein intake	Protein may affect the initiation phase of carcinogenesis and the subsequent growth and development of the tumor
Vitamin A	In animal studies, vitamin A deficiency generally increases the susceptibility to chemically induced neoplasia	An increased intake of vitamin A appears to protect against carcinogenesis in most cases
Iron	Increases risk for the Plummer–Vinson syndrome in humans, which is associated with cancer of the upper gastrointestinal tract and possibly gastric cancer	
Iodine	May be associated with cancer of the thyroid in humans	Excessive iodine intake may also increase the risk for thyroid cancer
Cholesterol (in blood)	An inverse correlation between low blood cholesterol levels and colon cancer in men has been noted in some but not all studies	It is not clear whether lower than normal blood cholesterol levels are a cause or whether they reflect the metabolic consequences of cancer; the data suggest that a low blood cholesterol may be a clue to some unknown factor

of alcohol, kilocalories, animal protein, and fat, has been associated in epidemiologic studies with cancer of the gastrointestinal tract and reproductive systems. In many instances, it is difficult to pinpoint the effect of specific factors, especially the effects of an excessive intake of kilocalories, animal protein, and fat, since the excesses often occur simultaneously. The epidemiology of various cancers, especially cancer of the colon and breast, demonstrates a prevalence that essentially parallels the prevalence of heart attacks. Although this fact does not prove that the same factors (such as diet patterns) are causally related to both cancer and heart attack, it does provide an attractive hypothesis for study. Both breast and colon cancers are relatively rare in primitive societies and increase with affluence and the adoption of the Western-type diet.

Excessive alcohol consumption in combination with cigarette smoking may be an important etiologic factor in the development of cancer of the head and neck (especially of the oral cavity, pharynx, larynx, and esophagus) and the respiratory tract. The effect of alcohol and tobacco combined appears to be greater than the sum of their individual effects. Some investigators relate the effect of alcohol and cigarettes on cancer to associated nutritional deficiencies (particularly of riboflavin), which appear to make the epithelial cells more susceptible to carcinogens. Cancer of the liver occurs more commonly in those with cirrhosis, and excessive alcohol consumption may lead to cirrhosis.

Body mass is related to the risk of developing cancer. Epidemiologic data have shown that obesity or increased body mass may be related to cancer of the breast, endometrium, and kidney in females and cancer of the colon in men. Diets high in fat tend to be associated with cancer of the large bowel and hormone-dependent cancers, especially cancer of the breast and prostate. However, the literature on dietary constituents and cancer incidence provides contradictory arguments. Total fat content, saturated fat, and polyunsaturated fat have all been implicated, although total fat and saturated fat have been associated most frequently in humans. In contrast, data from animal studies suggest that when total fat intake is low, polyunsaturated fats are more effective than saturated fat in enhancing carcinogenesis.

The incidence of cancer of the colon has been related to a high-calorie diet that is high in animal protein (especially beef) and fat. It is difficult to distinguish between the effects of dietary fat and meat, however, since a large proportion of dietary fat is derived from meat, and beef is a high-fat meat. The hypothesis that saturated fat, especially beef fat, is particularly harmful has been criticized as attention has been called to discrepancies in the data—e.g., some population groups with a high level of consumption of animal products have a low incidence of colon cancer, and vice versa.

An association has been uncovered between obesity and a high-fat diet and endocrine-dependent tumors such as malignancy of the endometrium and the breast. Although a high-fat diet may be associated with a high kilocalorie intake and obesity, modification of hormones by dietary factors may be important. One hypothesis is that a high-fat diet changes the prolactin:estrogen ratio. Prolactin production increases, bringing a high prolactin:estrogen ratio.[9] A high prolactin:estrogen ratio has been shown to be important in enhancing breast cancer induced by carcinogens in rats. Another possibility is that a high-fat diet induces early sexual maturity in girls, and since dietary fat is known to influence sterol metabolism, it may also influence steroid hormones or their effects on susceptible tissues. Among overweight postmenopausal women, the increased risk of developing endometrial cancer has been attributed to an increased conversion in adipose tissue of estrone from androstenedione. This may affect the risk of developing breast cancer as well. Thus obesity may accelerate estrogen synthesis from non-estrogenic precursors. Whereas these nutritional–hormonal relationships remain to be convincingly established, it appears that age of menarche and body fatness during postmenopausal years may influence susceptibility to breast and endometrial cancer. Although severe kilocalorie restriction (which has been shown to restrict the growth of most tumors in animals) may not be practical in humans, efforts to prevent overweight throughout the life-span are indicated.

Potential Inhibitors of Carcinogenesis. There is some evidence that certain nutritive and nonnutritive substances contained in food may protect against the development of cancer in certain body sites.

A nutritive substance that appears promising in preventing certain epithelial tumors (skin, lung, bladder, and breast) is vitamin A either in its preformed state, retinol (found in animal sources of the vitamin), as its precursor, B-carotene (found in dark green and deep yellow vegetables), or as synthetic analogs, the **retinoids**.[10] The retinoids appear to be more effective and are less toxic than retinol. In general, the studies point to an inverse relationship between dietary intakes of vitamin A and B-carotene and the incidence of cancer. In the studies, however, it has not been possible to differentiate between the effects of B-carotene and vitamin A. Moreover, since vitamin A in large doses is toxic, caution clients against increasing vitamin A intake by the use of supplements for the purpose of preventing cancer.

Vitamin C, vitamin E, the mineral selenium, and the synthetic food additive BHA have been reported to decrease the incidence of certain types of cancer. All of these substances have antioxidant properties, and vitamin C and vitamin E appear to inhibit the formation of *N*-nitroso compounds. Consumption of vitamin C-containing foods has been associated with a lower risk of cancer of the esophagus and stomach. Because of its effect on formation of *N*-nitroso compounds, suggest to clients that they consume foods rich in vitamin C when consuming foods containing nitrate or nitrite, such as cured ham or bacon.

Cruciferous vegetables, such as cabbage, cauliflower, broccoli, and brussels sprouts, contain various chemicals, including indoles, that stimulate enzymes that provide a protective effect against the development of chemically induced tumors of the breast and forestomach of animals.[11] Epidemiologic studies also support a protective effect for humans. Information on this subject is not complete, however, and it is possible that large amounts of the chemicals may have adverse effects.

ROLE OF DIET IN CANCER PREVENTION

The correlation of diet with certain forms of cancers does not mean there exists an exclusive etiologic link. Nutritional imbalances coupled with other environmental hazards, such as pollution and psychologic stress, may provide a continuous low-level insult that, over time, can weaken the natural defense mechanism. Diet may play a modifying rather than a causative role.

Although many factors may contribute to cancer incidence, the modification of one, e.g., diet, may be sufficient to stop or retard the chain of events. Ideally, it is desirable to eliminate all potential toxins from the diet, although it is unlikely that any food is totally free of toxic or carcinogenic substances. At present, the evidence is too fragmentary and inconclusive to recommend specific changes in the American diet for the specific purposes of cancer control. However, given the current evidence, encourage clients to eat a varied diet that curtails excessive kilocalories, total fat, refined sugar, alcohol, foods that are smoked, salt-cured or salt-pickled, and that contain food additives. Encourage a diet that provides adequate amounts of fruits, vegetables, and whole grains. Eating a varied diet is important to minimize the possible hazards that may be associated with any one food.

EFFECT OF NEOPLASTIC DISEASE AND ITS TREATMENT ON NUTRITIONAL STATUS

Assessment

Nutritional status is negatively affected by three aspects of the disease process: (1) systemic effects of cancer, (2) localized effects resulting from cancer occurring in a specific body site, and (3) effects of cancer therapy. The resulting catabolism and malnutrition are a component of a vicious cycle that induces secondary complications as a result of malnutrition per se.

The systemic effects arise from generalized metabolic changes that result in reduced food intake and changes in tissue and endocrine function produced by the tumor, whereas the localized effects are due to alteration in food intake and use associated with the specific tumor site, e.g., the gastrointestinal tract. The catabolism and negative effects on nutritional status are further intensified by each of the various therapies—surgery, radiation therapy, and chemotherapy. The combined result of ▶ these influences is **cachexia**, a syndrome characterized by generalized malnutrition and progressive tissue wasting and debilitation. The cachexia potentiates a cycle of malnutrition. Observe for signs and symptoms, such as muscle weakness that necessitates prolonged bed rest, loss of respiratory muscle power that may lead to pneumonia, skin breakdown with decubitus ulcers, fluid and electrolyte abnormalities, apathy, and further disinterest in food. Altered replication of intestinal villi cells brings malabsorption, and reduced immunocompetence leads to a decreased resistance to infection. No simple correlation exists between the degree of cachexia and tumor cell type, anatomic site of involvement, tumor burden, or kilocalorie intake.

Cachexia, one of the hallmarks of advanced cancer, was the most frequent single cause of death in cancer clients before the introduction of aggressive radiotherapeutic and chemotherapeutic management. Usually, it is the cancer itself that initiates and contributes most to the syndrome, which has been observed in one third to two thirds of clients with various cancers, and which is managed only by surgical, radiotherapeutic, or chemotherapeutic cure or control of the disease. However, prevention or control of the complications of cancer—and of the complications of the treatment regimens—may arrest or delay the development of the cachexia syndrome.

Systemic Effects of Cancer. The etiology of the gradual tissue wasting that occurs as a systemic response to cancer in a significant number of clients is unknown. However, it has been hypothesized that the tumor produces small metabolites, such as peptides and oligonucleotides, that result in chaotic metabolic reactions and may be responsible for such components of the cachexia syndrome as anorexia and mobilization of body fat. The components of the systemic response to cancer that contribute to cachexia are described below.

Weight Loss. The weight loss does not correlate with the type or duration of the cancer nor with the degree of metastasis. Moreover, weight loss can be observed even with a small tumor and occasionally in the presence of adequate food intake. An early clue to weight loss in a client is finding that clothing fits more loosely or having to tighten one's belt. While the cause of weight loss is not completely clear, it is associated with a loss of the appetite control mechanism, a decreased dietary intake, an increase in the metabolic rate, and loss of body protein

and fat. Decrease in dietary intake alone does not entirely account for the progressive weight loss. Even with forced feeding and use of total parenteral nutrition, the wasting may be only temporarily reversed.

A decrease in dietary intake may occur because of anorexia, early satiety, and alterations in the taste and odor of food, with the development of food aversions. Anorexia and weight loss may be one of the presenting symptoms that leads the client to seek medical help. Anorexia is most commonly manifest and noticeable in clients with cancer of the alimentary tract and in those with widely disseminated disease. However, nurses may see profound anorexia in clients with relatively small tumors. The cause of the anorexia is uncertain. It has been proposed that metabolites produced by the tumor may exert a direct effect on the hypothalamic and other central nervous system sensor and receptor cells and may also exert a peripheral effect on neuroendocrine cells and neuroreceptors. Observe for other factors, such as emotional and psychologic stresses, and mechanical problems, such as pain, nausea, and dry mouth, that may be contributing to anorexia. Sometimes mistaken for anorexia is a conditional aversion to eating because of pain or nausea associated with eating. This aversion may persist even after the causative factor has been removed or alleviated. Unless anorexia is associated with such factors as medications or other therapy, the degree of appetite may aid in judging the activity of the tumor, i.e., a decrease in tumor activity may be associated with an increase in appetite, and vice versa.

Observe for early satiety leading to decreased food intake that occurs in a significant number of cancer clients. The client may feel hungry at the beginning of a meal, but there is a feeling of fullness after only a small quantity is consumed. Changes in eating behavior (anorexia or early satiety) increase in incidence and degree with progression of cancer.

Sensory abnormalities, i.e., alterations in the taste or odor of food, may occur, and clients may complain that food "doesn't taste right." Sweet foods may taste excessively sweet to some clients with cancer, although some studies have shown that there is an elevated threshold for the sweet taste and a lowered threshold for the bitter taste in some clients with cancer. Check with clients to determine the liking for meat, since there is often an aversion to meat that may produce a bitter or rotten taste. Alterations have been noted in taste for sour and salt. Taste abnormalities appear to increase with the extent of the disease, and they may be one of the determinants of the anorexia associated with the malignancy. However, not all findings of studies on taste abnormalities are consistent, and taste sensations may range from normal to abnormal even in those with disseminated disease. It has been suggested that differences in sex, type of cancer, extent of the disease, and smoking habits may account for the different findings. Assess for nutrient deficiency. Deficiency of vitamin A, thiamine, zinc, copper, magnesium, or nickel may be associated with taste abnormalities. Taste abnormalities may be reversed with vigorous nutritional therapy, and reduction in tumor size by therapy also tends to return taste acuity to normal. Provide supplements if nutritional deficiencies are found.

Alteration in Carbohydrate, Protein, Fat, and Energy Metabolism. The metabolic rate of the tumor itself is significantly increased, although in general the overall metabolic rate of the host may be normal or only slightly increased. However, appetite control mechanisms do not function properly, and voluntary intake of food fails to meet the demands of both the host and the growing tumor.

Although it remains unclear if mechanisms involved in the production, trapping, and use of energy are altered in cancer, it appears that gluconeogenesis (from lactic acid produced by the tumor and muscle tissue) is an important mechanism for maintaining the blood glucose level. Tumors have a high rate of anaerobic (occurring in the absence of oxygen) glycolysis, with production of lactic acid. It has been proposed that the increased rate or resynthesis of glucose from lactate results in an energy drain on host tissues. Another source of energy cost that has been suggested is an increased conversion of glucose to fat before being metabolized. Assess for insulin sensitivity; a greater proportion of cancer clients have a decreased sensitivity to insulin, with a glucose tolerance curve characteristic of diabetics, than do control subjects. Most cancer cells concentrate and incorporate nutrients, such as amino acids and glucose, better than normal cells and successfully compete with the host for nutrients.

A tumor is often referred to as a "nitrogen trap," drawing nitrogen from the host and successfully competing with the host for protein. Significant amounts of protein are lost, but the mechanism is unknown. Normal tissues are deprived of amino acids, and catabolic processes exceed metabolic processes, leading to a state of negative nitrogen balance. Normal cells frequently die because of unavailability of nutrients that have been used by the tumor, and the tumor may continually break down normal tissue for its use. Observe for depletion of muscle mass, especially skeletal muscle. Depletion of the muscle mass of the shoulder girdle, the intercoastal muscles, the diaphragm, and the abdominal wall lead to cachetic wasting. When edema is observed, it may be due to hypoalbuminemia, caused by decreased albumin synthesis by the liver (because of the disease or the associated malnutrition), or secondary to losses such as protein-losing enteropathy. A leakage of plasma proteins into the intestinal tract (protein-losing enteropathy) is common in some types of cancer and may be due to blockage of the lymphatic channels of the gastrointestinal tract by tumor cells. Body fat is mobilized,

and it is speculated that tumor cells may produce and secrete a lipid-mobilizing substance. If the client has edema, body weight may remain the same even though protein and fat have been lost.

Marked Weakness. Weakness is associated with progressive muscle loss. In some instances, the degree of weakness is out of proportion to the degree of muscle atrophy. For example, marked weakness may be associated with loss of a large or a small amount of muscle.

Alterations in Vitamin, Mineral, Water, and Electrolyte Metabolism. The concentrations and metabolism of certain vitamins (e.g., folic acid, vitamin B_6, and vitamin B_{12}) may be altered in clients with certain cancers, and those with advanced cancer frequently develop vitamin deficiencies. However, the significance of these changes to the cachexia syndrome is not known. Iron metabolism is thought to be affected, and there are reduced levels of iron-containing enzymes and decreased hemoglobin synthesis and anemia. A normochromic, normocytic anemia, which does not respond to nutritional factors, is frequently associated with cancer. Iron deficiency also interferes with folic acid metabolism. Assess for nutritional deficiency as a cause of anemia; radiation and chemotherapy may also be contributing factors. Water retention (in both the intracellular and extracellular compartments) is seen in clients with advanced cancer, and this water retention may obscure actual weight loss. Although hyponatremia is the most common electrolyte abnormality seen with advancing cancer, abnormalities of other electrolytes and acid–base disturbances may occur secondary to the disease or its treatment.

Impaired Immunologic Competence. Both humoral and cell-mediated immunity are impaired, especially in those receiving radiotherapy or chemotherapy or in association with malnutrition, resulting in a decreased resistance to infection, which is the leading cause of death in cancer clients.

In the past, depressed immunity has frequently been attributed to the effects of cancer per se, although both malnutrition and the oncologic treatment (surgery, radiation, and chemotherapy) also lead to immunosuppression. Suspect depressed immunity even with as little as 5 to 10 lb of weight loss. Reestablish immunity by nutritional means. Appropriate support can restore immunocompetence to normal, as measured by several parameters, within approximately 2 weeks. Be aware that clients who are immunocompetent have an improved survival rate, fewer complications, and a better response to cancer therapy.

Localized Effects of Cancer. In addition to the systemic effects of cancer, there are a number of localized effects leading to malnutrition. Observe for the specific effects (which depend on the location of the tumor) summarized below.[12]

1. Impaired food intake secondary to gastrointestinal obstruction
2. Malabsorption associated with
   a. Deficiency of pancreatic enzymes or bile salts
   b. Infiltration of the small bowel by neoplasms, such as lymphoma or carcinoma
   c. Fistulous bypass of the small bowel with bacterial overgrowth into the colon
   d. Blind loop secondary to partial upper small bowel obstruction with resultant bacterial overgrowth, bile acid deconjugation, and vitamin B_{12} malabsorption
   e. Villous hypoplasia secondary to malnutrition
3. Protein-losing enteropathy (e.g., in gastrointestinal carcinoma, lymphoma, or with lymphatic obstruction) and loss of blood proteins via the gastrointestinal tract
4. Fluid and electrolyte imbalances associated with
   a. Persistent vomiting secondary to gastrointestinal obstruction or increased intracranial pressure
   b. Small bowel fluid losses from fistula
   c. Diarrhea associated with hormone-secreting tumors (e.g., carcinoid tumor of the intestine and bronchus, medullary carcinoma of the thyroid, gastrin-secreting pancreatic islet cell adenomas—Zollinger–Ellison syndrome—and villous adenoma of the colon)
   d. Hypercalcemia secondary to secretion of parathormone-like substances by a variety of tumors or secondary to bone destruction
   e. Hyperadrenalism secondary to excessive corticotropin or corticosteroid production by tumors (e.g., in bronchogenic tumors)
   f. Inappropriate secretion of antidiuretic hormone associated with certain tumors (e.g., in bronchogenic tumors)
5. Other problems associated with secretion of hormones by tumors—diabetes, ulcers, hypertension, or osteoporosis secondary to secretion of corticotropin or corticosteroids by certain tumors (e.g., lung tumors) and hypoglycemia secondary to hyperinsulinism as in adenomas of the islets of Langerhans of the pancreas

Reversal of the undesirable metabolic and nutritional changes secondary to systemic and localized effects of cancer for any significant period depends primarily upon eliminating, entirely or in part, the malignant lesion.

EFFECTS OF TREATMENT ON NUTRITIONAL STATUS

Assessment

The three major modalities of treatment—radiation, chemotherapy, and surgery—all have adverse effects, including a profound catabolic effect, on nutritional status.

Radiation Therapy. Radiation exerts its antineoplastic effect by disrupting mitosis, and actively dividing cells are most susceptible to the effects of radiation. Normal cells, as well as abnormal cells, in the treatment field are affected. The side effects of radiation therapy are related to the type and dosage of radiation used, the body area being irradiated, the size of the treatment field, and the status of the client. A variety of nutritional problems may arise—generalized effects include nausea, vomiting, and anorexia, and localized effects depend upon the site of irradiation, i.e., head and neck area, the mediastinum, or the abdomen or pelvic area. Any of the complications of radiation therapy may be intesified by associated therapy, such as chemotherapy. Radiation therapy is associated with a catabolic response, often greater, longer lasting, and from which recovery is slower than the catabolic response associated with surgery.

Radiation to the head and neck area may result in destruction of the taste buds, producing mouth blindness (loss of taste) and alteration in smell. Assess for other effects, such as inflammation and ulceration of the oral and pharyngeal mucosa (mucositis, stomatitis, and pharyngitis), damage to the salivary glands producing **xerostomia** (dry mouth), dental decay, and tooth loss, dysphagia secondary to xerostomia, mucositis, sore throat, or motor damage, osteoradionecrosis (bone loss) and trismus (inability to fully open the mouth—this condition is often seen with combined surgery and radiation).

Radiation to the mediastinal area produces a transient esophagitis with dysphagia. Observe that there may be delayed effects, such as fibrosis, stenosis, and esophageal stricture. Irradiation to the stomach can interfere with acid secretion, causing ulcer formation with secondary effects of anorexia and weight loss. Internal or external radiation to the abdominal or pelvic area leads to radiation enteritis, with both acute and chronic changes in intestinal function. The epithelium of the gastrointestinal tract is second only to the bone marrow in its sensitivity to radiation as well as to chemotherapeutic agents. Assess for such problems as mucositis, acute or chronic enteritis (involving both the small and large bowel), diarrhea, malabsorption, ileus, ulcer, fistula formation, endoarteritis (inflammation of inner coat of an artery) of the small blood vessels, stenosis, stricture formation, obstruction, ulceration

TABLE 35-2
POTENTIAL SIDE EFFECTS OF
RADIATION THERAPY

Body Area	Side Effects
Head and neck	Altered taste and smell
	Mucositis, stomatitis, pharyngitis
	Xerostomia
	Dental decay, tooth loss
	Dysphagia
	Sore throat
	Osteoradionecrosis
	Trismus
Mediastinum	Esophaghitis
	Esophageal fibrosis, stenosis, stricture
Abdomen and pelvis	Mucositis
	Acute and chronic enteritis
	Diarrhea, malabsorption
	Ileus
	Ulcer and fistula formation
	Endoarteritis
	Intestinal stenosis, stricture, obstruction, ulceration, perforation, hemorrhage, colic, constipation

or perforation, and hemorrhage. Colic and constipation may occur if there is intestinal motor damage. Acute changes in intestinal function usually disappear after therapy, but in a significant number of cases, chronic changes develop. Chronic changes—in which symptoms recur usually within 1 year, although they may be delayed for 10 years or more—appear when the radiation tolerance doses have been exceeded. Acute or chronic damage to the bladder mucosa may occur.

With total body irradiation that includes the bone marrow system, there are effects on the erythropoietic, granulopoietic, and thrombopoietic tissue. The overall effects depend on the amount of irradiation delivered and the amount of bone marrow affected. Other effects on the blood elements depend on the amount of injury to the blood vessels and the degree of hemorrhage involved. A summary of side effects of radiation therapy is given in Table 35-2.

Chemotherapy. A wide variety of chemotherapeutic agents is currently used for the treatment of neoplasms, and the number is constantly growing. Chemotherapeutic drugs produce numerous side effects that may lead to diminished oral food intake, fluid and electrolyte abnormalities, generalized weakness, and weight loss. Since many clients receive a combination of chemotherapy, radiation therapy, and surgery, they are thus subjected to combined insults to nutritional status.

Chemotherapeutic drugs are broadly classified as hormones, alkylating agents, antimetabolites, antibiotics, and alkaloids. Most of the chemotherapeutic agents in current use (except hormones) inhibit one or more key steps in the intermediary metabolism of cells. They unavoidably affect normal host cells as well as those of the target tissue. Rapidly dividing tissues, such as bone marrow and the epithelial cells of the gastrointestinal tract, are those most likely to be affected. New concepts in chemotherapy, involving multicombination, high-dose, cyclical (at 4 to 6 week intervals) administration, increase the effectiveness of drugs against malignant lesions. A drug-free interval is usually scheduled between courses to allow time for repair of normal tissue, resolution of side effects, and nutritional build-up.

In clients who receive corticosteroid hormones, observe for fluid and electrolyte imbalance (e.g., retention of sodium and loss of potassium), a negative nitrogen and calcium balance (leading to diminished growth in children), abnormally high blood sugar levels, and gastric bleeding and ulceration. These hormones also stimulate the appetite.

The side effects of the alkylating agents, antimetabolites, antibiotics, and alkaloids that affect nutrient intake are summarized in Table 35-3. Virtually all cause nausea and vomiting, and anorexia and mucosal ulceration (including such conditions as mucositis, cheilosis, glossitis, stomatitis, and esophagitis) are commonly seen. Many cause diarrhea, although some lead to constipation. Various other side effects, such as altered taste, fever, or hepatic dysfunction, may be noted with specific drugs. Anemia is a common complication of those chemotherapeutic agents that interfere with DNA synthesis.

Immunotherapy. Immunotherapy is being used in combination with radiation, surgery, or chemotherapy. This therapy assumes that there are characteristic antigens in or on tumor cells that distinguish them from normal host cells and that are capable of eliciting humoral and cell-mediated immune responses. The immunotherapy is directed toward manipulating these responses to reject tumors. Side effects of some types of immunotherapy include a flu-like syndrome of chills, fever, malaise, nausea, and body aches.

Surgical Procedures. Many of the surgical procedures used for cancer are the same as for other diseases and involve the same nutritional considerations. Catabolic effects of the surgical procedure itself and inadequate nutrient intake during the surgical period add to the overall catabolic state of the client. Table 35-4 provides a summary of nutritional problems to assess for secondary to some of the major surgical procedures performed for cancer and the diet considerations for managing the problems listed.

TABLE 35-3
SIDE EFFECTS OF COMMONLY USED ANTINEOPLASTIC AGENTS

Name of Drug	Category	Side Effects						Other Effects
		Oral Mucosal Ulceration or Inflammation	Anorexia	Nausea	Vomiting	Diarrhea	Constipation	
Actinomycin D	Antibiotic	+	+	+	+			Hepatic dysfunction
Asparaginase	Enzyme		+	+	+	+		Hepatic, pancreatic, renal, and CNS dysfunction
Bleomycin	Antibiotic	+	+	+	+			Fever, pulmonary toxicity
Busulfan	Alkylating agent		+	+	+			
Cyclophosphamide	Alkylating agent		+	+	+			Hemorrhagic cystitis
Cytarabine	Antimetabolite	+	+	+	+			
Daunorubicin	Antibiotic	+	+	+	+	+		Cardiac toxicity, fever
Doxorubicin	Antibiotic	+	+	+	+			Cardiac toxicity
5-Fluorouracil	Antimetabolite	+ +	+	+	+	+ +		
Hydroxyurea	Antimetabolite	+	+	+	+			Renal dysfunction
Melphalan	Alkylating agent			+	+			
6-Mercaptopurine	Antimetabolite	+	+	+	+	+ +		Fever, hepatic dysfunction
Methotrexate	Antimetabolite	+ +	+	+	+	+		Hepatic dysfunction
Mithramycin	Antibiotic		+	+	+	+		Hepatic and renal dysfunction
Nitrogen mustard	Alkylating agent		+	+	+			Metallic taste, fever
Nitrosureas (BCNU, CCNU, MeCCNU)	Alkylating agents	+	+	+	+			Prolonged anorexia
Procarbazine	Miscellaneous (methylhydrazine)	+	+	+	+			Mental depression
Vinblastine	Vinca alkaloid		+	+	+		+	Areflexia
Vincristine	Vinca alkaloid			+	+		+	Areflexia

TABLE 35-4
NUTRITIONAL PROBLEMS ENCOUNTERED SECONDARY TO MAJOR SURGICAL PROCEDURES AND ASSOCIATED DIET CONSIDERATIONS

Surgical Procedure	Effect of Surgery that Alters Nutritional Status	Diet Considerations
Radical resection of the oropharyngeal area	Chewing and swallowing difficulties	Long-term dependence on tube feeding or liquid feedings of a thick consistency may be necessary
Esophagectomy (includes a bilateral vagotomy)	Effects that appear to be secondary to the vagotomy, including gastric stasis, hypoacidity with bacterial overgrowth in the upper small bowel, malabsorption with diarrhea and steatorrhea, fistula development or stenosis	Individualized to client need, e.g., a diet of liquid, soft, semisoft, or pureed consistency, tube feeding, or DFD[a] (see Chap. 21), small, frequent feedings, medium-chain triglycerides (for steatorrhea)
Gastrectomy	Problems are related to the extent of the resection and may include the dumping syndrome, hypoglycemia secondary to the dumping syndrome, intrinsic factor deficiency, afferent loop syndrome, malabsorption (acute and chronic) of fat, fat-soluble vitamins, vitamin B_{12}, iron, magnesium, and calcium, and reflux gastritis	To control the dumping syndrome: A ↑ protein, ↑ fat (especially MCT)[b], ↓ carbohydrate (especially sugars) diet is served in small, frequent feedings with avoidance of fluid with meals (fluid is offered between meals). The food must be eaten slowly and the client advised to recline after meals; with extensive resection, vitamin B_{12} injections are necessary; vitamin and mineral (especially iron) supplements may be necessary
Intestinal resection Jejunum	Decreased absorption of all nutrients, except vitamin B_{12}. However, the ileum compensates by increasing its absorptive capacity	Individualized to client need, e.g., vitamin B_{12} injection if needed; fat restriction or substitution with MCT if bile salt losses result in diarrhea and steatorrhea; administration of cholestyramine to chelate bile salts; use of DFD or total parenteral nutrition (TPN) if malabsorption is severe; following enterostomy the diet gradually progresses to normal, eliminating only those foods not tolerated by the client; vitamin and mineral supplements as indicated (e.g., vitamin D and calcium)
Terminal ileum	Decreased absorption of vitamin B_{12}, bile salt losses leading to diarrhea and steatorrhea, hyperoxaluria leading to renal oxalate stones	
Massive bowel resection (a functional residual of less than 3 ft)	Malabsorption of life-threatening severity, metabolic acidosis, and gastric hypersecretion leading to diarrhea	
Ileostomy and colostomy	Complications of fluid and electrolyte balance in the early stages	
Pancreatectomy	Malabsorption and diabetes mellitus	For malabsorption: ↓ fat diet and pancreatic enzyme replacement; diabetic diet and insulin replacement for diabetes mellitus
Ureterosigmoidostomy	Hyperchloremic acidosis and potassium depletion (these complications occur with significantly less frequency with ileal conduit formation)	Fluid and electrolyte management

[a] Defined formula diets.
[b] Medium-chain triglycerides.
(Source: Adapted from Goodhart RS, Shils ME, eds: Modern Nutrition in Health and Disease, ed 6. Philadelphia, Lea & Febiger, 1980, pp 1182–1184.)

INTERVENTION

The malnutrition associated with cancer and its treatment places the client in jeopardy. Weight loss reflects protein–energy malnutrition, which is the most serious type of malnutrition affecting the cancer client. The individual who is deficient in protein and energy quickly succumbs to infections, heals wounds slowly, and so on. Kilocalories are equally important to protein, since with insufficient kilocalories, available protein is used for energy. The human body can tolerate only a limited amount of starvation before death occurs; therefore, prevention of weight loss should be a primary goal.

There are several potential advantages of a good nutritional status. These are:

1. A reversal of the catabolic state to an anabolic state
2. An increase in strength and an improved sense of well-being
3. An improved tolerance to therapy, e.g., the ability to tolerate surgery or a complete course of radiation therapy or chemotherapy involving larger doses over a shorter period

of time with a reduction in side effects and at least initially a more positive therapeutic response

4. An improved immune response necessary for combating tumor growth and secondary infections

In the past physicians were reluctant to force-feed cancer clients for fear that this would further stimulate tumor growth. Although the question is not totally clarified and differences of opinion remain, there is some convincing evidence that improved nutrition of the client will cause an increased rate of tumor growth. There is no evidence, however, that the tumor growth is disproportionate to the weight gain of the host. This growth is not necessarily undesirable, since newly formed cells are more responsive to radiation and cytotoxic agents. Malignant lesions are most sensitive to treatment when a large percentage of the cells are in the process of division. Provide nutritional support and appropriate antitumor therapy concurrently to obviate the possibility of further proliferation of the tumor. Many physicians are becoming more aggressive in providing nutritional support for those who are candidates for therapy.

Consider diet therapy as part of the nursing care plan during each of the three phases of treatment:

1. The period preceding treatment: Provide nutritional build-up to prevent complications; prevention is easier than rehabilitation. It may be necessary to delay aggressive therapy until appropriate nutritional support has been provided
2. The period during treatment: Provide supportive and symptomatic relief
3. The period following treatment: Provide nutritional build-up to reverse the damage

Effective nutritional support during each of these phases involves a team approach—doctor, nurse, dietitian–nutritionist, pharmacist, social worker, surgeon, and radiation therapist. The nursing care plan should be based on a careful assessment of the client's individual needs. With aggressive support, weight loss can be prevented. Those who fail to gain weight with aggressive support frequently have a poor response to therapy. In order to evaluate the effectiveness of intervention techniques, keep records not only of kilocaloric and protein intake but also of alterations in body weight.

Methods of Feeding

When the gastrointestinal tract functions, use either oral or tube feedings, since enteral alimentation is safer than parenteral feeding. If feeding via the gastrointestinal tract is contraindicated or unsuccessful or if rapid nutritional repletion is necessary in order for a client to be a candidate for treatment, give parenteral feeding. Total parenteral nutrition via a peripheral or central vein may be indicated.

First, consider oral feeding, since the food is tastier in this manner. Further, clients with cancer often object to tubes because of prior experience, sometimes associated with aspiration.

The type of oral feeding, which may be solid or liquid, will depend on the particular needs of the client. If a solid diet is used, it may be pureed, soft, semisoft, or low-residue and should be supplemented with beverages, such as milkshakes, eggnogs, or commercial liquid preparations. However, since commercially prepared formulas are flavored to appeal to normal taste, they may not be accepted by the client. Consider the client's taste preferences and provide flavorings, such as coffee or lemon juice. The choice of liquids may be the conventional clear or full liquid diets or nutritionally complete preparations, e.g., blenderized, liquefied conventional foods or commercial preparations, such as Ensure (Ross Labs), defined formula diets (DFD), or preparations containing medium-chain triglycerides. Use clear liquid diets for only a limited period, since they are nutritionally inadequate. In contrast, full liquid diets, if appropriately planned, can be more nutritionally adequate.

Long-term feeding by nasogastric tube may be undesirable because of the propensity to produce esophageal inflammation and esophageal strictures if large rubber or polyvinylchloride tubes are used. In addition, the client with cancer may be debilitated and have a poor cough reflex, and aspiration may thus be a problem. In general, Silastic or polyurethane tubes of a medium or fine bore may be tolerated. When these tubes are used, be sure that the feeding is in a finely dispersed form, such as a commercially prepared canned formula. Refer to Chapter 21 for a more detailed discussion of tube feeding, parenteral feeding, and special feeding formulas that are available.

Some clients with myelosuppression secondary to cancer therapy must be placed in a protected environment to reduce the risk of infection while the client's host defenses are impaired. The food, beverages, and trays entering the room must be sterile. Since nutrient losses may result from food sterilization procedures, recommend multivitamin preparations.

Specific modifications may be necessary to deal with anorexia, nausea and vomiting, oral problems, diarrhea, or constipation associated with the disease or its treatment. Some general considerations for nourishing the client are given below, along with specific tips for dealing with each of the above problems.

Client Education

Nurses should develop a close communication with the cancer client in the early stages of treatment to facilitate a working relationship should dietary complications of therapy arise. Obtain a nutritional history at the beginning of treatment in order to collect baseline data on food consumption and body weight, and monitor changes in nutritional status to serve as a basis for specific diet instructions. For psychologic reasons, it is of prime importance that the client consume as near normal foods as possible by the oral route. Allow the client to decide specific foods to be eaten and how they are to be seasoned. If possible, the client should be allowed to select the diet from the hospital menu. Should oral feeding be inadequate or contraindicated, initiate tube feeding or total parenteral nutrition early to prevent significant malnutrition.

Upon discharge from the hospital, provide follow-up counseling on an outpatient basis to assure that the program of nutritional therapy will not be neglected. Booklets for clients listed at the end of the chapter include tips for dealing with specific feeding problems, and some recipes are provided.

The health team must assist the client to understand the importance of nutrition as it relates to the course of the illness. Use simple, persuasive techniques to encourage eating even when the desire is lacking or when eating causes pain. Energy conservation becomes very important; assess the time of day when the energy level is highest and provide substantial meals at this time. It is not uncommon for clients to ingest the morning meal fairly well and to eat progressively less well at succeeding meals, although for some the best meal may be the evening meal. To conserve energy, encourage the use of convenience foods in home situations. Serve small meals at frequent intervals, e.g., six to eight times per day. Keep a high-calorie liquid supplement in a thermos or ice bath at the bedside (or suggest that the client keep one in the refrigerator at home), and encourage the client to sip it at intervals throughout the day. Offer foods of high-calorie density and those that are easy to digest.

Provide adequate mouth care, not only to improve the appetite but also to increase salivation, reduce dental problems, and numb the pain if oral lesions are present. Give attention to food preferences, taste alterations, service of food in its most palatable form, and maximum social interaction at mealtime. Recognize that there may be differences in response to food (such as degrees of anorexia and taste alterations) by clients with cancer, and each client will benefit from individualized care.

Some authors suggest that behavior modification techniques, e.g., giving rewards contingent upon weight gain, may be useful, whereas others feel that these techniques are not suitable for use with the physically ill. They may be useful, however, if there is a conditioned aversion to eating that persists after the causative factor has been removed or alleviated.

Assist the client to maintain a high fluid intake, especially if nausea, vomiting, or diarrhea is associated with the disease or its treatment. The presence of a secondary infection also increases fluid needs, as do chemotherapy and radiation therapy. For instance, some drugs produce fever, whereas others are toxic to the kidney or bladder. The excretion of the waste products of cell breakdown associated with radiation therapy or chemotherapy requires a high fluid intake.

Anorexia is controlled only by control of the disease process and disappears with curative or control measures. There are no drugs that are uniformly useful for dealing with this problem. Although some drugs used in cancer chemotherapy produce a transient increase in appetite (e.g., the adrenal steroids) others used as supportive therapy (e.g., sedatives and analgesics) may further reduce the appetite. In the presence of anorexia and taste alterations that occur secondary to the disease or in the presence of mouth blindness, highlight for the client other attributes of food, such as appearance, odor, texture, temperature, and seasonings. Suggest garnishes and seasonings that the client can experiment with. Unless the mouth is sore, provide foods that are more highly seasoned by use of herbs, spices, extra salt, or use of salty foods. Extra sugar, lemon, or other tart flavors may be helpful for those who report food to be tasteless. For example, cured meat, such as ham or cold cuts, may be tastier than other types of meat when the threshold for salt is elevated. Encourage the client to keep a record of responses to different food flavors. Acid foods, such as lemonade, or moderate amounts of wine with meals may stimulate the appetite. The greatest meat aversions are usually associated with beef and pork; fewer problems generally are noted with chicken and fish. Substitute milk, cheese, eggs, and vegetable sources of protein, including nuts and peanut butter, and legumes as sources of protein when meat is not well accepted. Serve protein-containing foods cold to make them more acceptable. For example, meat salads, meat sandwiches, deviled eggs, and cold plates of luncheon meat with cheese and cold fruits may be more acceptable than hot main dishes. Celery stuffed with cheese spreads or peanut butter, ice cream, milkshakes, gelatin, pudding, and custard may be acceptable snacks or desserts. The high-protein desserts may be more appealing when served with fresh fruit.

Nausea and vomiting are side effects of both radiation therapy and chemotherapy. However, the acute symptoms usually subside within 24 to 48 hours after treatment. Antiemetics (given one-half hour before meals) sometimes help to control the discomfort. For those who are prone to develop nausea during treatment, it may be best to avoid eating several hours prior to treatment. The smell of food may increase the discomfort, and if this is the case, do not deliver the meal tray (or suggest that the individual stay away from the kitchen while food is being prepared). Hot foods and their odors may aggravate nausea, and cold foods (such as cold meat or fruit plates, cottage cheese, icy cold drinks, flavored ices, or Jello) may be better tolerated. Overly sweet or greasy foods may increase discomfort, as may mixing hot and cold foods. In the absence of stomatitis, offer sour foods (such as sour pickles or lemon) or salty foods (such as broth and crackers) to aid in curbing nausea. Advise the client to drink liquids slowly and to lie down after meals, since activity can stimulate vomiting. A cold cloth applied to the head may be helpful. If the nausea is mild, foods that are acceptable to the client should be offered at times when he or she appears willing to accept them. Emphasize good nutrition during periods when drug or radiation reactions are not being experienced.

When the mouth or esophagus is sore in conjunction with chemotherapy or radiation, eliminate spicy and acid foods and serve a moist diet of smooth consistency. A combination of blended or pureed foods and liquids is usually preferred over a full liquid diet. Hot foods are not well tolerated, and foods served cold or at room temperature may be more acceptable. Try frozen foods, such as popsicles or ice cream, to numb the pain from the mouth ulceration, although in come cases frozen foods may be irritating. Rinsing the mouth with a local anesthetic (such as lidocaine) before meals may be of help. Clients sometimes request watermelon, grapes, and peeled cucumbers, all of which may aggravate oral lesions less than does apple or grape juice. Other measures that may require consideration when mucositis is severe are the restriction of smoking and alcohol consumption, removal of dentures, or use of a nutritionally complete liquid formula diet.

Exposure of the salivary glands to radiation produces a decrease in salivation. Not only is the volume of saliva decreased, but the quality changes to a tenacious, semiopaque substance of greater acidity than normal. The saliva reduction begins 1 to 2 weeks after radiation therapy is initiated and persists for a long period of time. The consequences of the scanty saliva are alteration in taste, difficulty in chewing, swallowing, and talking, and a tendency toward dental decay. The teeth, which are usually protected by the salivary flow, become covered with the sticky, tenacious saliva that provides an excellent substrate for bacterial growth.

Use the following measures to counteract the dry mouth: (1) provide sugarless gum or sugarless hard candy or lemon slices to increase salivation, (2) increase total fluid intake, (3) provide artificial saliva and saliva substitutes (the client can keep a plastic squeeze bottle for use throughout the day), and (4) serve a moist diet, i.e., increasing fluid intake with meals and moistening foods with sauces, milk, gravy, broth, butter, or salad dressing. Increase the air humidity of the room to provide some systemic relief.

A higher incidence of dental decay has long been recognized as a consequence of radiation therapy, and formerly it was customary to extract all of the client's teeth in the area to be treated to avoid the dental decay and other problems, such as osteoradionecrosis. This practice has been replaced by prophylactic dental care to prevent these complications. Prophylactic measures include a dental evaluation, daily fluoride treatments with a mouthwash or gel, brushing and flossing the teeth, and restriction of dietary sucrose. Because of the oral ulcerations and thickened oral secretions, good oral hygiene is essential to prevent bacterial or fungal infections. This can be achieved by teeth and gum brushing with a soft toothbrush, use of dental floss, and frequent irrigations with dilute hydrogen peroxide or salt and soda solutions. Commercial mouthwashes may cause a burning sensation and may upset the balance of the oral flora, leading to fungal infections.

Diarrhea and malabsorption may be a result of cancer localized in the gastrointestinal tract or may be secondary to chemotherapy or radiation of the abdominal or pelvic area or secondary to malnutrition. Treat the condition by administrating paragoric or an antidiarrheal drug and provide a diet restricted in residue. Sometimes exclusion of lactose from the diet halts the diarrhea. If the diarrhea persists, a defined formula diet may be ordered. A diet restricted in residue, fat, gluten, and lactose has been found effective in children who developed delayed radiation enteritis with small bowel obstruction. The children showed radiographic and histologic reversal of severe bowel damage coincident with the specific diet therapy alone. The rationale for the therapy is to limit gluten and lactose because of intestinal villous atrophy, to limit fat because of lymphatic dilatation, and to limit residue to prevent further mechanical irritation.

Constipation is not a frequent problem in individuals with cancer, but it can result from the use of certain drugs (Table 35–3). Avoid harsh laxatives and follow the dietary guidelines for treating constipation given in Chapter 27.

Nutritional Care for the Terminally Ill Client

Use a balanced judgment that gives consideration to comfort and dignity to guide the nutritional support of the terminally ill client. Do not force treatments that impose undue discomfort or interfere with family relationships.

USE OF SPECIFIC NUTRIENTS AS A FORM OF CANCER THERAPY

Studies are being conducted on the use of various diet manipulations as a mode of cancer therapy,[13] but as yet the inhibition of tumorgenesis by dietary means is a very complex and poorly understood phenomenon. Different malignancies have different growth characteristics and differing responses, and the effects change with the changing state of the disease. Further, dietary restriction or a specific deficiency leads to many changes in the body.

Manipulations that have been used include attempts to starve the tumor of its amino acid supply selectively, to create amino acid imbalances by providing excesses of some amino acids, and to alter the supply of various minerals or vitamins. It has been shown in studies with experimental animals that reducing the dietary intake of the amino acids, phenylalanine, valine, or isoleucine, reduces tumor growth without affecting host weight. In contrast, reducing the intake of tryptophan, threonine, leucine, and methionine inhibits both tumor growth and host weight, and lysine restriction affects neither tumor growth nor host weight. There have been a limited number of clinical trials in humans using diets low in phenylalanine and tyrosine, and the results are inconclusive.

Attempts have been made to deprive the tumor cells of amino acids by injecting enzymes that degrade specific amino acids. This mode of treatment carries the risk of antibody formation to the injected protein, however, and toxic responses have been noted in some instances. Enzymes that have been ▶ used include **asparaginase,** the enzyme that degrades asparagine, an amino acid that is an essential nutrient for some tumors although not considered ▶ an essential amino acid for humans, and **methioninase,** which degrades methionine. Asparaginase has been used to some extent in the treatment of acute lymphocytic leukemia, and methioninase may have some usefulness in humans, since methionine deficiency has been shown in some studies to reduce tumor growth.

Amino acid analogs have been tested as inhibitors of tumor growth, and some of these have been toxic. Other experimental uses of amino acid therapy involve creating an imbalance by adding excessive amounts of amino acids, such as phenylalanine and tyrosine.

The use of salts of minerals, such as platinum and gallium, is being investigated. Gallium nitrate has some antitumor effect, and platinum salts have been effective, especially in testicular and ovarian cancer.

▶ **Methotrexate,** a potent cytotoxic drug that is an antimetabolite of the B-vitamin folic acid, rapidly depletes folic acid supplies, leads to failure of cell replication, and results in significant inhibition of the growth of certain tumors. This compound is important in the treatment of acute leukemias and metastatic choriocarcinoma. Antimetabolites are more effective against rapidly growing cells. Thus the addition of specific nutrients to augment the growth rate of malignant cells may be useful in situations where tumor growth has reached a plateau, presumably because of nutritional deficiency. The provision of adequate nutrients can thus lead to improved activity of the antimetabolite.

▶ **Laetrile** (amygdalin) is a cyanide-containing compound found in the pits of apricots, peaches, plums, bitter almonds, and other plant products. It has been incorrectly called a vitamin (vitamin B_{17}) and promoted both as a preventive and a therapeutic agent in cancer. However, the compound has been studied extensively, and there is no evidence that it performs either a vitamin function or a role in the prevention or treatment of cancer.[14] There have been reports of cyanide poisoning among Laetrile users, including the accidental death of a child who ingested from one to five tablets. An additional hazard is that it may prevent the cancer client who uses it from receiving proven therapy until the chance of effective treatment is past. The interstate shipment of Laetrile in the United States for the treatment of cancer in humans is illegal. Although there is no evidence that Laetrile is effective against cancer in animals or humans or that it is useful for any purpose, a number of states have legalized its use.

REVIEW QUESTIONS AND ACTIVITIES

1. List two mechanisms whereby foods and nutrients may be involved in the etiology of cancer.
2. Discuss the possible role of food additives, environmental contaminants, and naturally occurring toxic substances in food in the etiology of cancer.
3. Identify the possible role of an imbalanced intake of each of the following nutrient factors in the etiology of cancer: (a) vitamin A, (b) iron, (c) iodine, (d) fiber, (e) alcohol, (f) kilocalories, (g) fat.
4. Discuss the etiology of breast cancer and colon cancer as it relates to the diet.
5. Describe possible inhibitors of cancer that are present in foods.
6. Discuss the use of amino acids and vitamin antagonists as specific forms of therapy in the treatment of cancer.
7. List three mechanisms whereby cancer may negatively affect nutritional status.
8. Describe the mechanisms that may lead to weight loss in cancer clients.
9. Identify the relationship between nutritional status, cancer therapy, and immunity in cancer clients.
10. Describe four potential advantages of good nutritional status in cancer clients.
11. Identify the effects of radiation therapy administered to the following body sites: (a) head and neck, (b) mediastinum, and (c) abdominal and pelvic region.
12. List four side effects that may occur secondary to the use of the common chemotherapeutic agents.
13. Identify two overall effects of surgery on nutritional status.
14. Identify interventions that may be useful in assisting cancer clients to meet their nutritional needs in the presence of each of the following problems: (a) anorexia, (b) nausea and vomiting, (c) sore mouth and esophagus, (d) dry mouth, and (e) diarrhea.

15. *Case study:* Your client is 8-year-old Mary, who was admitted to the hospital with symptoms that included a persistent fever, anorexia, weight loss, bruising tendencies, and bone and joint pain. Laboratory results revealed anemia; bone marrow results were consistent with a diagnosis of acute lymphoblastic leukemia. Chemotherapy was begun using the drugs prednisone, asparaginase, and vincristine. Normal weight for a child of Mary's age and height is 28 kg, height is 132 cm.

a. Identify systemic effects of cancer that may be contributing to Mary's anorexia and weight loss.

b. What recommendations would you make to encourage Mary to increase her food intake?

c. Calculate the RDA for protein and energy for a healthy child of Mary's age and height. What adjustments would you make in the intake of protein and energy in Mary's case?

d. What side effects of the medications would you anticipate?

e. What dietary manipulations would you suggest to counter the side effects of the medications?

f. Plan a day's menu for Mary taking into account both her nutritional requirements and the side effects of the disease and its treatment.

REFERENCES

1. Lyon JL, Gardner JW, West DW: Cancer risk and life style: Cancer among Mormons from 1967–1975. In J Cairns, JL Lyon, M Skolnick, eds: Cancer Incidence in Defined Populations. Banbury Report 4, Cold Spring Harbor, NY, Cold Spring Harbor Laboratory, 1980, pp 3–27.
2. Phillips RL, Kuzma JW, Beeson WL, Lotz T: Influences of selection versus lifestyle on risk of fatal cancer and cardiovascular disease among Seventh-Day Adventists. Am J Epidemiol 112:296, 1980.
3. Committee on Diet, Nutrition, and Cancer, National Research Council: Diet, Nutrition, and Cancer. Washington, DC, National Academy Press, 1982, pp 1–14.
4. Howe GR, Burch JD, Miller AB, et al.: Artificial sweeteners and human bladder cancer. Lancet 2:578, 1977.
5. Howe GR, Burch JD, Miller AB, et al.: Tobacco use, occupation, coffee, various nutrients, and bladder cancer. J Natl Cancer Inst 64:701, 1980.
6. MacMahon BS, Yen S, Trichopoulos D, et al.: Coffee and cancer of the pancreas. N Eng J Med 304:630, 1981.
7. Oace SM: Diet and cancer. J Nutr Educ 10:106, 1978.
8. Malhotra SL: Dietary factors in a study of colon cancer from Cancer Registry with special reference to the role of saliva, milk and fermented milk products and vegetable fibre. Med Hypotheses 3:122, 1977.
9. Wynder EL: The dietary environment and cancer. J Am Diet Assoc 71:385, 1977.
10. Hennekens CH, Lipnick RJ, Mayrent SL, Willett W: Vitamin A and risk of cancer. J Nutr Educ 14:135, 1982.
11. Wattenberg LW, Loub WD: Inhibition of polycyclic hydrocarbon-induced neoplasia by naturally occurring indoles. Cancer Res 38:1410, 1978.
12. Shils ME: Nutrition and neoplasia. In RS Goodhart, ME Shils, eds: Modern Nutrition in Health and Disease, ed 6. Philadelphia, Lea & Febiger, 1980, p 1176.
13. Bertino JR: Nutrients, vitamins, and minerals as therapy. Nutr Today 13:28, 1978.
14. Young VR, Newberne PM: Vitamins and cancer prevention—Issues and dilemmas. Cancer 47:1235, 1981.

BIBLIOGRAPHY

Ames BN: Dietary carcinogens, oxygen radicals and degenerative disease. Science 221:1256, 1983.
Darbinian JA: Parenteral nutrition in cancer therapy: A useful adjunct? J Am Diet Assoc 82:493, 1983.
Jeeranadam M, Horwitz GD, Lowry SF, Breenan MF: Cancer cachexia and protein metabolism. Lancet 1:1423, 1984.
Larsen GL: Rehabilitation for the patient with head and neck cancer. Am J Nurs 81:119, 1981.
Markley EJ, Mattes-Kulig DA, Henkin RI: A classification of dysgeusia. J Am Diet Assoc 83:578, 1983.
Morrison AS, Buring JE: Artificial sweeteners and cancer of the lower urinary tract. N Engl J Med 302:537, 1980.
Nielson SS, Theologides A, Vickers ZM: Influence of food odors on food aversions and preferences in patients with cancer. Am J Clin Nutr 33:2253, 1980.
Pizzo PA, Purvis DS, Waters C: Microbiological evaluation of food items. J Am Diet Assoc 81:272, 1982.
Proceedings of the American Cancer Society and National Cancer Institute National Conference on Nutrition in Cancer. Cancer 45(5)[Suppl] 1979.
Rivers JM, Collins KK: Planning meals that lower cancer risk. Washington, DC, American Institute of Cancer Research, 1984.
Shils ME: How to nourish the cancer patient. Nutr Today 16:4, 1981.
Snowden DD, Phillips RL: Coffee consumption and risk of fatal cancers. Am J Pub Health 74:820, 1984.
Trant AS, Serin J, Douglas HO: Is taste related to anorexia in cancer patients? Am J Clin Nutr 36:45, 1982.
Vitamin A and cancer. Lancet 2:325, 1984.
Welch D: Nutritional consequences of carcinogenesis and radiation therapy. J Am Diet Assoc 78:467, 1981.

CLIENT RESOURCES

A Guide to Proper Nutrition for the Patient Undergoing Cancer Therapy. Evansville, Ill, Mead Johnson & Co, 1974.

Aker S, Lenssen P: A Guide to Good Nutrition During and After Chemotherapy and Radiation, ed 2. Seattle, Wash, Fred Hutchison Cancer Research Center, 1979.

American Cancer Society: Nutrition for Patients Receiving Chemotherapy and Radiation Treatment. New York, 1974.

Bukoff M, Carlson S, Cleland B, et al.: Nutrition Guidance for the Cancer Patient. Iowa City, University of Iowa Press, 1981.

Mouth Care Instructions for the Chemotherapy Patient. Columbus, Ohio, Ross Labs, 1981.

Nutrition, A Helpful Ally in Cancer Therapy. Columbus, Ohio, Ross Labs, 1978.

Sherman M: Feeding the Sick Child. U.S. DHEW, NIH Publication No. 79–795, Bethesda, Md, 1979.

U.S. DHEW: Diet and Nutrition, A Resource for Parents of Children with Cancer. NIH Publication No. 80–2038, Bethesda, Md, 1979.

U.S. DHHS: Eating Hints, Recipes and Tips for Better Nutrition During Cancer Treatment. Bethesda, Md, National Cancer Institute, 1980.

Cancer Information Clearinghouse. To request assistance or to submit information for cancer, contact:

Cancer Information Clearinghouse, Office of Cancer Communications, National Cancer Institute, 7910 Woodmont Avenue, Suite 1320, Bethesda, MD 20014.

CHAPTER 36

Nutrition and Alcoholism

Objectives

After completion of this chapter, the student will be able to:

1. Differentiate between primary and secondary malnutrition as they occur in alcoholic clients.

2. Compare and contrast the metabolism of alcohol in clients who drink occasionally and chronic alcoholics.

3. Distinguish between the clinical manifestations of Wernicke's and Korsakoff's syndromes and plan their dietary management.

4. Manage the diet of a chronic alcoholic client and adapt it for each of the following complications: (a) anemia, (b) cardiomyopathy, (c) intestinal malabsorption due to nutrient deficiency, and (d) nutritional amblyopia.

5. Assess the potentially positive benefits of moderate alcohol consumption.

Alcohol abuse is a health problem of considerable significance in American society because of the widespread use of alcohol and its multiple effects—physiologic, psychologic, economic, and social. Although reliable statistical data are not available on the prevalence of problem drinking, alcoholism is thought to affect approximately 10 percent of the adult drinking American population, or approximately 10 million Americans, and 15 to 20 percent of hospitalized clients are thought to suffer from chronic alcoholism. The disorder affects all socioeconomic groups, both sexes, and all professions. Also of concern is the trend toward increased consumption of alcohol by adolescents. Only about 5 percent of the alcoholic population falls into the stereotyped skid row classification.

There is a complex interaction between nutrition and alcohol that may result in malnutrition, and alcoholism remains one of the major causes of nutritional deficiency syndromes in the adult population of the United States. Moreover, alcoholism is a major cause of malnutrition among hospitalized clients. Yet, while the nutritional status of alcoholics is generally considered to be poor, severe symptoms of malnutrition affect only a small percentage. The spread of alcoholism to various socioeconomic classes, the greater availability of food, and the bread enrichment program are all considered to be related to the low incidence of overt nutritional deficiency states. However, with alcohol abuse, which is defined by some as consumption of an excess of 20 percent of daily kilocaloric intake as alcohol, comes the potential for developing such medical problems as hepatic, neurologic, gastrointestinal, and cardiac disease. Malnutrition may contribute to the development of these diseases, and diet modifications are often necessary in their treatment.

This chapter focuses on factors implicated in the etiology of alcoholism, the synergistic relationship between alcohol and malnutrition, the metabolism of alcohol and its effects on overall body metabolism, associated nutritional deficiency, and nutritional managment of the alcoholic.

ASSESSMENT

Factors Implicated in the Etiology of Alcoholism

The precise cause of alcoholism is not completely understood, but most authorities agree that alcoholism develops as a result of complex interactions among biologic, psychologic, and sociocultural factors. From a biologic perspective, it has been suggested that specific endocrine, biochemical, or nutritional factors—either hereditary or acquired—may be important in the development of a predisposition to the disease. Although many experts think that there may be important antecedent biologic differences between alcoholics and nonalcoholics, to date no physiologic cause for excessive alcohol consumption has been unequivocally established. Genetic factors may have implications to be sure. Observe for the familial incidence of the disease, but whether this characteristic is explained by an inherited physiologic predisposition or associated environmental influences is not yet clear. According to some, a genetic etiology appears more promising than it has in the past. One study points to a different metabolism of alcohol in children of alcoholics and in matched controls with no familial alcoholism.[1]

A number of different psychologic theories have been proposed to explain the etiology of alcoholism. Although certain personality traits or other psychologic factors may influence the onset and course of the illness, it has not been possible to pinpoint a specific personality type or a single area of unresolved conflict to explain alcoholism.

Assess for certain attitudes and customs surrounding drinking that seem to be important environmental determinants. For example, social and cultural factors that favor drinking increase the exposure of the population at risk of alcoholism. Cultural factors thought to encourage alcoholism include poorly agreed-upon norms for drinking as opposed to ritualized alcohol use, use of distilled spirits in contrast to beverages with a lower alcohol content, cultural conflict and moralization surrounding alcohol use, encouragement of drinking for its own sake rather than as an accompaniment of eating or other activity, acceptance of drunkenness as a tolerable (or admirable) state, and encouragement of alcohol use as a remedy for emotional distress.

Synergistic Relation Between Alcohol and Malnutrition

► **Alcohol,** also called ethyl alcohol or ethanol, is produced by the fermentation of glucose in the presence of enzymes from yeast and in the absence of oxygen.

It is at once a food, a drug, and a toxin. As a food, alcoholic beverages provide little nutritive value except kilocalories. However, beer and wine contain some carbohydrate and trace quantities of vitamins and minerals, and table wines provide some iron. In contrast, distilled spirits (i.e., whiskey, gin, vodka, and rum) provide only kilocalories from the alcohol per se. The kilocaloric value of alcohol and the alcohol content (i.e., weight per volume) of various alcoholic beverages are summarized below:

Kcal value of alcohol	7.1 kcal/g
Alcohol content	Beer—3.5 percent
	Wine—10–15 percent
	Distilled spirits (100 proof) —42 percent

Alcoholics may consume as much as 50 percent or more of kilocalories as alcohol. A pint of 80 proof whiskey represents 183 g of pure alcohol or 1300 kcal at normal efficiency. However, kilocalories derived from alcohol do not appear to be as efficient as those from other sources. Less weight gain has been observed with the addition of alcohol than with the addition of equivalent kilocalories from other sources. Several explanations have been proposed for this phenomenon, including: (1) chronic alcoholism may be associated with a hypermetabolic state, such as that seen in hyperthyroidism, and (2) one of the metabolic pathways for the oxidation of alcohol (the microsomal ethanol-oxidizing system), which is activated by high concentrations or prolonged exposure to alcohol, results in energy wastage through dissipation as heat rather than conserving chemical energy. For this reason, heavy drinkers may not gain weight; in fact, observe that they may lose weight. For the chronic alcoholic whose intake is large, kilocalories from alcohol may not fully count.

As a drug, alcohol acts as a generalized cell depressant, affecting all body organs, and alcohol is directly toxic to many body organs and tissues. The hepatic toxicity of alcohol has been most convincingly established. The toxic effects are due to alcohol itself, possibly acting on cell membranes, and to its first metabolite, acetaldehyde. Impairment occurs in many organs and tissues, and the body's ability to maintain homeostasis is therefore altered. For example, notice that wound healing is impaired, fractures heal more slowly, and there is a decreased resistance to infection.

The malnutrition associated with alcoholism may be primary or secondary. Primary malnutrition results from the displacement of nutrient-containing foods by the nutrient-deficient alcohol. The money required to purchase alcohol to maintain the habit may limit the amount of money available to purchase food. Secondary malnutrition results from the toxicity of alcohol on body organs (including the gastrointestinal organs) in combination with functional impairment of the gastrointestinal organs caused

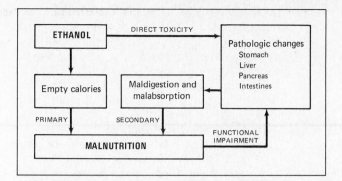

Figure 36–1
The synergistic relationship between alcohol and malnutrition.

by the primary malnutrition. Toxic effects on the gastrointestinal tract result in disturbances in digestion and absorption. The ensuing maldigestion and malabsorption potentiate a cycle of malnutrition. Through its effects on other organs, especially the liver, alcohol may alter the transport, activation, catabolism, use, and storage of nutrients. However, the synergistic relationship between alcohol and malnutrition (Fig. 36–1) remains to be fully clarified. When symptoms arise, they may be the result of the combined effects of alcohol and malnutrition.

Metabolism of Alcohol and Its Effects on Overall Body Metabolism

Alcohol, which requires no digestion, is absorbed by diffusion from both the stomach and small intestine, with the major absorption occurring in the small intestine. In the stomach, the rate of absorption depends on such factors as the presence or absence of food or a high or low concentration of alcohol. Soluble carbohydrate causes a greater delay in alcohol absorption than protein or fat.[2] The small intestine absorbs alcohol rapidly and completely, regardless of the presence of food. If the client's history indicates a gastrectomy, anticipate that the client will become intoxicated more quickly than others.

Being soluble in both water and fat, alcohol diffuses rapidly through all membranes and into cells and becomes distributed in the total body water. Its concentration in any one tissue parallels the water content of the tissue. In most localities, a blood alcohol concentration of 100 to 150 mg percent is evidence of excessive drinking, and the individual is in danger of respiratory arrest at 400 to 500 mg percent.

Alcohol is disposed of by metabolism and excretion. The liver is the main organ that metabolizes alcohol, and liver metabolism accounts for the disposal of approximately 90 percent of the amount ingested. Alcohol becomes the preferred fuel for the liver, displacing up to 90 percent of other energy-producing substances normally used by the liver.[3] Some alcohol is excreted by the lungs and kidneys, and the amount excreted is directly proportional

to the blood concentration. The breath test to determine driver intoxication is an example of a practical application of this fact.

In the liver, alcohol is oxidized to acetate, which is oxidized to carbon dioxide and water by the liver and peripheral tissue or follows other pathways of acetate metabolism. Liver oxidation of alcohol, which is shown in Figure 36–2, uses the enzyme alcohol dehydrogenase and the oxidized form of the niacin-containing coenzyme, NAD+. This reaction leads to the formation of acetaldehyde and the reduced form of NAD+ (NADH) and hydrogen ions. The NADH produced is oxidized back to NAD+ in the electron transport chain, with production of ATP. The excessive production of hydrogen resulting from generation of NADH and subsequent increase in the NADH:NAD+ ratio is thought to contribute to some of the important sequelae of alcohol metabolism, including a decrease in degradation and an increase in synthesis of fatty acids, resulting in the eventual deposition of fat in the liver. Moreover, the complete oxidation of alcohol uses not only niacin but other B-complex vitamins, such as thiamine and pantothenic acid, whose lack may help explain some of the neurologic complications sometimes seen in alcoholics. Whereas the alcohol dehydrogenase pathway of metabolism predominates at low ethanol concentrations, other pathways including the microsomal ethanol-oxidizing system are activated at high concentrations.

Liver metabolism proceeds at a slow, constant rate, leading to a linear fall in blood alcohol concentration that is a function of time. The limiting factor is the level of alcohol dehydrogenase available, which is limited only by the availability of NAD+.[4] The rate of metabolism varies widely in individuals and may range from 60 to 200 mg/kg of body weight/hour, with 100 mg/kg per hour being the usual rate. Thus approximately 4½ hours would be required

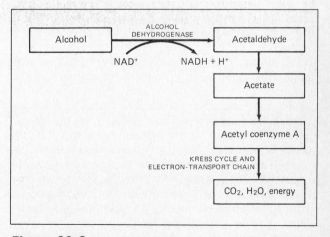

Figure 36–2
Liver oxidation of alcohol and release of acetate, which is oxidized by the tissues—similar to acetate derived from carbohydrate, protein, or fat.

for a 65 kg man to metabolize 30 g of alcohol. If the client's protein intake is low, the rate of alcohol metabolism will be reduced.

In clients who use alcohol on a chronic basis, metabolic tolerance may be evident. The rate of liver metabolism may increase by 30 to 50 percent by virtue of the development of the compensatory enzyme systems. Since these enzymes not only metabolize ethanol but also metabolize other substances, including some drugs, aromatic hydrocarbons, and other foreign substances, expect alcohol use and rate of clearance of those substances from the body to be related. Because of metabolic adaptation in chronic alcoholics, the clearance rate for these substances may be enhanced, and because of the associated drug tolerance, nurses may have to administer higher than normal doses of many drugs to achieve the desired effect. This may be the case with such drugs as barbiturates, anesthetics, phenothiazines, anticoagulants, and oral hypoglycemics. However, when the chronic alcoholic is drinking, expect drug metabolism to be inhibited and clearance delayed because of competition between ethanol and the drugs for metabolism by liver enzyme systems. For example, the sedative effect of barbiturates and anticonvulsants and the action of anticoagulants may be potentiated by alcohol ingestion. With prolonged drinking in susceptible clients, however, progressive liver injury may decrease the organ's ability to metabolize alcohol, drugs, and other toxic compounds.

Since the liver is the target organ of metabolism—for nutrients as well as for alcohol—many of the deleterious effects of alcohol abuse are concentrated in this organ. The metabolism of practically every nutrient is affected. Since ethanol alters nutrient storage, mobilization, activation, and metabolism, significant effects are noted in all body organs. The liver is the primary storage site for nutrients, such as iron and fat-soluble vitamins. Further, some vitamins, such as thiamine, pyridoxine, and vitamin D, are converted to metabolically active forms by the liver prior to use by the body. Each of these functions is compromised by excess alcohol consumption, particularly in those who develop liver damage.

Although maintenance of good nutritional status should theoretically provide protection against the toxic effect of alcohol on body organs, few body tissues are exempt from alcohol toxicity. An adequate nutrient intake will not prevent the metabolic changes resulting from alcohol toxicity, but be aware that malnutrition may potentiate these effects. Evaluate for the effects of acute or chronic alcohol use on the appetite, alterations in the metabolism of specific nutrients, and alterations in specific organ function as summarized below. Many of these effects may be potentiated by the synergistic effect between malnutrition and alcohol toxicity.

A. Altered appetite and food intake. Observe for appetite depression and reduction in food intake due to the drug effect of alcohol, gastritis associated with alcohol toxicity, nausea secondary to diminished gastric motility and delayed gastric emptying, and depressed consciousness in acute situations. Expect food tolerance in intoxicated clients to be similar to that of any acutely ill client and food intake to be erratic.

B. Altered nutrient metabolism
1. Carbohydrate. Gluconeogenesis is impaired. Observe for hypoglycemia in alcoholics whose food intake is severely restricted; if the client is diabetic and receiving insulin, severe hypoglycemia can lead to death. Conversely, chronic alcoholics may develop impaired glucose tolerance and hyperglycemia when alcohol is consumed in large doses in the nonfasting state.
2. Fat. Fatty acid oxidation is decreased, intestinal and hepatic synthesis of fat is increased, and there is mobilization of fat stores secondary to hormonal stimulation. Evaluate for deposition of fat in the liver (fatty liver), excretion of ketones, hypertriglyceridemia, and elevated levels of very low-density lipoprotein (VLDL) (see Chap. 29). Clients with type IV hyperlipoproteinemia may accentuate the hyperlipidemia by ingestion of even small amounts of alcohol.
3. Protein. Protein synthesis is impaired in all body cells (e.g., heart and skeletal muscle), and such rapidly dividing cells as blood cells may show pronounced impairment. Transport, uptake, and clearance of amino acids may also be altered; branched-chain amino acids may be increased.[2] Alcohol inhibits the synthesis of certain visceral proteins, such as albumin, transferrin, and complement. Observe for increased susceptibility to infection in alcoholics with complement deficiency. The effects of alcohol on protein synthesis may be potentiated by nutritional deficiency.
4. Water and electrolytes. The antidiuretic hormone is inhibited, causing a diuretic effect; as the blood alcohol concentration rises, observe for dehydration. When the blood alcohol concentration is stabilized or falling, however, the opposite is true. Because of the antidiuretic effect, evaluate for overhydration. Overhydration tends to be more common than dehydration. Acute alcohol intoxication may be accompanied by abnormal electrolyte balance. Study the results of laboratory tests to determine the state of fluid and electrolyte balance.

C. Altered gastrointestinal function

1. Stomach. The secretion of hydrochloric acid is increased, causing an increase in absorption of ferric iron; gastric emptying is delayed; the mucosal barrier is disrupted. Observe for nausea and anorexia and evaluate for acute gastritis and hemorrhage.

2. Liver. Liver metabolism is distorted, leading to liver injury, which may progress from a benign reversible stage (fatty liver) to an inflammatory necrotic stage (alcoholic hepatitis) and finally to advanced scarring (cirrhosis). Alcohol may produce cirrhosis without first producing alcoholic hepatitis, however. There are indications that even in the benign fatty liver stage, more severe lesions are developing. Evaluate for reduction in liver cell functioning in clients with alcoholic hepatitis, which in some cases may cause death. Not all alcoholics develop liver damage; this occurs in only about 20 percent of heavy drinkers. Although liver injury appears to be related to the duration and amount of alcohol consumed, genetic, immunologic, and nutritional factors may interact. With liver disease, a decrease in secretory function may lead to a bile salt deficiency; observe for malabsorption, steatorrhea, and weight loss. The incidence of gallstones is increased in alcoholic liver disease.

3. Pancreas. Toxic effects on the pancreas lead to a tendency to develop acute and chronic pancreatitis and pancreatic insufficiency; observe for malabsorption, steatorrhea, and weight loss with severe pancreatitis.

4. Small intestine. Erosions of the intestinal mucosa are induced, blocking the absorption of such nutrients as long-chain fatty acids, D-xylose, folic acid, vitamin B_{12}, thiamine, water, and salt. Even in the absence of gastrointestinal lesions, heavy alcohol use induces a deficiency of intestinal enzymes, including lactase, resulting in abdominal pain and diarrhea following milk ingestion. Concurrent malnutrition (especially of folate and, to a lesser extent, protein) and alterations in the bacterial flora may also contribute to malabsorption. Calcium absorption may be decreased secondary to decreased conversion of vitamin D_3 to 25-hydroxyvitamin D_3.

D. Altered urinary excretion. Urinary excretion of some nutrients (especially magnesium, calcium, and zinc) is increased, and the excretion of uric acid is decreased. Alcohol ingestion leads to an accumulation of lactic acid, which impairs uric acid excretion and may precipitate an acute attack of gout. Hyperuricemia may result from an increase in uric acid synthesis.[5] Deficiencies of calcium, with concomitant alteration in vitamin D metabolism, place the alcoholic at high risk for bone disorders, such as fractures, osteoporosis, osteomalacia, and bone necrosis.

E. Altered muscle function. Skeletal and heart muscle appears to be affected adversely by chronic alcohol consumption, malnutrition, or a combination of both, although alcohol appears to have a direct toxic effect on cardiac and skeletal muscle, independent of nutritional deficiency. Ethanol is a myocardial depressant, producing a reduction in myocardial contractility and cardiomyopathy (disorder of heart muscle), which may lead to congestive heart failure accompanied by a low cardiac output. Heart failure in the alcoholic may result from an associated thiamine deficiency (beriberi heart disease) in which the failure is accompanied by a high cardiac output. Magnesium deficiency may contribute to both types of cardiomyopathy.

Acute or chronic effects on skeletal muscle are also associated with alcohol ingestion. Acute myopathy (disease of muscle) produces painful muscle cramps, tenderness with diffuse muscle weakness, and myoglobinuria (excretion of myoglobin from muscle tissue in urine). With chronic myopathy, diffuse muscle wasting occurs, and there is a gradual onset of weakness.

F. Elevated blood pressure. Epidemiologic and clinical studies in several countries have shown an association between alcohol consumption and blood pressure, with some showing a progressive increase in blood pressure with increasing alcohol consumption. This association is independent of age, sex, relative body weight, serum cholesterol level, educational achievement, and social class. Complications of hypertension, especially cerebrovascular disease, also appear to be more common in heavy drinkers.[6] Obtain a detailed history of alcohol ingestion from hypertensive clients, especially when the condition does not respond to treatment.

G. Altered hematologic function

1. Evaluate for anemia and altered platelet and leukocyte function, which are common in alcoholics. The anemia may be associated with diminished intake, absorption, storage, conversion to active forms, or use of the nutrients most directly associated with blood cell formation—folic acid, vitamin B_{12}, pyridoxine, or iron. Alcohol appears to have a direct toxic action on the bone marrow. Folic acid deficiency is probably the most com-

mon cause of anemia among alcoholics. In addition to decreasing the absorption of folic acid, alcohol also appears to alter the hepatic metabolism of folic acid or inhibit the release of the vitamin from storage for use by the bone marrow in DNA synthesis. The anemia of folic acid deficiency (which is macrocytic) may occur even with an adequate dietary intake. Metabolic alterations in pyridoxine metabolism induced by acetaldehyde also contribute to anemia.

2. Iron deficiency anemia is relatively uncommon in alcoholics. If it is present, assess for a history of blood loss through the gastrointestinal tract, dietary extremes, or chronic infection. Actually the alcoholic has a propensity to develop increased stores of iron due to its increased absorption with elevated gastric acid secretion, the iron content of some wines, the inadvertent administration of some iron-containing vitamin preparations, and other factors.

3. Coagulation may be abnormal due to impaired synthesis of clotting factors secondary to liver injury, vitamin K deficiency, the toxic effect of alcohol on platelet production and function, or other factors.

H. Altered neurologic function. Acute and chronic abnormalities in the central, peripheral, or autonomic nervous system are associated with chronic alcohol abuse. Although the etiology (malnutrition vs alcohol toxicity) is clearer for some abnormalities than for others, for most a specific delineation has not been made. Deficiencies of the B vitamins (e.g., thiamine, riboflavin, and niacin) are commonly implicated in the neurologic manifestations of alcoholism, although recently the nutritional etiology of some of the disorders has been questioned. Protein intolerance in the alcoholic with cirrhosis accounts for acute manifestations under some circumstances. Many neurologic manifestations are nonspecific. They may be related to associated conditions (such as aging, diabetes mellitus, spinal cord tumors, and the like) as well as malnutrition or alcohol toxicity.

1. Acute neurologic manifestations
   a. Depression of the central nervous system—symptoms of acute intoxication.
   b. Development of dependence, physical tolerance and the acute withdrawal syndrome, delirium tremens, and convulsions in those physically dependent upon alcohol. Nutritional factors are felt to be unrelated to acute alcoholic intoxication and withdrawal. Al-

though magnesium deficiency has been associated with the acute withdrawal syndrome because of associated low serum magnesium in some clients with withdrawal illness, the low magnesium levels are thought to be a result (and not a cause) of the symptoms. During the withdrawal syndrome, there occurs an acute, temporary shift of magnesium in the fluid compartments. Dietary deficiency may also contribute to hypomagnesemia.

c. Hepatic encephalopathy. In clients with cirrhosis, toxic products of protein digestion in the intestine gain access to the systemic circulation by virtue of being shunted around the liver. Symptoms of encephalopathy ensue (see Chap. 28).

d. Wernicke's syndrome. This syndrome, in which symptoms may develop over a period of days or weeks, has a grave prognosis unless quickly diagnosed and treated. It is an acute manifestation of a deficiency of the B vitamin, thiamine, although there is no clear explanation for the finding that few thiamine-deficient clients develop Wernicke's encephalopathy in the absence of alcoholism. The hypothesis has been promoted that the syndrome is associated with an otherwise benign enzyme defect that may become deleterious when affected individuals are stressed, as by alcohol, or that the impact of alcohol on dietary kilocalories may be involved. The manifestations arise from acute diffuse bleeding into the central gray structures of the brain associated with thiamine deficiency. Observe for ocular muscle paralysis (inability to move the eyes laterally), nystagmus (jerky, cyclical movements of the eyeball), ataxia (uncoordinated gait), mental confusion, memory loss, and coma leading to death. The mental confusion may persist and contribute to Korsakoff's psychosis, a chronic condition. The association between the two disorders has led to their classification as one syndrome: Wernicke–Korsakoff syndrome. The relationship between thiamine deficiency and Korsakoff's psychosis is less clearly delineated than for the Wernicke's syndrome.

2. Chronic neurologic manifestations
   a. Organic brain syndromes
      (1) Korsakoff's syndrome. This syndrome, characterized by intellectual impairment, disorientation,

loss of recent memory, and fabricated stories, may follow an episode of acute, temporary clouding of consciousness (as in Wernicke's syndrome), or it may arise insidiously. The etiology is not clear and may result from combined effects of alcohol toxicity, nutritional deficiencies, or associated diseases not uncommon in the alcoholic population.

(2) Dementia. The condition is characterized by a decline in intellectual function (including the ability to solve problems that involve the acquisition, storage, and retrieval of information) and adequate attention. Dementia is often associated with aging, presumably due to loss of nerves that do not regenerate. Severe alcoholism may accentuate the neuronal loss that accompanies aging. However, a functional decline in the surviving neurons has not been discounted. Associated nutritional deficiency may contribute to dementia. For example, a B vitamin deficiency (niacin in particular) leading to pellagra may contribute to the disorder. The incidence of chronic brain syndromes in alcoholics appears to be increasing.

b. Other neurologic manifestations

(1) Peripheral polyneuropathy. In polyneuropathy, abnormalities of sensory, motor, and autonomic nerve functions may be evident. Clinical symptoms, which are usually progressive, include the symmetrical involvement of nerves, beginning in the lower extremities. Assess for symptoms of sensory nerve involvement that include tingling sensations in the extremities, pain, numbness, and increased sensitivity to pressure. Motor nerve involvement is evidenced by weakness, muscle wasting, foot drop, and ataxia. Reflexes are impaired (e.g., tendon reflexes are depressed), as are vibratory and position sense. Visual impairment and weakness of eye, facial, and throat muscles occur with cranial involvement in extreme cases. Evidence of autonomic nerve involvement includes a persistent low blood pressure, incontinence (from paralysis of uretheral and rectal sphincters), and hoarseness and a weak voice from vocal cord involvement. Although polyneuropathy in an alcoholic client may have its etiology in diseases unrelated to the alcoholism, nutritional deficiency and alcohol toxicity may be implicated. Deficiencies of the B vitamins, particularly thiamine and pyridoxine, have been strongly implicated.

(2) Nutritional amblyopia. This disorder, which may complicate all forms of malnutrition is associated with blurred vision, photophobia, retrobulbar (behind the eyeballs) pain, and central or paracentral scotomata (islandlike gaps in the visual field).

(3) Rare conditions of unknown etiology. On rare occasions, degeneration of certain well-defined areas of the brain, such as the cerebellum, central pons, or corpus callosum, occurs. The role of malnutrition or alcohol toxicity in the conditions remains speculative. However, administration of thiamine has resulted in a positive response in cerebellar degeneration.

I. Carcinogenesis. Epidemiologic data support an association of alcoholism with cancers of the head, neck, esophagus, liver, and colon (see Chap. 35). Further, the induction of microsomal enzymes (which are known to activate a variety of procarcinogens) by alcohol ingestion may lead to an increased conversion of procarcinogens to carcinogens. The possibility exists that carcinogenesis may be influenced by the nutritional consequences of alcoholism, and the respective role of alcohol and associated nutritional deficiency in carcinogenesis is currently being studied.

J. Teratogenesis. Alcoholic women are at high risk of giving birth to infants with congenital malformations, mental deficiency, and growth retardation. The growth failure in these children occurs both prenatally and postnatally, and catch-up growth does not occur (see Chap. 14).

Nutritional Deficiencies Associated with Alcoholism

Nutritional deficiencies occur as a result of decreased food intake, altered absorption and use, and increased urinary excretion of nutrients. The alcoholic hospitalized client may not be readily identified because of the associated social stigma and other social considerations. Thus, when taking a diet history, question the client in a nonthreatening manner regarding alcohol consumption.

The extent of malnutrition in the alcoholic depends on the stage of progression of the disease and is influenced by the degree of drinking, the amount of food ingested while drinking, and dietary adequacy between drinking bouts. Alcoholic clients who eat an adequate diet when sober may store nutrients sufficient to prevent overt malnutrition when drinking.

Chronic alcoholics are likely to be severely malnourished, since many do not or cannot afford to eat. Even in those who do consume food, the interference with nutrient digestion, absorption, and use may nonetheless result in malnutrition. Assess for food preferences in alcoholics. Often there is a preference for high-carbohydrate, easy-to-prepare foods and snack foods. Weight loss may not be a problem in the early stages because of the kilocaloric value of the alcohol. In the later stages, energy wastage may result in weight loss.

Nutrient deficiencies to which alcoholics are most prone are those of protein, the B-complex vitamins (especially thiamine, riboflavin, niacin, pyridoxine, and folic acid), and minerals (especially potassium, calcium, zinc, and magnesium). Symptoms of vitamin A deficiency, such as impaired spermatogenesis, occur in alcoholics, but the relationship between alcoholism, serum vitamin A, and liver vitamin A is not known.[7]

INTERVENTION

Treat acute alcohol intoxication by infusing glucose, B-complex vitamins, and electrolytes, particularly sodium, potassium, and magnesium. When oral intake is possible, give high-calorie beverages, fruit juices, and sweetened soft drinks. As soon as it is feasible, gradually progress to a normal diet. Following detoxification, the client's appetite usually returns.

Correct nutritional deficiencies through use of supplements. Do not expect to offset the toxic effects of alcohol with diet, but do expect to prevent the additive affects of malnutrition and possibly some of the vitamin deficiency states, such as Wernicke's syndrome, with adequate nutrition. Prompt thiamine administration corrects the ocular muscle paralysis of Wernicke's syndrome, although the ataxia and confusion respond more slowly. The rapidity of response depends on the conversion of thiamine to its active form in the liver. Although some improvement occurs when thiamine is administered to clients with Korsakoff's psychosis, some of the damage may be irreversible. Beriberi heart disease also responds dramatically to thiamine administration, and concomitant administration of magnesium may be necessary. Since a positive response to the administration of B vitamins has been observed in clients with other neurologic manifestations, such as nutritional amblyopia, consider this therapy as a prudent intervention for clients with neurologic disorders secondary to alcoholism.

Stress the importance of abstaining from alcohol in addition to consuming an adequate diet, since some of the conditions, such as cardiomyopathy and the erosive effects on the intestine, respond to those approaches unless the condition is advanced.

Administer folic acid supplements to correct the anemia; it is sometimes necessary to supplement with vitamin B_6 as well. Do not administer iron supplements unless it is clear that anemia is complicated by a deficiency of iron—iron-free vitamin–mineral supplements should be considered. Correction of folic acid deficiency may alleviate the intestinal malabsorption unless the malabsorption is complicated by hepatic or pancreatic insufficiency. Provide vitamin A supplements with caution, since it is theoretically possible that even moderate doses may produce toxicity.

Encourage the client to maintain a high fluid intake to prevent uric acid stone formation.

Client Education

The basic goal of nutritional counseling for the alcoholic client is to prevent or correct nutritional deficiencies. Give the client and family information about the components of the Basic Four Food Groups, meal planning, food selection, and food preparation (see Chap. 2).

Include information in counseling sessions about the toxic effects of alcohol on body organs and the interrelationships with specific nutrients. Although a moderate level of alcohol consumption may be safe in a number of individuals, a no-effect dose level has not been established clinically. Stress to the client that lesions can develop despite an adequate nutrient intake. In particular, stress the importance of consuming food on a regular basis to avoid the possibility of alcohol-induced hypoglycemia. Explain the interactions between alcohol and drugs, and outline the hazards of combining drugs and alcohol.

Inform women of childbearing age of the potential consequences of drinking during pregnancy, and provide intensive counseling for the alcoholic obstetric client. With regard to the fetal alcohol syndrome, no danger has been demonstrated from the daily consumption of less than 1 ounce of ethanol by pregnant women.[8] However, the best advice for pregnant and lactating women may be abstinence from alcohol. Be cautious of overstatement, however, to avoid unfounded guilt.

Provide counseling of a more specific nature for clients who have developed medical conditions as a consequence of alcoholism. Refer to Chapter 28 for interventions for clients with fatty liver, alcoholic hepatitis, cirrhosis, and pancreatitis and to Chapter 26 for the dietary management of gastritis. Provide nutrition counseling in the follow-up care of the alcoholic. For those at a high risk of returning to heavy drinking, stress simple dietary practices. Encourage them to eat at least one nutritious meal a day and to eat as many nutritious foods as possible between drinking episodes. Those clients who follow the nutritional recommendations made during a previous hospitalization are generally in a better state of health upon returning for subsequent treatment than they were on initial hospitalization.

POTENTIAL BENEFITS OF MODERATE ALCOHOL CONSUMPTION

Although continuous alcohol abuse has clearly been demonstrated to have deleterious effects on health, little is known about the long-term consequences of moderate consumption on a daily basis or infrequent episodes of heavy alcohol use. Current evidence suggests, however, that moderate consumption is not only safe but in some instances may be beneficial to the health and enjoyment of life for those whose lifestyles include alcohol use. Moderate alcohol consumption has been defined as 10 percent of the total kilocalorie allowance, or roughly two drinks per day for the average woman and three drinks per day for the average man.[9] Suggested benefits of moderate consumption of alcoholic beverages include these:[9]

1. Useful as an analgesic, sedative, and appetite stimulant for medical purposes.
2. Enhanced nutrient absorption and improved nutrient balance (calcium, phosphorus, magnesium, and zinc) by wine; the improved balance may result from the effects of nonalcoholic constituents of the wine.
3. Alcoholic beverages with a low sodium content, a high potassium content, and a favorable potassium:sodium ratio may enhance the flavor and appeal of sodium-restricted diets used to treat hypertension (unless contraindicated because of other medications and diagnosis); wine (unless treated with ion exchanged resins) and beer both have favorable potassium:sodium ratios, but beer may have more sodium than wine.
4. May improve glucose tolerance in clients with mild diabetes (to avoid hypoglycemia associated with fasting or adverse reactions in clients receiving sulfonyl compounds, the alcohol should be consumed in close proximity to meals).
5. May protect against coronary heart disease (when compared with abstinence or excessive consumption) by increasing high-density lipoprotein (HDL) (see Chap. 29).
6. May have social and psychologic benefits among geriatric and other adult clients in institutionalized settings and among older clients in community settings.

There are studies that show that people with moderate consumption patterns have lower mortality rates than either nondrinkers or heavy drinkers.[10] Since these studies, as well as others such

as those related to heart disease, have shortcomings, available evidence does not permit recommending alcohol as a preventive or intervention measure to promote health.

REVIEW QUESTIONS AND ACTIVITIES

1. Explain the rationale for describing alcohol as a food, a drug, and a toxin.
2. Describe the metabolic pathways involved in alcohol metabolism.
3. Describe the phenomenon of metabolic tolerance observed in chronic alcoholics.
4. Relate the rate of clearance of some drugs from the body to metabolic tolerance in chronic alcoholics and differentiate between the rate of clearance observed in acute vs chronic drinking.
5. List two metabolic factors that may explain the weight loss sometimes seen in individuals who consume a large percentage of kilocalories as alcohol on a chronic basis.
6. Describe the factors involved in primary and secondary malnutrition in chronic alcoholics.
7. List four factors that may lead to a decrease in appetite in alcoholics.
8. Identify the effects of excessive alcohol consumption on the metabolism of (a) carbohydrate, (b) protein, (c) fat, and (d) water.
9. Describe the damage that may occur in the gastrointestinal tract, heart, and muscles in association with chronic alcoholism.
10. Identify the relationship between alcohol consumption and neurologic disorders in chronic alcoholics.
11. Describe the symptoms of Wernicke's syndrome and Korsakoff's syndrome.
12. Explain the rationale for anemia in chronic alcoholics.
13. List the nutrient deficiencies to which alcoholics are particularly susceptible.
14. Describe the appropriate use of nutrient supplements in chronic alcoholics.
15. Identify six positive benefits that may potentially accrue from moderate alcohol use.

REFERENCES

1. Ethanol ingestion: Differences in blood acetaldehyde concentrations in relatives of alcoholics and controls. Science 203:54, 1979.
2. Eisenstein AB: Nutritional and metabolic effects of alcohol. J Am Diet Assoc 81:247, 1982.
3. Lieber CS: Alcohol, protein metabolism, and liver injury. Gastroenterology 79:373, 1980.
4. Boeker EA: Metabolism of alcohol. J Am Diet Assoc 76:550, 1980.
5. Faller J, Fox IH: Ethanol-induced hyperuricemia. Evidence for increased urate production by activation of

adenine nucleotide turnover. N Engl J Med 307:1598, 1982.

6. Larbi EB, Cooper RS, Stamler J: Alcohol and hypertension. Arch Intern Med 143:28, 1983.

7. Leo MA, Lieber CS: Hepatic vitamin A depletion in hepatic liver injury. N Engl J Med 307:597, 1982.

8. Rosett HL: Strategies for prevention of fetal alcohol effects. Obstet Gynecol 57:1, 1981.

9. McDonald J: Moderate use of alcoholic beverages and clinical nutrition. J Nutr Educ 14:58, 1982.

10. Kreitman N: The perils of abstention?" Br Med J 284:444, 1982.

BIBLIOGRAPHY

Alcohol and the enterohepatic circulation of folate. Nutr Rev 38:220, 1980.

Brodsley L: Avoiding a crisis: The assessment. Am J Nurs 82:1865, 1982.

Bunout D, Gattás V, Iturriaga H, et al.: Nutritional status of alcoholic patients: Its possible relationship to alcoholic liver damage. Am J Clin Nutr 38:469, 1983.

Cohn L: The hidden diagnosis. Am J Nurs 82:1822, 1982.

Deykin D, Janson JB, McMahon L: Ethanol potentiation of aspirin-induced prolongation of the bleeding time. N Engl J Med 306:852, 1982.

Eckardt MJ, Harford TC, Kaelber CT, et al.: Health hazards associated with alcohol consumption. JAMA 246:648, 1981.

Gordon T, Kannel WB: Drinking and its relation to smoking, blood pressure, blood lipids, and uric acid. Arch Intern Med 143:1366, 1983.

Hurt RD: Nutritional status of a group of alcoholics before and after admission to an alcoholic treatment unit. Am J Clin Nutr 34:386, 1981.

Immune response and host defense in alcoholics. Nutr Rev 38:206, 1980.

Lillien LJ, Huber AM, Rajala MM: Diet and ethanol intake during pregnancy. J Am Diet Assoc 81:252, 1982.

Roe DA: Nutritional concerns of the alcoholic. J Am Diet Assoc 78:17, 1981.

Visocan BJ: Nutritional management of alcoholism. J Am Diet Assoc 83:693, 1983.

Windham CT, Wyse BW, Hansen RG: Alcohol consumption and nutrient density of diets in the nationwide food consumption survey. J Am Diet Assoc 82:364, 1983.

Clearinghouse for Alcohol Information. A variety of information related to alcoholism may be obtained from: National Clearinghouse for Alcohol Information, P.O. Box 2345, Rockville, MD 20852.

CHAPTER 37

Nutrition and Musculoskeletal Disorders

Objectives

After completion of this chapter, the student will be able to:

1. Develop a nursing care plan for the nutritional management of a client during the acute and chronic stages of gout.

2. Compare and contrast rheumatoid arthritis and osteoarthritis in relation to clinical manifestations and dietary treatment.

3. Assess the relationship between nutritional factors in the etiology and management of periodontal disease.

4. Develop a nursing care plan for the nutritional management of a client with postmenopausal osteoporosis, and adjust the plan so that it is appropriate to use in preventive teaching related to this form of osteoporosis.

Diseases of the musculoskeletal system may affect nutritional status by altering dietary intake. For instance, food preparation and eating may be painful for clients with advanced gout, arthritis, or osteoporosis, and chewing may be difficult for clients with periodontal disease. Nutritional imbalances have been implicated in the etiology of osteoporosis, and dietary manipulations may be important in treatment of this disorder as well as gout. These disorders are discussed below, and more specific dietary interventions for clients with physical disabilities are included in Chapter 39.

GOUT

Assessment

▶ Gout is a disorder of **purine** (nitrogenous components of nucleic acids) metabolism with clinical manifestations that resemble arthritis. The condition has a familial tendency and occurs in stages. Observe for these clinical manifestations in affected clients:

1. Hyperuricemia (a serum uric acid level of 6 mg/100 ml in males and 5.5 mg/100 ml in females is considered hyperuricemia. On occasion, the level may be as high as 20 mg/100 ml)

2. Deposition of sodium urate crystals in soft and bony tissue, commonly in cartilage and bone and near or in joints, bursae, ligaments, and tendons; the deposits may be nodular ▶ (called **tophi**) or diffuse; the fingers, toes (often the big toes), knees, wrists, elbows, and the helix of the ear are involved; urate crystals may be deposited in the kidney

3. Recurrent attacks of acute gouty arthritis

4. Eventual degenerative and destructive changes in the joints

Gout is seen predominantly in males over the age of 35 and occasionally in postmenopausal women. Although it may occur at any age, its occurrence is rare before puberty in males and before menopause in females.

Uric acid is the normal end product of the catabolism of the purine bases, adenine and guanine, and

539

their metabolic intermediates, hypoxanthine and xanthine. Purines are constituents of all cells as structural elements of DNA and RNA. The metabolic pool of purines (and its end product, uric acid) arises from exogenous sources (the diet) and endogenous sources (body protein catabolism). In these conditions, the purine is in a preformed state. The liver also synthesizes purines from simple metabolites present in the metabolic pool, i.e., carbon and nitrogen compounds, such as glycine, carbon dioxide, and ammonia.

The hyperuricemia of gout may be due to overproduction or inadequate excretion of uric acid by the kidney. The cause may be primary or it may be secondary to other disease processes or to the use of medications that alter uric acid production or excretion. If the client's history includes starvation, alcoholism, diseases that impair renal excretion or lead to overproduction of uric acid, or the use of drugs that decrease uric acid excretion, gout may occur as a secondary phenomenon. In starvation (such as in fasting regimens used in treating obesity), ketoacids possibly compete with uric acid for renal tubular transport, and the accumulation of lactic acid in association with alcohol abuse inhibits uric acid excretion. Lead toxicity, toxemia of pregnancy, and chronic beryllium poisoning also cause lactic acidemia. With alcoholism, other possible causes of hyperuricemia are alcohol-induced hyperlipemia and ketogenesis and starvation-induced ketosis. The excretion of uric acid is impaired in chronic renal failure, whereas its production is accelerated in such conditions as leukemia, polycythemia, and psoriasis. Clients who take diuretics, such as the thiazides, acetazolamide (Diamox), furosemide (Lasix), and ethacrynic acid (Edecrin), may develop hyperuricemia as a side effect. The hyperuricemia is believed to occur secondary to shrinkage of extracellular fluid volume and nonspecific stimulation of proximal tubular reabsorption. Assess the client's dietary pattern. The ingestion of a high-fat diet also leads to diminished urinary uric acid excretion. Gout is a frequent complication of such chronic conditions as obesity, hypertension, and hypertriglyceridemia.

Clients with hyperuricemia are at a risk of developing uric acid stones in the urinary tract. Stone formation in some cases may be due to the secretion of a persistently acid urine due to a defect in ammonium excretion. Moreover, excessive excretion of uric acid appears to play a causal role in calcium oxalate stone formation (see Chap. 30).

Intervention

With the development of improved pharmacologic therapy, the need for the purine-restricted diet traditionally used in gout management has diminished. Nonetheless, certain nutritional principles remain important. Surgery may be a component of management in removal of bulky, draining tophi, particularly if they are impeding movement.

Drugs used to treat gout include those that block the formation of uric acid from its precursors (xanthine and hypoxanthine) and those that block urate absorption in the renal tubule and thus increase its excretion. Concurrent with the use of these drugs, advise the client to consume a minimum of 2 quarts of fluid daily with a volume sufficient to necessitate voiding at least once during the night to prevent the precipitation of xanthine and uric acid crystals in the kidney. It is essential that the client maintain an alkaline urine (with the use of alkalinizing agents, such as sodium bicarbonate) to prevent stone formation. Potassium supplements may be needed when sodium bicarbonate is used. Anti-inflammatory agents are used to relieve the joint pain of acute gouty arthritis.

Advise the client to follow a nutritionally balanced diet that is high in complex carbohydrates and moderate in protein (not to exceed 1 g/kg recommended body weight) and that avoids excessive amounts of fat. Complex carbohydrates tend to increase uric acid excretion. Fats, in contrast, lead to uric acid retention and can actually precipitate an acute gouty attack. Tell the client to avoid excessive amounts of fructose, however, since this sugar appears to increase uric acid production and excretion.[1] Although a high purine load can significantly elevate the serum urate level and a high protein intake may accelerate endogenous uric acid biosynthesis by increasing the availability of amino acids in the metabolic pool, drastic restriction of either protein or purine intake is of little value; this regimen decreases serum uric acid levels only slightly. Their restriction reduces only the exogenous sources of uric acid precursors, which accounts for less than half of the uric acid present in the blood. Rather than advise drastic purine restriction, tell the client to avoid foods extremely high in purine content, such as liver, sweetbreads, anchovies, sardines, shrimp, kidney, mackerel, and meat extracts (Table 37–1) in order to avoid any unnecessary metabolic stress on the body. This measure may be particularly important for clients being managed by drugs that increase uric acid excretion. Monitor the effectiveness of the dietary regimen by having the client keep a food diary for 3 or more days and assess the kilocalorie, protein, purine, and oxalate content of the diet and make adjustments as necessary.

There is some preliminary evidence that the individual purines, although closely related biochemically, are metabolized differently and produce different alterations in uric acid metabolism. These findings suggest that evaluation of individual purine components of food may provide better guidelines for recommending safe maximum purine levels in the human diet. For example, studies have shown that foods high in DNA-related purines have a lesser effect on the serum uric acid than those high in RNA content.[2,3] The investigators found that all purines except guanine and xanthine caused an eleva-

TABLE 37–1
PURINE CONTENT OF FOODS PER 100 G

Group 1 0–15 mg (Negligible)	Group 2 50–150 mg	Group 3 150 mg +
Vegetables and vegetable soups (except as noted in Group 2)	Meat, poultry, fish and seafood (except as noted in Group 3)	Organ meats
Fruits		Liver
Milk	Legumes	Kidney
Custard and puddings	Lentils	Sweetbreads
Ice cream	Dry peas	Brains
Rennet desserts	Dry beans	Heart
Cheese	Whole grain cereals	Fish
Eggs	Asparagus	Mussels
Cereal and cereal products (refined)	Cauliflower	Anchovies
	Mushrooms	Sardines
Butter and fats (in moderation)	Spinach	Fish roe
Sugars and sweets		Herring
Carbonated beverages		Shrimp
Chocolate		Mackerel
Coffee		Miscellaneous
Tea		Meat extracts
Gelatin desserts		Bouillon
Herbs		Consomme
Condiments		Gravies
Nuts		Mincemeat
		Yeast

tion in the uric acid level. Although a limited number of foods have been analyzed for their purine content, comprehensive tables are lacking, and it is not currently possible to take advantage of these findings.

When the client experiences an acute attack of gouty arthritis, it may be necessary to restrict purine intake temporarily to 100 to 150 mg/day and to provide protein in the form of cheese, milk, and eggs.

Although weight control is extremely important, stress to the client that drastic dieting or fasting should be avoided, since this may lead to an increase in the serum uric acid level. If the client consumes alcohol, stress that it should be used sparingly and diluted, as in highballs. Tell the client that the combined effects of alcohol and fasting are mutually potentiating. In the event of an acute illness that curtails food intake, urge the intake of high-carbohydrate foods to prevent starvation ketosis. Although coffee, tea, and chocolate contain methyl xanthines that are metabolized to methyl urates, these compounds are not deposited in the gouty tophi, and their intake need not be curtailed.

Provide appropriate dietary advice to control any associated disorders, such as hyperlipoproteinemia, obesity, or renal insufficiency.

ARTHRITIS

▶ The terms **arthritis** and **rheumatism** are applied to many diseases of the joints. Rheumatic disease is called "arthritis" when it attacks the joints, and diseases that involve the muscle tendons, ligaments, and bursae, are grouped under the term "rheumatism." In general, arthritis may be acute or chronic, and acute attacks can be of short duration but may recur and develop into a chronic condition. Moreover, arthritis may occur secondary to other diseases, such as ulcerative colitis or gout.

There are numerous forms of arthritis, but the two most common are rheumatoid arthritis and osteoarthritis. Differentiate between the incidence and etiology of these forms of arthritis. Of the two, osteoarthritis is more common but less damaging to tissues than is rheumatoid arthritis. Rheumatoid ar-
▶ thritis (also called **atrophic arthritis**) is three times more common in women than in men and usually has its onset between the ages of 25 and 50, although it can occur at any age. The peak age of onset of arthritis in children (juvenile arthritis) is in the preschool years. In juveniles the clinical course of the disease is variable, and many children recover completely within 1 to 2 years. The occurrence of
▶ osteoarthritis, sometimes referred to as **degenera-**
▶ **tive** or **hypertrophic arthritis,** is almost universal among older people, and its incidence increases with age.

The etiology of rheumatoid arthritis is unknown, and both autoimmunity and an infectious process have been implicated. A characteristic antibody, the rheumatoid factor, is usually present in the plasma. Osteoarthritis probably does not have a single cause but may follow repeated mechanical stress to the joints as a result of overweight, poor posture, injury, or unusual strain from one's occupation or recreation. Congenital and mechanical derangements of the joints may be contributing factors.

Rheumatoid Arthritis

▶ _Assessment._ Rheumatoid arthritis is a chronic, progressive, inflammatory disorder leading to inflammation and thickening of the synovial membrane of the joints. Observe its insidious onset; muscular stiffness develops first and is followed by pain, stiffness, and swelling of various joints—the latter frequently beginning with the small joints of the hands and feet. The swelling is a result of fluid accumulation in the lining membrane of the joints and inflammation of the surrounding tissues. Soreness and stiffness may be more severe upon first arising in the morning than later in the morning. After some years, the space between the joints may become bridged by bands of fibrous tissue that harden and cause the joints to fuse together. When this occurs, deformity and limited motion result.

The disorder is characterized by remissions and exacerbations. Even a client in an apparently complete remission is subject to a relapse. When the disease is in an active stage, assess for signs and symptoms including malaise and fatigue, poor appetite and weight loss, some degree of anemia, and sometimes fever. The anemia is due to a hemolytic process that is not amenable to iron therapy. Some authorities have observed a decrease in carbohydrate tolerance during the active stage of inflammation, although this finding is not universal.

Other characteristics of the disease process are negative nitrogen and calcium balances, muscle atrophy, and decalcification of bone. The observed lower serum albumin and elevated globulin may denote hypersensitivity, chronic inflammation, or malnutrition. Low levels of vitamin B$_6$ have been observed in clients with rheumatoid arthritis, and low levels of ascorbic acid in white blood cells are frequently seen. These changes may be associated with drug therapy. Because of the influence of the disease on the epiphyseal plate, growth disturbances are not uncommon in juvenile arthritics.

Assess the dietary intake of affected clients. There is evidence to indicate that the diets of arthritic clients are at least marginally inadequate in selected nutrients, some of which (vitamin E and zinc) may relate to immunologic events that may be important in perpetuating the disease.[4]

Intervention. Treatment of rheumatoid arthritis involves a combination of physical and emotional rest, physical therapy and corrective exercises, antiinflammatory and antirheumatic drugs, orthopedic surgery, and nutritional support. Encourage the client to remain as physically active as possible and to balance rest and exercise.

Although there are few well-controlled studies to demonstrate the effectiveness of dietary manipulation in treating the disorder, it is generally considered that there is no specific diet that will consistently be of benefit. There is some evidence that zinc supplements may be beneficial[5] and that large doses of vitamin E may be effective in decreasing the inflammation associated with the disease.[6] Affected clients are often the victims of quackery related to diet or nutritional supplements.

Instruct the client to follow a nutritionally adequate diet. Encourage an increase in the kilocalories and protein content of the diet until a good nutritional status is attained. Provide a multivitamin supplement, avoiding massive doses. Although oral iron supplements may assist in correction of the anemia, blood transfusions are usually necessary. Discourage quackery, including phony diets and devices, and explain the danger associated with taking large doses of vitamins, which are sometimes promoted for treatment. Since pain and stiffness may be greatest in the early morning and late in the day, plan for the largest meal at noon, with midmorning and mid-afternoon supplements. Adapt feeding methods to the client's ability and provide for independence in eating as much as possible. If adaptive equipment is needed for eating (see Chap. 39), provide training in its use. Give simple suggestions for accomplishing activities of daily living, such as food preparation, with a minimum of effort. In some cases, rearrangement of kitchen equipment will suffice, but in other instances, modification of the design of the kitchen may be necessary in order for the client to prepare food. Observe for side effects of drug therapy that may necessitate dietary modifications. For instance, a diet high in protein, calcium, and potassium, restriction of sodium, and possibly a diabetic diet may be needed when steroids are used on a prolonged basis. To counteract the gastrointestinal irritation associated with chronic aspirin ingestion, advise the client to take aspirin with food or antacids.

Monitor the rate of growth in children affected with the disorder. Supportive management is necessary in dealing with the food behavior arising from frustration and anxiety of children with arthritis. During acute phases of inflammation, food may serve as a means of asserting control.

Osteoarthritis

▶ _Assessment._ Osteoarthritis is a chronic, progressive, noninflammatory disorder characterized by degeneration of the articular cartilage and the formation of bony outgrowths (spurs) at the edges of the joint surfaces. The degenerative changes are particularly pronounced in joints exposed to major weightbearing trauma, i.e., the knees, hips, and spine. The terminal joints of the fingers and joints at the base of the thumb and big toe are also frequently involved. Enlargement of the last joint of the fingers occurs frequently, and although it is permanent, this type of enlargement seldom leads to disability. At times, osteoarthritis can be troublesome in the joints of the jaw and in the second row of finger joints.

Common symptoms manifested as the disease progresses are aches, pains, stiffness, and loss of mobility. Observe for the progressive occurrence of symptoms in affected clients. Pain, at first intermittent and aching in nature, occurs when certain joints, such as the fingers and those that bear the body's weight, are used. The pain is relieved by rest. As the disease progresses, movement in the affected joints becomes increasingly limited, at first by muscular spasm and later by the loss of joint cartilage and formation of bony outgrowths. Since activity may be curtailed, there is a tendency to become overweight, and this condition places additional stress on the weightbearing joints. In general, symptoms are confined to the affected parts. In this respect, osteoarthritis differs from rheumatoid arthritis, which is a systemic disease in which overall health is affected.

Intervention. The goals of treatment are similar to those for treating rheumatoid arthritis. In contrast to clients with rheumatoid arthritis who are often underweight, clients with osteoarthritis are often overweight, and the excess weight aggravates the condition by posing a burden for the weightbearing joints. Weight reduction may significantly relieve symptoms and prevent progressive degenerative changes. Since activity and mobility may be limited, however, weight reduction for these clients may be difficult. Use the education guidelines for weight reduction given in Chapter 23 to aid clients. Advise them to avoid crash diets and other forms of rapid weight reduction as they rarely result in sustained control of the overweight condition. Refer to the section on rheumatoid arthritis for the nutritional implications of drug therapy.

PERIODONTAL DISEASE

Assessment

▶ **Periodontal disease,** or **pyorrhea,** is a disease affecting the periodontal tissue—the gingiva (gums) and other supporting structures, including the periodontal ligament (located between the alveolar bone and teeth), the alveolar bone (which supports the teeth) and the cementum of the teeth roots. Suspect periodontal disease in clients who have gingivitis, with redness, swelling, occasional bleeding of the gums, and gum recession. In the absence of treatment, infection and toxins develop that invade and undermine the supporting periodontal tissue, causing periodontitis. As the disease progresses, teeth become loosened, and some or all may fall out or require extraction. In this event, nutrient intake may be adversely affected.

Although dental caries is the major cause of tooth loss in children, periodontal disease is the major cause of tooth loss in adults after the age of 35.

Although adults are more susceptible to periodontal disease, gingivitis is seen in approximately 80 percent of children by the age of 15 years. In a small percentage of clients, the disorder is seen in an advanced stage.

Unlike dental caries, which is closely associated with Western civilization and dietary sucrose intake, periodontal disease tends to be more prevalent in populations where poverty and malnutrition are extensive. As with dental caries, the etiology of periodontal disease is multifactorial. However, it appears to be predominantly inflammatory in origin and caused mainly by local irritating factors. Systemic and environmental factors may condition the susceptibility of the periodontal tissues to the disease.

The chief local irritant associated with periodontal disease appears to be dental plaque, which progresses to tartar or dental calculus. Dental plaque is a bacterial system composed of a sticky, colorless, nearly transparent film that is continuously formed on the teeth. It is composed of water, saliva, bacteria, bacterial toxins, and enzymes. Unless plaque is removed daily, it accumulates and eventually forms a hard deposit of calculus or tartar. If calculus is allowed to accumulate, the teeth, gums, and other supporting structures may become infected and eventually destroyed. Assess the status of oral hygiene in affected clients. Improper cleaning and poor oral hygiene with food impaction contribute to the problem. Tartar or calculus that cannot be brushed away tends to build up and requires professional removal. Other local irritating factors that may contribute to the initiation of periodontal disease are faulty restorations, malocclusion, and other chemical, mechanical, or thermal extremes.

Various systemic factors, such as age, nutritional and hormonal imbalances, and emotional and medical problems, may contribute to a lesser degree to the disease. Systemic conditions, such as diabetes mellitus, alterations in parathyroid secretion, estrogen imbalances, and hematologic disturbances, such as leukemia, may predispose the periodontal tissues to breakdown.

Much remains to be learned about the effect of nutrients on lesions of the oral mucosa and supporting structures of the teeth. However, food and nutrients may exert both local and systemic effects on the tooth-supporting structures and thus affect their resistance to breakdown. Assess the client's dietary pattern. Food composition and consistency appear to exert local effects. For example, foods that are soft in consistency and high in sucrose content may lead to an increase in the rate and amount of plaque formation. One theory on the action of sucrose in producing plaque is that this sugar is an excellent substrate for oral bacteria, which convert sucrose to dextran, a sticky material that makes plaque adhere to tooth surfaces. Although no longer considered "nature's toothbrush," there is some evidence that foods of a firm or fibrous consistency, such as raw fruits and vegetables, improve periodontal tissue integrity by stimulating salivary flow, which aids in the oral clearance of food debris. The chewing of firm foods aids in the maintenance of proper balance between alveolar bone resorption and new bone formation. The mechanical act of chewing can strengthen the periodontal ligament, increase the density of the alveolar bone, and may prevent atrophy and degneration of the oral tissue, hard and soft. Soft foods may disturb this balance and lead to atrophic changes. Further, selecting fibrous foods rather than soft, retentive, sweet foods may indirectly reduce plaque formation because there will be less sucrose available for conversion to substances that promote the accumulation of plaque and its adherence to the teeth.

The systemic effects of nutrients on periodontal disease are controversial. Although there is no evidence that gingivitis or periodontitis can be induced by nutritional imbalances alone, there is a relationship among nutrition, resistance to infection, and healing of the periodontium, as with other body tissues. For example, nutrient intake and nutritional status may affect the defense mechanisms of the gingival fluid, epithelial barrier, and saliva, although it is likely that nutrient imbalances may be secondary contributors or modifiers that alter the rate of development, severity, or progression of the disease.

The oral epithelial tissues and fluids play a protective role by virtue of their capacity to replace themselves rapidly, to act as a functional barrier to the passage of antigenic material (such as bacterial endotoxins and other metabolic by-products) from the surface to the underlying connective tissue, and to produce host defense factors, such as antibodies and other components of the immune system. The ability of the periodontal tissues to repair themselves is influenced by several factors, including the integrity of the inflammatory immune response, hormones, and an adequate supply of nutrients, particularly amino acids, vitamin C, vitamin A, vitamin D, riboflavin, folic acid, iron, and zinc. A breakdown of periodontal collagen has been observed in vitamin C deficiency, and various vitamin deficiency states can lead to gingival and periodontal alterations, resulting in an increased susceptibility to ulceration and secondary infection. A recent study provides the first concrete evidence that a subclinical vitamin C deficiency significantly influences susceptibility to periodontal disease.[7] In the study, vitamin C deficiency altered host defense mechanisms and permeability of the oral epithelial tissues.

The maintenance of normal calcium and phosphorus levels in the blood may have a bearing on the development of periodontal disease. The alveolar bone is susceptible to osteoporosis, and some researchers have postulated that alveolar bone resorption may be due to dietary calcium deficiency or phosphorus excess. A low ratio of calcium to phosphorus in the diet may produce secondary hyperparathyroidism, leading to mobilization of calcium from the alveolar bone. However, this theory has not been proved. Although no direct cause–effect relationship has been established between a low calcium intake or an altered calcium:phosphorus ratio and periodontal disease, it is possible that the resulting secondary hyperparathyroidism may contribute significantly to the progression of the disease process.

Intervention

If detected early, periodontal disease can be controlled by professional dental care and appropriate home care. Assist the client with plaque control, which includes mechanical cleansing of the teeth, stimulation of the gums, and dietary control. Tell the client to brush and floss the teeth daily. Other useful devices for plaque control are interdental rubber tips, water irrigation under pressure, and oral rinses. Assist the client with planning a well-balanced diet that contains sufficient fibrous foods and a minimum of sucrose-containing foods. If sucrose-containing foods are consumed, their intake should be confined to mealtimes.

Conflicting results have been reported in studies in which supplements of calcium and vitamin C have been given, and prevention or reversal of this disease by short-term nutritional therapy has not been demonstrated. In light of the potential role of nutrition in the etiology and progression of periodontal disease, consider the use of nutrient supplements if optimal dental care fails to control the disease. Since the disease may have its onset in childhood or puberty, initiate preventive measures early in life. Because the integrity of oral tissues and their subsequent ability to resist attack and maintain themselves are closely related to the consumption of adequate nutrients, provide appropriate dietary counseling for clients at all stages of the life cycle. This counseling is particularly important for pregnant women and young children in order to take advantage of both the preeruptive and posteruptive stages of tooth development.

OSTEOPOROSIS

Assessment

▶ **Osteoporosis** is a metabolic bone disorder characterized by a reduction in the bone mass without known concomitant changes in the chemical composition or histologic structure of the bone. The disorder is characterized by weakness, pain in the back and hips, muscle tenderness and cramping, and fractures (particularly of the thoracic and lumbar vertebrae, femoral neck, and distal forearm) as a result of normal stresses or trauma. Kyphosis (humpback) is frequently present, and the individual may lose height over a period of years due to vertebral collapse. The disorder is acquired slowly. The symptomatic client with a fracture is expressing evidence of a long history of bone loss.

Bone is a dynamic tissue that is important for maintaining the homeostasis of calcium and other ions in the blood and soft tissue. Skeletal calcium not only maintains skeletal rigidity but also provides a large reserve for maintaining the normal serum calcium level. In osteoporosis, the bone mass is decreased as a result of increased bone resorption. Bone formation is generally normal unless there is an associated fracture or significant bedrest or immobilization.

The balance between bone formation and bone resorption tips in favor of bone loss in adult life. Be alert to the fact that by the age of 35 to 40, both men and women begin to lose bone. With aging there is an increasing prevalence of the disabling symptoms of osteoporosis. The disorder is encountered particularly in clients after the age of 50 years and especially in women following the menopause (including women who have had surgical removal of the ovaries). Osteoporosis is more common in women than in men. Assess the family history of postmenopausal clients. If their mother, aunts, or sisters have osteoporosis, their risk is increased further. The total bone mass achieved at maturity influences the timing of development of symptoms of osteoporosis. Thus those with a smaller bone mass at maturity are prone to reach the stage of fracture risk before those with a considerably greater bone mass at maturity. Women typically have less bone mass than men at any age, and this may contribute to the higher incidence of the disorder in females. In general, small-boned Caucasian and Oriental women are most susceptible, whereas the risk for black women is much lower due to their tendency to have a greater bone mass.

Observe for osteoporosis as a manifestation of other disorders. For example, osteoporosis may occur secondary to other diseases, including renal disease (renal osteodystrophy), endocrine disorders (hyperthyroidism, hyperparathyroidism, hyperadrenocorticism, and acromegly), and gastrointestinal disorders (gastrectomy, celiac disease, liver cirrhosis, and steatorrhea). Osteoporosis may be a complication of idiopathic hypercalciuria, multiple myeloma, and as a side effect of drug therapy, including heparin and steroids. However, osteoporosis is believed to result most commonly from primary factors, including estrogen deficiency, inactivity and immobilization, and nutrient imbalances. Age-related osteoporosis (senile, occurring in men over the age of 75 years, and postmenopausal, occurring in women after the menopause) is the most common type of the disease.

The importance of nutritional factors in the etiology, prevention, and treatment of primary osteoporosis is receiving increased attention. In particular, the level of dietary calcium and phosphorus intake and the ratio of calcium:phosphorus consumption are being studied. Protein deficiency is a rare cause of osteoporosis, although some authorities consider osteoporosis to be a disease of the protein matrix and have associated the disorder with a low protein intake.

Calcium homeostasis and normal serum calcium levels are regulated by the parathyroid gland. A decrease in the serum ionized calcium or an increase in the serum phosphorus level (the latter bringing a decrease in the serum level of ionized calcium as the phosphorus combines with calcium in the blood) stimulates the secretion of parathyroid hormone. The increased secretion of parathyroid hormone in turn leads to activation of vitamin D by the kidney, which in turn stimulates the intestinal absorption of calcium, mobilization of calcium and phosphorus from the bone, and retention of calcium and excretion of phosphorus by the kidney, thus bringing the calcium blood level back to normal. The mobilization of calcium from the bone, however, leads to bone resorption. Data suggest that some clients with symptomatic osteoporosis have elevated levels of parathyroid hormone, leading to an increase in the rate of bone resorption, although this finding is not universal.[8]

It has been suggested that a prolonged inadequate dietary intake of calcium may be an etiologic factor in osteoporosis. Although this has not been proved, there are some epidemiologic data to support this contention.[9] Some investigators feel that the level of calcium intake in the diet is inadequate and that most adults are in a state of negative calcium balance. The RDA for calcium for adults is 800 mg. In older adults an even greater amount may be required to prevent negative balance, e.g., up to 1.2 to 1.5 g daily in postmenopausal women. However, the average daily calcium intake of adults is generally less than the recommended amount. Findings from the most recent government survey reveal that on any given day, 50 percent of women 15 years of age and above consume three fourths or less of the RDA for calcium and that after age 35, more than 75 percent of U.S. women have calcium intakes below the RDA of 800 mg.[10] Although adaptation to a low calcium intake occurs by an increase in the efficiency of calcium absorption from the intestine, this adaptation rarely is sufficient to compensate for a low calcium intake, and, in the aged, the efficiency of calcium absorption may increase relatively little and may actually decrease.

A high phosphorus intake and a low calcium:phosphorus ratio have both been mentioned as important nutritional influences in the etiology of osteoporosis. Phosphorus is prevalent in common foods, such as milk, meat, grain products, and potatoes, and is widely used as an additive in food processing. The current level of phosphorus intake approaches nearly 50 percent above the RDA of 800 mg for this mineral. Moreover, the calcium:phosphorus ratio has changed in recent decades in association with the decline in calcium intake and increase in phosphorus intake. Although the optimal ratio of calcium to phosphorus is not known, a ratio of 1:1 to 2:1 is considered acceptable; the ratio of current diets is 1:1.6.

Although high phosphorus diets and diets with a low ratio of calcium to phosphorus have been shown to cause bone loss and soft tissue calcification in some lower animal species, there is no direct evidence that a high intake of phosphorus causes a deterioration in calcium balance or bone loss in humans. Whereas an elevation in plasma phosphorus and an increase in the secretion of parathyroid hormone occur in response to excessive phosphorus intake, urinary excretion of calcium decreases. Since a high phosphorus intake also leads to an increase in the loss of calcium into the intestine, calcium balance remains unchanged.

Use the following list of factors that may potentially lead to a negative calcium balance to aid in assessing a client's degree of risk of developing osteoporosis:

1. A decrease in dietary calcium consumption with age (this may be due to a change in dietary consumption patterns with age or to adherence to diets that restrict the ingestion of foods high in calcium, such as a low-cholesterol diet)
2. A decrease in calcium absorption with age beginning at about 45 years of age in females and 60 years of age in males (the reason for this is not known, but it may be caused by inadequate vitamin D resulting from less exposure to sunlight or by decreased renal function, which impairs the activation of vitamin D)
3. A spontaneous decrease in consumption of milk due to lactase deficiency
4. A decrease in absorption, an increase in urinary excretion, and a decrease in intake of dietary calcium in association with alcoholism
5. A high intake of caffeine, dietary fiber, oxalates, and cigarette smoking
6. An increase in urinary excretion of calcium secondary to consumption of a high-protein diet (postulated mechanisms for this phenomenon are (1) a change in acid–base balance that necessitates the use of bone calcium as a buffering agent with a high-protein intake and (2) a high-protein diet increases the glomerular filtration rate leading to an increase in calcium clearance and decreased renal reabsorption of calcium. Dietary proteins differ in their effect on urinary calcium excretion and some studies show that a high-protein diet, when given as meat, does not increase urinary calcium excretion or result

in a negative calcium balance.[11] A rationale for this finding is that meat is rich in phosphorus as well as protein; since phosphorus decreases the urinary loss of calcium, it tends to offset the effect of protein on urinary calcium loss)
7. A low level of physical activity (with lack of exercise there is a lack of mechanical stimulation to maintain calcium in the bone)
8. Estrogen deficiency (e.g., following menopause; estrogens appear to slow down the bone destruction process and to improve the intestinal absorption of calcium)

Intervention

Direct interventions toward both the prevention of osteoporosis and reversal of the process in those in whom symptomatic bone disease is present. Treatment modalities include the use of nutrient supplements, exercise regimens, and hormonal therapy.

An important aspect of treatment is to reduce or stop the rate of bone loss, since by the time of diagnosis, affected clients may have lost a significant portion of skeletal calcium. Advise the client to increase the calcium content of the diet and provide supplements to amount to a total daily calcium intake of approximately 1000 to 1500 mg; an increase in calcium intake can retard the rate of bone loss. Remind the client of the best sources of calcium: an 8-ounce glass of milk or its equivalent as yoghurt or cheese contains about 300 mg calcium; other good sources are green, leafy vegetables, fish and shellfish, such as canned salmon and sardines, scallops, oysters, and shrimp, and legumes, such as kidney beans. Suggest that dry milk be added to baked goods and casseroles to increase calcium intake. Assess for the presence of lactose intolerance and suggest alternative calcium sources for these clients. Although an adequate protein intake is also important, stress to the client that the protein intake should not be excessive to prevent the possibility of precipitating urinary calcium loss. The physician may prescribe vitamin D supplements in addition to supplemental calcium. Monitor clients receiving vitamin D closely because of its potential toxicity.

Concurrent with the high calcium intake, assist the client to develop a regular exercise program. There is no clear evidence that exercise will prevent the disorder, but there is evidence to show that lack of physical activity hastens bone loss. Although the best exercises involve working the muscles against gravity, such as walking and running, even standing quietly may be valuable for clients with severe disabilities. Encourage clients with fractures to sustain an exercise program designed to accommodate their particular disabilities. Advise middle-age women to avoid lifting objects while bending forward. Rather, they should carry weight close to the body and should squat and lift straight up, using the hips and not the back.

The physician may prescribe estrogen therapy; estrogen helps preserve bone tissue from further loss but does not strengthen bones already weakened by osteoporosis. When estrogen therapy is used, monitor the client carefully, since this hormone increases the risk of uterine cancer.[12]

Regardless of treatment, the outlook for clients with osteoporosis is uncertain. Some may improve and enjoy a relatively comfortable life, whereas others experience little or no improvement, or even deterioration of their condition. Research is continuing to unveil more effective forms of treatment. The biologically active form of vitamin D (calcitriol) is being tested but as yet it appears to have no particular advantage over direct calcium supplementations for the average client.[12] Other drugs such as calcitonin, a synthetic form of a male sex hormone (stanozolol), and a combination of fluoride and calcium supplements are also being studied as therapy for osteoporotic clients. At present, only a calcium–fluoride combination offers the prospect of actually increasing bone mass. The other drugs tend to stabilize the bone tissue and prevent further loss. Some clients treated with the fluoride–calcium combination have experienced serious side effects, including stomach pain, nausea, inflamed joints, and anemia caused by gastrointestinal bleeding. These side effects may be controlled with a lower dosage should the lower dosage prove effective. Moreover, with high doses, the resulting bone has a high fluoride content, which tends to be more crystalline, less elastic, and therefore not as strong as normal bone.[12] Other combination regimens are being tested for their effectiveness.[13]

For clients who develop osteoporosis secondary to other medical disorders, it is unlikely that calcium or estrogen therapy can be efficacious in the same manner as with postmenopausal osteoporosis. Nonetheless, it is prudent to maintain an adequate dietary intake of calcium for clients with these conditions.

Measures toward preventing osteoporosis should be instituted early in life. Although the disorder may not be preventable by increasing calcium intake, a nutritionally adequate diet that includes adequate calcium is necessary for the development and maintenance of normal bone structure. Instruct pregnant and lactating women of their need for extra calcium, and encourage an adequate calcium intake for children throughout childhood to achieve an adequate bone mass at skeletal maturity. Since physical exercise stimulates production of bone tissue and increases its density, stress the importance of regular exercise. Encourage older clients to maintain an adequate intake of calcium. Postmenopausal females in particular may need an amount of calcium in excess of 800 mg to maintain the normal integrity of bone. Stress the need to avoid excessive protein, caffeine, and alcohol intake, as well as excessive smoking.

REVIEW QUESTIONS AND ACTIVITIES

1. *Case study:* Your client is a 45-year-old male (Mr. A) who has recently been diagnosed with gout. You are preparing a care plan to guide your nursing care. Consider the following as they relate to gout and its management:
   a. Identify the four major clinical manifestations of gout.
   b. Explain the two basic mechanisms that lead to hyperuricemia.
   c. Explain the rationale for the occurrence of hyperuricemia to each of the following conditions: (1) fasting, (2) alcoholism, (3) chronic renal failure, and (4) use of certain diuretics.
   d. Differentiate between endogenous and exogenous sources of purines.
   e. What would you tell Mr. A regarding the following aspects of his diet? (1) Carbohydrate, protein, and fat, (2) purines, (3) fluid, (4) alcohol, and (5) coffee, tea, and cocoa.
   f. Plan a menu for 1 day that would be suitable should Mr. A have an acute gouty attack.
2. Describe the clinical manifestations of rheumatoid arthritis and compare them with the manifestations of osteoarthritis.
3. Outline the dietary considerations, including nutritional implications of associated drug therapy, for treating rheumatoid arthritis and osteoarthritis.
4. Visit a local health food store and identify special remedies that may be offered for treatment of arthritis.
5. Differentiate between the local and systemic effects of food and nutrients in maintaining the integrity of oral structures.
6. Describe dietary adjustments that should accompany professional dental care in treating periodontal disease.
7. Describe the bone changes and the end result of these changes that are characteristic of osteoporosis.
8. Discuss the significance of long-term calcium deficiency as an etiologic factor in postmenopausal osteoporosis.
9. Discuss the significance of the ratio of dietary calcium to phosphorus intake as a possible etiologic factor in postmenopausal osteoporosis.
10. Describe the role of hormones and physical activity in the etiology of postmenopausal osteoporosis.
11. List six additional factors that may place menopausal women at risk of developing osteoporosis.

12. Describe the role of nutrient supplements, exercise, and hormonal therapy in treating osteoporosis.

13. Discuss the potential for prevention of age-related osteoporosis.

REFERENCES

1. American Dietetic Association: Handbook of Clinical Dietetics. New Haven, Yale University Press, 1981, p C-47.
2. Clifford AJ, Riumello JA, Young VR, Scrimshaw NS: Effect of oral purines on serum uric acid of normal, hyperuricemic, and gouty humans. J Nutr 106:428, 1976.
3. Clifford AJ, Story DL: Levels of purines in foods and their metabolic effect in rats. J Nutr 106:435, 1976.
4. Kowsari B, Finnie SK, Carter RL, et al.: Assessment of the diet of patients with rheumatoid arthritis and osteoarthritis. J Am Diet Assoc 82:657, 1983.
5. Simkin RA: Oral zinc sulfate in rheumatoid arthritis. Lancet 2:539, 1976.
6. Goodson WH: Nutrition and wound healing. Audio Cassette Series No 5, Chicago, American Dietetic Association, 1982.
7. Primate studies indicate that subclinical and acute vitamin C deficiency may lead to periodontal disease. JAMA 246:730, 1981.
8. Osteoporosis and calcium balance. Nutr Rev 41:83, 1983.
9. Matkovic V, Kostial K, Simonovic I, et al.: Bone status and fracture rates in two regions of Yugoslavia. Am J Clin Nutr 32:540, 1979.
10. Abraham S, Carroll MD, Dresser CM, Johnson CL: Dietary Intake Source Data, United States 1976–1980. National Center for Health Statistics, Hyattsville, Md, U.S. Department of Human Services, 1983.
11. Spencer H, Kramer L, DeBartolo M, et al.: Further studies on the effect of a high protein diet as meat on calcium metabolism. Am J Clin Nutr 37:924, 1983.
12. National Institutes of Arthritis, Diabetes, and Digestive and Kidney Diseases: Osteoporosis; Cause, Treatment, Prevention, U.S. DHHS, NIH Publication No 83–2226, Bethesda, Md, 1983.
13. Aloia JE, Zanzi I, Vaswani A, et al.: Combination therapy for osteoporosis with estrogen, fluoride, and calcium. J Am Geriatr Soc 30:13, 1982.

BIBLIOGRAPHY

Avioli LV: Postmenopausal osteoporosis: Prevention versus cure. Fed Proc 40:2418, 1981.

Barzel US: Osteoporosis in young men. Arch Intern Med 142:2079, 1982.

Chesnut CH III: Treatment of postmenopausal osteoporosis: Some current concepts. Scot Med J 26:72, 1981.

Draper HH, Scythes CA: Calcium, phosphorus, and osteoporosis. Fed Proc 40:2434, 1981.

Heaney RP, Recker RR: Effects of nitrogen, phosphorus, and caffeine on calcium balance in women. J Lab Clin Med 99:46, 1982.

Hormones, nutrients, and postmenopausal bone loss. Nutr Rev 40:13, 1982.

Horowitz M, Need AG, Philcox JC, Nordin BEC: Effect of calcium supplementation on urinary hydroxyproline in osteoporotic postmenopausal women. Am J Clin Nutr 39:857, 1984.

Jacobs HH: Nutrition and the development of oral tissues. J Am Diet Assoc 83:51, 1983.

Lee CJ, Lawler GS, Johnson GH: Effects of supplementation of the diet with calcium and calcium-rich foods on bone density of elderly females with osteoporosis. Am J Clin Nutr 34:819, 1981.

Linkswiler HM: Protein-induced hypercalciuria. Fed Proc 40:2429, 1981.

Madans J, Kleinman JC, Cornoni-Huntley J: The relationship between hip fracture and water fluoridation: An analysis of national data. Am J Public Health 73:296, 1983.

National Institutes of Arthritis, Diabetes, and Digestive and Kidney Diseases: Consensus conference: Osteoporosis. JAMA 252:799, 1984.

Raisz LG: Osteoporosis. J Am Geriatr Soc 30:127, 1982.

Wasnich RD, Benfante RJ, Yano K, et al.: Thiazide effect on the mineral content of bone. N Engl J Med 309:344, 1983.

Wical K, Brussee P: Effects of a calcium and vitamin D supplement on alveolar ridge resorption. J Prosthet Dent 41:6 1979.

CHAPTER 38

Nutrition and Nervous and Mental Disorders

Objectives

After completion of this chapter, the student will be able to:

1. Distinguish between the neurologic manifestations of an imbalance of glucose, protein, and selected vitamins and minerals.

2. Compare and contrast the nutritional implications regarding etiology and treatment of migraine headache and the hyperkinetic behavior syndrome.

3. Develop a nursing care plan for the nutritional management of a client with multiple sclerosis.

4. Develop a nursing care plan for the nutritional management of a client with mental illness.

5. Manage the diet of an infant with each of the following disorders: (a) Down's syndrome, (b) spastic cerebral palsy, and (c) athetoid cerebral palsy.

6. Manage the diet of a 3-year-old epileptic client who is following a ketogenic diet.

Nutrition plays an important role in the development and functioning of the nervous system, and nutritional deficiencies or imbalances may be related to central nervous system dysfunction. Psychiatric or neurologic disorders may lead to malnutrition, and nutritional support is a necessary component of the management of the disorders. Diet therapy is sometimes used to treat neurologic disorders that have a nonnutritional etiology. These aspects of nutrition and nervous system function and dysfunction are discussed in this chapter. Aspects of feeding the mentally and physically handicapped are discussed in more detail in Chapter 39.

RELATIONSHIP OF NUTRITION TO MENTAL FUNCTION

Assessment and Intervention

The preservation of the functioning of the central nervous system and the peripheral nerves is dependent upon adequate intake and availability of nutrients. The nutrient supply must be continuous, since, unlike other organs, such as the liver, the brain has a limited nutrient storage capacity. The highly specialized functions of the brain and the fact that the brain accounts for approximately one fifth of the basal metabolism make it particularly vulnerable to altered metabolism, especially to altered levels of glucose and oxygen. Since glucose is the primary source of energy for the brain, be aware that a sudden reduction in the blood glucose concentration can lead to convulsions and coma and that irreversible brain damage may result from a lack of glucose, even for a few minutes. An adequate supply of vitamins, particularly those of the B-complex category, must be available, since they are essential for metabolism of the glucose that plays such a predominant role in metabolism of the nervous system. Imbalances of minerals, including such electrolytes as sodium, potassium, calcium, and magnesium, can affect nervous system function, the latter by their effect on the composition of the cerebrospinal fluid and excitability of nerve cells. For example,

549

deficits of calcium and magnesium cause hyperirritability, while excesses have a depressant effect.

An adequate supply and proper balance of amino acids are also important. Recall that severe mental retardation may accompany the amino acid imbalances associated with certain inborn errors of metabolism, such as phenylketonuria. The brain achieves most of its growth during fetal life and the early postnatal period. The capacity for growth after this time is extremely limited. Thus the nutrient supply, particularly the amount of protein and kilocalories, at this time of rapid growth is especially critical.

During the brain growth spurt, brain growth and development are the result of complex interacting factors involving not only nutrient availability but also hormonal factors and sensory input from the environment. Although much evidence has been presented to implicate severe undernutrition in defective structure and functioning of the brain, it is often difficult to isolate the effects imposed on the developing brain by sensory and nutrient deprivation. Furthermore, defective brain functioning induced by nutritional inadequacy may under certain conditions be offset by increased sensory stimulation. The nervous system in an adult is generally more resilient to altered nutrition than is the developing nervous system.

Chronic alcoholism and its associated malnutrition (see Chap. 36) account for a large majority of nutritional disorders of the nervous system in Western societies. Not only is nutrient intake likely to be diminished with chronic heavy drinking, but also the intestinal absorption, tissue storage, use, and conversion of nutrients, such as vitamins, to metabolically active forms may be curtailed. Even so, alcohol-induced nutritional deficiency syndromes of the nervous system are found in only a small

TABLE 38–1
NEUROLOGIC MANIFESTATIONS OF NUTRIENT IMBALANCES

Nutrient	Neurologic Manifestation of Imbalance
B-complex vitamins	
Thiamine	*Deficiency.* Wernicke–Korsakoff syndrome and peripheral neuropathy (see Chap. 36)
Riboflavin and niacin	*Deficiency.* Peripheral neuropathy. Neurologic manifestations of mental confusion, hallucinations, and acute psychosis (pellagra may be due to a combined deficiency of preformed niacin and its precursor, tryptophan)
Pyridoxine	*Deficiency.* Convulsive disorders, peripheral neuropathy, and possibly depression
Folic acid	*Deficiency.* Vague neurologic manifestations (pathology is poorly understood)
Vitamin B$_{12}$	*Deficiency.* Peripheral neuropathy and degeneration of the spinal cord, which may lead to mental deterioration and psychosis
Pantothenic acid	*Deficiency.* Paresthesias of the feet and legs (burning foot syndrome)
Vitamin C	*Deficiency.* Depression, hysteria, hypochondriasis, peripheral neuropathy, postural dizziness
Vitamin A	*Deficiency.* Increased cerebrospinal fluid pressure and loss of vestibular function, loss of dark adaptation, and impairment of the sense of taste and smell
	Excess. Increased cerebrospinal fluid pressure and hydrocephalus; malformation of the central nervous system of the fetus if excessive amounts are consumed during pregnancy
Vitamin D	*Deficiency.* Microcephaly in infant; muscular weakness in adults
Zinc	*Deficiency.* Impairment of the senses of taste and smell and anorexia
Copper	*Excess.* Neurologic manifestations of Wilson's disease (see Chap. 22)
Selenium	*Deficiency.* Muscle pain and tenderness, muscle wasting, and difficulty in walking
Magnesium	*Deficiency.* Manifestations of organic brain syndrome and hallucinations

proportion of alcoholics. Consider these additional categories of clients to be at a high risk of developing neural manifestations of nutritional deficiency: clients who are malnourished from any cause, such as those with debilitating illnesses including malabsorption syndromes, renal disease, and neoplastic diseases, or those whose malnutrition is a result of food faddism, poverty, or ignorance. Stressful situations, such as chronic infection, can deplete the body of nutrients even in the presence of an adequate nutrient intake. Finally, a nutrient–drug interaction—e.g., a vitamin B_6 deficiency occurring secondary to isoniazid therapy used to treat tuberculosis—may lead to neurologic complications.

With the possible exception of deficient glucose in the blood and the altered amino acid metabolism that is characteristic of certain inborn errors of metabolism, expect neurologic manifestations of nutrient imbalance to demonstrate an insidious onset. For example, clinical manifestations of vitamin B_{12} deficiency may be delayed for several years, and secondary deficiencies that result from drug–nutrient interactions may have an even longer latent period. The disorders are likely to be less severe in adults than in children. Neurologic manifestations of nutrient imbalance are summarized in Table 38–1.

Monitor closely the nutritional status of clients who are at a high risk of developing neurologic manifestations of nutritional deficiency so that the nutrient imbalance can be corrected while it is still in a reversible stage. Replenishing the missing nutrients may not always result in cure, however. In some instances, the tissue structure or functioning may have degenerated beyond repair. Some conditions, such as peripheral neuropathy, may require a period of treatment ranging from several months to a year before any improvement is seen. Be especially aggressive in monitoring high-risk infants and children in whom neurologic manifestations may develop more rapidly and be more severe.

Since many of the effects of deficiency of the B-complex vitamins are nonspecific for a particular vitamin, consider the need for supplementing with the entire group in treatment. Although supplementation with deficient vitamins is essential in the management of neurologic disease induced by nutritional deficiency, also take measures to establish a nutritional regimen that meets the nutritional requirements of each individual client in order to prevent relapses and to correct the multiple nutritional deficiencies often associated with such conditions. When the vitamin deficiency results from gastrointestinal malabsorption, administer the vitamins by the parenteral route. In general, larger doses of vitamin B_{12} are required to treat the neurologic complications of vitamin B_{12} deficiency than are needed to treat uncomplicated pernicious anemia.

Another relationship between nutrition and mental function is the notion that the concentration of some of the brain's neurotransmitters is influenced by diet. There is active investigation of the theory that diet therapy can alter neurotransmitter synthesis. These findings may have promise in treating certain neurologic disorders.[1,2]

MIGRAINE

Assessment and Intervention

Although migraine headache, a familial disorder that is vascular in origin, is a multifactorial condition, dietary factors may be important in triggering the symptoms in some susceptible clients. Four mechanisms have been studied whereby food may serve as a migraine trigger[3]:

1. An allergic reaction (foods including wheat, citrus fruit, tea, coffee, pork, chocolate, milk, grapes, nuts, beef, corn, cane sugar, legumes, yeast, pineapple, coconut, and cola drinks have all been mentioned as migraine-associated allergens)
2. The presence of specific chemical components in foods (e.g., tyramine, phenylethylamine, sodium, sodium nitrite, monosodium glutamate, alcohol, certain chemicals—cogeners—found in alcoholic beverages, and excessive amounts of vitamin A)
3. Hypoglycemia (e.g., reactive hypoglycemia following fasting or the presence of hunger itself)
4. Taste aversion (e.g., a psychologic rather than physiologic response due to a learned taste aversion)

Although none of these mechanisms is accepted by all researchers in the field as food-related triggering mechanisms and sensitivity to foods and beverages varies with each client, ascertain if specific food offenders or food-related patterns exist in affected clients. Ask the client if he or she can name specific foods that appear to trigger a migraine headache. It may also be useful to have the client keep a food–symptom diary similar to that described for detecting food sensitivities in Chapter 32. Probe for the use of vitamin A supplements and question the client about symptoms that are experienced in association with hunger and fasting. If the client relates consumption of specific foods to the occurrence of headaches, the physician may perform tests similar to those described in Chapter 32 to determine if the foods are indeed related to the causation of migraine.

If specific food sensitivities are identified, advise the client to omit these foods from the diet, but avoid admonitions to eliminate all foods that have been implicated in triggering migraine attacks. This approach may lead to apprehension about eating that can itself serve as a psychologic stressor that may aggravate the condition or lead to malnutrition as the result of an overly restricted diet. If concurrent hypoglycemia is present, use the guidelines given in Chapter 24 to establish an anti-hypoglycemia regimen in accordance with the physician's orders and the client's lifestyle.

HYPERKINETIC BEHAVIOR SYNDROME

Assessment and Intervention

Recently, a great deal of clinical and research interest has centered around a commonly occurring syndrome of disorders creating behavior and learning problems in children. Officially termed the "attention deficit disorder with hyperactivity," the disorders are variously referred to as "hyperkinetic reaction of childhood," "hyperactive child syndrome," "minimal brain damage," "minimal brain dysfunction," and "minimal or minor cerebral dysfunction." At present there is little agreement on the extent to which several seemingly related syndromes overlap.

▶ Although there is disagreement on the precise definition of the **hyperkinetic behavior syndrome,** look for the any or all of the following clinical features in children suspected of having the disorder: (1) excessive gross motor activity (i.e., hyperactivity), (2) short attention span and poor powers of concentration, and (3) emotional lability (e.g., impulsive behavior with an inability to delay gratification, a low tolerance for frustration, a diminished ability to experience pleasure, and a refractoriness to disciplinary measures). Although most affected clients demonstrate average or above average intelligence, learning ability is affected in varying ways, as are neural functions and muscular coordination. In school the syndrome may contribute to significant underachievement as well as to classroom disruption, and it is disruptive to family relations at home.

The ambiguous nature of the disorder has led to much confusion about its diagnosis and incidence. In many cases the diagnosis is based solely on anecdotal observations of the child's behavior. The incidence of the hyperkinetic behavior syndrome in U.S. schools is reported by different investigators to vary from 3 to 10 percent.[4]

The syndrome is more common in males than in females, and the behavioral manifestations appear in early to midchildhood (ages 2 to 6 years). Although the hyperactive behavior per se appears to diminish with age, problems related to attention and concentration persist. Observe for feelings of underachievement, low self-esteem, depression, and a sense of failure in adults who had the disorder as a child.

In order to provide the appropriate treatment, assess for its etiology. It may consist of a group of disorders resulting from a synergism of the following predisposing factors: (1) genetic predisposition, (2) organic factors, such as trauma, infection, lead intoxication, and significant perinatal hypoxia, and (3) psychosocial factors, such as anxiety, inadequate parenting, and environmental stresses. In addition, there is evidence that the blood levels of the neurotransmitter serotonin (5-HT) are lower in hyperkinetic children than in nonhyperkinetic children or that there is a reduction in turnover of dopamine,

a catecholamine neurotransmitter. This suggests that there may be a structural, physiologic or biochemical cause for the hyperkinetic behavior syndrome, although the basic cause remains to be shown. If the condition is related to such factors as anxiety, a subclinical seizures disorder, or lead intoxication, direct treatment toward control of these disorders.

In 1973, Dr. Benjiman Feingold, a pediatric allergist, proposed that sensitivity to salicylates, to compounds that cross-react with salicylates, and to certain food additives, particularly artificial food flavors and food colors, is associated with hyperactivity in childhood. Feingold hypothesized that hyperkinesis could be controlled by dietary methods, i.e., removal from the diet of all artificial flavors and colors and all salicylate-containing foods. Feingold subsequently applied his hypothesis in treating children with hyperkinetic behavior. His clinical observations led him to postulate that one half to two thirds of hyperactive children, when managed with his elimination diet (referred to as the Kaiser-Per-
▶ manente or the **K-P diet**), demonstrate significant improvement in behavior, often quite dramatically and in a short period of time. The younger the child, the more rapid and extensive the response. Feingold published a popular book in which he described his hypothesis and his method of dietary treatment.[5] The basic diet described by Feingold eliminates two groups of foods: Group I, consisting of foods containing high levels of naturally occurring salicylates (Table 38–2), and Group II, consisting of foods known or thought to contain artificial colors and flavors. Additionally, drugs containing salicylates are excluded. With a favorable response to the diet, food intake is liberalized by reintroducing, one at a time, foods containing naturally occurring salicylates at intervals of about 4 days between individual trials. With the exception of butylated hydroxytoluene

---

TABLE 38–2
FOODS HIGH IN NATURAL SALICYLATE CONTENT

Fruits	Vegetables
Almonds	Cucumbers and pickles
Apples	Tomatoes and tomato products
Apricots	
Blackberries, boysenberries, gooseberries, raspberries, strawberries	
Cherries	
Currants	
Grapes and raisins (and all products made from grapes: wine, wine vinegar, jelly)	
Nectarines	
Oranges	
Peaches	
Plums and prunes	

(BHT), foods containing preservatives were not excluded from the original Feingold diet, but later modifications excluded butylated hydroxyanisole (BHA) and sodium benzoate, although certain Group I foods containing artificial preservatives were not excluded.

Actually, Feingold and his followers propose more than just adherence to a diet—they advocate a change in lifestyle. For example, they require that the entire family, not just the child, be placed on the diet to ensure adherence, and they urge parents to develop a close rapport with their children by spending more time with them. Parents are instructed to spend Saturday mornings making additive-free candy and cake with their children. The diet is widely used, and many parents report dramatic improvement in their children.

The findings described by Feingold have prompted much attention in the lay press and controversy in professional circles. The validity of Feingold's theory has been questioned by many professionals. Many of the criticisms are summarized in a report by the National Advisory Committee on Hyperkinesis and Food Additives.[6] In 1980 this body concluded that sufficient evidence is now available to refute the claims that the use of artificial food flavors, colorings, and salicylates is associated with hyperactivity and learning disability.[7] After examining the Feingold treatment, the supporting data, and the results of various studies, the Committee found no consistent pattern of improvement with use of the Feingold diet. The Committee contended, however, that the need exists to remain vigilant regarding the overall safety of food coloring and recommended that experimental studies in this area continue. Since the food additive-free diet has no apparent harmful effects and the placebo effects of the dietary treatment are frequently beneficial to families, the Committee saw no reason to discourage families who wish to pursue this type of treatment provided they follow other treatment that is helpful. In a later review of controlled studies on the effectiveness of diet in hyperkinesis,[8] it was noted that a small subset of hyperactive children demonstrated less evidence of hyperactivity on a controlled diet than on a noncontrolled diet and that some hyperactive children on the controlled diet experienced an increase in hyperactivity when given a moderate dose of artificial food dyes. These observations were not noted consistently, however, and involved only a small group of children. Moreover, it was not possible to identify beforehand the small group who may respond favorably.

Although scientific data do not provide the basis for the universal use of the K-P diet for treating hyperkinesis, its use may be warranted after appropriate evaluation of the child and parent and after full consideration of all therapeutic options. Assist parents who express confidence and enthusiasm in the dietary regimen to incorporate the aspects of the K-P diet into their dietary patterns. Advise

them, however, that existing law does not require that all ingredients contained in food be listed on the label and that they may have to contact food processors to detect sources of food additives. Further, stress to them that many pediatric medications, including some vitamins, contain artificial colorings and flavorings and must be carefully selected for this reason. Mouthwashes, toothpastes, cough syrups, and antacids are also artificially colored and flavored and must be eliminated.

Monitor the nutritional adequacy of the diet on an ongoing basis. Although the modified K-P diet that does not eliminate foods containing naturally occurring salicylates appears to be nutritionally adequate, nutritional inadequacies may appear in some children if a strict diet is followed over a long period of time without proper monitoring.

Whereas diet therapy is a current and well-publicized treatment for the hyperkinetic behavior syndrome, many clinicians advocate multiple modalities of treatment, including the use of stimulant drugs. Assess for anorexia and suppression of growth in height and weight as side effects of these drugs. The degree of suppression appears to be related to the specific drug used (methylphenidate appears to have a lesser effect than dextroamphetamine), the dosage (suppression increases with increasing drug use), and the duration of drug therapy (rebound growth occurs with discontinuation of the drug). To minimize these side effects, administer the minimal drug dosage needed to modify the most disruptive behavior and consider the desirability of discontinuing the drug on weekends and summer vacations from school.

Because appetite is affected with stimulant therapy, do not use the appetite as a guideline for consumption of an appropriate amount of food. Advise parents that appetite suppression may be offset if the medication is given during or after meals rather than before meals and that foods of high nutrient density should be provided when the appetite relative to the time of drug administration is likely to be optimal. Stress the importance of taking advantage of an expressed appetite, even if small, to provide nutritious food.

MULTIPLE SCLEROSIS

Assessment and Intervention

▶ **Multiple sclerosis** is a disease of the central nervous system characterized by widespread destruction of myelin surrounding the nerve fibers of the brain and spinal cord and its replacement by scar tissue. The disease usually appears early in adult life (most often between the ages of 20 and 40) in an acute form and follows an intermittent course characterized by a series of isolated attacks affecting different parts of the central nervous system. Although each attack is followed by some degree of remission, the overall picture is one of progressive deterioration. The disease affects not only the my-elinated nerve fibers but also the muscles they inner-vate. Evaluate for the presence of sensory disorders, such as paresthesias, visual complaints including blurred vision and nystagmus, spastic weakness of the limbs and ataxia, bladder dysfunction, and disorders of mood.

The etiology of the disorder is unknown and consequently the subject of much speculation. An infectious etiology (probably viral) has been suggested; i.e., a virus contracted early in life may become activated later, causing an autoimmune reaction that attacks myelin. Epidemiologic studies have related the etiology to nutritional factors. The disorder tends to be more prevalent in countries consuming large amounts of animal fat. Thus there is a possible correlation between the incidence of the disease and total fat consumption as well as the percentage of kilocalories derived from foods of animal origin. Evaluate serum levels of the essential fatty acid linoleic acid, which tends to be low in affected clients.

Although there is no conclusive evidence that diet manipulation is effective in improving the prognosis for multiple sclerosis clients, some evidence suggests that manipulating the fat intake over a prolonged period may slow the disease process and reduce the incidence of new attacks. The effects of dietary management appear to be much better in those clients in whom treatment is initiated early in the course of the disease than in those in whom it is started later. If a fat-restricted diet is ordered, assist the client with planning a diet that includes 40 to 50 g polyunsaturated fat and 10 g saturated fat, while keeping the protein content at a normal level and using sufficient carbohydrate to satisfy the kilocalorie requirement. Polyunsaturated fatty acids (linoleic and arachidonic acids) inhibit the lymphocyte–antigen interaction—the mechanism that may be responsible for the demyelination. Since meat intake is severely restricted in this regimen, assess the diet for its content of protein, iron, zinc, and B-complex vitamins in particular and provide supplements as indicated. Polyunsaturated fats are found in highest concentration in plant oils.

Wheat gluten has been implicated in the etiology, and some physicians suggest that the use of a gluten-free, milk-free regimen (see Chap. 27), supplemented with minerals including magnesium, may be effective in management.

Since the principles of diet therapy for clients with multiple sclerosis are not definitive, help multiple sclerosis clients to evaluate the relative merits of the proposed regimen so that hopes may not be falsely raised. Assist clients who are not following a modified dietary regimen to select a nutritionally balanced diet that can be easily assimilated. Assess the client's level of physical activity, ability to swallow, and ability for self-feeding. With limited activity, adjust the kilocalorie content of the diet to the activity level. If disabilities, such as poor hand grasp,

poor hand-to-mouth coordination, or poor control of the trunk and upper extremities, are present, provide feeding aids (see Chap. 39) so that the client can maintain independence in eating. Provide a blenderized diet regimen for clients who have difficulty swallowing. Constipation and fecal impaction are not uncommon in the chronic phase of the disorder. Suggest the inclusion of adequate fluids and laxative foods, including prune juice, to aid in managing these problems.

RELATIONSHIP OF NUTRITION TO EMOTIONAL OR PSYCHIATRIC DISORDERS

Assessment and Intervention
Food has many emotional connotations, such as providing a sense of security and pleasurable feelings, that may become more pronounced in mentally ill clients. Distortion in food intake may lead to kilocaloric and nutrient imbalances in those with emotional or psychiatric disturbances, and malnutrition (either undernutrition or obesity) may be the end result. Disturbances of food intake (either anorexia or excessive eating) are characteristic of psychiatric clients with psychoneurotic or hysterical states; thus the possibility of malnutrition is ever present. Some clients ease their anxiety with excessive eating, whereas others lose their appetite when anxious. Many psychiatric illnesses follow prolonged periods of tension and anxiety during which food intake may be altered.

Observe for the presence of food refusal and reluctant or bizarre eating habits as behavior patterns that may be manifest in mentally ill clients. When food is refused, determine the reason, which may be conscious or unconscious, e.g., depression, a wish to commit suicide, feelings of guilt or personal unworthiness, suspicion that the food has been poisoned, or because of hallucinations or catatonic states. Also determine whether there is a pattern of refusal relative to particular foods or particular meals. Anorexia nervosa (see Chap. 17) represents an extreme form of food refusal. Food refusal may also result from an underlying physical illness about which the client does not complain because of a withdrawn or mute state. Assess the anxiety level of clients who have difficulty making decisions about eating—about eating per se, about specific food choices, or about amounts of food that should be eaten. Other tactics, such as hiding food or giving it away, may also be used by the client to avoid the pressures of decision making regarding food. Other abnormal food-related behaviors that may be seen in clients who are mentally ill include a general untidiness related to food (such as dropping food on the floor or playing with it) or destructive behaviors (such as throwing food or dishes and utensils).

Include nutritional assessment as part of the periodic evaluation of mentally ill clients. Evaluate the adequacy of the client's diet, since the undernutrition associated with the altered behavior pattern may further complicate mental status. Weigh the client weekly and use weight deviations as a basis for further investigation so that corrective action can be taken before marked changes occur.

Provide nutritional support aimed at prevention of malnutrition, restoration of eating ability, and restoration of the emotional satisfaction that results from eating to accompany the basic treatment of the underlying disorder. The use of vitamin supplements and the provision of a nutritionally balanced diet may relieve some of the neurologic symptoms. Nutritional deficiency, when present, is likely to be multiple in origin.

In order to accomplish the nutritional goals, the client must feel a sense of confidence and trust in those who provide his or her food. Thus the feeding experience must not only provide food as a vehicle for satisfying a basic human need but also allow for its use as a vehicle for rebuilding relationships with others. Use a consistent, sympathetic, and nonthreatening approach, involve the client directly in establishing the nutritional care plan, and explain to the client the unmet needs that are possibly being communicated by particular food behaviors. Serve food in an attractive and pleasant environment and in the presence of others to stimulate the client to eat. Cafeteria-type food service is useful not only in allowing some choice in food selection but also in providing an opportunity for the client to develop confidence in the ability to make decisions about food choices. Moreover, a group eating experience provides the opportunity to relate to others. Food served family style and shared with staff provides an opportunity for developing closer staff–client rapport. Participation in food preparation may be another useful therapeutic device. Give particular attention to special occasions, such as birthdays and holidays.

If the client refuses to eat, spoon feeding or even tube feeding may be necessary initially. Approach tube feeding in a therapeutic, rather than punitive, manner, however. Give support and reassurance as the client assumes more responsibility for his or her own eating. For those who have suspicions that the food is poisoned, it may be necessary to taste the food in the client's presence or to serve food in unopened packages. If destructive behaviors are evident, use paper food containers. Orient confused clients to mealtimes, the particular meal being served, and the foods on the tray.

Give consideration to all foods consumed by clients who exhibit marked weight gain. This includes not only food served at mealtimes but also food purchased from snack bars and vending machines, food received as gifts from relatives or friends, and food that may be eaten from the trays of other clients.

Give consideration to the nutritional implications of the basic therapy. Shock therapy, for example, increases the kilocalorie needs, and there are interactions between the drugs administered and nutrient intake or use. Many tranquilizers and antipsychotic drugs cause the mouth to become dry and may lead to a decrease in food intake. Monoamine oxidase inhibitors used to treat depression may lead to a hypertensive crisis if consumed concomitantly with tyramine-containing foods (see Chap. 21).

ORTHOMOLECULAR PSYCHIATRY

Since the etiology and pathophysiology of a significant number of neurologic disorders are poorly understood, it is not always possible to devise definitive therapy. This void has led to scientifically undocumented and sometimes irrational use of vitamins and other nutritional approaches in treatment. Large doses of the B vitamins, such as thiamine and vitamin B_{12}, are sometimes used in treating neuropathies, neuralgias, peripheral nerve injuries, and the demyelinating disorders. Although administration of vitamins may have a placebo effect, there is no definitive evidence to show that vitamin therapy influences nerve metabolism unless a particular vitamin deficiency exists. Nor is there evidence to substantiate the efficacy of a nutritional approach in chronic neurologic diseases affecting intellectual function, such as dementia and mental retardation.

Megavitamin therapists or orthomolecular psychiatrists advocate the use of large doses of vitamins in treating some disorders, such as chronic alcoholism, learning disorders, childhood autism, hyperkinesis, schizophrenia, and depression. Pauling has ▶ coined the term **orthomolecular psychiatry** to denote "the treatment of mental disease by provision of the optimum molecular environment for the mind, especially the optimum concentration of substances normally present in the human body."[9] According to Pauling some people require larger amounts of vitamins than others to achieve optimal mental functioning. Orthomolecular psychiatry employs a combination of conventional drugs and nutritional management, including large doses (10 to 500 times the RDA) of water soluble-vitamins, such as vitamins C, B_6, B_{12}, and niacin, trace minerals, and special diets, such as an antihypoglycemia diet. Some psychiatrists practicing orthomolecular psychiatry adjust the vitamin dosage to suit the individual client, making it possible to reduce the level of intake of the drugs.

Orthomolecular psychiatry is used by some psychiatrists in treating schizophrenia. Because a schizoid-type of mental aberration is a component of pellagra (a niacin-deficiency disease), it is not surprising that the effects of this vitamin would be tested in schizophrenics. Proponents of this type of treatment claim that there are significant benefits for a modest number of the clients treated. Numerous clinical controlled trials have failed to substantiate these findings, however. Moreover, a Task Force of the American Psychiatric Association found no evidence to support the theory and practice of orthomolecular psychiatry in treating schizophrenia.[10] The report was challenged by advocates of orthomolecular psychiatry, and at present the value of orthomolecular psychiatry is a controversial issue, awaiting the findings of further studies.

RELATIONSHIP OF NUTRITION TO PHYSICAL HANDICAPS AND MENTAL RETARDATION

Assessment and Intervention

The nervous system is vulnerable to insult at all stages of the life cycle, although the vulnerability is greatest during the period of the brain's development. The causes of insults to the brain are many and varied. The results are varying degrees of physical handicaps, in some instances accompanied by mental retardation. These physical handicaps post many problems, such as the inability to suck and close the lips, the inability to bite, chew, or swallow, poor grasp, poor hand–mouth coordination, poor control of the trunk and upper extremities, and lack of bowel and bladder control. Many of these disorders may be evident in those who are severely mentally retarded.

Assess for the cause of the handicap in affected clients. Handicapping conditions in the infant may be the result of genetic or congenital abnormalities (e.g., inborn errors of metabolism, Down's syndrome, or congenital anomalies, such as myelomeningocele—a defect in the closure of the vertebral column) or prenatal complications, such as fetal malnutrition, circulatory insufficiency, toxemia, use of certain drugs, birth trauma, or hypoglycemia. Infection or brain or spinal cord injury or tumor may create neurologic complications in later childhood. In the adult, progressive neurologic disease, such as multiple sclerosis, Parkinson's disease, muscular dystrophy, and myesthenia gravis, and brain or spinal cord damage cause various neurologic complications.

These conditions pose many feeding problems, and often special feeding techniques are required to assure adequate nutrient intake. Factors contributing to feeding problems may be present in the handicapped child at birth and may persist as mechanical problems that interfere with adequate nutrition. The handicapping condition may pose obstacles to the accomplishment of the developmental milestones necessary for acquiring independence in self-feeding, i.e., development of head and trunk support, sitting balance, hand–eye coordination, and the ability to grasp, hold, and release objects. Use the achievement of these developmental tasks as evidence of the handicapped child's readiness to progress in feeding skills when setting goals for developing some degree of feeding independence.

Assess the physical growth of handicapped children and compare their growth with that of normal children of comparable age. Numerous studies show that in general, handicapped children do not attain the physical growth norms of the general population. Children with chromosomal aberrations appear to be particularly stunted in linear growth and skeletal development. Children with Down's syndrome display the most severe form of growth retardation, and those with multiple congenital anomalies and cerebral palsy exhibit significant but lesser growth retardation. Physical growth in children with minimal brain damage more nearly parallels normal growth. Although there are many recognized causes of the growth retardation, an inability to eat and consumption of an inadequate diet are usually regarded as major contributing factors. Evaluate the nutritional intake on an ongoing basis in affected clients.

Direct rehabilitative measures for clients who have nutritional imbalances as a result of their particular handicapping condition not only toward restoration and maintenance of adequate nutrition but also toward dealing with the emotional aspects of the disease. The rehabilitative process may be hindered by defense mechanisms associated with such emotions as anger, frustration, embarrassment, and isolation.

Abnormal weight patterns (either overweight or obesity) are problems that most frequently necessitate nutritional intervention in handicapped clients. Determine the cause of the abnormal weight pattern, which may be (1) an altered activity level (e.g., inactivity or excessive activity), (2) inappropriate care (e.g., neglect or oversolicitousness), and (3) disturbed interpersonal relationships between the caretaker and the client. Obesity may be a problem for those who use eating as an outlet for frustration or boredom. With regard to activity level, use the degree of ambulation possible as a major determinant of the kilocalorie requirement. For example, it has been shown that children whose motor dysfunction is severe enough to prevent ambulation require only approximately 75 percent of the kilocalories required by ambulatory children of comparable height.

Evaluate for the presence of these additional problems, which have nutritional implications: elimination difficulties associated with neuromuscular deficits affecting the bowel or bladder, the effects of prolonged immobility on nutritional status, the effect of intercurrent illness on nutritional status, and problems associated with ingestion of foods of various textures.

Neuromuscular deficits affecting the bowel or bladder may lead to constipation (necessitating a diet high in food fibers) or urinary tract infections (necessitating an increase in fluid intake, the use of urine acidifiers, and possibly an acid ash diet). In those with mechanical feeding difficulties, with an inability to express needs, or with an inability to respond to thirst, monitor fluid and nutrient intake carefully when there are increased metabolic demands, such as those imposed by fever or infection. Determine the consistency of foods to serve to handicapped clients by the degree of motor impairment and individual food tolerance. Provide vitamin and mineral supplements for any handicapped client in whom the adequacy of nutrient intake is questionable.

Special therapeutic diets may be used to treat the underlying disease or disorder that precipitates the handicapping condition. For instance, a low-fat, low-cholesterol diet may be used for clients who have suffered a stroke and a low-fat diet may sometimes be prescribed for clients with multiple sclerosis. Down's syndrome and cerebral palsy are specific conditions that present many of these feeding problems. These conditions are described here, and overall nutritional considerations for the mentally and physically handicapped are discussed in greater detail in Chapter 39.

DOWN'S SYNDROME AND CEREBRAL PALSY

Assessment

▶ **Down's syndrome** (or **mongolism**) is a chromosomal abnormality resulting from the presence of an extra chromosome in one chromosomal pair, yielding a total chromosome number of 47. Cells of the human body generally contain 46 chromosomes or 23 pairs: 22 pairs of autosomes (numbered from 1 to 22) plus a pair of sex chromosomes (X and Y). In Down's syndrome, also referred to as trisomy 21, 3 chromosomes appear in the so-called 21 position. The basic problem stems from failure of the separation of one chromosome pair that occurs in the development of the ovum. Counsel older women about the increased risk of occurrence of Down's syndrome in their children.

Evaluate for these clinical manifestations in affected clients: mild to moderate mental retardation, hypotonic musculature, delayed tooth development, periodontal disease, bridged palate, and narrow nasal passages. These characteristics frequently interfere with food ingestion, and nutritional management may be further complicated by the increased incidence of internal anatomic abnormalities, such as pyloric stenosis, tracheoesophageal fistula (a fistula between the trachea and the esophagus), and cardiac abnormalities. Examine the client's muscle tone and observe for problems associated with eating. The degree of muscle hypotonicity and weakness varies considerably from child to child but may lead to altered activity patterns, feeding problems associated with poor sucking and chewing, projecting of the tongue, and diminished gastrointestinal peristalsis and constipation. Sucking problems may be induced by the narrow palate's interference with the proper seal for sucking. Food may accumulate in the narrow palate. Mouth breathing is common because of the narrow nasal passage, and nasal secretions are heavy.

Follow the child's growth on an ongoing basis. Retardation of growth in stature is marked, and the incidence of obesity increases with advancing age. The flaccid musculature affects the activity level, and the client usually requires fewer total kilocalories than do normal children of the same height and age. Moreover, overfeeding may be a problem, since some clients may not recognize satiety and food may be used as a social reinforcer in these children. The incidence of diabetes mellitus is increased in clients with Down's syndrome.

▶ **Cerebral palsy,** one of the most common causes of crippling conditions in childhood, is actually a group of neurologic disorders resulting from damage to the motor centers of the brain. The condition occurs secondary to precipitating events that may occur in either the prenatal or perinatal periods. Cerebral anoxia, mechanical trauma to the brain at birth, congenital malformation of the brain, and cerebral vascular occlusion during fetal life have all been implicated in the etiology.

Interference with neuromotor control brings several types of neuromuscular problems, which may be mild or severe; distinguish among these four types:

1. Spasticity (increased muscle stretch reflexes and increased irritability of the muscles)
2. Athetosis (involuntary motor activity)
3. Ataxia (disturbances in balance)
4. Flaccidity (decreased muscle tone)

Spasticity and athetosis are the most common types.

Evaluate for mental retardation, which may or may not be present. There may be impairment in vision, speech, or hearing. Assess the child's ability to close the lips, suck, bite, chew, and swallow. Impairment of the tongue or throat muscles may lead to difficulties in feeding. The ability to suck and swallow may be impaired, and the persistence of the primitive reflexes (root, suck, swallow, bite, and gag) may prevent an adequate nutrient intake. Frequently there is a reversal of the swallowing wave— the wave of the tongue motion that normally takes food down the throat and pushes it back on the tongue is reversed so that all food put in the child's mouth tends to be pushed outward. Loss of food from the mouth through dribbling, the time involved with eating, and fatigue may contribute to inadequate nutrient intake. The extent of involvement of muscles in the area of the mouth tends to be closely associated with the amount of food consumed and thus with the general rate of growth. Sensitivity to tactile stimuli around the oral area may lead to difficulty in feeding without stimulating gagging. Poor occlusion and dental caries may also adversely affect nutritional status.

Assess the child's growth pattern and weight status. Growth deficits may be marked; athetoid children are smaller than spastic children. Affected children may be overweight, underweight, or of normal weight. The hyperactivity of the muscle stretch reflexes and increased irritability of muscles that are characteristic of spastic children lead to limited physical activity, and these children frequently become overweight for their height. If the client is nonambulatory, there is the risk of obesity, especially as the child approaches the teen years. In contrast, the involuntary motor activity observed in children with athetoid cerebral palsy increases the total energy requirement, and underweight may be the problem.

Intervention

Nutritional care planning for clients with Down's syndrome and cerebral palsy requires a knowledge of their feeding capabilities and their height and weight pattern. Intervene early in order to normalize the feeding experience as much as possible and to promote a growth pattern that deviates as little as possible from normal.

The energy requirement differs with the type of motor abnormality. If activity is limited, the total kilocalorie intake should be below the RDA for normal children of similar height and weight. Base the energy requirements on the child's height (kcal/cm of height) rather than on the RDA (kcal/kg body weight) and allow 10 kcal/cm of height. With this regimen, plan the diet carefully to ensure an adequate nutrient intake. Allow 15 kcal/cm of height for clients with athetoid cerebral palsy whose activity level is increased.

Use feeding techniques designed to facilitate sucking, swallowing, and chewing. Drooling may be reduced by thickening fluids with cereal or yoghurt. Assist clients who drool to keep the lips closed to avoid pushing food from the mouth or allowing food to fall from the mouth. For clients who are hypersensitive in the oral area, avoid excessive stimulation of the mouth during feeding. Counsel the parents regarding the normal sequence of developmental milestones in feeding, and encourage movement to the next milestone as each one is achieved. In particular, discourage parents from keeping the child on a liquid and strained food diet too long. Rather, encourage them to advance the diet from liquid to strained foods to foods that require chewing, and finally to independent eating when the child provides cues that he or she is ready for changes in consistency of the diet and for advancement to self-feeding. Assure parents that this approach supports the child's developmental progress. Parents, however, may be reluctant to relinquish dependence in feeding.

Assess the client's readiness to progress to pureed foods. When the infant can move food from the front to the back of the mouth and voluntary movements of the lips and tongue become coordinated, pureed foods may be gradually introduced. To decrease the possibility of choking, advise the parents to hold the infant in a semireclining posi-

tion, or to tilt the head back slightly, while placing a small spoonful of liquid, such as milk, into the mouth. Once the infant is accustomed to the feel of the spoon, the milk can be replaced with a dilute pureed mixture. As motor skills develop further and the infant can sit upright, demonstrates the ability to chew by moving the jaws vertically in a controlled way, and demonstrates the ability to grasp objects with the hand, tell the parents to introduce zwieback into the diet. As the child learns to bring the zwieback to the mouth, soft finger foods can be substituted. Foods that are hard to chew may cause choking and should be avoided. Cup feeding can be introduced when the child can bring small pieces of food to the mouth without difficulty. If the child experiences difficulty drinking from a cup, tell the parents to stand behind him or her and cup the jaws firmly in one hand while holding the cup in the other. Once chewing ability has progressed to the point that complete mastication of foods by the use of rotary chewing action is possible, family foods can be offered, although the child will continue to need assistance with feeding. Coordination of swallowing occurs gradually as lip, tongue, and jaw action become coordinated.

The age at which self-feeding is possible will vary. To prevent fatigue and frustration, tell parents to keep trials brief initially. When spoon feeding is initiated, a small amount of soft food should be placed on the tip of the spoon and the spoon placed on the front of the tongue with the spoon tip directed toward the throat. Pressure of the spoon on the tongue should be maintained until the lips begin to close slightly. The spoon should then be scraped against the upper lip (and not the teeth) so that the infant can gradually learn to use the upper lip. With spoon removal, the jaw should be closed. By applying pressure on the tongue and closing the jaw, it is possible to coordinate swallowing and block the tongue thrust that is a problem in some children.

Proper positioning for feeding is important to reduce fatigue and to prevent slipping or leaning to the side. Moreover, special techniques or exercises may be required to strengthen jaw control and chewing ability, and to reduce other problems related to eating. Finally, various feeding aids, including special utensils, dishes, and cups, are available or can be made to meet the needs of the particular child (see Chap. 39).

When weight deviations are noted, ask the parents to keep a record of food intake for several days to determine the feeding pattern and to determine if factors related to the feeding process may be contributing to the weight deviation. For instance, obesity may result from the parents' use of food as a method of rewarding achievement or from permissiveness of the parents, who may allow the child to eat whatever is desired. Fatigue associated with eating, a short attention span, and being fed too rapidly may be factors contributing to inadequate food intake and underweight. Stress to the parents the need to avoid obesity, since this will interfere with other aspects of rehabilitation. Avoid, however, overconcern about weight and strict diet control, which can lead to nutritional deficiency. If the child is not able to consume an adequate volume of food and underweight is manifest, recommend the use of foods of high nutrient density so that the child can consume adequate nutrients before becoming fatigued or distracted. Evaporated or dry skim milk powder can be added to some foods. Provide a vitamin and mineral supplement.

Control constipation by the judicious use of laxative foods, including prune juice, and adequate fluids.

EPILEPSY

Assessment and Intervention

▶ **Epilepsy** is a disease of the central nervous system characterized by recurrent loss of consciousness and seizures of varying intensity produced by excessive neuronal discharges in various parts of the brain.

▶ Differentiate between two categories of seizures: **petit mal seizures** produce momentary loss of consciousness, whereas the loss of consciousness is of longer duration and accompanied by convulsions in

▶ **grand mal seizures.** The disease occurs more frequently in children than in adults.

Although epilepsy may result from a variety of lesions in the central nervous system, cerebral trauma is a frequent cause. The disease itself does not affect mental ability, although drowsiness and dulling of mental function may be a side effect of the drugs used in treatment.

Drug therapy is the treatment of choice for epileptics. Drugs used are sedatives, e.g., phenobarbital, and anticonvulsants, e.g., phenytoin (Dilantin). With drug therapy, no particular diet modifications are indicated, and a normal diet for the client's age and activity is prescribed. However, prolonged use of drugs to control epilepsy is associated with a deficiency of several nutrients, especially folic acid and vitamin D. Vitamin D imbalance can lead to rickets and osteomalacia. The probability of developing these disorders increases with large doses of several drugs, little vitamin D in the diet, little exposure to sunlight, or dark skin. Dark skin allows less penetration of ultraviolet light and thus less synthesis of vitamin D in the skin. For this reason, blacks are more susceptible to rickets than are whites. Vitamin D supplementation (usually as the active form of the vitamin) may be prescribed in conjunction with the anticonvulsant therapy. Assess the folic acid content of the diet. If supplements are given, they should be administered with caution. In some cases, folic acid supplementation alleviates the deficiency, but it actually may precipitate seizures in others.

Should drug therapy be ineffective, a ketogenic

▶ diet may be tried. A **ketogenic diet,** which is high

TABLE 38–3
KETOGENIC AND ANTIKETOGENIC POTENTIAL OF CARBOHYDRATE, PROTEIN, AND FAT

Nutrient	Ketogenic Potential (% of weight)	Antiketogenic Potential (% of weight)
Carbohydrate (digestible)	0	100
Protein	~42	~ 58
Fat	90	10

in fat content and low in carbohydrate content, stimulates the production of large quantities of ketone bodies. The resulting acidosis (ketosis) has an anticonvulsant action, and restlessness, irritability, and hypermobility may be reduced in some clients with convulsive disorders. The exact mechanism of the anticonvulsant action of the diet is uncertain. The ketogenic diet is most effective in the young preschool child. Older children respond to the diet with less marked ketonuria. The energy-producing nutrients (carbohydrate, protein, and fat) are classified

▶ as **ketogenic** or **antiketogenic** depending on their ability, when oxidized, to stimulate or inhibit the production of ketones. Fatty acids and certain amino acids are precursors of ketone bodies and are thus called "ketogenic substances." In contrast, carbohydrate and those substances that are convertible to glucose in the body (the glycerol component of the fat molecule and certain amino acids) are antiketogenic. An estimate of the ketogenic and antiketogenic potential of carbohydrate, protein, and fat is shown in Table 38–3.

Basic Principles of the Diet. In the typical American diet, the percentage of kilocalories provided by fat, carbohydrate, and protein are approximately 42, 46, and 12 percent. This represents a ratio of grams of fat (ketogenic) to grams of protein and carbohydrate (antiketogenic) of approximately 1:3. To control seizures, this ketogenic:antiketogenic (K:AK) ratio is reversed. When the ratio of fatty acids to available glucose exceeds 2:1, ketosis occurs. To control seizures, however, a ratio of 3 or 4 g of fat to 1 g of protein and carbohydrate is necessary (K:AK ratio of 3:1 or 4:1). The diet is initially formulated to provide a K:AK ratio of 4:1 and usually liberalized to a 3:1 ratio once ketosis is established.

Initiate the diet after ketosis has been induced by a period of fasting for 24 to 72 hours. Fasting quickly depletes glycogen stores that would otherwise retard the onset of ketosis. During the fast, give 500 to 1000 ml of water daily. With the development of ketosis, notice that the client will not experience hunger. Some medical centers initiate the diet gradually by allowing a period of 3 to 4 days to reverse the K:AK ratio. However, a K:AK ratio of 4:1 may be used as soon as oral feeding is begun. Occasionally, it may be desirable to precede this with a 3:1 ratio for a couple of days. Assess for nausea and vomiting initially, but this disappears. Monitor the urine daily for ketones. Continual maintenance of a high level of ketosis is necessary to obtain the maximum effect. The ingestion of sugar or carbohydrate beyond the ratio required to produce ketosis can precipitate seizures.

The diet contains a high level of fat (75 percent or more of kilocalories) and a low level of carbohydrate and protein. The major part of the diet is provided by fat, such as butter, margarine, whipping cream, bacon, oils, and mayonnaise. The amount of protein-containing foods, such as meat, eggs, and cheese, is carefully regulated. Milk is omitted because of its carbohydrate content. The carbohydrate-containing foods allowed on the diet are limited to small amounts of vegetables and fruits; high-carbohydrate foods, such as bread, cereal, sugar-containing beverages, baked desserts, and concentrated sweets, are omitted.

Diet Calculation and Sample Menu. Precise calculation of the total kilocaloric level and the number of grams of fat, protein, and carbohydrate allowed for the day and for each meal is required. Meals are divided into three parts to avoid wide fluctuations in ketogenesis.

The kilocaloric level of the diet is adjusted to the rate of growth, body weight, and appetite. The protein content should provide the minimum needs for growth. The specific number of grams of fat, protein, and carbohydrate is determined by the total kilocalorie level and the particular K:AK ratio desired, e.g., 3:1 or 4:1. A simple food calculation table has been devised by Mike that lists the amount of fat, protein, and carbohydrate necessary to provide a 3:1 and 4:1 K:AK ratio for various kilocalorie levels.[11]

The nutrient values for the diet may be calculated from a food composition table (see Appendix 1) or by using exchange groupings of foods that have been especially designed for ketogenic diets.[12] The Food Exchange Lists developed for diabetic diets are

unsuitable with the traditional ketogenic diet. The nutritive value of one available exchange food groupings is shown in Table 38–4, and a sample calculation using the exchange values from Table 38–4 is illustrated in Table 38–5. The diet provides approximately 1400 kcal, 4:1 K:AK ratio, 140 g fat, 20 g protein, 15 g carbohydrate, and meals of approximately equal nutrient composition.

Implementing the Diet. The high level of accuracy required in calculating and preparing the diet and its monotony and unpalatability limit its usefulness to a small group of carefully screened clients. Since strict discipline is required for maintaining the diet, assess parents for their intelligence, willingness to cooperate, and emotional stability. An initial period of hospitalization is required for adjustment to and instruction about the diet.

Teach the parents to weigh food on a gram scale, since household measures are not sufficiently precise. However, the water consumed does not have to be weighed, and noncaloric beverages are not restricted. Stress the importance of eating meals at approximately the same time each day and of eating all food planned for the meal to avoid fluctuations in ketogenesis. Medications or other preparations that may contain carbohydrates should not be taken without consulting the physician. Provide recipes for using cream, butter, oil, and other high-fat foods and a Food Exchange List. If the child is old enough to comprehend, include him or her in the diet counseling sessions. Since alcohol tends to reduce the effectiveness of anticonvulsant medication, stress the necessity for excluding its use.

The unbalanced nature of the diet and wide deviation from customary eating patterns make it difficult to follow for extended periods. Nausea may be induced by the high fat content. The diet is severely limited in bulk, and bowel movements may occur no more frequently than every 2 to 3 days. The high level of serum cholesterol in some clients may be of concern. Be aware of the nutritional inadequacies of the diet: it provides only 65 percent of the RDA for protein and is inadequate in calcium, iron, and

TABLE 38–4
EXCHANGE FOOD GROUPING FOR KETOGENIC DIETS

Food Equivalent List	Kcal	Protein (g)	Fat (g)	Carbohydrate (g)
Meat	9	1.0	0.5	0
Vegetable A	5	0.2	0	1.0
Vegetable B	7	0.5	0	1.0
Fruit	4	0	0	1.0
Fat	45	0	5.0	0
Whipping cream (at least 32% fat)	160	1.0	17.0	1.5

(*Source:* Lasser JL, Brush MK: An improved ketogenic diet for treatment of epilepsy. *J Am Diet Assoc* 62:282, 1973.)

TABLE 38–5
SAMPLE CALCULATION FOR KETOGENIC DIET

Food	Number of Units	Household Measure	Protein (g)	Fat (g)	Carbohydrate (g)
Breakfast					
Orange juice (canned unsweetened)	2½ fruit	⅛ c			2.50
Frankfurter	6 meat	¾ frankfurter	6.0	12.0	
Butter	2 fat	2¼ tsp		10.0	
Whipping cream	1½ whipping cream	¼ c	1.5	25.5	2.25
Low-calorie wafer (Cellu brand)					
Blackberry jelly (Cellu brand)	½ miscellaneous	1 tsp	___	___	0.50
Total			7.5	47.5	5.25
Lunch					
Cheddar cheese	5 meat	⅔ oz	5.0	5.0	
Asparagus	2 B vegetable	⅛ c	1.0		2.0
Butter	3 fat	3½ tsp		15.0	
Whipping cream	1½ whipping cream	¼ c	1.5	25.5	2.25
Low-calorie wafer (Cellu brand)					
Apricot spread (Cellu brand)	½ miscellaneous	1 tsp	___	___	0.50
Total			7.5	45.5	4.75
Dinner					
Lean pork	6 meat	⅔ oz	6.0	3.0	
Carrots (cooked)	1 A vegetable	⅛ c	0.2		1.0
Applesauce (unsweetened)	1 fruit	2 tsp			1.0
Butter	4 fat	4¾ tsp		20.0	
Whipping cream	1½ whipping cream	¼ c	1.5	25.5	2.25
Low-calorie wafer (Cellu brand)					
Apricot spread (Cellu brand)	½ miscellaneous	1 tsp	___	___	0.50
Total			7.7	48.5	4.75

(Source: Based on calculations described by Lasser JL, Brush MK: An improved ketogenic diet for the treatment of epilepsy. J Am Diet Assoc 62:281, 1973.)

the B vitamins. Supplement with a multivitamin preparation, iron, and a carbohydrate-free form of calcium. Monitor growth in children on an ongoing basis.

The effectiveness of the diet in controlling seizures can be determined within approximately 6 weeks. If no improvement occurs within this period, the diet can be discontinued. If it is successful, it should be followed for a period of 1 to 3 years. After this time, the diet can be gradually returned to normal by decreasing the fat content and increasing protein and carbohydrate over a period of time. The anticonvulsant effect of diet, as with some types of medications, appears to diminish over time.

Ketogenic Diet Using Medium-chain Triglycerides. Medium-chain triglycerides (MCT) appear to be more ketogenic than equivalent amounts of traditional fats (long-chain triglycerides). Because of their rapid digestion and metabolism, less fat is required to produce ketogenesis, and because less fat is required, the diet can contain more protein and

carbohydrate and is thus more palatable. The percentage of kilocalories provided by the usual diet, the traditional ketogenic diet, and the MCT ketogenic diet are compared in Table 38–6.

In addition to being more palatable, the MCT ketogenic diet can be implemented with less rigid control of portion sizes and meal patterns. Food does not have to be weighed, household measures can be used, and the client can consume a greater variety of foods. The six Food Exchange Lists (see Appendix 2) can be used to establish the meal pattern, and again, the intake of noncaloric fluids need not be restricted. Serum cholesterol levels are lower when using the MCT diet.

Assess for gastrointestinal side effects, including nausea, diarrhea, and abdominal cramps, in clients who follow the MCT diet. These side effects may be attributed to the rapid hydrolysis of the MCT and build-up of fatty acids in the gastrointestinal system, hormonal changes, or other factors. Prevent these symptoms by advising the client to consume the MCT oil slowly and with a sufficient quantity

TABLE 38–6
PERCENTAGE OF KILOCALORIES PROVIDED BY CARBOHYDRATE, PROTEIN, AND FAT IN VARIOUS DIETS

Nutrient Factor	Usual Diet % kcal	MCT Ketogenic Diet % kcal	Traditional Ketogenic Diet % kcal (3:1 ratio)
Protein	12	10	7
Carbohydrate	46	19	6
Fat	42	11	87
MCT	0	60	0

(*Source: Figures for the percentage of the nutrients provided by the MCT diet and traditional ketogenic diet obtained from Signore JM: Ketogenic diet containing medium-chain triglycerides. J Am Diet Assoc 62:286, 1973.*)

of other food. Improperly planned MCT ketogenic diets that do not include adequate food sources of linoleic acid may lead to essential fatty acid deficiency.

For the diet to be effective in producing the desired degree of ketosis, 50 to 70 percent of the kilocalories are given as MCT. No less than 11 percent of total kilocalories are given in the form of fats exclusive of MCT.[13] The method for calculating the diet is given in Table 38–7, and Table 38–8 gives an example of the food exchanges included in a keto-

genic diet using MCT oil for a 2-year-old toddler weighing 12 kg. The MCT oil can be divided into three or four servings throughout the day, depending on the client's needs. Some children respond more favorably when a bedtime feeding containing MCT is included.

If the MCT-based ketogenic diet is being used, assist the parents in planning menus based on the six Food Exchange Lists to achieve flexibility and variety. Suggest ways of adding the MCT oil into the diet, including its incorporation into milk or

TABLE 38–7
CALCULATION OF A KETOGENIC DIET USING MCT FOR A 2-YEAR-OLD CHILD WITH EPILEPSY

1. Estimate kcal need according to the RDA:
   12 kg × 100 kcal/kg/day = 1200 kcal/day
2. Determine the amount of MCT oil to be given (50–70% of total kcal, depending on the amount needed to induce ketosis in the individual child):
   60% of 1200 = 720 kcal from MCT
   1 g MCT = 8.3 kcal
   720 ÷ 8.3 = approximately 87 g MCT (86.7)
   1 tbsp (15 ml) MCT = 14 g
   87 ÷ 14 = 6.2 tbsp (6 tbsp + ½ tsp) MCT
3. Determine kcal to be provided by foods exclusive of MCT:
   1200 − 720 = 480 kcal
4. Establish protein intake according to RDA and client's desires:
   RDA = 1.77 g/kg/day
   12 kg × 1.77 = 21 g/day
   For this child, protein content was established at 30 g/day
   30 × 4 = 120 kcal from protein
5. Estimate maximum kcal to be given in the form of carbohydrates:
   19% of 1200 = no more than 228 kcal
   228 ÷ 4 = no more than 57 g carbohydrate
6. Estimate maximum kcal to be given in the form of protein and carbohydrate combined:
   29% of 1200 = 348 kcal from protein and carbohydrate
7. Estimate minimum kcal to be given in form of fats exclusive of MCT oil:
   11% of 1200 kcal = at least 132 kcal from other fats
   15 × 9 = 135 kcal fat exclusive of MCT
8. After determining the above dietary requirements, the dietary pattern can be calculated using the Food Exchange Lists (see Table 38–8)

(*Source: Adapted from Signore JM: Ketogenic diet containing medium-chain triglycerides. J Am Diet Assoc 62:285, 1973.*)

TABLE 38–8
EXCHANGE VALUE FOR A 1200 KCAL KETOGENIC DIET USING MCT OIL FOR A 2-YEAR-OLD CHILD WITH EPILEPSY

Food	Exchanges	Carbohydrate (g)	Protein (g)	Fat (g)
Skim milk	1½	18	12	
Meat (medium fat)	2		14	10
Fruit	1	15		
Bread	1	15	2	
Vegetable	1½	8	3	
Fat	1			5
MCT oil	87 g (6 tbsp + ½ tsp)			
TOTAL		56	31	15

Total kcal from food exclusive of MCT = 483
Total kcal including MCT   = 1205

milkshakes, fruit juice, casseroles, tomato sauce, pizza, ice cream, salad dressing, and sandwich spreads. Artificial flavoring may be used as desired. However, a type that has less than 5 kcal/tsp should be used. Assess the diet for each particular child for nutritional adequacy, and supplement with vitamins and minerals as needed.

REVIEW QUESTIONS AND ACTIVITIES

1. Explain the neurologic manifestations of a below-normal blood glucose level.
2. Discuss the effects of protein deficiency on the developing nervous system and compare these effects with the neurologic manifestations of amino acid imbalances that accompany certain inborn errors of protein metabolism.
3. List 10 vitamins whose imbalance is associated with neurologic problems and compare the signs and symptoms of their imbalance.
4. Compare and contrast the neurologic manifestations of an imbalance of copper, zinc, selenium, and magnesium.
5. List four nutrition-related factors that have been implicated in the etiology of migraine.
6. Describe techniques for (a) identifying foods as migraine triggers and (b) treating migraine headache of nutritional origin.
7. Examine the postulated relationship among food additives, salicylates, and the hyperkinetic behavior syndrome.
8. What advice would you give to the mother of a hyperkinetic child who is following the K-P diet?
9. Identify the clinical manifestations of multiple sclerosis and discuss its dietary treatment.
10. Identify problems that may be encountered in feeding clients who are mentally ill, and list interventions that may be applied in assisting these clients to meet their nutritional needs.
11. Examine the use of orthomolecular psychiatry in treating neurologic disorders.
12. Identify the manifestations of Down's syndrome.
13. Recognize the two most common types of cerebral palsy and the major manifestation of each type.
14. Compare the relative kilocalorie requirements of children with Down's syndrome, spastic-type cerebral palsy, and athetoid-type cerebral palsy.
15. Identify techniques for feeding children with Down's syndrome or cerebral palsy who experience the following problems: (a) hypersensitivity to oral stimulation, (b) drooling tendency, (c) difficulty in drinking from a cup, (d) tendency of the parents to maintain the child on strained food for a prolonged period, (e) consumption of an inadequate volume of food, (f) obesity, and (g) constipation.
16. Describe techniques for introducing solid foods into the diet of children with Down's syndrome and cerebral palsy.
17. Identify the rationale for using a ketogenic diet in treating epilepsy.
18. Describe the meaning of a ketogenic:antiketogenic ratio of 3:1 and 4:1.
19. Discuss the characteristics of the traditional ketogenic diet with regard to its relative content of carbohydrate, protein, and fat and nutritional adequacy.
20. Describe the advice that you would give to the mother of a 3-year-old child who is following the traditional ketogenic diet.

21. Identify the advantages of using medium-chain triglycerides in lieu of traditional fats as the basis for the ketogenic diet.

REFERENCES

1. Wurtman RJ: Behavioral effects of nutrients. Lancet 1:1145, 1983.
2. Dubick MA: Dietary supplements and health aids—A critical evaluation. Part 2. Macronutrients and dietary fiber. J Nutr Educ 15:89–92, 1983.
3. Perkin JE, Hartje J: Diet and migraine: A review of the literature. J Am Diet Assoc 83:459, 1983.
4. Lipton MA, Mayo JP: Diet and hyperkinesis—An update. J Am Diet Assoc 83:132, 1983.
5. Feingold BJ: Why Your Child Is Hyperactive. New York, Random House, 1974.
6. The National Advisory Committee on Hyperkinesis and Food Additives: Final Report to the Nutrition Foundation. New York, Nutrition Foundation, 1975.
7. The National Advisory Committee on Hyperkinesis and Food Additives: Final Report to the Nutrition Foundation. New York, Nutrition Foundation, 1980.
8. U.S. DHHS: Defined Diets and Childhood Hyperactivity. Bethesda, Md, National Institutes of Health, Concensus Development Conference Summary, Vol 4, No. 3, 1982.
9. Pauling L: Orthomolecular psychiatry. Science 160: 265, 1968.
10. American Psychiatric Association, Task Force on Vitamin Therapy in Psychiatry: Megavitamins and Orthomolecular Therapy in Psychiatry. Washington, DC, American Psychiatric Assoc, 1973.
11. Mike EM: Practical guide and dietary management of children with seizures using the ketogenic diet. Am J Clin Nutr 17:393, 1965.
12. Lasser JL, Brush MK: An improved ketogenic diet for treatment of epilepsy. J Am Diet Assoc 62:281, 1973.
13. Signore JM: Ketogenic diet containing medium-chain triglycerides. J Am Diet Assoc 62:285, 1973.

BIBLIOGRAPHY

Bartus RT, Dean RL, Goas JA, Lippa HS: Age-related changes in passive avoidance retention: Modulation with dietary choline. Science 209:301, 1980.
Borkowski JM, Emmerich AL: Nutritional Care of the Young Child with Cerebral Palsy. Boston, Developmental Evaluation Clinic, The Children's Hospital Medical Center, 1980.
Dubick M, Rucker RB: Dietary supplements and health aids—A critical evaluation. Part 1. Vitamins and minerals. J Nutr Educ 15:47, 1983.
Finsand MJ: Caring and Cooking for the Hyperactive Child. New York, Sterling Publishing, 1981.
Goodwin JS, Goodwin JM, Garry PJ: Association between nutritional status and cognitive functioning in a healthy elderly population. JAMA 249:2917, 1983.
Hadley J: Facts about childhood hyperactivity. Children Today 13:8, 1984.
Hanington E: Diet and migraine. J Human Nutr 34:175, 1980.
Harner IC, Foiles RA: Effect of Feingold's K-P diet on a residential mentally handicapped population. J Am Diet Assoc 76:575, 1980.
Harper PH, Goyette CH, Conners CK: Nutrient intakes of children on the hyperkinesis diet. J Am Diet Assoc 73:515, 1978.
Pipes PL, Holm VA: Feeding children with Down's syndrome. J Am Diet Assoc 77:277, 1980.
Robb P: Cooking for Hyperactive and Allergic Children. Fort Wayne, Ind, Cedar Creek Publishers, 1980.
Slowie LA, Paige MS, Antel JP: Nutritional considerations in the management of patients with amyotrophic lateral sclerosis (ALS). J Am Diet Assoc 83:44, 1983.
Statement of the Resource Conference on Diet and Behavior. Nutr Rev 42:200, 1984.
Wood JL, Allison RG: Effects of consumption of choline and lecithin on neurological and cardiovascular systems. Fed Proc 41:3105, 1982.
Wurtman J: The involvement of brain serotonin in excessive carbohydrate snacking by obese carbohydrate cravers. J Am Diet Assoc 84:1004, 1984.

CHAPTER 39

Nutritional Considerations in Feeding the Mentally and Physically Handicapped

Objectives

After completion of this chapter, the student will be able to:

1. Assess the feeding skills of a brain-damaged infant.

2. Develop a teaching plan for the nutritional management of a brain-damaged infant with the following problems: (a) poor head control, (b) weak suck reflex, (c) poor control of the jaw, tongue, and lips, leading to difficulty in biting, chewing, and swallowing and a tendency to drool, and (d) a hyperactive gag reflex.

3. Develop a nursing care plan for the nutritional management of an adult client who is paralyzed in both the upper and lower extremities following a stroke.

4. Teach the mother of a 4-year-old child who exhibits abnormal mealtime behavior secondary to a neurologic disease techniques for meeting the child's nutritional needs.

Physical and mental handicaps may occur at any point in the life cycle, and handicapped clients are by no means a homogeneous group. Rather, they represent a diverse population with physical or mental abnormalities that include varying degrees of sensory or motor dysfunction or other impairment limiting normal activity, and many clients with handicapping conditions are unable to maintain a satisfactory nutritional status. Some of the most common disabling conditions are neuromuscular defects, such as those that accompany cerebral palsy, chromosomal aberrations, such as Down's syndrome, and orthopedic problems, such as spinal cord injury, leading to paralysis and other physical handicaps. Other types of handicapping conditions include blindness, arthritis, and cardiac and respiratory disorders that limit normal activity.

This chapter provides an introduction to the nutritional problems encountered by handicapped clients and intervention techniques for dealing with these problems.

ASSESSMENT

Conduct a complete assessment of the handicapped client's nutritional needs, physical capacity for meeting nutrition needs, nutritional status, and intervening psychosocial factors that affect nutritional status before developing a nursing care plan. Assess nutritional needs on the basis of age, sex, height, weight, growth history, activity level, medications used, and the extent and duration of the handicap. Bear in mind that the RDA are not specifically intended for the handicapped population. Attempt to estimate nutritional needs on an individual basis.

Assess the client's physical capacity for meeting nutritional needs in order to set realistic goals for self-feeding or a feeding training program for affected clients. Ask questions such as these: Is the problem one that involves motor activity, such as fine or gross motor movements? What muscles are involved? What muscle training or self-help devices are needed? Although different concepts must be borne in mind when dealing with adults and children, in many areas, the types of problems as well as the approaches to rehabilitation are similar.

The normal infant goes through a progressive series of motor performances in achieving the ability to feed himself or herself as a young child. The continuing ability to feed oneself throughout life depends on the normal development and maintenance of these skills. The prerequisites to self-feeding are listed in Table 39–1. Although complete mastery of each skill is not necessary for self-feeding, the achievement of self-feeding is dependent on some evidence of skill or readiness at each level. Children with handicapping conditions often have difficulty reaching the milestones, and conditions acquired in later life, such as stroke or arthritis, may result in the loss of one or more of these skills. For example, brain damage may lead to such problems as weakness of the arm and hand; muscle spasticity; impaired ability to execute precise movements (paralysis); vision, balance, and sensory disturbances; loss of intellectual acuity; and chewing problems resulting from poor tongue control and weakness of the facial muscles.

In developmentally delayed children, the development and sequence of feeding behaviors occur in the same orderly, predictable sequence as in the normal child. The chronologic age at which the developmental stage occurs, however, is unpredictable, and wide ranges are seen in both the timing and the ultimate level of function achieved.

In order to develop the best therapeutic interventions for an individualized feeding training program, give particular attention to evaluating these physical factors: (1) upper trunk and head control, (2) muscle tone, (3) the persistence of the primitive oral reflexes, (4) the response to stimulation around the mouth, (5) jaw control, (6) lip control, (7) swallowing ability, and (8) hand-to-mouth skills.

In the infant, the development of postural control and independent movement is contingent upon normal muscle tone. Moreover, the primitive oral reflexes must be integrated in order for more advanced feeding patterns to develop. Central nervous system dysfunction may lead to abnormal sensorimotor abilities, abnormal muscle tone (preventing head and trunk control), and persistence of the primitive oral reflexes. The persistence of the primitive reflexes in handicapped children may delay the progressive acquisition of self-feeding skills. For example, persistence of the rooting reflex interferes with maintenance of the appropriate head position for feeding, and a persistent suckle–swallow reflex interferes with taking food from a spoon with the lips, with cup drinking, and with chewing. In the primitive suckle–swallow reflex, the tongue normally protrudes and draws liquid back into the mouth. With retention of this reflex, oral stimulation brings tongue protrusion and consequent pushing of food from the mouth. If the bite reflex persists, there may be interference with mouthing activities, with ingesting food, with developing a more mature biting pattern, and with chewing.

Brain-injured children and adults often have an exaggerated or hyperactive gag reflex that interferes with the ingestion of solid food. The increased oral sensitivity associated with a hyperactive gag reflex may cause food to be constantly pushed from the mouth. In contrast, a hypoactive gag reflex can cause food to passively enter the esophagus or trachea and increase the danger of choking and food aspiration. Rumination is a common problem among clients with physical or mental impairment. In this situation, there is reverse peristalsis and the swallowed food is returned to the mouth, and reswallowed or evacuated.

Handicapped children may have had very little or abnormal oral experience, and, as a consequence, the face, mouth, and lips may be overly sensitive to stimulation. In the child with **hypertonia** (increased muscle tone), the muscles in the oral area will feel tight and stiff when the inside and the outside of the mouth, the tongue, and gums are touched with a finger. Conversely, with **hypotonia** (decreased muscle tone), the oral area may feel flaccid, giving little response to stimulation.

Handicapped children frequently have poor control of the jaws. At rest, the jaws may be halfway or totally open due to lack of muscle tone or hypertonicity. In some cases, the normal rotary and horizontal jaw movements may be absent. A child cannot learn to bite if he or she cannot guide jaw movements. Lack of control of the lips and tongue make it difficult to control food within the mouth. With lack of fine lip control, the ability to clear food from a spoon with the upper lip may be impaired. Furthermore, dribbling from the corners of the mouth will result from lack of lip closure around a cup. Swallowing difficulties may be encountered in those in whom the lips do not close properly but are partly or widely separated. The tongue may protrude with abnormal muscle tone as well as with a persistent suckle–swallow reflex. Hyperextension and rigidity in the legs sometimes lead to tongue thrusting. Malformation of the teeth and jaws can result from abnormal muscle tone in the tongue and oral area. An inflexible tongue whose movements tend to follow the gross movements of the jaw may result in

---

TABLE 39–1
MOTOR SKILLS NEEDED FOR SELF-FEEDING

Head and trunk control
Ability to remove food from spoon with lips
Ability to suck, bite, chew, swallow, and use the tongue
Ability to sip and take liquids
Sufficient upper extremity control to bring the hand to the mouth
Eye–hand coordination
Ability to grasp

abnormal pressure on the oral structures. Problems of sucking, swallowing, and coordination of sucking and breathing may be life threatening in some children with abnormal motor patterns and muscle tone.

The child with abnormal muscle tone associated with central nervous system dysfunction may not develop the skill of easily bringing the hand to the mouth. For example, the primitive hand grasp (palmar grasp) may persist, making the handling of food and utensils difficult. Persistence of the tonic neck reflex (also referred to as the "fencing" position) may interfere with the development of head and neck control, and thus sitting balance, as well as hand-to-mouth activities. For example, the head turns away as the child attempts to bring the hand to the mouth. Deficiency of upper trunk control and head control and abnormalities of muscle tone also impede self-feeding.

There are many reasons why nurses should be concerned about children who are not progressing adequately in developing feeding skills. One major reason is that the mouth movements used for the development of speech are based on the chewing, sucking, and swallowing movements used in eating. The child with poor physical control of eating usually does not develop the well-coordinated mouth movements necessary for clear speech.

Adults who have had a cerebrovascular accident or a severe accident resulting in quadriplegia or whose mobility is limited due to rheumatoid arthritis may have somewhat different problems from children. Most often their problems involve weakness, paralysis, or incoordination, and their task is to maintain or relearn the process of self-feeding.

Use anthropometric, dietary, biochemical, and clinical data to assess nutritional status. These assessments should be performed at routine intervals in order to evaluate the effectiveness of nutritional care. Include measurements of height, weight, and skinfolds, although these measurements may be difficult to obtain in some cases. Techniques for segmental measurement of height and for weighing nonambulatory physically handicapped clients have been published.[1] Comparison of the data obtained from standard growth charts or height–weight data has limited value in many cases because of gross anatomic defects, however. Nevertheless, serial measurements taken at regular intervals are a useful technique—the past pattern of growth and weight status aids in interpreting current status and indicates changes that occur over time. Growth retardation is common in handicapped children, and an altered activity level—excessive, as in athetoid cerebral palsy, or insufficient, as in a child or adult confined to a wheelchair—contributes to these weight abnormalities.

Include an assessment of the dietary pattern. The inability to eat an adequate diet is regarded as a major contributing factor to growth retardation and an underweight condition. While assessing dietary intake, determine factors that influence the actual amount of food consumed, such as the food consistency that is best handled, the physical effort and time required for eating, or food lost from the mouth or utensils due to poor motor control.

During the clinical assessment, observe not only for the usual clinical signs that may be reflective of malnutrition but also for the physical problems discussed above that may pose feeding problems. Observe the results of laboratory tests, such as the hemoglobin and hematocrit level, to detect further clues to malnutrition.

Assess also for psychosocial factors that may affect nutritional status. Factors that may contribute to malnutrition include inappropriate care (either oversolicitousness or neglect) or disturbed interpersonal relationships associated with the handicap. Be aware that developmentally delayed children may present the same food-related behaviors as normal children. For example, normal children exhibit clues to developmental readiness in progressing from a milk diet to table foods. Toddlers and preschool children often reduce the intake of milk and vegetables, go on food jags, and have very unpredictable appetites, and normal children as well as developmentally delayed children can control their parents by food acceptance or rejection. Since clues related to developmental readiness may be subtle and thus missed by parents, developmentally delayed children may be kept on a milk or pureed diet too long. Since many of these children have to be fed, parents may become overwhelmed by the tedious process of feeding and continue to serve soft foods that do not support developmental progress. Some parents may even deliberately limit food intake in those who cannot walk in order to limit weight gain. In these cases obesity may be prevented, but nutrient intake may be inadequate. Moreover, the child who lacks experience with foods of different tastes and textures is missing an opportunity to learn to discriminate differences. Finally, children as well as adults who have uncoordinated eating patterns may be rejected by others and thus become isolated.

INTERVENTION

Use the skills of the interdisciplinary health team in the rehabilitation of the handicapped client and work with each team member to assist the client to improve his or her feeding skills. The dentist corrects dental caries and malocclusion; occupational, physical, and speech therapists provide exercises for retraining affected muscles and self-help devices for eating; the behavior modification specialist designs techniques for changing behavior; the dietitian–nutritionist provides a diet of a consistency that can be best handled. Because handicapped clients experience so many failures in their efforts, design the nursing care plan to provide for some success, and reinforce the client for each gain, no matter how small. Many nutritional problems can be averted by anticipating potential problems based on the assessment and providing the appropriate intervention.

During the rehabilitative process, use adaptive feeding devices or even tube feeding as necessary in the initial stages. Work toward assisting the client to progress toward independent feeding skills as soon as the situation permits. A wide variety of therapeutic feeding techniques has been devised to assist the mentally and physically handicapped individual in eating as normally as possible. Continuously direct efforts toward stimulating normal motor patterning of the structures involved with eating. Feeding should not be stressful to the client. Provide a pleasant, calm atmosphere and approach changes with patience and persistence. For handicapped children, it may be desirable for the family to feed the child separately for one meal a day in order to practice the therapeutic approach. Eating with the family at other meals allows for participation in the socializing aspects of meals and for modeling of eating behavior.

Approaches for dealing with many of the eating problems encountered by physically and mentally handicapped clients are discussed below.

Difficulty in Maintaining an Upright Position for Eating

For clients who lack head and neck control or who have other alterations in feeding skills, give attention to the feeding position used. Base the position on the client's ability to hold himself or herself upright. Take precautions against aspiration of food or fluid into the lungs for clients who cannot maintain head balance. Use these guidelines for positioning affected clients for eating:

1. Maintain the client in an upright position (e.g., sitting in a chair rather than in bed) if possible. Except for small infants, lap feeding is not recommended, since with lap feeding the hands are not free to assist and there is difficulty in attaining the correct position.
2. Assist the client to hold the head in a slightly flexed position or bring it slightly forward. Tilting the head back makes swallowing difficult and creates the possibility of aspiration.
3. Assist the client to bring the shoulders and arms forward slightly, to keep the elbows level with the table top or tray surface, to keep the hips, knees, and ankles flexed to 90 degrees, and to have the feet supported on a flat surface, such as the floor, a footstool, or a footrest.
4. Use an infant seat, highchair, straight chair, cutout table, wheelchair, or armchair depending on the age and ability of the client to hold himself or herself upright. The edges of the chair may need to be padded to protect

the backs of the knees. Lapboards, when used, should have a raised edge to prevent dishes and utensils from sliding to the floor.
5. Provide stabilizers as needed for the head, trunk, arms, and feet. For example, head supports may be necessary to prevent excessive motion or to hold the head in proper position. Head rests, helmets, or specialized types of supports may be used. If supported manually, the head should be held at the base of the ears or on top rather than supported from the back. The latter technique encourages the client to push the head back against the hand. To stabilize the trunk, a binder or straps may be placed at the pelvis (rather than under the arm, which constricts the chest), or a harness or a posture jacket may be used. Trunk support can also be provided by placing pillows or blankets between the hips and sides of the chair. When the client is seated in a wheelchair, pillows may be placed under the arms.
6. Place food in front of the individual being fed. The feeder should be seated at the same level or slightly lower to prevent the client from looking up and holding the head back.

Problems with Sucking, Biting, Chewing, and Swallowing

Clients with dysfunction of the central nervous system, gross anatomic defects, or acute infections may have sucking and swallowing problems, and there may also be severe problems associated with coordinating sucking, swallowing, and breathing. Swallowing difficulties may lead to failure of the glottis to close, causing passage of some food into the trachea, reflux of food into the nose, or passage of air into the esophagus during breathing. Drooling may occur secondary to weak swallowing, uncoordinated lip movements, and inability of the anterior portion of the tongue to form a trough to hold saliva. Poor lip control may result in leakage of food while drinking, and lack of coordination between the jaws and tongue can result in ineffective swallowing.

Sucking skill involves closure of the lips around a nipple or straw and creating negative pressure inside the mouth through tongue and mouth movements. In a neurologically damaged infant with a weak sucking reflex, use tube feeding initially to maintain nutrition. Various means are used to stimulate sucking in the infant; strawdrinking (a form of sucking) may be used for a neurologically handicapped child or adult. Strawdrinking also facilitates chewing, lip closure, and swallowing by aiding in the development of the facial and oral musculature. Use these guidelines to facilitate sucking:

1. Hold the infant securely in the lap with the head in an upright position tilted slightly downward.
2. Use various stimuli to initiate sucking (e.g., tactile, extreme cold temperature, and sweet

taste). Provide tactile stimulation by touching or gently stroking the lips, the area above and below the lips, and the cheeks before and during feeding. Gently move the nipple up, down, and sideways in the mouth during feeding to stimulate the sucking reflex. Apply cold substances to the oral area (e.g., rub the lips with ice, provide a cloth soaked in cold water or milk to suck) to stimulate sucking. Sweet, cold substances, such as cold water sweetened with honey, or rubbing the gums and tongue with a Q-tip dipped in fruit, or putting honey or pureed fruit on a pacifier have been found helpful in stimulating the sucking reflex.

3. Encourage the sucking motion by manually puckering the lips around the nipple (gently pulling the lips outward or downward) and by closing the lips with the thumb and index finger after removal of the nipple or spoon from the mouth.

4. Experiment with nipples of various shapes and hole sizes to determine which is most suitable; return to a nipple with a smaller hole as sucking ability improves.

5. Encourage strawdrinking after weaning. Strawdrinking reinforces lip closure and the use of other oral structures necessary for speech. Initially, use a short straw of small diameter, with a gradual transition to longer straws of a larger diameter. For some, a plastic straw with an inch or two of rubber tubing attached to the mouth end to prevent crushing may be necessary. Feed clear liquids initially, with a gradual transition to thicker fluids. If difficulty in use of the straw is encountered, the straw may be first dipped in honey or other sweet, sticky substance; candy straws have also been used. Light pressure may be applied around the lips to hold them closed.

6. Have the client practice sucking on soda bottles and imitate noises made by the nurse or therapist, such as smacking and rounding the lips or making suction noises with the tongue.

The ability to bite, chew, and swallow is dependent on the functioning of many muscles, including those involved with the stability of the jaw, tongue control, and lip closure. Clients with cerebral palsy may have a tonic bite reflex (strong closure of the jaw following oral stimulation), leading to an impairment of the ability to release the bite and open the mouth. In brain-damaged clients, persistence of the early phasic biting reflex interferes with the development of lateral chewing movements. Moreover, dental or neuromuscular disorders may interfere with biting and chewing, bringing maldigestion. To strengthen jaw control and stimulate biting and chewing, use these techniques:

1. Apply jaw control exercises to improve oral motor patterns. Just before feeding, hold the jaw closed while stroking the outer gums on one side. After swallowing has occurred, stroke the other side of the gums. Finally, stroke the inside of the gums and the hard palate. Following this stroking, apply firm pressure with the middle finger held just under the chin while holding the thumb against the jaw joint and the index finger just between the chin and lower lip (Fig. 39-1) to block the gag reflex. If the child has poor head control, sit beside the child and apply jaw control techniques from the side (Fig. 39-1A). If the child has good head control and does not have a strong tendency to push the head back, sit in front of the child and apply jaw control techniques from the front (Fig. 39-1B).

2. Allow the client to observe and feel the jaw movements of the feeder as he or she chews.

3. Place a small amount of food between the back teeth and manually move the jaw up and down; encourage the client to feel the jaws as they move and observe the action in a mirror.

4. Stimulate chewing with the following exercises:
   a. Place a thin strip of meat or dried fruit into the mouth while holding onto one end; encourage chewing by aiding the client in the up and down movements of the jaw. Since this procedure is tiring, it should be done at the beginning of the meal before other foods are offered. Small bits of crisp food, such as dry cereal or pretzels or other foods that the child can bite off, are also effective in stimulating chewing movements. Encourage the child to bite on both the left and right sides. Chewing movements may be stimulated by placing a strip of dried fruit or rare

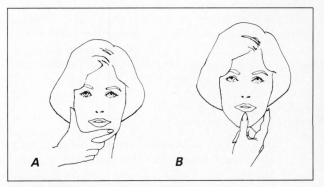

Figure 39–1
*Jaw control exercises applied from the side (**A**) and the front (**B**). (Source: Ross Laboratories: Developmental Disabilities: Mental and Physical. Columbus, Ohio, 1982, p 11.)*

cooked meat on one side of the mouth between the biting surface of the teeth in the premolar or molar area.[2]

b. Provide chewing practice with a gum bag (or a tea bag with gum inside) attached to a string; soften the gum with warm water.

c. Encourage the client to bite off small pieces of soft or semisolid food, such as small pieces of cooked potato, cooked vegetables, or banana. Place the food on the side of the mouth to stimulate chewing and to encourage the tongue to move the food to the side. Alternate the side of the mouth on which the food is placed. Each bite should be chewed and swallowed before more food is taken. With improvement, lumpy foods and others with increased texture can be gradually introduced. For example, lumpy foods, such as scrambled eggs, may stimulate munching movements of the jaw. Soft meats, such as chicken and fish, should be introduced before very chewy meats, such as beef or pork. At mealtime provide chewing practice by placing firm bits of meat or other food between the back teeth with the fingers.

5. Stimulate reflex closure of the mouth by tapping under the chin or pressing back on the chin while firmly rubbing the cheek at the back of the jaw in a rotating manner. Pressure exerted on the chin may also close the jaw.

6. Refrain from wiping food from the chin while chewing and swallowing activity is in process, since the entire mouth should be free for eating.

Lip closure and tongue movement are essential to proper eating. Lip closure is necessary to prevent drooling, and closing the lips keeps air from being sucked into the mouth and makes chewing and swallowing easier. The proper placement of the tongue while eating is within the mouth and behind the teeth; when sucking, drawn back and slightly grooved; when swallowing, moving up behind the upper teeth. Tongue thrust and the reversed swallowing wave—in which the tongue motion that normally transfers food from the front of the mouth to the throat is reversed—result in food being pushed out of the mouth.

Stimulate lip closure by:

1. Manually holding the lips together or having the client brush the lips together to close them.

2. Brushing and icing the affected muscles.

3. Using strawdrinking (with a short plastic straw or a piece of plastic tubing) to develop better lip closure and lip pressure and encouraging the client to keep the lips closed

around the straw. If this is difficult, pinch the lips closed with the thumb and forefinger.

4. Encouraging lip action, rather than the teeth, to remove food from a spoon. Use a spoon with a fairly flat bowl, pressing down on the tongue with the spoon and applying gentle but firm pressure to help the client get better action of the upper lip to remove the food from the spoon.

5. Using a cutout cup for drinking liquids (i.e., cutting out a side piece in a paper, Styrofoam, or plastic cup). The client drinks from the high side of the cup—the cutout section provides space for the child's nose when the cup is tipped. This procedure not only allows the nurse to observe the lips as the client drinks but also reduces problems associated with forcing the head into a hyperextended position.

6. Preceding each bite of food by a verbal command to "open."

7. Stimulating lip closure action by using such activities as throwing kisses, kissing the straw, and blowing bubbles. These activities should stress lip closure rather than teeth closure.

8. Creating interest in lip closure by making a paper impression of the closed lips painted with lipstick.

Neurologically handicapped individuals must be constantly reminded to use the tongue, and opportunities must be provided for this. Use these guidelines for stimulating normal tongue action and preventing tongue thrust:

1. Place food between the tip and middle of the tongue and exert a slight downward pressure on the tongue with the spoon, holding the pressure briefly. The mouth should remain closed after spoon removal until swallowing occurs. This practice not only may aid in reducing the tendency of the tongue to push food out of the mouth but also will encourage upper lip activity and chewing.

2. Place a tongue depressor under the tongue to stimulate return of the tongue to the mouth.

3. Experiment with food consistency; for example there may be less tongue thrusting in some clients when thicker foods are served than with purees.

4. Serve small spoonfuls of food, since this practice encourages a more advanced sucking or chewing movement.

5. Position the client in such a manner that the head is not pushed or tilted back. Hyperextending the head makes it easier to push foods out of the mouth with the tongue.

6. Provide muscle-building exercises for the tongue. For example, have the client use the tongue to reach for sticky foods, such as pea-

nut butter placed on the roof of the mouth or inside the cheek, or well-liked foods held 1½ to 2 inches from the mouth, or have the client try touching the upper lip, nose, or cheeks with the tongue.

Difficulty in swallowing is often due to inability of the tongue to move food or fluid to the back of the mouth. Swallowing ability frequently improves with improved sucking ability and with the ability to close the mouth and lips. Provide tube feeding initially for clients who cannot swallow. As swallowing ability develops—a test swallow of water can be used to determine whether or not aspiration is a problem and whether the client has a good cough—offer food and fluids by mouth. Although the consistency, texture, and type of food used initially will depend on individual tolerance, provide small bites of easy-to-swallow items, such as ice chips, Jello, and custards initially. Position the client properly to prevent aspiration.

Use these techniques to improve swallowing ability:

1. Use the upright, sitting position when possible. For the client in a supine position, heel-pounding results in excessive joint compression, which activates the neck muscles, including those involved with swallowing.
2. Use strawdrinking as an aid in teaching swallowing.
3. Stroke the throat gently in an upward direction toward the chin with the fingertips or a small brush, rub the cheek from the ear to the corner of the mouth, or gently pinch the larynx. Note, however, that stimulation of the laryngopharyngeal muscles of the neck tends to cause a person's head to tilt backwards, and swallowing is more difficult with the head back. Moreover, the danger of choking and aspirating food into the lungs is greatly increased. With the head held back, however, food will slide down the digestive tract if it is soft or semiliquid in consistency.
4. Use an ice collar, quickly stroke the throat with ice, or ice the sternal notch while briskly rubbing the back of the neck near the occiput with a terrycloth washcloth.
5. Encourage the client to observe and feel the movement of the throat as you swallow, to practice swallowing while looking in the mirror, and to feel the throat when he or she swallows, so as to become conscious of the act.
6. Encourage the client to take small sips or bites and swallow immediately; additional food should be delayed until swallowing is completed.
7. Refrain from allowing the client's head to tilt back when swallowing, since this encourages gulping rather than voluntary swallowing. Rather, the head should be held in a slightly downward position.
8. Observe for the consistency of food most easily swallowed. For example, following a stroke, thick liquids and semisolids (such as blenderized food thinned with milk, juice, or soup; thinned cooked cereal; soft ice cream; soupy mashed potato; pudding; applesauce; pureed or mashed fruit; gelatin; thick nectars; and thick milkshakes) are usually more easily swallowed than plain milk and clear liquids.
9. Allow the client to see and smell the food to stimulate salivary flow and prepare for swallowing. Fork-mashed food and finely cut meat may have a greater sensory appeal than purees.
10. In paralyzed clients, place food on the unaffected side of the mouth beyond the tip of the tongue.

The functioning of the jaw, tongue, and lip muscles may be improved by gentle brushing, application of ice to the affected muscles, and then providing resistance to muscle action. Techniques have been described to facilitate jaw stability, lip closure, tongue control, and swallowing in this manner.[3]

Gagging and Drooling

Normally, the gag reflex protects the esophagus and prevents food from being swallowed inappropriately or inhaled. In some brain-injured clients, the gag reflex may be exaggerated or hyperactive and may interfere with the introduction of solid foods. Hyperactivity in the oral area, particularly around the tongue, may induce vomiting when lumpy foods are swallowed. In others, the reflex may be slow or inactive; this in turn increases the danger of choking and aspiration.

If hypersensitivity exists, increase stimulation to the oral area, on a graduated basis beginning in the lower parts of the body, to increase the amount of tactile stimulation tolerated by the client. Monitor clients with an abnormal gag reflex while eating to prevent choking and aspiration. Use a progressive approach in dietary management, advancing from pureed to soft to regular foods to help correct the abnormal reflex pattern.

In some instances, gagging and vomiting may be used by developmentally delayed children as a means of manipulation or as an attention-getting device. This should be managed calmly and matter of factly. When gagging occurs, place your hands under the client's mouth and close it, being cautious not to tip the head backward. Should vomiting occur, Morris[4] suggests that the child, if he or she is old enough and physically able, should assist with the clean-up process, and no food should be given until the next meal.

Poor sucking and swallowing movements will often cause ineffective swallowing of saliva. Efforts directed toward correcting the poor jaw, tongue, and lip movements described above may reduce the problem of drooling. As the client's feeding skills improve, drooling will often spontaneously diminish. The problem of drooling throughout the day can be approached by occasionally applying firm, continuous pressure between the upper lip and nose with the finger. Some children seem to be unaware of the sensory or perceptual cues that tell them that the face is wet. In these cases, emphasize the feeling of dryness (for example, by blowing warm air on the face with a portable hair dryer) and make positive comments when swallowing occurs and the face is dry.[5] Drooling, like gagging, may be used as a manipulating device.

Adaptations for Poor Grasp

Various grasping and holding devices are available for clients with a poor grasp. Many of these can be easily constructed in the hospital or home to fit the needs of the client.

A loop handle (hand cuff with a palm pocket) can be made of wide elastic to hold eating utensils. If hand-to-mouth coordination is good, a fork may be more desirable to use than a spoon, since food can then be speared. A combination of a knife and spoon is also available, and tongs can be used. For those with hand weakness or use of only one hand, a knife with a curved blade (rocker knife) is useful for cutting meat or other food. When range of motion is limited, the handles of utensils can be lengthened or the tines of a fork or bowl of a spoon can be twisted inward. Handles on eating utensils can be built up with tape, foam rubber, sponge, wood, bicycle handgrips, or even hair curlers.

Lightweight cups, with large handles on both sides or with a handle large enough for the entire hand, should be made of nonbreakable material that does not conduct heat. Paper cups are generally unsatisfactory. Provide jackets or coasters made of a rough material, such as straw or crocheted material, for glasses. Again, the containers should be as lightweight as possible, and drinking straws and strawholders should be provided for those who have difficulty grasping and lifting a glass. For drinking straws, plastic tubing can be cut to the desired length, bent to the most satisfactory angle for approach to the mouth, and attached to the glass with a common pencil clip. For those with a poor grasp, give consideration to foods that can be eaten with the fingers, such as bite-size pieces of meat and cheese and bits of cooked or raw vegetables or fruit.

Adaptations for Poor Upper Extremity Strength

For those with poor upper extremity strength, it may be helpful to raise the height of the feeding tray or table. It is also helpful to properly position the client's body for support and balance, provide arm support, and use lightweight feeding equipment and utensils and drinking straws.

Adaptations for Poor Coordination of Hand-to-Mouth Movements

To reduce spills, anchor feeding equipment such as plates and bowls with nonslip mats or attach adhesive tape, sponge, foam rubber, or a suction cup to the bottom. Provide cup holders and straw holders to stabilize these items. Alternatively, a hole can be cut in a lapboard or tray to fit the plate, bowl, or cup, or a rim can be constructed to hold the dish. Cups with weighted bottoms and trays with depressions and straight sides help to reduce spills. Deep dishes with steep, high sides help contain the food when eating. Special utensils, such as plate guards and scoop plates, are available, but baking-type dishes available in the home may be just as satisfactory. For the visually impaired, it is useful to place meat and vegetables consistently in the same areas of the plate. If the client eats slowly, an insulated dish with a hot water compartment helps to keep the food hot.

Finger foods are appropriate when coordination is poor. Foods that stick together and to the utensils (such as mashed potatoes, applesauce, or firm pudding—not peas) may also be easy to eat. A spoon may be easier to manage than a knife and fork until coordination can be improved with retraining. Games and activities are useful to help develop hand-to-mouth and hand–eye coordination. For example, children can pour sand, play with a ball, and use push–pull objects.

IMMOBILIZATION

Assessment and Intervention

The integrity of the muscle and bone mass (i.e., a balance between accretion and withdrawal) is maintained by a combination of weight bearing and muscle tension. The muscle tension comes from the natural pull on the origin and insertion of muscles produced by normal motion and activity. Immobilization, even in healthy individuals consuming an adequate kilocalorie, protein, and calcium intake, results in a negative calcium and nitrogen balance. The nitrogen is lost primarily from the muscle mass, and the calcium from the long bones. Conditions requiring prolonged enforced immobilization, such as paralytic disorders, immobilizing injuries, and treatment with extensive body casting, result in increased losses. At full bedrest the nitrogen loss is approximately 2 to 3 g (13 to 20 g protein), and the calcium loss approximates 200 to 300 mg/day. Not only is calcium lost from the bone, but there also occurs a decrease in the intestinal absorption of calcium secondary to suppression of parathyroid hormone and 1,25-dihydroxyvitamin D_3 activity.[6,7] Observe for effects of the negative nitrogen balance, which include weight loss, skin breakdown, decubitus ulcers, and infection, and for the effects of the negative calcium balance, which include hypercalcemia, hypercalciuria, and concomitant danger of metastatic calcification of soft tissue and renal calculi. Observe the blood albumin level in immunobilized clients. Problems related to hypercalcemia are more common in clients whose serum albumin is low, since albumin normally binds calcium in the blood. Because of the accelerated rate of bone metabolism in children and adolescents, hypercalcemia may pose a particular problem when they are immobilized.

The negative nitrogen and calcium balances can be reversed by muscle activity combined, when possible, with weight bearing on the long bones. Therefore, for physically handicapped clients, provide as much physical activity as possible to improve the efficiency of the nutrient intake and offset the protein and calcium losses during the period of immobilization itself and to repair the losses during recovery.

Counteract the negative nitrogen balance in immobilized clients by increasing the dietary protein intake to approximately 1.2 g/kg of recommended body weight. Provide sufficient kilocalories to maintain body weight and adequate vitamins (particularly ascorbic acid) and minerals to offset the effects of the negative nitrogen balance and the potential for skin breakdown and infection. To maintain a dilute urine and thus limit the possibility of stone crystallization, provide a fluid intake in excess of 3000 ml daily. A urine acidifier may be prescribed by the physician.

While an increased calcium intake alone does not appreciably alter the basic pattern of bone loss, when it is given with extra phosphate, the rate of loss may be somewhat diminished.[8] However, a calcium intake in excess of the RDA may be needed to achieve a positive calcium balance during recovery. Calcium restriction is commonly recommended as a means of reducing hypercalcemia and hypercalciuria in immobilized clients. A recent study, however, noted no difference in serum or urine calcium levels with restricted and unrestricted calcium intake, suggesting that calcium restriction with its comcomitant limitations in intake of protein and other foods should not have a role in the management of immobilization-induced hypercalcemia and hypercalciuria.[9]

FLUID INTAKE AND FOOD CONSISTENCY

Assessment and Intervention
Maintenance of an adequate fluid intake in some handicapped clients, especially those who can take only sips of water slowly by mouth, can present a problem. An adequate fluid intake is essential to prevent dehydration, urinary tract infection, and for some, renal stones. Include an accurate record of fluid intake and output as a part of the nursing assessment.

Fluid requirements of normal individuals are discussed in Chapter 10. Assuming an adequate renal function, 2 to 3 liters of fluid daily are usually sufficient. When a high-protein diet or a high-protein tube feeding is administered, provide additional fluid to compensate for water lost in excreting the waste products of protein metabolism. If the client cannot help himself or herself, offer fluids frequently, or place a drinking tube attached to a plastic water bottle within easy reach. Some rehabilitation centers use a bottle filled with water that includes a 1-inch layer of water initially frozen at the bottom to keep it cool. This water bottle is attached to the bedside.

The consistency of the food served is important. Make every attempt to serve a diet that is as nearly normal in consistency as possible. Assess the client's ability to eat foods of varying textures, and adjust the consistency of the food to individual needs. For example, in the early stages following a cerebrovascular accident, the client may not be able to swallow liquids but may be able to swallow semisolids, such as thick milkshakes or thin mashed potatoes. A child with a swallowing problem may not be able to manage lumpy or dry foods initially but may be able to take liquids or soft foods. Introduce firmer textured foods that stimulate biting and chewing when the appropriate skills are mastered.

Blenderized foods are sometimes diluted with liquids, such as water and broth, to attain a consistency that the client can manage. When this practice is used, be aware that the kilocalorie and nutritive values of the food are correspondingly diminished.

ELIMINATION

Assessment and Intervention
Constipation and fecal impaction are not uncommon problems in clients with paralysis or muscle hypotonia. Contributing factors are immobility and a diet low in residue. Relieve constipation by promoting physical activity to the degree possible and providing a high-fiber diet, prune juice, and increased fluid intake. The physician may order additional elimination aids, such as wetting agents to soften the stool or bulk-producing agents if the intake of natural bulk-containing foods is impossible.

Evaluate the client's ability to control bowel and bowel function. Bowel and bladder control may be absent in clients with some types of neuromuscular disorders, such as spinal cord injury or disease. Provide a well-regulated schedule of fluid intake to aid in reestablishing bladder control (i.e., give fluid at regularly spaced intervals throughout the day, and record routinely the time, amount, and type of fluids given). With a bowel training program, give attention to both fluid and food intake. Assist the client to establish regular evacuation by following this regimen:

1. Include a diet high in fiber to stimulate peristalsis (too much fiber may cause fecal impaction, however).
2. Include adequate fluids (2 to 3 liters daily); record intake and output to establish the optimum amount.
3. Schedule a regular time for evacuation; this time may be morning or evening.
4. Ingest ½ c of prune juice (a natural laxative) approximately 12 hours before the scheduled evacuation (for morning evacuation, the juice is drunk the night before; for evening evacuation, in the morning).
5. Insert a glycerine suppository 20 to 30 minutes before the scheduled time of evacuation.
6. Evacuate the bowel while sitting in a relaxed position on the toilet or bedside commode.
7. Maintain the schedule without resorting to enemas, and record results.

WEIGHT CONTROL

Assessment and Intervention

Both excessive and inadequate weight gain may pose nutritional problems in some handicapped clients. Diminished kilocaloric requirements in those whose disability limits physical activity may result in excessive weight gain unless appropriate kilocaloric control is maintained. Excess weight in those with severe disabilities may impair progress (such as the ability to walk) and also add to the physical burden of those providing care. Obesity also adds to problems related to self-image. In contrast, inadequate weight gain may occur in those whose physical abilities limit food intake. Keep ongoing records of anthropometric data in affected clients, and when growth or weight deviations are noted, ask the client to keep a record of food intake for several days to determine the types and amounts of food consumed.

Assist clients who are overweight (10 to 20 percent above recommended weight) or obese (20 percent or more above recommended weight) to control their kilocalorie intake by such dietary measures as (1) consuming skim milk, unsweetened fruits, and such low-kilocalorie snacks as raw vegetables, (2) decreasing portion sizes, and (3) restricting fried foods, gravies, fats, and sauces to allow for gradual weight reduction. Develop a diet plan for adults that allows for a loss of 1 to 2 lb per week. For children, strive to limit the rate of weight gain rather than achieve a weight loss per se. Severe kilocalorie restriction in children may result in retarded growth.

Assist the client to plan daily physical activities compatible with the level of functioning. Participation in games may serve as a replacement for eating to relieve boredom. Reinforce positive patterns of weight control with activities, not food, and provide continuing support for weight control efforts. Counsel all persons who provide food for the client about the weight control program. If the client is under-

weight, advise him or her to increase the frequency of eating and to use high-calorie, high-nutrient snacks, such as milkshakes and peanut butter and dried fruit on crackers, to increase kilocalorie intake.

ABNORMAL BEHAVIOR PATTERNS

Assessment and Intervention

Evaluate for abnormal behavior patterns that may alter food intake in children with neurologic damage or other types of developmental delays. Appetite disorders (including lack of appetite, excessive appetite, and bizarre eating patterns, including pica), hypoactivity, limited attention span at meals, and disruptive mealtime behavior are examples of these behavior patterns.

Some children with central nervous system damage have no appetite. The volume of food consumed is limited, since these children never express hunger. Parents become discouraged by the child's lack of response to their feeding efforts, which may even involve setting an alarm clock to remind them to feed, and, as a result, continued motivation for helping the child consume food may be adversely affected. A lack of positive interplay between parent and child adversely affects the child's motivation to consume food as well. Counsel parents of these clients on a continued basis regarding the child's need for food. Advise them to serve small portions of food and to provide high-nutrient snacks at intervals that do not interfere with the appetite for meals. Suggest that a quiet period be planned before meals and that parents give reinforcement for food acceptance. Eating with the child will provide a role model.

If the client has hypothalamic damage, look for the opposite effect—an insatiable appetite. Children thus affected gorge, steal food, and even eat pet food. Behavior modification techniques are not effective in the control of this type of food behavior. To prevent obesity, extreme measures, such as locking the refrigerator and cupboards, are sometimes necessary.[10]

Developmentally delayed children may demonstrate behavior patterns not totally dissimilar to those of some normal children, such as refusing specific groups of food or refusing to eat table food. When major food groups, such as vegetables and fruits, are rejected, encourage the parents to continue to expose the child to small amounts of the food. Suggest that the parents act as role models by letting the child see them eating the food. With acceptance of the food, suggest that reinforcement be provided in a positive manner.

When a child insists on eating strained food and refuses table food, make an assessment to determine whether a critical stage in the development of the progression of feeding has been ignored, whether hypersensitivity exists in the oral area or in the gag reflex, or whether the correct feeding position is being used. To initiate the use of table foods, Morris[11] suggests eliminating prepared baby foods from the diet and using table foods blenderized to the consistency of strained baby food. Encourage the parents to expose the child to as many different tastes as possible over a period of several weeks. As the new foods are accepted, advise the parents to begin to introduce thicker foods, starting first with foods that do not contain lumps (for example, foods can be thickened with mashed potatoes or cereal) and then gradually increasing the lumpiness of the diet.

If the child is hypoactive, determine if food consumption is used as a method of relieving boredom. If this is the case, suggest alternatives to food to keep the child occupied. On the other hand, the limited attention span of hyperactive children often results in inadequate intake at mealtime. Suggest that small, frequent feedings be provided for these children to maintain their nutrient intake.

Disruptive mealtime behavior, such as throwing food or utensils, spitting out food, stuffing the mouth, or whining, often serves as an attention-getting device for the child. When this occurs, encourage the parents to approach this behavior in a consistent manner. Aid the parents to eliminate the behavior by ignoring it, removing the child from the situation and withholding food (except fluids) until the next meal, and providing positive reinforcement for all appropriate mealtime behavior.[12]

REVIEW QUESTIONS AND ACTIVITIES

1. Identify the seven prerequisites to self-feeding.
2. Compare normal and developmentally delayed children with regard to the development of food-related behaviors.
3. Describe the significance of evaluating the following physical factors in an infant with neurologic damage: (a) upper trunk and head control, (b) muscle tone, (c) presence of the primitive reflexes (rooting, suckle–swallow, biting, gag), (d) response to stimulations around the mouth, (e) jaw, lip, and tongue control, (f) swallowing ability, and (g) hand-to-mouth skills.
4. Identify the correct position of the head when it is held in the normal eating position.
5. During a meal hour, visit the pediatric ward of a hospital or visit a hospital that specializes in caring for children with handicaps. Observe the various devices that are used to position older infants who have difficulty in maintaining an upright position for eating.
6. *Case study:* Your client today is a 6-month-old infant with a neurologic disorder that has resulted in a weak sucking reflex, difficulty in biting, chewing, and swallowing, a tendency to drool, and a hypoactive gag reflex.
   a. What tactile stimulation could you use to stimulate sucking?
   b. What other types of stimuli or manipulations could be used to stimulate sucking?
   c. Describe the role of jaw control, lip closure, and tongue movements in the eating process.
   d. How can poor jaw control, inability to close the lips, and improper placement of the tongue in the mouth create problems related to biting, chewing, swallowing, and drooling?
   e. Describe techniques for strengthening jaw control, lip closure, and proper tongue movements.
   f. What techniques could you use to stimulate swallowing?
   g. What effect would improved oral motor patterns have on drooling?
   h. What hazard related to feeding does the hypoactive gag reflex pose?
   i. Compare the problems related to a hypoactive gag reflex with those related to a hyperactive gag reflex.
7. *Case study:* Mr. A, a 68-year-old client has been hospitalized for a long period of time following a stroke. He has lost sensation and movement in both the upper and lower extremities, including loss of bowel and bladder control. He is slowly recovering some muscle strength, although he still has a poor hand grasp, poor strength in the upper extremities, and poor hand-to-mouth coordination. Initially he was given a tube feeding but he is now ready to progress to oral food intake.
   a. Explain the effects of immobilization on Mr. A's metabolism and its dietary implications.
   b. Describe the consistency of food that should be used for Mr. A's initial feedings, and state the rationale for using foods of this type.
   c. Discuss techniques that could be used to stimulate swallowing.
   d. Visit the occupational therapy department and discuss with the therapist adaptations that can be made in feeding equipment (utensils, cups, glasses, plates, and bowls) to facilitate self-feeding.
   e. When foods of differing textures can be tolerated, how should these foods be served in order to facilitate self-feeding?
   f. Discuss techniques that can be used to assure that Mr. A's fluid intake is adequate.
   g. Describe the components of a bowel and bladder training program.
   h. What weight control problems would you anticipate that Mr. A might have over a period of time?

8. Bruce, a 4-year-old boy, had brain damage at birth. His mother brings to your attention that he prefers strained food, refuses table food, refuses vegetables, and is very disruptive at mealtimes. What advice would you give to Bruce's mother for dealing with these problems?

REFERENCES

1. Smith MA, Connolly B, McFadden S, et al.: Feeding Management of a Child With a Handicap: A Guide for Professionals. Memphis, Tenn, University of Tennessee Center for the Health Sciences, Child Development Center, 1982, pp 25–26.
2. Morris SE: Program Guidelines for Children with Feeding Problems. Edison, NJ, Childcraft Education Corporation, 1977, pp. 34–35.
3. Smith MAH, ed: Feeding the Handicapped Child. Memphis, Tenn, University of Tennessee Child Development Center, 1976, pp 48–49.
4. Morris SE, op cit, p 12.
5. Morris SE, op cit, pp 38–39.
6. Heaney RP, Gallager JC, Johnston CC, et al.: Calcium nutrition and bone health in the elderly. Am J Clin Nutr 36:993, 1982.
7. Stewart AF, Adler M, Byers CM, et al.: Calcium homeostasis in immobilization: An example of resorptive hypercalciuria. N Engl J Med 306:1136, 1982.
8. Heany RP, Gallager JC, Johnston CC, et al., op cit, p 993.
9. Stewart AF, Adler M, Byers CM, et al., op cit, p 1137.
10. Pipes PL: Nutrition in Infancy and Childhood, ed 2. St. Louis, Mo, CV Mosby, 1981, p 285.
11. Morris SE, op cit, pp 4–5.
12. Pipes PL, op cit, pp 285–286.

BIBLIOGRAPHY

Ashley BM, Blackburn GL: Nutritional needs of a paraplegic patient. JAMA 248:2180, 1982.
Caliendo MA, Booth G, Moser P: Iron intakes and serum ferritin levels in developmentally delayed children. J Am Diet Assoc 81:401, 1982.
Furse A, Levine E: Food, Nutrition and the Disabled: An Annotated Bibliography. Ontario, Canada, Library Publications Office, Ryerson Polytechnical Institute, 1981.
Nutrition Handbook for Caretakers of the Handicapped Child. Baltimore, John F. Kennedy Institute for Handicapped Children, 1981.
Rogers JC: Assistive devices: Aids to functional independence. Am Health Care Assoc J 9:31, 1983.
Roueche JR: An Assessment and Management Program for Adults. Minneapolis, Sister Kenney Institute, 1981.
Shinnar SE: Use of adaptive equipment in feeding the elderly. J Am Diet Assoc 83:321, 1983.
Springer NS: Nutrition Casebook on Developmental Disorders. Syracuse, NY, Syracuse University Press, 1982.
Tilton CN Maloof M: Diagnosing the problems in stroke. Am J Nurs 82:596, 1982.
Warpula D: Meeting the nutritional needs of the mentally retarded. J Can Diet Assoc 42:310, 1981.

CLIENT RESOURCES

Adaptations and Techniques for the Disabled Homemaker. Minneapolis, Sister Kenney Institute.
Do It Yourself Again—Self-Help Devices for the Stroke Patient. Dallas, Texas, American Heart Association.
Klinger JL, with the Institute of Rehabilitation Medicine, New York Medical Center and Campbell Soup Co: Mealtime Manual for People with Disabilities and the Aging, ed 2. Camden NJ, Campbell Soup Co., 1978.

Appendices

APPENDIX 1
NUTRITIVE VALUES OF THE EDIBLE PART OF FOODS

					Fatty Acids		

Item No.	Foods, Approximate Measures, Units, and Weight (edible part unless footnotes indicate otherwise)	(g)	Water (%)	Food Energy (kcal)	Protein (g)	Fat (g)	Saturated (total) (g)	Oleic (g)	Linoleic (g)
	Dairy Products (Cheese, Cream, Imitation Cream, Milk; Related Products)								
	Butter (see Fats, oils; related products, items 103–108)								
	Cheese								
	Natural								
1	Blue	1 oz	28	42	100	6	8	5.3	1.9	0.2
2	Camembert (3 wedges per 4 oz container)	1 wedge	38	52	115	8	9	5.8	2.2	0.2
	Cheddar								
3	Cut pieces	1 oz	28	37	115	7	9	6.1	2.1	0.2
4		1 in³	17.2	37	70	4	6	3.7	1.3	0.1
5	Shredded	1 c	113	37	455	28	37	24.2	8.5	0.7
	Cottage (curd not pressed down)								
	Creamed (cottage cheese, 4% fat)								
6	Large curd	1 c	225	79	235	28	10	6.4	2.4	0.2
7	Small curd	1 c	210	79	220	26	9	6.0	2.2	0.2
8	Low fat (2%)	1 c	226	79	205	31	4	2.8	1.0	0.1
9	Low fat (1%)	1 c	226	82	165	28	2	1.5	0.5	0.1
10	Uncreamed (cottage cheese dry curd, less than ½% cottage fat)	1 c	145	80	125	25	1	0.4	0.1	trace
11	Cream	1 oz	28	54	100	2	10	6.2	2.4	0.2
	Mozzarella, made with								
12	Whole milk	1 oz	28	48	90	6	7	4.4	1.7	0.2
13	Part skim milk	1 oz	28	49	80	8	5	3.1	1.2	0.1
	Parmesan, grated								
14	Cup, not pressed down	1 c	100	18	455	42	30	19.1	7.7	0.3
15	Tbsp	1 tbsp	5	18	25	2	2	1.0	0.4	trace
16	Oz	1 oz	28	18	130	12	9	5.4	2.2	0.1
17	Provolone	1 oz	28	41	100	7	8	4.8	1.7	0.1
	Ricotta, made with								
18	Whole milk	1 c	246	72	430	28	32	20.4	7.1	0.7
19	Part skim milk	1 c	246	74	340	28	19	12.1	4.7	0.5
20	Romano	1 oz	28	31	110	9	8	—	—	—
21	Swiss	1 oz	28	37	105	8	8	5.0	1.7	0.2
	Pasteurized process cheese								
22	American	1 oz	28	39	105	6	9	5.6	2.1	0.2
23	Swiss	1 oz	28	42	95	7	7	4.5	1.7	0.1
24	Pasteurized process cheese food, American	1 oz	28	43	95	6	7	4.4	1.7	0.1
25	Pasteurized process cheese spread, American	1 oz	28	48	80	5	6	3.8	1.5	0.1
	Cream, sweet								
26	Half-and-half (cream and milk)	1 c	242	81	315	7	28	17.3	7.0	0.6
27		1 tbsp	15	81	20	trace	2	1.1	0.4	trace
28	Light, coffee, or table	1 c	240	74	470	6	46	28.8	11.7	1.0
29		1 tbsp	15	74	30	trace	3	1.8	0.7	0.1

(Dashes (—) denote lack of reliable data for a constituent believed to be present in measurable amount)
(Source: U.S. Department of Agriculture: Nutritive Value of Foods. Home and Garden Bulletin No. 72, Washington, DC, U.S. Government Printing Office, 1981.)

Carbohydrate (g)	Calcium (mg)	Phosphorus (mg)	Iron (mg)	Potassium (mg)	Vitamin A Value (IU)	Thiamine (mg)	Riboflavin (mg)	Niacin (mg)	Ascorbic Acid (mg)
1	150	110	0.1	73	200	0.01	0.11	0.3	0
trace	147	132	0.1	71	350	0.01	0.19	0.2	0
trace	204	145	0.2	28	300	0.01	0.11	trace	0
trace	124	88	0.1	17	180	trace	0.06	trace	0
1	815	579	0.8	111	1200	0.03	0.42	0.1	0
6	135	297	0.3	190	370	0.05	0.37	0.3	trace
6	126	277	0.3	177	340	0.04	0.34	0.3	trace
8	155	340	0.4	217	160	0.05	0.42	0.3	trace
6	138	302	0.3	193	80	0.05	0.37	0.3	trace
3	46	151	0.3	47	40	0.04	0.21	0.2	0
1	23	30	0.3	34	400	trace	0.06	trace	0
1	163	117	0.1	21	260	trace	0.08	trace	0
1	207	149	0.1	27	180	0.01	0.10	trace	0
4	1376	807	1.0	107	700	0.05	0.39	0.3	0
trace	69	40	trace	5	40	trace	0.02	trace	0
1	390	229	0.3	30	200	0.01	0.11	0.1	0
1	214	141	0.1	39	230	0.01	0.09	trace	0
7	509	389	0.9	257	1210	0.03	0.48	0.3	0
13	669	449	1.1	308	1060	0.05	0.46	0.2	0
1	302	215	—	—	160	—	0.11	trace	0
1	272	171	trace	31	240	0.01	0.10	trace	0
trace	174	211	0.1	46	340	0.01	0.10	trace	0
1	219	216	0.2	61	230	trace	0.08	trace	0
2	163	130	0.2	79	260	0.01	0.13	trace	0
2	159	202	0.1	69	220	0.01	0.12	trace	0
10	254	230	0.2	314	260	0.08	0.36	0.2	2
1	16	14	trace	19	20	0.01	0.02	trace	trace
9	231	192	0.1	292	1730	0.08	0.36	0.1	2
1	14	12	trace	18	110	trace	0.02	trace	trace

(continued)

Item No.	Foods, Approximate Measures, Units, and Weight (edible part unless footnotes indicate otherwise)		(g)	Water (%)	Food Energy (kcal)	Protein (g)	Fat (g)	Fatty Acids		
								Saturated (total) (g)	Unsaturated	
									Oleic (g)	Linoleic (g)
	Dairy Products (Cheese, Cream, Imitation Cream, Milk; Related Products)—Cont									
	Cream—Cont									
	Whipping, unwhipped (volume about double when whipped)									
30	Light	1 c	239	64	700	5	74	46.2	18.3	1.5
31		1 tbsp	15	64	45	trace	5	2.9	1.1	0.1
32	Heavy	1 c	238	58	820	5	88	54.8	22.2	2.0
33		1 tbsp	15	58	80	trace	6	3.5	1.4	0.1
34	Whipped topping (pressurized)	1 c	60	61	155	2	13	8.3	3.4	0.3
35		1 tbsp	3	61	10	trace	1	0.4	0.2	trace
36	Cream, sour	1 c	230	71	495	7	48	30.0	12.1	1.1
37		1 tbsp	12	71	25	trace	3	1.6	0.6	0.1
	Cream products, imitation (made with vegetable fat)									
	Sweet									
	Creamers									
38	Liquid (frozen)	1 c	245	77	335	2	24	22.8	0.3	trace
39		1 tbsp	15	77	20	trace	1	1.4	trace	0
40	Powdered	1 c	94	2	515	5	33	30.6	0.9	trace
41		1 tsp	2	2	10	trace	1	0.7	trace	0
	Whipped topping									
42	Frozen	1 c	75	50	240	1	19	16.3	1.0	0.2
43		1 tbsp	4	50	15	trace	1	0.9	0.1	trace
44	Powdered, made with whole milk	1 c	80	67	150	3	10	8.5	0.6	0.1
45		1 tbsp	4	67	10	trace	trace	0.4	trace	trace
46	Pressurized	1 c	70	60	185	1	16	13.2	1.4	0.2
47		1 tbsp	4	60	10	trace	1	0.8	0.1	trace
48	Sour dressing (imitation sour cream) made with nonfat dry milk	1 c	235	75	415	8	39	31.2	4.4	1.1
49		1 tbsp	12	75	20	trace	2	1.6	0.2	0.1
	Ice cream (see Milk desserts, frozen, items 75–80)									
	Ice milk (see Milk desserts, frozen, items 81–83)									
	Milk									
	Fluid									
50	Whole (3.3% fat)	1 c	244	88	150	8	8	5.1	2.1	0.2
	Lowfat (2%)									
51	No milk solids added	1 c	244	89	120	8	5	2.9	1.2	0.1
	Milk solids added									
52	Label claim less than 10 g of protein per c	1 c	245	89	125	9	5	2.9	1.2	0.1

[1] Vitamin A value is largely from beta-carotene used for coloring. Riboflavin value for items 40–41 apply to products with added riboflavin.
[2] Applies to product without added vitamin A. With added vitamin A, value is 500 International Units (IU).

Carbohydrate (g)	Calcium (mg)	Phosphorus (mg)	Iron (mg)	Potassium (mg)	Vitamin A Value (IU)	Thiamine (mg)	Riboflavin (mg)	Niacin (mg)	Ascorbic Acid (mg)
7	166	146	0.1	231	2690	0.06	0.30	0.1	1
trace	10	9	trace	15	170	trace	0.02	trace	trace
7	154	149	0.1	179	3500	0.05	0.26	0.1	1
trace	10	9	trace	11	220	trace	0.02	trace	trace
7	61	54	trace	88	550	0.02	0.04	trace	0
trace	3	3	trace	4	30	trace	trace	trace	0
10	268	195	0.1	331	1820	0.08	0.34	0.2	2
1	14	10	trace	17	90	trace	0.02	trace	trace
28	23	157	0.1	467	220[1]	0	0	0	0
2	1	10	trace	29	10[1]	0	0	0	0
52	21	397	0.1	763	190[1]	0	0.16[1]	0	0
1	trace	8	trace	16	trace[1]	0	trace[1]	0	0
17	5	6	0.1	14	650[1]	0	0	0	0
1	trace	trace	trace	1	30[1]	0	0	0	0
13	72	69	trace	121	290[1]	0.02	0.09	trace	1
1	4	3	trace	6	10[1]	trace	trace	trace	trace
11	4	13	trace	13	330[1]	0	0	0	0
1	trace	1	trace	1	20[1]	0	0	0	0
11	266	205	0.1	380	20[1]	0.09	0.38	0.2	2
1	14	10	trace	19	trace[1]	0.01	0.02	trace	trace
11	291	228	0.1	370	310[2]	0.09	0.40	0.2	2
12	297	232	0.1	377	500	0.10	0.40	0.2	2
12	313	245	0.1	397	500	0.10	0.42	0.2	2

(continued)

Item No.	Foods, Approximate Measures, Units, and Weight (edible part unless footnotes indicate otherwise)		(g)	Water (%)	Food Energy (kcal)	Protein (g)	Fat (g)	Saturated (total) (g)	Unsaturated	
									Oleic (g)	Linoleic (g)
	Dairy Products (Cheese, Cream, Imitation Cream, Milk; Related Products)—Cont									
	Milk—Cont									
	Fluid—Cont									
53	Label claim 10 or more g of protein per C (protein fortified)	1 c	246	88	135	10	5	3.0	1.2	0.1
	Lowfat (1%)									
54	No milk solids added	1 c	244	90	100	8	3	1.6	0.7	0.1
	Milk solids added									
55	Label claim less than 10 g of protein per c	1 c	245	90	105	9	2	1.5	0.6	0.1
56	Label claim 10 or more g of protein per c (protein fortified)	1 c	246	89	120	10	3	1.8	0.7	0.1
	Nonfat (skim)									
57	No milk solids added	1 c	245	91	85	8	trace	0.3	0.1	trace
	Milk solids added									
58	Label claim less than 10 g of protein per c	1 c	245	90	90	9	1	0.4	0.1	trace
59	Label claim 10 or more g of protein per c (protein fortified)	1 c	246	89	100	10	1	0.4	0.1	trace
60	Buttermilk	1 c	245	90	100	8	2	1.3	0.5	trace
	Canned									
	Evaporated, unsweetened									
61	Whole milk	1 c	252	74	340	17	19	11.6	5.3	0.4
62	Skim milk	1 c	255	79	200	19	1	0.3	0.1	trace
63	Sweetened, condensed	1 c	306	27	980	24	27	16.8	6.7	0.7
	Dried									
64	Buttermilk	1 c	120	3	465	41	7	4.3	1.7	0.2
	Nonfat instant									
65	Envelope, net wt, 3.2 oz[5]	1 envelope	91	4	325	32	1	0.4	0.1	trace
66	Cup[7]	1 c	68	4	245	24	trace	0.3	0.1	trace
	Milk beverages									
	Chocolate milk (commercial)									
67	Regular	1 c	250	82	210	8	8	5.3	2.2	0.2
68	Lowfat (2%)	1 c	250	84	180	8	5	3.1	1.3	0.1
69	Lowfat (1%)	1 c	250	85	160	8	3	1.5	0.7	0.1

[3] Applies to product without vitamin A added.
[4] Applies to product with added vitamin A. Without added vitamin A, value is 20 IU.
[5] Yields 1 qt of fluid milk when reconstituted according to package directions.
[6] Applies to product with added vitamin A.
[7] Weight applies to product with label claim of 1⅓ c equal 3.2 oz.

Carbohydrate (g)	Calcium (mg)	Phosphorus (mg)	Iron (mg)	Potassium (mg)	Vitamin A Value (IU)	Thiamine (mg)	Riboflavin (mg)	Niacin (mg)	Ascorbic Acid (mg)
14	352	276	0.1	447	500	0.11	0.48	0.2	3
12	300	235	0.1	381	500	0.10	0.41	0.2	2
12	313	245	0.1	397	500	0.10	0.42	0.2	2
14	349	273	0.1	444	500	0.11	0.47	0.2	3
12	302	247	0.1	406	500	0.09	0.34	0.2	2
12	316	255	0.1	418	500	0.10	0.43	0.2	2
14	352	275	0.1	446	500	0.11	0.48	0.2	3
12	285	219	0.1	371	80[3]	0.08	0.38	0.1	2
25	657	510	0.5	764	610[3]	0.12	0.80	0.5	5
29	738	497	0.7	845	1000[4]	0.11	0.79	0.4	3
166	868	775	0.6	1136	1000[3]	0.28	1.27	0.6	8
59	1421	1119	0.4	1910	260[3]	0.47	1.90	1.1	7
47	1120	896	0.3	1552	2160[6]	0.38	1.59	0.8	5
35	837	670	0.2	1160	1610[6]	0.28	1.19	0.6	4
26	280	251	0.6	417	300[3]	0.09	0.41	0.3	2
26	284	254	0.6	442	500	0.10	0.42	0.3	2
26	287	257	0.6	426	500	0.10	0.40	0.2	2

(continued)

| | | | | | | | Fatty Acids | | |
| | | | | | | | Saturated | Unsaturated | |
Item No.	Foods, Approximate Measures, Units, and Weight (edible part unless footnotes indicate otherwise)	(g)	Water (%)	Food Energy (kcal)	Protein (g)	Fat (g)	(total) (g)	Oleic (g)	Linoleic (g)
	Dairy Products (Cheese, Cream, Imitation Cream, Milk; Related Products)—Cont								
	Milk beverages—Cont								
70	Eggnog (commercial)	1 c	254	74	340	10	19	11.3	5.0	0.6
	Malted milk, home-prepared with 1 c of whole milk and 2 to 3 heaping tsp of malted milk powder (about ¾ oz)									
71	Chocolate	1 c of milk plus ¾ oz of powder	265	81	235	9	9	5.5	—	—
72	Natural	1 c of milk plus ¾ oz of powder	265	81	235	11	10	6.0	—	—
	Shakes, thick[8]									
73	Chocolate, container, net wt, 10.6 oz	1 container	300	72	355	9	8	5.0	2.0	0.2
74	Vanilla, container, net wt, 11 oz	1 container	313	74	350	12	9	5.9	2.4	0.2
	Milk desserts, frozen									
	Ice cream									
	Regular (about 11% fat)									
75	Hardened	½ gal	1064	61	2155	38	115	71.3	28.8	2.6
76		1 c	133	61	270	5	14	8.9	3.6	0.3
77		3-fl oz container	50	61	100	2	5	3.4	1.4	0.1
78	Soft serve (frozen custard)	1 c	173	60	375	7	23	13.5	5.9	0.6
79	Rich (about 16% fat), hardened	½ gal	1188	59	2805	33	190	118.3	47.8	4.3
80		1 c	148	59	350	4	24	14.7	6.0	0.5
	Ice milk									
81	Hardened (about 4.3% fat)	½ gal	1048	69	1470	41	45	28.1	11.3	1.0
82		1 c	131	69	185	5	6	3.5	1.4	0.1
83	Soft serve (about 2.6% fat)	1 c	175	70	225	8	5	2.9	1.2	0.1
84	Sherbet (about 2% fat)	½ gal	1542	66	2160	17	31	19.0	7.7	0.7
85	Milk desserts, other	1 c	193	66	270	2	4	2.4	1.0	0.1
86	Custard, baked	1 c	265	77	305	14	15	6.8	5.4	0.7
	Puddings									
	From home recipe									
	Starch base									
87	Chocolate	1 c	260	66	385	8	12	7.6	3.3	0.3
88	Vanilla (blancmange)	1 c	255	76	285	9	10	6.2	2.5	0.2

(Dashes (—) denote lack of reliable data for a constituent believed to be present in measurable amount)

[8] Applies to products made from thick shake mixes and that do not contain added ice cream. Products made from milkshake mixes are higher in fat and usually contain added ice cream.

Carbohydrate (g)	Calcium (mg)	Phosphorus (mg)	Iron (mg)	Potassium (mg)	Vitamin A Value (IU)	Thiamine (mg)	Riboflavin (mg)	Niacin (mg)	Ascorbic Acid (mg)
34	330	278	0.5	420	890	0.09	0.48	0.3	4
29	304	265	0.5	500	330	0.14	0.43	0.7	2
27	347	307	0.3	529	380	0.20	0.54	1.3	2
63	396	378	0.9	672	260	0.14	0.67	0.4	0
56	457	361	0.3	572	360	0.09	0.61	0.5	0
254	1406	1075	1.0	2052	4340	0.42	2.63	1.1	6
32	176	134	0.1	257	540	0.05	0.33	0.1	1
12	66	51	trace	96	200	0.02	0.12	0.1	trace
38	236	199	0.4	338	790	0.08	0.45	0.2	1
256	1213	927	0.8	1771	7200	0.36	2.27	0.9	5
32	151	115	0.1	221	900	0.04	0.28	0.1	1
232	1409	1035	1.5	2117	1710	0.61	2.78	0.9	6
29	176	129	0.1	265	210	0.08	0.35	0.1	1
38	274	202	0.3	412	180	0.12	0.54	0.2	1
469	827	594	2.5	1585	1480	0.26	0.71	1.0	31
59	103	74	0.3	198	190	0.03	0.09	0.1	4
29	297	310	1.1	387	930	0.11	0.50	0.3	1
67	250	255	1.3	445	390	0.05	0.36	0.3	1
41	298	232	trace	352	410	0.08	0.41	0.3	2

(continued)

Item No.	Foods, Approximate Measures, Units, and Weight (edible part unless footnotes indicate otherwise)		(g)	Water (%)	Food Energy (kcal)	Protein (g)	Fat (g)	Saturated (total) (g)	Oleic (g)	Linoleic (g)
								Fatty Acids		
								Saturated	**Unsaturated**	
								(total) (g)	Oleic (g)	Linoleic (g)

Item No.	Foods, Approximate Measures, Units, and Weight (edible part unless footnotes indicate otherwise)	(g)	Water (%)	Food Energy (kcal)	Protein (g)	Fat (g)	Saturated (total) (g)	Oleic (g)	Linoleic (g)
	Dairy Products (Cheese, Cream, Imitation Cream, Milk; Related Products)—Cont								
	Milk desserts, other—Cont								
89	Tapioca cream	1 c	165	72	220	8	8	4.1	2.5	0.5
	From mix (chocolate) and milk								
90	Regular (cooked)	1 c	260	70	320	9	8	4.3	2.6	0.2
91	Instant	1 c	260	69	325	8	7	3.6	2.2	0.3
	Yogurt								
	With added milk solids								
	Made with lowfat milk								
92	Fruit-flavored[9]	1 container, net wt, 8 oz	227	75	230	10	3	1.8	0.6	0.1
93	Plain	1 container, net wt, 8 oz	227	85	145	12	4	2.3	0.8	0.1
94	Made with nonfat milk	1 container, net wt, 8 oz	227	85	125	13	trace	0.3	0.1	trace
	Without added milk solids								
95	Made with whole milk	1 container, net wt, 8 oz	227	88	140	8	7	4.8	1.7	0.1
	Eggs								
	Eggs, large (24 oz per dozen)								
	Raw								
96	Whole, without shell	1 egg	50	75	80	6	6	1.7	2.0	0.6
97	White	1 white	33	88	15	3	trace	0	0	0
98	Yolk	1 yolk	17	49	65	3	6	1.7	2.1	0.6
	Cooked								
99	Fried in butter	1 egg	46	72	85	5	6	2.4	2.2	0.6
100	Hard-cooked, shell removed	1 egg	50	75	80	6	6	1.7	2.0	0.6
101	Poached	1 egg	50	74	80	6	6	1.7	2.0	0.6
102	Scrambled (milk added) in butter. Also omelet	1 egg	64	76	95	6	7	2.8	2.3	0.6
	Fats, Oils; Related Products								
	Butter								
	Regular (1 brick or 4 sticks per lb)								
103	Stick (½ c)	1 stick	113	16	815	1	92	57.3	23.1	2.1
104	Tablespoon (about ⅛ stick)	1 tbsp	14	16	100	trace	12	7.2	2.9	0.3

[9] Content of fat, vitamin A, and carbohydrate varies. Consult the label when precise values are needed for special diets.
[10] Applies to product made with milk containing no added vitamin A.
[11] Based on year-round average.

Carbohydrate (g)	Calcium (mg)	Phosphorus (mg)	Iron (mg)	Potassium (mg)	Vitamin A Value (IU)	Thiamine (mg)	Riboflavin (mg)	Niacin (mg)	Ascorbic Acid (mg)
28	173	180	0.7	223	480	0.07	0.30	0.2	2
59	265	247	0.8	354	340	0.05	0.39	0.3	2
63	374	237	1.3	335	340	0.08	0.39	0.3	2
42	343	269	0.2	439	120[10]	0.08	0.40	0.2	1
16	415	326	0.2	531	150[10]	0.10	0.49	0.3	2
17	452	355	0.2	579	20[10]	0.11	0.53	0.3	2
11	274	215	0.1	351	280	0.07	0.32	0.2	1
1	28	90	1.0	65	260	0.04	0.15	trace	0
trace	4	4	trace	45	0	trace	0.09	trace	0
trace	26	86	0.9	15	310	0.04	0.07	trace	0
1	26	80	0.9	58	290	0.03	0.13	trace	0
1	28	90	1.0	65	260	0.04	0.14	trace	0
1	28	90	1.0	65	260	0.04	0.13	trace	0
1	47	97	0.9	85	310	0.04	0.16	trace	0
trace	27	26	0.2	29	3470[11]	0.01	0.04	trace	0
trace	3	3	trace	4	430[11]	trace	trace	trace	0

(continued)

								Fatty Acids		
									Unsaturated	
Item No.	Foods, Approximate Measures, Units, and Weight (edible part unless footnotes indicate otherwise)		(g)	Water (%)	Food Energy (kcal)	Protein (g)	Fat (g)	Saturated (total) (g)	Oleic (g)	Linoleic (g)
	Fats, Oils; Related Products—Cont									
	Butter—Cont									
	Regular—Cont									
105	Pat (1 in square, ⅓ in high; 90 per lb)	1 pat	5	16	35	trace	4	2.5	1.0	0.1
	Whipped (6 sticks or two 8-oz containers per lb)									
106	Stick (½ c)	1 stick	76	16	540	1	61	38.2	15.4	1.4
107	Tablespoon (about ⅛ stick)	1 tbsp	9	16	65	trace	8	4.7	1.9	0.2
108	Pat (1¼ in square, ⅓ in high; 120 per lb)	1 pat	4	16	25	trace	3	1.9	0.8	0.1
109	Fats, cooking (vegetable shortenings)	1 c	200	0	1770	0	200	48.8	88.2	48.4
110		1 tbsp	13	0	110	0	13	3.2	5.7	3.1
111	Lard	1 c	205	0	1850	0	205	81.0	83.8	20.5
112		1 tbsp	13	0	115	0	13	5.1	5.3	1.3
	Margarine									
	Regular (1 brick or 4 sticks per lb)									
113	Stick (½ c)	1 stick	113	16	815	1	92	16.7	42.9	24.9
114	Tablespoon (about ⅛ stick)	1 tbsp	14	16	100	trace	12	2.1	5.3	3.1
115	Pat (1 in square, ⅓ in high; 90 per lb)	1 pat	5	16	35	trace	4	0.7	1.9	1.1
116	Soft, two 8 oz containers per lb	1 container	227	16	1635	1	184	32.5	71.5	65.4
117		1 tbsp	14	16	100	trace	12	2.0	4.5	4.1
	Whipped (6 sticks per lb)									
118	Stick (½ c)	1 stick	76	16	545	trace	61	11.2	28.7	16.7
119	Tablespoon (about ⅛ stick)	1 tbsp	9	16	70	trace	8	1.4	3.6	2.1
	Oils, salad or cooking									
120	Corn	1 c	218	0	1925	0	218	27.7	53.6	125.1
121		1 tbsp	14	0	120	0	14	1.7	3.3	7.8
122	Olive	1 c	216	0	1910	0	216	30.7	154.4	17.7
123		1 tbsp	14	0	120	0	14	1.9	9.7	1.1
124	Peanut	1 c	216	0	1910	0	216	37.4	98.5	67.0
125		1 tbsp	14	0	120	0	14	2.3	6.2	4.2
126	Safflower	1 c	218	0	1925	0	218	20.5	25.9	159.8
127		1 tbsp	14	0	120	0	14	1.3	1.6	10.0
128	Soybean oil, hydrogenated (partially hardened)	1 c	218	0	1925	0	218	31.8	93.1	75.6

(Dashes (—) denote lack of reliable data for a constituent believed to be present in measurable amount)

[12] Based on average vitamin A content of fortified margarine. Federal specifications for fortified margarine require a minimum of 15,000 IU of vitamin A per pound.

Carbohydrate (g)	Calcium (mg)	Phosphorus (mg)	Iron (mg)	Potassium (mg)	Vitamin A Value (IU)	Thiamine (mg)	Riboflavin (mg)	Niacin (mg)	Ascorbic Acid (mg)
trace	1	1	trace	1	150[11]	trace	trace	trace	0
trace	18	17	0.1	20	2310[11]	trace	0.03	trace	0
trace	2	2	trace	2	290[11]	trace	trace	trace	0
trace	1	1	trace	1	120[11]	0	trace	trace	0
0	0	0	0	0	—	0	0	0	0
0	0	0	0	0	—	0	0	0	0
0	0	0	0	0	0	0	0	0	0
0	0	0	0	0	0	0	0	0	0
trace	27	26	0.2	29	3750[12]	0.01	0.04	trace	0
trace	3	3	trace	4	470[12]	trace	trace	trace	0
trace	1	1	trace	1	170[12]	trace	trace	trace	0
trace	53	52	0.4	59	7500[12]	0.01	0.08	0.1	0
trace	3	3	trace	4	470[12]	trace	trace	trace	0
trace	18	17	0.1	20	2500[12]	trace	0.03	trace	0
trace	2	2	trace	2	310[12]	trace	trace	trace	0
0	0	0	0	0	—	0	0	0	0
0	0	0	0	0	—	0	0	0	0
0	0	0	0	0	—	0	0	0	0
0	0	0	0	0	—	0	0	0	0
0	0	0	0	0	—	0	0	0	0
0	0	0	0	0	—	0	0	0	0
0	0	0	0	0	—	0	0	0	0
0	0	0	0	0	—	0	0	0	0
0	0	0	0	0	—	0	0	0	0

(continued)

Item No.	Foods, Approximate Measures, Units, and Weight (edible part unless footnotes indicate otherwise)		(g)	Water (%)	Food Energy (kcal)	Protein (g)	Fat (g)	Saturated (total) (g)	Oleic (g)	Linoleic (g)
									Unsaturated	
	Fats, Oils; Related Products—Cont									
	Oils, salad or cooking—Cont									
129		1 tbsp	14	0	120	0	14	2.0	5.8	4.7
130	Soybean-cotton-seed oil blend, hydrogenated	1 c	218	0	1925	0	218	38.2	63.0	99.6
131		1 tbsp	14	0	120	0	14	2.4	3.9	6.2
	Salad dressings Commercial Blue cheese									
132	Regular	1 tbsp	15	32	75	1	8	1.6	1.7	3.8
133	Low calorie (5 kcal per tsp)	1 tbsp	16	84	10	trace	1	0.5	0.3	trace
	French									
134	Regular	1 tbsp	16	39	65	trace	6	1.1	1.3	3.2
135	Low calorie (5 kcal per tsp)	1 tbsp	16	77	15	trace	1	0.1	0.1	0.4
	Italian									
136	Regular	1 tbsp	15	28	85	trace	9	1.6	1.9	4.7
137	Low calorie (2 kcal per tsp)	1 tbsp	15	90	10	trace	1	0.1	0.1	0.4
138	Mayonnaise	1 tbsp	14	15	100	trace	11	2.0	2.4	5.6
	Mayonnaise type									
139	Regular	1 tbsp	15	41	65	trace	6	1.1	1.4	3.2
140	Low calorie (8 kcal per tsp)	1 tbsp	16	81	20	trace	2	0.4	0.4	1.0
141	Tartar sauce, regular	1 tbsp	14	34	75	trace	8	1.5	1.8	4.1
	Thousand Island									
142	Regular	1 tbsp	16	32	80	trace	8	1.4	1.7	4.0
143	Low calorie (10 kcal per tsp)	1 tbsp	15	68	25	trace	2	0.4	0.4	1.0
	From home recipe									
144	Cooked type[13]	1 tbsp	16	68	25	1	2	0.5	0.6	0.3
	Fish, Shellfish, Meat, Poultry; Related Products									
	Fish and shellfish									
145	Bluefish, baked with butter or margarine	3 oz	85	68	135	22	4	—	—	—
	Clams									
146	Raw, meat only	3 oz	85	82	65	11	1	—	—	—
147	Canned, solids and liquid	3 oz	85	86	45	7	1	0.2	trace	trace
148	Crabmeat (white or king), canned, not pressed down	1 c	135	77	135	24	3	0.6	0.4	0.1
149	Fish sticks, breaded, cooked, frozen (stick, 4 by 1 by ½ in)	1 fish stick or 1 oz	28	66	50	5	3	—	—	—
150	Haddock, breaded fried[14]	3 oz	85	66	140	17	5	1.4	2.2	1.2

(Dashes (—) denote lack of reliable data for a constituent believed to be present in measurable amount)

[13] Fatty acid values apply to product made with regular-type margarine.

[14] Dipped in egg, milk or water, and breadcrumbs; fried in vegetable shortening.

Carbohydrate (g)	Calcium (mg)	Phosphorus (mg)	Iron (mg)	Potassium (mg)	Vitamin A Value (IU)	Thiamine (mg)	Riboflavin (mg)	Niacin (mg)	Ascorbic Acid (mg)
0	0	0	0	0	—	0	0	0	0
0	0	0	0	0	—	0	0	0	0
0	0	0	0	0	—	0	0	0	0
1	12	11	trace	6	30	trace	0.02	trace	trace
1	10	8	trace	5	30	trace	0.01	trace	trace
3	2	2	0.1	13	—	—	—	—	—
2	2	2	0.1	13	—	—	—	—	—
1	2	1	trace	2	trace	trace	trace	trace	—
trace	trace	1	trace	2	trace	trace	trace	trace	—
trace	3	4	0.1	5	40	trace	0.01	trace	—
2	2	4	trace	1	30	trace	trace	trace	—
2	3	4	trace	1	40	trace	trace	trace	—
1	3	4	0.1	11	30	trace	trace	trace	trace
2	2	3	0.1	18	50	trace	trace	trace	trace
2	2	3	0.1	17	50	trace	trace	trace	trace
2	14	15	0.1	19	80	0.01	0.03	trace	trace
0	25	244	0.6	—	40	0.09	0.08	1.6	—
2	59	138	5.2	154	90	0.08	0.15	1.1	8
2	47	116	3.5	119	—	0.01	0.09	0.9	—
1	61	246	1.1	149	—	0.11	0.11	2.6	—
2	3	47	0.1	—	0	0.01	0.02	0.5	—
5	34	210	1.0	296	—	0.03	0.06	2.7	2

(continued)

Item No.	Foods, Approximate Measures, Units, and Weight (edible part unless footnotes indicate otherwise)		(g)	Water (%)	Food Energy (kcal)	Protein (g)	Fat (g)	Saturated (total) (g)	Unsaturated	
									Oleic (g)	Linoleic (g)

Fish, Shellfish, Meat, Poultry; Related Products—Cont

Fish and shellfish—Cont

Item No.	Food	Measure	(g)	Water (%)	Food Energy (kcal)	Protein (g)	Fat (g)	Saturated (total) (g)	Oleic (g)	Linoleic (g)
151	Ocean perch, breaded, fried[14]	1 fillet	85	59	195	16	11	2.7	4.4	2.3
152	Oysters, raw, meat only (13–19 medium Selects)	1 c	240	85	160	20	4	1.3	0.2	0.1
153	Salmon, pink canned, solids and liquid	3 oz	85	71	120	17	5	0.9	0.8	0.1
154	Sardines, Atlantic, canned in oil, drained solids	3 oz	85	62	175	20	9	3.0	2.5	0.5
155	Scallops, frozen, breaded, fried, reheated	6 scallops	90	60	175	16	8	—	—	—
156	Shad, baked with butter or margarine, bacon	3 oz	85	64	170	20	10	—	—	—
	Shrimp									
157	Canned meat	3 oz	85	70	100	21	1	0.1	0.1	trace
158	French fried[16]	3 oz	85	57	190	17	9	2.3	3.7	2.0
159	Tuna, canned in oil, drained solids	3 oz	85	61	170	24	7	1.7	1.7	0.7
160	Tuna salad[17]	1 c	205	70	350	30	22	4.3	6.3	6.7
	Meat and meat products									
161	Bacon (20 slices per lb, raw), broiled or fried, crisp	2 slices	15	8	85	4	8	2.5	3.7	0.7
	Beef,[18] cooked									
	Cuts braised, simmered or pot roasted									
162	Lean and fat (piece, 2½ by 2½ by ¾ in)	3 oz	85	53	245	23	16	6.8	6.5	0.4
163	Lean only from item 162	2.5 oz	72	62	140	22	5	2.1	1.8	0.2
	Ground beef, broiled									
164	Lean with 10% fat	3 oz or patty 3 by ⅝ in	85	60	185	23	10	4.0	3.9	0.3
165	Lean with 21% fat	2.9 oz or patty 3 by ⅝ in	82	54	235	20	17	7.0	6.7	0.4

(Dashes (—) denote lack of reliable data for a constituent believed to be present in measurable amount)

[15] If bones are discarded, value for calcium will be greatly reduced.
[16] Dipped in egg, breadcrumbs, and flour or batter.
[17] Prepared with tuna, celery, salad dressing (mayonnaise type), pickle, onion, and egg.
[18] Outer layer of fat on the cut was removed to within approximately ½ in of the lean. Deposits of fat within the cut were not removed.

Carbohydrate (g)	Calcium (mg)	Phosphorus (mg)	Iron (mg)	Potassium (mg)	Vitamin A Value (IU)	Thiamine (mg)	Riboflavin (mg)	Niacin (mg)	Ascorbic Acid (mg)
6	28	192	1.1	242	—	0.10	0.10	1.6	—
8	226	343	13.2	290	740	0.34	0.43	6.0	—
0	167[15]	243	0.7	307	60	0.03	0.16	6.8	—
0	372	424	2.5	502	190	0.02	0.17	4.6	—
9	—	—	—	—	—	—	—	—	—
0	20	266	0.5	320	30	0.11	0.22	7.3	—
1	98	224	2.6	104	50	0.01	0.03	1.5	—
9	61	162	1.7	195	—	0.03	0.07	2.3	—
0	7	199	1.6	—	70	0.04	0.10	10.1	—
7	41	291	2.7	—	590	0.08	0.23	10.3	2
trace	2	34	0.5	35	0	0.08	0.05	0.8	—
0	10	114	2.9	184	30	0.04	0.18	3.6	—
0	10	108	2.7	176	10	0.04	0.17	3.3	—
0	10	196	3.0	261	20	0.08	0.20	5.1	—
0	9	159	2.6	221	30	0.07	0.17	4.4	—

(continued)

Item No.	Foods, Approximate Measures, Units, and Weight (edible part unless footnotes indicate otherwise)	(g)	Water (%)	Food Energy (kcal)	Protein (g)	Fat (g)	Fatty Acids		
							Saturated (total) (g)	Unsaturated	
								Oleic (g)	Linoleic (g)
	Fish, Shellfish, Meat, Poultry; Related Products—Cont								
	Meat and meat products —Cont								
	Beef,[18] cooked—Cont								
	Roast, oven cooked, cooked, no liquid added								
	Relatively fat, such as rib								
166	Lean and fat, (2 pieces, 4⅛ by 2¼ by ¼ in)	3 oz	85	40	375	17	33	14.0	13.6	0.8
167	Lean only from item 166	1.8 oz	51	57	125	14	7	3.0	2.5	0.3
	Relatively lean, such as heel of round								
168	Lean and fat (2 pieces, 4⅛ by 2¼ by ¼ in)	3 oz	85	62	165	25	7	2.8	2.7	0.2
169	Lean only from item 168	2.8 oz	78	65	125	24	3	1.2	1.0	0.1
	Steak								
	Relatively fat —sirloin, broiled								
170	Lean and fat (piece, 2½ by 2½ by ¾ in)	3 oz	85	44	330	20	27	11.3	11.1	0.6
171	Lean only from item 170	2.0 oz	56	59	115	18	4	1.8	1.6	0.2
	Relatively lean —round, braised								
172	Lean and fat (piece, 4⅛ by 2¼ by ½ in)	3 oz	85	55	220	24	13	5.5	5.2	0.4
173	Lean only from item 172	2.4 oz	68	61	130	21	4	1.7	1.5	0.2
	Beef, canned								
174	Corned beef	3 oz	85	59	185	22	10	4.9	4.5	0.2
175	Corned beef hash	1 c	220	67	400	19	25	11.9	10.9	0.5
176	Beef, dried, chipped	2½ oz jar	71	48	145	24	4	2.1	2.0	0.1
177	Beef and vegetable stew	1 c	245	82	220	16	11	4.9	4.5	0.2
178	Beef potpie (home recipe), baked[19] (piece, ⅓ of 9 in diam pie)	1 piece	210	55	515	21	30	7.9	12.8	6.7

(Dashes (—) denote lack of reliable data for a constituent believed to be present in measurable amount)
[19] Crust made with vegetable shortening and enriched flour.

Carbohydrate (g)	Calcium (mg)	Phosphorus (mg)	Iron (mg)	Potassium (mg)	Vitamin A Value (IU)	Thiamine (mg)	Riboflavin (mg)	Niacin (mg)	Ascorbic Acid (mg)
0	8	158	2.2	189	70	0.05	0.13	3.1	—
0	6	131	1.8	161	10	0.04	0.11	2.6	—
0	11	208	3.2	279	10	0.06	0.19	4.5	—
0	10	199	3.0	268	trace	0.06	0.18	4.3	—
0	9	162	2.5	220	50	0.05	0.15	4.0	—
0	7	146	2.2	202	10	0.05	0.14	3.6	—
0	10	213	3.0	272	20	0.07	0.19	4.8	—
0	9	182	2.5	238	10	0.05	0.16	4.1	—
0	17	90	3.7	—	—	0.01	0.20	2.9	—
24	29	147	4.4	440	—	0.02	0.20	4.6	—
0	14	287	3.6	142	—	0.05	0.23	2.7	0
15	29	184	2.9	613	2400	0.15	0.17	4.7	17
39	29	149	3.8	334	1720	0.30	0.30	5.5	6

(continued)

Item No.	Foods, Approximate Measures, Units, and Weight (edible part unless footnotes indicate otherwise)		(g)	Water (%)	Food Energy (kcal)	Protein (g)	Fat (g)	Saturated (total) (g)	Unsaturated	
									Oleic (g)	Linoleic (g)
	Fish, Shellfish, Meat, Poultry; Related Products—Cont									
	Meat and meat products —Cont									
179	Chili con carne with beans, canned	1 c	255	72	340	19	16	7.5	6.8	0.3
180	Chop suey with beef and pork (home recipe)	1 c	250	75	300	26	17	8.5	6.2	0.7
181	Heart, beef, lean, braised	3 oz	85	61	160	27	5	1.5	1.1	0.6
	Lamb, cooked Chop, rib (cut 3 per lb with bone), broiled									
182	Lean and fat	3.1 oz	89	43	360	18	32	14.8	12.1	1.2
183	Lean only from item 182	2 oz	57	60	120	16	6	2.5	2.1	0.2
	Leg, roasted									
184	Lean and fat (2 pieces, 4⅛ by 2¼ by ¼ in)	3 oz	85	54	235	22	16	7.3	6.0	0.6
185	Lean only from item 184	2.5 oz	71	62	130	20	5	2.1	1.8	0.2
	Shoulder, roasted									
186	Lean and fat (3 pieces, 2½ by 2½ by ¼ in)	3 oz	85	50	285	18	23	10.8	8.8	0.9
187	Lean only from item 186	2.3 oz	64	61	130	17	6	3.6	2.3	0.2
188	Liver, beef fried[20] (slice, 6½ by 2⅜ by ⅜ in)	3 oz	85	56	195	22	9	2.5	3.5	0.9
	Pork, cured, cooked									
189	Ham, light cure, lean and fat, roasted (2 pieces, 4⅛ by 2¼ by ¼ in)[22]	3 oz	85	54	245	18	19	6.8	7.9	1.7
	Luncheon meat									
190	Boiled ham, slice (8 per 8 oz pkg)	1 oz	28	59	65	5	5	1.7	2.0	0.4
	Canned, spiced or unspiced									
191	Slice, approx 3 by 2 by ½ in	1 slice	60	55	175	9	15	5.4	6.7	1.0

(Dashes (—) denote lack of reliable data for a constituent believed to be present in measurable amount)

[20] Regular-type margarine used.

[21] Value varies widely.

[22] About one fourth of the outer layer of fat on the cut was removed. Deposits of fat within the cut were not removed.

Carbohydrate (g)	Calcium (mg)	Phosphorus (mg)	Iron (mg)	Potassium (mg)	Vitamin A Value (IU)	Thiamine (mg)	Riboflavin (mg)	Niacin (mg)	Ascorbic Acid (mg)
31	82	321	4.3	594	150	0.08	0.18	3.3	—
13	60	248	4.8	425	600	0.28	0.38	5.0	33
1	5	154	5.0	197	20	0.21	1.04	6.5	1
0	8	139	1.0	200	—	0.11	0.19	4.1	—
0	6	121	1.1	174	—	0.09	0.15	3.4	—
0	9	177	1.4	241	—	0.13	0.23	4.7	—
0	9	169	1.4	227	—	0.12	0.21	4.4	—
0	9	146	1.0	206	—	0.11	0.20	4.0	—
0	8	140	1.0	193	—	0.10	0.18	3.7	—
5	9	405	7.5	323	45,390[21]	0.22	3.56	14.0	23
0	8	146	2.2	199	0	0.04	0.15	3.1	—
0	3	47	0.8	—	0	0.12	0.04	0.7	—
1	5	65	1.3	133	0	0.19	0.13	1.8	—

(continued)

| | | | | | | | Fatty Acids | | |
| | | | | | | | | Unsaturated | |
Item No.	Foods, Approximate Measures, Units, and Weight (edible part unless footnotes indicate otherwise)	(g)	Water (%)	Food Energy (kcal)	Protein (g)	Fat (g)	Saturated (total) (g)	Oleic (g)	Linoleic (g)
	Fish, Shellfish, Meat, Poultry; Related Products—Cont								
	Pork, cured, cooked —Cont								
	Pork, fresh,[18] cooked								
	Chop, loin (cut 3 per lb with bone), broiled								
192	Lean and fat	2.7 oz	78	42	305	19	25	8.9	10.4	2.2
193	Lean only from item 192	2 oz	56	53	150	17	9	3.1	3.6	0.8
	Roast, oven cooked, no liquid added								
194	Lean and fat (piece, 2½ by 2½ by ¾ in)	3 oz	85	46	310	21	24	8.7	10.2	2.2
195	Lean only from item 194	2.4 oz	68	55	175	20	10	3.5	4.1	0.8
	Shoulder cut, simmered								
196	Lean and fat (3 pieces, 2½ by 2½ by ¼ in)	3 oz	85	46	320	20	26	9.3	10.9	2.3
197	Lean only from item 196	2.2 oz	63	60	135	18	6	2.2	2.6	0.6
	Sausages (see also Luncheon meat, items 190–191)								
198	Bologna, slice (8 per 8 oz pkg)	1 slice	28	56	85	3	8	3.0	3.4	0.5
199	Braunschweiger, slice (6 per 6 oz pkg)	1 slice	28	53	90	4	8	2.6	3.4	0.8
200	Brown and serve (10–11 per 8 oz pkg), browned	1 link	17	40	70	3	6	2.3	2.8	0.7
201	Deviled ham, canned	1 tbsp	13	51	45	2	4	1.5	1.8	0.4
202	Frankfurter (8 per 1 lb pkg), cooked (reheated)	1 frankfurter	56	57	170	7	15	5.6	6.5	1.2
203	Meat, potted (beef, chicken, turkey), canned	1 tbsp	13	61	30	2	2	—	—	—
204	Pork link (16 per 1 lb pkg), cooked	1 link	13	35	60	2	6	2.1	2.4	0.5
	Salami								
205	Dry type, slice (12 per 4 oz pkg)	1 slice	10	30	45	2	4	1.6	1.6	0.1

(Dashes (—) denote lack of reliable data for a constituent believed to be present in measurable amount)

Carbohydrate (g)	Calcium (mg)	Phosphorus (mg)	Iron (mg)	Potassium (mg)	Vitamin A Value (IU)	Thiamine (mg)	Riboflavin (mg)	Niacin (mg)	Ascorbic Acid (mg)
0	9	209	2.7	216	0	0.75	0.22	4.5	—
0	7	181	2.2	192	0	0.63	0.18	3.8	—
0	9	218	2.7	233	0	0.78	0.22	4.8	—
0	9	211	2.6	224	0	0.73	0.21	4.4	—
0	9	118	2.6	158	0	0.46	0.21	4.1	—
0	8	111	2.3	146	0	0.42	0.19	3.7	—
trace	2	36	0.5	65	—	0.05	0.06	0.7	—
1	3	69	1.7	—	1850	0.05	0.41	2.3	—
trace	—	—	—	—	—	—	—	—	—
0	1	12	0.3	—	0	0.02	0.01	0.2	—
1	3	57	0.8	—	—	0.08	11	1.4	—
0	—	—	—	—	—	trace	0.03	0.2	—
trace	1	21	0.3	35	0	0.10	0.04	0.5	—
trace	1	28	0.4	—	—	0.04	0.03	0.5	—

(continued)

Item No.	Foods, Approximate Measures, Units, and Weight (edible part unless footnotes indicate otherwise)	(g)	Water (%)	Food Energy (kcal)	Protein (g)	Fat (g)	Fatty Acids		
							Saturated (total) (g)	Unsaturated	
								Oleic (g)	Linoleic (g)
	Fish, Shellfish, Meat, Poultry; Related Products—Cont								
	Sausages—Cont								
	Salami—Cont								
206	Cooked type, slice (8 per 8 oz pkg)	28	51	90	5	7	3.1	3.0	0.2
207	Vienna sausage (7 per 4 oz can)	16	63	40	2	3	1.2	1.4	0.2
	Veal, medium fat, cooked, bone removed								
208	Cutlet (4⅛ by 2¼ by ½ in), braised or broiled	85	60	185	23	9	4.0	3.4	0.4
209	Rib (2 pieces, 4⅛ by 2¼ by ¼ in), roasted	85	55	230	23	14	6.1	5.1	0.6
	Poultry and poultry products								
	Chicken, cooked								
210	Breast, fried,[23] bones removed, ½ breast (3.3 oz with bones)	79	58	160	26	5	1.4	1.8	1.1
211	Drumstick, fried,[23] bones removed (2 oz with bones)	38	55	90	12	4	1.1	1.3	0.9
212	Half broiler, broiled, bones removed (10.4 oz with bones)	176	71	240	42	7	2.2	2.5	1.3
213	Chicken, canned, boneless	85	65	170	18	10	3.2	3.8	2.0
214	Chicken à la king, cooked (home recipe)	245	68	470	27	34	2.7	14.3	3.3
215	Chicken and noodles, cooked (home recipe)	240	71	365	22	18	5.9	7.1	3.5
	Chicken chow mein								
216	Canned	250	89	95	7	trace	—	—	—
217	From home recipe	250	78	255	31	10	2.4	3.4	3.1
218	Chicken potpie (home recipe), baked,[19] piece (⅓ or 9 in diam pie)	232	57	545	23	31	11.3	10.9	5.6
	Turkey, roasted, flesh without skin								
219	Dark meat, piece, 2½ by 1⅝ by ¼ in	85	61	175	26	7	2.1	1.5	1.5

(Dashes (—) denote lack of reliable data for a constituent believed to be present in measurable amount)

[23] Vegetable shortening used.

Carbohydrate (g)	Calcium (mg)	Phosphorus (mg)	Iron (mg)	Potassium (mg)	Vitamin A Value (IU)	Thiamine (mg)	Riboflavin (mg)	Niacin (mg)	Ascorbic Acid (mg)
trace	3	57	0.7	—	—	0.07	0.07	1.2	—
trace	1	24	0.3	—	—	0.01	0.02	0.4	—
0	9	196	2.7	258	—	0.06	0.21	4.6	—
0	10	211	2.9	259	—	0.11	0.26	6.6	—
1	9	218	1.3	—	70	0.04	0.17	11.6	—
trace	6	89	0.9	—	50	0.03	0.15	2.7	—
0	16	355	3.0	483	160	0.09	0.34	15.5	—
0	18	210	1.3	117	200	0.03	0.11	3.7	3
12	127	358	2.5	404	1130	0.10	0.42	5.4	12
26	26	247	2.2	149	430	0.05	0.17	4.3	trace
18	45	85	1.3	418	150	0.05	0.10	1.0	13
10	58	293	2.5	473	280	0.08	0.23	4.3	10
42	70	232	3.0	343	3090	0.34	0.31	5.5	5
0	—	—	2.0	338	—	0.03	0.20	3.6	—

(continued)

Item No.	Foods, Approximate Measures, Units, and Weight (edible part unless footnotes indicate otherwise)	(g)	Water (%)	Food Energy (kcal)	Protein (g)	Fat (g)	Saturated (total) (g)	Unsaturated Oleic (g)	Unsaturated Linoleic (g)
	Fish, Shellfish, Meat, Poultry; Related Products—Cont								
	Poultry and poultry products—Cont								
	Turkey—Cont								
220	Light meat, piece, 4 by 2 by ¼ in	2 pieces	85	62	150	28	3	0.9	0.6	0.7
	Light and dark meat								
221	Chopped or diced	1 c	140	61	265	44	9	2.5	1.7	1.8
222	Pieces (1 slice white meat, 4 by 2 by ¼ in with 2 slices dark meat, 2½ by 1⅝ by ¼ in)	3 pieces	85	61	160	27	5	1.5	1.0	1.1
	Fruits and Fruit Products								
	Apples, raw, unpeeled, without cores								
223	2¾-in diam (about 3 per lb with cores)	1 apple	138	84	80	trace	1	—	—	—
224	3¼ in diam (about 2 per lb with cores)	1 apple	212	84	125	trace	1	—	—	—
225	Applejuice, bottled or canned[24]	1 c	248	88	120	trace	trace	—	—	—
	Applesauce, canned								
226	Sweetened	1 c	255	76	230	1	trace	—	—	—
227	Unsweetened	1 c	244	89	100	trace	trace	—	—	—
	Apricots								
228	Raw, without pits (about 12 per lb with pits)	3 apricots	107	85	55	1	trace	—	—	—
229	Canned in heavy syrup (halves and syrup)	1 c	258	77	220	2	trace	—	—	—
	Dried								
230	Uncooked (28 large or 37 medium halves per c)	1 c	130	25	340	7	1	—	—	—
231	Cooked, unsweetened, fruit and liquid	1 c	250	76	215	4	1	—	—	—
232	Apricot nectar, canned	1 c	251	85	145	1	trace	—	—	—

(Dashes (—) denote lack of reliable data for a constituent believed to be present in measurable amount)

[24] Also applies to pasteurized apple cider.

[25] Applies to product without added ascorbic acid. For value of product with added ascorbic acid, refer to label.

[26] Based on product with label claim of 45% of U.S. RDA in 6 fl oz.

Carbohydrate (g)	Calcium (mg)	Phosphorus (mg)	Iron (mg)	Potassium (mg)	Vitamin A Value (IU)	Thiamine (mg)	Riboflavin (mg)	Niacin (mg)	Ascorbic Acid (mg)
0	—	—	1.0	349	—	0.04	0.12	9.4	—
0	11	351	2.5	514	—	0.07	0.25	10.8	—
0	7	213	1.5	312	—	0.04	0.15	6.5	—
20	10	14	0.4	152	120	0.04	0.03	0.1	6
31	15	21	0.6	233	190	0.06	0.04	0.2	8
30	15	22	1.5	250	—	0.02	0.05	0.2	2[25]
61	10	13	1.3	166	100	0.05	0.03	0.1	3[25]
26	10	12	1.2	190	100	0.05	0.02	0.1	2[25]
14	18	25	0.5	301	2890	0.03	0.04	0.6	11
57	28	39	0.8	604	4490	0.05	0.05	1.0	10
86	87	140	7.2	1273	14,170	0.01	0.21	4.3	16
54	55	88	4.5	795	7500	0.01	0.13	2.5	8
37	23	30	0.5	379	2380	0.03	0.03	0.5	36[26]

(continued)

Item No.	Foods, Approximate Measures, Units, and Weight (edible part unless footnotes indicate otherwise)		(g)	Water (%)	Food Energy (kcal)	Protein (g)	Fat (g)	Saturated (total) (g)	Unsaturated	
									Fatty Acids	
									Oleic (g)	Linoleic (g)
	Fruits and Fruit Products—Cont									
	Avocados, raw, whole, without skins and seeds									
233	California, mid- and late-winter (with skin and seed, 3⅛ in diam; wt, 10 oz)	1 avocado	216	74	370	5	37	5.5	22.0	3.7
234	Florida, late summer and fall (with skin and seed, 3⅝ in diam; wt, 1 lb)	1 avocado	304	78	390	4	38	6.7	15.7	5.3
235	Banana without peel (about 2.6 per lb with peel)	1 banana	119	76	100	1	trace	—	—	—
236	Banana flakes	1 tbsp	6	3	20	trace	trace	—	—	—
237	Blackberries, raw	1 c	144	85	85	2	1	—	—	—
238	Blueberries, raw	1 c	145	83	90	1	1	—	—	—
	Cantaloupe (see Muskmelons, item 271)									
	Cherries									
239	Sour (tart), red, pitted, canned, water pack	1 c	244	88	105	2	trace	—	—	—
240	Sweet, raw, without pits and stems	10 cherries	68	80	45	1	trace	—	—	—
241	Cranberry juice cocktail, bottled, sweetened	1 c	253	83	165	trace	trace	—	—	—
242	Cranberry sauce, sweetened, canned, strained	1 c	277	62	405	trace	1	—	—	—
	Dates									
243	Whole, without pits	10 dates	80	23	220	2	trace	—	—	—
244	Chopped	1 c	178	23	490	4	1	—	—	—
245	Fruit cocktail, canned, in heavy syrup	1 c	255	80	195	1	trace	—	—	—
	Grapefruit Raw, medium, 3¾ in diam (about 1 lb 1 oz)									
246	Pink or red	½ grapefruit with peel[28]	241	89	50	1	trace	—	—	—

(Dashes (—) denote lack of reliable data for a constituent believed to be present in measurable amount)

[27] Based on product with label claim of 100% of U.S. RDA in 6 fl oz.

[28] Weight includes peel and membranes between sections. Without these parts, the weight of the edible portion is 123 g for item 246 and 118 g for item 247.

Carbohydrate (g)	Calcium (mg)	Phosphorus (mg)	Iron (mg)	Potassium (mg)	Vitamin A Value (IU)	Thiamine (mg)	Riboflavin (mg)	Niacin (mg)	Ascorbic Acid (mg)
13	22	91	1.3	1303	630	0.24	0.43	3.5	30
27	30	128	1.8	1836	880	0.33	0.61	4.9	43
26	10	31	0.8	440	230	0.06	0.07	0.8	12
5	2	6	0.2	92	50	0.01	0.01	0.2	trace
19	46	27	1.3	245	290	0.04	0.06	0.6	30
22	22	19	1.5	117	150	0.04	0.09	0.7	20
26	37	32	0.7	317	1660	0.07	0.05	0.5	12
12	15	13	0.3	129	70	0.03	0.04	0.3	7
42	13	8	0.8	25	trace	0.03	0.03	0.1	81[27]
104	17	11	0.6	83	60	0.03	0.03	0.1	6
58	47	50	2.4	518	40	0.07	0.08	1.8	0
130	105	112	5.3	1153	90	0.16	0.18	3.9	0
50	23	31	1.0	411	360	0.05	0.03	1.0	5
13	20	20	0.5	166	540	0.05	0.02	0.2	44

(continued)

Item No.	Foods, Approximate Measures, Units, and Weight (edible part unless footnotes indicate otherwise)	(g)	Water (%)	Food Energy (kcal)	Protein (g)	Fat (g)	Saturated (total) (g)	Unsaturated Oleic (g)	Unsaturated Linoleic (g)
	Fruits and Fruit Products—Cont								
	Grapefruit—Cont								
	Raw—Cont								
247	White	241	89	45	1	trace	—	—	—
248	Canned, sections with syrup	254	81	180	2	trace	—	—	—
	Grapefruit juice								
249	Raw, pink, red, or white	246	90	95	1	trace	—	—	—
	Canned, white								
250	Unsweetened	247	89	100	1	trace	—	—	—
251	Sweetened	250	86	135	1	trace	—	—	—
	Frozen, concentrate unsweetened								
252	Undiluted, 6 fl oz can	207	62	300	4	1	—	—	—
253	Diluted with 3 parts water by volume	247	89	100	1	trace	—	—	—
254	Dehydrated crystals, prepared with water (1 lb yields about 1 gal)	247	90	100	1	trace	—	—	—
	Grapes, European type (adherent skin), raw								
255	Thompson seedless	50	81	35	trace	trace	—	—	—
256	Tokay and Emperor, seeded types	60	81	40	trace	trace	—	—	—
	Grapejuice								
257	Canned or bottled	253	83	165	1	trace	—	—	—
	Frozen concentrate, sweetened								
258	Undiluted, 6 fl oz can	216	53	395	1	trace	—	—	—
259	Diluted with 3 parts water by volume	250	86	135	1	trace	—	—	—
260	Grape drink, canned	250	86	135	trace	trace	—	—	—
261	Lemon, raw, size 165, without peel and seeds (about 4 per lb with peels and seeds)	74	90	20	1	trace	—	—	—

Note on measures: item 247 = ½ grapefruit with peel[28]; items 248, 250, 251, 253, 254, 257, 259, 260 = 1 c; items 249 = 1 c; items 252, 258 = 1 can; items 255, 256 = 10 grapes; item 261 = 1 lemon.

(Dashes (—) denote lack of reliable data for a constituent believed to be present in measurable amount)

[29] For white-fleshed varieties, value is about 20 IU per c; for red-fleshed varieties, 1080 IU.

[30] Weight includes seeds. Without seeds, weight of the edible portion is 57 g.

[31] Applies to product without added ascorbic acid. With added ascorbic acid, based on claim that 6 fl oz of reconstituted juice contain 45% or 50% of the U.S. RDA, value in milligrams is 108 or 120 for a 6 fl oz can (item 258), 36 or 40 for 1 c of diluted juice (item 259).

[32] For products with added thiamine and riboflavin but without added ascorbic acid, values in milligrams would be 0.60 for thiamine, 0.80 for riboflavin, and trace for ascorbic acid. For products with only ascorbic acid added, value varies with the brand. Consult the label.

Carbohydrate (g)	Calcium (mg)	Phosphorus (mg)	Iron (mg)	Potassium (mg)	Vitamin A Value (IU)	Thiamine (mg)	Riboflavin (mg)	Niacin (mg)	Ascorbic Acid (mg)
12	19	19	0.5	159	10	0.05	0.02	0.2	44
45	33	36	0.8	343	30	0.08	0.05	0.5	76
23	22	37	0.5	399	([29])	0.10	0.05	0.5	93
24	20	35	1.0	400	20	0.07	0.05	0.5	84
32	20	35	1.0	405	30	0.08	0.05	0.5	78
72	70	124	0.8	1250	60	0.29	0.12	1.4	286
24	25	42	0.2	420	20	0.10	0.04	0.5	96
24	22	40	0.2	412	20	0.10	0.05	0.5	91
9	6	10	0.2	87	50	0.03	0.02	0.2	2
10	7	11	0.2	99	60	0.03	0.02	0.2	2
42	28	30	0.8	293	—	0.10	0.05	0.5	trace[25]
100	22	32	0.9	255	40	0.13	0.22	1.5	32[31]
33	8	10	0.3	85	10	0.05	0.08	0.5	10[31]
35	8	10	0.3	88	—	0.03[32]	0.03[32]	0.3	([32])
6	19	12	0.4	102	10	0.03	0.01	0.1	39

(continued)

Item No.	Foods, Approximate Measures, Units, and Weight (edible part unless footnotes indicate otherwise)		(g)	Water (%)	Food Energy (kcal)	Protein (g)	Fat (g)	Saturated (total) (g)	Unsaturated Oleic (g)	Unsaturated Linoleic (g)
	Fruits and Fruit Products—Cont									
	Lemon juice									
262	Raw	1 c	244	91	60	1	trace	—	—	—
263	Canned, or bottled, unsweetened	1 c	244	92	55	1	trace	—	—	—
264	Frozen, single strength, un-sweetened, 6 fl oz can	1 can	183	92	40	1	trace	—	—	—
	Lemonade concentrate, frozen									
265	Undiluted, 6 fl oz can	1 can	219	49	425	trace	trace	—	—	—
266	Diluted with 4⅓ parts water by volume	1 c	248	89	105	trace	trace	—	—	—
	Limeade concentrate, frozen									
267	Undiluted, 6 fl oz can	1 can	218	50	410	trace	trace	—	—	—
268	Diluted with 4⅓ parts water by volume	1 c	247	89	100	trace	trace	—	—	—
	Limejuice									
269	Raw	1 c	246	90	65	1	trace	—	—	—
270	Canned, un-sweetened	1 c	246	90	65	1	trace	—	—	—
	Muskmelons, raw, with rind, without seed cavity									
271	Cantaloupe, orange-fleshed (with rind and seed cavity, 5 in diam, 2⅓ lb)	½ melon with rind[33]	477	91	80	2	trace	—	—	—
272	Honeydew (with rind and seed cavity, 6½ in diam, 5¼ lb)	⅒ melon with rind[33]	226	91	50	1	trace	—	—	—
	Oranges, all commercial varieties raw									
273	Whole, 2⅝ in diam, without peel and seeds (about 2½ per lb with peel and seeds)	1 orange	131	86	65	1	trace	—	—	—
274	Sections without membranes	1 c	180	86	90	2	trace	—	—	—
	Orange juice									
275	Raw, all varieties	1 c	248	88	110	2	trace	—	—	—
276	Canned, un-sweetened	1 c	249	87	120	2	trace	—	—	—

(Dashes (—) denote lack of reliable data for a constituent believed to be present in measurable amount)

[33] Weight includes rind. Without rind, the weight of the edible portion is 272 g for item 271 and 149 g for item 272.

Carbohydrate (g)	Calcium (mg)	Phosphorus (mg)	Iron (mg)	Potassium (mg)	Vitamin A Value (IU)	Thiamine (mg)	Riboflavin (mg)	Niacin (mg)	Ascorbic Acid (mg)
20	17	24	0.5	344	50	0.07	0.02	0.2	112
19	17	24	0.5	344	50	0.07	0.02	0.2	102
13	13	16	0.5	258	40	0.05	0.02	0.2	81
112	9	13	0.4	153	40	0.05	0.06	0.7	66
28	2	3	0.1	40	10	0.01	0.02	0.2	17
108	11	13	0.2	129	trace	0.02	0.02	0.2	26
27	3	3	trace	32	trace	trace	trace	trace	6
22	22	27	0.5	256	20	0.05	0.02	0.2	79
22	22	27	0.5	256	20	0.05	0.02	0.2	52
20	38	44	1.1	682	9240	0.11	0.08	1.6	90
11	21	24	0.6	374	60	0.06	0.04	0.9	34
16	54	26	0.5	263	260	0.13	0.05	0.5	66
22	74	36	0.7	360	360	0.18	0.07	0.7	90
26	27	42	0.5	496	500	0.22	0.07	1.0	124
28	25	45	1.0	496	500	0.17	0.05	0.7	100

(continued)

							Fatty Acids		
							Saturated (total) (g)	Unsaturated	
Item No.	Foods, Approximate Measures, Units, and Weight (edible part unless footnotes indicate otherwise)	(g)	Water (%)	Food Energy (kcal)	Protein (g)	Fat (g)		Oleic (g)	Linoleic (g)
	Fruits and Fruit Products—Cont								
	Orange juice—Cont								
	Frozen concentrate								
277	Undiluted, 6 fl oz can	1 can	213	55	360	5	trace	—	—	—
278	Diluted with 3 parts water by volume	1 c	249	87	120	2	trace	—	—	—
279	Dehydrated crystals, prepared with water (1 lb yields about 1 gal)	1 c	248	88	115	1	trace	—	—	—
	Orange and grape-fruit juice								
	Frozen concentrate								
280	Undiluted, 6 fl oz can	1 can	210	59	330	4	1	—	—	—
281	Diluted with 3 parts water by volume	1 c	248	88	110	1	trace	—	—	—
282	Papayas, raw, ½ in cubes	1 c	140	89	55	1	trace			
	Peaches								
	Raw								
283	Whole, 2½ in diam, peeled, pitted (about 4 per lb with peels and pits)	1 peach	100	89	40	1	trace	—	—	—
284	Sliced	1 c	170	89	65	1	trace	—		—
	Canned, yellow-fleshed, solids and liquid (halves or slices)								
285	Syrup pack	1 c	256	79	200	1	trace	—	—	—
286	Water pack	1 c	244	91	75	1	trace	—	—	—
	Dried								
287	Uncooked	1 c	160	25	420	5	1	—	—	—
288	Cooked, un-sweetened, halves and juice	1 c	250	77	205	3	1	—	—	—
	Frozen, sliced, sweetened								
289	10 oz container	1 con-tainer	284	77	250	1	trace	—	—	—
290	Cup	1 c	250	77	220	1	trace	—	—	—
	Pears								
	Raw, with skin, cored								
291	Bartlett, 2½ in diam (about 2½ per lb with cores and stems)	1 pear	164	83	100	1	1	—	—	—

(Dashes (—) denote lack of reliable data for a constituent believed to be present in measurable amount)

[34] Represents yellow-fleshed varieties. For white-fleshed varieties, value is 50 IU for 1 peach, 90 IU for 1 c of slices.

[35] Value represents products with added ascorbic acid. For products without added ascorbic acid, value in milligrams is 116 for a 10 oz container, 103 for 1 c.

Carbohydrate (g)	Calcium (mg)	Phosphorus (mg)	Iron (mg)	Potassium (mg)	Vitamin A Value (IU)	Thiamine (mg)	Riboflavin (mg)	Niacin (mg)	Ascorbic Acid (mg)
87	75	126	0.9	1500	1620	0.68	0.11	2.8	360
29	25	42	0.2	503	540	0.23	0.03	0.9	120
27	25	40	0.5	518	500	0.20	0.07	1.0	109
78	61	99	0.8	1308	800	0.48	0.06	2.3	302
26	20	32	0.2	439	270	0.15	0.02	0.7	102
14	28	22	0.4	328	2450	0.06	0.06	0.4	78
10	9	19	0.5	202	1330[34]	0.02	0.05	1.0	7
16	15	32	0.9	343	2260[34]	0.03	0.09	1.7	12
51	10	31	0.8	333	1100	0.03	0.05	1.5	8
20	10	32	0.7	334	1100	0.02	0.07	1.5	7
109	77	187	9.6	1520	6240	0.02	0.30	8.5	29
54	38	93	4.8	743	3050	0.01	0.15	3.8	5
64	11	37	1.4	352	1850	0.03	0.11	2.0	116[35]
57	10	33	1.3	310	1630	0.03	0.10	1.8	103[35]
25	13	18	0.5	213	30	0.03	0.07	0.2	7

(continued)

Item No.	Foods, Approximate Measures, Units, and Weight (edible part unless footnotes indicate otherwise)		(g)	Water (%)	Food Energy (kcal)	Protein (g)	Fat (g)	Fatty Acids		
								Saturated (total) (g)	Unsaturated	
									Oleic (g)	Linoleic (g)
	Fruits and Fruit Products—Cont									
	Pears—Cont									
	Raw, with skin, cored—Cont									
292	Bosc, 2½ in diam (about 3 per lb with cores and stems)	1 pear	141	83	85	1	1	—	—	—
293	D'Anjou, 3 in diam (about 2 per lb with cores and stems)	1 pear	200	83	120	1	1	—	—	—
294	Canned, solids and liquid, syrup pack, heavy (halves or slices)	1 c	255	80	195	1	1	—	—	—
	Pineapple									
295	Raw, diced	1 c	155	85	80	1	trace	—	—	—
	Canned, heavy syrup pack, solids and liquid									
296	Crushed, chunks, tidbits	1 c	255	80	190	1	trace	—	—	—
	Slices and liquid									
297	Large	1 slice; 2¼ tbsp liquid	105	80	80	trace	trace	—	—	—
298	Medium	1 slice; 1¼ tbsp liquid	58	80	45	trace	trace	—	—	—
299	Pineapple juice, unsweetened, canned	1 c	250	86	140	1	trace	—	—	—
	Plums									
	Raw, without pits									
300	Japanese and hybrid (2⅛ in diam, about 6½ per lb with pits)	1 plum	66	87	30	trace	trace	—	—	—
301	Prune-type (1½ in diam, about 15 per lb with pits)	1 plum	28	79	20	trace	trace	—	—	—
	Canned, heavy syrup pack (Italian prunes), with pits and liquid									
302	Cup	1 c[36]	272	77	215	1	trace	—	—	—
303	Portion	3 plums; 2¾ tbsp liquid[36]	140	77	110	1	trace	—	—	—
	Prunes, dried, "softenized," with pits									
304	Uncooked	4 extra large or 5 large prunes[36]	49	28	110	1	trace	—	—	—

(Dashes (—) denote lack of reliable data for a constituent believed to be present in measurable amount)

[36] Weight includes pits. After removal of the pits, the weight of the edible portion is 258 g for item 302, 113 g for item 303, 43 g for item 304, and 213 g for item 305.

Carbohydrate (g)	Calcium (mg)	Phosphorus (mg)	Iron (mg)	Potassium (mg)	Vitamin A Value (IU)	Thiamine (mg)	Riboflavin (mg)	Niacin (mg)	Ascorbic Acid (mg)
22	11	16	0.4	83	30	0.03	0.06	0.1	6
31	16	22	0.6	260	40	0.04	0.08	0.2	8
50	13	18	0.5	214	10	0.03	0.05	0.3	3
21	26	12	0.8	226	110	0.14	0.05	0.3	26
49	28	13	0.8	245	130	0.20	0.05	0.5	18
20	12	5	0.3	101	50	0.08	0.02	0.2	7
11	6	3	0.2	56	30	0.05	0.01	0.1	4
34	38	23	0.8	373	130	0.13	0.05	0.5	80[27]
8	8	12	0.3	112	160	0.02	0.02	0.3	4
6	3	5	0.1	48	80	0.01	0.01	0.1	1
56	23	26	2.3	367	3130	0.05	0.05	1.0	5
29	12	13	1.2	189	1610	0.03	0.03	0.5	3
29	22	34	1.7	298	690	0.04	0.07	0.7	1

(continued)

Item No.	Foods, Approximate Measures, Units, and Weight (edible part unless footnotes indicate otherwise)		(g)	Water (%)	Food Energy (kcal)	Protein (g)	Fat (g)	Saturated (total) (g)	Unsaturated Oleic (g)	Linoleic (g)
	Fruits and Fruit Products—Cont									
	Prunes—Cont									
305	Cooked, unsweetened, all sizes, fruit and liquid	1 c[36]	250	66	255	2	1	—	—	—
306	Prune juice, canned or bottled	1 c	256	80	195	1	trace	—	—	—
	Raisins, seedless									
307	Cup, not pressed down	1 c	145	18	420	4	trace	—	—	—
308	Packet, ½ oz (1½ tbsp)	1 packet	14	18	40	trace	trace	—	—	—
	Raspberries, red									
309	Raw, capped, whole	1 c	123	84	70	1	1	—	—	—
310	Frozen, sweetened, 10 oz container	1 container	284	74	280	2	1	—	—	—
	Rhubarb, cooked, added sugar									
311	From raw	1 c	270	63	380	1	trace	—	—	—
312	From frozen, sweetened	1 c	270	63	385	1	1	—	—	—
	Strawberries									
313	Raw, whole berries, capped	1 c	149	90	55	1	1	—	—	—
	Frozen, sweetened									
314	Sliced, 10 oz container	1 container	284	71	310	1	1	—	—	—
315	Whole, 1 lb container (about 1¾ c)	1 container	454	76	415	2	1	—	—	—
316	Tangerine, raw, 2⅜ in diam, size 176, without peel (about 4 per lb with peels and seeds)	1 tangerine	86	87	40	1	trace	—	—	—
317	Tangerine juice, canned, sweetened	1 c	249	87	125	1	trace	—	—	—
318	Watermelon, raw, 4 by 8 in wedge with rind and seeds (1/16 of 32⅔ lb melon, 10 by 16 in)	1 wedge with rind and seeds[37]	926	93	110	2	1	—	—	—
	Grain Products									
	Bagel, 3 in diam									
319	Egg	1 bagel	55	32	165	6	2	0.5	0.9	0.8
320	Water	1 bagel	55	29	165	6	1	0.2	0.4	0.6
321	Barley, pearled, light, uncooked	1 c	200	11	700	16	2	0.3	0.2	0.8

(Dashes (—) denote lack of reliable data for a constituent believed to be present in measurable amount)

[37] Weight includes rind and seeds. Without rind and seeds, weight of the edible portion is 426 g.

Carbohydrate (g)	Calcium (mg)	Phosphorus (mg)	Iron (mg)	Potassium (mg)	Vitamin A Value (IU)	Thiamine (mg)	Riboflavin (mg)	Niacin (mg)	Ascorbic Acid (mg)
67	51	79	3.8	695	1590	0.07	0.15	1.5	2
49	36	51	1.8	602	—	0.03	0.03	1.0	5
112	90	146	5.1	1106	30	0.16	0.12	0.7	1
11	9	14	0.5	107	trace	0.02	0.01	0.1	trace
17	27	27	1.1	207	160	0.04	0.11	1.1	31
70	37	48	1.7	284	200	0.06	0.17	1.7	60
97	211	41	1.6	548	220	0.05	0.14	0.8	16
98	211	32	1.9	475	190	0.05	0.11	0.5	16
13	31	31	1.5	244	90	0.04	0.10	0.9	88
79	40	48	2.0	318	90	0.06	0.17	1.4	151
107	59	73	2.7	472	140	0.09	0.27	2.3	249
10	34	15	0.3	108	360	0.05	0.02	0.1	27
30	44	35	0.5	440	1040	0.15	0.05	0.2	54
27	30	43	2.1	426	2510	0.13	0.13	0.9	30
28	9	43	1.2	41	30	0.14	0.10	1.2	0
30	8	41	1.2	42	0	0.15	0.11	1.4	0
158	32	378	4.0	320	0	0.24	0.10	6.2	0

(continued)

Item No.	Foods, Approximate Measures, Units, and Weight (edible part unless footnotes indicate otherwise)		(g)	Water (%)	Food Energy (kcal)	Protein (g)	Fat (g)	Saturated (total) (g)	Unsaturated	
									Oleic (g)	Linoleic (g)
	Grain Products—Cont									
	Biscuits, baking powder, 2 in diam (enriched flour, vegetable shortening)									
322	From home recipe	1 biscuit	28	27	105	2	5	1.2	2.0	1.2
323	From mix	1 biscuit	28	29	90	2	3	0.6	1.1	0.7
	Breadcrumbs (enriched)[38]									
324	Dry, grated	1 c	100	7	390	13	5	1.0	1.6	1.4
	Soft (see white bread, items 339–356)									
	Breads									
325	Boston brown bread, canned, slice, 3¼ by ½ in[38]	1 slice	45	45	95	2	1	0.1	0.2	0.2
	Cracked-wheat bread (¾ enriched wheat flour, ¼ cracked wheat)[38]									
326	Loaf, 1 lb	1 loaf	454	35	1195	39	10	2.2	3.0	3.9
327	Slice (18 per loaf)	1 slice	25	35	65	2	1	0.1	0.2	0.2
	French or Vienna bread, enriched[38]									
328	Loaf, 1 lb	1 loaf	454	31	1315	41	14	3.2	4.7	4.6
	Slice									
329	French (5 by 2½ by 1 in)	1 slice	35	31	100	3	1	0.2	0.4	0.4
330	Vienna (4¾ by 4 by ½ in)	1 slice	25	31	75	2	1	0.2	0.3	0.3
	Italian bread, enriched									
331	Loaf, 1 lb	1 loaf	454	32	1250	41	4	0.6	0.3	1.5
332	Slice, 4½ by 3¼ by ¾ in	1 slice	30	32	85	3	trace	trace	trace	0.1
	Raisin bread, enriched[38]									
333	Loaf, 1 lb	1 loaf	454	35	1190	30	13	3.0	4.7	3.9
334	Slice (18 per loaf)	1 slice	25	35	65	2	1	0.2	0.3	0.2
	Rye bread									
	American, light (⅔ enriched wheat flour, ⅓ rye flour)									
335	Loaf, 1 lb	1 loaf	454	36	1100	41	5	0.7	0.5	2.2
336	Slice (4¾ by 3¾ by ⁷⁄₁₆ in)	1 slice	25	36	60	2	trace	trace	trace	0.1
	Pumpernickel (⅔ rye flour, ⅓ enriched wheat flour)									
337	Loaf, 1 lb	1 loaf	454	34	1115	41	5	0.7	0.5	2.4

[38] Made with vegetable shortening.
[39] Applies to product made with white cornmeal. With yellow cornmeal, value is 30 IU.

Carbohydrate (g)	Calcium (mg)	Phosphorus (mg)	Iron (mg)	Potassium (mg)	Vitamin A Value (IU)	Thiamine (mg)	Riboflavin (mg)	Niacin (mg)	Ascorbic Acid (mg)
13	34	49	0.4	33	trace	0.08	0.08	0.7	trace
15	19	65	0.6	32	trace	0.09	0.08	0.8	trace
73	122	141	3.6	152	trace	0.35	0.35	4.8	trace
21	41	72	0.9	131	0[39]	0.06	0.04	0.7	0
236	399	581	9.5	608	trace	1.52	1.13	14.4	trace
13	22	32	0.5	34	trace	0.08	0.06	0.8	trace
251	195	386	10.0	408	trace	1.80	1.10	15.0	trace
19	15	30	0.8	32	trace	0.14	0.08	1.2	trace
14	11	21	0.6	23	trace	0.10	0.06	0.8	trace
256	77	349	10.0	336	0	1.80	1.10	15.0	0
17	5	23	0.7	22	0	0.12	0.07	1.0	0
243	322	395	10.0	1057	trace	1.70	1.07	10.7	trace
13	18	22	0.6	58	trace	0.09	0.06	0.6	trace
236	340	667	9.1	658	0	1.35	0.98	12.9	0
13	19	37	0.5	36	0	0.07	0.05	0.7	0
241	381	1039	11.8	2059	0	1.30	0.93	8.5	0

(continued)

Item No.	Foods, Approximate Measures, Units, and Weight (edible part unless footnotes indicate otherwise)		(g)	Water (%)	Food Energy (kcal)	Protein (g)	Fat (g)	Saturated (total) (g)	Unsaturated	
									Oleic (g)	Linoleic (g)
	Grain Products—Cont									
	Rye bread—Cont									
	Pumpernickel—Cont									
338	Slice (5 by 4 by ⅜ in)	1 slice	32	34	80	3	trace	0.1	trace	0.2
	White bread, enriched[38]									
	Soft-crumb type									
339	Loaf, 1 lb	1 loaf	454	36	1225	39	15	3.4	5.3	4.6
340	Slice (18 per loaf)	1 slice	25	36	70	2	1	0.2	0.3	0.3
341	Slice, toasted	1 slice	22	25	70	2	1	0.2	0.3	0.3
342	Slice (22 per loaf)	1 slice	20	36	55	2	1	0.2	0.2	0.2
343	Slice, toasted	1 slice	17	25	55	2	1	0.2	0.2	0.2
344	Loaf, 1½ lb	1 loaf	680	36	1835	59	22	5.2	7.9	6.9
345	Slice (24 per loaf)	1 slice	28	36	75	2	1	0.2	0.3	0.3
346	Slice, toasted	1 slice	24	25	75	2	1	0.2	0.3	0.3
347	Slice (28 per loaf)	1 slice	24	36	65	2	1	0.2	0.3	0.2
348	Slice, toasted	1 slice	21	25	65	2	1	0.2	0.3	0.2
349	Cubes	1 c	30	36	80	3	1	0.2	0.3	0.3
350	Crumbs	1 c	45	36	120	4	1	0.3	0.5	0.5
	Firm-crumb type									
351	Loaf, 1 lb	1 loaf	454	35	1245	41	17	3.9	5.9	5.2
352	Slice (20 per loaf)	1 slice	23	35	65	2	1	0.2	0.3	0.3
353	Slice, toasted	1 slice	20	24	65	2	1	0.2	0.3	0.3
354	Loaf, 2 lb	1 loaf	907	35	2495	82	34	7.7	11.8	10.4
355	Slice (34 per loaf)	1 slice	27	35	75	2	1	0.2	0.3	0.3
356	Slice, toasted	1 slice	23	24	75	2	1	0.2	0.3	0.3
	Whole-wheat bread									
	Soft-crumb type[38]									
357	Loaf, 1 lb	1 loaf	454	36	1095	41	12	2.2	2.9	4.2
358	Slice (16 per loaf)	1 slice	28	36	65	3	1	0.1	0.2	0.2
359	Slice, toasted	1 slice	24	24	65	3	1	0.1	0.2	0.2
	Firm-crumb type[38]									
360	Loaf, 1 lb	1 loaf	454	36	1100	48	14	2.5	3.3	4.9
361	Slice (18 per loaf)	1 slice	25	36	60	3	1	0.1	0.2	0.3
362	Slice, toasted	1 slice	21	24	60	3	1	0.1	0.2	0.3
	Breakfast cereals									
	Hot type, cooked									
	Corn (hominy) grits, degermed									
363	Enriched	1 c	245	87	125	3	trace	trace	trace	0.1
364	Unenriched	1 c	245	87	125	3	trace	trace	trace	0.1
365	Farina, quick-cooking, enriched	1 c	245	89	105	3	trace	trace	trace	0.1

[40] Applies to white varieties. For yellow varieties, value is 150 IU.
[41] Applies to products that do not contain disodium phosphate. If disodium phosphate is an ingredient, value is 162 mg.

Carbohydrate (g)	Calcium (mg)	Phosphorus (mg)	Iron (mg)	Potassium (mg)	Vitamin A Value (IU)	Thiamine (mg)	Riboflavin (mg)	Niacin (mg)	Ascorbic Acid (mg)
17	27	73	0.8	145	0	0.09	0.07	0.6	0
229	381	440	11.3	476	trace	1.80	1.10	15.0	trace
13	21	24	0.6	26	trace	0.10	0.06	0.8	trace
13	21	24	0.6	26	trace	0.08	0.06	0.8	trace
10	17	19	0.5	21	trace	0.08	0.05	0.7	trace
10	17	19	0.5	21	trace	0.06	0.05	0.7	trace
343	571	660	17.0	714	trace	2.70	1.65	22.5	trace
14	24	27	0.7	29	trace	0.11	0.07	0.9	trace
14	24	27	0.7	29	trace	0.09	0.07	0.9	trace
12	20	23	0.6	25	trace	0.10	0.06	0.8	trace
12	20	23	0.6	25	trace	0.08	0.06	0.8	trace
15	25	29	0.8	32	trace	0.12	0.07	1.0	trace
23	38	44	1.1	47	trace	0.18	0.11	1.5	trace
228	435	463	11.3	549	trace	1.80	1.10	15.0	trace
12	22	23	0.6	28	trace	0.09	0.06	0.8	trace
12	22	23	0.6	28	trace	0.07	0.06	0.8	trace
455	871	925	22.7	1097	trace	3.60	2.20	30.0	trace
14	26	28	0.7	33	trace	0.11	0.06	0.9	trace
14	26	28	0.7	33	trace	0.09	0.06	0.9	trace
224	381	1152	13.6	1161	trace	1.37	0.45	12.7	trace
14	24	71	0.8	72	trace	0.09	0.03	0.8	trace
14	24	71	0.8	72	trace	0.07	0.03	0.8	trace
216	449	1034	13.6	1238	trace	1.17	0.54	12.7	trace
12	25	57	0.8	68	trace	0.06	0.03	0.7	trace
12	25	57	0.8	68	trace	0.05	0.03	0.7	trace
27	2	25	0.7	27	trace[40]	0.10	0.07	1.0	0
27	2	25	0.2	27	trace[40]	0.05	0.02	0.5	0
22	147	113[41]	([42])	25	0	0.12	0.07	1.0	0

(continued)

[42] Value may range from less than 1 mg to about 8 mg depending on the brand. Consult the label.

Item No.	Foods, Approximate Measures, Units, and Weight (edible part unless footnotes indicate otherwise)		(g)	Water (%)	Food Energy (kcal)	Protein (g)	Fat (g)	Saturated (total) (g)	Oleic (g)	Linoleic (g)
								Fatty Acids		
									Unsaturated	
	Grain Products—Cont									
	Breakfast cereals—Cont									
	Hot type—Cont									
366	Oatmeal or rolled oats	1 c	240	87	130	5	2	0.4	0.8	0.9
367	Wheat, rolled	1 c	240	80	180	5	1	—	—	—
368	Wheat, whole-meal	1 c	245	88	110	4	1	—	—	—
	Ready-to-eat									
369	Bran flakes (40% bran), added sugar, salt, iron, vitamins	1 c	35	3	105	4	1	—	—	—
370	Bran flakes with raisins, added sugar, salt, iron, vitamins	1 c	50	7	145	4	1	—	—	—
	Corn flakes									
371	Plain, added sugar, salt, iron, vitamins	1 c	25	4	95	2	trace	—	—	—
372	Sugar-coated, added salt, iron, vitamins	1 c	40	2	155	2	trace	—	—	—
373	Corn, oat flour, puffed, added sugar, salt, iron, vitamins	1 c	20	4	80	2	1	—	—	—
374	Corn, shredded, added sugar, salt, iron, thiamin, niacin	1 c	25	3	95	2	trace	—	—	—
375	Oats, puffed, added sugar, salt, minerals, vitamins	1 c	25	3	100	3	1	—	—	—
	Rice, puffed									
376	Plain, added iron, thiamin, niacin	1 c	15	4	60	1	trace	—	—	—
377	Presweetened, added salt, iron, vitamins	1 c	28	3	115	1	0	—	—	—
378	Wheat flakes, added sugar, salt, iron, vitamins	1 c	30	4	105	3	trace	—	—	—
	Wheat, puffed									
379	Plain, added iron, thiamin, niacin	1 c	15	3	55	2	trace	—	—	—
380	Presweetened, added salt, iron, vitamins	1 c	38	3	140	3	trace	—	—	—
381	Wheat, shredded, plain	1 oblong biscuit or ½ c spoon-size biscuits	25	7	90	2	1	—	—	—

(Dashes (—) denote lack of reliable data for a constituent believed to be present in measurable amount)

[43] Applies to product with added nutrient. Without added nutrient, value is trace.

[44] Value varies with the brand. Consult the label.

[45] Applies to product with added nutrient. Without added nutrient, value is trace.

Carbohydrate (g)	Calcium (mg)	Phosphorus (mg)	Iron (mg)	Potassium (mg)	Vitamin A Value (IU)	Thiamine (mg)	Riboflavin (mg)	Niacin (mg)	Ascorbic Acid (mg)
3	3	70	0.5	57	10	0.11	0.05	0.3	1
78	11	86	1.0	314	0	0.08	0.04	0.4	0
44	27	263	1.9	151	0	0.08	0.05	4.1	0
377	603	756	2.5	381	0	0.37	0.95	3.6	0
32	50	63	0.2	32	0	0.03	0.08	0.3	0
225	262	748	6.9	469	690	0.82	0.91	7.7	1
38	44	125	1.2	78	120	0.14	0.15	1.3	trace
14	40	59	0.3	21	40	0.05	0.05	0.4	trace
21	47	71	0.4	42	60	0.05	0.06	0.4	trace
645	653	1162	16.6	1439	1660	1.06	1.65	10.1	1
40	41	72	1.0	90	100	0.07	0.10	0.6	trace
20	21	37	0.5	46	50	0.03	0.05	0.3	trace
291	513	570	8.6	1562	trace	0.84	1.00	7.4	trace
32	57	63	0.9	173	trace	0.09	0.11	0.8	trace
716	1129	2041	11.4	1322	680	1.50	1.77	12.5	2
45	70	127	0.7	82	40	0.09	0.11	0.8	trace
638	1008	2017	12.2	1208	1550	1.24	1.67	10.6	2
40	63	126	0.8	75	100	0.08	0.10	0.7	trace
412	553	833	8.2	734[48]	1730	1.04	1.27	9.6	2

(continued)

[48] Applies to product made with a sodium aluminum-sulfate type baking powder. With a low-sodium type baking powder containing potassium, value would be about twice the amount shown.

					Food			Fatty Acids		
									Unsaturated	
Item No.	Foods, Approximate Measures, Units, and Weight (edible part unless footnotes indicate otherwise)		(g)	Water (%)	Food Energy (kcal)	Protein (g)	Fat (g)	Saturated (total) (g)	Oleic (g)	Linoleic (g)
	Grain Products—Cont									
	Cakes—Cont									
401	Piece, 1/12 of cake	1 piece	69	35	210	3	6	1.9	2.5	1.3
	Fruitcake, dark									
402	Loaf, 1 lb (7½ by 2 by 1½ in)	1 loaf	454	18	1720	22	69	14.4	33.5	14.8
403	Slice, 1/30 of loaf	1 slice	15	18	55	1	2	0.5	1.1	0.5
	Plain, sheet cake									
	Without icing									
404	Whole cake (9 in square)	1 cake	777	25	2830	35	108	29.5	44.4	23.9
405	Piece, 1/9 of cake	1 piece	86	25	315	4	12	3.3	4.9	2.6
	With uncooked white icing									
406	Whole cake (9 in square)	1 cake	1096	21	4020	37	129	42.2	49.5	24.4
407	Piece, 1/9 of cake	1 piece	121	21	445	4	14	4.7	5.5	2.7
	Pound[49]									
408	Loaf, 8½ by 3½ by 3¼ in	1 loaf	565	16	2725	31	170	42.9	73.1	39.6
409	Slice, 1/17 of loaf	1 slice	33	16	160	2	10	2.5	4.3	2.3
	Spongecake									
410	Whole cake (9¾ in diam tube cake)	1 cake	790	32	2345	60	45	13.1	15.8	5.7
411	Piece, 1/12 of cake	1 piece	66	32	195	5	4	1.1	1.3	0.5
	Cookies made with enriched flour[50, 51]									
	Brownies with nuts:									
	Home-prepared, 1¾ by 1¾ by ⅞ in									
412	From home recipe	1 brownie	20	10	95	1	6	1.5	3.0	1.2
413	From commercial recipe	1 brownie	20	11	85	1	4	0.9	1.4	1.3
414	Frozen, with chocolate icing,[52] 1½ by 1¾ by ⅞ in	1 brownie	25	13	105	1	5	2.0	2.2	0.7
	Chocolate chip									
415	Commercial, 2¼ in diam, ⅜ in thick	4 cookies	42	3	200	2	9	2.8	2.9	2.2
416	From home recipe 2⅓ in diam	4 cookies	40	3	205	2	12	3.5	4.5	2.9
417	Fig bars, square (1⅝ by 1⅝ by ⅜ in) or rectangular (1½ by 1¾ by ½ in)	4 cookies	56	14	200	2	3	0.8	1.2	0.7
418	Gingersnaps, 2 in diam, ¼ in thick	4 cookies	28	3	90	2	2	0.7	1.0	0.6
419	Macaroons, 2¾ in diam, ¼ in thick	2 cookies	38	4	180	2	9	—	—	—
420	Oatmeal with raisins, 2⅝ in diam, ¼ in thick	4 cookies	52	3	235	3	8	2.0	3.3	2.0
421	Plain, prepared from commercial chilled dough, 2½ in diam, ¼ in thick	4 cookies	48	5	240	2	12	3.0	5.2	2.9

(Dashes (—) denote lack of reliable data for a constituent believed to be present in measurable amount)

[49] Equal weights of flour, sugar, eggs, and vegetable shortening.
[50] Products are commercial unless otherwise specified.
[51] Made with enriched flour and vegetable shortening except for macaroons, which do not contain flour or shortening.
[52] Icing made with butter.

Carbohydrate (g)	Calcium (mg)	Phosphorus (mg)	Iron (mg)	Potassium (mg)	Vitamin A Value (IU)	Thiamine (mg)	Riboflavin (mg)	Niacin (mg)	Ascorbic Acid (mg)
34	46	70	0.7	61[48]	140	0.09	0.11	0.8	trace
271	327	513	11.8	2250	540	0.72	0.73	4.9	2
9	11	17	0.4	74	20	0.02	0.02	0.2	trace
434	497	793	8.5	614[48]	1320	1.21	1.40	10.2	2
48	55	88	0.9	68[48]	150	0.13	0.15	1.1	trace
694	548	822	8.2	669[48]	2190	1.22	1.47	10.2	2
77	61	91	0.8	74[48]	240	0.14	0.16	1.1	trace
273	107	418	7.9	345	1410	0.90	0.99	7.3	0
16	6	24	0.5	20	80	0.05	0.06	0.4	0
427	237	885	13.4	687	3560	1.10	1.64	7.4	trace
36	20	74	1.1	57	300	0.09	0.14	0.6	trace
10	8	30	0.4	38	40	0.04	0.03	0.2	trace
13	9	27	0.4	34	20	0.03	0.02	0.2	trace
15	10	31	0.4	44	50	0.03	0.03	0.2	trace
29	16	48	1.0	56	50	0.10	0.17	0.9	trace
24	14	40	0.8	47	40	0.06	0.06	0.5	trace
42	44	34	1.0	111	60	0.04	0.14	0.9	trace
22	20	13	0.7	129	20	0.08	0.06	0.7	0
25	10	32	0.3	176	0	0.02	0.06	0.2	0
38	11	53	1.4	192	30	0.15	0.10	1.0	trace
31	17	35	0.6	23	30	0.10	0.08	0.9	0

(continued)

Item No.	Foods, Approximate Measures, Units, and Weight (edible part unless footnotes indicate otherwise)		(g)	Water (%)	Food Energy (kcal)	Protein (g)	Fat (g)	Saturated (total) (g)	Unsaturated	
									Oleic (g)	Linoleic (g)
	Grain Products—Cont									
	Cookies—Cont									
422	Sandwich type (chocolate or vanilla), 1¾ in diam, ⅜ in thick	4 cookies	40	2	200	2	9	2.2	3.9	2.2
423	Vanilla wafers, 1¾ in diam, ¼ in thick	10 cookies	40	3	185	2	6	—	—	—
	Cornmeal									
424	Whole-ground, unbolted, dry form	1 c	122	12	435	11	5	0.5	1.0	2.5
425	Bolted (nearly whole-grain), dry form	1 c	122	12	440	11	4	0.5	0.9	2.1
	Degermed, enriched									
426	Dry form	1 c	138	12	500	11	2	0.2	0.4	0.9
427	Cooked	1 c	240	88	120	3	trace	trace	0.1	0.2
	Degermed, unenriched									
428	Dry form	1 c	138	12	500	11	2	0.2	0.4	0.9
429	Cooked	1 c	240	88	120	3	trace	trace	0.1	0.2
	Crackers[38]									
430	Graham, plain, 2½ in square	2 crackers	14	6	55	1	1	0.3	0.5	0.3
431	Rye wafers, whole-grain, 1⅞ by 3½ in	2 wafers	13	6	45	2	trace	—	—	—
432	Saltines, made with enriched flour	4 crackers or 1 packet	11	4	50	1	1	0.3	0.5	0.4
	Danish pastry (enriched flour), plain without fruit or nuts[54]									
433	Packaged ring, 12 oz	1 ring	340	22	1435	25	80	24.3	31.7	16.5
434	Round piece, about 4¼ in diam by 1 in	1 pastry	65	22	275	5	15	4.7	6.1	3.2
435	Ounce	1 oz	28	22	120	2	7	2.0	2.7	1.4
	Doughnuts, made with enriched flour[38]									
436	Cake type, plain, 2½ in diam, 1 in high	1 doughnut	25	24	100	1	5	1.2	2.0	1.1
437	Yeast-leavened, glazed 3¾ in diam, 1¼ in high	1 doughnut	50	26	205	3	11	3.3	5.8	3.3
	Macaroni, enriched, cooked (cut lengths, elbows, shells)									
438	Firm stage (hot)	1 c	130	64	190	7	1	—	—	—
	Tender stage									
439	Cold macaroni	1 c	105	73	115	4	trace	—	—	—
440	Hot macaroni	1 c	140	73	155	5	1	—	—	—
	Macaroni (enriched) and cheese									
441	Canned[55]	1 c	240	80	230	9	10	4.2	3.1	1.4
442	From home recipe (served hot)[56]	1 c	200	58	430	17	22	8.9	8.8	2.9

(Dashes (—) denote lack of reliable data for a constituent believed to be present in measurable amount)
[53] Applies to yellow varieties; white varieties contain only a trace.
[54] Contains vegetable shortening and butter.
[55] Made with corn oil.
[56] Made with regular margarine.

Carbohydrate (g)	Calcium (mg)	Phosphorus (mg)	Iron (mg)	Potassium (mg)	Vitamin A Value (IU)	Thiamine (mg)	Riboflavin (mg)	Niacin (mg)	Ascorbic Acid (mg)
28	10	96	0.7	15	0	0.06	0.10	0.7	0
30	16	25	0.6	29	50	0.10	0.09	0.8	0
90	24	312	2.9	346	620[53]	0.46	0.13	2.4	0
91	21	272	2.2	303	590[53]	0.37	0.10	2.3	0
108	8	137	4.0	166	610[53]	0.61	0.36	4.8	0
26	2	34	1.0	38	140[53]	0.14	0.10	1.2	0
108	8	137	1.5	166	610[53]	0.19	0.07	1.4	0
26	2	34	0.5	38	140[53]	0.05	0.02	0.2	0
10	6	21	0.5	55	0	0.02	0.08	0.5	0
10	7	50	0.5	78	0	0.04	0.03	0.2	0
8	2	10	0.5	13	0	0.05	0.05	0.4	0
155	170	371	6.1	381	1050	0.97	1.01	8.6	trace
30	33	71	1.2	73	200	0.18	0.19	1.7	trace
13	14	31	0.5	32	90	0.08	0.08	0.7	trace
13	10	48	0.4	23	20	0.05	0.05	0.4	trace
22	16	33	0.6	34	25	0.10	0.10	0.8	0
39	14	85	1.4	103	0	0.23	0.13	1.8	0
24	8	53	0.9	64	0	0.15	0.08	1.2	0
32	11	70	1.3	85	0	0.20	0.11	1.5	0
26	199	182	1.0	139	260	0.12	0.24	1.0	trace
40	362	322	1.8	240	860	0.20	0.40	1.8	trace

(continued)

Item No.	Foods, Approximate Measures, Units, and Weight (edible part unless footnotes indicate otherwise)		(g)	Water (%)	Food Energy (kcal)	Protein (g)	Fat (g)	Saturated (total) (g)	Oleic (g)	Linoleic (g)
									Fatty Acids	
										Unsaturated

Grain Products—Cont

Muffins made with enriched flour[38]
From home recipe

Item No.	Food	Measure	(g)	Water (%)	Food Energy (kcal)	Protein (g)	Fat (g)	Saturated (total) (g)	Oleic (g)	Linoleic (g)
443	Blueberry, 2⅜ in diam, 1½ in high	1 muffin	40	39	110	3	4	1.1	1.4	0.7
444	Bran	1 muffin	40	35	105	3	4	1.2	1.4	0.8
445	Corn (enriched degermed cornmeal and flour), 2⅜ in diam, ½ in high	1 muffin	40	33	125	3	4	1.2	1.6	0.9
446	Plain, 3 in diam, 1½ in high	1 muffin	40	38	120	3	4	1.0	1.7	1.0
	From mix, egg, milk;									
447	Corn, 2⅜ in diam, 1½ in high[58]	1 muffin	40	30	130	3	4	1.2	1.7	0.9
448	Noodles (egg noodles), enriched, cooked	1 c	160	71	200	7	2	—	—	—
449	Noodles, chow mein, canned	1 c	45	1	220	6	11	—	—	—
	Pancakes (4 in diam)[38]									
450	Buckwheat, made from mix (with buckwheat and enriched flours), egg and milk added	1 cake	27	58	55	2	2	0.8	0.9	0.4
	Plain									
451	Made from home recipe using enriched flour	1 cake	27	50	60	2	2	0.5	0.8	0.5
452	Made from mix with enriched flour, egg and milk added	1 cake	27	51	60	2	2	0.7	0.7	0.3
	Pies, piecrust made with enriched flour vegetable shortening (9 in diam)									
	Apple									
453	Whole	1 pie	945	48	2420	21	105	27.0	44.5	25.2
454	Sector, ⅐ of pie	1 sector	135	48	345	3	15	3.9	6.4	3.6
	Banana cream									
455	Whole	1 pie	910	54	2010	41	85	26.7	33.2	16.2
456	Sector, ⅐ of pie	1 sector	130	54	285	6	12	3.8	4.7	2.3
	Blueberry									
457	Whole	1 pie	945	51	2285	23	102	24.8	43.7	25.1
458	Sector, ⅐ of pie	1 sector	135	51	325	3	15	3.5	6.2	3.6
	Cherry									
459	Whole	1 pie	945	47	2465	25	107	28.2	45.0	25.3
460	Sector, ⅐ of pie	1 sector	135	47	350	4	15	4.0	6.4	3.6
	Custard									
461	Whole	1 pie	910	58	1985	56	101	33.9	38.5	17.5
462	Sector, ⅐ of pie	1 sector	130	58	285	8	14	4.8	5.5	2.5
	Lemon meringue									
463	Whole	1 pie	840	47	2140	31	86	26.1	33.8	16.4
464	Sector, ⅐ of pie	1 sector	120	47	305	4	12	3.7	4.8	2.3

(Dashes (—) denote lack of reliable data for a constituent believed to be present in measurable amount)
[57] Applies to product made with yellow cornmeal.
[58] Made with enriched degermed cornmeal and enriched flour.

Carbohydrate (g)	Calcium (mg)	Phosphorus (mg)	Iron (mg)	Potassium (mg)	Vitamin A Value (IU)	Thiamine (mg)	Riboflavin (mg)	Niacin (mg)	Ascorbic Acid (mg)
17	34	53	0.6	46	90	0.09	0.10	0.7	trace
17	57	162	1.5	172	90	0.07	0.10	1.7	trace
19	42	68	0.7	54	120[57]	0.10	0.10	0.7	trace
17	42	60	0.6	50	40	0.09	0.12	0.9	trace
20	96	152	0.6	44	100[57]	0.08	0.09	0.7	trace
37	16	94	1.4	70	110	0.22	0.13	1.9	0
26	—	—	—	—	—	—	—	—	—
6	59	91	0.4	66	60	0.04	0.05	0.2	trace
9	27	38	0.4	33	30	0.06	0.07	0.5	trace
9	58	70	0.3	42	70	0.04	0.06	0.2	trace
360	76	208	6.6	756	280	1.06	0.79	9.3	9
51	11	30	0.9	108	40	0.15	0.11	1.3	2
279	601	746	7.3	1847	2280	0.77	1.51	7.0	9
40	86	107	1.0	264	330	0.11	0.22	1.0	1
330	104	217	9.5	614	280	1.03	0.80	10.0	28
47	15	31	1.4	88	40	0.15	0.11	1.4	4
363	132	236	6.6	992	4160	1.09	0.84	9.8	trace
52	19	34	0.9	142	590	0.16	0.12	1.4	trace
213	874	1028	8.2	1247	2090	0.79	1.92	5.6	0
30	125	147	1.2	178	300	0.11	0.27	0.8	0
317	118	412	6.7	420	1430	0.61	0.84	5.2	25
45	17	59	1.0	60	200	0.09	0.12	0.7	4

(continued)

Item No.	Foods, Approximate Measures, Units, and Weight (edible part unless footnotes indicate otherwise)		(g)	Water (%)	Food Energy (kcal)	Protein (g)	Fat (g)	Fatty Acids: Saturated (total) (g)	Fatty Acids: Unsaturated: Oleic (g)	Fatty Acids: Unsaturated: Linoleic (g)
	Grain Products—Cont									
	Pies—Cont									
	Mince									
465	Whole	1 pie	945	43	2560	24	109	28.0	45.9	25.2
466	Sector, ⅐ of pie	1 sector	135	43	365	3	16	4.0	6.6	3.6
	Peach									
467	Whole	1 pie	945	48	2410	24	101	24.8	43.7	25.1
468	Sector, ⅐ of pie	1 sector	135	48	345	3	14	3.5	6.2	3.6
	Pecan									
469	Whole	1 pie	825	20	3450	42	189	27.8	101.0	44.2
470	Sector, ⅐ of pie	1 sector	118	20	495	6	27	4.0	14.4	6.3
	Pumpkin									
471	Whole	1 pie	910	59	1920	36	102	37.4	37.5	16.6
472	Sector, ⅐ of pie	1 sector	130	59	275	5	15	5.4	5.4	2.4
473	Piecrust (home recipe) made with enriched flour and vegetables shortening, baked	1 pie shell, 9 in diam	180	15	900	11	60	14.8	26.1	14.9
474	Piecrust mix with enriched flour and vegetable shortening, 10 oz pkg prepared and baked	Piecrust for 2-crust pie, 9 in diam	320	19	1485	20	93	22.7	39.7	23.4
475	Pizza (cheese) baked, 4 ¾ in sector; ⅛ of 12 in diam pie[19]	1 sector	60	45	145	6	4	1.7	1.5	0.6
	Popcorn, popped									
476	Plain, large kernel	1 c	6	4	25	1	trace	trace	0.1	0.2
477	With oil (coconut) and salt added, large kernel	1 c	9	3	40	1	2	1.5	0.2	0.2
478	Sugar coated	1 c	35	4	135	2	1	0.5	0.2	0.4
	Pretzels, made with enriched flour									
479	Dutch twisted, 2¾ by 2⅝ in	1 pretzel	16	5	60	2	1	—	—	—
480	Thin, twisted, 3¼ by 2¼ by ¼ in	10 pretzels	60	5	235	6	3	—	—	—
481	Stick, 2¼ in long	10 pretzels	3	5	10	trace	trace	—	—	—
	Rice, white, enriched									
482	Instant, ready-to-serve, hot	1 c	165	73	180	4	trace	trace	trace	trace
	Long grain									
483	Raw	1 c	185	12	670	12	1	0.2	0.2	0.2
484	Cooked, served hot	1 c	205	73	225	4	trace	0.1	0.1	0.1
	Parboiled									
485	Raw	1 c	185	10	685	14	1	0.2	0.1	0.2
486	Cooked, served hot	1 c	175	73	185	4	trace	0.1	0.1	0.2
	Rolls, enriched[38]									
	Commercial									
487	Brown-and-serve (12 per 12 oz pkg), browned	1 roll	26	27	85	2	2	0.4	0.7	0.5
488	Cloverleaf or pan, 2½ in diam, 2 in high	1 roll	28	31	85	2	2	0.4	0.6	0.4

(Dashes (—) denote lack of reliable data for a constituent believed to be present in measurable amount)

[59] Product may or may not be enriched with riboflavin. Consult the label.

Carbohydrate (g)	Calcium (mg)	Phosphorus (mg)	Iron (mg)	Potassium (mg)	Vitamin A Value (IU)	Thiamine (mg)	Riboflavin (mg)	Niacin (mg)	Ascorbic Acid (mg)
389	265	359	13.3	1682	20	0.96	0.86	9.8	9
56	38	51	1.9	240	trace	0.14	0.12	1.4	1
361	95	274	8.5	1408	6900	1.04	0.97	14.0	28
52	14	39	1.2	201	990	0.15	0.14	2.0	4
423	388	850	25.6	1015	1320	1.80	0.95	6.9	trace
61	55	122	3.7	145	190	0.26	0.14	1.0	trace
223	464	628	7.3	1456	22,480	0.78	1.27	7.0	trace
32	66	90	1.0	208	3210	0.11	0.18	1.0	trace
79	25	90	3.1	89	0	0.47	0.40	5.0	0
141	131	272	6.1	179	0	1.07	0.79	9.9	0
22	86	89	1.1	67	230	0.16	0.18	1.6	4
5	1	17	0.2	—	—	—	0.01	0.1	0
5	1	19	0.2	—	—	—	0.01	0.2	0
30	2	47	0.5	—	—	—	0.02	0.4	0
12	4	2	0.2	21	0	0.05	0.04	0.7	0
46	13	79	0.9	78	0	0.20	0.15	2.5	0
2	1	4	trace	4	0	0.01	0.01	0.1	0
40	5	31	1.3	—	0	0.21	[59]	1.7	0
149	44	174	5.4	170	0	0.81	0.06	6.5	0
50	21	57	1.8	57	0	0.23	0.02	2.1	0
150	111	370	5.4	278	0	0.81	0.07	6.5	0
41	33	100	1.4	75	0	0.19	0.02	2.1	0
14	20	23	0.5	25	trace	0.10	0.06	0.9	trace
15	21	24	0.5	27	trace	0.11	0.07	0.9	trace

(continued)

							Fatty Acids		
								Unsaturated	
Item No.	Foods, Approximate Measures, Units, and Weight (edible part unless footnotes indicate otherwise)	(g)	Water (%)	Food Energy (kcal)	Protein (g)	Fat (g)	Saturated (total) (g)	Oleic (g)	Linoleic (g)
	Grain Products—Cont								
	Rolls—Cont								
489	Frankfurter and hamburger (8 per 11½ oz pkg)	1 roll	40	31	120	3	2	0.5	0.8	0.6
490	Hard, 3¾ in diam, 2 in high	1 roll	50	25	155	5	2	0.4	0.6	0.5
491	Hoagie or submarine, 11½ by 3 by 2½ in	1 roll	135	31	390	12	4	0.9	1.4	1.4
	From home recipe								
492	Cloverleaf, 2½ in diam, 2 in high	1 roll	35	26	120	3	3	0.8	1.1	0.7
	Spaghetti, enriched, cooked								
493	Firm stage, al dente, served hot	1 c	130	64	190	7	1	—	—	—
494	Tender stage, served hot	1 c	140	73	155	5	1	—	—	—
	Spaghetti (enriched) in tomato sauce with cheese								
495	From home recipe	1 c	250	77	260	9	9	2.0	5.4	0.7
496	Canned	1 c	250	80	190	6	2	0.5	0.3	0.4
	Spaghetti (enriched) with meat balls and tomato sauce								
497	From home recipe	1 c	248	70	330	19	12	3.3	6.3	0.9
498	Canned	1 c	250	78	260	12	10	2.2	3.3	3.9
499	Toaster pastries	1 pastry	50	12	200	3	6	—	—	—
	Waffles, made with enriched flour, 7 in diam[38]								
500	From home recipe	1 waffle	75	41	210	7	7	2.3	2.8	1.4
501	From mix, egg and milk added	1 waffle	75	42	205	7	8	2.8	2.9	1.2
	Wheat flours								
	All-purpose or family flour, enriched								
502	Sifted, spooned	1 c	115	12	420	12	1	0.2	0.1	0.5
503	Unsifted, spooned	1 c	125	12	455	13	1	0.2	0.1	0.5
504	Cake or pastry flour, enriched, sifted, spooned	1 c	96	12	350	7	1	0.1	0.1	0.3
505	Self-rising, enriched, unsifted, spooned	1 c	125	12	440	12	1	0.2	0.1	0.5
506	Whole-wheat, from hard wheats, stirred	1 c	120	12	400	16	2	0.4	0.2	1.0
	Legumes (Dry), Nuts, Seeds; Related Products								
	Almonds, shelled								
507	Chopped (about 130 almonds)	1 c	130	5	775	24	70	5.6	47.7	12.8
508	Slivered, not pressed down (about 115 almonds)	1 c	115	5	690	21	62	5.0	42.2	11.3
	Beans, dry								
	Common varieties as Great Northern, navy, and others								
	Cooked, drained								
509	Great Northern	1 c	180	69	210	14	1	—	—	—

(Dashes (—) denote lack of reliable data for a constituent believed to be present in measurable amount)

Carbohydrate (g)	Calcium (mg)	Phosphorus (mg)	Iron (mg)	Potassium (mg)	Vitamin A Value (IU)	Thiamine (mg)	Riboflavin (mg)	Niacin (mg)	Ascorbic Acid (mg)
21	30	34	0.8	38	trace	0.16	0.10	1.3	trace
30	24	46	1.2	49	trace	0.20	0.12	1.7	trace
75	58	115	3.0	122	trace	0.54	0.32	4.5	trace
20	16	36	0.7	41	30	0.12	0.12	1.2	trace
39	14	85	1.4	103	0	0.23	0.13	1.8	0
32	11	70	1.3	85	0	0.20	0.11	1.5	0
37	80	135	2.3	408	1080	0.25	0.13	2.3	13
39	40	88	2.8	303	930	0.35	0.28	4.5	10
39	124	236	3.7	665	1590	0.25	0.30	4.0	22
29	53	113	3.3	245	1000	0.15	0.18	2.3	5
36	54[60]	67[60]	1.9	74[60]	500	0.16	0.17	2.1	([60])
28	85	130	1.3	109	250	0.17	0.23	0.14	trace
27	179	257	1.0	146	170	0.14	0.22	0.9	trace
88	18	100	3.3	109	0	0.74	0.46	6.1	0
95	20	109	3.6	119	0	0.80	0.50	6.6	0
76	16	70	2.8	91	0	0.61	0.38	5.1	0
93	331	583	3.6	—	0	0.80	0.50	6.6	0
85	49	446	4.0	444	0	0.66	0.14	5.2	0
25	304	655	6.1	1005	0	0.31	1.20	4.6	trace
22	269	580	5.4	889	0	0.28	1.06	4.0	trace
38	90	266	4.9	749	0	0.25	0.13	1.3	0

[60] Value varies with the brand. Consult the label.

Item No.	Foods, Approximate Measures, Units, and Weight (edible part unless footnotes indicate otherwise)		(g)	Water (%)	Food Energy (kcal)	Protein (g)	Fat (g)	Fatty Acids		
								Saturated (total) (g)	Unsaturated	
									Oleic (g)	Linoleic (g)
	Legumes (Dry), Nuts, Seeds—Cont									
	Beans—Cont									
	Cooked—Cont									
510	Pea (navy)	1 c	190	69	225	15	1	—	—	—
	Canned, solids and liquid									
	White with									
511	Frankfurters (sliced)	1 c	255	71	365	19	18	—	—	—
512	Pork and tomato sauce	1 c	255	71	310	16	7	2.4	2.8	0.6
513	Pork and sweet sauce	1 c	255	66	385	16	12	4.3	5.0	1.1
514	Red kidney	1 c	255	76	230	15	1	—	—	—
515	Lima, cooked, drained	1 c	190	64	260	16	1	—	—	—
516	Blackeye peas, dry, cooked (with residual cooking liquid)	1 c	250	80	190	13	1	—	—	—
517	Brazil nuts shelled (6–8 large kernels)	1 oz	28	5	185	4	19	4.8	6.2	7.1
518	Cashew nuts, roasted in oil	1 c	140	5	785	24	64	12.9	36.8	10.2
	Coconut meat, fresh									
519	Piece, about 2 by 2 by ½ in	1 piece	45	51	155	2	16	14.0	0.9	0.3
520	Shredded or grated, not pressed down	1 c	80	51	275	3	28	24.8	1.6	0.5
521	Filberts (hazelnuts), chopped (about 80 kernels)	1 c	115	6	730	14	72	5.1	55.2	7.3
522	Lentils, whole, cooked	1 c	200	72	210	16	trace	—	—	—
523	Peanuts, roasted in oil, salted (whole, halves, chopped)	1 c	144	2	840	37	72	13.7	33.0	20.7
524	Peanut butter	1 tbsp	16	2	95	4	8	1.5	3.7	2.3
525	Peas, split, dry, cooked	1 c	200	70	230	16	1	—	—	—
526	Pecans, chopped or pieces (about 120 large halves)	1 c	118	3	810	11	84	7.2	50.5	20.0
527	Pumpkin and squash kernels, dry, hulled	1 c	140	4	775	41	65	11.8	23.5	27.5
528	Sunflower seeds, dry, hulled	1 c	145	5	810	35	69	8.2	13.7	43.2
	Walnuts									
	Black									
529	Chopped or broken kernels	1 c	125	3	785	26	74	6.3	13.3	45.7
530	Ground (finely)	1 c	80	3	500	16	47	4.0	8.5	29.2
531	Persian or English, chopped (about 60 halves)	1 c	120	4	780	18	77	8.4	11.8	42.2
	Sugars and Sweets									
	Cake icings									
	Boiled, white									
532	Plain	1 c	94	18	295	1	0	0	0	0

(Dashes (—) denote lack of reliable data for a constituent believed to be present in measurable amount)

Carbohydrate (g)	Calcium (mg)	Phosphorus (mg)	Iron (mg)	Potassium (mg)	Vitamin A Value (IU)	Thiamine (mg)	Riboflavin (mg)	Niacin (mg)	Ascorbic Acid (mg)
40	95	281	5.1	790	0	0.27	0.13	1.3	0
32	94	303	4.8	668	330	0.18	0.15	3.3	trace
48	138	235	4.6	536	330	0.20	0.08	1.5	5
54	161	291	5.9	—	—	0.15	0.10	1.3	—
42	74	278	4.6	673	10	0.13	0.10	1.5	—
49	55	293	5.9	1163	—	0.25	0.11	1.3	—
35	43	238	3.3	573	30	0.40	0.10	1.0	—
3	53	196	1.0	203	trace	0.27	0.03	0.5	—
41	53	522	5.3	650	140	0.60	0.35	2.5	—
4	6	43	0.8	115	0	0.02	0.01	0.2	1
8	10	76	1.4	205	0	0.04	0.02	0.4	2
19	240	388	3.9	810	—	0.53	—	1.0	trace
39	50	238	4.2	498	40	0.14	0.12	1.2	0
27	107	577	3.0	971	—	0.46	0.19	24.8	0
3	9	61	0.3	100	—	0.02	0.02	2.4	0
42	22	178	3.4	592	80	0.30	0.18	1.8	—
17	86	341	2.8	712	150	1.01	0.15	1.1	2
21	71	1602	15.7	1386	100	0.34	0.27	3.4	—
29	174	1214	10.3	1334	70	2.84	0.33	7.8	—
19	trace	713	7.5	575	380	0.28	0.14	0.9	—
12	trace	456	4.8	368	240	0.18	0.09	0.6	—
19	119	456	3.7	540	40	0.40	0.16	1.1	2
75	2	2	trace	17	0	trace	0.03	trace	0

(continued)

Item No.	Foods, Approximate Measures, Units, and Weight (edible part unless footnotes indicate otherwise)		(g)	Water (%)	Food Energy (kcal)	Protein (g)	Fat (g)	Saturated (total) (g)	Unsaturated	
									Oleic (g)	Linoleic (g)
	Sugars and Sweets—Cont									
	Cake icings—Cont									
	Boiled—Cont									
533	With coconut	1 c	166	15	605	3	13	11.0	0.9	trace
	Uncooked									
534	Chocolate made with milk and butter	1 c	275	14	1035	9	38	23.4	11.7	1.0
535	Creamy fudge from mix and water	1 c	245	15	830	7	16	5.1	6.7	3.1
536	White	1 c	319	11	1200	2	21	12.7	5.1	0.5
	Candy									
537	Caramels, plain or chocolate	1 oz	28	8	115	1	3	1.6	1.1	0.1
	Chocolate									
538	Milk, plain	1 oz	28	1	145	2	9	5.5	3.0	0.3
539	Semisweet, small pieces (60 per oz)	1 c or 6 oz pkg	170	1	860	7	61	36.2	19.8	1.7
540	Chocolate-coated peanuts	1 oz	28	1	160	5	12	4.0	4.7	2.1
541	Fondant, uncoated (mints, candy corn, other)	1 oz	28	8	105	trace	1	0.1	0.3	0.1
542	Fudge, chocolate, plain	1 oz	28	8	115	1	3	1.3	1.4	0.6
543	Gum drops	1 oz	28	12	100	trace	trace	—	—	—
544	Hard	1 oz	28	1	110	0	trace	—	—	—
545	Marshmallows	1 oz	28	17	90	1	trace	—	—	—
	Chocolate-flavored beverage powders (about 4 heaping tsp per oz)									
546	With nonfat dry milk	1 oz	28	2	100	5	1	0.5	0.3	trace
547	Without milk	1 oz	28	1	100	1	1	0.4	0.2	trace
548	Honey, strained or extracted	1 tbsp	21	17	65	trace	0	0	0	0
549	Jams and preserves	1 tbsp	20	29	55	trace	trace	—	—	—
550		1 packet	14	29	40	trace	trace	—	—	—
551	Jellies	1 tbsp	18	29	50	trace	trace	—	—	—
552		1 packet	14	29	40	trace	trace	—	—	—
	Syrups									
	Chocolate-flavored syrup or topping									
553	Thin type	1 fl oz or 2 tbsp	38	32	90	1	1	0.5	0.3	trace
554	Fudge type	1 fl oz or 2 tbsp	38	25	125	2	5	3.1	1.6	0.1
	Molasses, cane									
555	Light (first extraction)	1 tbsp	20	24	50	—	—	—	—	—
556	Blackstrap (third extraction)	1 tbsp	20	24	45	—	—	—	—	—
557	Sorghum	1 tbsp	21	23	55	—	—	—	—	—
558	Table blends, chiefly corn, light and dark	1 tbsp	21	24	60	0	0	0	0	0
	Sugars									
559	Brown, pressed down	1 c	220	2	820	0	0	0	0	0

(Dashes (—) denote lack of reliable data for a constituent believed to be present in measurable amount)

Carbohydrate (g)	Calcium (mg)	Phosphorus (mg)	Iron (mg)	Potassium (mg)	Vitamin A Value (IU)	Thiamine (mg)	Riboflavin (mg)	Niacin (mg)	Ascorbic Acid (mg)
124	10	50	0.8	277	0	0.02	0.07	0.3	0
185	165	305	3.3	536	580	0.06	0.28	0.6	1
183	96	218	2.7	238	trace	0.05	0.20	0.7	trace
260	48	38	trace	57	860	trace	0.06	trace	trace
22	42	35	0.4	54	trace	0.01	0.05	0.1	trace
16	65	65	0.3	109	80	0.02	0.10	0.1	trace
97	51	255	4.4	553	30	0.02	0.14	0.9	0
11	33	84	0.4	143	trace	0.10	0.05	2.1	trace
25	4	2	0.3	1	0	trace	trace	trace	0
21	22	24	0.3	42	trace	0.01	0.03	0.1	trace
25	2	trace	0.1	1	0	0	trace	trace	0
28	6	2	0.5	1	0	0	0	0	0
23	5	2	0.5	2	0	0	trace	trace	0
20	167	155	0.5	227	10	0.04	0.21	0.2	1
25	9	48	0.6	142	—	0.01	0.03	0.1	0
17	1	1	0.1	11	0	trace	0.01	0.1	trace
14	4	2	0.2	18	trace	trace	0.01	trace	trace
10	3	1	0.1	12	trace	trace	trace	trace	trace
13	4	1	0.3	14	trace	trace	.01	trace	1
10	3	1	0.2	11	trace	trace	trace	trace	1
24	6	35	0.6	106	trace	0.01	0.03	0.2	0
20	48	60	0.5	107	60	0.02	0.08	0.2	trace
13	33	9	0.9	183	—	0.01	0.01	trace	—
11	137	17	3.2	585	—	0.02	0.04	0.4	—
14	35	5	2.6	—	—	—	0.02	trace	—
15	9	3	0.8	1	0	0	0	0	0
212	187	42	7.5	757	0	0.02	0.07	0.4	0

(continued)

Item No.	Foods, Approximate Measures, Units, and Weight (edible part unless footnotes indicate otherwise)		(g)	Water (%)	Food Energy (kcal)	Protein (g)	Fat (g)	Saturated (total) (g)	Unsaturated	
									Oleic (g)	Linoleic (g)
	Sugars and Sweets—Cont									
	Sugars—Cont									
	White									
560	Granulated	1 c	200	1	770	0	0	0	0	0
561		1 tbsp	12	1	45	0	0	0	0	0
562		1 packet	6	1	23	0	0	0	0	0
563	Powdered, sifted, spooned into cup	1 c	100	1	385	0	0	0	0	0
	Vegetables and Vegetable Products									
	Asparagus, green									
	Cooked, drained									
	Cuts and tips, 1½ to 2 in lengths									
564	From raw	1 c	145	94	30	3	trace	—	—	—
565	From frozen	1 c	180	93	40	6	trace	—	—	—
	Spears, ½ in diam at base									
566	From raw	4 spears	60	94	10	1	trace	—	—	—
567	From frozen	4 spears	60	92	15	2	trace	—	—	—
568	Canned, spears, ½ in diam at base	4 spears	80	93	15	2	trace	—	—	—
	Beans									
	Lima, immature seeds, frozen, cooked, drained									
569	Thick-seeded types Fordhooks)	1 c	170	74	170	10	trace	—	—	—
570	Thin-seeded types (baby limas)	1 c	180	69	210	13	trace	—	—	—
	Snap									
	Green									
	Cooked, drained									
571	From raw (cuts and French style)	1 c	125	92	30	2	trace	—	—	—
	From frozen									
572	Cuts	1 c	135	92	35	2	trace	—	—	—
573	French style	1 c	130	92	35	2	trace	—	—	—
574	Canned, drained solids (cuts)	1 c	135	92	30	2	trace	—	—	—
	Yellow or wax									
	Cooked, drained									
575	From raw (cuts and French style)	1 c	125	93	30	2	trace	—	—	—
576	From frozen (cuts)	1 c	135	92	35	2	trace	—	—	—
577	Canned, drained solids (cuts)	1 c	135	92	30	2	trace	—	—	—
	Beans, mature (see Beans, dry, items 509–515, and Black-eye peas, dry, item 516)									
	Bean sprouts (mung)									
578	Raw	1 c	105	89	35	4	trace	—	—	—
579	Cooked, drained	1 c	125	91	35	4	trace	—	—	—

(Dashes (—) denote lack of reliable data for a constituent believed to be present in measurable amount)

Carbohydrate (g)	Calcium (mg)	Phosphorus (mg)	Iron (mg)	Potassium (mg)	Vitamin A Value (IU)	Thiamine (mg)	Riboflavin (mg)	Niacin (mg)	Ascorbic Acid (mg)
199	0	0	0.2	6	0	0	0	0	0
12	0	0	trace	trace	0	0	0	0	0
6	0	0	trace	trace	0	0	0	0	0
100	0	0	0.1	3	0	0	0	0	0
5	30	73	0.9	265	1310	0.23	0.26	2.0	38
6	40	115	2.2	396	1530	0.25	0.23	1.8	41
2	13	30	0.4	110	540	0.10	0.11	0.8	16
2	13	40	0.7	143	470	0.10	0.08	0.7	16
3	15	42	1.5	133	640	0.05	0.08	0.6	12
32	34	153	2.9	724	390	0.12	0.09	1.7	29
40	63	227	4.7	709	400	0.16	0.09	2.2	22
7	63	46	0.8	189	680	0.09	0.11	0.6	15
8	54	43	0.9	205	780	0.09	0.12	0.5	7
8	49	39	1.2	177	690	0.08	0.10	0.4	9
7	61	34	2.0	128	630	0.04	0.07	0.4	5
6	63	46	0.8	189	290	0.09	0.11	0.6	16
8	47	42	0.9	221	140	0.09	0.11	0.5	8
7	61	34	2.0	128	140	0.04	0.07	0.4	7
7	20	67	1.4	234	20	0.14	0.14	0.8	20
7	21	60	1.1	195	30	0.11	0.13	0.9	8

(continued)

Item No.	Foods, Approximate Measures, Units, and Weight (edible part unless footnotes indicate otherwise)		(g)	Water (%)	Food Energy (kcal)	Protein (g)	Fat (g)	Saturated (total) (g)	Unsaturated	
									Oleic (g)	Linoleic (g)
	Vegetable and Vegetable Products—Cont									
	Beets									
	Cooked, drained, peeled									
580	Whole beets 2 in diam	2 beets	100	91	30	1	trace	—	—	—
581	Diced or sliced	1 c	170	91	55	2	trace			
	Canned, drained solids									
582	Whole beets, small	1 c	160	89	60	2	trace	—	—	—
583	Diced or sliced	1 c	170	89	65	2	trace	—	—	—
584	Beet greens, leaves and stems, cooked, drained	1 c	145	94	25	2	trace	—	—	—
	Blackeye peas, immature seeds, cooked and drained									
585	From raw	1 c	165	72	180	13	1	—	—	—
586	From frozen	1 c	170	66	220	15	1	—	—	—
	Broccoli, cooked, drained									
	From raw									
587	Stalk, medium size	1 stalk	180	91	45	6	1	—	—	—
588	Stalks cut into ½ in pieces	1 c	155	91	40	5	trace	—	—	—
	From frozen									
589	Stalk, 4 ½ to 5 in long	1 stalk	30	91	10	1	trace	—	—	—
590	Chopped	1 c	185	92	50	5	1	—	—	—
	Brussels sprouts, cooked, drained									
591	From raw, 7–8 sprouts (1¼ to 1½ in diam)	1 c	155	88	55	7	1	—	—	—
592	From frozen	1 c	155	89	50	5	trace	—	—	—
	Cabbage									
	Common varieties									
	Raw									
593	Coarsely shredded or sliced	1 c	70	92	15	1	trace	—	—	—
594	Finely shredded or chopped	1 c	90	92	20	1	trace	—	—	—
595	Cooked, drained	1 c	145	94	30	2	trace	—	—	—
596	Red, raw, coarsely shredded or sliced	1 c	70	90	20	1	trace	—	—	—
597	Savory, raw, coarsely shredded or sliced	1 c	70	92	15	2	trace	—	—	—
598	Cabbage, celery (also called pe-tsai or wongbok), raw, 1 in pieces	1 c	75	95	10	1	trace	—	—	—
599	Cabbage, white mustard (also called bokchoy or pakchoy), cooked, drained	1 c	170	95	25	2	trace	—	—	—
	Carrots									
	Raw, without crowns and tips, scraped									
600	Whole, 7½ by 1⅛ in, or strips, 2½ to 3 in long	1 carrot or 18 strips	72	88	30	1	trace	—	—	—

(Dashes (—) denote lack of reliable data for a constituent believed to be present in measurable amount)

Carbohydrate (g)	Calcium (mg)	Phosphorus (mg)	Iron (mg)	Potassium (mg)	Vitamin A Value (IU)	Thiamine (mg)	Riboflavin (mg)	Niacin (mg)	Ascorbic Acid (mg)
7	14	23	0.5	208	20	0.03	0.04	0.3	6
12	24	39	0.9	354	30	0.05	0.07	0.5	10
14	30	29	1.1	267	30	0.02	0.05	0.2	5
15	32	31	1.2	284	30	0.02	0.05	0.2	5
5	144	36	2.8	481	7400	0.10	0.22	0.4	22
30	40	241	3.5	625	580	0.50	0.18	2.3	28
40	43	286	4.8	573	290	0.68	0.19	2.4	15
8	158	112	1.4	481	4500	0.16	0.36	1.4	162
7	136	96	1.2	414	3880	0.14	0.31	1.2	140
1	12	17	0.2	66	570	0.02	0.03	0.2	22
9	100	104	1.3	392	4810	0.11	0.22	0.9	105
10	50	112	1.7	423	810	0.12	0.22	1.2	135
10	33	95	1.2	457	880	0.12	0.16	0.9	126
4	34	20	0.3	163	90	0.04	0.04	0.2	33
5	44	26	0.4	210	120	0.05	.05	0.3	42
6	64	29	0.4	236	190	0.06	.06	0.4	48
5	29	25	0.6	188	30	0.06	.04	0.3	43
3	47	38	0.6	188	140	0.04	0.06	0.2	39
2	32	30	0.5	190	110	0.04	0.03	0.5	19
4	252	56	1.0	364	5270	0.07	0.14	1.2	26
7	27	26	0.5	246	7930	0.04	0.04	0.4	6

(continued)

Item No.	Foods, Approximate Measures, Units, and Weight (edible part unless footnotes indicate otherwise)		(g)	Water (%)	Food Energy (kcal)	Protein (g)	Fat (g)	Saturated (total) (g)	Unsaturated	
									Oleic (g)	Linoleic (g)
	Vegetable and Vegetable Products—Cont									
	Carrots—Cont									
	Raw—Cont									
601	Grated	1 c	110	88	45	1	trace	—	—	—
602	Cooked (crosswise cuts), drained	1 c	155	91	50	1	trace	—	—	—
	Canned									
603	Sliced, drained solids	1 c	155	91	45	1	trace	—	—	—
604	Strained or junior (baby food)	1 oz (1¾ to 2 tbsp)	28	92	10	trace	trace	—	—	—
	Cauliflower									
605	Raw, chopped	1 c	115	91	31	3	trace	—	—	—
	Cooked, drained									
606	From raw (flower buds)	1 c	125	93	30	3	trace	—	—	—
607	From frozen (flowerets)	1 c	180	94	30	3	trace	—	—	—
	Celery, Pascal type, raw									
608	Stalk, large outer, 8 by 1½ in, at root end	1 stalk	40	94	5	trace	trace	—	—	—
609	Pieces, diced	1 c	120	94	20	1	trace	—	—	—
	Collards, cooked, drained									
610	From raw (leaves without stems)	1 c	190	90	65	7	1	—	—	—
611	From frozen (chopped)	1 c	170	90	50	5	1	—	—	—
	Corn, sweet									
	Cooked, drained									
612	From raw, ear 5 by 1¾ in	1 ear[61]	140	74	70	2	1	—	—	—
	From frozen									
613	Ear, 5 in long	1 ear[61]	229	73	120	4	1	—	—	—
614	Kernels	1 c	165	77	130	5	1	—	—	—
	Canned									
615	Cream style	1 c	256	76	210	5	2	—	—	—
	Whole kernel									
616	Vacuum pack	1 c	210	76	175	5	1	—	—	—
617	Wet pack, drained solids	1 c	165	76	140	4	1	—	—	—
	Cowpeas (see Blackeye Peas, items 585–586)									
	Cucumber slices, ⅛ in thick (large, 2⅛ in diam; small, 1¾ in diam)									
618	With peel	6 large or 8 small slices	28	95	5	trace	trace	—	—	—
619	Without peel	6½ large or 9 small pieces	28	96	5	trace	trace	—	—	—

(Dashes (—) denote lack of reliable data for a constituent believed to be present in measurable amount)

[61] Weight includes cob. Without cob, weight is 77 g for item 612, 126 g for item 613.

[62] Based on yellow varieties. For white varieties, value is trace.

Carbohydrate (g)	Calcium (mg)	Phosphorus (mg)	Iron (mg)	Potassium (mg)	Vitamin A Value (IU)	Thiamine (mg)	Riboflavin (mg)	Niacin (mg)	Ascorbic Acid (mg)
11	41	40	0.8	375	12,100	0.07	0.06	0.7	9
11	51	48	0.9	344	16,280	0.08	0.08	0.8	9
10	47	34	1.1	186	23,250	0.03	0.05	0.6	3
2	7	6	0.1	51	3690	0.01	0.01	0.1	1
6	29	64	1.3	339	70	0.13	0.12	0.8	90
5	26	53	0.9	258	80	0.11	0.10	0.8	69
6	31	68	0.9	373	50	0.07	0.09	0.7	74
2	16	11	0.1	136	110	0.01	0.01	0.1	4
5	47	34	0.4	409	320	0.04	0.04	0.4	11
10	357	99	1.5	498	14,820	0.21	0.38	2.3	144
10	299	87	1.7	401	11,560	0.10	0.24	1.0	56
16	2	69	0.5	151	310[62]	0.09	0.08	1.1	7
27	4	121	1.0	291	440[62]	0.18	0.10	2.1	9
31	5	120	1.3	304	580[62]	0.15	0.10	2.5	8
51	8	143	1.5	248	840[62]	0.08	0.13	2.6	13
43	6	153	1.1	204	740[62]	0.06	0.13	2.3	11
33	8	81	0.8	160	580[62]	0.05	0.08	1.5	7
1	7	8	0.3	45	70	0.01	0.01	0.1	3
1	5	5	0.1	45	trace	0.01	0.01	0.1	3

(continued)

Item No.	Foods, Approximate Measures, Units, and Weight (edible part unless footnotes indicate otherwise)		(g)	Water (%)	Food Energy (kcal)	Protein (g)	Fat (g)	Fatty Acids		
								Saturated (total) (g)	Unsaturated	
									Oleic (g)	Linoleic (g)
	Vegetable and Vegetable Products—Cont									
	Cucumber slices—Cont									
620	Dandelion greens, cooked, drained	1 c	105	90	35	2	1	—	—	—
621	Endive, curly (including escarole), raw, small pieces	1 c	50	93	10	1	trace	—	—	—
	Kale, cooked, drained									
622	From raw (leaves without stems and midribs)	1 c	110	88	45	5	1	—	—	—
623	From frozen (leaf style)	1 c	130	91	40	4	1	—	—	—
	Lettuce, raw									
	Butterhead, as Boston types									
624	Head, 5 in diam	1 head[63]	220	95	25	2	trace	—	—	—
625	Leaves	1 outer or 2 inner or 3 heart leaves	15	95	trace	trace	trace	—	—	—
	Crisphead, as Iceberg									
626	Head, 6 in diam	1 head[64]	567	96	70	5	1	—	—	—
627	Wedge, ¼ of head	1 wedge	135	96	20	1	trace	—	—	—
628	Pieces, chopped or shredded	1 c	55	96	5	trace	trace	—	—	—
629	Looseleaf (bunching varieties including romaine or cos), chopped or shredded pieces	1 c	55	94	10	1	trace	—	—	—
630	Mushrooms, raw, sliced or chopped	1 c	70	90	20	2	trace	—	—	—
631	Mustard greens, without stems and midribs, cooked, drained	1 c	140	93	30	3	1	—	—	—
632	Okra pods, 3 by ⅝ in, cooked	10 pods	106	91	30	2	trace	—	—	—
	Onions									
	Mature									
	Raw									
633	Chopped	1 c	170	89	65	3	trace	—	—	—
634	Sliced	1 c	115	89	45	2	trace	—	—	—
635	Cooked (whole or sliced), drained	1 c	210	92	60	3	trace	—	—	—
636	Young green, bulb (⅜ in diam) and white portion of top	6 onions	30	88	15	trace	trace	—	—	—
637	Parsley, raw, chopped	1 tbsp	4	85	trace	trace	trace	—	—	—
638	Parsnips, cooked (diced or 2 in lengths)	1 c	155	82	100	2	1	—	—	—
	Peas, green									
	Canned									
639	Whole, drained solids	1 c	170	77	150	8	1	—	—	—

(Dashes (—) denote lack of reliable data for a constituent believed to be present in measurable amount)

[63] Weight includes refuse of outer leaves and core. Without these parts, weight is 163 g.

[64] Weight includes core. Without core, weight is 539 g.

[65] Value based on white-fleshed varieties. For yellow-fleshed varieties, value in IU is 70 for item 633, 50 for item 634, and 80 for item 635.

Carbohydrate (g)	Calcium (mg)	Phosphorus (mg)	Iron (mg)	Potassium (mg)	Vitamin A Value (IU)	Thiamine (mg)	Riboflavin (mg)	Niacin (mg)	Ascorbic Acid (mg)
7	147	44	1.9	244	12,290	0.14	0.17	—	19
2	41	27	0.9	147	1650	0.04	0.07	0.3	5
7	206	64	1.8	243	9130	0.11	0.20	1.8	102
7	157	62	1.3	251	10,660	0.08	0.20	0.9	49
4	57	42	3.3	430	1580	0.10	0.10	0.5	13
trace ·	5	4	0.3	40	150	0.01	0.01	trace	1
16	108	118	2.7	943	1780	0.32	0.32	1.6	32
4	27	30	0.7	236	450	0.08	0.08	0.4	8
2	11	12	0.3	96	180	0.03	0.03	0.2	3
2	37	14	0.8	145	1050	0.03	0.04	0.2	10
3	4	81	0.6	290	trace	0.07	0.32	2.9	2
6	193	45	2.5	308	8120	0.11	0.20	0.8	67
6	98	43	0.5	184	520	0.14	0.19	1.0	21
15	46	61	0.9	267	trace[65]	0.05	0.07	0.3	17
10	31	41	0.6	181	trace[65]	0.03	0.05	0.2	12
14	50	61	0.8	231	trace[65]	0.06	0.06	0.4	15
3	12	12	0.2	69	trace	0.02	0.01	0.1	8
trace	7	2	0.2	25	300	trace	0.01	trace	6
23	70	96	0.9	587	50	0.11	0.12	0.2	16
29	44	129	3.2	163	1170	0.15	0.10	1.4	14

(continued)

Item No.	Foods, Approximate Measures, Units, and Weight (edible part unless footnotes indicate otherwise)		(g)	Water (%)	Food Energy (kcal)	Protein (g)	Fat (g)	Saturated (total) (g)	Unsaturated	
									Oleic (g)	Linoleic (g)
	Vegetable and Vegetable Products—Cont									
640	Strained (baby food)	1 oz (1¾ to 2 tbsp)	28	86	15	1	trace	—	—	—
641	Frozen, cooked, drained	1 c	160	82	110	8	trace	—	—	—
642	Peppers, hot, red, without seeds, dried (ground chili powder, added seasonings)	1 tsp	2	9	5	trace	trace	—	—	—
	Peppers, sweet (about 5 per lb, whole), stem and seeds removed									
643	Raw	1 pod	74	93	15	1	trace	—	—	—
644	Cooked, boiled, drained	1 pod	73	95	15	1	trace	—	—	—
	Potatoes, cooked									
645	Baked, peeled after baking (about 2 per lb, raw)	1 potato	156	75	145	4	trace	—	—	—
	Boiled (about 3 per lb, raw)									
646	Peeled after boiling	1 potato	137	80	105	3	trace	—	—	—
647	Peeled before boiling	1 potato	135	83	90	3	trace	—	—	—
	French-fried, strip, 2 to 3½ in long									
648	Prepared from raw	10 strips	50	45	135	2	7	1.7	1.2	3.3
649	Frozen, oven heated	10 strips	50	53	110	2	4	1.1	0.8	2.1
650	Hashed brown, prepared from frozen	1 c	155	56	345	3	18	4.6	3.2	9.0
	Mashed, prepared from Raw									
651	Milk added	1 c	210	83	135	4	2	0.7	0.4	trace
652	Milk and butter added	1 c	210	80	195	4	9	5.6	2.3	0.2
653	Dehydrated flakes (without milk), water, milk, butter, and salt added	1 c	210	79	195	4	7	3.6	2.1	0.2
654	Potato chips, 1¾ by 2½ in oval cross section	10 chips	20	2	115	1	8	2.1	1.4	4.0
655	Potato salad, made with cooked salad dressing	1 c	250	76	250	7	7	2.0	2.7	1.3
656	Pumpkin, canned	1 c	245	90	80	2	1	—	—	—
657	Radishes, raw (pre-packaged) stem ends, rootlets cut off	4 radishes	18	95	5	trace	trace	—	—	—
658	Sauerkraut, canned, solids and liquid	1 c	235	93	40	2	trace	—	—	—
	Southern peas (see Blackeye peas, items 585–586)									
	Spinach									
659	Raw, chopped	1 c	55	91	15	2	trace	—	—	—

(Dashes (—) denote lack of reliable data for a constituent believed to be present in measurable amount)

Carbohydrate (g)	Calcium (mg)	Phosphorus (mg)	Iron (mg)	Potassium (mg)	Vitamin A Value (IU)	Thiamine (mg)	Riboflavin (mg)	Niacin (mg)	Ascorbic Acid (mg)
3	3	18	0.3	28	140	0.02	0.03	0.3	3
19	30	138	3.0	216	960	0.43	0.14	2.7	21
1	5	4	0.3	20	1300	trace	0.02	0.2	trace
4	7	16	0.5	157	310	0.06	0.06	0.4	94
3	7	12	0.4	109	310	0.05	0.05	0.4	70
33	14	101	1.1	782	trace	0.15	0.07	2.7	31
23	10	72	0.8	556	trace	0.12	0.05	2.0	22
20	8	57	0.7	385	trace	0.12	0.05	1.6	22
18	8	56	0.7	427	trace	0.07	0.04	1.6	11
17	5	43	0.9	326	trace	0.07	0.01	1.3	11
45	28	78	1.9	439	trace	0.11	0.03	1.6	12
27	50	103	8	548	40	0.17	0.11	2.1	21
26	50	101	0.8	525	360	0.17	0.11	2.1	19
30	65	99	0.6	601	270	0.08	0.08	1.9	11
10	8	28	0.4	226	trace	0.04	0.01	1.0	3
41	80	160	1.5	798	350	0.20	0.18	2.8	28
19	61	64	1.0	588	15,680	0.07	0.12	1.5	12
1	5	6	0.2	58	trace	0.01	0.01	0.1	5
9	85	42	1.2	329	120	0.07	0.09	0.5	33
2	51	28	1.7	259	4460	0.06	0.11	0.3	28

(continued)

| | | | | | | | Fatty Acids | | |
| | | | | | | | Saturated (total) (g) | Unsaturated | |
Item No.	Foods, Approximate Measures, Units, and Weight (edible part unless footnotes indicate otherwise)	(g)	Water (%)	Food Energy (kcal)	Protein (g)	Fat (g)		Oleic (g)	Linoleic (g)
	Vegetable and Vegetable Products—Cont								
	Spinach—Cont								
	Cooked, drained								
660	From raw	1 c	180	92	40	5	1	—	—	—
	From frozen								
661	Chopped	1 c	205	92	45	6	1	—	—	—
662	Leaf	1 c	190	92	45	6	1	—	—	—
663	Canned, drained solids	1 c	205	91	50	6	1	—	—	—
	Squash, cooked								
664	Summer (all varieties), diced, drained	1 c	210	96	30	2	trace	—	—	—
665	Winter (all varieties), baked, mashed	1 c	205	81	130	4	1	—	—	—
	Sweetpotatoes								
	Cooked (raw, 5 by 2 in; about 2½ per lb)								
666	Baked in skin, peeled	1 potato	114	64	160	2	1	—	—	—
667	Boiled in skin, peeled	1 potato	151	71	170	3	1	—	—	—
668	Candied, 2½ by 2 in piece	1 piece	105	60	175	1	3	2.0	0.8	0.1
	Canned								
669	Solid pack (mashed)	1 c	255	72	275	5	1	—	—	—
670	Vacuum pack, piece 2¾ by 1 in	1 piece	40	72	45	1	trace	—	—	—
	Tomatoes								
671	Raw, 2⅗ in diam (3 per 12 oz pkg)	1 tomato[66]	135	94	25	1	trace	—	—	—
672	Canned, solids and liquid	1 c	241	94	50	2	trace	—	—	—
673	Tomato catsup	1 c	273	69	290	5	1	—	—	—
		1 tbsp	15	69	15	trace	trace	—	—	—
674	Tomato juice, canned								
675	Cup	1 c	243	94	45	2	trace	—	—	—
676	Glass (6 fl oz)	1 glass	182	94	35	2	trace	—	—	—
677	Turnips, cooked, diced	1 c	155	94	35	1	trace	—	—	—
	Turnip greens, cooked drained								
678	From raw (leaves and stems)	1 c	145	94	30	3	trace	—	—	—
679	From frozen (chopped)	1 c	165	93	40	4	trace	—	—	—
680	Vegetables, mixed, frozen, cooked	1 c	182	83	115	6	1	—	—	—
	Miscellaneous Items								
	Baking powders for home use								
	Sodium aluminum sulfate								
681	With monocalcium phosphate monohydrate	1 tsp	3.0	2	5	trace	trace	0	0	0

(Dashes (—) denote lack of reliable data for a constituent believed to be present in measurable amount)

[66] Weight includes cores and stem ends. Without these parts, weight is 123 g.

[67] Based on year-round average. For tomatoes marketed from November through May, value is about 12 mg; from June through October, 32 mg.

[68] Applies to product without calcium salts added. Value for products with calcium salts added may be as much as 63 mg for whole tomatoes, 241 mg for cut forms.

Carbohydrate (g)	Calcium (mg)	Phosphorus (mg)	Iron (mg)	Potassium (mg)	Vitamin A Value (IU)	Thiamine (mg)	Riboflavin (mg)	Niacin (mg)	Ascorbic Acid (mg)
6	167	68	4.0	583	14,580	0.13	0.25	0.9	50
8	232	90	4.3	683	16,200	0.14	0.31	0.8	39
7	200	84	4.8	688	15,390	0.15	0.27	1.0	53
7	242	53	5.3	513	16,400	0.04	0.25	0.6	29
7	53	53	0.8	296	820	0.11	0.17	1.7	21
32	57	98	1.6	945	8610	0.10	0.27	1.4	27
37	46	66	1.0	342	9230	0.10	0.08	0.8	25
40	48	71	1.1	367	11,940	0.14	0.09	0.9	26
36	39	45	0.9	200	6620	0.06	0.04	0.4	11
63	64	105	2.0	510	19,890	0.13	0.10	1.5	36
10	10	16	0.3	80	3120	0.02	0.02	0.2	6
6	16	33	0.6	300	1110	0.07	0.05	0.9	28[67]
10	14[68]	46	1.2	523	2170	0.12	0.07	1.7	41
69	60	137	2.2	991	3820	0.25	0.19	4.4	41
4	3	8	0.1	54	0.210	0.01	0.01	0.2	2
10	17	44	2.2	552	1940	0.12	0.07	1.9	39
8	13	33	1.6	413	1460	0.09	0.05	1.5	29
8	54	37	0.6	291	trace	0.06	0.08	0.5	34
5	252	49	1.5	—	8270	0.15	0.33	0.7	68
6	195	64	2.6	246	11,390	0.08	0.15	0.7	31
24	46	115	2.4	348	9010	0.22	0.13	2.0	15
1	58	87	—	5	0	0	0	0	0

(continued)

				Fatty Acids		
					Unsaturated	
Item No.	Foods, Approximate Measures, Units, and Weight (edible part unless footnotes indicate otherwise)	(g)	Water (%)	Food Energy (kcal)	Protein (g)	Fat (g)	Saturated (total) (g)	Oleic (g)	Linoleic (g)

Item No.	Foods, Approximate Measures, Units, and Weight	(g)	Water (%)	Food Energy (kcal)	Protein (g)	Fat (g)	Saturated (total) (g)	Oleic (g)	Linoleic (g)
	Miscellaneous Items—Cont								
	Baking powders for home use—Cont								
	Sodium aluminum sulfate—Cont								
682	With monocalcium phosphate monohydrate, calcium sulfate	1 tsp	2.9	1	5	trace	trace	0	0	0
683	Straight phosphate	1 tsp	3.8	2	5	trace	trace	0	0	0
684	Low sodium	1 tsp	4.3	2	5	trace	trace	0	0	0
685	Barbecue sauce	1 c	250	81	230	4	17	2.2	4.3	10.0
	Beverages, alcoholic								
686	Beer	12 fl oz	360	92	150	1	0	0	0	0
	Gin, rum, vodka, whisky								
687	80 proof	1½ fl oz jigger	42	67	95	—	—	0	0	0
688	86 proof	1½ fl oz jigger	42	64	105	—	—			
689	90 proof	1½ fl oz jigger	42	62	110	—	—	0	0	0
	Wines								
690	Dessert	3½ fl oz glass	103	77	140	trace	0	0	0	0
691	Table	3½ fl oz glass	102	86	85	trace	0	0	0	0
	Beverages, carbonated, sweetened, nonalcoholic								
692	Carbonated water	12 fl oz	366	92	115	0	0	0	0	0
693	Cola type	12 fl oz	369	90	145	0	0	0	0	0
694	Fruit-flavored sodas and Tom Collins mixer	12 fl oz	372	88	170	0	0	0	0	0
695	Ginger ale	12 fl oz	366	92	115	0	0	0	0	0
696	Root beer	12 fl oz	370	90	150	0	0	0	0	0
	Chili powder (see Peppers, hot, red, item 642)								
	Chocolate								
697	Bitter or baking Semisweet (see Candy, chocolate, item 539)	1 oz	28	2	145	3	15	8.9	4.9	0.4
698	Gelatin, dry	1 7 g en-velope	7	13	25	6	trace	0	0	0
699	Gelatin dessert pre-pared with gelatin dessert powder and water	1 c	240	84	140	4	0	0	0	0
700	Mustard, prepared, yellow	1 tsp or individual serving pouch or cup	5	80	5	trace	trace	—	—	—

(Dashes (—) denote lack of reliable data for a constituent believed to be present in measurable amount)

Carbohydrate (g)	Calcium (mg)	Phosphorus (mg)	Iron (mg)	Potassium (mg)	Vitamin A Value (IU)	Thiamine (mg)	Riboflavin (mg)	Niacin (mg)	Ascorbic Acid (mg)
1	183	45	—	—	0	0	0	0	0
1	239	359	—	6	0	0	0	0	0
2	207	314	—	471	0	0	0	0	0
20	53	50	2.0	435	900	0.03	0.03	0.8	13
14	18	108	trace	90	—	0.01	0.11	2.2	—
trace	—	—	—	1	—	—	—	—	—
trace	—	—	—	1	—	—	—	—	—
trace	—	—	—	1	—	—	—	—	—
8	8	—	—	77	—	0.01	0.02	0.2	—
4	9	10	0.4	94	—	trace	0.01	0.1	—
29	—	—	—	—	0	0	0	0	0
37	—	—	—	—	0	0	0	0	0
45	—	—	—	—	0	0	0	0	0
29	—	—	—	0	0	0	0	0	0
39	—	—	—	0	0	0	0	0	0
8	22	109	1.9	235	20	0.01	0.07	0.4	0
0	—	—	—	—	—	—	—	—	—
34	—	—	—	—	—	—	—	—	—
trace	4	4	0.1	7	—	—	—	—	—

(continued)

Item No.	Foods, Approximate Measures, Units, and Weight (edible part unless footnotes indicate otherwise)		(g)	Water (%)	Food Energy (kcal)	Protein (g)	Fat (g)	Fatty Acids		
								Saturated (total) (g)	Unsaturated	
									Oleic (g)	Linoleic (g)
	Miscellaneous Items—Cont									
	Olives, pickled, canned									
701	Green	4 medium or 3 extra large or 2 giant[69]	16	78	15	trace	2	0.2	1.2	0.1
702	Ripe, Mission	3 small or 2 large[69]	10	73	15	trace	2	0.2	1.2	0.1
	Pickles, cucumber									
703	Dill, medium, whole, 3¾ in long, 1¼ in diam	1 pickle	65	93	5	trace	trace	—	—	—
704	Fresh-pack, slices 1½ in diam, ¼ in thick	2 slices	15	79	10	trace	trace	—	—	—
705	Sweet, gherkin, small, whole, about 2½ in long, ¾ in diam	1 pickle	15	61	20	trace	trace	—	—	—
706	Relish, finely chopped, sweet	1 tbsp	15	63	20	trace	trace	—	—	—
	Popcorn (see items 476–478)									
707	Popsicle, 3 fl oz size	1 popsicle	95	80	70	0	0	0	0	0
	Soups									
	Canned, condensed									
	Prepared with equal volume of milk									
708	Cream of chicken	1 c	245	85	180	7	10	4.2	3.6	1.3
709	Cream of mushroom	1 c	245	83	215	7	14	5.4	2.9	4.6
710	Tomato	1 c	250	84	175	7	7	3.4	1.7	1.0
	Prepared with equal volume of water									
711	Bean with pork	1 c	250	84	170	8	6	1.2	1.8	2.4
712	Beef broth, bouillon, consomme	1 c	240	96	30	5	0	0	0	0
713	Beef noodle	1 c	240	93	65	4	3	0.6	0.7	0.8
714	Clam chowder, Manhattan type (with tomatoes, without milk)	1 c	245	92	80	2	3	0.5	0.4	1.3
715	Cream of chicken	1 c	240	92	95	3	6	1.6	2.3	1.1
716	Cream of mushroom	1 c	240	90	135	2	10	2.6	1.7	4.5
717	Minestrone	1 c	245	90	105	5	3	0.7	0.9	1.3
718	Split pea	1 c	245	85	145	9	3	1.1	1.2	0.4
719	Tomato	1 c	245	91	90	2	3	0.5	0.5	1.0
720	Vegetable beef	1 c	245	92	80	5	2	—	—	—
721	Vegetarian	1 c	245	92	80	2	2	—	—	—
	Dehydrated									
722	Bouillon cube, ½ in	1 cube	4	4	5	1	trace	—	—	—
	Mixes									
	Unprepared									
723	Onion	1½ oz pkg	43	3	150	6	5	1.1	2.3	1.0

(Dashes (—) denote lack of reliable data for a constituent believed to be present in measurable amount)
[69] Weight includes pits. Without pits, weight is 13 g for item 701, 9 g for item 702.

Carbohydrate (g)	Calcium (mg)	Phosphorus (mg)	Iron (mg)	Potassium (mg)	Vitamin A Value (IU)	Thiamine (mg)	Riboflavin (mg)	Niacin (mg)	Ascorbic Acid (mg)
trace	8	2	0.2	7	40	—	—	—	—
trace	9	1	0.1	2	10	trace	trace	—	—
1	17	14	0.7	130	70	trace	0.01	trace	4
3	5	4	0.3	—	20	trace	trace	trace	1
5	2	2	0.2	—	10	trace	trace	trace	1
5	3	2	0.1	—	—	—	—	—	—
18	0	—	trace	—	0	0	0	0	0
15	172	152	0.5	260	610	0.05	0.27	0.7	2
16	191	169	0.5	279	250	0.05	0.34	0.7	1
23	168	155	0.8	418	1200	0.10	0.25	1.3	15
22	63	128	2.3	395	650	0.13	0.08	1.0	3
3	trace	31	0.5	130	trace	trace	0.02	1.2	—
7	7	48	1.0	77	50	0.05	0.07	1.0	trace
12	34	47	1.0	184	880	0.02	0.02	1.0	—
8	24	34	0.5	79	410	0.02	0.05	0.5	trace
10	41	50	0.5	98	70	0.02	0.12	0.7	trace
14	37	59	1.0	314	2350	0.07	0.05	1.0	—
21	29	149	1.5	270	440	0.25	0.15	1.5	1
16	15	34	0.7	230	1000	0.05	0.05	1.2	12
10	12	49	0.7	162	2700	0.05	0.05	1.0	—
13	20	39	1.0	172	2940	0.05	0.05	1.0	—
trace	—	—	—	4	—	—	—	—	—
23	42	49	0.6	238	30	0.05	0.03	0.3	6

(continued)

Item No.	Foods, Approximate Measures, Units, and Weight (edible part unless footnotes indicate otherwise)		(g)	Water (%)	Food Energy (kcal)	Protein (g)	Fat (g)	Saturated (total) (g)	Unsaturated Oleic (g)	Unsaturated Linoleic (g)
	Miscellaneous Items—Cont									
	Prepared with water									
724	Chicken noodle	1 c	240	95	55	2	1	—	—	—
725	Onion	1 c	240	96	35	1	1	—	—	—
726	Tomato vegetable with noodles	1 c	240	93	65	1	1	—	—	—
727	Vinegar, cider	1 tbsp	15	94	trace	trace	0	0	0	0
728	White sauce, medium, with enriched flour	1 c	250	73	405	10	31	19.3	7.8	0.8
	Yeast									
729	Baker's dry, active	1 pkg	7	5	20	3	trace	—	—	—
730	Brewer's, dry	1 tbsp	8	5	25	3	trace	—	—	—

(Dashes (—) denote lack of reliable data for a constituent believed to be present in measurable amount)

[70] Value may vary from 6 to 60 mg.

Carbohydrate (g)	Calcium (mg)	Phosphorus (mg)	Iron (mg)	Potassium (mg)	Vitamin A Value (IU)	Thiamine (mg)	Riboflavin (mg)	Niacin (mg)	Ascorbic Acid (mg)
8	7	19	0.2	19	50	0.07	0.05	0.5	trace
6	10	12	0.2	58	trace	trace	trace	trace	2
12	7	19	0.2	29	480	0.05	0.02	0.5	5
1	1	1	0.1	15	—	—	—	—	—
22	288	233	0.5	348	1150	0.12	0.43	0.7	2
3	3	90	1.1	140	trace	0.16	0.38	2.6	trace
3	17[70]	140	1.4	152	trace	1.25	0.34	3.0	trace

APPENDIX 2
FOOD EXCHANGE LISTS

LIST 1. MILK EXCHANGES (One exchange contains carbohydrate 12 g, protein 8 g, and 80 kcal)

	Amount to Use
Milk, nonfat, fortified[a]	
Skim or nonfat milk	1 c
Powdered (nonfat dry before adding liquid)	⅓ c
Canned, evaporated, skim	½ c
Buttermilk made from skim milk	1 c
Yoghurt, made from skim milk, plain, unflavored	1 c
Milk, low-fat, fortified	
1% fat, fortified (omit ½ fat exchange)	1 c
2% fat, fortified (omit 1 fat exchange)	1 c
Yoghurt made from 2% fortified, plain, unflavored (omit 1 fat exchange)	1 c
Milk, whole (omit 2 fat exchanges)	
Whole milk	1 c
Canned evaporated whole milk	½ c
Buttermilk made from whole milk	1 c
Yoghurt made from whole milk, plain, unflavored	1 c

[a] For diets restricted in saturated fat and cholesterol, select nonfat milk exchanges. If other types of milk are used, eliminate the indicated number of fat exchanges.

LIST 2. VEGETABLE EXCHANGES (One exchange contains carbohydrate 5 g, protein 2 g, and 25 kcal)

½ c equals 1 exchange

Asparagus[a]	Greens[a,b]	Rhubarb
Bean sprouts	Beet greens	Rutabaga[a]
Beets	Chard	Sauerkraut
Broccoli[a,b]	Collards	String beans, green or yellow
Brussels sprouts[a]	Dandelion greens	Summer squash
Cabbage[a]	Kale	Tomatoes[a]
Carrots[b]	Mustard greens	Tomato juice[a]
Cauliflower[a]	Spinach	Turnips[a]
Celery	Turnip greens	Vegetable juice cocktail
Cucumbers	Mushrooms	Zucchini
Eggplant	Okra	
	Onions	

Note: Starchy vegetables are found in List 4 (bread exchanges)

[a] Good source of ascorbic acid.
[b] Good source of vitamin A.

(continued)

LIST 3. FRUIT EXCHANGES (*One exchange contains carbohydrate 10 g and 40 kcal*)

	Amount to Use
Apple	1 small
Apple juice	⅓ c
Applesauce (unsweetened)	½ c
Apricots, fresh[a]	2 medium
Apricots, dried[a]	4 halves
Banana	½ small
Berries	
Blackberries	½ c
Blueberries	½ c
Raspberries[b]	½ c
Strawberries[b]	¾ c
Cherries	10 large
Cider	⅓ c
Dates	2
Figs, fresh	1
Figs, dried	1
Grapefruit[b]	½
Grapefruit juice[b]	½ c
Grapes	12
Grape juice	¼ c
Mango[a,b]	½ small
Melon	
Cantaloupe[a,b]	¼ small
Honeydew[b]	⅛ medium
Watermelon[b]	1 c
Nectarine[b]	1 small
Orange[b]	1 small
Orange juice[b]	½ c
Papaya[a,b]	¾ c
Peach[a]	1 medium
Pear	1 small
Persimmon, native[a]	1 medium
Pineapple	½ c
Pineapple juice	⅓ c
Plums	2 medium
Prunes	2 medium
Prune juice	¼ c
Raisins	2 tbsp
Tangerine[b]	1 large
Cranberries may be used as desired if no sugar is added	

[a] Good source of vitamin A.
[b] Good source of ascorbic acid.

LIST 4. BREAD EXCHANGES (*Includes bread, cereal, and starchy vegetables. One exchange contains carbohydrate 15 g, protein 2 g, and 70 kcal*)

	Amount to Use
Bread	
White (including French and Italian)	1 slice
Whole wheat	1 slice
Rye or pumpernickel	1 slice
Raisin	1 slice
Bagel, small	½
English muffin, small	½
Plain roll (bread)	1
Frankfurter roll	½
Hamburger bun	½
Dry bread crumbs	3 tbsp
Tortillas, 6 in	1
Cereal	
Bran flakes	½ c
Other ready-to-eat unsweetened cereal	¾ c
Puffed cereal, unfrosted	1 c
Cereal, cooked	½ c
Grits, cooked	½ c

LIST 4. BREAD EXCHANGES (Continued)

	Amount to Use
Rice or barley, cooked	½ c
Pastas, cooked: macaroni, noodles, spaghetti	½ c
Popcorn, popped (no fat added)	3 c
Cornmeal, dry	2 tbsp
Flour	2½ tbsp
Wheat germ	¼ c
Crackers	
Arrowroot	3
Graham, 2½ in square	2
Matzo, 4 × 6 in	½
Oyster	20
Pretzels, 3⅛ in × ⅛ in	25
Rye wafers, 2 × 3½ in	3
Saltines	6
Soda, 2½ in square	4
Dried beans, peas, and lentils	
Dried beans, peas, and lentils, cooked	½ c
Baked beans, no pork (canned)	¼ c
Starchy vegetables	
Corn	⅓ c
Corn on cob	1 small
Lima beans	½ c
Parsnips	⅔ c
Peas, green, fresh, canned, or frozen	½ c
Potato, white	1 small
Potato, mashed	½ c
Pumpkin	¾ c
Winter squash, acorn or butternut*a*	½ c
Yam or sweet potato*a*	¼ c
Prepared foods	
Biscuit, 2 in diameter (omit 1 fat exchange)	1
Cornbread, 2 x 2 x 1 in (omit 1 fat exchange	1
Corn muffin, 2 in diameter (omit 1 fat exchange)	1
Crackers, round, butter type (omit 1 fat exchange)	5
Muffin, plain, small (omit 1 fat exchange)	1
Potatoes, French fried, 2 in to 3½ in (omit 1 fat exchange)	8 pieces
Potato or corn chips (omit 2 fat exchanges)	15
Pancake, 5 x ½ in (omit 1 fat exchange)	1
Waffle, 5 x ½ in (omit 1 fat exchange)	1

a Good source of vitamin A.

LIST 5. MEAT EXCHANGES

	Amount to Use
Lean meat*a* (One exchange contains protein 7 g, fat 3 g, and 55 kcal)	
Beef: baby beef (very lean), chipped beef, chuck, flank steak, tenderloin, plate ribs, plate skirt steak, round (bottom, top), all cuts rump, spare ribs, tripe	1 oz
Lamb: leg, rib, sirloin, loin (roast and chops), shank, shoulder	1 oz
Pork: leg (whole rump, center shank), smoked ham (center slices)	1 oz
Veal: leg, loin, rib, shank, shoulder, cutlets	1 oz
Poultry: without skin of chicken, turkey, cornish hen, guinea hen, pheasant	1 oz
Fish: any fresh or frozen	
Canned crab, lobster, mackerel, salmon, tuna	¼ c
Clams, oysters, scallops, shrimp	5 or 1 oz
Sardines, drained	3
Cheeses: containing less than 5% butterfat	1 oz
Cottage cheese: dry and 2% butterfat	¼ c
Dried peas and beans (omit 1 bread exchange)	½ c
Medium-fat meat—omit ½ fat exchange (One exchange contains protein 7 g, fat 5 g, and 75 kcal)	
Beef: ground, 15% fat; corned beef, canned; rib eye; round (ground commercial)	1 oz

(continued)

LIST 5. MEAT EXCHANGES (Continued)

	Amount to Use
Pork: loin (all cuts tenderloin), shoulder arm (picnic), shoulder blade, Boston Butt, Canadian bacon, boiled ham	1 oz
Liver, heart, kidney, and sweetbreads (all high in cholesterol)	1 oz
Cottage cheese, creamed	¼
Cheese: Mozzarella, ricotta, farmer's, Neufchatel, parmesan	3 tbsp
Eggs (high in cholesterol)	1
Peanut butter (omit 2 additional fat exchanges)	2 tbsp
High-fat meat—omit 1 fat exchange (One exchange contains protein 7 g, fat 8 g, and 100 kcal)	
Beef: brisket, corned beef brisket, ground beef (over 20% fat), hamburger (commercial), chuck (ground commercial), rib roast, club and rib steak	1 oz
Lamb: breast	1 oz
Pork, spare ribs, loin (back ribs), ground pork, country style ham, deviled ham	1 oz
Veal: breast	1 oz
Poultry: capon, duck (domestic), goose	1 oz
Cheese: cheddar type	1 oz
Cold cuts, 4½ x ⅛ in	1 slice
Frankfurter	1 small

[a] For diets restricted in saturated fat and cholesterol, select lean meat exchanges. If medium-fat or high-fat meat exchanges are used, eliminate the indicated number of fat exchanges.

LIST 6. FAT EXCHANGES (One exchange contains fat 5 g and 45 kcal)

	Amount to Use
Polyunsaturated fat[a]	
Margarine: soft, tub, or stick (made with corn, cottonseed, safflower, soy, or sunflower oil)	1 tsp
Avocado, 4 in diam[b]	⅛
Oil: corn, cottonseed, safflower, soy, sunflower	1 tsp
Oil: olive or peanut[b]	1 tsp
Olives[b]	5 small
Nuts	
Almonds[b]	10 whole
Pecans[b]	2 large whole
Peanuts[b]	
Spanish	20 whole
Virginia	10 whole
Walnuts	6 small
Other nuts[b]	6 small
Salad dressings (if made with corn, cottonseed, safflower, soy, or sunflower oil)	
French or Italian dressing	1 tbsp
Mayonnaise	1 tsp
Salad dressing, mayonnaise type	2 tsp
Saturated fat	
Margarine, regular stick	1 tsp
Butter	1 tsp
Bacon fat	1 tsp
Bacon, crisp	1 strip
Cream, light	2 tbsp
Cream, sour	2 tbsp
Cream, heavy	1 tbsp
Cream cheese	1 tbsp
Lard	1 tsp
Salt pork	¾ in cube
Salad dressing made with oils other than corn, cottonseed, safflower, soy, sunflower, peanut, or olive	
French or Italian dressing	1 tbsp
Mayonnaise	1 tsp
Salad dressing, mayonnaise type	2 tsp

[a] For diets restricted in saturated fat and cholesterol with substitution of polyunsaturated fat, select only from this list.
[b] Fat content is primarily monounsaturated.

FREE FOODS ALLOWED AS DESIRED (*Carbohydrate, protein, fat negligible*)

Coffee	Saccharin	Endive
Tea	Vinegar	Escarole
Clear broth	Lemon	Lettuce
Bouillon, fat free	Mustard, dry	Parsley
Pickle, dill, unsweetened	Calorie-free diet beverages	Radishes
Herbs	Vegetables	Watercress
Spices	Chicory	Fruit
Gelatin, unsweetened	Chinese cabbage	Unsweetened cranberries

(*Source: Adapted from* Exchange Lists for Meal Planning, *prepared by Committees of the American Dietetic Association and the American Diabetes Association in cooperation with the National Institute of Arthritis, Metabolism, and Digestive Diseases, the National Heart and Lung Institute, National Institutes of Health, Public Health Service, and U.S. Department of Health, Education, and Welfare.*)

APPENDIX 3
LIBERAL FOOD PLAN

Quantities of Food for a Week[a]

Food Group	Child (Years)				Male (Years)				Female[b] (Years)		
	1-2	3-5	6-8	9-11	12-14	15-19	20-50	51 or More	12-19	20-50	51 or More
	Pounds[c]										
Vegetables, fruit											
Potatoes (fresh weight)	0.70	0.78	1.13	1.48	1.57	2.44	2.06	1.74	1.20	1.18	1.10
High-nutrient vegetables	0.78	0.81	1.24	1.22	1.57	1.78	2.79	2.77	1.89	3.90	2.81
Other vegetables	1.03	0.87	1.47	1.61	2.08	2.04	3.02	3.14	2.00	3.72	2.89
Mixtures, mostly vegetable; condiments	0.10	0.11	0.18	0.19	0.24	0.29	0.49	0.36	0.19	0.34	0.28
Vitamin C-rich fruit[d]	1.65	2.28	2.32	3.26	2.79	3.08	2.72	2.50	2.21	2.47	2.63
Other fruit[d]	3.24	2.47	2.68	3.38	2.54	2.29	2.44	3.02	2.09	2.15	3.13
Grain products											
Whole grain/high-fiber breakfast cereals	0.53[e]	0.25	0.32	0.37	0.51	0.48	0.27	0.19	0.45	0.20	0.24
Other breakfast cereals	0.54[e]	0.26	0.34	0.40	0.56	0.52	0.30	0.21	0.46	0.20	0.17
Whole-grain/high-fiber flour, meal, rice, pasta	0.05	0.06	0.09	0.09	0.08	0.10	0.11	0.11	0.07	0.09	0.09
Other flour, meal, rice, pasta	0.85	0.89	1.26	1.35	1.20	1.40	1.48	1.54	0.93	1.22	0.81
Whole-grain/high-fiber bread	0.13	0.20	0.25	0.33	0.45	0.52	0.60	0.43	0.34	0.21	0.28
Other bread	0.45	0.76	0.94	1.26	1.71	1.94	2.22	1.61	1.24	1.38	0.86
Bakery products, not bread	0.29	0.62	0.81	0.64	0.95	0.98	0.91	0.97	0.55	0.56	0.41
Grain mixtures	0.23	0.29	0.34	0.38	0.46	0.43	0.35	0.18	0.42	0.31	0.15
Milk, cheese, cream											
Milk, yoghurt (quarts)[f]	4.14	3.64	5.05	5.13	6.12	5.30	2.46	1.87	5.44	2.05	2.42
Cheese	0.23	0.24	0.41	0.38	0.34	0.50	0.45	0.41	0.43	0.45	0.45
Cream, mixtures mostly milk	0.17	0.57	0.61	0.77	0.69	0.33	0.19	0.68	0.96	0.15	0.76
Meat and alternates											
Lower-cost red meats, variety meats	0.60	0.54	0.98	1.07	1.21	1.23	1.46	1.35	1.15	1.95	1.36
Higher-cost red meats, variety meats	0.61	0.73	1.13	1.44	1.66	1.65	2.00	1.80	1.42	1.64	1.69
Poultry	0.38	0.79	0.89	1.18	1.06	1.05	1.17	1.20	0.89	1.28	1.31
Fish, shellfish	0.22	0.26	0.27	0.36	0.38	0.34	0.74	0.77	0.66	0.91	0.89
Bacon, sausage, luncheon meats	0.18	0.53	0.51	0.62	0.68	0.70	0.36	0.43	0.27	0.19	0.22
Eggs (number)	3.51	2.72	2.48	3.73	2.87	3.11	3.55	3.84	3.86	3.90	4.27
Dry beans, peas, lentils (dry weight)[g]	0.07	0.13	0.14	0.20	0.26	0.17	0.30	0.20	0.26	0.27	0.16
Mixtures, mostly meat, poultry, fish, egg, legume	0.10	0.13	0.15	0.19	0.31	0.26	0.19	0.21	0.24	0.28	0.19
Nuts (shelled weight), peanut butter	0.03	0.20	0.26	0.22	0.21	0.26	0.21	0.04	0.03	0.01	0.06
Other foods[h]											
Fats, oils	0.10	0.25	0.34	0.48	0.56	0.65	0.82	0.68	0.34	0.43	0.30
Sugar, sweets	0.20	0.47	0.71	0.84	0.89	0.94	1.06	1.01	0.43	0.48	0.67
Soft drinks, punches, ades (single-strength)	1.65	3.20	3.14	4.10	4.84	5.95	4.46	1.46	5.07	3.83	1.28

[a] Quantities are for food as purchased or brought into the houshold from garden of farm. Food is for preparation of all meals and snacks for a week. About 30% of the edible parts of food above quantities needed to meet caloric needs is included to allow for food assumed to be discarded as plate waste, spoilage, and so on.
[b] Pregnant and lactating females usually require added nutrients and should consult a doctor for recommendations about diet and supplements.
[c] Quantities in pounds, except milk which is in quarts, and eggs which are by number.
[d] Frozen concentrated juices are included as single-strength juice.
[e] Cereal fortified with iron is recommended.
[f] Quantities of dry and evaporated milk and yoghurt included as their fluid whole milk equivalents in terms of calcium content.
[g] Count 1 pound of canned dry beans—pork and beans, kidney beans, etc.—as 0.33 pound.
[h] Two small food groups—coffee and tea, and seasonings—are not shown. Their cost is a part of the estimated cost for the food plan.
(Source: U.S. Department of Agriculture, Consumer and Food Economics Institute, Agricultural Research Service: Family Economics Review, No. 2, 1983.)

APPENDIX 4
MODERATE-COST FOOD PLAN

Quantities of Food for a Week[a]

Food Group	Child (Years)				Male (Years)				Female[b] (Years)		
	1–2	3–5	6–8	9–11	12–14	15–19	20–50	51 or More	12–19	20–50	51 or More
	Pounds[c]										
Vegetables, fruit											
Potatoes (fresh weight)	0.68	0.81	1.34	1.90	1.69	2.17	2.11	1.81	1.31	1.31	1.03
High-nutrient vegetables	0.78	1.00	0.88	1.48	1.33	1.55	2.22	2.17	1.56	2.51	2.76
Other vegetables	1.06	0.81	1.38	1.82	1.65	2.11	2.51	2.76	1.86	2.71	2.52
Mixtures, mostly vegetable; condiments	0.10	0.12	0.17	0.22	0.21	0.26	0.32	0.34	0.20	0.29	0.23
Vitamin C-rich fruit[d]	1.60	1.92	2.61	2.47	2.10	2.32	2.26	2.15	1.96	2.22	2.51
Other fruit[d]	1.98	2.19	2.32	2.44	2.88	2.42	1.99	3.12	1.81	1.91	2.78
Grain products											
Whole grain/high-fiber breakfast cereals	0.53[e]	0.24	0.35	0.42	0.42	0.38	0.19	0.22	0.41	0.23	0.23
Other breakfast cereals	0.43[e]	0.26	0.38	0.47	0.46	0.43	0.21	0.25	0.42	0.24	0.17
Whole grain/high-fiber flour, meal, rice, pasta	0.07	0.06	0.07	0.07	0.09	0.08	0.11	0.10	0.06	0.08	0.11
Other flour, meal, rice, pasta	0.81	0.81	0.87	0.86	1.19	1.03	1.53	1.38	0.86	1.10	0.85
Whole grain/high-fiber bread	0.11	0.19	0.25	0.31	0.34	0.50	0.46	0.34	0.30	0.32	0.26
Other bread	0.41	0.82	1.07	1.34	1.52	2.18	2.02	1.48	1.24	1.27	0.87
Bakery products, not bread	0.21	0.53	0.76	0.65	0.78	0.86	0.93	0.80	0.59	0.53	0.31
Grain mixtures	0.14	0.18	0.26	0.46	0.43	0.46	0.30	0.15	0.32	0.25	0.18
Milk, cheese, cream											
Milk, yoghurt (quarts)[f]	3.79	3.58	4.72	5.16	6.07	5.38	2.62	1.93	5.09	1.89	2.24
Cheese	0.18	0.18	0.29	0.21	0.26	0.46	0.39	0.40	0.38	0.44	0.40
Cream, mixtures mostly milk	0.28	0.34	0.71	0.99	1.08	0.75	0.59	0.61	0.70	0.25	0.58
Meat and alternates											
Lower-cost red meats, variety meats	0.51	0.60	0.85	1.11	1.36	1.19	1.48	1.37	1.12	1.60	1.58
Higher-cost red meats, variety meats	0.46	0.64	0.90	1.17	1.43	1.35	1.60	1.46	1.04	1.35	1.50
Poultry	0.57	0.59	0.82	1.00	1.15	0.74	1.12	1.03	0.94	1.06	1.03
Fish, shellfish	0.10	0.16	0.22	0.29	0.40	0.36	0.41	0.51	0.41	0.41	0.56
Bacon, sausage, luncheon meats	0.26	0.42	0.59	0.50	0.26	0.72	0.50	0.43	0.32	0.24	0.22
Eggs (number)	3.64	3.40	2.52	3.08	2.42	2.73	3.10	3.83	3.23	4.37	4.12
Dry beans, peas, lentils (dry weight)[g]	0.10	0.07	0.16	0.21	0.20	0.18	0.23	0.20	0.24	0.35	0.19
Mixtures, mostly meat, poultry, fish, egg, legume	0.08	0.10	0.14	0.16	0.17	0.23	0.29	0.19	0.17	0.19	0.17
Nuts (shelled weight), peanut butter	0.05	0.13	0.18	0.15	0.28	0.13	0.16	0.04	0.06	0.03	0.02
Other foods[h]											
Fats, oils	0.11	0.30	0.31	0.46	0.52	0.57	0.65	0.62	0.28	0.36	0.29
Sugar, sweets	0.17	0.49	0.60	0.68	0.79	0.84	0.92	0.91	0.42	0.47	0.44
Soft drinks, punches, ades (single-strength)	1.57	2.37	2.86	3.69	3.90	4.84	3.73	1.06	4.26	3.71	1.18

[a] Quantities are for food as purchased or brought into the household from garden or farm. Food is for preparation of all meals and snacks for a week. About 20% of the edible parts of food above quantities needed to meet caloric needs is included to allow for food assumed to be discarded as plate waste, spoilage, and so on.

[b] Pregnant and lactating females usually require added nutrients and should consult a doctor for recommendations about diet and supplements.

[c] Quantities in pounds, except milk which is in quarts, and eggs which are by number.

[d] Frozen concentrated juices are included as single-strength juice.

[e] Cereal fortified with iron is recommended.

[f] Quantities of dry and evaporated milk and yoghurt included as their fluid whole milk equivalents in terms of calcium content.

[g] Quantities of dry and evaporated milk and yoghurt included as their fluid whole milk equivalents in terms of calcium content.

[g] Count 1 pound of canned dry beans—pork and beans, kidney beans, etc.—as 0.33 pound.

[h] Two small food groups—coffee and tea, and seasonings—are not shown. Their cost is a part of the estimated cost for the food plan.

(Source: U.S. Department of Agriculture, Consumer and Food Economics Institute, Agricultural Research Service: Family Economics Review, No. 2, 1983.)

APPENDIX 5
LOW-COST FOOD PLAN

Quantities of Food for a Week[a]

Food Group	Child (Years)				Male (Years)				Female[b] (Years)		
	1–2	3–5	6–8	9–11	12–14	15–19	20–50	51 or More	12–19	20–50	51 or More
					Pounds[c]						
Vegetables, fruit											
Potatoes (fresh weight)	0.50	0.73	1.16	1.28	1.55	1.88	1.97	1.71	1.19	1.19	1.11
High-nutrient vegetables	0.55	0.50	0.86	0.98	1.30	1.34	1.91	2.00	1.19	1.86	2.17
Other vegetables	0.82	0.88	1.20	1.41	1.41	1.54	2.12	2.19	1.54	2.30	2.04
Mixtures, mostly vegetable; condiments	0.06	0.10	0.14	0.17	0.18	0.20	0.29	0.30	0.15	0.24	0.15
Vitamin C-rich fruit[d]	1.51	1.43	1.79	1.94	2.03	2.16	1.62	1.75	1.76	1.79	1.91
Other fruit[d]	1.97	1.58	2.30	2.44	2.07	1.45	1.98	2.21	1.81	1.53	2.19
Grain products											
Whole grain— high-fiber breakfast cereals	0.35[e]	0.27	0.31	0.35	0.36	0.28	0.14	0.22	0.33	0.21	0.31
Other breakfast cereals	0.38[e]	0.26	0.33	0.38	0.39	0.31	0.16	0.25	0.36	0.23	0.22
Whole grain/high-fiber flour, meal, rice, pasta	0.11	0.07	0.08	0.09	0.10	0.10	0.11	0.10	0.09	0.09	0.12
Other flour, meal, rice, pasta	0.86	0.83	1.04	1.17	1.32	1.34	1.40	1.34	0.95	1.01	0.83
Whole grain/high-fiber bread	0.12	0.17	0.22	0.26	0.31	0.39	0.42	0.30	0.28	0.30	0.25
Other bread	0.41	0.79	1.08	1.28	1.52	1.95	2.08	1.45	1.19	1.24	0.84
Bakery products, not bread	0.09	0.36	0.62	0.75	0.96	0.85	0.86	0.71	0.44	0.46	0.19
Grain mixtures	0.15	0.20	0.18	0.30	0.33	0.34	0.29	0.13	0.23	0.22	0.14
Milk, cheese, cream											
Milk, yoghurt (quarts)[f]	3.41	3.23	4.26	4.69	5.02	4.86	2.49	2.07	4.64	1.85	2.16
Cheese	0.17	0.17	0.20	0.19	0.22	0.30	0.36	0.28	0.34	0.34	0.35
Cream, mixtures mostly milk	0.13	0.44	0.57	0.69	0.67	0.75	0.51	0.50	0.65	0.34	0.55
Meat and alternates											
Lower-cost red meats, variety meats	0.71	0.52	0.60	0.74	0.99	1.23	1.65	1.23	1.13	1.57	1.67
Higher-cost red meats, variety meats	0.37	0.38	0.47	0.57	0.79	0.94	0.86	1.04	0.70	0.95	1.21
Poultry	0.42	0.43	0.63	0.67	0.85	0.77	0.94	0.98	0.83	0.91	0.95
Fish, shellfish	0.09	0.07	0.14	0.11	0.16	0.14	0.25	0.23	0.17	0.21	0.19
Bacon, sausage, luncheon meats	0.15	0.39	0.48	0.51	0.58	0.57	0.34	0.58	0.29	0.41	0.21
Eggs (number)	3.34	3.24	2.50	2.99	3.02	2.97	3.38	3.93	3.82	4.23	4.02
Dry beans, peas lentils (dry weight)[g]	0.22	0.09	0.12	0.15	0.20	0.19	0.27	0.19	0.24	0.34	0.14
Mixtures, mostly meat, poultry fish, egg, legume	0.08	0.08	0.11	0.15	0.20	0.20	0.22	0.15	0.16	0.17	0.16
Nuts (shelled weight), peanut butter	0.09	0.20	0.20	0.22	0.20	0.22	0.14	0.08	0.11	0.07	0.04
Other foods[h]											
Fats, oils	0.09	0.27	0.43	0.50	0.55	0.54	0.68	0.54	0.25	0.32	0.26
Sugar, sweets	0.15	0.46	0.57	0.62	0.74	0.77	0.84	0.83	0.43	0.35	0.43
Soft drinks, punches, ades (single-strength)	1.53	1.96	2.72	3.25	3.35	4.63	3.67	1.19	3.96	3.33	0.96

[a] Quantities are for food as purchased or brought into the household from garden or farm. Food is for preparation of all meals and snacks for a week. About 10% of the edible parts of food above quantities needed to meet caloric needs is included to allow for food assumed to be discarded as plate waste, spoilage, and so on.
[b] Pregnant and lactating females usually require added nutrients and should consult a doctor for recommendations about diet and supplements.
[c] Quantities in pounds, except milk which is in quarts, and eggs which are by number.
[d] Frozen concentrated juices are included as single-strength juice.
[e] Cereal fortified with iron is recommended.
[f] Quantities of dry and evaporated milk and yoghurt included as their fluid whole milk equivalents in terms of calcium content.
[g] Count 1 pound of canned dry beans—pork and beans, kidney beans, etc—as 0.33 pound.
[h] Two small groups—coffee and tea, and seasonings—are not shown. Their cost is a part of the estimated cost for the food plan.
(Source: U.S. Department of Agriculture, Consumer and Food Economics Institute, Agricultural Research Service: Family Economics Review, No. 2, 1983.)

APPENDIX 6
THRIFTY FOOD PLAN

Quantities of Food for a Week[a]

Food Group	Child (Years)				Male (Years)				Female[b] (Years)		
	1–2	3–5	6–8	9–11	12–14	15–19	20–50	51 or More	12–19	20–50	51 or More
	Pounds[c]										
Vegetables, fruit											
Potatoes (fresh weight)	0.47	0.82	1.04	1.11	1.29	2.22	1.50	1.55	1.27	1.16	0.90
High-nutrient vegetables	0.52	0.67	1.05	1.17	1.65	1.08	1.61	1.52	1.14	1.91	2.28
Other vegetables	0.60	0.70	0.97	1.25	1.35	1.15	1.86	1.33	1.08	2.68	2.03
Mixtures, mostly vegetable; condiments	0.01	0.02	0.05	0.07	0.02	0.06	0.13	0.06	0.07	0.02	0.02
Vitamin C-rich fruit[d]	1.19	1.24	1.32	1.62	1.08	1.17	1.13	1.00	2.02	1.73	1.35
Other fruit[d]	0.97	0.92	1.61	1.86	1.11	1.04	1.20	1.41	1.30	0.93	1.37
Grain products											
Whole grain/high-fiber breakfast cereals	0.44[e]	0.33	0.17	0.24	0.38	0.27	0.17	0.13	0.30	0.12	0.17
Other breakfast cereals	0.30[e]	0.27	0.19	0.26	0.05	0.12	0.21	0.12	0.39	0.19	0.27
Whole grain/high-fiber flour, meal, rice, pasta	0.11	0.14	0.12	0.11	0.20	0.22	0.15	0.21	0.16	0.15	0.18
Other flour, meal, rice, pasta	0.88	1.23	1.85	1.73	2.15	2.34	1.81	1.87	1.32	1.81	1.32
Whole grain/high-fiber bread	0.09	0.10	0.09	0.11	0.15	0.17	0.24	0.21	0.21	0.34	0.29
Other bread	0.38	0.65	1.01	1.27	1.68	1.33	1.85	1.33	1.04	0.59	0.29
Bakery products, not bread	0.06	0.10	0.42	0.58	0.19	0.43	0.56	0.30	0.36	0.12	0.10
Grain mixtures	0.08	0.06	0.07	0.11	0.02	0.13	0.23	0.15	0.31	0.37	0.19
Milk, cheese, cream											
Milk, yoghurt (quarts)[f]	3.42	3.06	3.39	4.17	3.99	3.91	2.00	1.63	4.36	2.37	2.17
Cheese	0.04	0.05	0.08	0.11	0.11	0.11	0.13	0.12	0.27	0.29	0.32
Cream, mixtures mostly milk	0.15	0.15	0.34	0.30	0.10	0.24	0.41	0.26	0.35	0.03	0.26
Meat and alternates											
Lower-cost red meats, variety meats	0.93	0.69	0.70	0.92	1.20	1.49	1.40	1.73	1.75	1.60	1.95
Higher-cost red meats, variety meats	0.15	0.11	0.13	0.19	0.18	0.26	0.39	0.54	0.20	0.35	0.55
Poultry	0.35	0.48	0.64	0.70	0.90	0.90	0.96	0.71	0.20	0.95	0.70
Fish, shellfish	0.02	0.02	0.02	0.03	0.03	0.02	0.04	0.04	0.04	0.04	0.04
Bacon, sausage, luncheon meats	0.18	0.32	0.31	0.24	0.26	0.27	0.56	0.49	0.24	0.45	0.45
Eggs (number)	3.00	2.90	1.90	2.50	2.20	3.10	4.10	4.30	4.10	4.40	4.10
Dry beans, peas, lentils (dry weight)[g]	0.27	0.18	0.18	0.24	0.59	0.58	0.45	0.59	0.35	0.41	0.43
Mixtures, mostly meat, poultry, fish, egg, legume	0.05	0.06	0.01	0.01	0.02	0.03	0.13	0.15	0.20	0.13	0.15
Nuts (shelled weight), peanut butter	0.09	0.24	0.13	0.15	0.37	0.14	0.17	0.22	0.09	0.28	0.08
Other foods[h]											
Fats, oils	0.14	0.33	0.58	0.67	0.73	0.93	0.76	0.60	0.22	0.28	0.21
Sugar, sweets	0.10	0.36	0.78	0.87	1.20	0.95	1.01	0.76	0.31	0.21	0.22
Soft drinks, punches, ades (single-strength)	0.39	0.57	0.65	0.87	0.87	1.51	1.17	0.32	1.12	0.40	0.38

[a] Quantities are for food as purchased or brought into the household from garden or farm. Food is for preparation of all meals and snacks for a week. About 5% of the edible parts of food is assumed to be discarded as plate waste, spoilage, and so on.

[b] Pregnant and lactating females usually require added nutrients and should consult a doctor for recommendations about diet and supplements.

[c] Quantities in pounds, except milk which is in quarts, and eggs which are by number.

[d] Frozen concentrated juices are included as single-strength juice.

[e] Cereal fortified with iron is recommended.

[f] Quantities of dry and evaporated milk and yoghurt included as their fluid whole milk equivalents in terms of calcium content.

[g] Count 1 pound of canned dry beans—pork and beans, kidney beans, etc—as 0.33 pound.

[h] Small quantities of coffee, tea, and seasonings are not shown. Their cost is a part of the estimated cost for the food plan.

(Source: U.S. Department of Agriculture, Consumer and Food Economics Institute, Agricultural Research Service: Family Economics Review, No. 1, 1984.)

APPENDIX 7
WEIGHTS OF ADULTS ASSOCIATED WITH THE LOWEST MORTALITY

HEIGHT AND WEIGHT TABLES[a]

		Men					Women		
Height		Small Frame	Medium Frame	Large Frame	Height		Small Frame	Medium Frame	Large Frame
Ft	In				Ft	In			
5	2	128–134	131–141	138–150	4	10	102–111	109–121	118–131
	3	130–136	133–143	140–153		11	103–113	111–123	120–134
	4	132–138	135–145	142–156	5	0	104–115	113–126	122–137
	5	134–140	137–148	144–160		1	106–118	115–129	125–140
	6	136–142	139–151	146–164		2	108–121	118–132	128–143
	7	138–145	142–154	149–168		3	111–124	121–135	131–147
	8	140–148	145–157	152–172		4	114–127	124–138	134–151
	9	142–151	148–160	155–176		5	117–130	127–141	137–155
	10	144–154	151–163	158–180		6	120–133	130–144	140–159
	11	146–157	154–166	161–184		7	123–136	133–147	143–163
6	0	149–160	157–170	164–188		8	126–139	136–150	146–167
	1	152–164	160–174	168–192		9	129–142	139–153	149–170
	2	155–168	164–178	172–197		10	132–145	142–156	152–173
	3	158–172	167–182	176–202		11	135–148	145–159	155–176
	4	162–176	171–187	181–207	6	0	138–151	148–162	158–179

[a] Weights at ages 25–59 based on lowest mortality. Weight in pounds according to frame (in indoor clothing weighing 5 lb for men and 3 lb for women; shoes with 1 in heels).
(*Source: Metropolitan Height and Weight Tables. Metropolitan Life Insurance Company, Health and Safety Education Division, 1983. Source of basic data: 1979 Build Study, Society of Actuaries and Association of Life Insurance Medical Directors of America, 1980.*)

APPENDIX 8
PHYSICAL GROWTH NCHS PERCENTILES

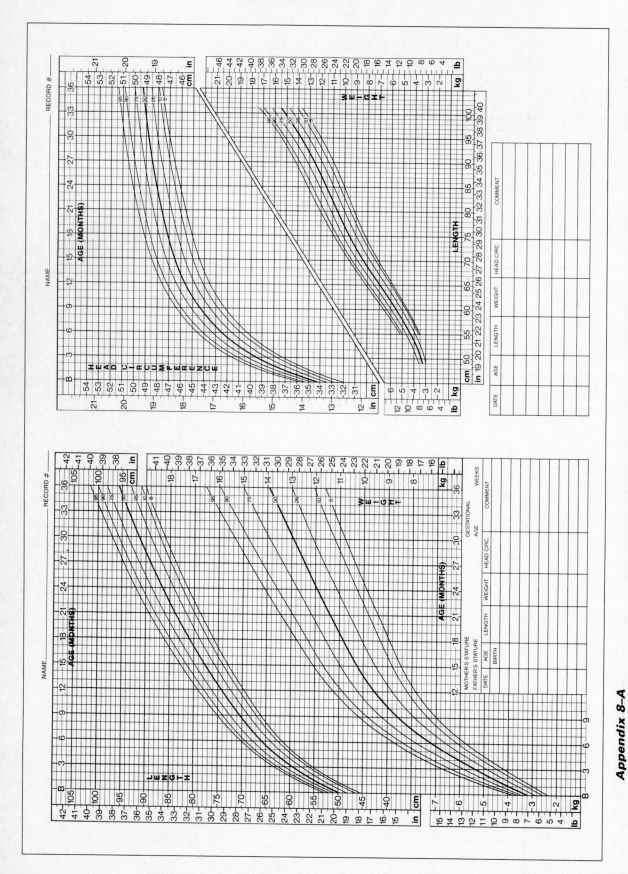

Appendix 8–A
Girls: Birth to 36 months. (Source: Adapted from Hamill PVV, Drizd TA, Johnson CL, et al.: Physical growth: National Center for Health Statistics percentiles. Am J Clin Nutr 32:607–629, 1979. Data from the Fels Research Institute, Wright State University School of Medicine, Yellow Springs, Ohio. Copyright 1982 Ross Laboratories.)

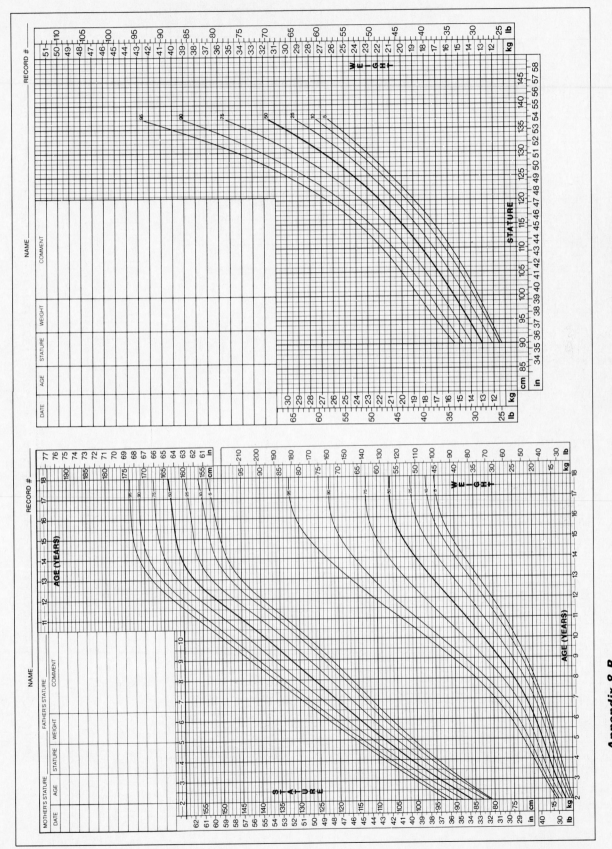

Appendix 8-B
Girls: 2 to 18 years. (Source: Adapted from Hamill PVV, Drizd TA, Johnson CL, et al.: Physical growth: National Center for Health Statistics percentiles. Am J Clin Nutr 32:607-629, 1979. Data from the National Center for Health Statistics [NCHS] Hyattsville, Md. Copyright 1982 Ross Laboratories.)

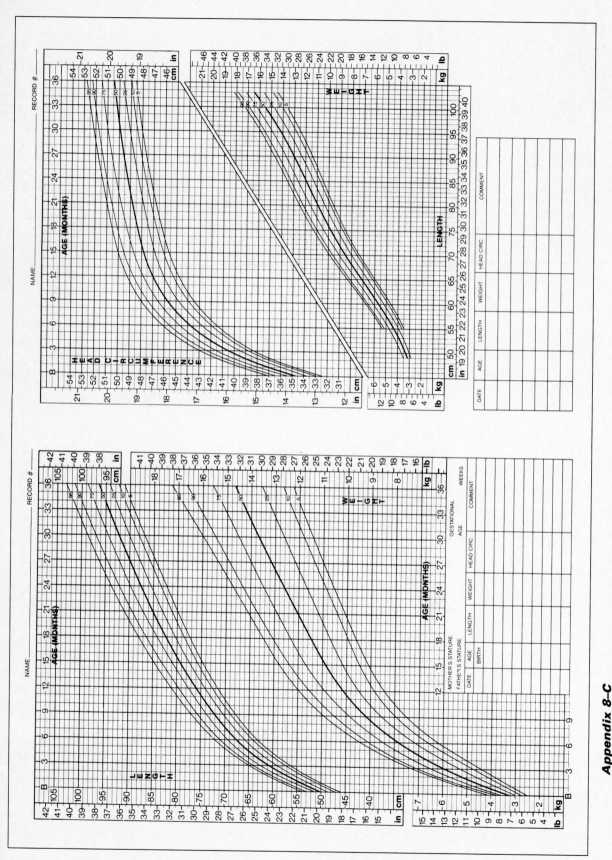

Appendix 8-C

Boys: Birth to 36 months. (Source: Adapted from Hamill PVV, Drizd TA, Johnson CL, et al.: Physical growth: National Center for Health Statistics percentiles. Am J Clin Nutr 32:607–629, 1979. Data from the Fels Research Institute, Wright State University School of Medicine, Yellow Springs, Ohio. Copyright 1982 Ross Laboratories.)

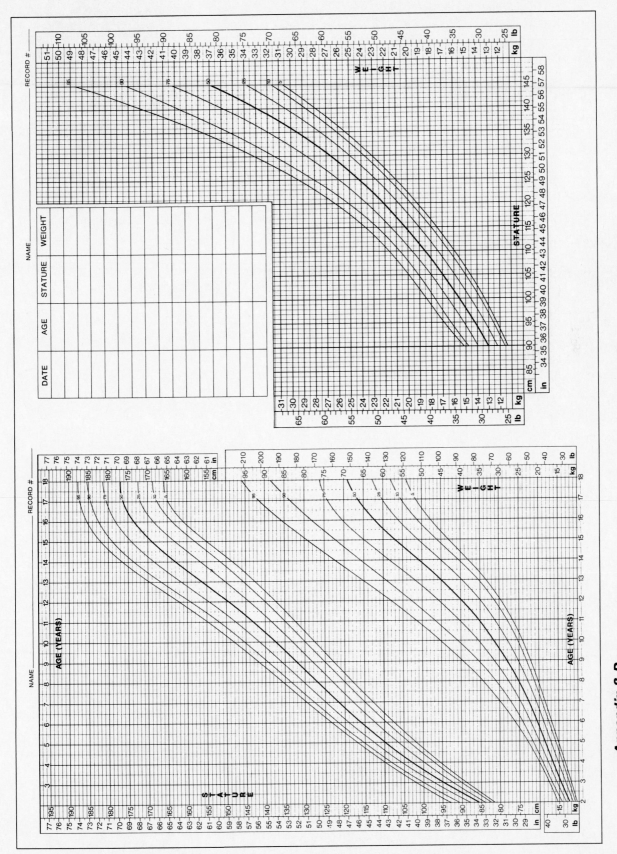

Appendix 8–D
Boys: 2 to 18 years. (Source: Adapted from Hamill PVV, Drizd TA, Johnson CL, et al.: *Physical growth: National Center for Health Statistics percentiles. Am J Clin Nutr 32:607–629, 1979. Data from the National Center for Health Statistics [NCHS], Hyattsville, Md. Copyright 1980 Ross Laboratories.*)

APPENDIX 9
MEASUREMENT OF TRICEPS SKINFOLD THICKNESS AND MIDARM MUSCLE CIRCUMFERENCE

APPENDIX 9–A

Triceps Skinfold Thickness

1. Locate and mark with a pen or adhesive label the midpoint of the bare upper right arm (the midpoint is located halfway between the acromial process of the scapula and the olecranon process of the ulna). While the midpoint is being located and marked, have the subject stand erect, bending the arm at a 90° angle with the forearm held across the stomach; make the mark on the back of the arm directly in line with the elbow (see Figure A).

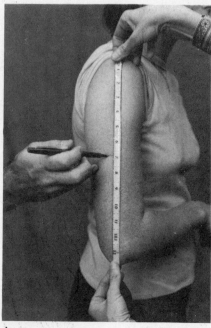
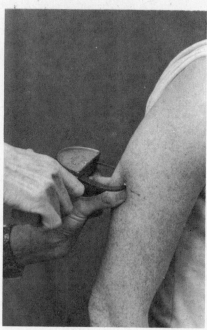

A   **B**

2. As the subject's arm hangs freely by the side, use the thumb and forefinger to grasp a lengthwise double fold of skin and fat about 1 cm above the midpoint mark and directly in line with the point of the olecranon process. Pull the fold away from the underlying muscle; have the subject contract and relax the triceps muscle several times to assure that muscle is excluded from the fold.

3. Apply a skin-gold caliper over the fatfold below the fingers at the midpoint at a depth about equal to the thickness of the fold (see Figure B).

4. Release the caliper while maintaining the fold; read measurement approximately 2 seconds after full pressure is applied to the skinfold; record reading to the nearest 0.1 mm.

5. Remove calipers and reapply for a total of three readings.

6. Average the three readings and record the average.

(*Source: Adapted from Lewis CM: Basic and Family Nutrition, A Self-Instructional Approach, ed 2. Philadelphia, FA Davis, 1984, pp 164–165.*)

APPENDIX 9–B

Midarm Muscle Circumference

1. Follow Step 1 of Appendix 9–A to locate the midpoint of the bare upper right arm.
2. Measure the circumference of the midarm at the midpoint with a tape as the arm hangs freely by the side; avoid constricting the skin with tape.
3. Record the measurement to the nearest 0.1 centimeter.
4. Calculate the midarm muscle circumference from the midarm circumference and triceps skinfold measurements by applying the following equation:

Arm muscle circumference (mm) = midarm circumference (cm) −
[3.14 × triceps skinfold (cm)[a]]

[a] Convert triceps skinfold measurement in mm to cm by dividing mm value by 10.
(*Source: Adapted from Lewis CM: Basic and Family Nutrition, A Self-Instructional Approach, ed 2. Philadelphia, FA Davis, 1984, pp 164–165.*)

APPENDIX 10
CURRENT GUIDELINES FOR CRITERIA OF NUTRITIONAL STATUS FOR LABORATORY EVALUATION

Nutrient and Units	Age of Subject (years)	Criteria of Status		
		Deficient	Marginal	Acceptable
Hemoglobin[a] (g/100 ml)	6–23 months	Up to 9.0	9.0– 9.9	10.0+
	2–5	Up to 10.0	10.0–10.9	11.0+
	6–12	Up to 10.0	10.0–11.4	11.5+
	13–16 M	Up to 12.0	12.0–12.9	13.0+
	13–16 F	Up to 10.0	10.0–11.4	11.5+
	16+ M	Up to 12.0	12.0–13.9	14.0+
	16+ F	Up to 10.0	10.0–11.9	12.0+
	Pregnant (after 6+ months)	Up to 9.5	9.5–10.9	11.0+
Hematocrit[a] (Packed cell volume in %)	Up to 2	Up to 28	28–30	31+
	2–5	Up to 30	30–33	34+
	6–12	Up to 30	30–35	36+
	13–16 M	Up to 37	37–39	40+
	13–16 F	Up to 31	31–35	36+
	16+ M	Up to 37	37–43	44+
	16+ F	Up to 31	31–37	33+
	Pregnant	Up to 30	30–32	33+
Serum albumin[a] (g/100 ml)	Up to 1		Up to 2.5	2.5+
	1–5		Up to 3.0	3.0+
	6–16		Up to 3.5	3.5+
	16+	Up to 2.8	2.8–3.4	3.5+
	Pregnant	Up to 3.0	3.0–3.4	3.5+
Serum protein[a] (g/100 ml)	Up to 1		Up to 5.0	5.0+
	1–5		Up to 5.5	5.5+
	6–16		Up to 6.0	6.0+
	16+	Up to 6.0	6.0–6.4	6.5+
	Pregnant	Up to 5.5	5.5–5.9	6.0+
Serum ascorbic acid[a] (mg/100 ml)	All ages	Up to 0.1	0.1–0.19	0.2+
Plasma vitamin A[a] (mcg/100 ml)	All ages	Up to 10	10–19	20+
Plasma carotene[a] (mcg/100 ml)	All ages	Up to 20	20–39	40+
	Pregnant		40–79	80+
Serum iron[a] (mcg/100 ml)	Up to 2	Up to 30		30+
	2–5	Up to 40		40+
	6–12	Up to 50		50+
	12+ M	Up to 60		60+
	12+ F	Up to 40		40+
Transferrin saturation[a] (%)	Up to 2	Up to 15.0		15.0+
	2–12	Up to 20.0		20.0+

(continued)

Nutrient and Units	Age of Subject (years)	Criteria of Status		
		Deficient	Marginal	Acceptable
	12+ M	Up to 20.0		20.0+
	12+ F	Up to 15.0		15.0+
Serum folacin[b] (ng/ml)	All ages	Up to 2.0	2.1–5.9	6.0+
Serum vitamin B_{12}[b] (pg/ml)	All ages	Up to 100		100+
Thiamine in urine[a] (μg/g creatinine)	1–3	Up to 120	120–175	175+
	4–5	Up to 85	85–120	120+
	6–9	Up to 70	70–180	180+
	10–15	Up to 55	55–150	150+
	16+	Up to 27	27– 65	65+
	Pregnant	Up to 21	21– 49	50+
Riboflavin in urine[a] (μg/g creatinine)	1–3	Up to 150	150–499	500+
	4–5	Up to 100	100–299	300+
	6–9	Up to 85	85–269	270+
	10–16	Up to 70	70–199	200+
	16+	Up to 27	27– 79	80+
	Pregnant	Up to 30	30– 89	90+
RBC transketolase-TPP effect (ratio)[b]	All ages	25+	15– 25	Up to 15
RBC glutathione reductase-FAD effect[b] (ratio)	All ages	1.2+		Up to 1.2
Tryptophan load[b] (mg xanthurenic acid excreted)	Adults (Dose: 100 mg/kg body weight)	25+(6 hr) 75+(24 hr)		Up to 25 Up to 75
Urinary pyridoxine[b] (μg/g creatinine)	1–3	Up to 90		90+
	4–6	Up to 80		80+
	7–9	Up to 60		60+
	10–12	Up to 40		40+
	13–15	Up to 30		30+
	16+	Up to 20		20+
Urinary N'methyl nicotinamide[a] (mg/g creatinine)	All ages	Up to 0.2	0.2–5.59	0.6+
	Pregnant	Up to 0.8	0.8–2.49	2.5+
Urinary pantothenic acid (μg)[b]	All ages	Up to 200		200+
Plasma vitamin E[b] (mg/100 ml)	All ages	Up to 0.2	0.2–0.6	0.6+
Transaminase[b] index (ratio)				
EGOT[c]	Adult	2.0 +		Up to 2.0
EGPT[d]	Adult	1.25+		Up to 1.25

[a] Adapted from the Ten-State Nutrition Survey.
[b] Criteria may vary with different methodology.
[c] Erythrocyte glutamic oxalacetic transaminase.
[d] Erythrocyte glutamic pyruvic transaminase.
(*Source: Nutritional assessment in health programs. Am J Public Health* [*Suppl*] *63:34–35, 1973.*)

APPENDIX 11
PHENYLALANINE-RESTRICTED DIETS

APPENDIX 11–A

Average Nutrient Content of Serving Lists for Phenylalanine-restricted Diets

List	Phenylalanine (mg)	Protein (g)	Energy (kcal)
Vegetables			
Strained and junior	15	0.5	20
Table	15	0.5	10
Fruits			
Strained and junior	15	0.6	150
Table and juices	15	0.6	70
Bread and cereals	30	0.6	30
Fats	5	0.1	60

When analyses were not available, the phenylalanine content was calculated on the following basis:

Breads and cereals	Phenylalanine 5% of protein
Fat	Phenylalanine 5% of protein
Fruits	Phenylalanine 2.6% of protein
Vegetables	Phenylalanine 3.3% of protein

(Source: Acosta PB, Wenz E: Diet Management of PKU for Infants and Preschool Children. DHEW Publication No. (HSA) 78-5209, Rockville, Md, 1978, p 16.)

APPENDIX 11–B

Serving Lists for Phenylalanine-restricted Diets

PART A—STRAINED AND JUNIOR FOODS					
Food	g per tbsp	Amount	Phenylalanine (mg)	Protein (g)	Energy (kcal)
Each Serving as Listed Below Contains 15 mg Phenylalanine					
Vegetables	14.3				
Mixed vegetables		3 tbsp	16	0.5	15
Garden vegetables		2 tbsp	16	0.5	8
Beets		6 tbsp	15	1.1	33
Carrots		5 tbsp	15	0.5	19
Creamed spinach		2 tbsp	15	0.9	14
Green beans		2 tbsp	15	0.3	7
Squash		3 tbsp	14	0.3	13
Peas		1 tbsp	17	0.5	6
Fruits	14.3				
Applesauce		11 tbsp	15	0.3	127
Applesauce and apricots		10 tbsp	15	0.4	124
Applesauce and cherries		18 tbsp	15	0.5	239
Applesauce and pineapple		10 tbsp	15	0.4	169
Apricots and tapioca		12 tbsp	14	0.7	138
Bananas and tapioca		8 tbsp	15	0.8	137
Peaches		5 tbsp	16	0.4	60
Pears		10 tbsp	15	0.6	99
Pears and pineapple		11 tbsp	15	0.6	111
Plums and tapioca		11 tbsp	15	0.5	154
Prunes and tapioca		8 tbsp	15	0.7	105
Bananas with pineapple and tapioca		11 tbsp	15	0.6	180
Apples and pears		18 tbsp	15	0.5	208
Note: Free food					
Applesauce and raspberries		10 tbsp	4	0.1	151
Applesauce and cherries		7 tbsp	6	0.2	93
Apples and cranberries		16 tbsp	5	0.2	213
Fruit juices	15.0				
Apple		16 oz	14	0.5	235
Apple—apricot		16 oz	14	0.5	336
Apple—cherry		10 oz	15	0.6	135
Apple—grape		16 oz	14	0.5	312
Apple—pineapple		16 oz	14	0.5	336
Mixed fruit		6 oz	14	0.5	106
Orange		4 oz	16	0.6	60
Orange—apple		6 oz	14	0.5	97
Orange—apple—banana		4 oz	16	0.6	78
Orange—apricot		3 oz	14	0.5	55
Orange—pineapple		4 oz	16	0.6	71
Pineapple		6 oz	14	0.5	99
Pineapple—grapefruit drink		6 oz	14	0.4	70
Prune—orange		4 oz	16	0.6	90
Apple—prune		10 oz	15	0.6	204
Each Serving as Listed Below Contains 30 mg of Phenylalanine					
Breads and cereals					
Dry cereals	2.4				
Barley		2 tbsp	28	0.5	18
Mixed cereal		2 tbsp	28	0.6	18
Oatmeal		2 tbsp	30	0.8	15
Rice cereal		4 tbsp	31	0.6	36
Mixed cereal with bananas		2 tbsp	29	0.6	21
Oatmeal with bananas		2 tbsp	30	0.6	19
Rice cereal with strawberries		4 tbsp	30	0.6	33
Barley with mixed fruit		3 tbsp	31	0.6	information not available

PART A—STRAINED AND JUNIOR FOODS (Continued)

Food	g per tbsp	Amount	Phenylalanine (mg)	Protein (g)	Energy (kcal)
Cereals in jars	14.3				
Strained					
Mixed with applesauce and bananas		3 tbsp	30	0.6	39
Oatmeal with applesauce and bananas		4 tbsp	30	0.5	47
Rice with applesauce and bananas		15 tbsp	30	0.6	148
Rice with mixed fruit		3 tbsp	30	0.6	37
Junior					
Mixed with applesauce and bananas		3 tbsp	30	0.6	39
Oatmeal with applesauce and bananas		4 tbsp	30	0.5	47
Strained vegetables	14.3				
Creamed corn		3 tbsp	30	0.7	30
Sweet potatoes		3 tbsp	29	0.6	30

PART B—TABLE FOODS

Food	g per tbsp	Amount	Phenylalanine (mg)	Protein (g)	Energy (kcal)
Each serving as Listed Below Contains 15 mg Phenylalanine					
Vegetables					
Asparagus, cooked	9	3 tbsp or 1½ stalks	17	0.6	5
Beans, green, cooked	8	3 tbsp	14	0.4	6
Beans, yellow, cooked	8	¼ c	16	0.4	7
Beans, sprouts, Mung, cooked	8	1 tbsp	16	0.3	3
Beets, cooked	10	⅔ c	16	1.2	34
Beet greens, cooked	13	3 tbsp	15	0.6	6
Broccoli, cooked, chopped	10	1 tbsp	14	0.4	3
Brussels sprouts, cooked	—	1 medium	13	0.4	4
Cabbage, raw, shredded	6	½ c	15	0.6	12
Cabbage, cooked	10	⅓ c	14	0.6	11
Carrots, raw	—	½ large or 1 small	18	0.6	21
Carrots, cooked	—	⅓ c	15	0.5	16
Cauliflower, cooked	7	3 tbsp	17	0.5	5
Celery, raw	6	6 tbsp or 2 stalks	15	0.3	6
Celery, cooked, diced	8	6 tbsp	18	0.4	7
Chard leaves, cooked	10	3 tbsp	14	0.5	5
Collards, cooked	11	1 tbsp	13	0.4	4
Cucumber, pared, raw	—	1 whole	14	0.6	14
Eggplant, diced, raw	13	2 tbsp	13	0.3	7
Eggplant, cooked	13	3 tbsp	17	0.4	7
Kale, cooked	7	2 tbsp	18	0.4	4
Lettuce	—	2 leaves	14	0.4	5
Mushroom, raw	4	3 small	17	0.8	8
Mushroom, canned	13	3 tbsp	16	0.7	7
Mushroom, sauteed	17	½ large	13	0.2	10
Mustard greens, cooked	13	2 tbsp	16	0.5	5
Okra, cooked	—	3 tbsp	17	0.7	10
Onion, raw, chopped	10	¼ c	15	0.6	15
Onion, cooked	13	¼ c	16	0.6	15
Onion, young, scallion	—	2 whole	15	0.6	14
Parsley, raw, chopped	3	4 tbsp	17	0.4	5
Parsnips, cooked, diced	13	3 tbsp	18	0.6	26
Peppers, raw, chopped	10	3 tbsp	17	0.4	7
Pickles, dill	—	1 large	16	0.7	11
Pickles, sweet	13	1 large	16	0.7	146
Pickles, sweet relish	13	8 tbsp	14	0.5	144
Pumpkin, cooked	14	4 tbsp	16	0.6	18
Radishes, raw	—	3 small	13	0.3	5
Sauerkraut	15	¼ c	15	0.6	11
Spinach, cooked	11	1 tbsp	15	0.3	3
Squash, summer, cooked	13	5 tbsp	16	0.6	9

PART B—TABLE FOODS (Continued)

Food	g per tbsp	Amount	Phenylalanine (mg)	Protein (g)	Energy (kcal)
Vegetables—Cont					
Squash, winter, cooked	13	¼ c	16	0.6	20
Tomato, raw	17	½ small	14	0.6	11
Tomato, canned	17	¼ c	17	0.7	14
Tomato juice	14	¼ c	16	0.6	13
Tomato catsup	17	2 tbsp	17	0.7	36
Tomato puree	6	6 tbsp	15	0.6	14
Tomato sauce	18	3 tbsp	18	0.7	52
Turnip greens, cooked	9	2 tbsp	18	0.4	4
Turnips, diced, cooked	10	9 tbsp	15	0.7	21
Soups (prepared with equal volume of water)					
Asparagus (Campbell's condensed)		3 tbsp	15	0.5	12
Beef broth (Campbell's condensed)		2 tbsp	17	0.6	4
Celery (Campbell's condensed)		3 tbsp	15	0.3	16
Minestrone (Campbell's condensed)		3 tbsp	18	0.8	17
Mushroom (Campbell's condensed)		2 tbsp	15	0.3	17
Onion (Campbell's condensed)		3 tbsp	19	0.9	11
Tomato (Campbell's condensed)		3 tbsp	17	0.4	16
Vegetarian vegetable (Campbell's condensed)		3 tbsp	14	0.3	12
Vegetable and beef broth (Campbell's condensed)		4 tbsp	16	0.5	15
Clam chowder and tomato (Campbell's condensed)		3 tbsp	14	0.4	15
Chicken gumbo (Campbell's condensed)		2 tbsp	14	0.4	7
Cream of chicken (Campbell's condensed)		2 tbsp	15	0.4	12
Beef noodle (Campbell's condensed)		2 tbsp	19	0.5	8

Each Serving as Listed Below Contains 30 mg of Phenylalanine

Food	g per tbsp	Amount	Phenylalanine (mg)	Protein (g)	Energy (kcal)
Fruits					
Apple, raw		2½ small	15	0.5	145
Applesauce	19	¾ c	14	0.5	207
Apricots, raw		1½ medium	14	0.6	31
Apricots, canned		3 halves	14	0.6	86
Apricots, dried		2 halves	14	0.6	31
Avocado, cubed or mashed	9.5	3 tbsp	14	0.6	48
Banana, raw sliced		½ small or ⅓ c sliced	17	0.6	43
Blackberries, canned, syrup	15.6	5 tbsp	16	0.6	71
Blackberries, raw	9	6 tbsp	17	0.6	31
Blueberries, raw	8.8	10 tbsp	16	0.6	55
Blueberries, frozen, unsweetened	10	9 tbsp	16	0.6	50
Blueberries, canned, syrup	15	10 tbsp	15	0.6	151
Cantaloupe, raw, diced	15	5 tbsp	16	0.5	23
Sour cherries	13	4 tbsp	16	0.6	30
Sweet cherries, canned, syrup	13	5 tbsp	15	0.6	53
Cranberries, raw	6	1½ c	14	0.6	66
Cranberry sauce	20	1⅔ c	16	0.5	780
Cranberry, sweetened, cooked	13	1½ c	16	0.6	555
Dates	11	2 tbsp	15	0.6	69
Figs, raw	—	1 large	15	0.6	40
Figs, canned, syrup	—	4 small	16	0.6	105
Figs, dried	—	1 small	16	0.6	41
Fruit cocktail	13	¾ c	16	0.6	119
Grapefruit, raw	12	¾ c or ½ large	14	0.7	59
Grapes, Thompson, seedless	10	½ c (12 grapes)	14	0.5	54
Guava, raw	—	1 small	16	0.6	47
Honeydew, raw, diced	13	5 tbsp	16	0.5	21
Mango, raw	—	½ medium	18	0.7	66
Nectarines, raw	—	2 large	15	0.8	80
Oranges, raw	—	1 medium (3 in diam)	18	1.5	74
Papaya, raw	16	⅓ medium or 6 tbsp	16	0.6	39
Peaches, raw	11	1 large or ¾ c sliced	16	0.8	50
Peaches, canned, syrup	16	4 medium halves	16	0.8	156
Peaches, dried	10	2½ tbsp	16	0.8	66
Pears, raw	—	½ medium (3 x 2½ in)	17	0.7	61

PART B—TABLE FOODS *(Continued)*

Food	g per tbsp	Amount	Phenylalanine (mg)	Protein (g)	Energy (kcal)
Fruits—Cont					
Pears, canned, syrup	16	5 small halves	15	0.5	190
Pears, dried	—	½ pear	12	0.4	35
Pineapple, raw	8	1 c diced	14	0.5	67
Pineapple, canned, syrup	16	2 large slices	16	0.6	148
Plums, Damson, raw	13	2 whole	13	0.5	66
Plums, prune-type, raw	13	1½ whole	17	0.4	38
Plums, canned, syrup	14	4 whole	13	0.5	110
Prunes, dried, medium	—	3 whole	18	0.4	54
Raisins, dried, seedless	10	2 tbsp	15	0.5	58
Raspberries, black, raw	11	¼ c	17	0.7	32
Raspberries, red, raw	8	6 tbsp	15	0.6	27
Raspberries, black, canned, syrup	13	4 tbsp	15	0.6	27
Raspberries, red, canned, syrup	13	7 tbsp	16	0.6	32
Rhubarb, cooked, added sugar	15	6 tbsp	15	0.5	141
Strawberries, raw	9	10 large	17	0.7	37
Strawberries, frozen, whole	15	15 large	15	0.6	138
Tangerine	—	1 small or ½ large	12	0.4	23
Watermelon, ball or cubes	12.5	⅔ c	17	0.7	36
Breads and cereals					
Prepared cereals					
Alpha Bits		3 tbsp	27	0.6	23
Apple Jacks		6 tbsp	32	0.7	47
Cap'n Crunch		5 tbsp	29	0.7	65
Cheerios		2 tbsp	27	0.5	15
Corn Chex		½ c	29	0.6	30
Cornflakes		¼ c	28	0.6	31
Froot Loops		5 tbsp	36	0.6	40
Kix		½ c	28	0.6	32
Lucky Charms		3 tbsp	29	0.5	23
Puffed Rice		10 tbsp	31	0.6	40
Puffed Wheat		¼ c	32	0.9	12
Cap'n Crunchberries		¼ c	31	0.5	47
Cap'n Crunch Peanut Butter Cereal		3 tbsp	32	0.6	38
Rice Chex		6 tbsp	31	0.6	44
Rice Krinkles		½ c	28	0.5	63
Rice Krispies		¼ c	28	0.5	30
Quisp		½ c	31	0.8	68
Shredded Wheat		¼ biscuit	29	0.6	21
Sugar Frosted Flakes		½ c	30	0.6	62
Sugar Pops		½ c	30	0.6	43
Sugar Smacks		7 tbsp	31	0.7	55
Trix		6 tbsp	30	0.7	47
Wheaties		¼ c	31	0.7	25
Wheat Chex		7 biscuits	31	0.7	25
Cocoa Krispies		½ c	29	0.5	48
Team Flakes		10 tbsp	30	0.6	39
Quaker Life		1 tbsp	30	0.6	12
King Vitamin		½ c	32	0.6	63
Special K		2 tbsp	29	0.6	11
Franken Berry		7 tbsp	30	0.6	50
Count Chocula		6 tbsp	28	0.6	42
Sir Grapefellow		5 tbsp	27	0.5	39
Boo Berry		5 tbsp	27	0.5	39
Granola		1 tbsp	32	0.6	19
Grapenuts		1 tbsp	27	0.6	26
Grapenut Flakes		3 tbsp	29	0.7	30
Cooked cereals					
Cornmeal		4 tbsp	29	0.7	30
Cream of Rice		5 tbsp	31	0.6	38
Cream of Wheat		2 tbsp	28	0.6	17
Farina		3 tbsp	31	0.6	19
Malt-O-Meal		2 tbsp	30	0.6	20
Oatmeal		2 tbsp	33	0.6	17
Pettijohns		2 tbsp	32	0.7	23
Ralston		2 tbsp	31	0.6	16
Rice, white		3 tbsp	28	0.5	29

PART B—TABLE FOODS (Continued)

Food	g per tbsp	Amount	Phenylalanine (mg)	Protein (g)	Energy (kcal)
Breads and Cereals—Cont					
Rice, brown		2 tbsp	28	0.5	25
Wheatena		2 tbsp	31	0.6	22
Wheat Hearts		2 tbsp	31	0.7	17
Crackers					
Animal Crackers		5	33	0.7	43
Arrowroot Cookies		2	30	0.6	45
Graham Crackers		1	28	0.6	21
Ritz Crackers		3	35	0.7	45
Saltines		2	27	0.5	26
Tortilla, corn		¼ (6 in diam)	33	0.7	27
Wheat Thins		4	34	0.7	32
Meal Mates		1	25	0.5	24
Miscellaneous					
Corn, cooked		2 tbsp	29	0.5	17
Hominy grits, cooked		6 tbsp	32	0.7	31
Macaroni, cooked		2 tbsp	32	0.6	20
Noodles, cooked		2 tbsp	32	0.7	20
Potato chips		6 (2 in diam)	29	0.6	68
Potato, Irish, cooked		⅓ potato (2¼ in diam)	29	0.6	21
Potatoes, French fried		3 (½ x ½ x 2 in)	30	0.6	41
Instant potatoes (dry) without milk		5 tbsp	33	0.7	36
Popcorn, popped, plain		5 tbsp	29	0.6	19
Spaghetti cooked		2 tbsp	32	0.6	20
Sweet potatoes, cooked		3 tbsp	28	0.6	38
Instant sweet potatoes, dry without milk		2 tbsp	29	0.6	53
Each Serving as Listed Below Contains 5 mg Phenylalanine					
Fats					
Butter		1 tbsp	4	0.1	100
French dressing, commercial		5 tbsp	5	0.2	442
Margarine		1 tbsp	5	0.1	108
Miracle Whip		1 tbsp	5	0.1	68
Olives, green		2 tbsp	5	0.2	16
Olives, ripe		2 tbsp	5	0.2	18
Mayonnaise		2 tbsp	5	0.1	72
Desserts—Comstock					
Apple pie filling		¼ c	1	<0.5	89
Apricot pie filling		¼ c	8	0.4	79
Blackberry pie filling		¼ c	1	<0.5	109
Blueberry pie filling		¼ c	6	0.2	83
Boysenberry pie filling		¼ c	11	0.4	93
Cherry pie filling		¼ c	11	0.4	83
Peach pie filling		¼ c	4	0.2	78
Pineapple pie filling		¼ c	4	0.1	70
Raspberry pie filling		¼ c	8	0.3	106
Strawberry pie filling		¼ c	5	0.2	79
Free foods					
(These foods contain little or no phenylalanine. May be used as desired.)					
Apple juice		6 oz			85
Candies					
Butterscotch		1 piece			20
Cream mints		1 piece			7
Fondant, patties or mint		1 piece			40
Gum drops		1 large			35
Hard candy		2 pieces			39
Jelly beans		10			110
Lollipops		1 medium (2½ in diam)			108
Carbonated beverages		6 oz			78
Corn syrup		1 tbsp			58
Danish dessert		½ c			123
Diet margarine		1 tbsp			50
Fruit butter		1 tbsp			37
Fruit ices		½ c			69

PART B—TABLE FOODS (Continued)

Food	g per tbsp	Amount	Phenylalanine (mg)	Protein (g)	Energy (kcal)
Free Foods—Cont					
Jellies		1 tbsp			55
Kool-Aid		4 oz			48
Lemonade		4 oz			53
Maple syrup		1 tbsp			50
Molasses		1 tbsp			46
Popsicle		1 twin bar			95
Shortening		1 tbsp			123
Start liquid		4 oz			60
Sugar, brown		1 tbsp			46
Sugar, granulated		1 tbsp			43
Sugar, white, powdered		1 tbsp			59
Tang liquid		4 oz			59
Miscellaneous					
Cake flour		1 tbsp	29	0.6	29
Cornstarch		1 tbsp	1	trace[a]	29
Tapioca, granulated		1 tbsp	2	0.1	35
Wheat starch		1 tbsp	1	trace	25
Nondairy creams					
Coffee rich		1 tbsp	3	trace	23
Cool whip		1 tbsp	2	trace	14
Dzert Whip, liquid		1 tbsp	9	0.2	44
Rich's topping		1 tbsp			43
Mocha mix		1 tbsp	2	trace	13

[a] Less than 0.04 g protein = trace
(*Source: Acosta PB, Wenz E: Diet Management of PKU for Infants and Preschool Children. DHEW Publication No. (HSA) 78-5209, Rockville, Md, 1978, pp 16–23.*)

Glossary

Achalasia—A neuromuscular disorder of the esophagus that causes dilatation of the esophagus, dysphagia, dyspepsia, esophageal regurgitation, and esophageal pain; cardiospasm.

Acidosis—Excess hydrogen ions in the blood; may result from an excess of carbonic acid (respiratory acidosis) or a deficit of bicarbonate (metabolic acidosis).

Acids—Substances that, in solution, give off hydrogen ions (protons).

Acne vulgaris—An inflammatory, papulo-pustular skin eruption occurring usually on the face, neck, shoulders, and upper back; its cause is unknown but involves bacterial breakdown of sebum into fatty substances irritating to surrounding subcutaneous tissue.

Active transport—Passage of substances across a membrane from an area of lower concentration to an area of higher concentration; the process involves the expenditure of energy and a special transport carrier.

Acute renal failure—An acute reduction in kidney function to a level in which the kidneys are unable to maintain normal biologic homeostasis.

Addison's disease—Adrenal insufficiency; deficiency in the secretion of adrenocortical hormones; manifestations include increased pigmentation of the skin and mucous membranes, hypotension, fasting hypoglycemia, electrolyte imbalance with excessive loss of sodium chloride in the urine, retention of potassium, and loss of appetite and body weight.

Adenosine triphosphate (ATP)—A compound of adenosine (a nucleotide containing adenine and ribose) that has three phosphoric acid groups; a high-energy phosphate compound important in energy exchange for cellular activity; the splitting off of the terminal phosphate bond of ATP to produce adenosine diphosphate (ADP) releases bond energy and transfers it to free energy available for body work; the reformation of ATP in cellular oxidation again stores energy in high-energy phosphate bonds for use as needed.

Adolescence—The period of development between the onset of puberty and adulthood, usually beginning between the ages of 10 and 13; the period spans the teen years, terminating at 18 to 20 years of age with the acquisition of completely developed adult form; extensive physical, psychologic, and emotional changes occur during the period.

Adrenal insufficiency—Decreased functioning of the adrenal gland, particularly the cortex; Addison's disease.

Alcohol—A group of compounds derived from carbohydrate fermentation; ethyl alcohol or ethanol.

Alcoholic hepatitis—Inflammation and necrosis of the liver caused by alcohol abuse.

Alkalosis—Deficit of hydrogen ions in the blood; may result from a deficit of carbonic acid (respiratory alkalosis) or an excess of bicarbonate (metabolic alkalosis).

Allergy—An abnormal and individual hypersensitivity to a substance that is ordinarily harmless; denotes adverse physiologic reactions resulting from the interaction of an antigen with humoral antibody and/or lymphoid cells.

Amylophagia—A type of pica in which starch is consumed.

695

Anabolism—The constructive (building up) reactions of metabolism characterized by the conversion of simple substances into the more complex compounds of living matter; the opposite of catabolism; together anabolism and catabolism constitute metabolism.

Anaphylactic shock—A profound state of shock resulting from hypersensitivity to an allergen such as a drug, foreign protein, or toxin; can be fatal unless emergency measures are taken.

Angina pectoris—Acute chest pain caused by interference with the oxygen supply to the heart; pain begins just under the sternum, sometimes radiating to the neck, throat, jaw, down the left arm, and more rarely to the stomach, back or to the right side of the chest.

Angioedema—An acute, transitory, localized swelling of the subcutaneous tissue or submucosa of the face, hands, feet, genitalia, or viscera.

Anions—Negatively charged ions; anions in body fluids include chloride, bicarbonate, phosphate, sulfate, lactate, pyruvate, and proteinates.

Anorexia nervosa—A psychoneurotic disorder characterized by a prolonged refusal to eat leading to emaciation, amenorrhea, altered body image, and an abnormal fear of becoming fat.

Anthropometric assessment—A technique for assessing nutritional status that involves measurement of physical dimensions of the body such as height, weight, arm and head circumferences, and skinfold thickness and comparing the figures with norms.

Antibodies—Protein substances that are produced in the body in response to invasion by foreign substances such as antigens; also referred to as immunoglobulins.

Antigen—Any substance not normally present in the body which, when introduced into it, elicits an immunologic response, such as the production of an antibody specific for that substance.

Antiketogenic—Property of a food component to inhibit production of ketone bodies when oxidized; carbohydrate, glycerol, and amino acids that are convertible to glucose are antiketogenic substances.

Arthritis—Inflammation of a joint, usually accompanied by pain, and frequently changes in structure of the joint.

Ascorbic acid—Vitamin C, a water-soluble vitamin that functions in formation and maintenance of collegen in connective tissue.

Asparaginase—An enzyme present in liver and other animal tissue that catalyzes the hydrolysis of asparagine to asparaginic acid and ammonia; has antileukemic activity.

Atherosclerosis—A type of arteriosclerosis characterized by the deposition of lipids, complex carbohydrates, calcium, fibrin, and the formed elements of the blood in the intimal layer of large- and medium-sized arteries that progressively occludes the vascular lumen; the medial layer of the arterial wall is also susceptible to pathologic changes.

Atrophic arthritis—See Rheumatoid arthritis.

Autoimmune disease—A condition in which an immune response is directed against a constituent of an organism's own body.

Azotemia—The presence of nitrogenous substances, especially urea, in the blood in increased amounts.

Basal metabolism—The minimum amount of energy required to maintain life in the resting state.

Bases—Substances that, in solution, accept hydrogen ions.

Biologically active vitamin—A vitamin that has been converted from its precursor state to the active form of the vitamin; an example is the conversion of β-carotene to vitamin A.

Bottle mouth caries—Rampant decay of the upper front teeth, and sometimes the lower molars, caused by prolonged pooling of fermentable carbohydrate around the teeth; also called nursing caries.

Brittle diabetes—A form of Type I diabetes mellitus that is difficult to control and is sensitive to both hypoglycemia and acidosis.

Buffer system—A pair of compounds (usually a weak acid and its alkali base) that, in solution, offset the changes in pH that would otherwise occur on adding an acid or a base; the major buffer system in maintaining the normal pH of body fluids is the carbonic acid–sodium bicarbonate system.

Bulimia—An eating disorder characterized by an insatiable craving for food; a clinical gorge–purge syndrome that may be associated with anorexia nervosa.

Cachexia—A state of malnutrition, emaciation, and debility, usually occurring in the course of a chronic illness.

Calorigenic effect—The increase in energy expenditure associated with food ingestion (digestion, nutrient absorption, and nutrient transport); also called the specific dynamic action of food or dietary thermogenesis.

Carbohydrates—The term was originally designated for compounds of hydrates of carbon with the general formula $C_N(H_2O)_N$; it now includes other compounds having the properties of carbohydrates but not the required 2:1 ratio of hydrogen to oxygen; examples of important carbohydrates are sugar, starch, and cellulose.

Carrier-facilitated diffusion—A type of diffusion in which a substance that is unable to cross a membrane on its own attaches to another substance that carries it across the membrane.

Caseation—A form of tissue necrosis in which there is loss of cellular outline and the appearance is that of crumbly cheese; it is typical of tuberculosis.

Catabolism—The destructive (breaking down) reactions of metabolism; the breakdown of complex substances by living cells into simpler compounds with the liberation of energy; the opposite of anabolism; together catabolism and anabolism constitute metabolism.

Cations—Positively charged ions; cations in body fluids include sodium, potassium, calcium, and magnesium.

Cerebral palsy—A group of congenital disorders characterized by a major disorder of motor function; mental retardation may or may not be present.

Cholecalciferol—Activated 7-dehydrocholesterol, or vitamin D_3.

Cholecystitis—Acute or chronic inflammation of the gallbladder.

Cholelithiasis—Formation or presence of calculi in the gallbladder or common bile duct.

Cholesterol—A fat-related sterol that is a precursor of various steroids such as sex hormones and adrenal corticoids; it is synthesized by the liver and occurs naturally in animal protein foods; a normal constituent of bile and a principal constituent of gallstones.

Chronic nonspecific diarrhea—A type of diarrhea occurring in late infancy or early childhood that may be related to consuming an inadequate amount of fat; malabsorption is not present and the disorder appears not to affect growth.

Chronic renal failure—Chronic reduction of kidney function to a level at which the kidneys are unable to maintain biologic homeostasis.

Chylomicrons—The largest and lightest of the lipoproteins; synthesized in the intestinal mucosal cell, they serve to transport absorbed dietary triglycerides to sites of utilization; consist chiefly of triglyceride and smaller amounts of cholesterol, phospholipid, and protein.

Cirrhosis—A chronic progressive disease of the liver in which fibrous connective tissue replaces the functioning liver cells; manifestations may include anorexia, weight loss, abdominal discomfort, portal hypertension, jaundice, ascites, esophageal varices, altered nutrient metabolism, hypoalbuminemia, endocrine change, fluid and electrolyte imbalance, hepatic coma, and kidney failure; in some instances severe malnutrition may be present.

Colic—A condition that may occur during early infancy associated with paroxysms of pain, crying, and irritability resulting from such factors as swallowed air, overfeeding, allergy, and emotional disturbances.

Colloidal osmotic pressure—Pressure produced by protein molecules in plasma and cells; as proteins are large molecules, they do not diffuse through the separating membranes of capillary cells and thus remain in their respective compartments exerting a constant osmotic pull that protects the vital plasma and cell fluid volumes in these compartments.

Colostrum—The first milk secreted by the mother's breasts after the birth of the child; a thick, yellowish, transparent fluid that is higher in protein and mineral content but lower in carbohydrate, fat, and kilocalories than the mature milk that follows.

Complete protein—A protein that contains the essential amino acids in the correct quantity and ratio for growth and maintenance; such proteins are said to have a high biologic value; examples are eggs, milk, cheese, and meat.

Compound lipids—Lipids that contain not only fatty acids and an alcohol, but other substances such as phosphorus, nitrogen, and carbohydrate as well; glycolipids are an example.

Complex carbohydrates—Polysaccharides that contain 10 or more monosaccharide units.

Congenital—Present at birth, as a congenital anomaly or defect.

Congestive heart failure—A condition characterized by shortness of breath, edema, and abdominal discomfort resulting from inadequate cardiac output.

Conjugated (compound) proteins—Proteins made up of combinations of simple proteins and nonprotein substances; lipoproteins are an example.

Constipation—A disorder of the colon characterized by infrequent or difficult bowel movements.

Coronary heart disease—A condition characterized by inadequate coronary circulation in which the heart is deprived of its oxygen and nutrient supply; narrowing or complete occlusion of the lumen of the coronary arteries occurs as a result of atherosclerosis, thrombus formation, or embolism; also called ischemic heart disease.

Crude fiber—Insoluble plant material remaining after chemical treatment with weak acid and alkali in laboratory nutrient analysis; chiefly composed of cellulose and lignin.

Deamination—The removal of the amino (NH_2) group from an amino acid.

Degenerative (hypertrophic) arthritis—See Osteoarthritis.

Dehydration—A condition resulting from excessive loss of body fluids; may be hypertonic, isotonic, or hypotonic.

Dental fluorosis—A condition of generalized increased density of the skeleton resulting from prolonged ingestion of excessive fluoride.

Derived lipids—Substances resulting from the breakdown of simple or compound lipids, such as fatty acids.

Derived proteins—Compounds formed during the various stages of breakdown of a protein molecule such as a dipeptide or tripeptide formed during digestion.

Development—Increased complexity of function of the organism, both physiologic and psychosocial.

Developmental obesity—A type of obesity that manifests itself over a period of time.

Dialysis—The process of diffusing blood across a semipermeable membrane for the purpose of removing toxic substances and maintaining fluid and electrolyte balance.

Diarrhea—A condition characterized by frequent passage of loose, watery, and unformed stools.

Dietary fiber—Undigestible polysaccharide and lignin components of plants.

Dietary thermogenesis—See Calorigenic effect.

Diet counseling—The process of providing individualized guidance to assist a person to adjust his or her daily consumption to meet health needs.

Dietetic foods—Foods in which the content of some nutrient, such as sodium or fat, or of kilocalories has been altered or reduced.

Diffusion—Passage of substances across a membrane from an area of higher concentration to an area of lower concentration.

Diglycerides—Glycerides containing two molecules of fatty acid.

Dipeptide—A product formed by the combination of two amino acids or by hydrolysis of proteins.

Direct/Indirect calorimetry—Direct calorimetry is a direct measure of heat lost from the body measured by placing the subject in an insulated boxlike chamber and noting the rise in the temperature of the water circulating in the tubes surrounding the chamber; indirect calorimetry is a measure of heat produced by a subject by calculating oxygen consumption and carbon dioxide elimination over a given period of time.

Disaccharidases—Enzymes that hydrolyze disaccharides; the most common are sucrase, maltase, and lactase.

Diverticulitis—An inflammatory condition of a diverticulum (or of diverticula) characterized by nausea, vomiting, fever, abdominal tenderness, distention, pain, and intestinal spasm.

Down's syndrome—A congenital condition associated with physical malformation and some degree of mental retardation; also called mongolism and trisomy 21.

Dumping syndrome—A complex of symptoms occurring after ingestion of food by clients who have had a total or subtotal gastrectomy; manifestations include a combination of vasomotor symptoms (such as sweating and faintness), diarrhea, and late postprandial hypoglycemia.

Dyspepsia—Gastric indigestion; typical symptoms are heartburn, nausea, epigastric pain, belching, distention, and flatulence.

Eclampsia—An acute complication of pregnancy occurring usually in the third trimester toward term, accompanied by hypertension, edema, proteinuria, convulsions, and coma.

Ectomorph—A description given to a tall, thin individual with underdeveloped muscles and large subcutaneous tissue and surface areas with respect to body mass.

Edema—A condition resulting from excess accumulation of body fluids.

Electrolytes—Substances that, in solution, dissociate into electrically charged particles called ions.

Electrolytic solutions—Solutions, such as body fluids, that contain large numbers of electrically charged ions.

Emulsification—The process of lowering surface tension or breaking up large particles of an immiscible liquid into smaller ones that remain suspended in another liquid; emulsification of fat by bile salts facilitates fat digestion.

Encopresis—Incontinence of feces not caused by an organic defect or illness.

Endomorph—A description given to a stocky, fat individual with round body features, prominent abdominal viscera, large trunk and thighs, and tapering extremities.

Enzyme induction—Stimulation of enzyme synthesis resulting from the presence of substrate, such as the stimulation of enzymes involved in alternate pathways of alcohol oxidation caused by chronic alcohol use.

Enzymes—Organic substances, usually protein in nature, that accelerate chemical reactions by catalytic action.

Epilepsy—A disorder of the nervous system characterized by a recurring excessive neuronal discharge leading to transient episodes of motor, sensory, and psychic dysfunction with or without convulsions or loss of consciousness.

Esophagitis—Inflammation of the esophagus.

Essential amino acids—The eight (nine in infants) amino acids that must be obtained from the diet because the body is not capable of synthesizing them: threonine, leucine, isoleucine, valine, lysine, methonine, phenylalanine, tryptophan, and in infants, histidine.

Essential fatty acids—Fatty acids that are essential for body metabolism or function, cannot be synthesized by the body, and thus must be supplied by the diet; the major essential fatty acid is linoleic acid.

Essential hypertension—Hypertension in which the cause cannot be determined; primary hypertension.

Extracellular fluid (ECF)—Body fluid contained outside of the cells; consists of plasma, lymph, spinal fluid, secretions, and interstitial fluid.

Extrinsic factor—Vitamin B_{12}; a term used by Castle to describe the substance prior to the identification of the nature of the compound.

Extrusion reflex—A normal response in infants to force the tongue outward when touched or depressed; begins to disappear about 3 to 4 months of age; constant protrusion of a large tongue may be a sign of Down's syndrome.

Failure to thrive—A general term used to describe an infant who fails to attain the minimal expected gains in growth and development.

Fasting hypoglycemia—A below normal blood glucose level that occurs after a period of fasting in persons with conditions that alter the mechanisms involved with maintaining glucose homeostasis.

Fatty acids—The structural component of fats; organic acids containing carbon, hydrogen, and oxygen with a methyl group at one end of the carbon chain and a carboxyl group at the other end.

Fatty infiltration (liver)—A relatively benign, reversible condition of the liver associated with the deposition of fat and enlargement of the organ.

Fetal alcohol syndrome—A syndrome of congenital anomalies, mental deficiency, and prenatal and postnatal growth retardation occurring in infants of mothers who consume excessive amounts of alcohol during pregnancy.

Fiber—Indigestible organic tissues such as ligaments and gristle in meat and indigestible carbohydrates such as cellulose, hemicellulose, and lignin found in vegetables, fruits, and cereals; a term often used synonymously with roughage.

Food allergy—Hypersensitivity that is caused by an immunologic reaction to specific constituents of food or their digestion products.

Food intolerance—Food-induced reactions caused by nonimmunologic mechanisms such as cow's milk intolerance resulting from lactase deficiency.

Food sensitivity—The preferred term for hypersensitivity caused by immunologic reactions associated with food ingestion.

Foremilk—A low-fat, low-protein secretion that is the milk first withdrawn at each nursing.

Gag reflex—The reflex normally present at birth that allows food to return from the back to the front of the mouth; it is protective in nature and can be stimulated by placing a finger at the back of the oral cavity and applying pressure on the tongue; present throughout adulthood but weakens when chewing begins.

Glactosemia—An inborn error of metabolism characterized by the inability to convert galactose to glucose because of the absence of the enzyme galactose-1-phosphate uridyl transferese.

Gastritis—Inflammation of the gastric mucosa; may be acute or chronic.

Geophagia—A type of pica in which clay or dirt is consumed.

Gestational diabetes—A disorder characterized by an impaired ability to metabolize carbohydrates that may be caused by insulin resistance, occurring in pregnancy and disappearing after delivery but, in some cases, returning years later.

Glomerulonephritis—An inflammatory disease of the kidneys affecting primarily the glomeruli; occurs in acute, subacute, and chronic forms; manifestations may include nitrogen retention, hematuria, proteinuria, edema, hypertension, oliguria or anuria, anorexia, lethargy, nausea and vomiting.

Glucagon—A hormone secreted by the alpha cells of the islets of Langerhans of the pancreas; it increases the blood sugar level by stimulating gluconeogenesis and the breakdown of glycogen and release of glucose by the liver.

Glucose—Dextrose; blood sugar; a monosaccharide, the form in which carbohydrate circulates in the blood.

Glucosuria—Presence of glucose in the urine.

Gluten-induced enteropathy—A disorder of the small intestine resulting from a sensitivity to gluten present in certain cereals; manifestations include generalized malabsorption, abdominal distention, weight loss, anemia, and other signs of malnutrition; in children it is sometimes called celiac disease and in adults, nontropical sprue.

Glycerol—A colorless, odorless, syrupy, sweet liquid that is chemically an alcohol; esterified with fatty acids to produce glycerides (monoglycerides, diglycerides, and triglycerides).

Glycogen—A branched-chain polysaccharide composed of glucose units; the chief carbohydrate storage material in animals; stored especially in the liver and muscles; also called animal starch.

Glycogen loading—A technique for increasing the amount of glycogen stored in muscles for the purpose of improving performance in endurance-type athletic events lasting 60 minutes or longer; the technique involves first depleting glycogen stores while consuming a low-carbohydrate diet, followed by consumption of a high-carbohydrate diet.

Glycolipids—Lipids composed of a carbohydrate, a fatty acid, and an alcohol; important components of nerve tissue.

Goiter—Enlargement of the thyroid gland.

Grand mal seizures—Seizures characterized by a sudden loss of consciousness and tonic, followed by clonic, contraction of muscles.

Growth—An increase in the size of the organism as a result of cell division and increase in cell size.

Growth and development—A general phrase that incorporates the complex physiologic and psychosocial changes that occur in persons throughout the life cycle.

Growth spurt—The most rapid phase of physical growth during adolescence; the spurt begins at about age 10 in females and 2 years later in males.

Haptens—Substances of low molecular weight that react with a specific antibody but that alone are unable to elicit the formation of that antibody.

Health food—An inclusive term that refers to organic, natural, dietetic, vegetarian and other foods, some of which may contain artificial chemicals.

Heme iron—The form of iron contained in hemoglobin and myoglobin of muscle meats.

Hemochromatosis—A genetic disorder resulting in excessive absorption and storage of iron with tissue damage, particularly in the liver.

Hemodialysis—The process of exposing blood to a semipermeable membrane for the purpose of removing or adding diffusable materials while the blood circulates outside the body.

Hemosiderosis—A condition of excessive body storage of iron without associated tissue damage.

Hepatomegaly—Enlargement of the liver.

Hiatus hernia—Diaphragmatic hernia; an outpouching of a portion of the stomach through the hiatus of the diaphragm and into the thoracic cavity; may be paraesophageal or gastroesophageal; manifestations include gastric reflux, esophagitis, and heartburn.

High biologic value—See Complete protein.

Hindmilk—A secretion that is higher in protein and fat content than foremilk (first withdrawn at the beginning of nursing) that is withdrawn shortly after nursing is initiated.

Homeostasis—A relative constancy in the internal environment of the body, naturally maintained by adaptive responses that promote healthy survival.

Hydramnios—An abnormal condition of pregnancy characterized by an excess of amniotic fluid.

Hyperalimentation—A type of parenteral feeding that provides complete nutritional support to clients who have increased nutritional requirements and who are unable to ingest foods by the external route for an extended period of time; nutrients including water, hypertonic glucose, amino acids, fat in the form of an emulsion, vitamins, and minerals are infused via an indwelling catheter into the superior vena cava; now called total parenteral nutrition.

Hypercalcemia—Abnormally high blood level of calcium.

Hyperglycemia—An above normal blood glucose level.

Hyperkalemia—A condition in which there is a greater than normal amount of potassium, the major intracellular cation, in the blood; occurs frequently in acute renal failure.

Hyperkinetic behavior syndrome—A complex of learning and behavioral disabilities seen primarily in children of near average to above average intelligence.

Hyperlipidemia—A general term that refers to an elevation of one or more lipid constituents in the blood.

Hypernatremia—A greater than normal concentration of sodium in the blood; may result from excessive sodium intake, deficient water intake, or water loss in excess of sodium loss.

Hyperplasia—An increase in the size of a tissue or organ as a result of cell division and an increase in cell number.

Hyperplastic obesity—A type of obesity associated with an increase in the number of fat cells.

Hypertension—Elevation of the blood pressure above normal; also called high blood pressure.

Hyperthyroidism—An endocrine disorder resulting from excessive secretion of thyroid hormones; characterized by thyroid enlargement, increased metabolic and pulse rate, weight loss, excessive sweating, heat intolerance, insomnia, nervousness and excitability; thyrotoxicosis; Graves' disease; toxic goiter; Basedow's disease; exophthalmic goiter.

Hypertonia—Abnormal tension of arteries or muscles.

Hypertonic dehydration—A condition resulting from net water loss that exceeds electrolyte loss.

Hypertrophy—An increase in the size of a tissue or organ as a result of enlargement of existing cells.

Hypertropic obesity—A type of obesity associated with an increase in fat cell size.

Hyperuricemia—An elevation in the blood levels of uric acid.

Hyperuricosuria—Elevated uric acid in the urine.

Hypocalcemia—Abnormally low blood level of calcium.

Hypoglycemia—A below normal blood glucose level.

Hypokalemia—A condition in which there is a below normal amount of potassium, the major intracellular cation in the blood.

Hyponatremia—A below normal concentration of sodium in the blood; may result from deficient sodium intake, sodium loss in excess of water loss, or water intake that exceeds sodium intake.

Hypothyroidism—An endocrine disorder resulting from a decreased activity of the thyroid gland; in its severe form it is called myxedema in adults and cretinism in children.

Hypotonia—Relaxation of arteries or loss of tonicity of muscles.

Hypotonic dehydration—A condition resulting from net electrolyte loss that exceeds water loss.

Iatrogenic malnutrition—Malnutrition produced inadvertently as a result of treatment by the medical team.

Inappropriate ADH syndrome—A disorder characterized by excessive secretion of the antidiuretic hormone; manifested by a low concentration of sodium in the blood.

Inborn errors of metabolism—Inherited biochemical disorders that results from a defect in the structure or function of a protein.

Incomplete protein—Food protein lacking sufficient amounts of one or more essential amino acids; such proteins are said to have a low biologic value; examples are cereal grains and vegetables.

Indigestion—See Dyspepsia.

Insulin—A hormone secreted by the beta cells of the islets of Langerhans of the pancreas; lowers blood glucose; increases liver and muscle glycogen, inhibits gluconeogenesis, and increases the rate of glucose use by the tissues.

Insulin-dependent diabetes—A type of diabetes in which endogenous insulin production is absent or very minimal.

Interdisciplinary team approach—An approach to health care delivery that combines the expertise of all members of the health team such as the physician, nurse, dietitian, social worker, pharmacist, and others.

Intracellular fluid (ICF)—Body fluid contained inside the cells.

Intravenous feeding—Provision of nutrients through a peripheral or central vein.

Intrinsic factor—An enzyme present in gastric secretions that facilitates the absorption of vitamin B_{12}.

Ions—Particles that carry an electrical charge; positively charged ions are called cations, negatively charged ions are called anions.

Iron deficiency anemia—A hematologic disorder associated with a decrease in the hemoglobin concentration because of a lack of iron.

Ischemic heart disease—See Coronary heart disease.

Isotonic dehydration—A condition resulting from loss of water and electrolytes in equal amounts.

Ketoacidosis—Acidosis accompanied by an accumulation of ketone bodies in the blood; occurs primarily as a complication of diabetes mellitus; also seen in starvation and following ingestion of low-carbohydrate, high-fat diet.

Ketoacids—Compounds that contain both a ketone or carbonyl group ($C{=}O$) and a carboxyl group ($COOH{-}$).

Ketogenic—Property of a food component to stimulate the production of ketone bodies when oxidized; fatty acids and amino acids that follow the metabolic pathways of fatty acids are precursors of ketone bodies and are ketogenic substances.

Ketogenic diet—A diet that is high in fat and low in carbohydrate, sometimes used in the treatment of epilepsy; the proportions of carbohydrates, proteins, and fat are regulated so that the ketogenic:antiketogenic ratio equals 2 or more; this ratio produces a state of ketosis, which is believed to be effective in controlling certain types of convulsive seizures.

Ketones—A collective term given to the intermediate products of fatty acid degradation; these are acetoacetic acid, beta-hydroxybutyric acid, and acetone; present in blood in very small amounts under normal conditions; tend to accumulate when the rate of production becomes excessive.

Ketosis—Accumulation of ketone bodies in the blood resulting from the incomplete oxidation of fatty acids in the absence of carbohydrate oxidation; occurs in carbohydrate deficiency or impaired carbohydrate metabolism.

Kilocalorie (kcalorie)—The amount of heat required to raise the temperature of one kilogram of water 1°C; the unit of measure for heat (energy).

Kilojoule (kjoule)—The unit of measure for heat (energy) in the metric system; one kilocalorie is equal to 4.184 kilogjoules.

Kosher—A term referring to foods that are used in accordance with the dietary laws of Orthodox Judaism; milk and meat are not consumed at the same meals; allowed meats must be prepared in a specified manner.

K-P diet—Kaiser-Permanente diet; a diet eliminating salicylates and certain food additives that is sometimes recommended for treating the hyperkinetic behavior syndrome.

Lacto-ovo-vegetarians—Vegetarians who consume milk and eggs but no meat.

Lactose—Milk sugar; a disaccharide found only in animal milk.

Lactose intolerance—A syndrome of diarrhea and other gastrointestinal manifestations induced by ingestion of lactose-containing foods by individuals with a congenital or acquired deficiency of the enzyme lactase in the intestinal secretions.

Laetrile—A cyanide-containing compound found in the pits of apricots, peaches, plums, bitter almonds, and other plant products that has been incorrectly called a vitamin and promoted both as a perventive and therapeutic agent in cancer.

Latent period—The school-age period of development.

Limiting amino acids—The amino acid in a test food that shows the greatest deviation from that in a reference standard.

Linoleic acid—An essential fatty acid that is polyunsaturated, containing 2 double bonds and 18 carbons.

Lipases—Enzymes that hydrolyze fats during digestion.

Lipids—Members of a large group of organic compounds that are insoluble in water and soluble in fat solvents such as ether; lipids of nutritional importance are fatty acids, triglycerides, phospholipids, terpenes (especially carotene), and steroids such as cholesterol.

Lipogenesis—Synthesis of lipids or formation of body fat from acetate.

Lipolysis—Breakdown or degradation of lipids into fatty acids and glycerol.

Lipoprotein—A compound protein formed when a simple protein unites with a lipid; it has solubility characteristics of protein and is thus involved in lipid transport; four types circulate in the blood.

Low biologic value—See Incomplete protein.

Low-birth-weight infants—Newborns weighing 2500 g or less; may be born prematurely (before the 38th week of gestation), or may be small for gestational age.

Lymphoid cells—Mononuclear cells that differentiate from stem cells and that may be either T-cells (which mediate cellular immunity) or B-cells (which mediate humoral immunity).

Macrocytic normochromic anemia—A hematologic disorder resulting from deficiency of either vitamin B_{12} or folic acid, in which the red blood cells are larger than normal size and normal in color.

Macronutrients—Mineral elements present in relatively large amounts in the body; calcium, phosphorus, sodium, potassium, magnesium, chloride, and sulfur.

Malabsorption syndrome—A group of symptoms indicating defective absorption; examples of disorders that show the malabsorption syndrome are celiac disease, chronic pancreatitis, and cystic fibrosis.

Maltose—Malt sugar; a disaccharide formed during the digestion of starch.

Megaloblastic anemia—A hematologic disorder characterized by the production and peripheral proliferation of large, immature, and dysfunctional erythrocytes; associated with a deficiency of vitamin B_{12} or folic acid.

Megavitamin therapy—The use of vitamins at dosage levels of at least 10 times the RDA as pharmacologic agents in the treatment of nonnutritional disorders.

Menadione—Vitamin K_3; synthetic vitamin K, which is about three times more potent biologically than naturally occurring vitamin K.

Menarche—The first menstruation and the beginning of cyclic menstrual function.

Metabolic pool—Body components indistinguishable in origin that may be employed for either synthetic or degradative processes; when the end products of digestion are absorbed they enter the metabolic pool and intermingle with other substances or are metabolized for various body functions.

Metabolic water—Water produced in the body as an end product of the oxidation of carbohydrate, protein, and fat.

Methionase—An enzyme that catalyzes the breakdown of the amino acid methionine.

Methotrexate—An antineoplastic antimetabolite of folic acid.

Micronutrients—Trace elements; mineral elements present in the body in relatively minute amounts; iron, copper, cobalt, zinc, manganese, iodine, molybdenum, fluorine, selenium, and chronium.

Midarm muscle circumference—An anthropometric measure of nutritional status that is an approximation of the skeletal muscle mass; the measure is mathematically derived from the midarm circumference and skinfold measures.

Middle childhood—The school-age period of development; begins at age 6 and terminates at puberty.

Mineral elements—Inorganic elements that remain as ash when food is burned; 21 minerals are essential to human nutrition; criteria for essentiality are: (1) a deficiency state occurs on a diet considered adequate except for the mineral under study, (2) there is a significant response when a supplement of the mineral is given, (3) the response is repeatedly demonstrable, and (4) the deficiency state correlates with a low level of the mineral in the blood or tissues.

Mixed micelles—Dispersed particles in a colloidal system that are held in a particulate form because of their special physiochemical properties; during digestion, the particles are formed by the combination of bile salts with fat substances to achieve the absorption of fat across the intestinal mucosal cell membrane.

Mongolism—See Down's syndrome.

Monoglyceride—A glyceride containing one molecule of fatty acid.

Monosaccharides—Carbohydrates consisting of one sugar molecule; major monoscaccharides are glucose, fructose, galactose, and ribose.

Monounsaturated fats—Triglycerides that are composed predominantly of monounsaturated fatty acids and glycerol.

Monounsaturated fatty acids—Fatty acids that have one double bond and consequently lack two hydrogen atoms.

Multiple sclerosis—A disease characterized clinically by episodes of focal disorder of the optic nerves, spinal cord, and brain, which remits to a varying extent and recurs over a period of many years; scattered, sharply defined demyelinative lesions in the white matter of the central nervous system are present.

Mutation—An unusual change in the genetic material occurring spontaneously or by induction.

Natural foods—Foods that are marketed as containing no added preservatives, emulsifiers, or artificial ingredients, and that have not been preserved or refined.

Necrosis—Localized tissue death that occurs in groups of cells in response to disease or injury.

Nephrogenic diabetes insipidus—A congenital disorder caused by failure of the renal tubules to reabsorb water; manifested by excessive thirst and passage of a large volume of urine.

Nephrolithiasis—The formation of renal calculi; the disease state characterized by the presence of renal calculi.

Nephrotic syndrome—Nephrosis; a condition in which there are degenerative changes in the kidneys, especially the renal tubules, without the occurrence of inflammation; characterized by marked proteinuria, hypoproteinemia, edema, and hyperlipidemia.

Nitrogen balance—A state of equilibrium that exists when nitrogen intake is equal to nitrogen excretion; if intake is greater, a positive nitrogen balance exists and if output is greater, a negative nitrogen balance exists.

Nonelectrolytes—Substances that do not ionize in solution; examples are urea and glucose.

Nonessential amino acids—The 12 (11 in infants) amino acids that the body is capable of synthesizing: glycine, alanine, aspartic acid, proline, glutamic acid, hydroxyproline, cystine, cysteine, tyrosine, serine, arginine, and histidine (essential in infants).

Nonheme iron—The form of iron present in nonmeat sources such as plant foods and eggs.

Noninsulin-dependent diabetes—A type of diabetes characterized by a relative (rather than absolute) deficiency of insulin.

Nonprotein nitrogen—Nitrogenous compounds such as ammonia and urea that are not components of proteins.

Nontoxic goiter—An enlargement of the thyroid gland caused by insufficient available iodine, which is needed to produce thyroid hormones; also called simple goiter.

Nursing caries—See Bottle mouth caries.

Nursing diagnosis—A statement that describes a health state or an actual or potential alteration in one's life processes (physiologic, psychologic, sociocultural, developmental, and spiritual); nurses use the nursing process to identify and synthesize clinical data and to order nursing interventions to reduce, eliminate, or prevent (health promotion) health alterations that are in the legal and educational domain of nursing.

Nursing process—An adaptation of the scientific method used by nurses as a basis for nursing care; also called the problem-solving method; the steps in the nursing process are: (1) assessment, (2) planning, (3) intervention, and (4) evaluation; some authors describe the process as having five steps, listing nursing diagnosis as the second step.

Nutrition—The study of food in relation to health; as defined by the Food and Nutrition Council (AMA), nutrition is the "science of food, the nutrients and other substances therein, their action, interaction and balance in relation to health and disease, and the processes by which the organism ingests, digests, absorbs, transports, utilizes, and excretes food substances."

Obesity—Excessive accumulation of body fat or adipose tissue; usually associated, but not synonymous with, the overweight state.

Oligosaccharides—A group of carbohydrates composed of 2 to 10 simple sugars or monosaccharides.

Organic compounds—Carbon-containing compounds; substances of animal and vegetable origin are generally organic in nature.

Organic foods—Foods that are allegedly grown without agricultural chemicals (pesticides or fertilizers) and processed without chemicals or additives.

Orthomolecular psychiatry—Treatment for a variety of mental disorders that advocates the use of large doses of vitamins, particularly the water-soluble vitamins, trace minerals, and special diets.

Osteoarthritis—A chronic disease involving the joints, particularly the weight-bearing joints, and characterized by degeneration of the articular cartilage, spur formation, and impaired functioning.

Osteoporosis—A bone disorder characterized by abnormal bone porosity and bone fractures as a result of a decrease in the amount of bone; the remaining bone is normal in chemical composition.

Osteosclerosis—Abnormal increased density of bone occurring in a variety of pathologic states.

Overweight—Excessive heaviness; may or may not include an abnormal amount of adipose tissue; a body weight that exceeds given weight standards.

Pagophagia—A type of pica in which an excessive amount of ice is consumed.

Parenteral nutrition—Provision of nutrients by routes other than through the mouth and digestive tract, such as subcutaneous, intramuscular, or intravenous feeding.

Pectin—A water-soluble component of dietary fiber that delays gastric emptying.

Peptic ulcers—Eroded lesions in the gastrointestinal tract that are a result, at least in part, of the digestive action of gastric juice; may occur in the lower part of the esophagus, in the stomach usually along the lesser curvature, in the duodenum, or on the jejunal side of a gastrojejunostomy; epigastric pain is the most characteristic manifestation and is characterized by its chronicity, periodicity, rhythm, and location.

Periodontal disease—A disease process affecting the tissues surrounding the teeth including the gums, the periodontal ligament, the alveolar bone, and the cementum of the teeth roots; the major cause of tooth loss after the age of 35.

Peritoneal dialysis—The use of the peritoneum surrounding the abdominal cavity as a dialyzing membrane for the purpose of removing waste products or toxic substances.

Pernicious anemia—Anemia that results from lack of secretion of intrinsic factor by the gastric mucous membrane leading to failure to absorb vitamin B_{12}.

Petit mal seizure—A seizure characterized by a momentary loss of consciousness.

pH (power of hydrogen ion concentration)—A scale representing the relative acidity (or alkalinity) of a solution in which a value of 7.0 is neutral, a value below 7.0 is acid, and a value above 7.0 is alkaline.

Phenylketones—Metabolites of phenylalanine that arise from alternate pathways of phenylalanine metabolism when the normal pathways are blocked in phenylketonuria.

Phospholipids—Any of a class of fat-related substances that contain phosphorus, fatty acids, and a nitrogenous base; essential elements in every cell.

Physiologic anemia of pregnancy—A drop in the hemoglobin concentration occurring in pregnancy as a result of a disproportionate increase in plasma volume and the red blood cell mass.

Physiologic anorexia—A normal decrease in appetite that accompanies a slowing of the growth rate in toddlers and preschoolers.

Pica—An appetite disorder associated with a craving for inappropriate items such as dirt, clay, starch, or chalk.

Pinocytosis—A type of absorption by cells in which the cell membrane invaginates to form a saccular structure that engulfs extracellular fluid and is then closed at the membrane so that the saccule remains as a vesicle or vacuole within the cell.

Pituitary diabetes—Abnormal glucose tolerance that results from excessive secretion of pituitary hormones, which have the property of increasing the blood glucose concentration.

Pituitary diabetes insipidus—An endocrine disorder resulting from deficient secretion of the antidiuretic hormone by the posterior portion of the pituitary gland; manifested by excessive thirst and passage of a large volume of urine.

Polypeptide—A combination of many amino acids joined by peptide linkages.

Polysaccharides—Carbohydrates consisting of 10 or more monosaccharide units; major polysaccharides are starch, glycogen, and dietary fiber.

Polyunsaturated fats—Triglycerides that contain predominantly polyunsaturated fatty acids and glycerol.

Polyunsaturated fatty acids—Fatty acids that contain two or more double bonds and consequently lack four or more hydrogen atoms.

Preeclampsia—An acute hypertensive disorder occurring after the 20th week of pregnancy; the hypertension is accompanied by edema and/or proteinuria.

Preformed vitamins—Vitamins present in foods in their biologically active forms.

Primary hypertension—See Essential hypertension.

Primary malnutrition—A type of malnutrition resulting from a deficit or excess of kilocalories or essential nutrients, which is not secondary to disease states.

Problem-solving method—See Nursing process.

Progressive hospital diets—Modifications of a regular diet in consistency such as liquid or soft diets.

Proteases—Enzymes that hydrolyze proteins during digestion.

Protein—An organic compound essential to all living organisms; composed of a polymer of amino acids linked together by peptide bonds; a protein molecule always contains carbon, hydrogen, oxygen, and nitrogen, and occasionally phosphorus, sulfur, copper, and iron.

Protein-sparing modified fast—A weight reduction strategy that utilizes a diet consisting of lean meat protein (1.0 to 1.5 g/kg body weight), noncaloric liquids, and mineral and vitamin supplements.

Proteinuria—Presence of protein in the urine.

Puberty—The developmental period characterized by a spurt in physical growth and appearance of the secondary sex characteristics.

Purine—A nitrogenous compound with a ring structure that is a component of nucleic acids; examples are adenosine and guanine.

Pyorrhea—See Periodontal disease.

Reactive hypoglycemia—A drop below normal of the blood glucose level that results from an exaggerated insulin response to the ingestion of carbohydrate-containing foods.

Reactive obesity—A type of obesity that follows a stressful situation such as a hospitalization.

Regional enteritis—A chronic, nonspecific, granulomatous, inflammatory bowel disease frequently involving the terminal ileum but occasionally extending into the colon or arising in the more proximal portions of the small intestine; manifestations include recurrent crampy abdominal pain accompanied by diarrhea, fever, anorexia, and weight loss; also referred to as Crohn's disease.

Regurgitation—The return of swallowed food into the mouth.

Residue—All material that remains in the lower intestinal tract after digestion and absorption; includes undigested and unabsorbed food and metabolic and bacterial residues.

Retinoic acid—The acid form of vitamin A, sometimes used in the treatment of acne.

Retinoids—Synthetic analogs of vitamin A.

Rheumatic heart disease—Heart disease that occurs as a complication of rheumatic fever.

Rheumatism—A general term used for acute and chronic conditions characterized by inflammation, soreness, and stiffness of muscles and pain in joints and associated structures.

Rheumatoid arthritis—A chronic systemic disease characterized by inflammatory changes in joints and related structures that result in crippling deformaties.

Rooting reflex—The reflex that causes an infant to turn the mouth and head toward the direction of a stimulus applied to the mouth or lips; enables infants to locate the breast or bottle; it is present at birth and gradually weakens and disappears at approximately 3 months of age.

Roughage—See Fiber.

Rumination—Regurgitation with little force and remastication of undigested food; occurs chiefly in emotionally disturbed and occasionally in mentally retarded and psychiatric clients.

Satiety reflex—A response indicating fullness beyond desire.

Saturated fats—Triglycerides that are composed of saturated fatty acids and glycerol.

Saturated fatty acids—Fatty acids that contain as many hydrogen atoms as each of the carbons in the chain can hold.

School-age period—The period of childhood development from the age of 6 until the onset of puberty; also referred to as middle childhood or the latent period.

Secondary hypertension—Hypertension that develops secondary to other disease conditions, such as renal disease.

Senescence—The process of aging or growing old.

Simple carbohydrates—Monosaccharides and disaccharides.

Simple goiter—See Nontoxic goiter.

Simple lipids—Lipids such as triglycerides that are composed only of fatty acids and an alcohol.

Simple proteins—Proteins that are made up entirely of amino acids or their derivatives; collagen and elastin are examples.

Skinfold thickness—An anthropometric measure of nutritional status that refers to the thickness of a double layer of pinched skin with its attached subcutaneous tissue; the measurement is taken with a caliper at one or several body sites, such as over the triceps muscle and in the subscapular area; useful for determining the amount of body fat and for differientiating between overweight and obesity.

Spastic colon diverticulitis—A noninflammatory condition characterized by an abnormal motor activity of the colon; manifestations include constipation or diarrhea, abdominal pain, anorexia, nausea, vomiting, distention, flatulence, and heartburn; also called mucous colitis and irritable colon syndrome; considered by some clinicians to be a forerunner of diverticular disease.

Specific dynamic action—See Calorigenic effect.

Sports anemia—Anemia that is sometimes seen during the early stages of strenuous athletic training; its cause is unclear.

Starch—A polysaccharide composed of many glucose units linked in a straight line (amylose) or with branches (amylopectin), which is the major storage form of carbohydrate in plants.

Starvation ketosis—Accumulation of ketone bodies in the blood resulting from excessive body fat breakdown secondary to lack of food intake; characterized by hypoglycemia and treated by administration of glucose.

Steatorrhea—Excessive fat in the stool.

Sucking reflex—The reflex that appears within the first to second day of life in normal infants, stimulating the infant to suck on objects such as a nipple or finger placed in the mouth; sucking stimulates swallowing (suckle–swallow reflex); it remains for the first 3 to 5 months of life.

Sucrose—Table sugar; a disaccharide present in many fruits, vegetables, and prepared foods.

Swallowing reflex—See Sucking reflex.

Teratogenic—Having the property of interferring with normal prenatal development, causing the formation of one or more developmental anomalies in the fetus.

Tetany—A disorder of generalized muscle hypertonicity with tremors and spasmodic muscle contraction caused by hypocalcemia.

Tocopherol—Any one of several related complex alcohols with antioxidant properties that has vitamin E activity; occurs naturally in vegetable germ oils and is also prepared by synthesis; the most potent form is alpha tocopherol.

Tophi—Deposits of sodium urate in tissues.

Total parenteral nutrition—See Hyperalimentation.

Toxemia—A generic term that includes preeclampsia and eclampsia; also called pregnancy-induced hypertension; see Eclampsia and Preeclampsia.

Trace contaminants—Trace elements with no known body functions.

Trace elements—See Micronutrients.

Triglyceride—Fat in which the glycerol molecule has three attached fatty acids.

Tripeptide—A product formed by the combination of three amino acids or by hydrolysis of proteins.

Uremia—A toxic condition associated with renal insufficiency; retention in the blood of nitrogenous substances normally excreted by the kidneys; characterized by azotemia, acidosis, fluid and electrolyte imbalance, anemia, and dysfunction of multiple body organs; end-stage renal disease.

Uric acid—The end product of purine metabolism in humans; increased uric acid in the blood is characteristic of gout.

Vegans—Vegetarians who consume no animal foods but subsist entirely on plant foods.

Vegetarians—A general term that refers to persons who eliminate animal foods from the diet and use plant foods; vegetarians utilize a variety of diet categories ranging from those who eat no animal food to those who eliminate only red meats, for example.

Villi—Small fingerlike projections on the surface of a mucous membrane, as in the walls of the small intestine where digestion takes place.

Viral hepatitis—An acute inflammatory disease of the liver caused by either type A, type B, or type non A–non B virus; can be transmitted by either the oral or parenteral route.

Vitamin—A general term given to a group of organic substances that are present in food in minute quantities and that perform specific functions for normal nutrition; it has been suggested that an organic compound should have all of the following characteristics in order to be considered a vitamin: (1) an organic compound in natural foods but distinct from carbohydrate, protein, and fat; (2) present in foods in extremely small concentrations; (3) essential for growth and health; (4) the cause of a specific deficiency disease when not adequately supplied in the diet; and (5) not synthesized in sufficient amounts by the host and therefore obtained exclusively from the diet.

Water intoxication—A type of sodium and water imbalance in which water intake exceeds sodium intake.

Xanthomas—Benign, fatty, fibrous, yellow plaques, nodules, or tumors that develop in the subcutaneous layer of the skin, often around tendons; the lesions are characterized by the intracellular accumulation of cholesterol and cholesterol esters.

Xerostomia—Dry mouth caused by insufficient secretion of saliva.

Index

Letters after page numbers represent figures (f) and tables (t).

Body weight (*cont.*)
  control of (*cont.*)
    gout and, 541
    in handicapped client, 574
   determination of recommended, 22f
   diabetes mellitus and, 348–349
   Down's syndrome and, 558–559
   excess in, osteoarthritis and, 543
   frame size and, 22t
   gain in
    glucocorticoids and, 366
    pregnancy and, 156–157, 157f
   of handicapped clients, 567
   hospital malnutrition and, 291
   hypertension and, 439
   imbalance of, 314t, 318t, 322, 320–332t, 326f, 328t, 329f
   kilocalorie restriction and, 319–322, 320–322t
   kilocalories and, 21
   lipoproteins and, 429
   loss of
    cancer and, 516–517
    cardiovascular disease and, 447
    client education in, 329–330
    delivery and, 167–168
    diabetes mellitus and, 348
    diet for, 319–325, 320–322t
    drugs for, 328t
    emphysema and, 509
    exercise and, 325
    fad diets and, 323–325
    fasting and, 323
    pharmacologic therapy for, 327, 328t
    psychotherapy for, 329
    starvation and, 290
    surgical management of, 327–329, 329f
    wound healing and, 282
   mental retardation and, 556
   peptic ulcers and, 374
   physical handicaps and, 556
   recommended energy intake and, 14t
   serum lipids and, 432
   sodium tolerance and, 463
   TPN and, 280
   vegetarian diet and, 254
Bone disease, chronic renal failure and, 464–465
Bottle mouth caries, 189
Brain
  alcoholism and, 535
  degenerative changes in, 535
  development of, 149
  gag reflex and, 566
  glucose and, 549
  growth of
   inborn errors of metabolism and, 300
   nutrition and, 550
  hypoglycemia and, 337
  injury of, 566
  metabolism in, 549
  nutrition and, 149
  social environment and, 149
Bran
  constipation and, 401
  inflammatory bowel disease and, 392–393
Bread–cereal food group, 19, 19f
Breakfast programs, 210
Breast
  cancer of, Western-type diet and, 514
  fibrocystic disease of, methylxanthine restriction and, 513
Breastfeeding, 177, 257
  advantages of, 168–170
  caffeine and, 171
  contraindications for, 170
  cystic fibrosis and, 421
  immunologic benefits of, 169–170
  iron deficiency anemia and, 485

  lactose intolerance and, 398
  maternal diet and, 171
  milk sensitivity and, 495
  nutrition and, 170–171
  supplements needed with, 181t
Breast milk, 179, 180t
  vs. cow's milk, 168t
  nutritional benefits of, 169
Buffer system, 115–116
Bulemia, 210, 212
BUN. *See* Blood urea nitrogen
Burn
  nutrition and, 283
  vitamin C therapy for, 84
Butylated hydroxyanisole, cancer and, 512–513, 515
Butylated hydroxytoluene, cancer and, 512–513

Cachexia, cancer and, 516
Cadmium, toxicity of, 106
Caffeine
  athletes and, 216
  breastfeeding and, 171
  coronary heart disease and, 428
  hypertension and, 439
  peptic ulcers and, 375t
Calcium
  absorption of, 96t
   Billroth II operation and, 378
  balance of, immobilization and, 572–573
  blood level of, 96
  blood pressure and, 99
  deficiency of, 97
   hypertension and, 439
  depletion of, steatorrhea and, 384
  dietary deficiency of, 97
  diet high in, 364
  functions of, 96
  imbalance of, 97
  ionic imbalance of, 99t
  kidney stones and, 474–476, 475t
  malabsorption of, drugs and, 284
  metabolism of, 96
   chronic renal failure and, 464–465
   glucocorticoids and, 364
  in milk and cheese groups, 18
  osteoporosis and, 545–546
  peridontal disease and, 544
  pregnancy and, 161–162
  requirement of
   in adolescents, 206
   in adults, 545
   breastfeeding and, 170
   in elderly persons, 227
  skeletal imbalance of, 98t
  sources of, 97
  steatorrhea and, 384
  supplementation of, in vegetarian diet, 257, 258t
Calcium–phosphorus ratio, 96, 97t
Calorimetry, 42
Cancer. *See also specific site*
  alcoholism and, 535
  effects of treatment, 518, 521
  etiology of, 512–515, 514t
  high protein diet and, 66
  incidence of, 511–512
  intervention, 521–524
  local effects of, 517–518
  nutritional care in (case study), 136
  nutrition and, 511–525, 514t, 519–521t
  prevention of, 515
  in Seventh-Day Adventists, 254
  systemic effects of, 515–517